Kathleen Ingram

Operative Obstetrics

Gary D.V. Hankins, MD
Professor and Chief, Maternal-Fetal Medicine
Department of Obstetrics and Gynecology
University of Texas Medical Branch at Galveston

Formerly
Chairman
Department of Obstetrics and Gynecology
Wilford Hall USAF Medical Center
San Antonio, Texas

Steven L. Clark, MD
Professor
Department of Obstetrics and Gynecology
University of Utah School of Medicine

Director
Intermountain Health Care Perinatal Centers
Latter Day Saints Hospital
Salt Lake City, Utah

F. Gary Cunningham, MD
Professor and Chairman
Jack A. Pritchard Professor
Department of Obstetrics & Gynecology
The University of Texas Southwestern Medical Center at Dallas

Chief of Obstetrics and Gynecology
Parkland Memorial Hospital
Dallas, Texas

Larry C. Gilstrap III, MD
Professor
Department of Obstetrics & Gynecology

Director
Maternal-Fetal Medicine Fellowship and Clinical Genetics
The University of Texas Southwestern Medical Center at Dallas

Attending Staff
Parkland Memorial Hospital
St. Paul Medical Center
Dallas, Texas

Operative Obstetrics

APPLETON & LANGE
Norwalk, Connecticut

Notice: The authors and the publisher of this volume have taken care to make certain that the doses of drugs and schedules of treatment are correct and compatible with the standards generally accepted at the time of publication. Nevertheless, as new information becomes available, changes in treatment and in the use of drugs become necessary. The reader is advised to carefully consult the instruction and information material included in the package insert of each drug or therapeutic agent before administration. This advice is especially important when using new and infrequently used drugs. The publisher disclaims any liability, loss, injury, or damage incurred as a consequence, directly or indirectly, of the use and application of any of the contents of this volume.

95 96 97 98 99 / 10 9 8 7 6 5 4 3 2 1

Prentice Hall International (UK) Limited, *London*
Prentice Hall of Australia Pty. Limited, *Sydney*
Prentice Hall Canada, Inc., *Toronto*
Prentice Hall Hispanoamericana, S.A., *Mexico*
Prentice Hall of India Private Limited, *New Delhi*
Prentice Hall of Japan, Inc., *Tokyo*
Simon and Schuster Asia Pte. Ltd., *Singapore*
Editora Prentice Hall do Brasil Ltda., *Rio de Janeiro*
Prentice Hall, *Englewood Cliffs, New Jersey*

Library of Congress Cataloging-in-Publication Data

Operative obstetrics / Gary D.V. Hankins . . . [et al.].
p. cm.
ISBN 0-8385-7409-2
1. Obstetrics—Surgery. I. Hankins, Gary D.V.
[DNLM: 1. Pregnancy Complications—surgery. WQ 400 0609 1995]
RG725.062 1995
618.8—dc20 95-1975
DNLM/DLC CIP
for Library of Congress

ISBN 0-8385-7409-2

Production Editor: Elizabeth C. Ryan

PRINTED IN THE UNITED STATES OF AMERICA

The first edition of Operative Obstetrics *is dedicated to our mentors, teachers, and to all those who have laid the foundation for the practice of obstetrics. While there are far too many to name individually, we would like to acknowledge some individuals who were very special teachers to us: Dr. Abe Michael, Dr. Jack Pritchard, Dr. Peggy Whalley, Dr. Alvin Brekken, Dr. Richard Paul, Dr. Frank Miller, and Dr. Robert Maier. Finally, we would be remiss if we did not dedicate this book to our residents and fellows-in-training, who continue to serve as our teachers.*

CONTRIBUTORS

Bill D. Atkinson, MD
Fellow and Instructor
Section of Maternal-Fetal Medicine
Department of Obstetrics and Gynecology
University of Oklahoma College of Medicine
Oklahoma City, Oklahoma
Chapter 32, Cervical Ripening

Hani K. Atrash, MD, MPH
Clinical Associate Professor of Community Medicine
Emory University School of Public Health

Chief, Pregnancy and Infant Health Branch
Centers for Disease Control
Atlanta, Georgia
Chapter 33, Pregnancy Termination: First and Second Trimesters

William H. Barth, Jr., MD
Chief of Obstetrics
Wilford Hall USAF Medical Center
San Antonio, Texas
Chapter 31, Operative Procedures on the Cervix

Richard L. Berkowitz, MD
Professor and Chair
Department of Obstetrics and Gynecology
Mt. Sinai School of Medicine
New York, New York
Chapter 34, Multifetal Reduction

Jeffrey D. Bloss, MD
Major, USAFMC
Division of Gynecologic Oncology
Department of Obstetrics and Gynecology
Wilford Hall USAF Medical Center
San Antonio, Texas
Chapter 27, Cancer
Chapter 37, Gestational Trophoblastic Diseases

Steven L. Clark, MD
Professor
Department of Obstetrics and Gynecology
University of Utah School of Medicine

Director
Intermountain Health Care Perinatal Centers
Latter Day Saints Hospital
Salt Lake City, Utah
Chapter 1, Needles, Sutures, and Knots
Chapter 3, Asepsis and Infection Control
Chapter 18, Cesarean Section
Chapter 26, Management of Postpartum Hemorrhage

Karoll Cortez-Austerlitz, MD
Research Assistant
Department of Obstetrics and Gynecology
Wayne State University/Hutzel Hospital
Detroit, Michigan
Chapter 39, The Fetus as a Surgical Patient

F. Gary Cunningham, MD
Professor and Chairman
Jack A. Pritchard Professor
Department of Obstetrics & Gynecology
The University of Texas Southwestern Medical Center at Dallas

Chief of Obstetrics and Gynecology
Parkland Memorial Hospital
Dallas, Texas
Chapter 20, Postoperative Complications
Chapter 21, Evaluation of the Surgical Abdomen

Mary E. D'Alton, MD
Associate Professor
Department of Obstetrics and Gynecology
Tufts University School of Medicine

Chief, Obstetrics and Maternal-Fetal Medicine
New England Medical Center
Boston, Massachusetts
Chapter 30, Invasive Prenatal Diagnostic Procedures

Alan DeCherney, MD
Louis E. Phaneuf Professor and Chairman
Department of Obstetrics and Gynecology
Tufts University School of Medicine
New England Medical Center
Boston, Massachusetts
Chapter 24, Ectopic Pregnancy

John O.L. Delancey, MD
Associate Professor
Department of Obstetrics and Gynecology
University of Michigan Medical School
Ann Arbor, Michigan
Chapter 7, Episiotomy

Gary A. Dildy, MD
Assistant Professor
Department of Obstetrics and Gynecology
University of Utah School of Medicine

Director, Perinatal Center
Utah Valley Regional Medical Center
Park City, Utah
Chapter 13, Shoulder Dystocia

Patrick Duff, MD
Professor and Residency Program Director
Division of Maternal-Fetal Medicine
Department of Obstetrics and Gynecology
University of Florida College of Medicine
Gainesville, Florida
Chapter 38, Prophylactic Antibiotics

Alice A. Frye, MPH
Faculty Associate
Women's and Children's Center
Emory University School of Public Health
Atlanta, Georgia
Chapter 33, Pregnancy Termination: First and Second Trimesters

Donald G. Gallup, MD
Professor and Director
Section of Gynecologic Oncology
Department of Obstetrics and Gynecology
The Medical College of Georgia
Augusta, Georgia
Chapter 4, Anatomy, Incisions, and Closures

Larry C. Gilstrap III, MD
Professor
Department of Obstetrics and Gynecology

Director
Maternal-Fetal Medicine Fellowship and Clinical Genetics
The University of Texas Southwestern Medical Center at Dallas

Attending Staff
Parkland Memorial Hospital
St. Paul Medical Center
Dallas, Texas
Chapter 10, Breech Delivery
Chapter 11, Multifetal Gestation
Chapter 23, Abdominal Pregnancy

W. Mark Grant, MD
Assistant Professor
Department of Obstetrics and Gynecology
University of Missouri Medical Center
Columbia, Missouri
Chapter 22, Adnexal Masses

Michael F. Greene, MD
Associate Professor
Department of Obstetrics, Gynecology and Reproductive Biology
Harvard Medical School

Chief, Maternal-Fetal Medicine
Vincent Memorial Obstetric Division
Massachusetts General Hospital
Boston, Massachusetts
Chapter 31, Operative Procedures on the Cervix

Gary D.V. Hankins, MD
Professor and Chief, Maternal-Fetal Medicine
Department of Obstetrics and Gynecology
University of Texas Medical Branch at Galveston

Formerly
Chairman
Department of Obstetrics and Gynecology
Wilford Hall USAF Medical Center
San Antonio, Texas
Chapter 7, Episiotomy
Chapter 8, Forceps Delivery
Chapter 14, Puerperal Hematomas and Lower Genital Tract Lacerations
Chapter 40, Circumcision

Robert H. Hayashi, MD
Director
Division of Maternal Fetal Medicine
J. Robert Willson Professor of Obstetrics
Department of Obstetrics and Gynecology
University of Michigan School of Medicine
Ann Arbor, Michigan
Chapter 9, Vacuum Delivery

L. Wayne Hess, MD
Associate Professor
Department of Obstetrics and Gynecology

Head
Maternal-Fetal Medicine
University of Missouri Medical Center
Columbia, Missouri
Chapter 22, Adnexal Masses

Gary H. Johnson, MD
Chairman
Department of Obstetrics and Gynecology
Latter Day Saints Hospital
Salt Lake City, Utah
Chapter 2, Surgical Instruments and Drains

Neil K. Kochenour, MD
Professor
Department of Obstetrics and Gynecology
University of Utah School of Medicine
Salt Lake City, Utah
Chapter 15, Diagnosis and Management of Uterine Inversion

Herschel W. Lawson, MD
Assistant Clinical Professor
Department of Gynecology and Obstetrics
Emory University School of Medicine

Medical Epidemiologist
Division of Cancer Prevention and Control
National Center for Chronic Disease Prevention and Health Promotion
Centers for Disease Control and Prevention
Atlanta, Georgia
Chapter 33, Pregnancy Termination: First and Second Trimesters

Joseph A. Lucci III, MD
Associate Professor
Division of Gynecologic Oncology
Department of Obstetrics and Gynecology
The University of Texas Southwestern Medical Center at Dallas
Dallas, Texas
Chapter 28, Urologic and Gastrointestinal Injuries

H. Trent MacKay, MD, MPH
Associate Clinical Professor
Department of Obstetrics and Gynecology
University of California, Davis

Medical Epidemiologist
Centers for Disease Control and Prevention
Atlanta, Georgia
Chapter 33, Pregnancy Termination: First and Second Trimesters

Robert C. Maier, MD
Associate Professor
Department of Obstetrics and Gynecology
Medical College of Georgia
Augusta, Georgia
Chapter 16, Uterine Packing for Control of Postpartum Uterine Hemorrhage

David Scott Miller, MD
Associate Professor
Division of Gynecologic Oncology
Department of Obstetrics and Gynecology
The University of Texas Southwestern Medical Center

Director of Gynecologic Oncology
Zale Lipsky University Hospital
Parkland Memorial Hospital
Dallas, Texas
Chapter 27, Cancer
Chapter 37, Gestational Trophoblastic Diseases

Mark D. Pearlman, MD
Assistant Professor
Department of Obstetrics and Gynecology
University of Michigan Medical School
Ann Arbor, Michigan
Chapter 35, Trauma

Herbert B. Peterson, MD
Clinical Professor
Department of Gynecology and Obstetrics
Emory University School of Medicine

Chief, Women's Health and Fertility Branch
Division of Reproductive Health
National Center for Chronic Disease and Health Promotion
Centers for Disease Control and Prevention
Atlanta, Georgia
Chapter 25, Female Sterilization

Marcello Pietrantoni, MD
Assistant Professor
Division of Maternal-Fetal Medicine
Department of Obstetrics and Gynecology
University of Louisville School of Medicine
Louisville, Kentucky
Chapter 29, Diagnostic and Operative Laparoscopy

Warren C. Plauché, MD
Professor
Department of Obstetrics and Gynecology
Louisiana State University School of Medicine in New Orleans

Executive Associate Dean for Clinical Affairs
Medical Center of Louisiana at Charity Hospital
New Orleans, Louisiana
Chapter 19, Obstetric Hysterectomy

David J. Quinlan, BS, MBBCH, MRCOG, FRCSC
Clinical Instructor
Department of Obstetrics and Gynecology
University of Utah School of Medicine
Salt Lake City, Utah
Chapter 2, Surgical Instruments and Drains
Chapter 6, Symphysiotomy

Ruben Quintero, MD
Assistant Professor
Department of Obstetrics and Gynecology
Wayne State University

Director
Fetal Endoscopy Unit
Department of Obstetrics and Gynecology
Hutzel Hospital
Detroit, Michigan
Chapter 39, The Fetus as a Surgical Patient

Susan M. Ramin, MD
Associate Professor
Department of Obstetrics and Gynecology
The University of Texas Southwestern Medical Center at Dallas

Attending Staff, Parkland Memorial Hospital
St. Paul Medical Center
Dallas, Texas
Chapter 23, Abdominal Pregnancy

William Rayburn, MD
John W. Records Chair
Professor and Chief
Section of Maternal-Fetal Medicine
Department of Obstetrics and Gynecology
University of Oklahoma College of Medicine
Oklahoma City, Oklahoma
Chapter 32, Cervical Ripening

John Read, MD
Professor
Department of Obstetrics and Gynecology
University of Kentucky College of Medicine

Director
Maternal-Fetal Medicine
University of Kentucky Chandler Medical Center
Lexington, Kentucky
Chapter 5, Pelvimetry

Joseph S. Sanfilippo, MD
Professor and Director
Division of Reproductive Endocrinology
Department of Obstetrics and Gynecology
University of Louisville School of Medicine
Louisville, Kentucky
Chapter 29, Diagnostic and Operative Laparoscopy

Andrew J. Satin, MD
Assistant Professor, Department of Obstetrics and Gynecology
Uniformed Services University of the Health Sciences
Bethesda, Maryland

Assistant Chief of Obstetrics
Wilford Hall USAF Medical Center
San Antonio, Texas
Chapter 40, Circumcision

Russell R. Snyder, MD
Associate Professor
Uniformed Services University of the Health Sciences
Bethesda, Maryland

Chairman
Department of Obstetrics and Gynecology
Wilford Hall USAF Medical Center
San Antonio, Texas
Chapter 36, Breast Disease During Pregnancy and Lactation

Kim L. Thornton, MD
Assistant Professor
Division of Reproductive Endocrinology and Fertility
Department of Obstetrics and Gynecology
University of Connecticut Health Center
Farmington, Connecticut
Chapter 24, Ectopic Pregnancy

J. Peter Van Dorsten, MD
Professor and Vice-Chairman
Department of Obstetrics and Gynecology
Medical University of South Carolina
Charleston, South Carolina
Chapter 12, External Cephalic Version

Jeffrey S. Warshaw, MD
Assistant Professor
Department of Gynecology and Obstetrics
Emory University School of Medicine
Atlanta, Georgia
Chapter 25, Female Sterilization

George Wendel, Jr., MD
Associate Professor
Department of Obstetrics and Gynecology
The University of Texas Southwestern
Medical Center
Dallas, Texas
Chapter 17, Surgical Treatment of Lower Genital Tract Infections

Edward R. Yeomans, MD
Associate Professor
Department of Obstetrics and Gynecology
University of Texas Medical School at Houston
Houston, Texas
Chapter 8, Forceps Delivery

Christopher M. Zahn, MD
Assistant Professor
Departments of Obstetrics and Gynecology
and Pathology
Wilford Hall USAF Medical Center
San Antonio, Texas
Chapter 14, Puerperal Hematomas and Lower Genital Tract Lacerations
Chapter 36, Breast Disease During Pregnancy and Lactation

CONTENTS

PREFACE

In writing this book, our goal was to construct a comprehensive source on operative obstetrics that would be useful to individuals in training as well as practicing obstetricians. Topics covered include anatomy, needles, sutures and knots, and virtually every major surgical procedure performed in obstetrics ranging from episiotomy to cesarean hysterectomy to shoulder dystocia management. While our primary goal was to present the surgical procedures and maneuvers in sufficient detail to serve as a self-instructional text, we believed it equally important to provide the scientific rationale and basis for the procedures.

After constructing a comprehensive table of contents, we identified individuals with notable expertise in the various areas and solicited their participation in the project. Each contributor not only had extensive experience, but also was actively practicing the techniques and surgical procedures described. We reviewed each submission in an effort to present a consensus viewpoint of sound clinical practice. In clinical circumstance in which more than one option was valid, we attempted to present them all rather than limit the presentation to the technique most preferred by the author.

Illustrations for all procedures were drawn especially for this text, and were reviewed carefully to insure anatomic and surgical accuracy of the presentation. Clinical material in the form of radiologic studies, histologic slides, etc. were also each individually selected to optimally illustrate important teaching points and concepts.

We have spent the past three years designing the text, and hope that you find it informative and timely. We invite your comments so that the next edition may be even better.

ACKNOWLEDGMENTS

The editors wish to acknowledge the contributions of the primary authors of each of the chapters, whose initial manuscripts served as the skeletal framework for this book.

We also gratefully acknowledge the contributions of our artists, who performed so capably in the creation of the comprehensive and extensive art program. The team assembled were simply outstanding and included Jan Redden, Carl Clingman, Tim Phelps, and David Rini. We further acknowledge the contributions of our administrative support staff whose many hours at the telephone and computer keyboard allowed the transformation of ideas into what we consider to be an outstanding textbook. Included are Karylyn Bliss, Lynne McDonnell and Connie Utterbach.

Finally, a special debt of gratitude is due Barbara Ohlstein, who served as administrative director of this project during the three years from its conception to its completion.

CHAPTER 1

Needles, Sutures, and Knots

Mastering the use of needles, sutures, and instruments, as well as the technique of knot tying, is the technical foundation of the surgeon's craft. A bewildering array of needles and sutures are available; some offer distinct advantages in specific situations while others are simply competitive equivalents. In this chapter, we describe the variety of available needles and sutures and provide guidelines for their selection and use.

NEEDLES

Surgical needles consist of three structural parts: the swage or eye, the body, and the point (Fig. 1–1). Needles are designed with different combinations of eye, body, and point types, depending upon their intended surgical use. Each variation has advantages and disadvantages.

The Swage (Eye)

Three types of eye are in common surgical use: **swaged, controlled release** ("pop-off"), and **open.** With a **swaged-on shank**, the suture is placed inside the hollowed end of the needle and crimped into place by the manufacturer (Bennett, 1988). The convenience and ease of surgical manipulation makes this design ideal for most obstetric applications. The diameter of the swaged-on needle end is larger than that of the rest of the needle and determines the size of the suture tract (Bennett, 1988). One exception is Prolene suture; its tapered end allows the suture to be swaged to a needle of similar diameter (Hochberg and Murray, 1991).

Controlled release needles are similar to swaged-on needles but are designed to be released ("pop-off") with a sharp tug of the needle holder. Controlled-release needles allow needle removal of interrupted sutures without the suture being cut.

The advantage of **open-eyed needles** is that they allow the use of a variety of suture types and diameters. Such needles generally are manufactured in uncommonly used sizes because prepackaging with a spectrum of suture types would be economically unfeasible. Open-eyed needles are rarely used in obstetric surgery, but occasionally are helpful in specialized situations such as uterine artery ligation or cerclage placement. The principal disadvantage of an open-eyed shank is that the increased eye diameter necessary for manual attachment or threading increases the total size of the suture tract. A second disadvantage is that for placing a running suture, open-eyed needles are less convenient and more difficult to handle than are those of the swaged-on design.

The Body

The needle body may be round, triangular, or ovoid and is tapered gradually to the point. **Triangular** needles have three cutting edges. **Ovoid** needles may be flattened on top and bottom with rounded sides, or flattened on all four sides, producing a square or rectangular body. Some needle bodies also are ribbed longitudinally on the inner curvature to allow them to be securely grasped by the needle holder.

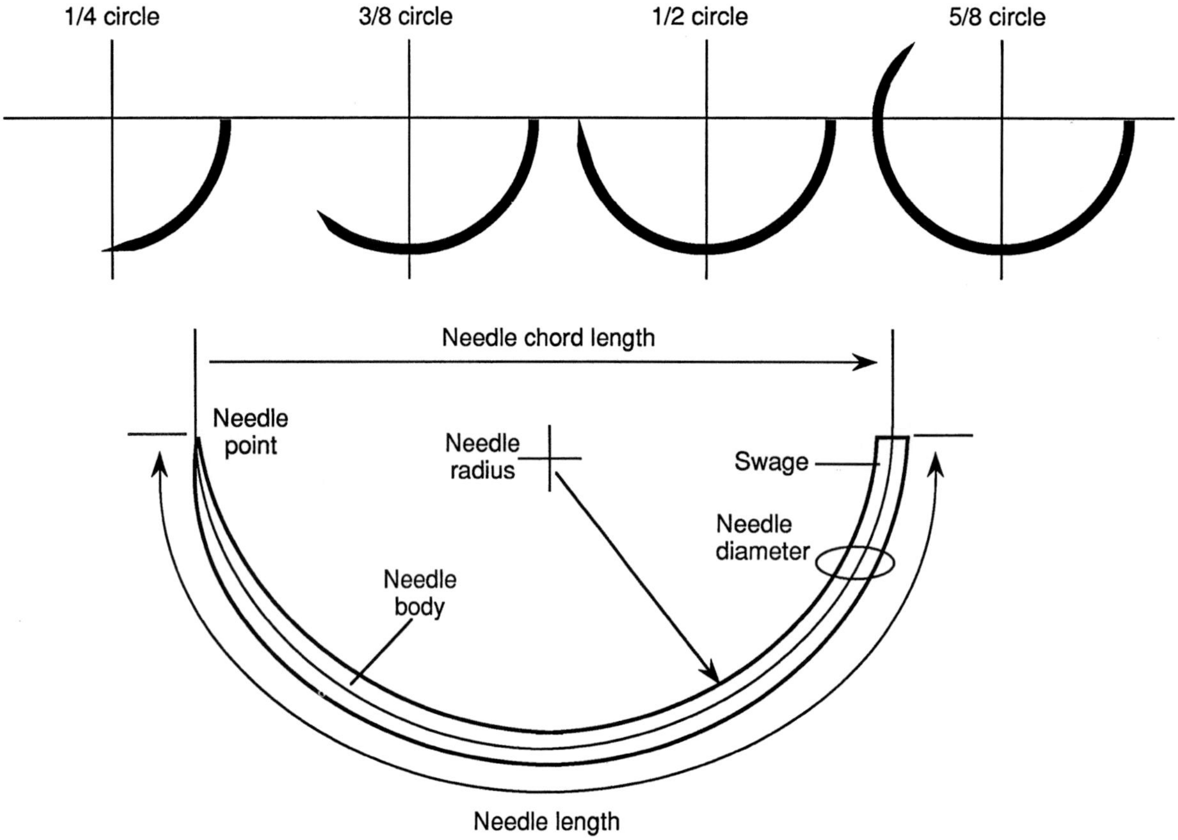

Figure 1–1. Parts of a curved surgical needle and various needle circle lengths. (Modified from Ethicon, Inc., 1993, with permission.)

The needle body may be either straight or curved. Most curved needles have either a 1/2 or 3/8 circle configuration, although a 5/8 circle needle is sometimes used in vaginal surgery (Fig. 1–1). The 3/8 circle needle is most commonly used in obstetrics; however, the 1/2 or 5/8 circle design facilities maneuvering in small spaces.

The Point

Needles are most commonly classified according to the cross section of their point (Fig. 1–2). Needle points may be either tapered, cutting, reverse cutting, or blunt. Cutting needles are most useful in suturing relatively tough tissues such as skin. However, they are more likely to pull through tissue than are tapered points, which are used for softer tissues such as uterus and fascia. The blunt point is used for very friable tissues, or occasionally for cannulating, and will not penetrate gloves.

Because conventional cutting needles have the cutting edge directed toward the wound edge, they have a greater tendency to pull through when tightened than does the reverse cutting needle, with its flat surface toward the wound (Fig. 1–2). However, conventional cutting needles may be useful for very fine skin suturing. Most commonly available cutting needles are of the reverse cutting design.

In obstetric surgery, cutting needles are used primarily for skin suturing. We have been surprised at the widespread availability of cutting needles on heavy, absorbable sutures in delivery suites and obstetric operating rooms. Suturing of uterus, peritoneal edges (if desired), and fascia are all best accomplished with taper point needles, which have less tendency to "pull through" than do cutting or reverse cutting points.

Using the Needle

Curved needles are designed to be grasped and driven through tissue with a needle holder. The placement of the needle in the

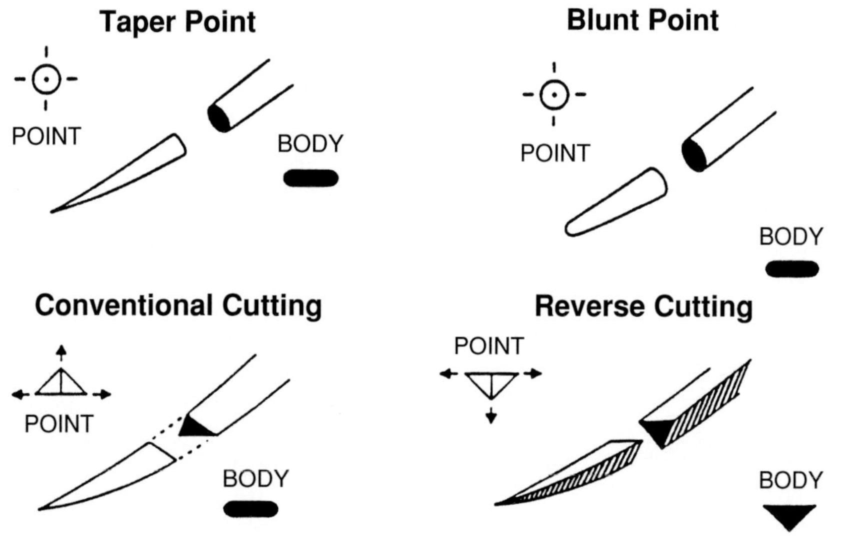

Figure 1–2. Surgical needle points and bodies. (Reprinted with permission from Ethicon, Inc., 1993.)

holder is dependent upon the tissue to be sutured. Where a long tract is planned or little resistance will be encountered (in uterine closure, for example), the needle may be grasped 2/3 or 3/4 of the distance from point to eye. Where tougher tissue is encountered (for example, the pubic periosteum), the needle is more appropriately grasped in the middle or even slightly toward the point, to facilitate needle passage and avoid deformation of the needle.

Curved needles should not be grasped with the hand. In a review of surgical glove perforation in obstetrics, Serrano and associates (1991) described a 13.3 percent rate of glove perforation. The majority of perforations occurred in the surgeon's nondominant hand, suggesting perforation due to direct grasping of the needle. Such technique increases the risk of infection transmission to both patient and physician (Dalgleish and Malkovsky, 1988). Longer, straight needles of the Keith type are sometimes used manually (without a needle holder) for mattress-type skin closures.

SUTURES

Sutures have been used for centuries either to approximate tissue or to ligate vessels. Wound suturing was described as early as 3500 BC in an Egyptian papyrus, and was used by Galen, physician to the gladiators, to stop their bleeding (Snyder, 1976; Stone, 1988). During the Middle Ages, however, many earlier advances were forgotten, and hemostasis was accomplished primarily through cauterization. With the Renaissance came renewed interest in the use of suture material; by the fifteenth century, horsehair, flaxen thread, and gut material were described. In the nineteenth century, both buckskin and silver wire were used in various types of gynecologic surgery (Snyder, 1976; Stone, 1988).

Joseph Lister, who pioneered the concept of antisepsis (1869), made the first major advance in suture material. His chromatization of gut suture in 1876 resulted in significant prolongation of suture tensile strength. In Lister's day, the violin was often referred to as a "kit." The most common source of gut material for suture was violin strings fashioned from sheep or ox intestines; thus the term "kitgut" was introduced, which later became "catgut" (Stone, 1988).

Table 1–1 describes various characteristics of suture material. The ideal suture would cost little, tie easily and securely, possess superb tensile strength, and have no adverse effect upon wound healing or infection rates. Unfortunately, no currently available suture meets all these requirements. Therefore, compromises must be made in selecting suture material because each type has both advantages and disadvantages.

Physical Characteristics

Physical configuration refers to mono- or multifilamentous construction of the suture material. Multifilamentous materials tie more easily, but also have an increased tendency to

TABLE 1–1. CHARACTERISTICS OF SUTURE MATERIAL

I. Physical Characteristics
  - Physical configuration
  - Capillarity
  - Fluid absorption ability
  - Diameter (caliber)
  - Tensile strength
  - Knot strength
  - Elasticity
  - Plasticity
  - Memory

II. Handling Characteristics
  - Pliability
  - Tissue drag
  - Knot tying
  - Knot slippage

III. Tissue Reaction Characteristics
  - Inflammatory and fibrous cell reaction
  - Absorption
  - Potentiation of infection
  - Allergic reaction

From Bennett (1988), with permission.

harbor bacteria in the braiding (Bennett, 1988).

Capillarity refers to a suture's ability to absorb fluid from a wet end to a dry end. **Fluid absorption ability** is the capacity of a suture to absorb fluid when immersed. Both of these characteristics also increase a suture's tendency to soak up and retain bacteria. For example, braided nylon, a material with high fluid absorption ability and capillarity, will absorb three times as many bacteria as the corresponding monofilament suture (Bucknall, 1983).

Diameter is determined in millimeters, but commonly expressed according to USP standards (3-0, 4-0, etc). However, USP terminology is affected by specific tensile strength as well as diameter; thus 4-0 catgut has a slightly larger diameter than 4-0 nylon (Fig. 1–3).

Tensile strength is defined as the amount of weight necessary to break a suture divided by the suture's cross-sectional area. Thus the breaking load will be quadrupled by a doubling of suture diameter. A knotted suture has roughly 1/3 the strength of unknotted suture; the strength depends to some degree upon the type of knot used (Rodeheaver and associates, 1981; Tera and Aberg, 1977). Table 1–2 lists relative tensile strengths of various knotted and unknotted suture materials. Note the dramatic decline in strength of knotted versus unknotted suture for all except metallic sutures. Figure 1–4 represents the relationship between suture diameter and tensile strength (Herrmann, 1971). Figures 1–5 and 1–6 represent tensile strength over time following suture placement (Salthouse, 1980).

Tensile strength also is affected by surgical technique. For example, a stray knot in prolene suture decreases tensile strength by

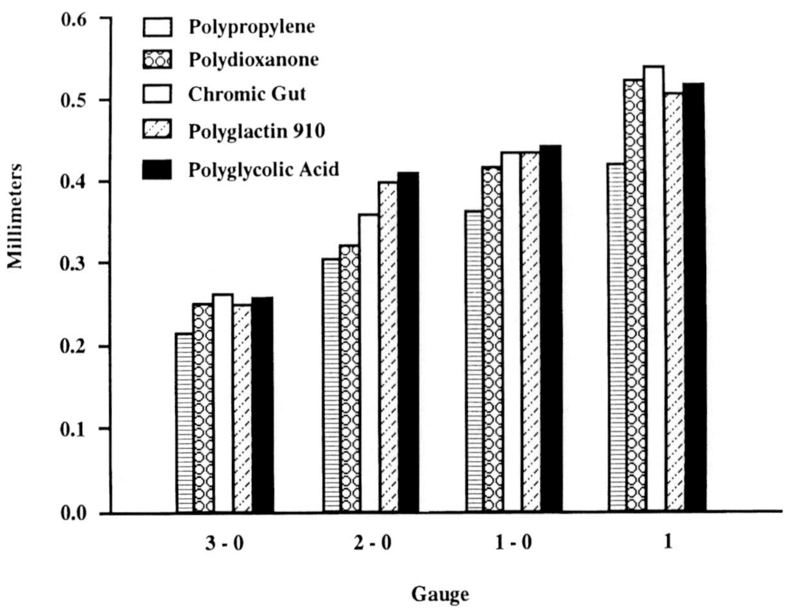

Figure 1–3. Suture diameters of five commonly used materials in four different gauges. (Adapted from Von Fraunhofer and associates, 1985, with permission.)

TABLE 1–2. PHYSICAL CHARACTERISTICS OF SURGICAL SUTURE MATERIALS (VALUES REPRESENT MEAN ± 1 STANDARD ERROR)

	Tensile Strength KgF/mm2	Effective Tensile Strength With 2 Throws
Metallic		
Steel, monofilament	162.6 ± 0.4	162.6 ± 0.4
Steel, multifilament	113.8 ± 1.2	113.8 ± 1.2
Tantalum, monofilament	131.4 ± 1.0	131.4 ± 1.0
Tantalum, multifilament	79.8 ± 0.9	79.8 ± 0.9
Synthetic		
Polyester		
Dacron, uncoated	86.4 ± 0.7	55.1 ± 3.8
Dacron, Teflon coated	87.1 ± 0.7	6.6 ± 0.8
Dacron, silicone coated	92.1 ± 0.6	18.4 ± 3.8
Polyglycolic acid	75.5 ± 0.4	37.1 ± 5.1
Polyolefin		
Polypropylene, monofilament	67.9 ± 2.2	32.3 ± 13.2
Polyethylene, monofilament	56.8 ± 1.4	14.8 ± 1.8
Polyamide		
Nylon, monofilament	78.6 ± 1.7	19.4 ± 3.3
Nylon, multifilament	70.9 ± 0.5	17.9 ± 2.8
Supramid extra	84.8 ± 1.0	26.5 ± 7.7
Natural fibers		
Silk	54.6 + 0.3	5.9 ± 0.7
Cotton	46.0 + 1.1	15.5 ± 3.8
Linen	65.7 + 0.7	25.8 ± 4.7
Catgut	49.5 + 0.5	42.4 ± 3.3
Collagen	47.8 + 1.9	36.0 ± 3.5

From Herrmann (1971), with permission.

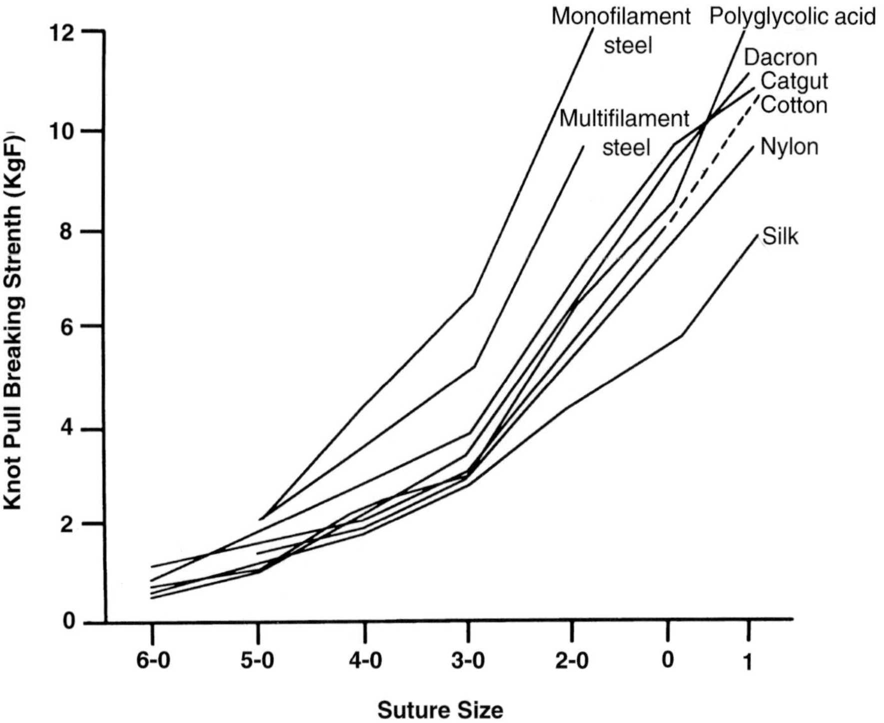

Figure 1–4. Knot pull breaking strength of various sizes of surgical sutures. Size and strength are not linearly related. (From Herrmann, 1971, with permission.)

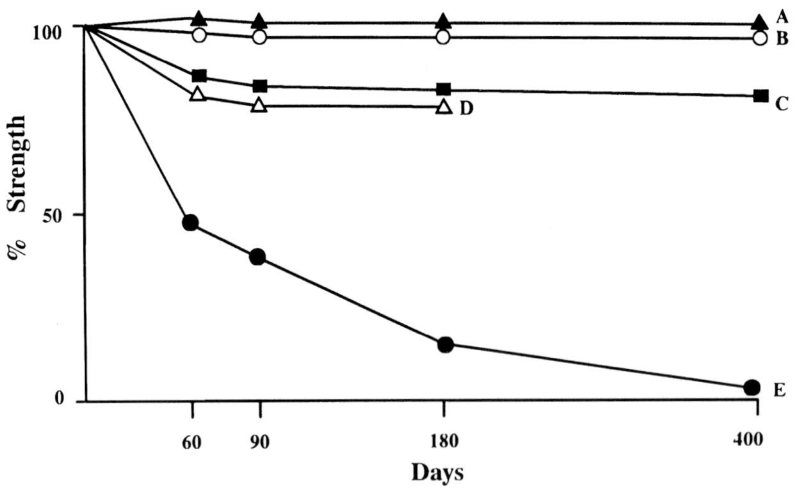

Figure 1–5. Nonabsorbable sutures, percentage strength remaining. Polyester (Ethibond and Mersilene) sutures (**A**) and polypropylene (Prolene) sutures (**B**) retained 100 percent of original breaking strength after 400 days. Monofilament nylon (Ethilon) sutures (**C**) retained about 80 percent. Multifilament nylon (**D**) lost slightly more of its original strength than the monofilament suture. Silk sutures (**E**) degrade and lose strength more rapidly, with usually less than 50 percent of the original strength remaining at two months. Data shown are from size 2-0 and 4-0 sutures implanted in rat subcutaneous sites. (From Salthouse, 1980, with permission.)

17 percent, and grasping suture with forceps or needle holders decreases suture strength in a dose-dependent fashion (Stamp and associates, 1988; Abidin and associates, 1989).

Knot strength refers to the force necessary to cause a given type of knot to slip, either partially or fully, and is dependent upon the material's coefficient of friction and its ability to stretch (Bennett, 1988).

Elasticity refers to a suture's tendency to return to its original form after stretching. With high elasticity, a suture will be easily stretched by tissue swelling and will not tend to cut into or through the tissue. **Plasticity**

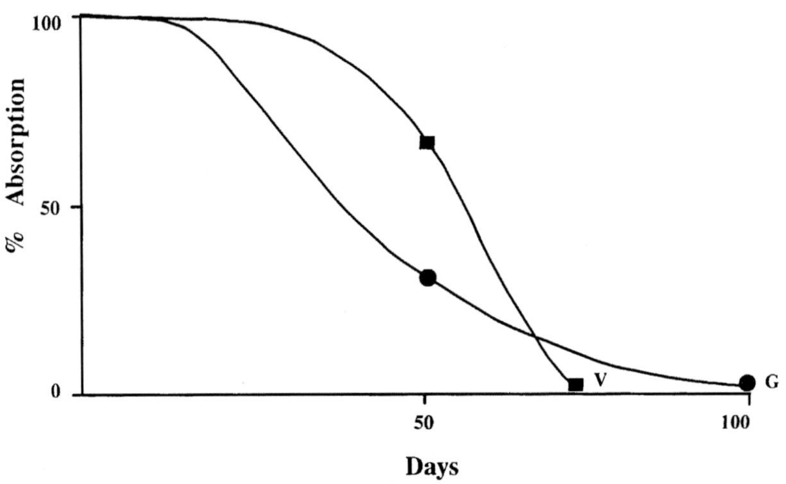

Figure 1–6. Absorption profile of chromic surgical gut (G) and synthetic absorbable polyglactin 910 (Vicryl) suture (V). Size 4-0 sutures were implanted in a rat gluteal muscle and absorption calculated from cross-sectional area remaining. Absorption of surgical gut is seen by 14 days, synthetic absorbable suture shows evidence of absorption at about 35 days, but is more rapid thereafter. (From Salthouse, 1980, with permission.)

refers to a suture's tendency to retain its new form after stretching. Thus a highly plastic suture will retain its larger form even after tissue swelling subsides, and may become loose. The tendency of suture material to cut through tissue is also directly related to tensile strength, inversely related to suture diameters and dependent upon tissue type. The tendency for suture to cut through tissue is least with fascia, followed by muscle, peritoneum and fat (Bennett, 1988; Tera and Aberg, 1976a).

The forces required for suture to tear various tissue types also changes with the duration of the healing process. From week 1 to week 2 following surgery, the tendency of suture to cut through tissue is less than in the immediate postoperative period (Aberg, 1976).

Memory refers to the tendency of a material to return to its original shape after deformation, for example, tying (Bennett, 1988). Suture with a high memory attempts to return to its original shape, and thus does not hold a knot well. Nylon is an example of a suture with a high degree of memory.

Handling Characteristics

Pliability is a subjective term related to how easily suture can be bent (Bennett, 1988). Relatively pliable sutures such as silk are easier to handle than stiffer, monofilament nylon sutures.

The **coefficient of friction** of a suture can be viewed as a measurement of "slipperiness" (Bennett, 1988). The inherent coefficient of friction of a given suture material may be altered by the application of special coatings. Sutures with high coefficients of friction are more difficult to pull through tissue. Materials with low coefficients of friction (monofilament nylon or coated polyglactin, for example) are easier to set by a slip knot, but may more easily come undone. For example, a simple square surgeon's knot with uncoated Dexon approaches maximum knot security, but the same knot tied with coated Vicryl is insecure (Trimbos, 1984).

Tissue Reaction Characteristics

All suture material is a foreign substance and will elicit a tissue reaction directly related to the amount of suture material present (Bennett, 1988). In this respect, the less suture used, the better. Further, the diameter of suture used under many circumstances is more closely linked to adhesion formation than the inherent reactivity of the material itself (Stone, 1988).

Three sequential histologic stages have been described in the normal reaction of tissue to suture material (Madsen, 1953; Postlethwait and colleagues, 1975). Stage I occurs during days 1–4, and consists of a leukocytic infiltrate including polymorphonuclear leukocytes, as well as lymphocytes and monocytes. During Stage II (days 4–7), infiltration with macrophages and fibroblasts occurs. Stage III, which occurs after the seventh day, consists primarily of a chronic inflammatory response and the appearance of additional fibrous tissue, with the formation of a fibrous capsule by day 28 (nonabsorbable suture) or a continued inflammatory response resulting in eventual complete absorption of the suture (absorbable suture).

Table 1–3 ranks suture material according to tissue reactivity. Within this ranking, multifilamentous suture elicits greater tissue reaction than monofilamentous material and increases the risk of infection to a greater degree (Alexander, 1967; James, 1961; Sharp, 1982; and their associates). In addition, infection is higher with braided suture material, which can harbor bacteria in the interstices where they are less susceptible to the action of leukocytes. Knots similarly provide interstices favorable to bacterial growth, suggesting that the number of knots placed should be minimized (Bennett, 1988; Osterberg, 1983a, b).

TABLE 1–3. RELATIVE TISSUE REACTIVITY TO SUTURES

	Nonabsorbable	Absorbable
Most Reactive	Silk, cotton	Catgut
↓	Polyester coated	Polyglactin 910
↓	Polyester uncoated	Polyglycolic acid
↓	Nylon	
Least Reactive	Polypropylene	

From Bennett (1988), with permission.

TABLE 1–4. COMPARISON OF ABSORBABLE SUTURES

Trade Name	Company	Material	Configuration	Tensile Strength	Tissue Reactivity
Collagen (plain)	Davis & Geck	Beef flexor tendon	Twisted	Poor (0% at 2–3 weeks)	Moderate
Collagen (chromic)	Davis & Geck	Beef flexor tendon	Twisted	Poor (0% at 2–3 weeks)	Moderate
Surgical gut (plain)	Ethicon; Davis & Geck	Animal collagen	Twisted	Poor (0% at 2–3 weeks)	High
Surgical gut (chromic)	Ethicon; Davis & Geck	Animal collagen	Twisted	Poor (0% at 2–3 weeks)	Moderately high
Coated Vicryl	Ethicon	Polyglactin 910 (coated with calcium stearate and polyglactin 370)	Braided	Good (50% at 2–3 weeks)	Low
Dexon "S"	Davis & Geck	Polyglycolic acid	Braided	Good (50% at 2–3 weeks)	Low
Dexon Plus	Davis & Geck	Polyglycolic acid (coated with poloxamer 188)	Braided	Good (50% at 2–3 weeks)	Low
PDS	Ethicon	Polydioxanone	Monofilamentous	Good (50% at 2–3 weeks)	Low

From Bennett (1988), with permission.

Specific Suture Types

Specific properties of absorbable and nonabsorbable sutures are detailed in Tables 1–4 and 1–5. The terms *absorbable* and *nonabsorbable* are in reality relative. Plain catgut, for example, an absorbable suture, may occasionally persist in tissue for many years (Postlethwait and colleagues, 1975), and with the exception of polyester (Dacron), polypropylene (Prolene), and stainless steel, all "nonabsorbable" sutures eventually degrade or are absorbed (Nilsson, 1982; Edlich and associates, 1974). However, those sutures that retain significant tensile strength beyond 60 days are commonly classified as "nonabsorbable" (Bennett, 1988).

Catgut

Catgut sutures are made from the submucosa of sheep or the intestinal serosa of cattle. "Chromic" catgut is treated with salts of chromium, which strengthen the suture. Catgut-based sutures are absorbed by lysosomal proteolytic enzymes in a process that is relatively unpredictable and is enhanced in the presence of local infection, which reduces the duration of tensile strength (Stone, 1988). In contrast, synthetic absorbable sutures dissolve by hydrolysis in a more predictable manner. With catgut sutures, degradation and phagocytosis begin 12 hours after implantation and reach a peak level 3 days later. Tensile strength is minimal after 10 days, and absorption is complete within 2–3 weeks (Bennett, 1988; Postlethwait and associates, 1975).

Plain catgut elicits a greater inflammatory response than chromic catgut. Catgut is slightly larger at each USP size than either Dexon or Vicryl (Fig. 1–3) (Stone, 1988). There is no evidence that catgut can induce an allergic response (Carroll, 1989).

Polyglycolic Acid (Dexon)

Polyglycolic acid is a high-molecular-weight linear chain polymer of hydroxyacetic (glycolic) acid. It is available as an uncoated (Dexon S) or coated (Dexon Plus) braided suture in either clear or green form. All synthetic absorbable sutures are non-antigenic and are degraded to CO_2 and H_2O by hydrolysis in the presence of tissue fluids in a predictable manner (Salthouse, 1980; Williams and Mort, 1977). One-third of breaking strength is lost at 7 days; complete absorption occurs in 90–120 days (Postlethwait, 1970; Eilert, 1971; Craig and associates, 1975; Frazza and Schmitt, 1971). While the prolonged retention of tensile strength would seem a theoretical advantage over chromic

Handling	Knot Security	Memory	Absorption	Degradation	Comments
Fair	Poor	Low	Unpredictable (12 weeks)	Proteolytic	Less impure than surgical gut
Fair	Poor	Low	Unpredictable (12 weeks)	Proteolytic	Less impure than surgical gut
Fair	Poor	Low	Unpredictable (12 weeks)	Proteolytic	May be ordered as "fast-absorbing gut" (Ethicon) for percutaneous sutures
Fair	Fair	Low	Unpredictable (14–80 days)	Proteolytic	Darker, more visible (Davis & Geck); mild or extra chromatization
Good	Fair	Low	Predictable (80 days)	Hydrolytic	Clear, violet, coated
Fair	Good	Low	Predictable (90 days)	Hydrolytic	Uncoated
Good	Fair	Low	Predictable (90 days)	Hydrolytic	Clear, green, coated
Poor	Poor	High	Predictable (180 days)	Hydrolytic	Violet, clear

catgut, any actual superiority is probably related more to the predictability of degradation compared to the more erratic enzymatic degradation seen with catgut.

Dexon evokes less tissue reaction than plain or chromic catgut (McGeehan and associates, 1980). Although its braided composition makes it less than ideal for heavily contaminated surgical sites, a study performed in Guinea pigs suggests superiority of this material to chromic catgut in avoiding infection following a bacterial inoculum (McGeehan and associates, 1980). However, the interstices in braided Dexon may potentiate infection, and its absorption is delayed in an infected environment (Foster and Hardcastle, 1978; Williams, 1980). Because Dexon is braided, it is inappropriate for use as a transcutaneous skin closure material.

Polyglactin 910 (Vicryl)

This material is a copolymer of lactide and glycolide, cyclic compounds derived from lactic and glycolic acids. Like polyglycolic acid, **polyglactin 910** is braided. The tensile strength of Vicryl is slightly less than Dexon, and thus Vicryl is manufactured in slightly larger diameters than Dexon at each USP specified size (Bennett, 1988; Stone, 1988). All currently manufactured Vicryl is coated, and available in either clear or purple. The inflammatory response to Vicryl is similar to that of Dexon. In rats, Vicryl is absorbed faster than Dexon. In two studies, 77 percent of Dexon remained after 63 days compared with 26 percent of Vicryl, which was completely absorbed in 60–90 days, compared to 90–120 for Dexon (Craig and associates, 1975; Conn and associates, 1974). In rats, Vicryl does not contribute to the strength of abdominal wounds after 15 days (Nilsson, 1981).

The Oxford Perinatal Database identified 14 controlled trials of perineal suturing following vaginal delivery. This survey concluded that polyglycolic acid or polyglactin sutures were superior to catgut derivatives because they produced significantly less pain, less need for analgesia, less late dyspareunia, and possibly less risk of dehiscence (Grant, 1989) (see Chapter 7). However, both Dexon and Vicryl have relatively high tensile strength and low elasticity compared to chromic catgut, and thus tend to cut through tissue more readily.

Polydioxanone (PDS II)

Polydioxanone is a polymer made from paradioxanone and is manufactured as a monofilamentous suture, unlike Dexon or Vicryl. In one study, PDS II was found to be

TABLE 1–5. COMPARISON OF NONABSORBABLE SUTURES

Generic Trade Name	Company	Material	Configuration	Tensile Strength
Cotton	—	Cotton	Twisted	Good
Silk	Ethicon; David & Geck	Silk	Braided	Good
Ethilon	Ethicon	Polyamide (nylon)	Monofilamentous	High
Dermalon	Davis & Geck	Polyamide (nylon)	Monofilamentous	High
Surgamid	Look	Polyamide (nylon)	Monofilamentous or braided	High
Nurolon	Ethicon	Polyamide (nylon)	Braided	High
Surgilon	Davis & Geck	Polyamide (nylon) (coated with silicone)	Braided	High
Prolene	Ethicon	Polyolefin (polypropylene)	Monofilamentous	Fair
Surgilene	Davis & Geck	Polyolefin (polypropylene)	Monofilamentous	Fair
Dermalene	Davis & Geck	Polyolefin (polypropylene)	Monofilamentous	Good
Novafil	Davis & Geck	Polybutester	Monofilamentous	High
Mersilene	Ethicon	Polyester	Braided	High
Dacron	DeKnatel; Davis & Geck	Polyester	Braided	High
Polyviolene	Look	Polyester	Braided	High
Ethibond	Ethicon	Polyester (coated with polybutilate)	Braided	High
Tri-Cron	Davis & Geck	Polyester (coated with silicone)	Braided	High
Polydek	DeKnatel	Polyester (coated with Teflon-light)	Braided	High
Tavdek	DeKnatel	Polyester (coated with Teflon-heavy)	Braided	High
Stainless steel	Ethicon	Stainless steel	Monofilamentous, twisted, or braided	High

From Bennett (1988), with permission.

completely absorbed in 180 days, as compared to 60–90 days for Vicryl and 120 days for Dexon (Ray and associates, 1981). PDS II also maintains 58 percent of breaking strength at 28 days, compared to 5 percent or less for either Dexon or Vicryl (Ray and associates, 1981). PDS II suture is capable of maintaining its integrity in the presence of bacterial infection (Schoetz and colleagues, 1988). The principal disadvantage of PDS II suture is its stiffness, a result of monofilament construction, which makes it more difficult to tie.

Silk

Silk is a natural protein, produced during cocoon construction by the silkworm larva. Silk is braided and dyed black for surgical use. "Dermal silk" sutures are silk sutures that are encased in protein to prevent epithelial ingrowth along the suture line, which would make removal more difficult. The widespread fear of painful suture removal probably originated with uncoated transcutaneous silk sutures, which allowed epithelial tissue ingrowth prior to suture removal (Bennett, 1988; Freeman and colleagues, 1970). Silk suture is absorbed after several months; this delay may occasionally result in granuloma formation. Thus silk suture is unsuitable for procedures requiring long-term stability (Salthouse, 1980; Postlethwait, 1970b).

The advantages of silk sutures include easy handling, little knot slippage, and a minimal tendency to tear through tissues. How-

Tissue Reactivity	Handling	Knot Security	Memory	Comments
High	Good	Good	Poor	Obsolete
High	Good	Good	Poor	Predisposes to infection; does not tear tissue; D & G suture is silicone treated; Ethicon is waxed
Low	Poor	Poor	High	Cuts tissue; nylon 6, 6; black, clear, or green
Low	Poor	Poor	High	Nylon 6, 6
Low	Poor	Poor	High	Nylon 6, 6
Moderate	Good	Fair	Fair	May predispose to infection; black or white; waxed; nylon 6, 6
Moderate	Fair	Fair	Fair	Nylon 6, 6
Low	Poor	Poor	High	Very low coefficient of friction; cuts tissue; blue or clear
Low	Poor	Poor	High	—
Low	Poor	Poor	High	—
Low	Fair	Poor	Low	Blue or clear
Moderate	Good	Good	Fair	Green or white
Moderate	Good	Good	Fair	—
Moderate	Good	Good	Fair	Green or white
Moderate	Good	Good	Fair	Green or white
Moderate	Poor	Poor	Fair	—
Moderate	Good	Good	Fair	—
Moderate	Poor	Poor	Fair	—
Low	Poor	Good	Poor	May kink

ever, it has great fluid and bacterial absorption ability and is not suitable for use in an infected surgical field. Further, quantitative investigations into knot strength suggest that compared to other materials, silk actually forms relatively weak knots (Tera and Aberg, 1976a).

Cotton

Cotton suture is constructed of braided cotton fibers. Unlike any other material, cotton is made stronger and the knot firmer by fluid absorption (Hochberg and Murray, 1991). Cotton is essentially identical to silk in its reactivity and infection-enhancing capacity (Hochberg and Murray, 1991). Cotton suture is rarely used in obstetric surgery.

Nylon

Nylon is a synthetic polyamide polymer and is manufactured as either a multi- or monofilament fiber. Tensile strength is great, but nylon sutures are stiff; they easily cut through thin tissue and require several well-placed knots to prevent untying. Such sutures are used primarily in cutaneous or subcutaneous suturing, and are rarely used for internal hemostasis or wound approximation (Goulbourne and associates, 1988). Nylon is eventually degraded and absorbed and has little remaining tensile strength after 6 months (Moloney, 1961). Birdsell and associates (1981) found that in human studies, there was no difference in the strength of cutaneous wounds closed with buried nylon as opposed to Vicryl sutures.

Polypropylene
These sutures are formed by **propylene polymerization** (Prolene, Surgilene) and are virtually identical to polyethylene sutures (Dermalene). The principal distinguishing feature of these sutures is an extremely small coefficient of friction, making them ideal for cutaneous intradermal closure with later removal (Freeman, 1970; Homsy, 1968; and their associates). This same feature, however, makes knots less secure. Polypropylene is also a very plastic suture, which stretches and deforms easily as a wound swells; thus these sutures rarely cut through tissue (Bennett, 1988).

Polypropylene is relatively noninflammatory (Salthouse and Matlaga, 1975). In rabbits, Prolene was found to have superior tensile strength over time compared to nylon (Nilsson, 1982). In vascular grafts, prolene sutures removed at 2–6 years showed no loss of tensile strength (Dobrin, 1989).

Polyester
Polyester suture material is a braided, multifilament polymerized permanent suture, manufactured in coated and uncoated forms. Merseline is the most common uncoated form used in obstetrics. Tevdek and the Ethibond are examples of polyester sutures coated with Teflon and polybutilate, respectively, resulting in much smoother passage through tissues. Polyester sutures are second only to metal sutures in tensile strength (Herrmann, 1971). Polyester sutures are truly nonabsorbable and retain their tensile strength indefinitely. Uncoated polyester suture evokes minimal inflammatory response (Hartko, 1982).

Stainless steel
Stainless steel suture is available in either mono- or multifilamentous form. It is inert and has excellent tensile strength and knot security. However, it is difficult to handle. Its use in obstetrics is generally limited to select cases of abdominal wall/fascia closure in women at extreme risk for infection and dehiscence.

Conclusion
As presented in the foregoing discussion, each type of suture material has both advantages and drawbacks. With the exception of the prospective studies examining perineal repair, convincing data does not exist to document clear and generalized superiority of any suture type for obstetric use. In the chapters that follow, examples of appropriate suture choice for specific indications are presented. Alternate choices may be equally acceptable.

KNOTS

Knot tying is the most important, but potentially weakest, part of suture technique. As Taylor observed, "The surgeon naturally feels that others may tie faulty knots but that his knots are beyond reproach" (Taylor, 1939). Unfortunately, this assumption is often invalid. When the knots of a group of board-certified general surgeons were subjected to mechanical performance tests, it was determined that only 25 percent used appropriate knot construction (Thacker and colleagues, 1977). Similarly, a poll of a group of 25 gynecologists, "well known . . . and selected on the grounds of their experience in, and contributions to, the field of gynecologic surgery," revealed that most were convinced they made square knots, even though the technique described resulted in slip knots (Trimbos, 1984). Batra and associates (1983) demonstrated that with minimal instruction, medical students consistently constructed stronger standard square knots than a cohort of practicing obstetrician/gynecologists using both monofilament and multifilament nylon sutures (Batra and associates, 1993). This data validates Haxton's observation

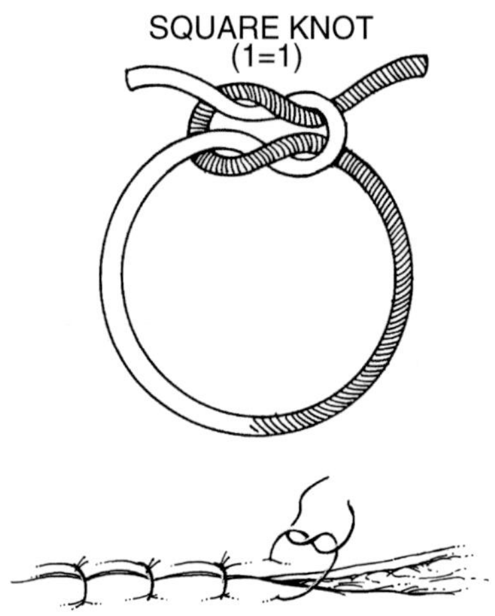

Figure 1–7. The components of a tied suture. (Modified from Edlich, 1991, with permission.)

(1965) that "the use of methods and materials for suturing is usually a matter of habit, guesswork or tradition."

Faulty knot tying may be devastating and lead to exsanguination or wound dehiscence. It is thus mandatory that the obstetrician thoroughly understand that certain knots are stronger than others, that different suture materials require different numbers of throws for knot security, and that these relationships have been defined biomechanically (Edlich, 1991). Such knowledge provides the foundation for the proper practice of the science of knot tying.

Terminology

A **tied suture** consists of three components: the **loop**, which affects hemostasis or wound approximation; the **knot**, which maintains security of the loop; and the **ears**, which act as "insurance" that the loop will not become untied because of knot slippage (Fig. 1–7) (Edlich, 1991).

An international code has been developed to describe surgical knots (Fig. 1–8). The number of wraps in a single throw is indicated by arabic numerals. Thus the common single throw is 1 and the double or "surgeon's" throw is 2. The slip configuration is designated by the letter S. If successive throws are parallel, or square, the symbol = is used, whereas the letter x signifies a crossed or "granny" configuration. Thus the common square knot is described as 1=1, a granny as 1x1, a square surgeon's knot as 2=2 and a simple slip knot as S=S.

Knot Slippage

Knot slippage is influenced by several factors: the coefficient of friction of the chosen suture material, the suture diameter, coating, moisture, knot configuration, and the final

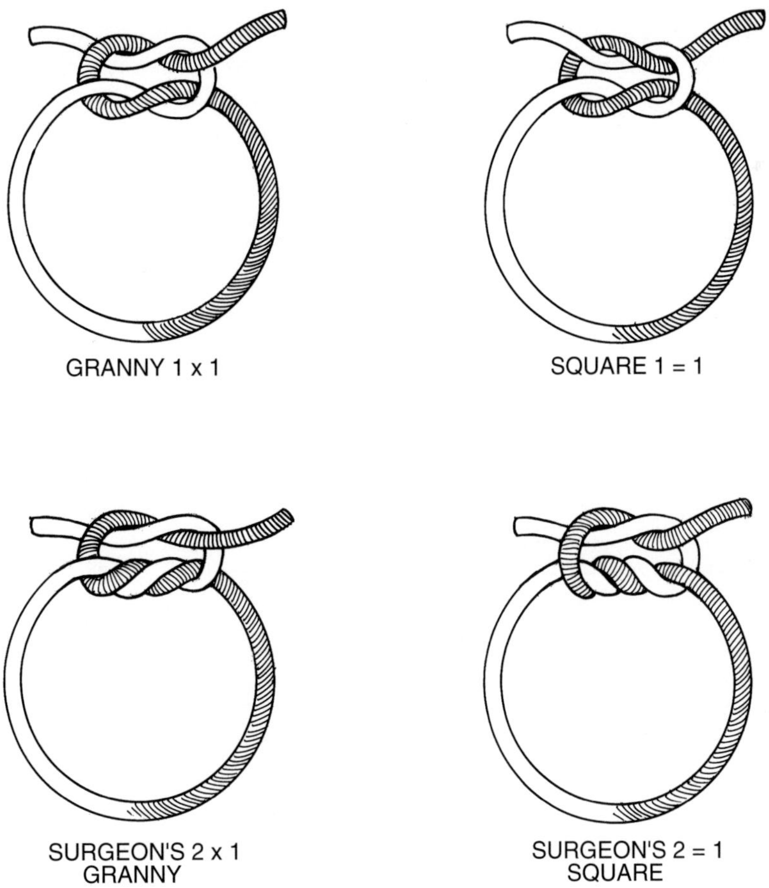

Figure 1–8. The configuration of surgical knots.

geometry of the finished knot; additional factors are the human element and tying technique (Edlich, 1991). In particular, the coefficient of friction for any suture is linearly related to and determines the number of throws needed for knot security (Herrmann, 1971). Knot slippage exceeding 2 mm (commonly accepted as the maximum allowable slippage of a properly tied knot) (Tera and Aberg, 1976a; Thacker and associates, 1975) varies from 0 to 100 percent depending upon the knot type alone (Madsen, 1953). For example, even in knots laid flat, the granny configuration always results in greater slippage than a square knot with the exception of the 2=2 and 2x2 configurations, which appear to be similar for most materials (Tera and Aberg, 1976a). Coated suture results in greater knot slippage than corresponding uncoated suture (Trimbos, 1984). Many types of suture also exhibit significant knot slackening in vivo, independent of inherent suture degradation. Notable exceptions to this principle are polyester sutures such as Ethibond (Tomita, 1992).

Each additional throw reduces knot slippage. After a certain number of throws (determined by the knot configuration and suture material), however, knot failure will occur by breakage, rather than slippage. At this point, additional throws only result in greater foreign body inflammatory reaction and encourage infection (Edlich, 1991).

The human element also greatly influences knot slippage (Thacker and associates, 1975). Two particularly important aspects of tying technique are the force and the direction in which tension is applied as the knot is tightened. A slip knot may be constructed in either a square or granny configuration. Such knots are often helpful in obtaining close approximation of tissues during the initial stage of knot formation, especially when tying one-handed knots and deep-seated ligatures (Zimmer, 1991; Thacker, 1975; and their associates). If such a knot is tightened by applying pressure to one ear only (Fig. 1–9), the knot will remain in an S configuration and will tend to fail by slippage rather than breakage even after five throws (Zimmer and associates, 1991). After the tissues have been appropriately coapted, however, the slip knot can be converted to a square or granny configuration by applying tension to both ears in opposite directions in a plane roughly horizontal to the tissue surface

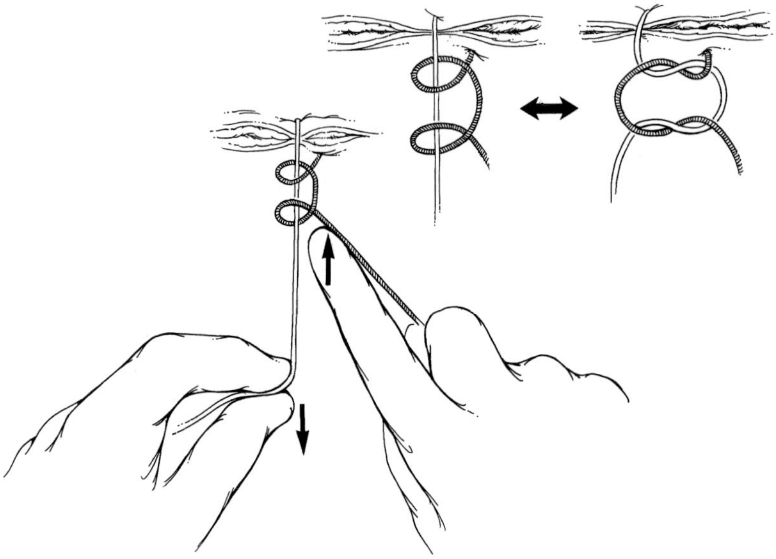

Figure 1–9. Advance slip knot (S = S) to wound surface. The tip of the right index finger slides (arrow) this second throw against the first throw, completing the slip knot (S = S), while the left hand maintains tension (arrow) on its suture end. The slip knot will become a square knot by applying tension to the suture end held by the right hand. The square knot can be converted to a slip knot by applying tension primarily to one suture end. (Modified from Edlich, 1991, with permission.)

for materials with lower coefficients of friction, additional parallel throws with these materials would seem prudent.

For monofilament nylon or silk in 0 and 000 gauges, significant additional strength is gained with a 2=2=2 or 1=1=1=1 knot, compared to a 1=1=1 construction. 0 Prolene demonstrated maximum knot strength with a 2=2=2 or 2x2x2 knot structure; such configurations are superior even to a 1=1=1=1=1 construction. For Tevdek, five throws of any configuration have been recommended (Table 1–8) (Haxton, 1965).

It is interesting to note that with most materials tested, a 1=2 configuration is significantly stronger than a 2=1 knot construction (Tera and Aberg, 1977). Further, a 2=2=2 configuration is stable with all types and gauges of suture, and is recommended if the specific suture characteristics are not known (Tera and Aberg, 1976a). In constructing a square knot, it is important to remember that such a knot cannot be constructed without crossing either the suture ends or the hands (Fig. 1–10) (Trimbos, 1984).

Wound security is, of course also dependent upon aspects of surgical technique other than knot and suture strength. For example, tight fascial approximation results in a significantly weaker incision line than looser closure technique, presumably due to ischemia and poor healing (Stone and associates, 1986).

STAPLES

The original surgical stapling device, developed in 1908, weighed 7.5 pounds (Hochberg and Murray, 1991; Nilsson, 1982; Stone and associates, 1986). Today's surgical staplers are much smaller and include instruments designed to divide and simultaneously close intestine as well as devices for skin approximation only (Hochberg and Murray, 1991). A device for placement of absorbable cuticular sutures is also available. Most devices currently used for skin approximation are disposable and are popular due to their speed as well as the excellent cosmetic appearance resulting from the precise everting of skin edges during closure.

Other significant advantages of staples are that when placed, they do not form a continuous tract from the skin surface into the wound, as do percutaneous sutures, and they do not form a foreign body within the wound, as do subcuticular sutures. Thus there is a decreased likelihood of infection using this method of skin closure (Bennett, 1988).

TABLE 1–8. RECOMMENDED KNOT CONFIGURATIONS FOR COMMONLY USED OBSTETRIC SUTURE MATERIAL

Suture	Recommended Knot Configuration
Chromic catgut	1=1=1 or 1x1x1
Dexon, Vicryl	1=1=1=1=1
Monofilament silk	1=1=1=1
Monofilament nylon	1=1=1=1=1
Prolene	2 = 2 = 2 or 2 x 2 x 2
Tevdek	1=1=1=1=1 or 1x1x1x1x1
All suture types	2 = 2 = 2

SKIN TAPES

Modern skin tapes are relatively non-occlusive, yet have excellent adhesive properties (Bennett, 1988). If the patient keeps the skin dry, skin tapes generally will not loosen for 3–7 days, a period long enough for most cutaneous wounds to heal. Using skin tapes precludes the need to puncture the skin surface, thus maintaining epidermal integrity, reducing the risk of tissue strangulation and wound infection, and avoiding suture marks (Bennett, 1988; Alexander and colleagues, 1967).

Commonly used microporous surgical tapes have a backing of rayon fibers coated with an adhesive copolymer, and are pervious to sweat but not to blood or pus (Hochberg and Murray, 1991). The principal disadvantages of these tapes is that they do not evert the wound edges and readily loosen when wet.

SUMMARY

From the forgoing discussion, the following principles may be drawn:

1. Cutting needles are rarely useful in obstetrics, except in placing a subcuticular skin closure. The use of cutting needles contributes to tearing soft tissue like uterus, vagina, hysterectomy

pedicles, and fascia. Cutting needles should be avoided.

2. When cutting needles are used, those with a reverse cutting design may reduce the risk of pull-through.
3. A curved needle should not be grasped with the fingers.
4. Vicryl or Dexon sutures are clearly superior in tensile strength to chromic catgut for the repair of vaginal lacerations and episiotomies.
5. Suture strength is reduced significantly by stray knots, and by grasping the suture with any instrument.
6. With appropriate knot-tying technique, knot ears exceeding 3 mm in length should be unnecessary regardless of suture type. Ears exceeding this length predispose to infection.
7. A square configuration is generally more secure than a crossed (granny) knot. However, either of these knots is preferable to a slip knot, which is insecure after any number of throws.
8. If slip knots are necessary, as in tying one-handed knots in deep spaces, or assisting in initial tissue approximation, they should be converted to square or granny configuration after placement (Fig. 1–9). If conversion is not technically possible, tying slip knots over alternate threads is an acceptable substitute.
9. Use the appropriate knot configuration for the suture material selected. In a properly tied knot, additional "insurance throws" do not contribute to knot security and may enhance infection (Table 1–8).

REFERENCES

Aberg C. Change in strength of aponeurotic tissue enclosed in the suture during the initial healing period. An experimental investigation in rabbits. Acta Chir Scand 1976; 142:429.

Abidin MR, Towler MA, Thacker JG, Nochimson GD, McGregor W, Edlich RF. New atraumatic rounded-edge surgical needle holder jaws. Am J Surg 1989; 157:241.

Alexander JW, Kaplan JZ, Altemeier WA. Role of suture materials in the development of wound infection. Ann Surg 1967; 165:192.

Batra EK, Taylor PT, Franz DA, et al. A portable tensiometer for assessing surgeon's knot tying technique. Gynecol Oncology 1993; 48:114.

Bennett RG. Selection of wound closure materials. J Am Acad Dermatol 1988; 18:619.

Birdsell DC, Gavelin GE, Kemsley GM, Hein KS. "Staying power"—absorbable vs. nonabsorbable. Plast Reconstr Surg 1981; 68:742.

Bucknall TE. Factors influencing wound complications: a clinical and experimental study. Ann R Coll Surg 1983; 65:71.

Carroll RE. Surgical catgut: the myth of allergy. J Hand Surg 1989; 14B:218.

Conn J Jr, Oyasu R, Welsh M, Beal JM. Vicryl (polyglactin 910) synthetic absorbable sutures. Am J Surg 1974; 128:19.

Craig PH, Williams JA, Davis KW, et al. A biologic comparison of polyglactin 910 and polyglycolic acid synthetic absorbable sutures. Surg Gynecol Obstet 1975; 141:1.

Dalgleish AG, Malkovsky M. Surgical gloves as a mechanical barrier against human immunodeficiency virus. Br J Surg 1988; 75:171.

Dobrin PB. Surgical manipulation and the tensile strength of polypropylene sutures. Arch Surg 1989; 124:665.

Edlich RF, Panek PH, Rodeheaver GT, Kurtz LD, Edgerton MT. Surgical sutures and infection: a biomaterial evaluation. J Biomed Mater Res 1974; 8:115.

Edlich RF. *USSC Surgical Knot Tying Manual,* United States Surgical Corporation, Norwalk, CT, 1991.

Eilert JB, Binder P, McKinney PW, Beal JM, Conn J Jr. Polyglycolic acid synthetic absorbable sutures. Am J Surg 1971; 121:561.

Ethicon, Inc. Ethicon Product Catolog, 1993.

Foster GE, Hardcastle JD. Polyglycolic acid as suture material [letter]. Lancet 1978; 1:154.

Frazza EJ, Schmitt EE. A new absorbable suture. J Biomed Mater Res 1971; 5:43.

Freeman BS, Homsy CA, Fissette J, Hardy SB. An analysis of suture withdrawal stress. Surg Gynecol Obstet 1970; 131:441.

Goulbourne IA, Nixon SJ, Naylor AR, Varma JS. Comparison of polyglactin 910 and nylon in skin closure. Br J Surg 1988; 75:586.

Grant A. The choice of suture materials and techniques for repair of perineal trauma: an overview of the evidence from controlled trials. Br J Obstet Gynecol 1989; 96:1281.

Hartko WJ, Ghanekar G, Kemmann E. Suture materials currently used in obstetric-gynecologic surgery in the United States: A questionnaire survey. Obstet Gynecol 1982; 59:241.

Haxton H. The influence of suture materials and methods on the healing of abdominal wounds. Br J Surg 1965; 52:372.

Herrmann JB. Tensile strength and knot security of surgical suture materials. Am Surg 1971 (April):209.

Herrmann JB. Changes in tensile strength and knot security of surgical sutures in vivo. Arch Surg 1973; 106:707.

Hochberg J, Murray GF. Principles of operative surgery. In Sabiston DC Jr (ed), *Textbook of Surgery*, 14th ed. Philadelphia: WB Saunders, 1991.

Homsy CA, McDonald KE, Akers WW. Surgical suture—canine tissue interaction for six common suture types. J Biomed Mater Res 1968; 2:215.

James RC, MacLeod CJ. Induction of staphylococcal infections in mice with small inocula introduced on sutures. Br J Exp Pathol 1961; 42:266.

Lister J. Observations on ligature of arteries on the antiseptic system. Lancet 1969; 6:289.

Madsen ET. An experimental and clinical evaluation of surgical suture materials—I and II. Surg Gynecol Obstet 1953; 97:73.

McGeehan D, Hunt D, Chaudhuri A, Rutter P. An experimental study of the relationship between synergistic wound sepsis and suture materials. Br J Surg 1980; 67:636.

Meade WH, Ochsner A. A relative value of catgut, silk, linen, and cotton as suture material. Surgery 1940; 7:485.

Moloney GE. The effect of human tissues on the tensile strength of implanted nylon sutures. Br J Surg 1961; 48:528.

Nilsson T. The relative importance of Vicryl and Prolene sutures to the strength of healing abdominal wounds. Acta Chir Scand 1981; 147:503.

Nilsson T. Mechanical properties of Prolene and Ethilon sutures after three weeks in vivo. Scand J Plast Reconstr Surg 1982; 16:11.

Osterberg B. Enclosure of bacteria within capillary multifilament sutures as protection against leukocytes. Acta Chir Scand 1983a; 149:663.

Osterberg B. Influence of capillary multifilament sutures on the antibacterial action of inflammatory cells in infected wounds. Acta Chir Scand 1983b; 149:751.

Postlethwait RW. Polyglycolic acid surgical suture. Arch Surg 1970a; 101:489.

Postlethwait RW. Long-term comparative study of non-absorbable sutures. Ann Surg 1970b; 171:892.

Postlethwait RW, Willigan DA, Ulin AW. Human tissue reaction to sutures. Ann Surg 1975; 181:144.

Ray JA, Doddi N, Regula D, et al. Polydioxanone (PDS), a novel monofilament synthetic absorbable suture. Surg Gynecol Obstet 1981; 153:497.

Rodeheaver GT, Thacker JG, Edlich RF. Mechanical performance of polyglycolic acid and polyglactin 910 synthetic absorbable sutures. Surg Gynecol Obstet 1981; 153:835.

Salthouse TN. Biologic response to sutures. Otolaryngol Head Neck Surg 1980 (Nov-Dec); 88:658.

Salthouse TN, Matlaga BF. Significance of cellular enzyme activity at nonabsorbable suture implant sites: silk, polyester, and polypropylene. J Surg Res 1975; 19:127.

Schoetz DJ, Coller JA, Veidenheimer MC. Closure of abdominal wounds with polydioxanone. Arch Surg 1988; 123:72.

Serrano CW, Wright JW, Newton ER. Surgical glove perforation in obstetrics. Obstet Gynecol 1991; 77:525.

Sharp WV, Belden TA, King PH, Teague PC. Suture resistance to infection. Surgery 1982; 92:61.

Snyder CC. On the history of the suture. Plast Reconstr Surg 1976; 58(4):401.

Stamp CV, McGregor W, Rodeheaver GT, et al. Surgical needle holder damage to sutures. Am Surg 1988; 54:300.

Stone IK, von Fraunhofer JA, Masterson BJ. The biomechanical effects of tight suture closure upon fascia. Surg Gynecol Obstet 1986; 163:448.

Stone IK. Suture materials. Clin Obstet Gynecol 1988; 31(3):712.

Taylor FW. Surgical knots and sutures. Surgery 1939; 5:499.

Tera H, Aberg C. Tensile strengths of twelve types of knot employed in surgery, using different suture materials. Acta Chir Scand 1976a; 142:1.

Tera H, Aberg C. Tissue strength of structures involved in musculo-aponeurotic layer sutures in laparotomy incisions. Acta Chir Scand 1976b; 142:349.

Tera H, Aberg C. Strength of knots in surgery in relation to type of knot, type of suture material and dimension of suture thread. Acta Chir Scand 1977; 143:75.

Thacker JG, Rodeheaver G, Moore JW, et al. Mechanical performance of surgical sutures. Am J Surg 1975; 130:374.

Thacker JG, Rodeheaver G, Kurtz L, et al. Mechanical performance of sutures in surgery. Am J Surg 1977; 133:713.

Tomita N, Tamai S, Shimaya M, et al. A study of elongation and knot slacking of various sutures. Bio-Medical Materials and Engineering 1992; 2:71.

Trimbos JB. Security of various knots commonly used in surgical practice. Obstet Gynecol 1984; 64:274.

Von Fraunhofer JA, Storey RS, Stone IK, Masterson BJ. Tensile strength of suture materials. J Biomed Mater Res 1985; 19:596.

Williams DF, Mort E. Enzyme-accelerated hydrolysis of polyglycolic acid. J Bioeng 1977; 1:231.

Williams DF. The effect of bacteria on absorbable sutures. J Biomed Mater Res 1980; 14:329.

Zimmer CA, Thacker JG, Powell DM, et al. Influence of knot configuration and tying technique on the mechanical performance of sutures. J Emerg Med 1991; 9:107.

CHAPTER 2

Surgical Instruments and Drains

"Give me what I need, not what I ask for," is a request commonly heard at a crucial time during a surgical procedure. Unfortunately adequate training in surgical instruments is lacking in many residency programs. Often the operating room nursing staff have more knowledge regarding the name, care, and purpose of surgical instruments than the surgeon. The purpose of this chapter is to provide an overview of the most common instruments and devices used in obstetrics.

INSTRUMENTS

A bewildering variety of instruments is available, many of which differ insignificantly from one another. For example, there are at least six different types of single-tooth tenaculum, including the Braun, Barrett, Deplay, Jarcho, Adair, and Skene variations. Regional differences in nomenclature are another complication, especially for obstetrical surgery because instruments are often prepacked for emergency use by a number of different physicians. Surgeons should review the instruments in these "packs" regularly. All surgeons should be aware of which instruments are available and be able to ask for them by their correct name and use them for their intended purpose.

Lighting Devices

Although operating room lighting is usually adequate for routine surgical procedures, this is not always the case in delivery rooms. If additional lighting is required for deep spaces, a **fiberoptic head light** can be invaluable, in both the delivery room and operating room (Fig. 2–1). Although lighted retractors can be used for abdominal and vaginal work (Fig. 2–2), a head light is a more versatile instrument.

INSTRUMENTS FOR SUTURING

Needle holders are available in several sizes; one catalogue of surgical instruments lists 19 varieties of needle holders in addition to those described for microsurgical procedures (Codman, 1990). Needle holders commonly used in obstetrics have either serrated or longitudinal teeth and are manufactured in both straight and curved (Heaney) configurations (Figs. 2–3, 2–4). The Heaney needle holder is especially valuable in placing needles in deep abdominal recesses and in performing vaginal surgery. The rings in the handles of needle holders assist the novice surgeon in manipulating the instrument. With time and experience, the surgeon acquires the ability to "palm" the instrument, ie, place and manipulate needles

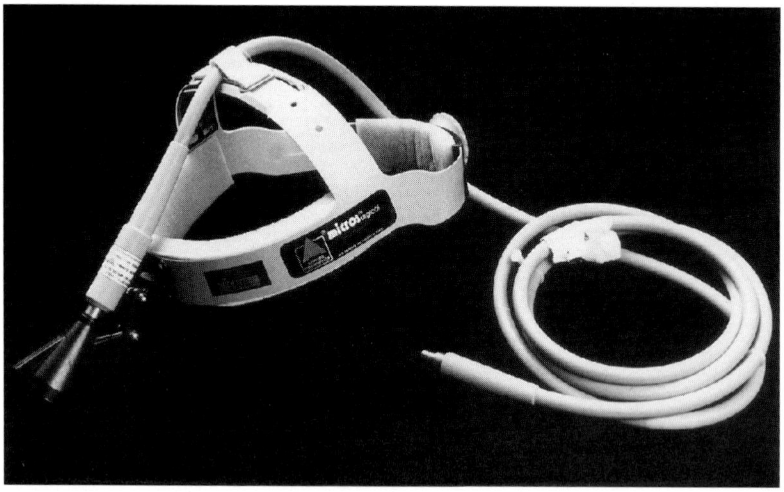

Figure 2–1. Surgical headlamp.

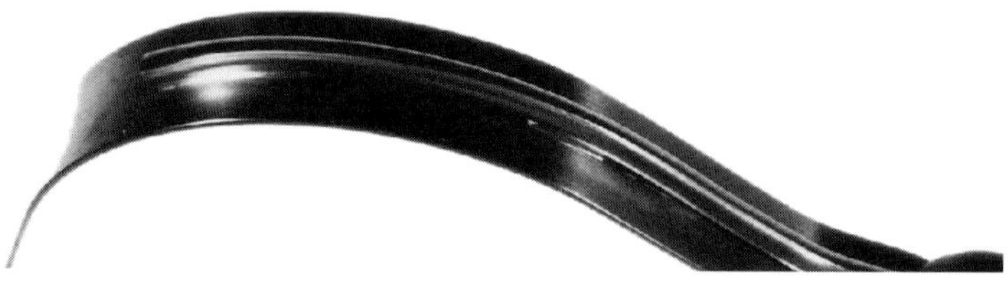

Figure 2–2. Illuminated retractor.

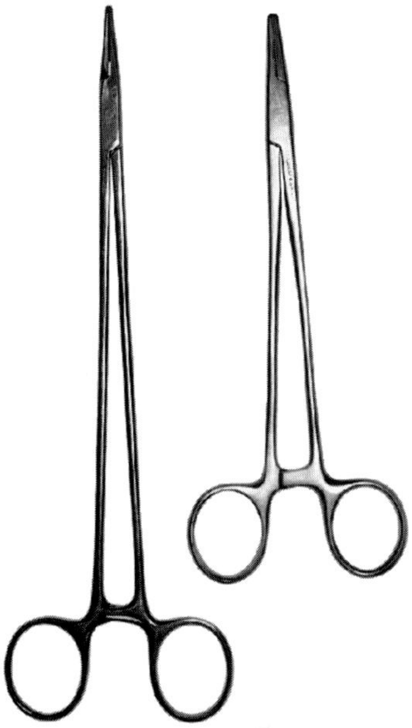

Figure 2–3. Straight needle holders.

as well as lock and unlock the needle holder without placing the fingers of the dominant hand through the rings (Figs. 2–5, 2–6). Using this technique, the surgeon can quickly run suture lines in tissues such as myometrium or fascia without the need to remove the fingers from the needle holder or reposition the needle manually after each stitch. The obstetric surgeon should strive to perfect this technique for use of needle holders, and extend it when possible to all instruments with ringed handles.

Clamps and scissors are not designed for ambidextrous use. The easy release of a clamp or use of standard right-handed scissors with the left hand therefore requires a different hand grip and technique than when these instruments are used with the right hand. The obstetrician should strive to become facile in the use of these instruments with either hand, using the appropriate grip and technique as demonstrated in Figure 2–7.

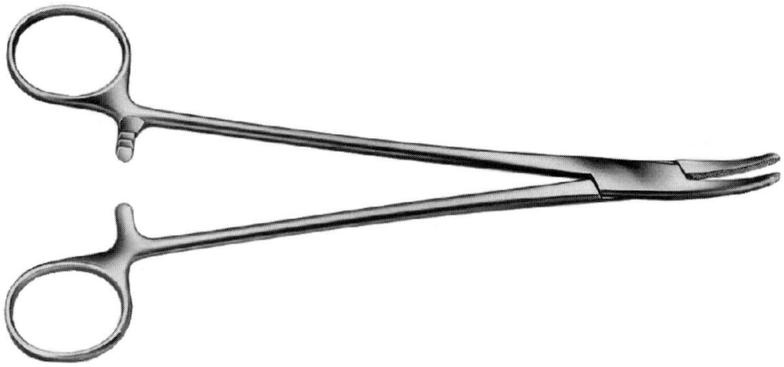

Figure 2–4. Curved (Heaney) needle holder. (Photo courtesy of Aesculap, Inc.)

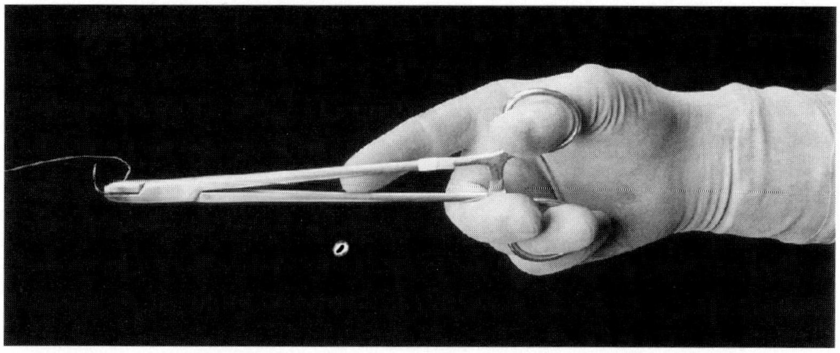

Figure 2–5. Technique of grasping the needle holder with the fingers through the rings. Manipulation of the instrument and resetting the needle is awkward using this grip.

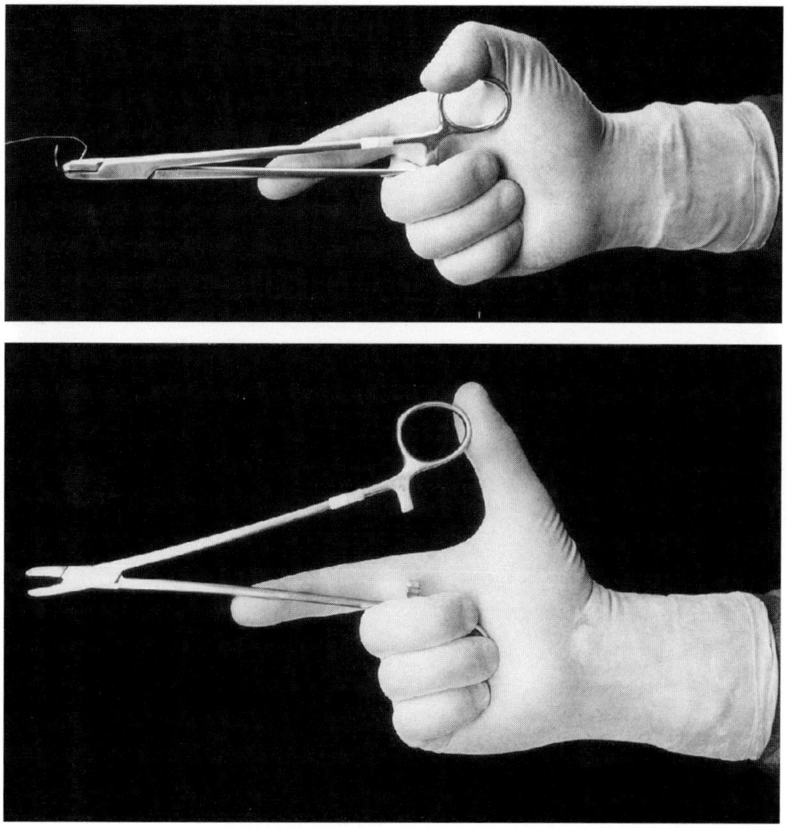

Figure 2–6. Technique of grasping the needle holder avoiding fingers through the rings. Manipulation is facilitated by using the instrument without placing the fingers through the rings.

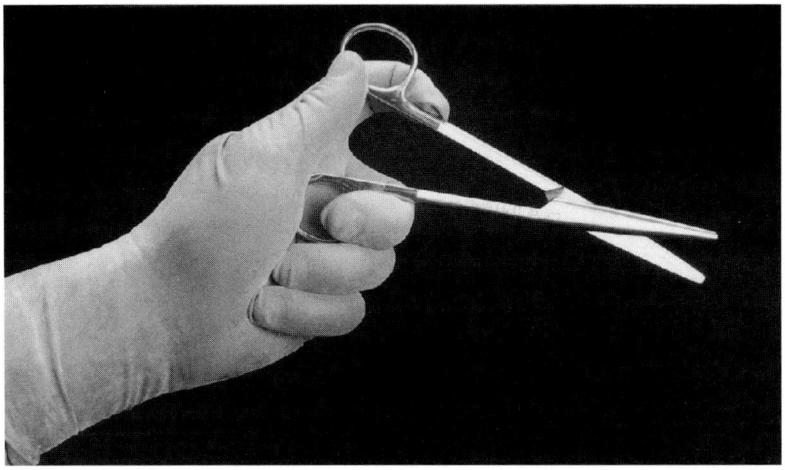

Figure 2–7. Left-handed use of scissors. The same technique is used for left-handed release of clamps.

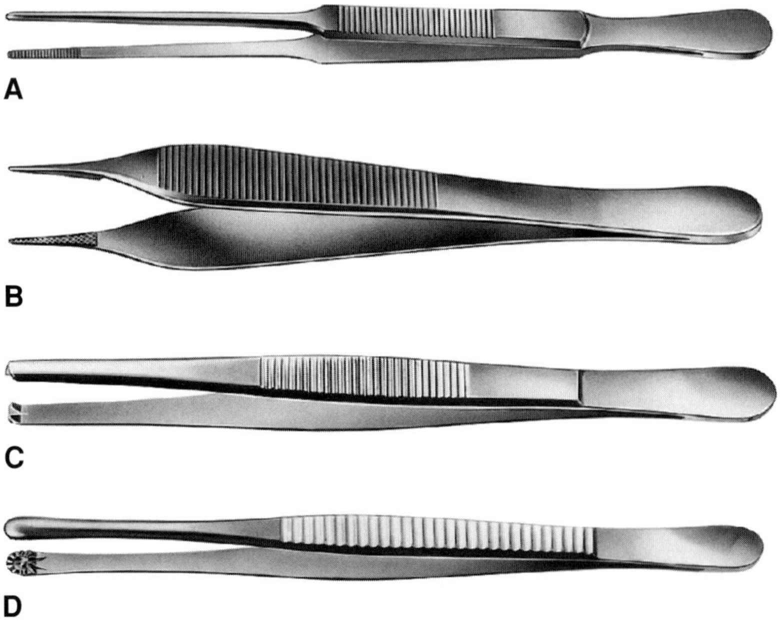

Figure 2–8. Forceps used in suture placement. **A.** Dressing ("smooth") forceps. **B.** Adson modification of dressing forceps. **C.** Tissue forceps ("rat-toothed"). **D.** Russian forceps. (Photo courtesy of Aesculap, Inc.)

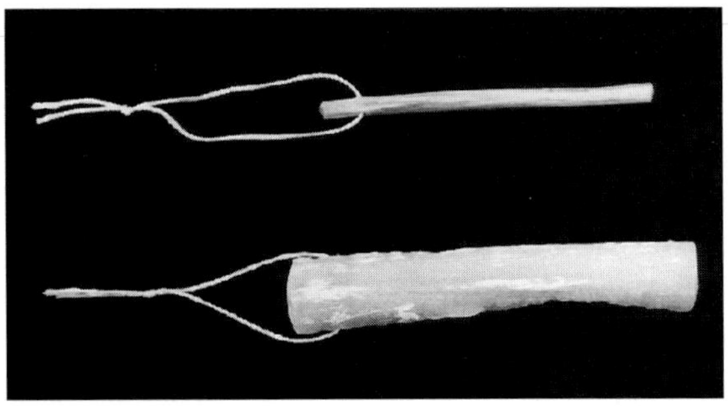

Figure 2–9. Laminaria cervical dilator. **Top.** Prior to insertion. **Bottom.** Following insertion and fluid absorption.

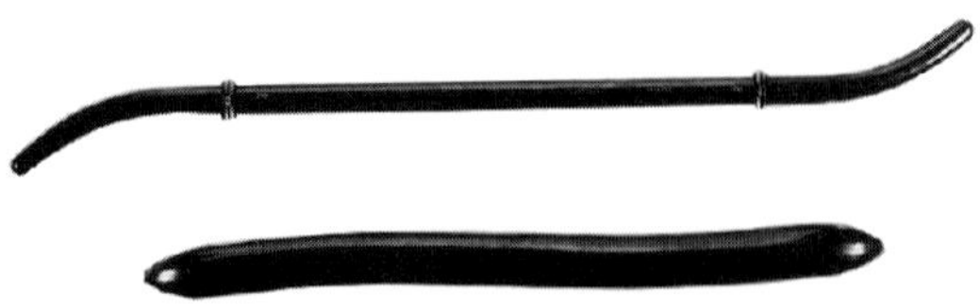

Figure 2–10. Mechanical cervical dilators. **Top.** Hanks. **Bottom.** Hegar.

Forceps for Suturing

Three types of forceps ("pickups") are commonly used for suture placement: **dressing forceps** ("smooth"), **tissue forceps** ("toothed") and **Russian** or **Mayo** forceps (Fig. 2–8). These instruments are available in various lengths. Forceps are designed to grasp tissue, not needles or suture. Although the occasional use of forceps to grasp the needle is of little consequence, the handling of suture with these instruments results in a significant decrease in suture tensile strength and should be avoided.

Dressing forceps are used to handle delicate tissue such as skin, peritoneum, mesosalpinx, or ovary. Tissue forceps have an interlocking tooth and socket configuration and are useful in obtaining a firm hold of tougher, relatively avascular tissue such as fascia. Russian or Mayo forceps have a broad, serrated tip and are most useful in grasping thicker, vascular tissues such as myometrium, where the use of a toothed instrument may cause penetration and bleeding.

Instruments for Evacuating the Uterus

If the cervix requires dilatation and urgent evacuation is not necessary, cervical dilatation with laminaria is advised. These expand slowly, and maximum dilation occurs within 6–8 hours (Fig. 2–9). Laminaria japonica is available in diameters from 2 to 6 mm. The largest diameter that passes easily into the cervical canal should be used. If additional dilatation is required, multiple devices may be inserted simultaneously. Synthetic osmotic dilators are also available and are discussed in more detail in Chapter 32 (Cervical Ripening).

If manual dilation is required, it should be performed gradually using either Hegar or Hank dilators (Fig. 2–10). These instruments come in graduated diameters and are commonly referred to in French gauge. One French = 3 mm. There is no one dilator type that offers a clear-cut advantage; the choice of instrument is based on availability and operator preference.

For exposure of the cervix, an Auvard vaginal weighted speculum (Fig. 2–11) is ideal. If the cervix is firm and closed, it should be grasped on the anterior lip with a single-toothed tenaculum such as the Barrett or Pozzi forceps (Fig. 2–12). In the postpartum patient it is preferable to grasp the ante-

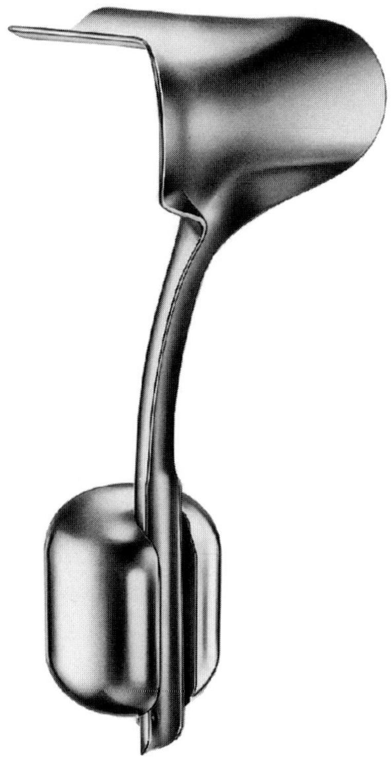

Figure 2–11. Auvard weighted vaginal speculum. (Photo courtesy of Aesculap, Inc.)

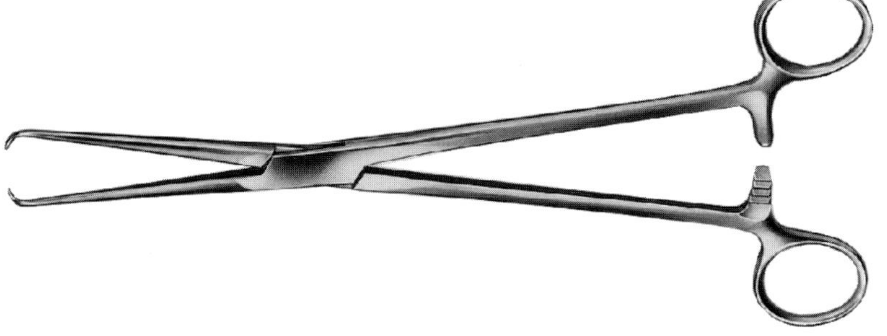

Figure 2–12. Pozzi uterine tenaculum forceps. (Photo courtesy of Aesculap, Inc.)

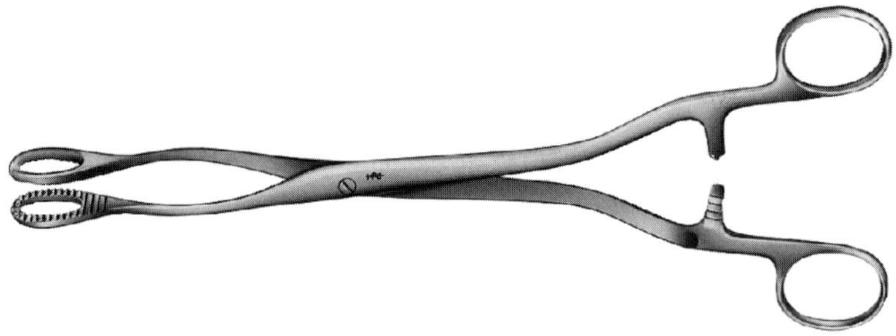

Figure 2–13. Noto or De Lee type cervical grasping forceps. (Photo courtesy of Aesculap, Inc.)

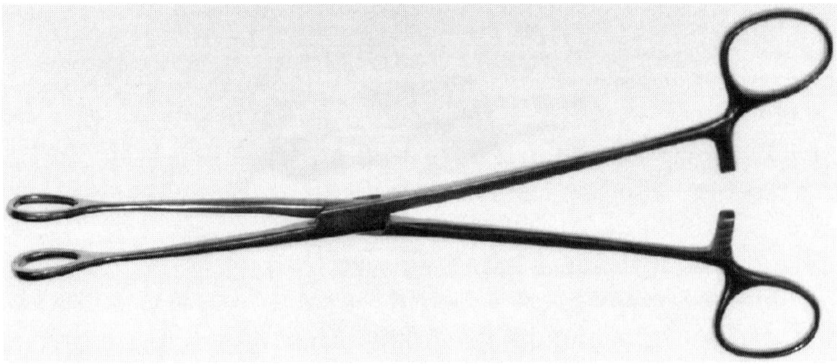

Figure 2–14. Foerster sponge forceps.

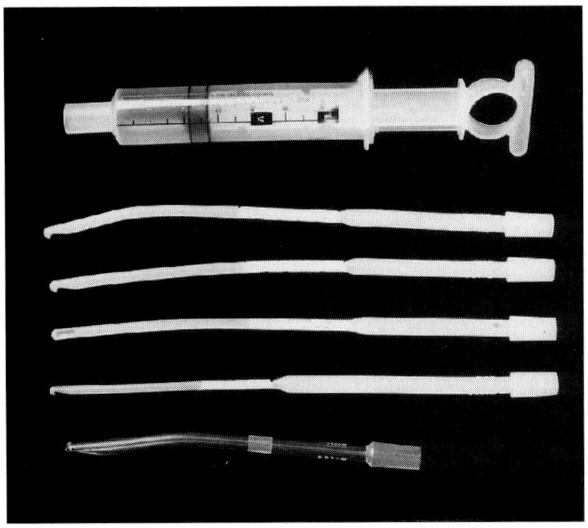

Figure 2–15. 50-cc self-locking suction device and cannulae.

rior lip of the cervix with a less traumatic instrument. A Noto or De Lee type cervical grasping forceps or the more commonly available Foerster sponge forceps ("ring forceps") are most suitable (Figs. 2–13, 2–14). These grasping or sponge forceps also are the instruments of choice to expose cervical tears following delivery.

The uterus can be evacuated with either suction curettage, sharp curettage, or forceps. Generally the largest curette that passes easily through the cervix should be selected. Suction is usually supplied by an electric suction pump connected via plastic tubing with an attached swivel handle to the rigid plastic suction curette. Curettes are available in up to 12-mm diameters. If an electric suction device is not available, a 50-cc self-locking syringe can be attached directly to suction cannulas from 2 mm to 7 mm in diameter (Fig. 2–15). The self-locking syringe is an extremely useful and versatile device.

De Lee type ovum forceps facilitate removal of loose tissue from the uterine cavity (Fig. 2–16). If uterine curettage is required, it may be performed with a sharp uterine curette (Fig. 2–17). Larger curettes may be more suitable for postpartum hemorrhage due to retained placental tissue (Fig. 2–18).

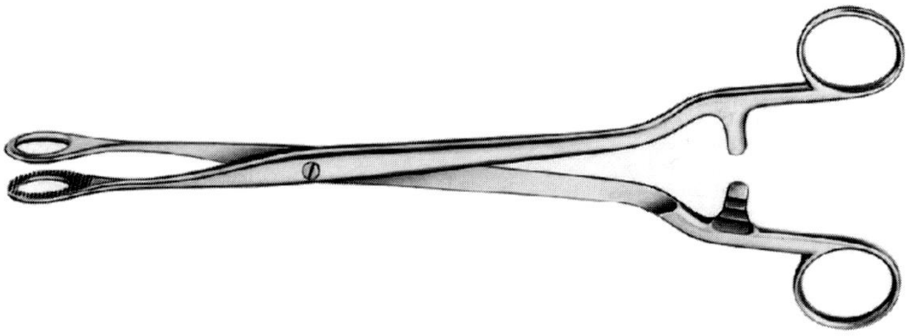

Figure 2–16. De Lee type ovum forceps. (Photo courtesy of Aesculap, Inc.)

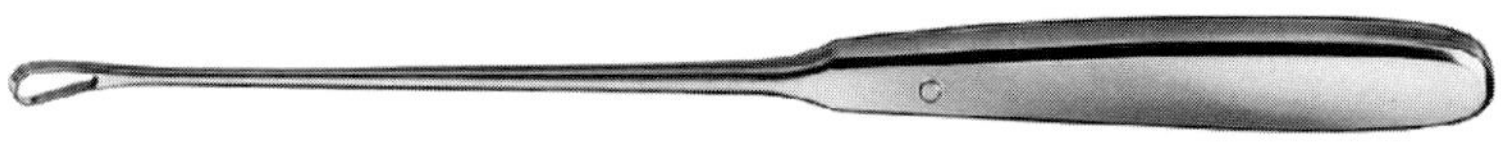

Figure 2–17. Small sharp uterine curette. (Photo courtesy of Aesculap, Inc.)

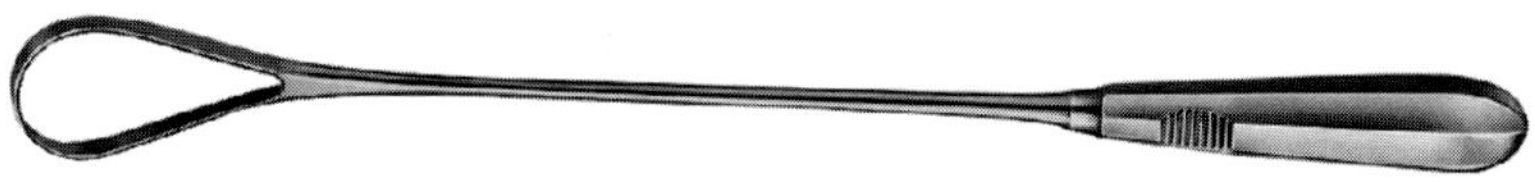

Figure 2–18. Larger diameter curette for use postpartum. (Photo courtesy of Aesculap, Inc.)

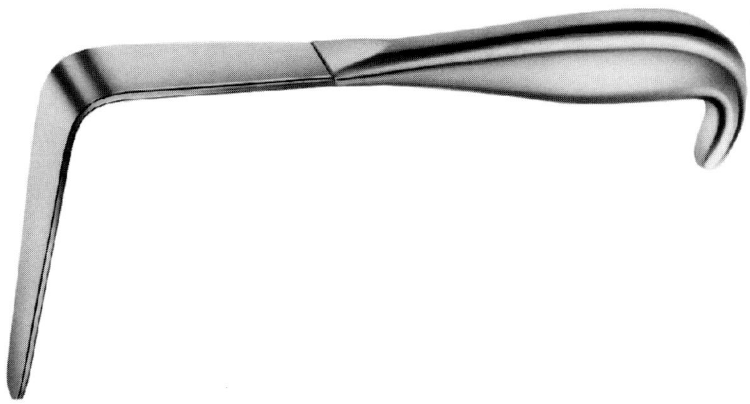

Figure 2–19. Right-angle vaginal speculum. (Photo courtesy of Aesculap, Inc.)

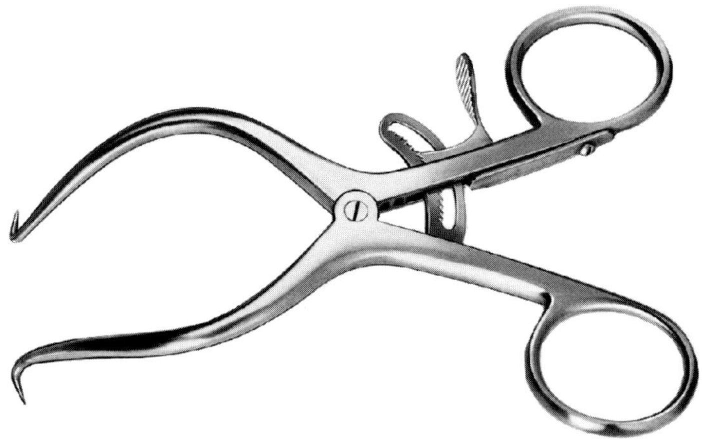

Figure 2–20. Gelpi self-retaining perineal retractor. (Photo courtesy of Aesculap, Inc.)

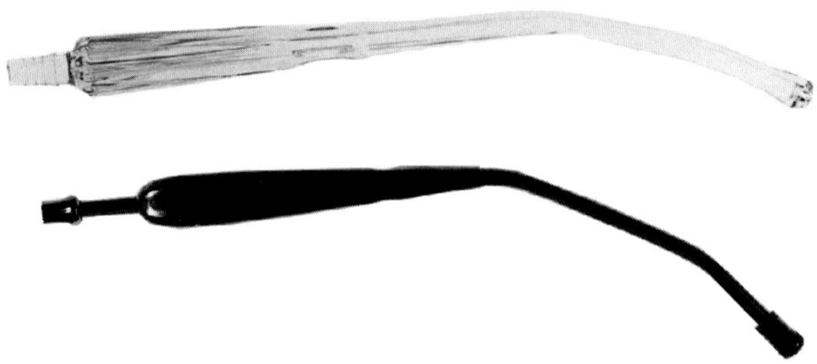

Figure 2–21. Yankauer suction device.

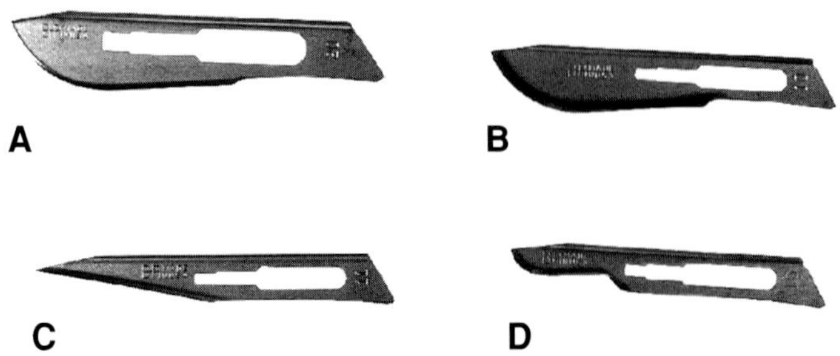

Figure 2–22. Commonly used scalpel blades. **A.** #20. **B.** #10. **C.** #11. **D.** #16.

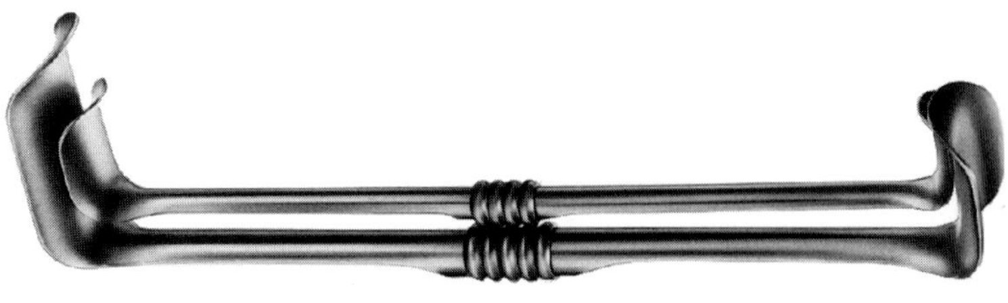

Figure 2–23. Richardson-Eastman type retractor. (Photo courtesy of Aesculap, Inc.)

Repair of Vaginal Tears

Adequate visualization may require retraction by a knowledgeable assistant and good lighting is mandatory. A right-angle vaginal retractor and Gelpi self-retaining perineal retractor may facilitate visualization (Figs. 2–19, 2–20). A suction device is often required to keep the operative field clear of blood; a metal Yankauer suction probe or a disposable plastic probe should be available (Fig. 2–21). A curved Heaney needle holder of adequate length with a 5/8 curved needle such as a UR4 or UR5 are well suited for repair of lacerations of the vaginal fornix.

Instruments for Abdominal Delivery

A No. 4 knife handle with a No. 21 blade is suitable for incising the skin at laparotomy. For smaller incisions, such as with postpartum sterilization, a No. 15 blade on a No. 3 handle is useful. Caution must be exercised when using a No. 11 blade because of the very sharp point (Fig. 2–22). It is not necessary to change knives for use on deeper tissues, the concept of a "skin knife" and "deep knife" as issues for wound infection having been proven a myth (Hasselgren and associates, 1984).

In making an abdominal incision, a Richardson-Eastman type retractor (Fig. 2–23) is used to retract the skin while a scalpel or electrocautery device is used to incise the subcutaneous fat to expose the fascia. The incision of the fascia can be made either with a scalpel or with curved Mayo scissors (Fig. 2–24). Straight Kocher hemostatic forceps are used to hold the edge of the rectus fascia to dissect it free from the underlying muscle (Fig. 2–25). The peritoneum is grasped with a more delicate hemostatic forceps such as a Kelly or Mixter (Fig. 2–26). The peritoneum may be cut with a scalpel and extended using either scalpel or curved Metzenbaum scissors (Fig.

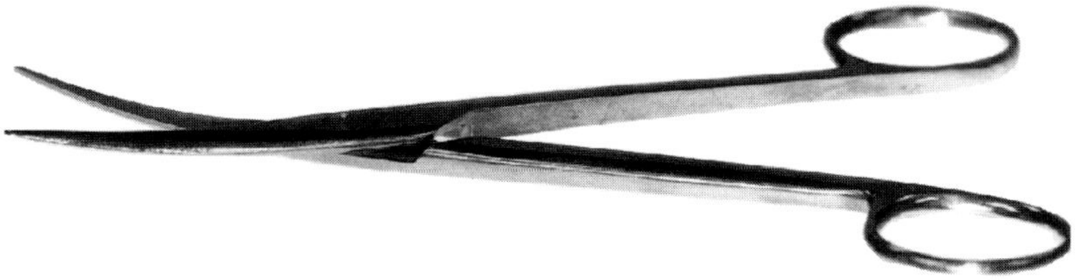

Figure 2–24. Curved Mayo scissors.

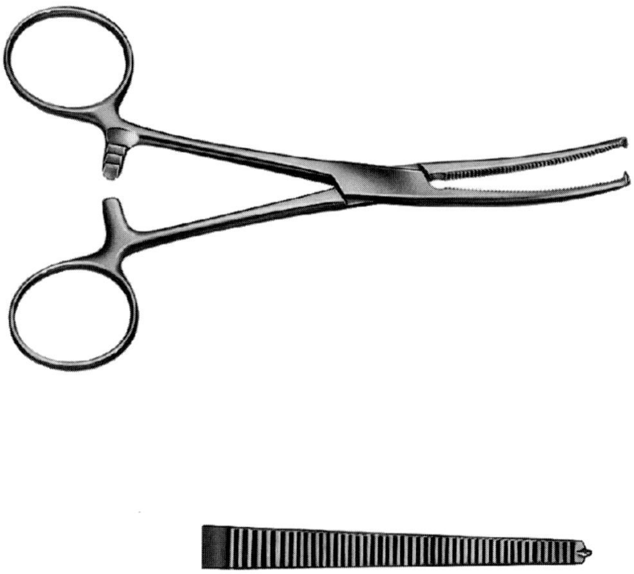

Figure 2–25. Kocher clamp. Note serrations perpendicular to direction of blade. (Photo courtesy of Aesculap, Inc.)

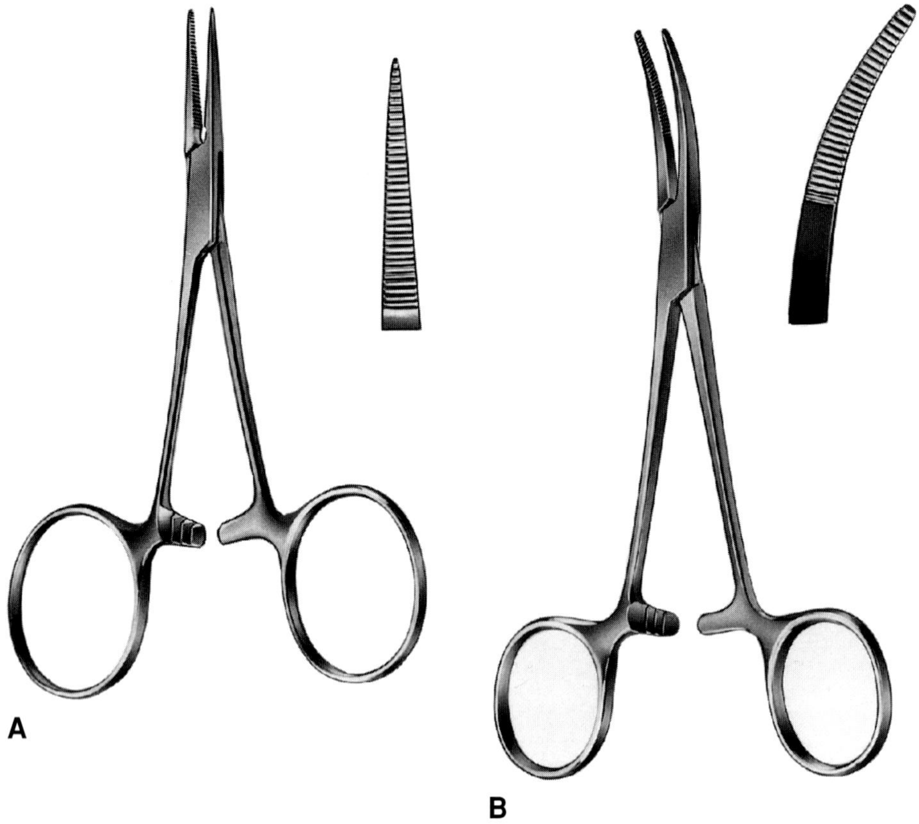

Figure 2–26. Kelly hemostatic clamp. **A.** Straight. **B.** Curved. (Photo courtesy of Aesculap, Inc.)

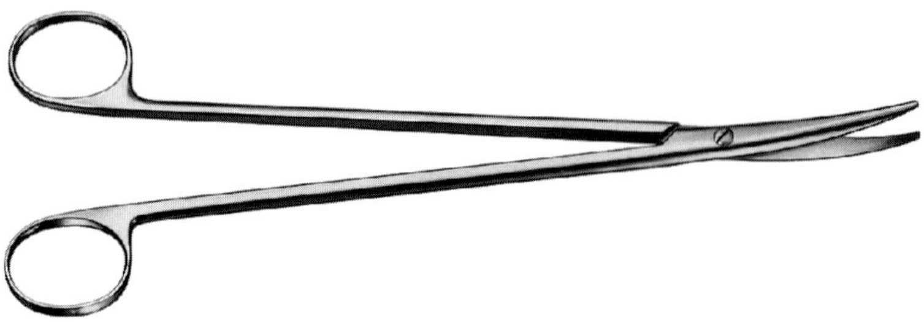

Figure 2–27. Metzenbaum scissors. (Photo courtesy of Aesculap, Inc.)

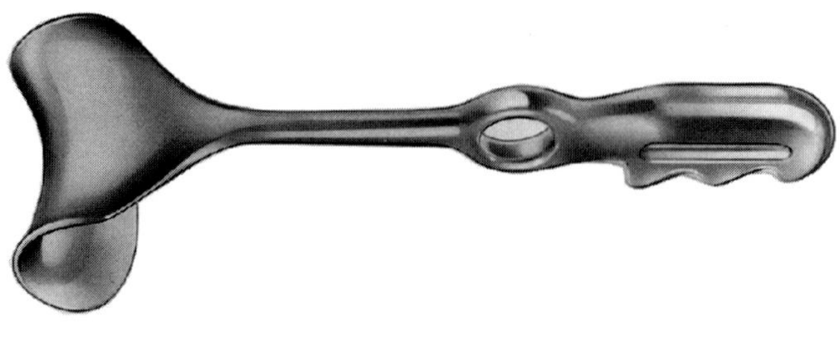

Figure 2–28. Fritsch bladder retractors. (Photo courtesy of Aesculap, Inc.)

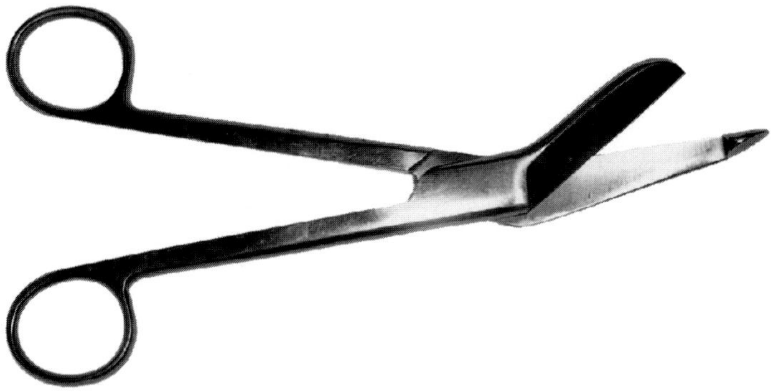

Figure 2–29. Lister bandage scissors.

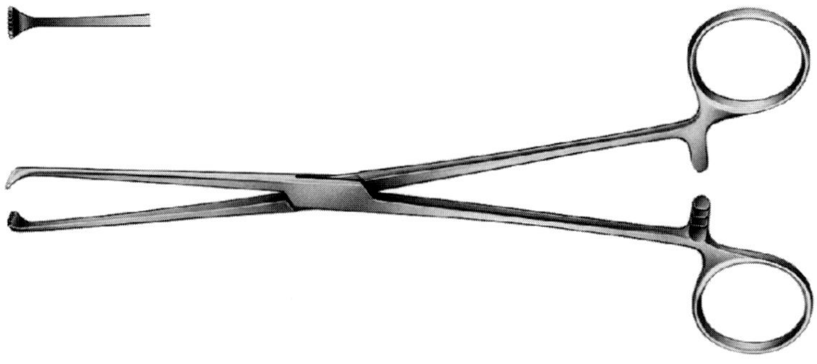

Figure 2–30. Allis clamp. (Photo courtesy of Aesculap, Inc.)

2–27). The lower uterine segment can be exposed with either a De Lee, Fritsch, or Rochard universal retractor ("bladder blade") (Fig. 2–28) or the lower central blade of a Balfour retractor. The curved Metzenbaum scissors also are used to cut the visceral peritoneum to reflect the bladder inferiorly. In performing cesarean section, the uterus is initially entered with a scalpel. If the uterine incision is to be extended using scissors, either curved Mayo scissors or Lister bandage scissors may be used (Fig. 2–29). A bandage scissors with a blunt tip on the lower blade provides added protection to the fetus; even so, it is imperative to place one or more fingers between the interior scissor blade and the fetus as the incision is extended. Allis forceps (Fig. 2–30) are useful to rupture the fetal membranes, if they have not been ruptured during uterine incision. The Allis clamp is also helpful in grasping the edges of the bladder during repair of incidental or planned cystotomy.

Following cesarean section, the uterine incision is closed in either one or two layers. The edges of the uterine incision are held with Green-Armytage or Pennington forceps (Fig. 2–31), which are designed for this purpose and are very hemostatic. Another suitable option is a sponge or "ring" forceps.

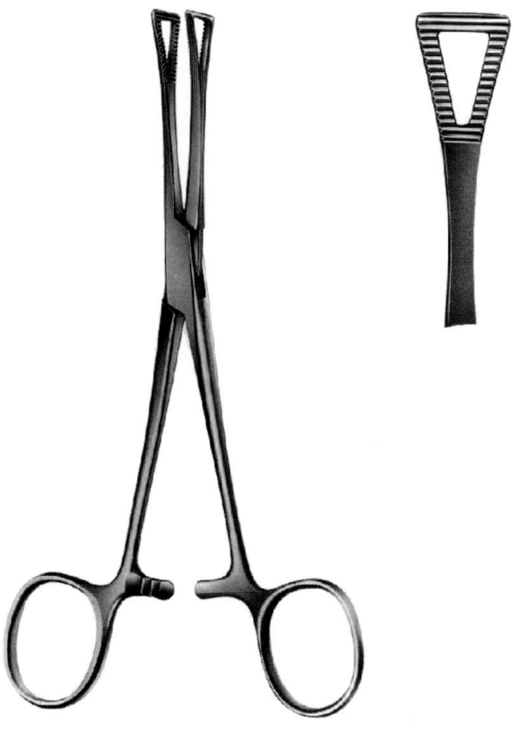

Figure 2–31. Pennington clamp. (Photo courtesy of Aesculap, Inc.)

Abdominal Retractors

When performing a laparotomy on a patient with a large gravid uterus or excess adipose tissue, retraction is often difficult. Under such circumstances a self-retaining retractor, such as the Balfour, Kirschner, or Semm (Fig. 2–32) may be used. Both the Kirschner and Semm retractors consist of rings around which a number of retractor blades can be attached. The Balfour retractor is normally configured with two lateral and fixed blades and a caudal central blade. A fourth arm converts the standard Balfour retractor into an invaluable instrument for obtaining exposure at the superior aspect of the incision. Further exposure can be achieved by use of surgical assistants and hand-held retractors of the Richardson, Tuffier, or Deaver variety (Fig. 2–33). The commonly used O'Connor-O'Sullivan four-way retractor (Fig. 2–34) does not usually give adequate exposure in the gravid patient.

In closing the abdomen, using a McNealy-Glassman viscera retainer ("fish") (Fig. 2–35) often helps to avoid bowel perforation with a

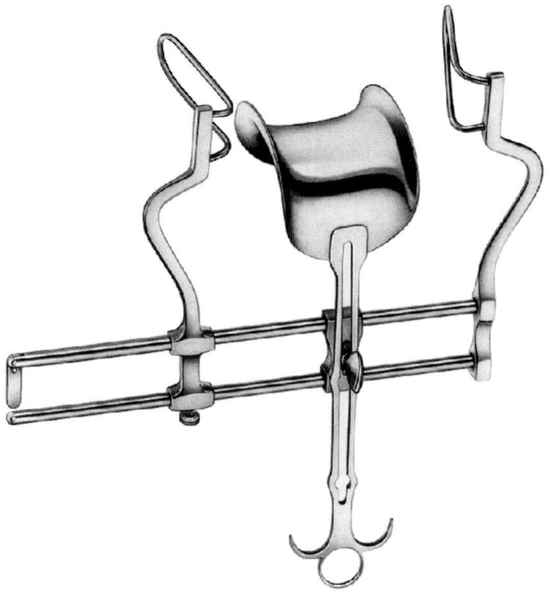

Figure 2–32. The Balfour abdominal retractor (standard three-blade configuration). (Photo courtesy of Aesculap, Inc.)

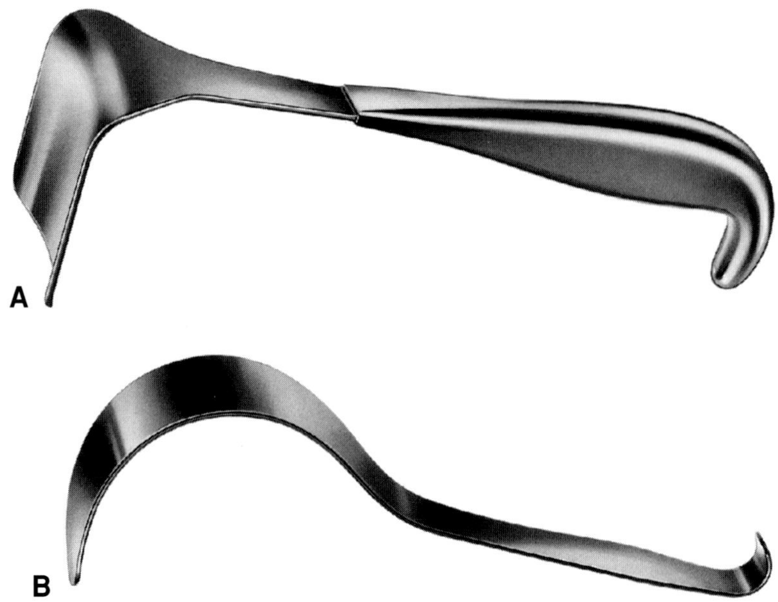

Figure 2–33. Hand-held abdominal retractors. **A.** Richardson type, shown is Tuffier. **B.** Deaver retractor. (Photo courtesy of Aesculap, Inc.)

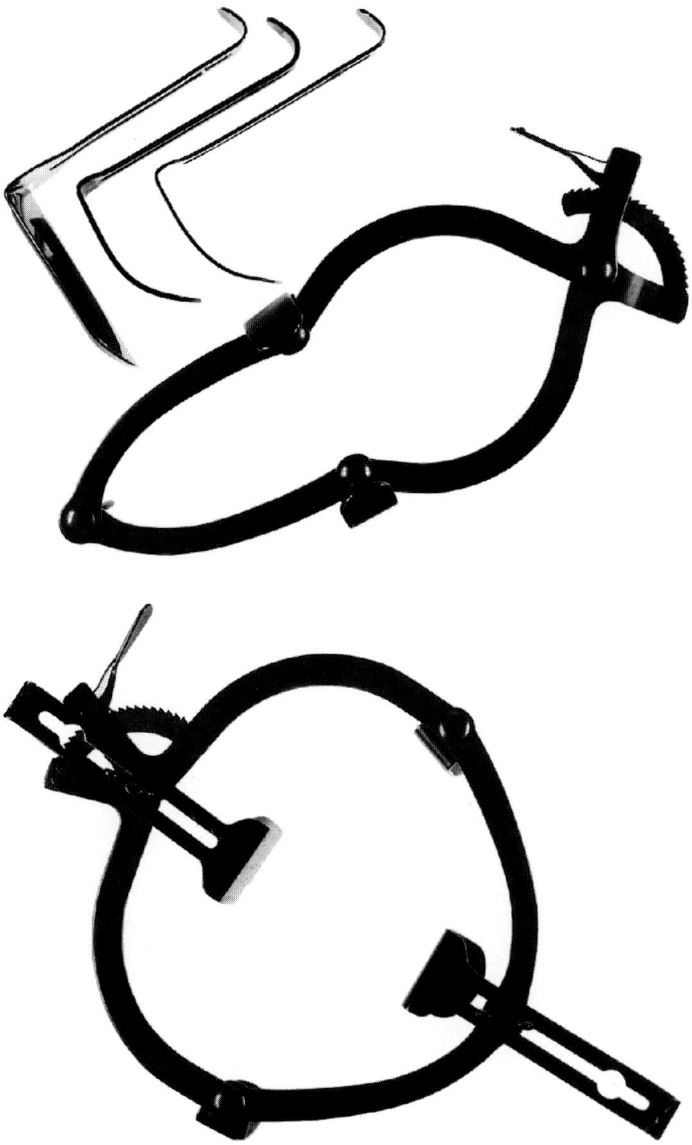

Figure 2–34. O'Sullivan-O'Connor abdominal retractor with lower blade attachments.

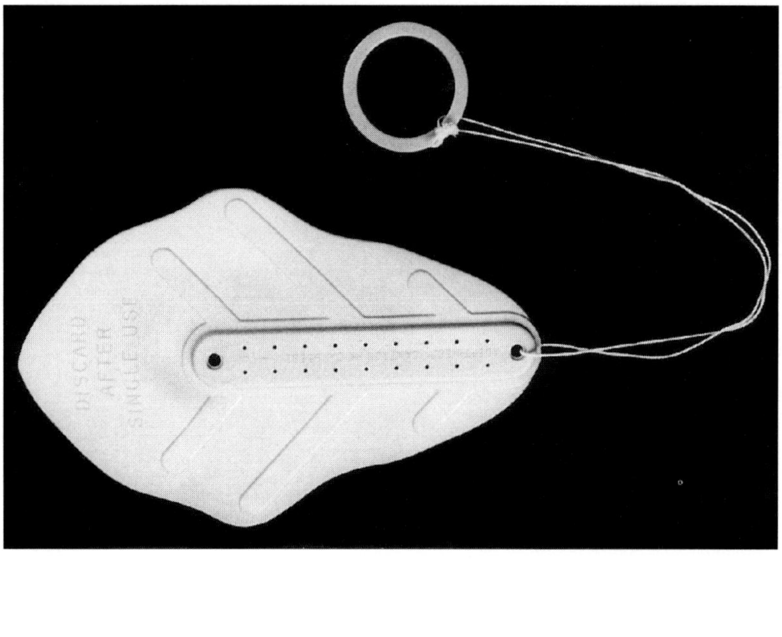

Figure 2–35. McNealy-Glasman visceral retainer ("fish").

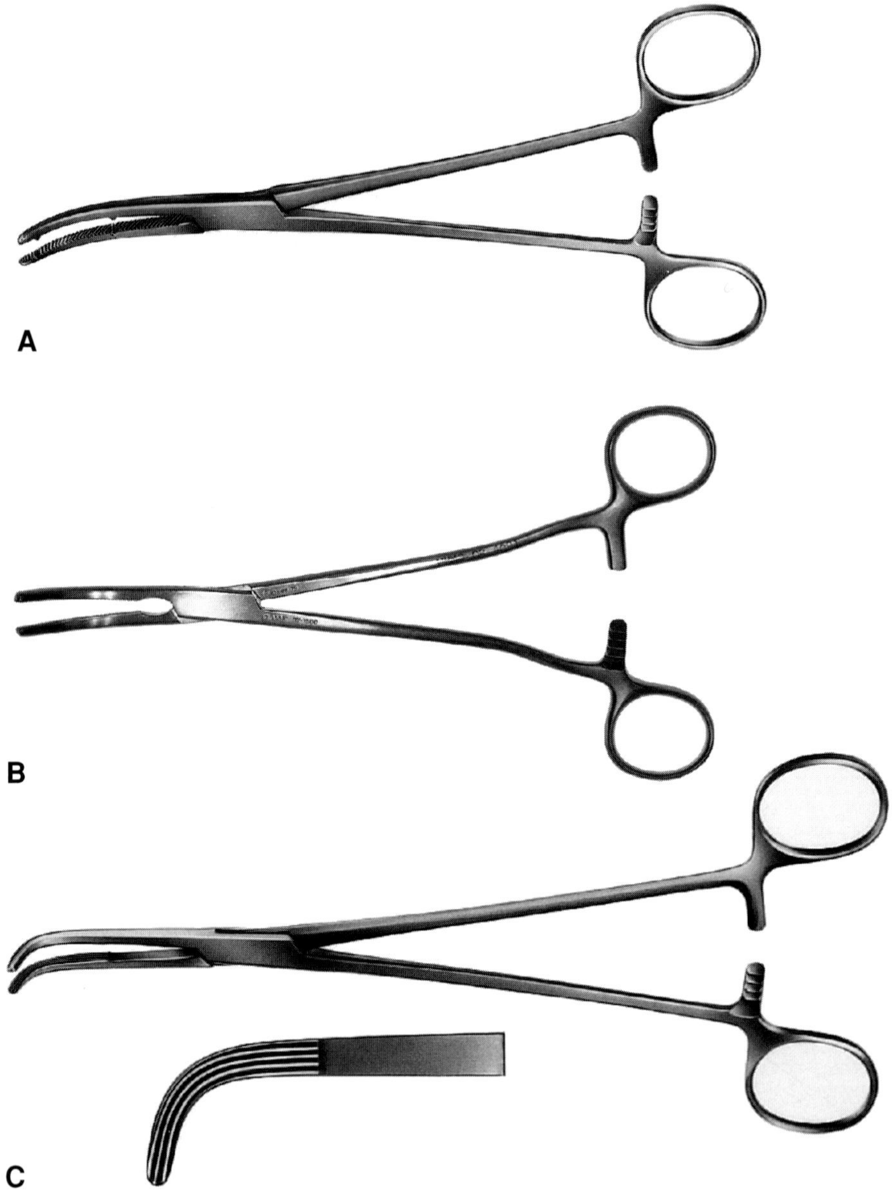

Figure 2–36. Vascular pedicle clamps. **A.** Heaney variations. Note serrations are tangential to direction of blade. **B.** Lahey clamp. **C.** Herrick clamp. In **B** and **C** note serrations are parallel to direction of blade. All these clamps are more secure and superior to the standard Kocher clamp (Fig. 2–25), whose serrations are perpendicular to the blade and thus parallel to the vascular pedicle upon which the clamp is placed. (**A** and **C** courtesy of Aesculap, Inc.)

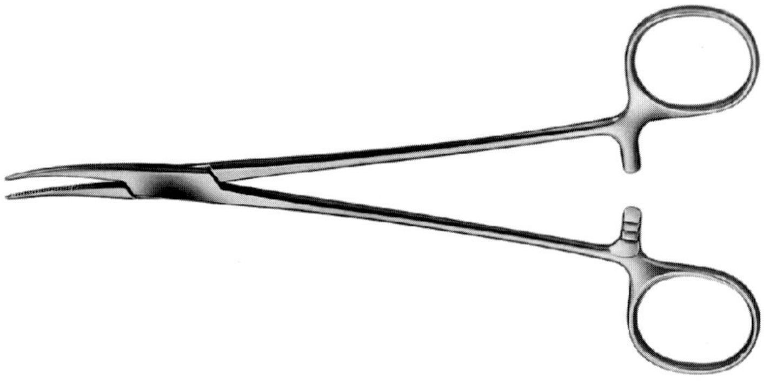

Figure 2–37. Schnidt hemostatic clamp. (Photo courtesy of Aesculap, Inc.)

needle, especially in obese patients or when anesthetic relaxation is less than ideal. This retainer is placed over the intestines beneath the fascia and left in place as a barrier to bowel perforation while the fascia is closed. Prior to closure of the final 2–3 cm of the fascia, the flexible retainer is removed by pulling on the attached ring.

Clamps

In obstetrical surgery clamps are used at cesarean hysterectomy or adnexectomy. A vast number of clamps are available. Clamps with a claw at the end are unnecessarily traumatic. The serrations should be either tangential or parallel to the jaws and therefore at right angles to the vessels clamped. Kocher clamps fail on both accounts and are therefore less than ideal for these purposes. Heaney clamps and modifications of this design often are useful as are the lighter Rogers and Wertheim clamps (Fig. 2–36). These latter instruments are available in both curved and straight models and come in a variety of lengths.

If bleeding is intractable and ligation of the internal iliac arteries is required, longer and more delicate instruments should be readily available. Schnidt hemostatic forceps (Fig. 2–37) are ideal for the delicate dissection required in this area. A pair of long Metzenbaum scissors also is required. A fine right-angled forceps such as the Mixter instrument (Fig. 2–38) is essential. A vein retractor (Fig. 2–39) often is useful to provide exposure of the internal iliac artery. Passage of the right-angle clamp beneath the artery is facilitated by elevating the artery with a large Babcock clamp (Fig. 2–40). This instrument is also valuable in retracting delicate tissues such as the fallopian tube without causing trauma.

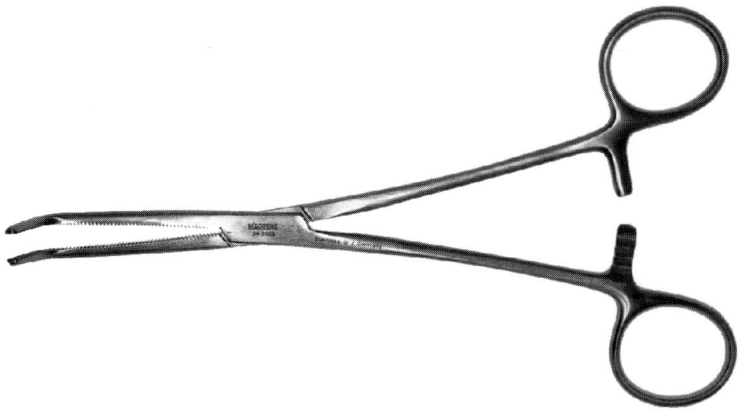

Figure 2–38. Mixter right-angle clamp.

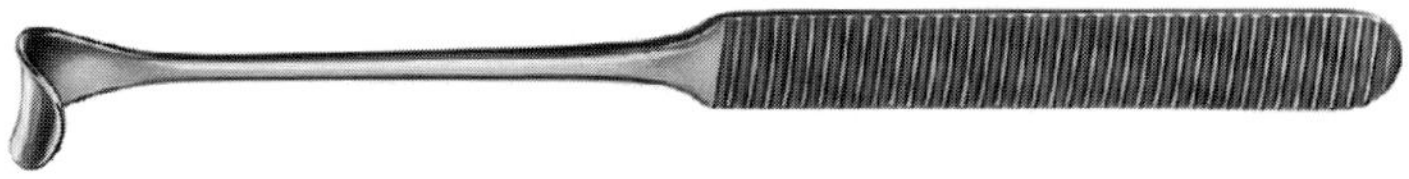

Figure 2–39. Konig vein retractor. (Photo courtesy of Aesculap, Inc.)

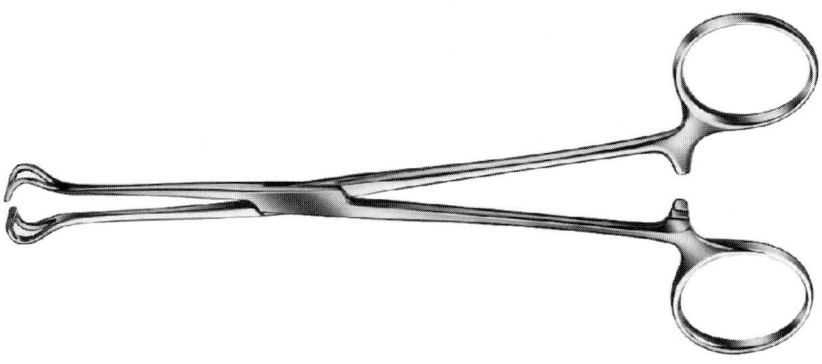

Figure 2–40. Atraumatic Babcock clamp. (Photo courtesy of Aesculap, Inc.)

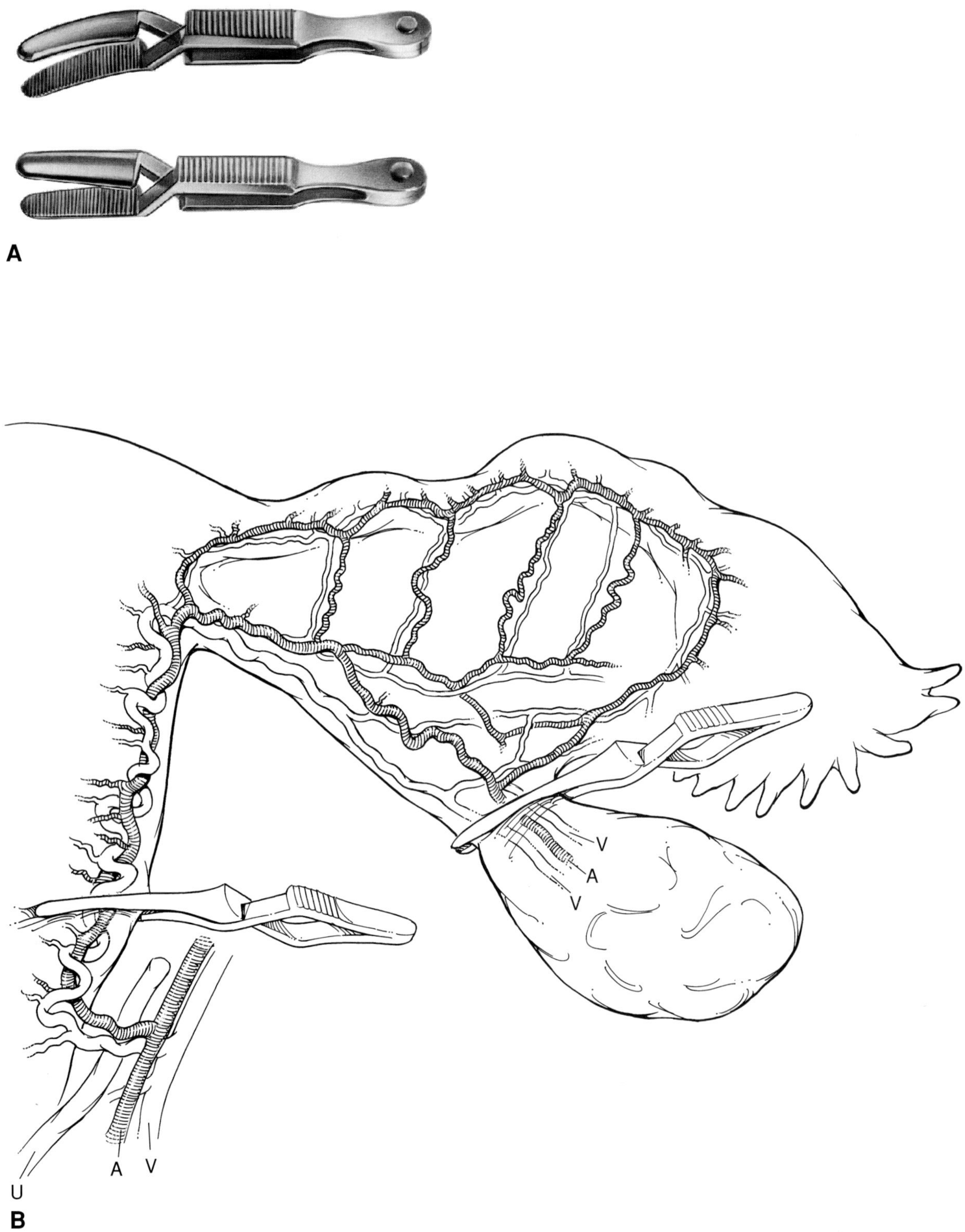

Figure 2–41. A. Atraumatic Dieffenbach bulldog clamps (curved and straight). (Courtesy of Aesculap, Inc.) **B.** Clamps have been placed on infundibulopelvic ligaments and uterine arteries without cutting the pedicles to achieve uterine hemostasis without injuring structures within the intact pedicles.

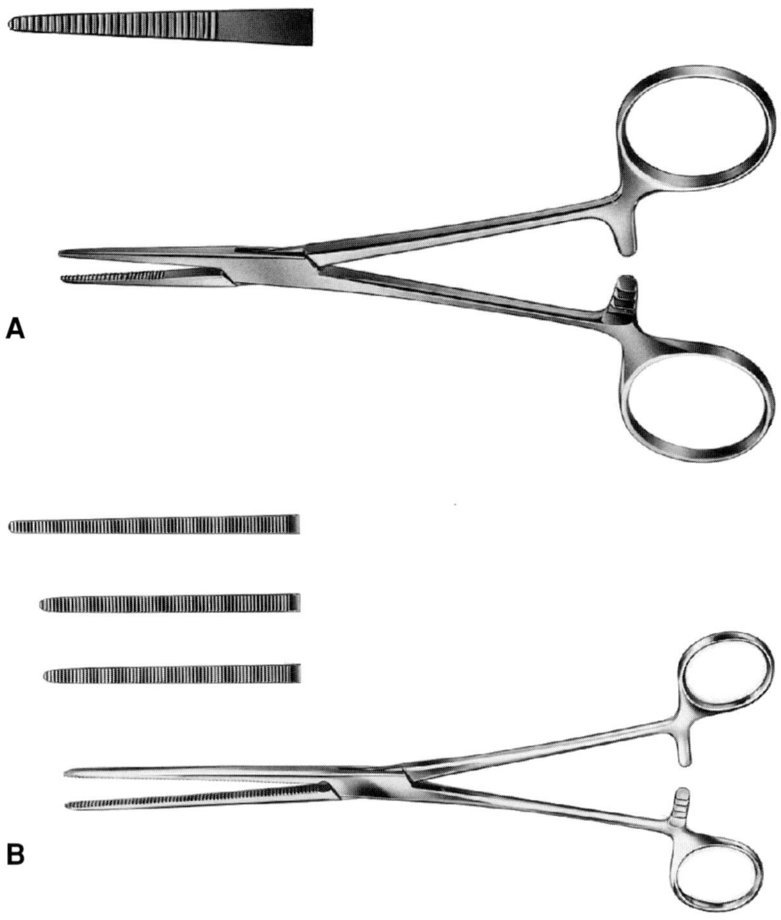

Figure 2–42. Additional hemostatic clamps. **A.** Fine mosquito clamp. **B.** Pean clamp.

If temporary clamps are required to stem blood flow while help is summoned or blood prepared, large, atraumatic DeBakey or Dieffenbach bulldog clamps (Fig. 2–41) are useful. These may be placed on one or both infundibulopelvic ligaments or uterine arteries to reduce blood flow to the uterus, but will not injure structures in these pedicles. Individual bleeding vessels may be grasped with hemostatic forceps. A variety of sizes (Figs. 2–26, 2–42) are available, depending upon the size of the vessel or pedicle.

Clearly there is a wide variety of instruments from which to choose. Although it is important to become familiar and comfortable with instruments used regularly, it is just as important to be open to new ideas. Therefore, the surgeon should make time to operate with a variety of colleagues, particularly those trained in other units. It is only with this attitude that surgery becomes an art, one that the surgeon should strive to perfect as long as he or she has the privilege to operate.

SURGICAL DRAINS

During the last 100 years, there have been great changes in the use of surgical drains; the majority of surgeons still debate the place of drains in the surgeon's armamentarium. In Price's words, "There are those who ardently advocate it; there are those who, in great part, reject it [the use of drains]; there are those who Laodicean-like, are lukewarm concerning it, and finally, some who, without convictions, are either for or against it, use it, or dispense with it, as chance or whim, not logic may determine." (Price, 1988)

According to Dougherty and Simmons (1992), the ideal drain should:

1. Efficiently evacuate the effluent.
2. Avoid damage to surrounding tissues.
3. Prevent the introduction of infection.
4. Be easily removed when drainage is no longer needed.

Types of Drainage

Conceptually there are three major categories of wound drainage: **therapeutic, prophylactic,** and **decompressive.** The type of drainage used can be either passive or active. Active drains may be open or closed. Closed active drains may be described as being low- or high-pressure systems.

The variability of drain usage was reported by Hilton in a survey of practices among 947 gynecologists in the British Isles (Hilton, 1988). In routine cases performed by generalists in obstetrics and gynecology, use of drains was limited; prophylactic drainage of the peritoneal cavity (0.4%), pelvis (1%), subcutaneous tissues (4%), and rectus sheath (20%) Specialists used drainage procedures more frequently, but this primarily reflected a difference in the operations performed by them. Drainage is most often used in procedures such as suprapubic incontinence procedures (51%), radical hysterectomy (55%), and radical vulvectomy (63%).

Therapeutic

Retained pus, urine, or hostility need to be released. The placement of drains following surgical extirpation of an intraabdominal abscess is a well established principle. Such drains function by creating a fistula from the abscess cavity to the outside. Few would question the need for some type of drainage following such surgery. Newer methods using percutaneous drainage of loculated fluids under radiographic guidance have decreased tissue damage, blood loss, anesthesia requirements, and open surgical interventions.

Prophylactic

Prophylactic drainage remains controversial with little documentation of benefit. Some have hypothesized that used prophylactically, drains decrease infection by reducing the accumulation of loculated fluid that could serve as a medium for bacterial growth. Loong (1988) reported the use of closed suction drainage of the rectus sheath in women undergoing Cesarean section with potentially contaminated wounds who had not been given prophylactic antibiotics. Subcutaneous drainage also was used in a portion of the patients reported. Closed suction drainage of the rectus sheath decreased the incidence of wound infection from 14 percent to 4 percent. In contrast, the subcutaneous drains may have increased the infection rate from 7 percent to 11 percent. Prophylactic antibiotics have been shown to decrease wound infection rates with a similar degree of efficiency; thus closed active or passive drains probably have little value when prophylactic antibiotics are used. Passive drains have been shown to increase the infection rate in clean wounds in some circumstances. Closed active drainage in potentially contaminated wounds may reduce the risk of infection if prophylactic antibiotics are not used.

Prophylactic drainage has been used following abdominal and vaginal hysterectomies. Comparison studies have been undertaken to evaluate outcomes with prophylactic antibiotics and/or drainage (Wijma, 1987; Poulsen, 1984; Swartz, 1986; Scotto, 1985). In general, prophylactic antibiotics appear to be more efficacious than suction drainage in preventing infection. When prophylactic antibiotics are not used, suction drainage provides some protection. The combined use of prophylactic antibiotics and suction drainage provides no benefit beyond that achieved with prophylactic antibiotics alone.

Decompressive

Decompressive drainage, as used beneath the skin flaps from the groin dissection of a radical vulvectomy, helps prevent fluid accumulation and bring about better apposition of the skin and underlying tissues. There is no evidence that such drainage prevents infection.

Drainage Devices

Passive Drains

Passive drains establish a path of decreased resistance from the surgical field or other site to be drained to the outside. The most popular passive drains are the Penrose and Malecot catheters (Fig. 2–43). These drains function as wicks to allow egress of fluid, blood, or abscess contents to the outside. Brigham Penrose, Professor of Gynecology at the University of Pennsylvania, used a condom with the end removed as the first drainage tube, which now bears his name. Passive drains function by capillary action and natural pressure differences, ie, posture and gravity. Passive drains like the Penrose use soft, pliable material and allow drainage of viscous and bulky fluid. Placement requires an exit large enough to avoid collapse of the pliable rubber catheter.

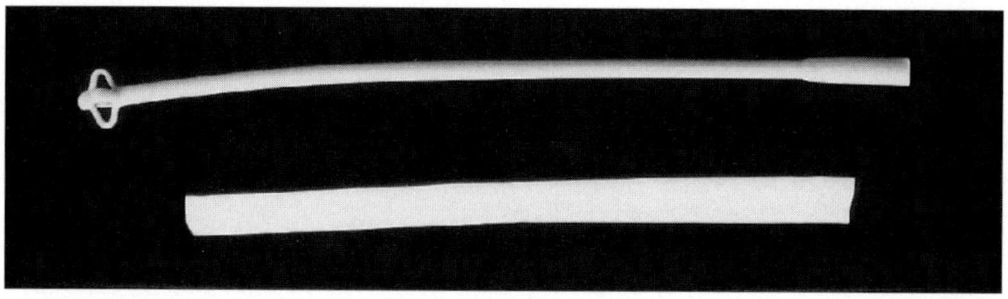

Figure 2–43. Passive drains. **Top.** Malecot drain. **Bottom.** Penrose drain (cut section).

Because of this passive nature, bacterial contamination from outside to inside is possible and the incidence of infections may be increased. When passive drains are used in any wound, they should be removed after no more than 3–4 days. Because dislodging of the drain is possible, it should be used with some type of radio-opaque marker (eg, a safety pin). Figures 2–44A and 2–44B show a large cul-de-sac abscess in a woman 4 days postpartum in longitudinal and transverse views. The abscess was drained through a posterior colpotomy and Malecot drain placed to ensure continued egress of the infected material (Fig.

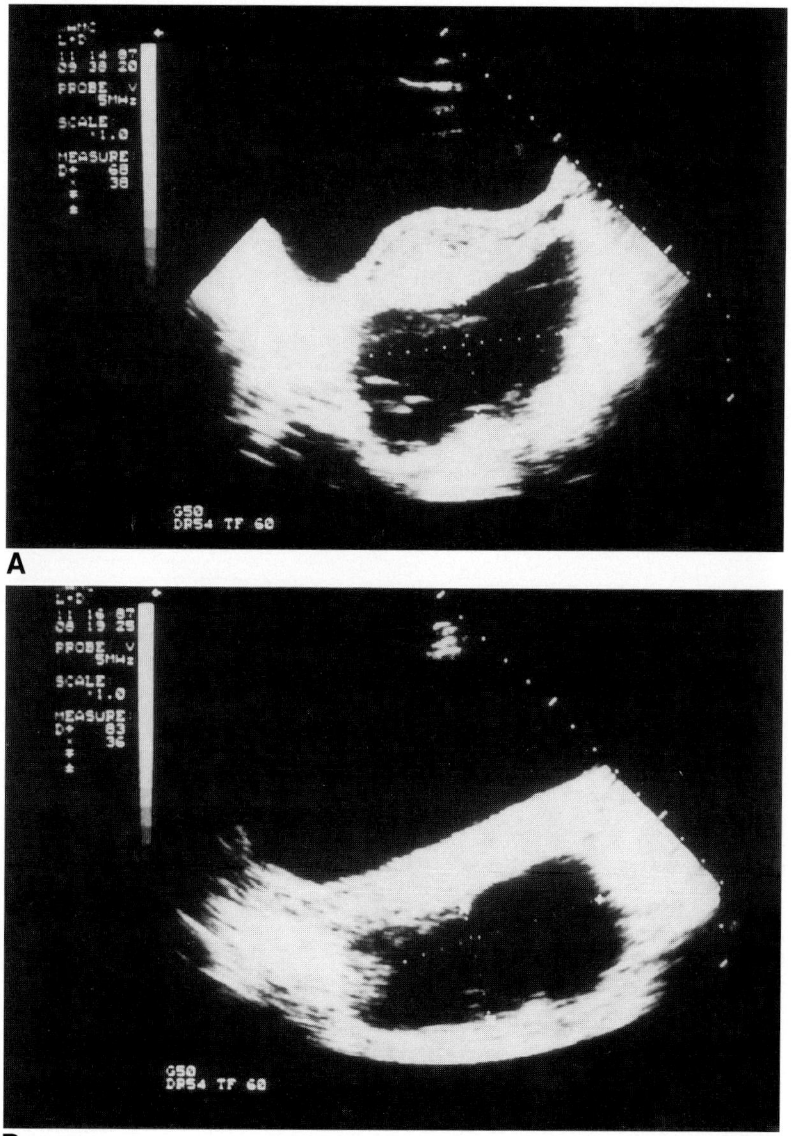

A

B

Figure 2–44. A. Sonogram in transverse orientation showing cross section of uterus and broad ligament with large posterior fluid accumulation. **B.** Sonogram in longitudinal orientation, showing a 4 x 9 cm abscess cavity.

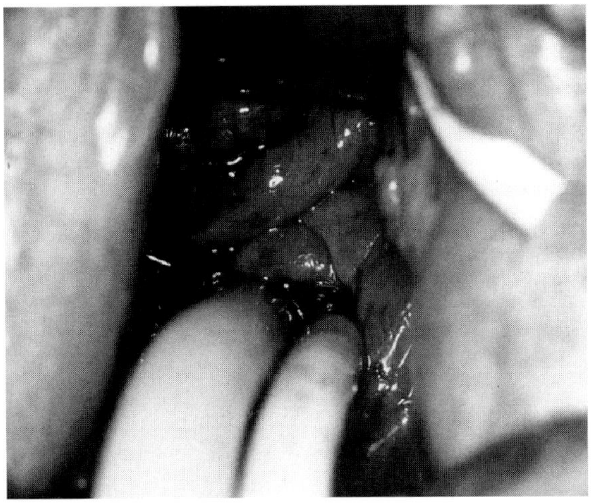

Figure 2–45. Two Malecot drains seen exiting from a posterior colpotomy incision. At 12 o'clock is seen a Deaver retractor with a patulous postpartum cervix immediately below the retractor.

2–45). The Malecot drains are visualized on sonogram, now with collapse of the abscess cavity (Fig. 2–46).

Active Closed Drains

Hemovac and Jackson Pratt drains are examples of active closed drainage systems (Figs. 2–47A, 2–47B). Most drain into an enclosed receptacle, which allows the system to remain sealed. Silastic tubing aids in preventing damage that might be caused by the mechanical irritation of more rigid evacuation tubes. In contrast to open systems, active closed drains allow better collection of effluent, protect the skin from irritating discharges, and are less vulnerable to retrograde bacterial infection. Low pressure (100–150 mm Hg) can be attained with rechargeable bulbs or canisters, although such devices may occasionally allow retrograde passage of fluid with bacterial contamination at the time of recharging. A nonreturn valve may prevent this complication.

Active drains are preferred beneath large skin flaps to promote rapid adherence and healing. High vacuum pressures are recommended. High-pressure systems (150–500 mm Hg) require little or no recharging, but have the disadvantage of frequent obstruction from blood clots or exudate.

Active Open Drains (Sump)

A typical active open drain is the Snyder system (Fig. 2–48). Sump drains are useful when large volumes of fluid must be removed from relatively spacious body cavities. Air vents are initially placed along the side of the main drain tube, allowing air to enter to keep omentum and intestine from blocking the drain holes. The air suctioned back through the larger drainage tube prevents the high vacuum responsible for the suction of adjacent structures into the openings of the tube. The air vent allows the entrance of bacteria unless

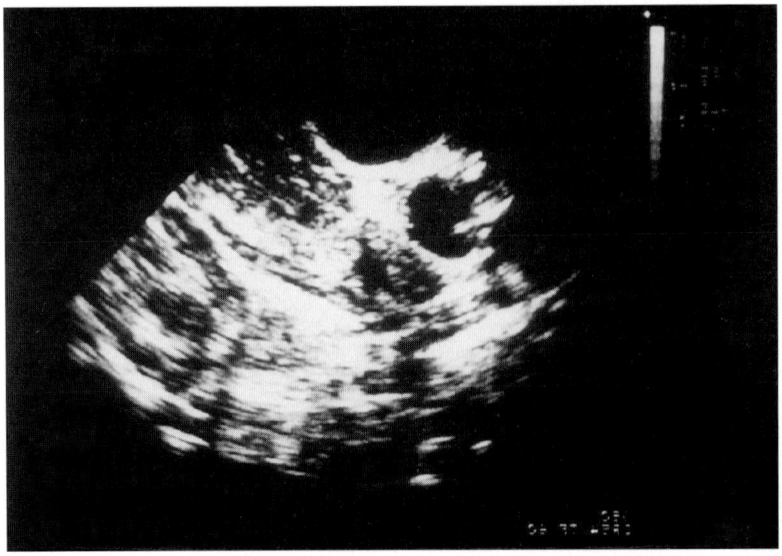

Figure 2–46. Sonogram showing collapse of the abscess cavity. Sono lucency at right is the tip of the Malecot drain.

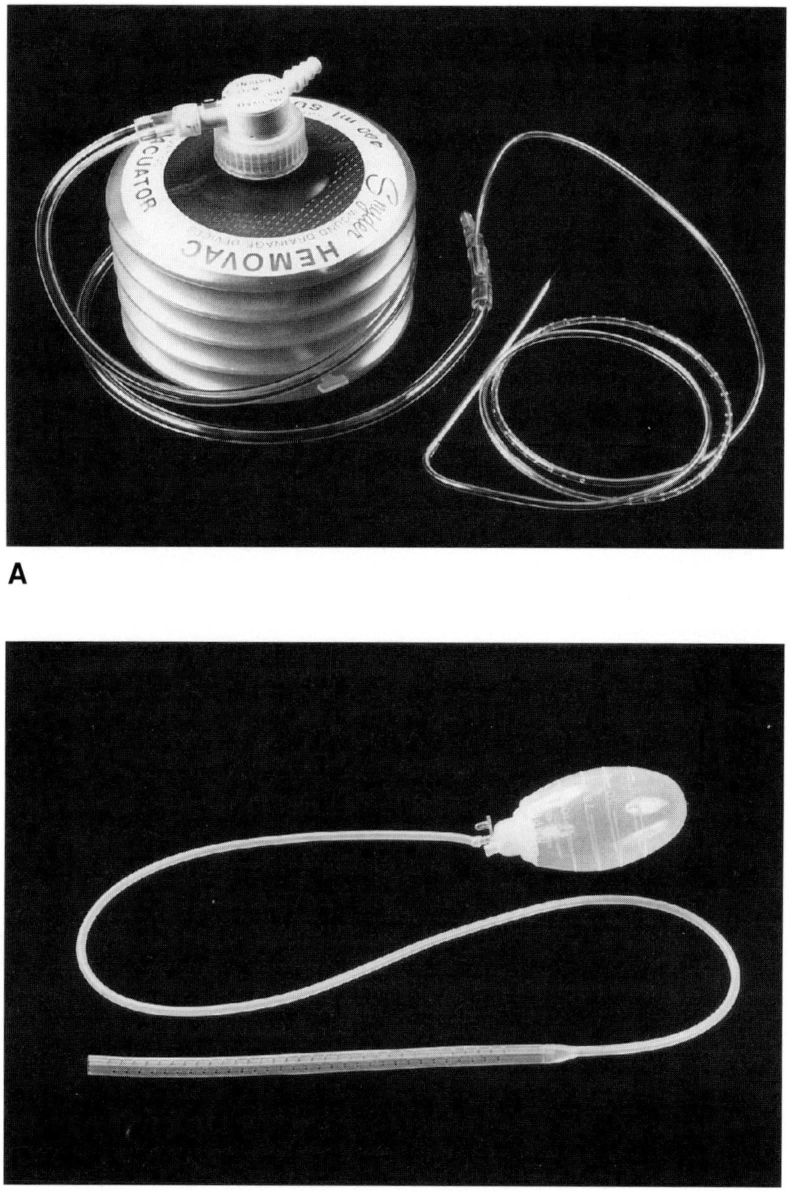

A

B

Figure 2–47. Active closed drains. **A.** Hemovac polyvinylchoride drain with collapsible reservoir. **B.** Jackson-Pratt silastic drain and bulb-type reservoir.

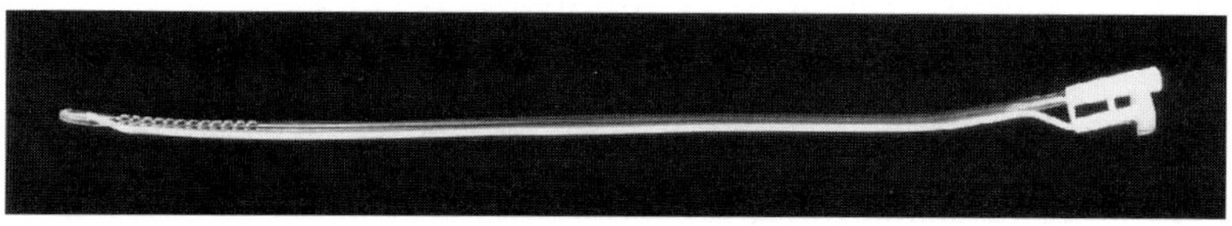

Figure 2–48. Functional components of an active open sump-style drain.

used with a bacterial air filter. The addition of a valve preventing retrograde flow of effluent fluid may also be of benefit.

Both active open and closed drainage systems are susceptible to occlusion from tissue fragments. Tissue erosion is also a risk, especially with higher pressures and more rigid tubes. One novel technique employs a sump tube threaded inside a regular Penrose drain. The Penrose drain is perforated on both sides and its distal end is tied around the shaft of the sump tube with a ligature proximal to the air vent (Hanna, 1970).

Complications

Mechanical drainage is not without the risks outlined in Table 2–1 (Dougherty and Simmons, 1992). Drains left in place more than 5–6 days should have surveillance cultures of the drain site to check for suprainfection. Prophylactic antibiotics may prevent infectious morbidity during short-term drain placement. Longer use of drains and antibiotics may lead to the development of resistant bacterial infections.

TABLE 2–1. POTENTIAL COMPLICATIONS OF SURGICAL DRAINS

I. FOREIGN BODY EFFECTS
- Chemical and/or mechanical effects
  - Erosion (hemorrhage, fistula, perforation, obstruction)
  - Torsion (bowel obstruction)
- Potentiation of infection
  - Tissue irritation (inflammation)
  - Bacterial surface adherence
  - Retrograde bacterial migration
- Impaired healing of intestinal suture lines

II. MECHANICAL PROBLEMS
- Drain entrapment (due to sutures, kinking, or tissue ingrowth)
- Herniation of viscera through drain tracts
- Drain loss (due to migration, breakage, fragmentation)
- Leakage due to incomplete drain tract formation

III. PHYSIOLOGIC DERANGEMENTS
- Decompression injury (lung, brain)
- Pain (eg, may lead to pulmonary atelectasis)
- Fluid and electrolyte loss
- Pneumoperitoneum, pneumothorax

IV. INADEQUATE DRAINAGE
- Faulty positioning, kinking, or obstruction
- Wrong type of drain or drainage method

Technical Considerations

A review of available literature concerning surgical drains suggests the following general technical principles (Dougherty and Simmons, 1992).

1. Drains should not exit through the incision site but through a separate stab wound.
2. Drains should be removed as soon as possible because of the risk of retrograde infection.
3. Silicone drainage tubes are preferred because silicone generates less tissue reaction than other materials used to make drainage tubes.
4. Air inlet filters should be used in nonclosed systems to prevent bacteria from entering from external sources.
5. If peritoneal drains are used, a closed passive system or an open active drain should be employed.
6. Closed-wound suction with high pressures should be used to obliterate dead spaces, as seen with skin flaps and potential collecting areas for wound fluids.
7. Primary surgical drainage of abscesses or hematomas may be augmented by:
   a. Open passive drains.
   b. Open active drains with air inlet filters and low pressures.
   c. Closed active drains with low pressures. High pressures tend to bring about obstruction of the drainage perforation.
8. If tubes are placed in proximity to blood vessels, bowel, or bladder, negative pressure drains should be of the open type and of low pressure or should be used with tubing holes of a small diameter.
9. Tube diameter is the largest determinant for flow. Large fluid volumes needing rapid removal will require an increased tubal lumen.
10. The stab wound for the drain exit should be of smaller diameter than the drain but not compromise its egress.

Finally, Tait's axiom (1887): "When in doubt, drain" should be modified; drains must not be considered as a substitute for hemostasis or a replacement for meticulous surgical technique. Halstead's axiom (1898) may be more germane: "No drainage at all is better than the ignorant employment of it."

SUMMARY

While there is a bewildering array of instruments available to the surgeon, many are simply minor variations of the same basic instrument. We have described those instruments and drains that we find most practical and well suited to obstetrics. Each surgeon will develop preferences as regards what constitutes their individual "instrument pack." A broader knowledge of available instrumentation will give further flexibility in the management of unique and unusual intraoperative events or complications.

REFERENCES

Codman Surgical Product Catalog, Codman & Shurtleff Inc., 1990.

Dougherty SH, Simmons RL. The biology and practice of surgical drains, part 1 & 2. Curr Probl Surg 1992; Aug: 539–623 (289 ref), Sept: 639–85.

Halstead WS. Concerning drainage and drainage tubes. Trans Am Surg Assoc 1898; 16:103.

Hanna E. Efficiency of peritoneal drainage. Surg Gynecol Obstet 1970; 131:983.

Hasselgren AO, Harbey E, Malmer H, et al. One instead of two knives for surgical incision. Arch Surg 1984; 118:917.

Hilton P. Surgical wound drainage: Survey of practices among gynecologists in the British Isles. Br Obstet Gynecol 1988; 95: 1063–9.

Loong, R. A controlled trial on wound drainage in cesarean section. Aust/NZ Obstet Gynecol 1988; 28:266.

Poulsen HK. Prophylactic metronidazole or suction drainage in abdominal hysterectomy. Obstet Gynecol 1984; 63:291–294.

Price J. Drainage in abdominal surgery. Trans Am Assoc Obstet Gynecol 1888; 1:84.

Scotto V. Cefoxitin, single-dose prophylaxis and/or T-tube suction drainage for vaginal and abdominal hysterectomy: Prospective randomized trial on 155 patients. Clin Exp Obstet Gynecol 1985; 12:75–81.

Swartz WH. T-tube suction drainage and/or prophylactic antibiotics. A randomized study of 451 hysterectomies. Obstet Gynecol 1976; 47:655–70.

Tait, Lawson, cited by: Robinson JO. Surgical drainage: An historical perspective. Br J Surg 1986; 73:422–6.

Wijma J. Antibiotics and suction drainage as prophylaxis in vaginal and abdominal hysterectomy. Obstet Gynecol 1987; 70:384–8.

CHAPTER 3

Asepsis and Infection Control

In the late nineteenth century, medicine was revolutionized by the observations of Holmes and Semmelweiss, Lister's publication of antiseptic principles, and acceptance of Pasteur's germ theory of disease (Lasson, 1988). These basic principles remain important today in the surgical specialties and have been further refined into specific procedural recommendations. This chapter will review the scientific foundation for current recommendations designed to minimize the risk of infection in surgical patients.

SURGICAL BARRIERS

Surgical barriers include gowns, gloves, masks, caps, and shoe covers, as well as surgical drapes. Surgical scrub suits are constructed of a material that is loosely woven for comfort; they are not designed to be barriers. These garments transmit bacteria freely and bidirectionally as air currents pass through the weave's interstices (Beck, 1981; Bernard and associates, 1965; Lidwell and MacIntosh, 1978). Scrub suits serve to prevent transmission and distribution of community-acquired organisms to the operating suite and vice versa.

Surgical gowns, on the other hand, are worn as barriers to microbial transmission during operative procedures and serve to separate sterile from nonsterile areas (Beck, 1981). Penetration of such barriers is dramatically affected by whether the barrier material is wet or dry. Older standard cloth drapes and gowns were constructed of cotton thread, woven to contain 140 threads per linear inch. Such material is comfortable and when dry is resistant to through transmission of microorganisms even in high humidity (Beck and associates, 1964). However, when such materials become wet with any aqueous liquid, microorganisms are transmitted freely in both directions (Beck and Carlson, 1963; Schwartz and Saunders, 1980; Laufman and associates, 1979). If liquid is wicked from a sterile to a nonsterile site, both sides become contaminated (Beck, 1981). Bacterial transmission through wet material is affected somewhat by the surface tension of the liquid (Laufman and colleagues, 1980). Although experimental transmission rates differ with blood, urine, amniotic fluid, or saline, from a clinical standpoint transmission through standard cloth drapes is instantaneous (Beck, 1981).

These observations have led to abandoning the use of standard cloth material as surgical barriers. Today, two types of material are used for gowns and drapes: one, a reusable, tightly woven (280 threads per inch) fabric treated chemically to render it non-wicking, and the second a disposable and impermeable material. Resistance to microbial penetration in the reusable gowns and drapes is lost after 75 launderings, and problems with spot failure with such materials may occur after penetration by towel clips, hemostats, or rubbing.

Two series have shown increased wound infection with the use of adhesive plastic drapes (Cruse and Foord, 1980; Paskini and Lerner, 1969). Although modern liquid-impervious materials do not "breathe" well and are less comfortable to the surgeon, their aseptic superiority over older materials is clear.

Face masks are designed to cover the mouth and nose of operating room personnel. Such masks do not form a barrier to microorganisms. Careful bacteriologic studies have found no difference in operating room bacterial counts regardless of whether masks are worn (Paskini and Lerner, 1969). Randomized clinical studies also have shown no difference in wound infection rate when masks were eliminated from all operating room personnel except those with upper respiratory infections (Ritter and associates, 1975). Rather than form a barrier to microorganisms, masks redirect them so that they flow out of the sides of the mask (Paskini and Lerner, 1969).

Gloves are designed to provide a true aseptic barrier. No studies exist to document the efficacy of gloves in reducing wound infection. In one series, no wound infections occurred in 141 instances of glove puncture. These authors concluded that organisms escaped in insufficient numbers to be a serious hazard to patients and speculated that the risk of wound infection would be minimal even without gloves (Dalgleish and Malkovsky, 1988). The importance of gloves, however, in preventing transmission of blood-borne disease to the surgeon is unquestioned (Tuneval, 1987; Dalgleish and Malkovsky, 1988). Unfortunately, gloves puncture in 11–38 percent of surgical procedures (Dalgleish and Malkovsky, 1988; Serrano and associates, 1991; Cohn and Seifer, 1990). In one series, 62 percent of such punctures were unrecognized, and most occurred in the fingers of the nondominant hand, suggesting that needle handling with fingers may be the cause (Serrano and associates, 1991). Double gloving appeared to reduce the risk of blood contamination on the hands of gynecologic surgeons from 38 percent to 2 percent (Cohn and Seifer, 1990).

Shoe covers do not affect surgical infection and are used mainly to prevent dissemination of body fluids to areas outside the operating room.

HAND WASHING/SURGICAL SCRUBBING

No difference in wound infection rate has been noted following hand washing with iodophor versus hexachlorophene solutions, nor is the rate of overall infection greater. There does not appear to be any difference between scrub times of 3–5 minutes and those that are longer (Dineen, 1969; Galle and associates, 1978). Water conservation considerations also apply in determining the appropriate length of scrub time, eg, a 10-minute scrub uses roughly 50 gallons of water (Galle and associates, 1978). Accepted practice calls for a 5-minute scrub before the first procedure of the day followed by 2- to 5-minute scrubs between consecutive operations (Polk and associates, 1983).

PATIENT PREPARATION

It is well established that the most important source of potential surgical infection is the patient herself, from bacteria colonizing the skin or, in obstetric surgery, the genital tract (Howard and colleagues, 1964). There is currently no effective method of diminishing colonization of the vagina or uterus other than limiting the number of intrapartum pelvic examinations. However, preoperative preparation of the patient's skin is of utmost importance (Edlich and associates, 1977). Hair removal is indicated only if essential for proper performance of the procedure because hair itself does not contribute to infection. Shaving hair at the operation site the night before surgery significantly increases the rate of wound infection (Polk and associates, 1983; Seropain and Reynolds, 1971). If hair removal is imperative, shaving the area in the operating room immediately prior to the procedure or using electric clippers or depilatory cream is recommended (Seropain and Reynolds, 1971; Cruse and Foord, 1980).

Proper skin cleansing involves scrubbing the incision site, most commonly with a complexed iodine solution. Iodine is released slowly and is active over a prolonged period of time against all common microbial organisms including fungi and viruses (Edlich, 1977; Branemark, 1966; and their associates). The incision area commonly is cleansed in a circular motion beginning at the incision site and extending to include the widest foreseeable operative field (Seropain and Reynolds, 1971).

Although intact skin is not damaged by iodophor or chlorhexidine, the introduction of such agents into subcutaneous tissues for irri-

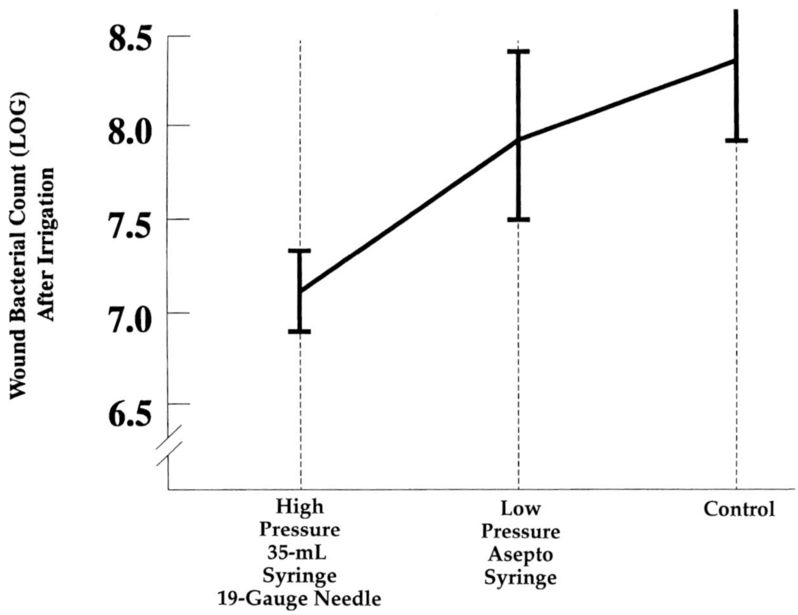

Figure 3–1. Bacterial removal efficiency of fluids delivered by an Asepto syringe or by a 35-mL syringe via a 19-gauge needle. (From Stevenson and associates, 1976.)

gation purposes causes tissue damage and actually increases the rate of wound infections (Cruse and Foord, 1980). Irrigation should be carried out only with crystalloid solution. High-pressure irrigation is extremely effective in producing up to a 10-fold decrease in wound bacterial count (Fig. 3–1). Such irrigation may be accomplished using normal saline with a 19-1 gauge needle and 35-cc syringe (Stevenson and associates, 1976). It is also important not to perform elective procedures on patients with ongoing bacterial infections or open sores (Polk and colleagues, 1983).

The longer a patient is in the hospital prior to operation, the greater the risk of wound infection (Fig. 3–2) (Cruse and Foord, 1980). These authors found a 1.2 percent infection rate with a 1-day stay, a 2.1 percent infection with a 1-week preoperative stay, and 3.4 percent infection with a preoperative hospital stay exceeding 2 weeks. They also documented a sixfold increase in wound infection in patients over age 66 compared to children and teens (Fig. 3–3). In clean wounds, infection increases directly with operating time; the rate of wound infection roughly doubles

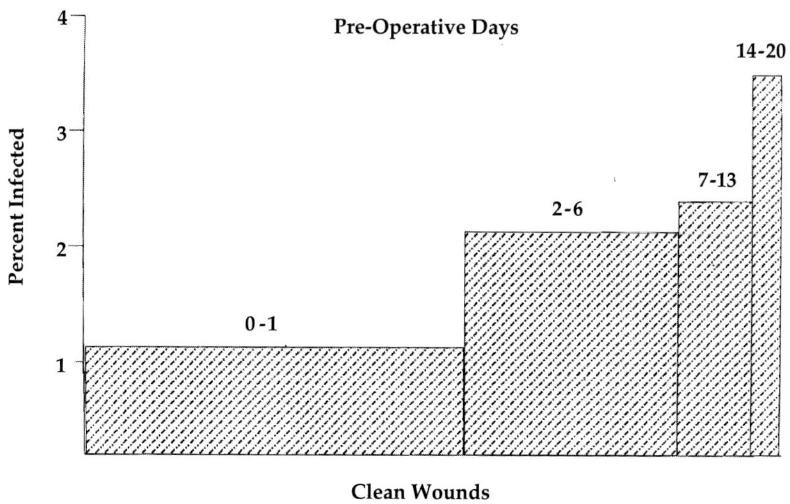

Figure 3–2. Relationship of the preoperative hospital stay to wound infection. (From Cruse and Foord, 1980.)

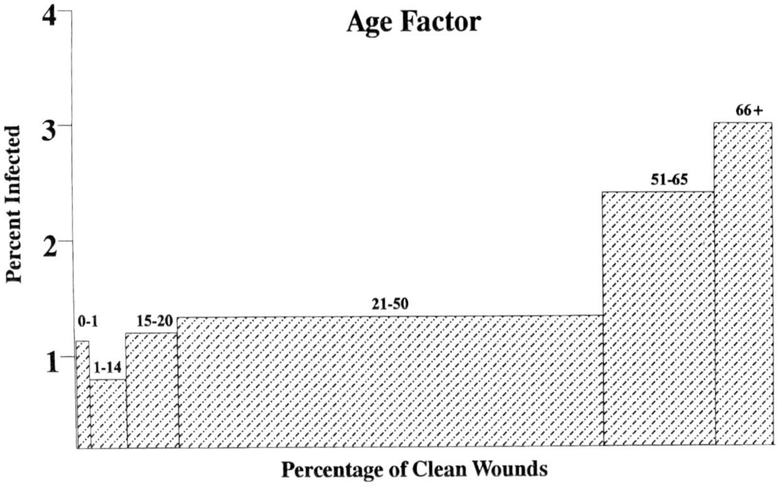

Figure 3–3. Relationship of age to wound infection. (From Cruse and Foord, 1980.)

with each half hour (Fig. 3–4) (Cruse and Foord, 1980; Stevenson and associates, 1976; Public Health Lab Service, 1960). Potential explanations for this increase include increasing dosage of bacterial contamination with time and progressive devitalization of tissue through drying and pressure from retractors. Longer operations also often involve more electrocoagulation and suture placement and a greater likelihood of blood loss and shock (Cruse and Foord, 1980).

Operating room preparation is also important in preventing infection. In many hospitals, concentrations of airborne bacteria are minimized through air flow systems, which change the air 20–25 times per hour or pass it through a high-efficiency particulate filter. Regardless of air flow or filtration systems, traffic flow through the operating room should be kept to a minimum; airborne bacteria counts correlate directly with the length of time operating room doors are open (Ritter and associates, 1975). On the other hand, redispersal of bacteria from the floor to air is not significant (Hochberg and Murray, 1991).

SURGICAL TECHNIQUE

Basic concepts of surgical technique originally established by Halsted remain valid today. These include principles of gentle tissue handling, meticulous hemostasis, and wound irrigation.

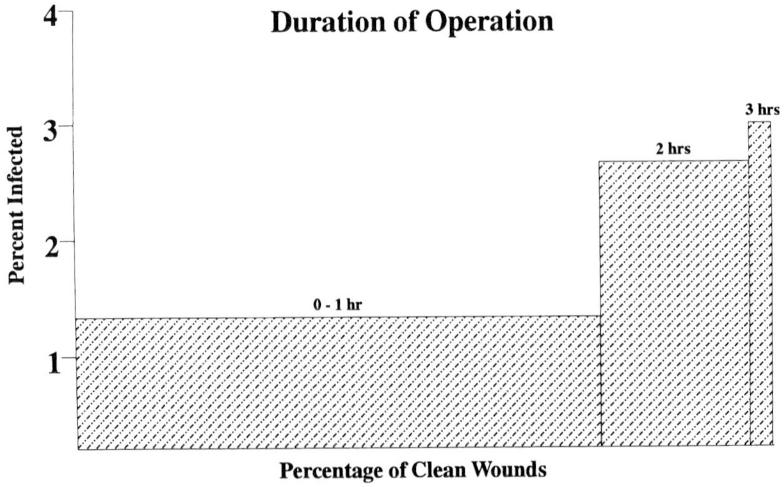

Figure 3–4. Influence of operative time on wound infection. (From Cruse and Foord, 1980.)

Gentle handling of skin edges is especially important in preventing incisional wound infection (Salasche and associates, 1989). The ideal surgeon has historically been described as one with "harte as the harte of a lyon, his eyes like the eyes of a hawke, and his handes the handes of a woman" (Cruse and Foord, 1980).

Electrocautery is a valuable surgical tool; however, care should be taken to minimize its use—especially in subcutaneous spaces—in order to limit devitalization of tissue and wound infection. Although hemostasis must be complete prior to skin closure, often direct pressure on bleeding points for 20–30 seconds will allow for hemostasis via platelet aggregation and avoid the need for cautery or suture ligation. The use of hot, wet sponges for hemostasis causes hyperthermic tissue injury, which enhances infection and should be avoided (Hochberg and Murray, 1991).

There is a direct relationship between the number of viable bacteria in an open wound and the ability to effect wound closure without infection (Cruse and Foord, 1980). Wounds containing less than 10^5 bacteria per gram of tissue generally heal well, whereas wounds containing more than this concentration of bacteria may have a wound infection rate of 50–100 percent (Hochberg and Murray, 1991). Contaminated wounds should be irrigated as outlined above. With heavy contamination, consideration should be given to delayed primary closure after four or more days (Verrier and associates, 1979). The placement of absorbable sutures in the subcutaneous tissue to close dead space increases the likelihood of wound infection and should generally be avoided, as the number of bacteria needed to establish a subcutaneous infection is decreased 10,000-fold or more by the presence of a suture (Edlich and associates, 1977; Elek and Conen, 1957; Howe and Marston, 1962).

Dressing is an important part of wound care and has a direct influence on the course of healing (Edlich and associates, 1977; Hochberg and Murray, 1991). During the first 48 hours of healing when epithelialization is incomplete, the incision should be covered with dry dressings (Hochberg and Murray, 1991). Soaked dressings enhance bacterial passage and should be promptly changed.

In 1964, the National Research Council established a classification of wounds based upon clinical estimate of wound contamination. Table 3–1 details this classification. Obstetrical wounds commonly range from clean contaminated (repeat cesarean section not in labor) to dirty (cesarean section, in the presence of gross amnionitis). As detailed in Table 3–1, the anticipated infection rate without antibiotic prophylaxis is directly related to this classification (Cruse and Foord, 1980). Table 3–2 summarizes strongly or moderately recommended guidelines for the prevention of surgical wound infection issued by an expert panel of the Centers for Disease Control (Polk and associates, 1983).

TABLE 3–1. NATIONAL RESEARCH COUNCIL CLASSIFICATION OF SURGICAL WOUNDS

			Anticipated Infection Rate %	
Classification	**Definition**	**Example**	*Without Antibiotic*	*With Antibiotic*
Clean	Intact technique; respiratory, GI, and genitourinary tract not entered; no inflammation	Oophorectomy; cystectomy	1–2	—
Clean-contaminated	Intact technique; respiratory, GI, or genitourinary tract entered; no inflammation	Hysterectomy	10–20	7
Contaminated	Major breakdown in technique; gross spillage from GI tract; inflamed biliary system	Cesarean section with labor	20–35	10–15
Dirty	Old traumatic wounds; perforated viscus; presence of pus	Perforated cecum; cesarean section with chorioamnionitis	25–50	15–35

TABLE 3–2. CDC RECOMMENDATIONS FOR INFECTION CONTROL

1. If the operation is elective, all bacterial infections that are identified, excluding ones for which the operation is performed, should be treated and controlled before the operation.
2. If the operation is elective and the patient is grossly malnourished, the patient should receive preoperative oral or parenteral hyperalimentation.
3. a. Unless hair near the operative site is thick enough to interfere with the surgical procedure, it should not be removed.
   b. If hair removal is necessary, it should be done as near the time of operation as possible, preferably immediately before.
4. a. The area around and including the operative site should be scrubbed with a detergent solution and then covered with an antiseptic solution. This area should include the entire incision and an adjacent area large enough for the surgeon to work during the operation without contacting unprepared skin.
   b. Tincture of chlorhexidine, iodophors, and tincture of iodine are the recommended antiseptic products for preparing a patient's operative site. Plain soap, alcohol, or hexachlorophene is not recommended as a single agent for operative site preparation, unless the patient's skin is sensitive to the recommended antiseptic products. Aqueous quaternary ammonium compounds should not be used.
5. For major operations involving an incision and requiring use of the operating room (OR), the patient should be covered with sterile drapes in such a manner that no part of the patient is uncovered except the operative field and those body parts necessary for the administration of anesthesia.
6. Everyone who enters the OR should wear at all times (1) a high-efficiency mask that fully covers the mouth and nose, (2) a cap or hood that fully covers the head hair, and (3) shoe covers. A beard should be fully covered by the mask and hood.
7. a. The surgical team (those who will touch the sterile surgical field, sterile instruments, or an incisional wound) should scrub their hands and arms to the elbows with an antiseptic before each operation. Scrubbing should be done before every procedure and for at least 5 minutes before the first procedure of the day.
   b. Chlorhexidine, iodophors, and hexachlorophene are the recommended active antimicrobial ingredients for the surgical hand scrub. Aqueous quaternary ammonium compounds (eg, benzalkonium chloride) should not be used.
   c. Hexachlorophene should not be used by pregnant women.
8. a. After the hands are scrubbed with an antiseptic and dried with a sterile towel, the surgical team should don sterile gowns.
   b. Gowns used in the OR should be made of reusable or disposable fabrics that have been shown to be nearly impermeable to bacteria, even when wet.
9. The surgical team should wear sterile gloves. If a glove is punctured during the operation, it should be promptly changed.

SUMMARY

Surgical barriers are important for the protection of the patient and the health care provider. Of these barriers the surgical gown and gloves afford the greatest level of protection from bacterial contamination. Hand washing by the surgeons and surgical field preparation are also important aspects of asepsis and infection control. Attention to details of surgical technique with minimization of tissue trauma and operating time further reduce the risk of infection.

REFERENCES

Beck WC, Carlson W. Aseptic barriers. Arch Surg 1963; 87:288.

Beck WC, Chandler HW, Carlson WW, et al. The bacterial permeability of humidity moistened textiles. Guthrie Clin Bull 1964; 34:102.

Beck WC. Aseptic barriers in surgery. Arch Surg 1981; 116:240.

Bernard HR, Speere R, O'Grady F, et al. Reduction of dissemination of skin bacteria by modification of operating room clothing and by ultraviolet irradiation. Lancet 1965; 2:458.

Branemark PI, Albrektsson B, Lindstrom F, Lundborg G. Local tissue effects of wound disinfectants. Acta Chir Scand (Suppl) 1966; 357:166.

Cohn GM, Seifer DB. Blood exposure in single versus double gloving during pelvic surgery. Am J Obstet Gynecol 1990; 162:715.

Cruse PJ, Foord R. The epidemiology of wound infection: a 10 year prospective study of 62,939 wounds. Surg Clin North Am 1980; 60:27.

Dalgleish AG, Malkovsky M. Surgical gloves as a mechanical barrier against human immunodeficiency virus. Br J Surg 1988; 75:171.

Dineen P. An evaluation of the duration of the surgical scrub. Surg Gynecol Obstet 1969; 129:1181.

Edlich RF, Rodeheaver G, Thacker JG, Edgerton MT. Technical factors in wound management. In: Fundamentals of Wound Management of Surgery. South Plainfield: Chirurgecom, Inc. 1977; p. 364.

Elek SD, Conen PE. The virulence of *Staphylococcus pyogenes* for man; a study of the problems of wound infection. Br J Exp Pathol 1957; 38:573.

Galle PC, Homesley HD, Rhyne AL. Assessment of the surgical scrub. Surg Gynecol Obstet 1978; 147:214.

Hochberg J, Murray GF. Principles of operative surgery. Antisepsis, technique, sutures, and drains. In: Textbook of Surgery, Sabiston DC Jr (ed), 14th ed. Philadelphia; WB Saunders, 1991.

Howard JM, Barker WF, Culbertson WR, et al. Factors influencing the incidence of wound infection. Ann Surg Suppl 1964; 160:32.

Howe CCW, Marston AT. A study on sources of postoperative staphylococcal infection. Surg Gynecol Obstet 1962; 115:266.

Lasson E. Innovations in health care: antisepsis as a case study. Am J Public Health 1988; 75:476.

Laufman H, Siegal JD, Edberg SC. Moist bacterial strike-through of surgical materials: confirmatory tests. Am Surg 1979; 189:68.

Laufman H, Montefusco C, Siegal JD, et al. Scanning electron microscopy of moist bacterial strike-through of surgical materials. Surg Gynecol Obstet 1980; 150:165.

Lidwell OM, MacIntosh CA. The evaluation of fabrics in relation to their use as protective garments in nursing and surgery: I. Physical measurements and bench tests. J Hyg Camb 1978; 433.

National Academy of Sciences—National Research Council. Division of Medical Sciences, Ad Hoc Committee of the Committee on Trauma: Postoperative wound infections: The influence of ultraviolet irradiation of the operating room and various other factors. Ann Surg 1964; 160 (Suppl. 2):1.

Paskini DL, Lerner HJ. A prospective study of wound infections. Am Surg 1969; 35:627.

Polk HC, Simpson CJ, Simmons BP, Alexander JW. Guidelines for prevention of surgical wound infection. Arch Surg 1983; 118:1213.

Public Health Laboratory Service. Incidence of surgical wound infection in England and Wales: A report of the Public Health Laboratory Service, Great Britain. Lancet 1960; 2:658.

Ritter MA, Eitzen H, French MLV, Hart JB. The operating room environment as affected by people and the surgical face mask. Clinical Orthopaedics and Related Research 1975; 3:147.

Salasche SJ, Winton GB, Adnot J. Surgical pearls. Dermatol Clin 1989; 7:75.

Schwartz JJ, Saunders DE. Microbial penetration of surgical gown material. Surg Gynecol Obstet 1980; 150:507.

Seropain R, Reynolds BM. Wound infections after pre-operative depilatory versus razor preparation. Am J Surg 1971; 121:251.

Serrano CW, Wright JW, Newton ER. Surgical glove perforation in obstetrics. Obstet Gynecol 1991; 77:525.

Stevenson TR, Thacker JG, Rodeheaver GT, et al. Cleansing the traumatic wound by high pressure syringe irrigation. J Am Coll Emerg Phys 1976; 5:17.

Tuneval TG. Surgical face mask: with or without. Abstracts of 32nd World Congress of Surgery, Sydney, Australia, 1987.

Verrier ED, Bossart KJ, Heer FW. Reduction of infection rates in abdominal incisions by delayed wound closure techniques. Am J Surg 1979; 138:22.

CHAPTER 4

Anatomy, Incisions, and Closures

With the obstetrical patient, the choice of abdominal incision and closure depends upon several factors: the urgency for operative intervention, the indications for the operation, associated preoperative conditions, the presence of previous abdominal scars, and the surgeon's prior experience. Incisions should be selected with the objectives of reasonably rapid entry, adequate exposure, and a closure that will reduce the likelihood of infection or dehiscence. This chapter compares and contrasts classical techniques with some recent modifications; the goal is to enable the surgeon to choose the incision most appropriate to each clinical situation.

ANTERIOR ABDOMINAL WALL ANATOMY

A thorough understanding of abdominal wall anatomy is essential to avoid injury to nerves and blood vessels and to close the incision with minimal chance of dehiscence. Superiorly, the anterior abdominal wall is bounded by the costal margins of the seventh, eighth, ninth, and tenth ribs and the xiphoid process of the sternum. Lateral boundaries are delineated by the iliac crests, while the inferior boundaries consist of the inguinal ligaments, the pubic crests, and the upper border of the symphysis pubis. Because the lines of tension—**Langer's lines**—of abdominal skin are almost transverse, the scars associated with transverse incisions tend to be more cosmetic as time passes; in contrast, vertical scars have a tendency to stretch.

Muscles and Fascia

The anterior abdominal wall has two groups of muscles, one with fibers running transversely and one with fibers running vertically. The transverse or flat muscles include the external oblique, the internal oblique, and the transverse abdominis. The vertical group is composed of the rectus and pyramidal muscles. The rectus muscle with its thin investing fascia is a muscle of locomotion and posture. The integrity of the anterior abdominal wall is not greatly associated with this muscle (Daversa and Landers, 1961).

The **external oblique muscle** and its aponeurosis form the most anterior layer of the flat muscles. Superiorly, its fibers run transversely; inferiorly, they assume an oblique downward course. A portion of the muscle gives rise to a broad fibrous aponeurosis, which courses medially, anterior to the rectus muscle. The next posterior fan-like muscle is the **internal oblique.** The midportion of the muscle runs an upward oblique course and gives rise to the aponeurosis of the internal oblique. At the lateral border of the rectus, the aponeurosis splits and forms a sheath around the rectus muscle, rejoining medial to the rectus to help form the linea alba (Fig. 4–1). The third "flat" muscle, the **transverse abdominis,** has a truly transverse course. Above the midway point between the umbilicus and pubis, the aponeurosis of this muscle passes behind the rectus muscle and contributes to the posterior rectus sheath. Below this point, the aponeurosis passes anterior to the rectus muscle, contributing to the anterior rectus sheath (Fig. 4–1). Medial to the rectus muscle, the fascia of all three flat muscles insert to form the linea alba.

The lower limit of the upper portion of the transverse aponeurosis, which is situated posterior to the rectus muscle, forms a crescentic border, the **arcuate** or **semilunar line.** Below the arcuate line, near the level of the anterior superior iliac spines, the posterior rectus sheath is absent. If proper closure methods are not used, hernias or fascial dehiscence is more likely to occur in this area. According to the study by Rees and Coller (1943), the force required to approximate the edges of a vertical incision in the lower abdomen is 30 times greater than that required to approximate a transverse incision.

The **rectus abdominis muscle** arises from the pubic crest (Fig. 4–1). Its upper attachment is three times as broad as its pubic insertion. It has three to four fibrous insertions, the **linea transversae.** One is at the level of the umbilicus; the other two are usually halfway between the umbilicus and the insertions. Importantly, the fibrous insertions are tightly adherent to the anterior rectus sheath, which limits its retraction when cut. The **pyramidalis,** a triangular muscle, usually lies anterior to the rectus. The midportion of this muscle usually has an avascular raphe, which can easily be incised for adequate exposure of the space of Retzius.

Arteries and Veins

The anterior abdominal wall has an excellent blood supply, with extensive collateral circulation. The medial abdominal wall receives blood from the **epigastric arteries,** while

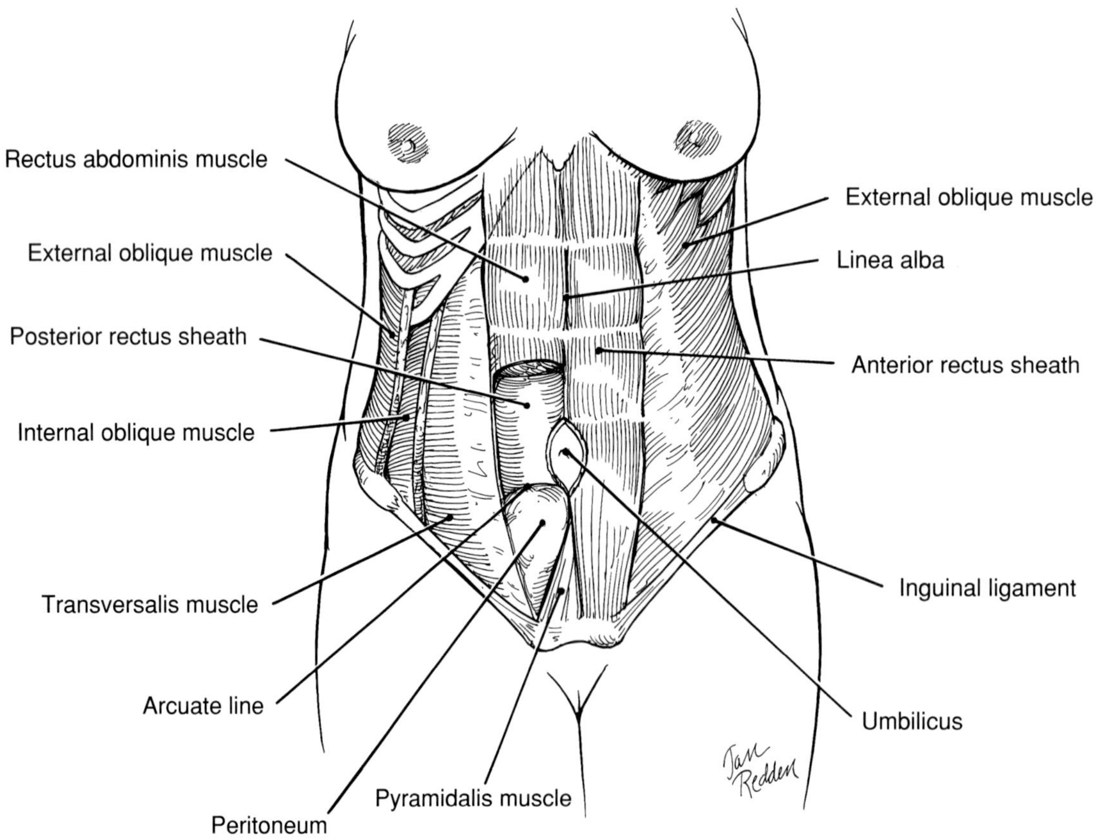

Figure 4–1. Anatomy of the anterior abdominal wall showing major muscle groups.

the lateral wall is supplied by the **musculophrenic** and **deep circumflex iliac arteries.** Because of their rich anastomoses, vascular deficiency is usually not a complication of abdominal wall surgery (Fig. 4–2). Since the linea is relatively bloodless, wound healing is thought to be somewhat impaired when midline incisions are used. In contrast, the epigastric vessels are subject to injury when a muscle splitting incision is used. Also, the deep circumflex or musculophrenic vessels can be injured when a transverse incision is carried too far laterally in the muscle bundles.

The **superior epigastric artery** is a continuation of the anterior thoracic artery, which enters the sheath of the rectus muscle from behind the seventh costal cartilage and descends posterior to the rectus muscle. It anastomoses with the inferior epigastric artery; these vessels supply multiple branches into the substance of the rectus muscle. Above the umbilicus, the superior epigastric artery tends to lie posterior to the midportion of the rectus muscle. The **inferior epigastric artery** arises from the external iliac artery near the midinguinal point and courses in a cephalad direction along the posterior lateral portion of the rectus muscle. Because the inferior epigastric artery course runs from **lateral** toward the midline (Fig. 4–2), a low transverse incision is unlikely to damage these vessels. The veins lie in close approximation to the main trunks of the epigastric arteries.

The **musculophrenic artery** runs along the costal margin behind the cartilages with anastomosis with the deep circumflex artery, which originates from the external iliac artery at about the same level as the inferior epigastric artery. The deep circumflex artery courses behind the inguinal ligament and along the iliac crest before piercing the transverse abdominis muscle and interdigitating between that muscle and the internal oblique. Prior to its anastomosis with the musculophrenic, it

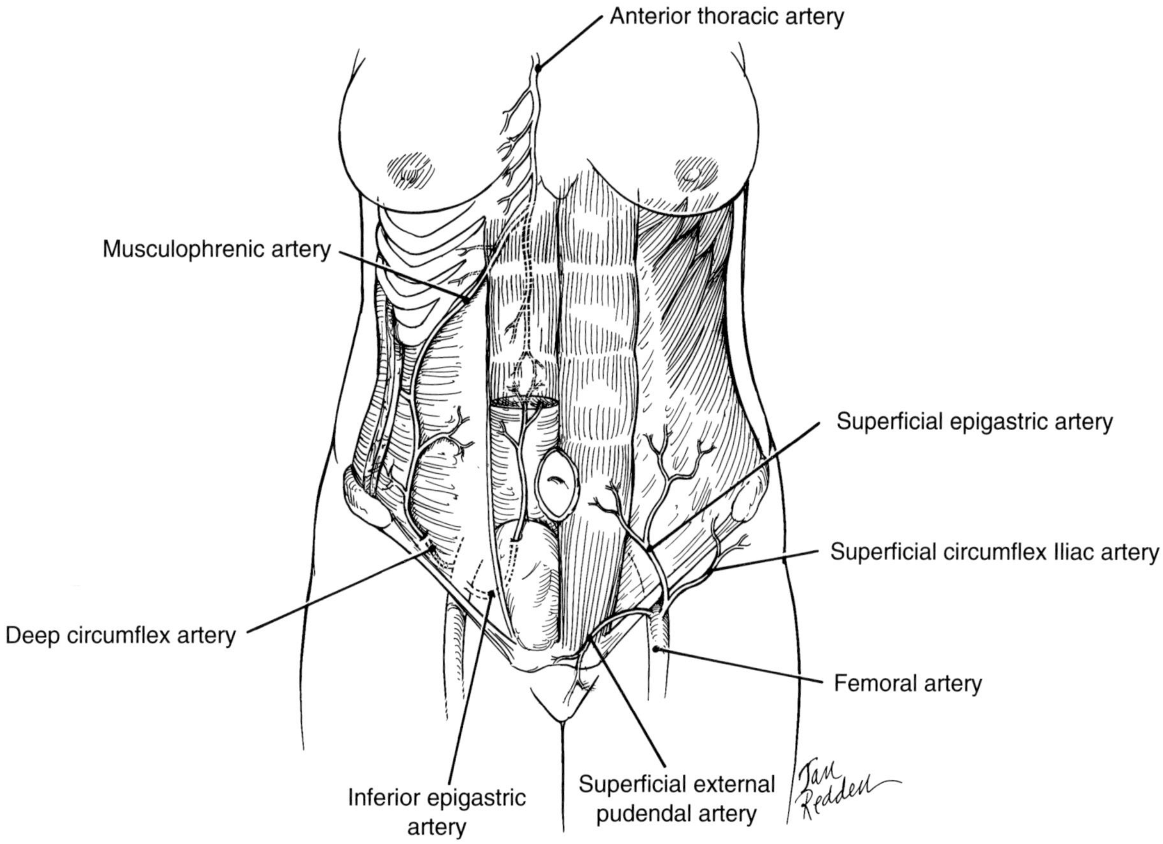

Figure 4–2. The major arterial blood supply of the anterior abdominal wall. The four major vessels, two medial and two lateral, contribute to the rich anastomoses. The superficial epigastric artery serves the superficial tissues of the lower abdominal wall.

can be relatively large and care must be taken when these muscles are incised laterally to avoid vessel injury.

Nerves

The anterior abdominal wall is supplied by the thoracoabdominal, the iliohypogastric, and the ilioinguinal nerves (Fig. 4–3). The **thoracoabdominal nerves,** consisting of the seventh to eleventh intercostal nerves, leave the intercostal spaces and travel caudad and anterior between the transverse abdominis and internal oblique muscles. They supply these muscles and the external oblique muscles. They also enter the sheath of the rectus and supply the rectus muscle and the overlying skin. The majority of these nerves are supplied by several trunks. When an incision is made lateral to the midline, a vertical type is more likely than a transverse incision to cause injury to these nerves. A vertical incision made lateral to the rectus muscle or through the muscle will denervate the tissues lying medial to the incision. The longer the incision, the greater the degree of denervation and the greater the risk of atony or atrophy of the underlying muscle. The **iliohypogastric** and **ilioinguinal nerves** (Fig. 4–3) are sensory nerves. Injury to the iliohypogastric nerve, when wide transverse incisions are used, may result in sensation changes in the skin over the mons pubis, whereas injury to the ilioinguinal nerve may result in sensation changes to the labia majora. Both nerves also supply the lower fibers of the internal oblique and transverse abdominis muscles. Damage to these nerves at the level of the anterior superior iliac spine will denervate these muscle fibers. A weakening of the normal inguinal canal controlling mechanism may also result, predisposing the woman to an inguinal hernia.

WOUND HEALING

Incisions resulting in an excellent cosmetic scar are desirable, although not always feasible. Abdominal wound infections, and occasionally the resulting dehiscence after obstet-

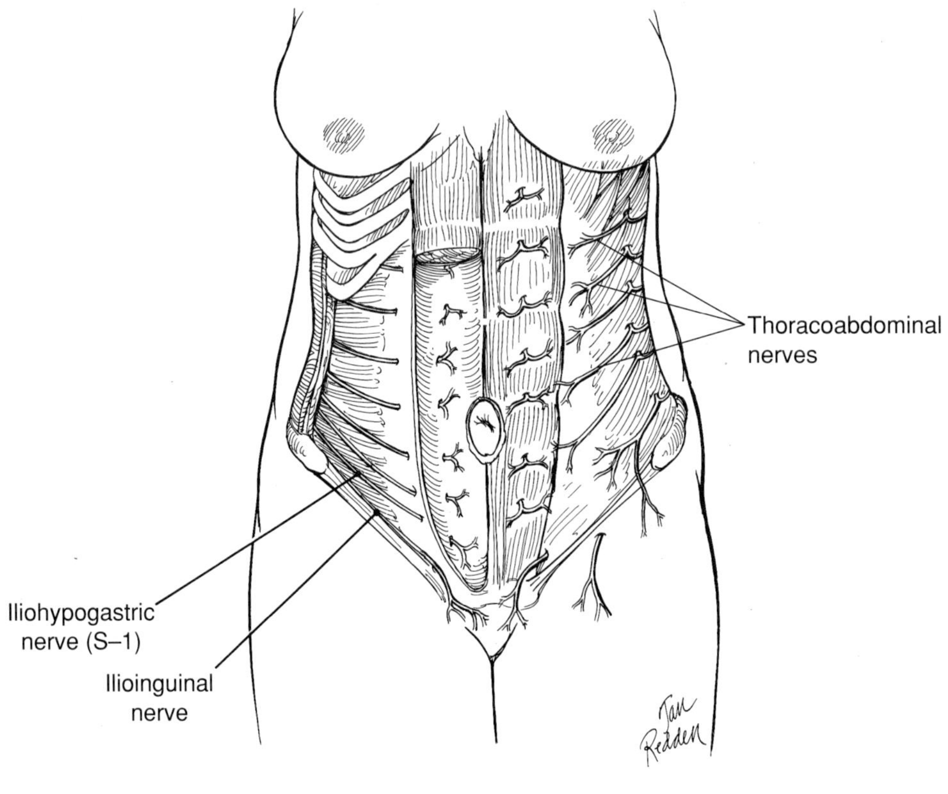

Figure 4–3. The major innervation of the anterior abdominal wall is via the thoracoabdominal, iliohypogastric, and ilioinguinal nerves.

rical operative procedures, are a psychologic and economic problem. Factors negatively affecting wound healing include diabetes, malnutrition, prior irradiation or chemotherapy, older age, alcoholism, preoperative shaving the evening before, duration of preoperative hospitalization, duration of the operation, the use of Penrose-type drains brought out through the incision, ascites, malignancy, immunosuppression (including long-term corticosteroid therapy), and obesity (Cruse, 1977; Cruse and Foord, 1973; Dineen, 1961). Additionally, factors contributing to wound disruption in the absence of infection include choice of suture material, closure technique, excessive coughing, retching and vomiting, and intestinal obstruction. Wound complication rates in obstetrical patients are also increased by factors that predispose to infection, including prematurely ruptured membranes and long labors.

The four phases of wound healing include **inflammation, migration, proliferation,** and **maturation.** Disruption can occur in any of these phases and depends on preexisting conditions. Importantly, the fibroblastic-proliferation phase from about day 5 through day 20 provides the most strength to the wound. By day 21, most wounds will have regained almost 30 percent of their original tensile strength. Any wound contamination or foreign bodies can cause chronic inflammation, sinuses, delayed incisional hernias, or early postoperative problems of infection and dehiscence. Yet cesarean section performed in a laboring woman would at best be classified as a clean-contaminated wound (class II); and in some cases will be even a higher risk procedure when there is overt chorioamnionitis and perhaps further wound contamination with meconium laden amniotic fluid.

TYPES OF ABDOMINAL INCISIONS

The four incisions that are most useful for obstetrical patients are shown in Figure 4–4: **midline** (vertical), **Pfannenstiel, Maylard,** and **supraumbilical** (transverse). The transverse incisions achieve the best cosmetic results. Proponents of transverse incisions have suggested that they are as much as 30 times stronger than midline incisions. Mowat and Bonnar (1971), for example, observed that

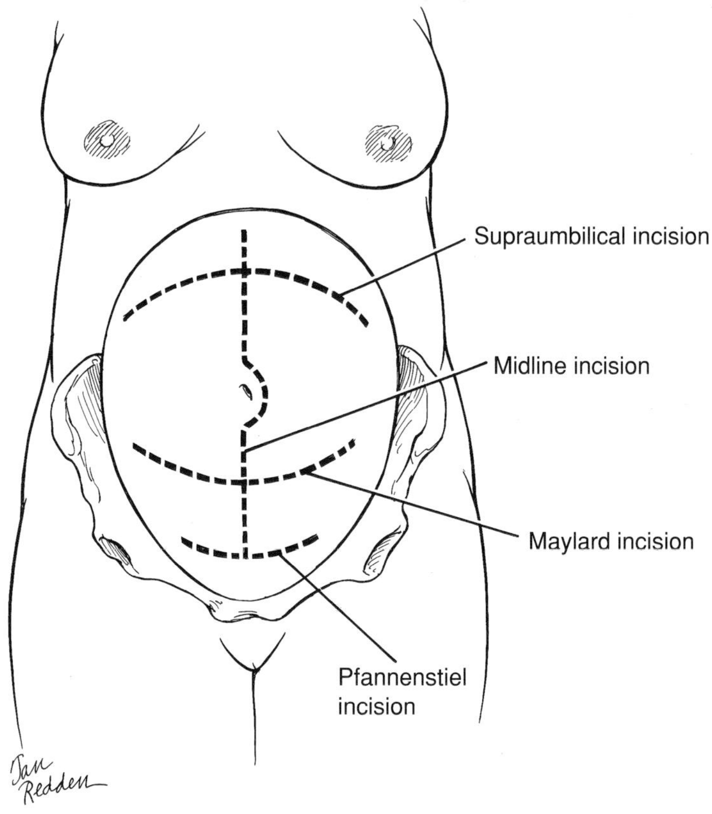

Figure 4–4. The four primary abdominal incisions used in the obstetrical patient, depending on the indications for operative intervention: (1) midline, (2) Pfannenstiel, (3) Maylard, and (4) supraumbilical.

abdominal wound dehiscence after cesarean delivery was eight times more common with a vertical incision than with a transverse. The older literature suggests that wound evisceration was three to five times more common; and hernias developed two to three times more often when midline incisions were used (Helmkamp, 1977; Thompson et al., 1949; Tollefson and Russell, 1954). Some studies indicated that this increased incidence of eviscerations with midline incisions was secondary to inappropriate closures. Conversely, more recent studies have shown an advantage of midline incisions over transverse incisions to avoid dehiscence, or have shown no difference (Farnell et al., 1986; Greenburg et al., 1979).

Transverse Incisions

Transverse incisions not only produce good cosmetic results but also are less painful. In addition, when these incisions are placed in the lower abdomen, they interfere less with postoperative respiratory movement. Transverse incisions, however, do have certain disadvantages: (1) The division of multiple layers of fascia and muscle may result in the formation of dead spaces. (2) There is relatively more bleeding. (3) Making the incision is relatively more time consuming. (4) Transverse incisions may result in division of nerves (Tollefson and Russell, 1954).

Pfannenstiel Incision

This is an excellent cosmetic incision and is indicated in nonobese women when the extra speed of delivery afforded by a vertical incision is not essential. The Pfannenstiel incision should not be used when exposure is critical, for example, in reexploration of a patient for hemorrhage. Exposure of the pregnant uterus often is marginal, particularly in the obese woman. Rapid extension of the incision is difficult and the extensive dissection involved often leads to diffuse small vessel injury, making hemostasis more difficult to obtain and necessitating a subfascial closed drainage system in some women.

The incision, which is made in semielliptical manner, should follow a curve of semilunar skin marking from one side to the other. The midportion of the incision should lie within the shaved area of pubic hair. Its length depends upon the amount of exposure required. The average incision begins and ends 2 or 3 cm below and medial to the anterior superior iliac crests. The scalpel blade should be kept perpendicular to the skin throughout so that the skin edges are not cut on a bevel. The adipose layer is likewise cut in a transverse manner. Bleeding can be minimized by use of electrocautery for this layer. Alternatively, blunt tearing through the adipose tissue also produces less bleeding than occurs with scalpel dissection. The anterior fascia of the recti muscles is exposed and incised transversely. Following blunt dissection underneath and laterally with the curved Mayo scissors, the aponeurosis of the external oblique, internal oblique, and transversus muscles is divided laterally as the continuation of the rectus fascia incision. After further blunt dissection with the forefinger, the upper and lower fascial flaps are elevated from underlying muscle. In the midline, however, they are fused to the conjoined rectus sheath and must be divided with scissors or scalpel. Thereafter, the recti muscles are bluntly separated from each other vertically in the midline. Incision in the underlying peritoneum is also made in a vertical direction, upward as high as the recti are divided and downward to the dome of the bladder. Danger of cutting into the bladder is remote if an open indwelling catheter is in place and the other usual precautions are exercised.

For fascial closure, a running suture can be used with clean or clean-contaminated wounds. Polyglycolic acid or a delayed absorbable suture material can be used. In assessing the use of running versus interrupted polyglycolic acid sutures in midline incisions, Fagniez and colleagues (1985) found no difference in dehiscence rate in a randomized prospective trial of 3135 patients. Drains should be used in the subfascial space if complete hemostasis is in doubt. Subcutaneous sutures are unnecessary, and the skin may be closed with staples or a subcuticular suture.

Modified Pfannenstiel Incision

Once the transverse subcutaneous incision is carried to the aponeurosis of the external oblique muscle and anterior sheath of the recti, the fascia is cleansed cephalad and caudad from the umbilicus to the symphysis in the midline. A vertical incision is then made in the linea alba. This modified incision is not expedient, and subcutaneous closed drainage is usually indicated.

Cherney Incision

Occasionally, a low transverse abdominal incision will not be large enough to deliver the infant safely and expediently or to obtain adequate exposure for hemostasis or to deal with other abnormal conditions. Under these circumstances, the best approach is to perform a modified Cherney incision rather than to "half-transect" the recti. This incision also affords excellent exposure of the pelvic sidewall when needed, for example, for internal iliac artery ligation. The incision is about 25 percent longer than a midline incision from the umbilicus to the symphysis (Cherney, 1941).

If the peritoneum is already incised, it is useful to develop the space of Retzius by blunt dissection prior to incising the recti to avoid bladder injury. This can be easily accomplished by downward traction and pressure in the relatively bloodless midline beneath the rectus muscle and its inferior fascia. The inferior epigastric vessels are easily located and injury avoided. These vessels course more laterally in the caudad portion of the pelvis. The finger of the operator is inserted in the space of Retzius, posterior to the muscle bundles for countertraction (Fig. 4–5). The pyramidalis muscles and the fibrous, tendinous recti are then sharply dissected from their insertion into the pubis. Bleeding is negligible in this area, and the inferior epigastric vessels do not need to be ligated. The peritoneal incision can be extended laterally, about 2 cm cephalad to the bladder.

The peritoneum is closed separately with a running polyglycolic acid suture. The need for drainage of the subfascial space should be assessed. The ends of the rectus tendons are affixed to the inferior portion of the rectus sheath with six to eight interrupted or horizontal mattress permanent sutures (Fig. 4–6). The recti should not be sutured to the symphysis pubis in order to avoid osteomyelitis. Fascial closure can be accomplished with a running continuous No. 1 or No. 2 delayed absorbable suture, as in the Pfannenstiel incision. The remaining portion of the incision is closed similarly.

Maylard Incision

The true transverse muscle-cutting incision, the Maylard or Maylard-Bardenheuer incision is a poor incision for cesarean delivery because of operating time (Maylard, 1907). This incision affords excellent pelvic exposure and is used for radical pelvic surgery, including exenterations and removal of large adnexal masses. For the obstetrical patient, this incision can be used for exploration for postpartum bleeding, internal iliac artery ligation, or hysterectomy. It is an excellent incision for the woman treated by radical hysterectomy for cervical cancer in early pregnancy. While it may be used for pregnant women with adnexal masses, exposure of the upper abdomen is limited. Some feel that a Pfannenstiel incision can be converted into a Maylard incision simply by incising the recti and avoiding the inferior epigastric vessels.

The Maylard begins with a transverse skin incision 3–8 cm above the symphysis, depending on the woman's weight and indications for surgery. Following a transverse fas-

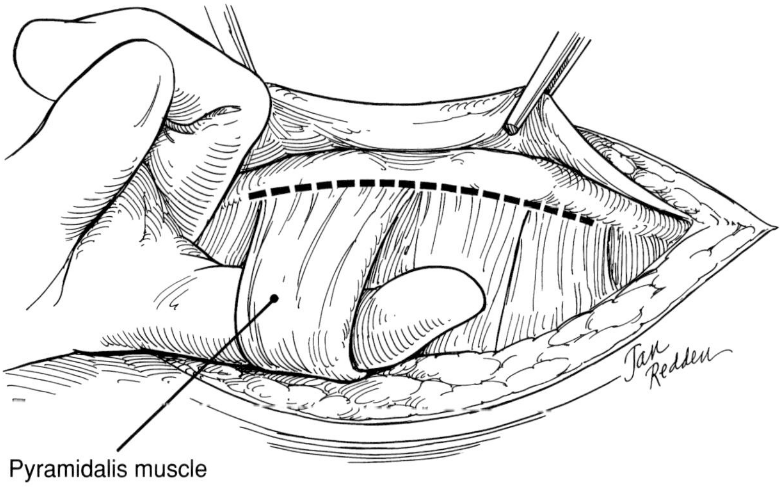

Figure 4–5. Countertraction with Kocher clamps is provided on the inferior fascia. The finger of the operator is placed in the space of Retzius, posterior to the pyramidalis and left rectus muscle. This maneuver easily exposes the fibrous insertion for transection with the cautery.

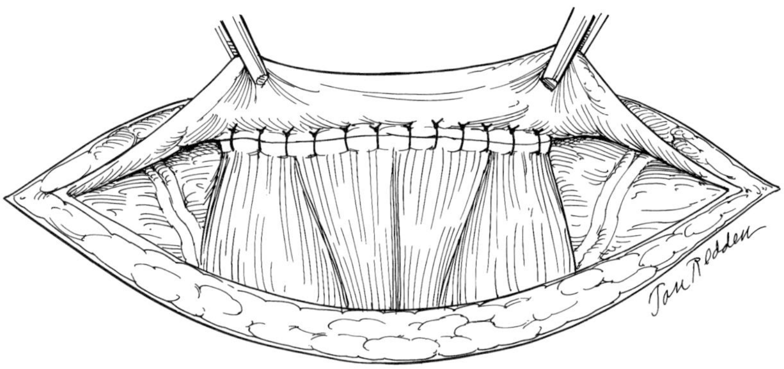

Figure 4–6. Reuniting the rectus tendons to the inferior portion of the rectus sheath. Note the lateral course of the inferior epigastric vessels. (Adapted from Gallup, 1988, with permission.)

cial incision carried well lateral to the borders of the rectus muscles, the inferior epigastric vessels are identified lying on the posterior lateral border of each muscle. With gentle finger dissection, the vessels are separated from their attachments. The vessels are ligated with permanent suture prior to incising the rectus muscles, in order to avoid tearing of the vessels, vessel retraction, and hematoma formation (Fig. 4–7). Worthy of note is that some gynecologic surgeons advocate preserving these vessels, even when the rectus muscles are transected (Parson and Ulfelder, 1968). Blunt dissection is used to separate the overlying rectus muscle from the peritoneum. The muscles are divided using the scalpel or electrocautery.

For better approximation of the recti during closure, the underlying muscle is sutured to the overlying fascia prior to entering the peritoneum (Fig. 4–8). The peritoneum is incised transversely. Closure of the fascia is similar to the technique for other transverse incisions. The muscles do not require approximation with individual sutures. A subfascial drain should be considered if hemostasis is not absolute.

Supraumbilical Incision

This curving incision, about 6 cm above the umbilicus in the midline (Fig. 4–4), is an excellent approach for the pregnant women with a large uterus or an adnexal mass. It can easily be extended caudad and medial to the iliac crests to locate the infundibulopelvic ligament prior to transection, helping to avoid ureteral injury (Gallup et al., 1993). A minimal staging operation for ovarian malignancy

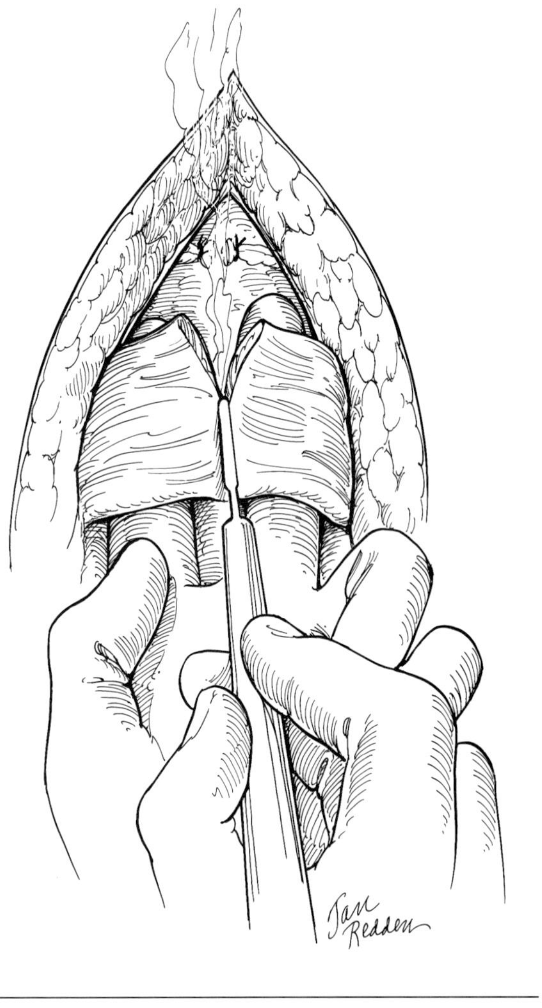

Figure 4–7. For the Maylard incision the rectus muscle is transected using a knife or cautery. The hand of the surgeon is withdrawn as the muscle is cut. The inferior epigastric vessels have been previously isolated, transected, and ligated.

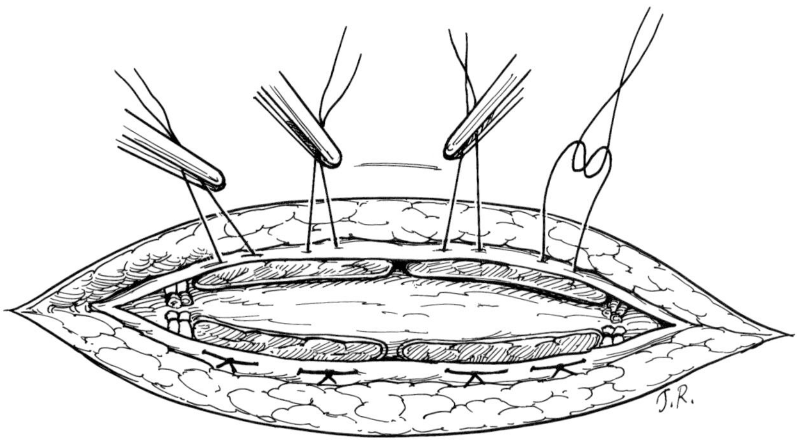

Figure 4–8. Prior to entering the peritoneum, the recti are sutured to the overlying fascia with 2-0 delayed absorbable suture. A *U-suture* is used, and the knots are placed anterior to the fascia. Note the inferior epigastric vessels which have been secured and separated.

can easily be done through this incision, which allows easy access to the omentum and hemidiaphragms.

As described on page 55, the epigastric vessels are posterior to the midportion of the recti in this area and are also richly anastomotic. Isolation is unnecessary and the muscles are transected using electrocautery. The peritoneum is incised transversely and closed separately as for other large transverse incisions. A subfascial drain may be needed.

Vertical Incisions

When exploratory laparotomy is needed and the diagnosis is uncertain, a vertical incision is almost always indicated. For instance, trauma in the pregnant woman should be managed by a vertical incision (see Chap. 35). In pregnant women, the two types of vertical incisions used are the paramedian and the midline.

Paramedian Incision

Proponents of **paramedian** incision claim that it is stronger than the **midline** incision. However, when Guillou and co-workers (1980) compared midline, medial paramedian, and lateral paramedian incisions in a prospective study, they did not identify significant differences in respiratory complications, wound infections, and dehiscence. No incisional hernias developed in patients with lateral paramedian incisions. They also found that the incidence of incisional hernias in patients with midline and medial paramedian incisions was the same. Relative disadvantages of the paramedian incision include greater rates of infection, intraoperative bleeding, and operating time; there also may be nerve damage and atrophy to the rectus muscle. In addition, long paramedian incisions may increase pain with respirations.

Midline Incision

This incision is rapid, easy to perform, and relatively bloodless and may be useful in obstetrical situations described in Table 4–1. In general, the lower midline incision is made from the umbilicus to the symphysis and can be extended around the umbilicus and more cephalad as needed. Because of the naturally occurring diastasis of the recti in pregnancy, there is little need to separate the muscles, thus affording rapid access to the peritoneal cavity.

With midline incisions, dehiscence and hernias are said to be more common, particularly in the area caudad to the arcuate line. Abdominal wound disruption is one of the most serious postoperative problems associated with surgery. **Evisceration** is seen more frequently in general surgical patients, but has a frequency of about 0.5 percent in obstet-

TABLE 4–1. POSSIBLE INDICATIONS FOR MIDLINE INCISIONS

Acute fetal distress
Prolapsed cord
Hypovolemic shock
Prior midline incision
Ovarian tumor highly suspicious for malignancy
Trauma
Bowel obstruction
Suspected perforated viscus
Preexisting midline incisional hernia
Obesity

rics and gynecology patients. It has an associated mortality of 10–35 percent (Alexander and Prudden, 1966; Pratt, 1973; Richards et al., 1983). The choice of incision is only one of several factors associated with evisceration. Wound infection is present in up to half of cases. Obstetric patients who have poorly controlled diabetes or who are receiving systemic corticosteroids are at increased risk. Use of chromic catgut for fascial closure is associated with a higher incidence of dehiscence than other suture materials. Mechanical factors, such as wound hematomas, coughing associated with chronic pulmonary disease, or gastrointestinal problems such as retching, vomiting, or ileus may lead to evisceration. Newer closure techniques can help avoid the problems with hernia and dehiscence, but the cosmetic result is relatively poor.

Many surgeons prefer the layered closure for midline incisions; this closure is unnecessary for most pregnant women. If used, the sutures should be loosely tied. The major cause of wound evisceration is too many sutures placed too closely together, too close to the fascial edge, and tied too tightly (Jurkiewicz and Morales, 1983). At reoperation for evisceration, the sutures and knots are often intact, but the sutures are found to have torn through the fascia. To avoid wound disruptions in high-risk patients, several investigators have advocated a Smead-Jones closure (Gallup, 1984; Morrow and colleagues, 1977; Wallace and associates, 1980). This is a far-far, near-near suturing technique, and only the anterior fascia is included in the near-near bite. A No. 1 nylon or No. 1 polypropylene suture is used. The key to the success of this closure is using wide far-far bites of at least 2–3 cm of tissue (Fig. 4–9). The Smead-Jones closure is time consuming.

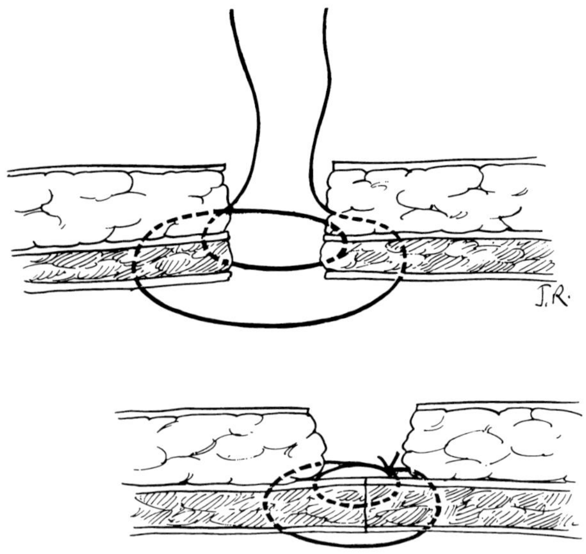

Figure 4–9. The Smead-Jones multilayered double loop suture. **A.** The first stitch is placed lateral and approximately 2–3 cm from the midline and incorporates all layers while the second stitch incorporates 1 cm of the anterior facia. **B.** Cross-sectional view after suture is tied.

Other investigators have advocated a single-layer running mass closure technique as expedient yet safe (Archie and Feldman, 1981; Knight and Griffen, 1983; Shepard and colleagues, 1983). Gallup and colleagues (1989) used this technique in 210 high-risk patients and observed no fascial dehiscences, although one woman later developed an incisional hernia. When these experiences are added to four other studies of patients who had running mass closures, the incidence of fascial dehiscence is only 0.5 percent (Table 4–2). Fagniez and associates (1985) reported that polyglycolic acid was effective when used

TABLE 4–2. FASCIAL DEHISCENCE AFTER CLOSURE WITH RUNNING SUTURES IN MIDLINE INCISIONS

Study	Number	Suture	Dehiscence
Archie and Feldman (1981)	120	No. 1 polypropylene	1
Murray and Blaisdell (1978)	255	No. 1 polyglycolic acid	1
Shepherd et al. (1983)	200	No. 2 polypropylene	0
Knight and Griffen (1983)	419	No. 1 polypropylene	4
Gallup et al. (1989)	210	No. 2 polypropylene	0
Total	1204		6 (0.5%)

in a running manner for midline incisions. Others have reported use of a running looped mono-filament permanent suture with excellent re-sults (Sutton and Morgan, 1992).

In the original study by Gallup and colleagues (1989), the midline incisions were closed with a continuous, No. 2 polypropylene suture. Bites about 1 cm apart were taken and placed 1.5–2 cm from the fascial edge. These bites should include the peritoneum, if easily located, the fascial layers, and the intervening muscle (Fig. 4–10). One suture is started from the cephalad pole, another from the caudad end, and both are tied in the middle. A double-strand of suture should never be tied to a single strand of suture. Sutures should not be pulled too tightly because the major advantage of the mass closure is that tension is equally distributed over a continuous line.

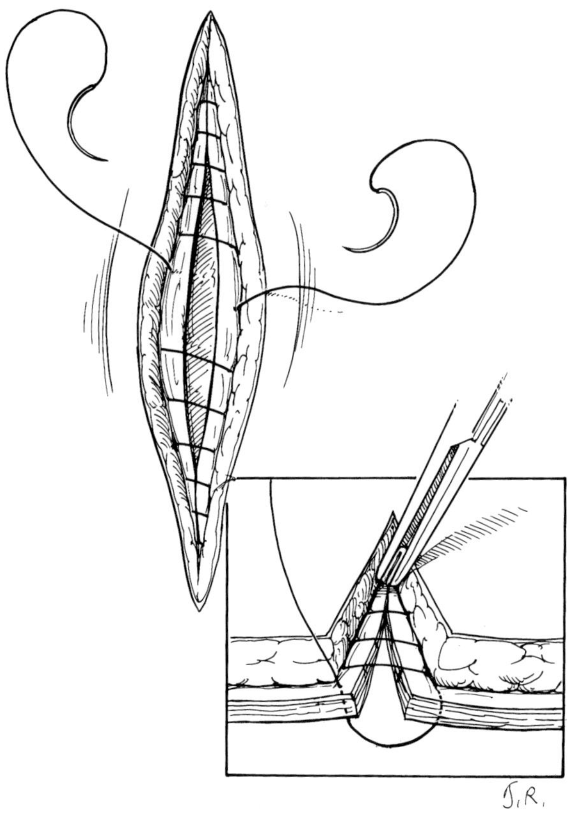

Figure 4–10. Closing the fascia and adjacent areas using a mass closure technique. A large-bore monofilament suture (No. 1 or No. 2) is run from each end and tied in the middle. If polypropylene is used, a hemoclip is placed on the short end. With Maxon the clip is not used. Six throws are placed and all knots are buried.

One problem with the use of large-bore permanent sutures for mass running closure is the occasional late occurring wound sinus formation (Gallup et al., 1989; Knight and Griffen, 1983). The development of delayed absorbable sutures (Maxon and PDS) avoid problems with large knots causing sinus formation. Because of its relatively easier handling and knot security, No. 1 Maxon can be used in a running closure similar to that done with polypropylene (Gallup et al., 1990). Seven throws are used for each knot, and the knots are buried. Of 285 patients with midline incisions who were at high risk for wound disruption, seven developed a superficial wound infection, one developed a ventral hernia, and one had an evisceration on the fourth postoperative day. The latter woman was found to have an intact suture line at reexploration, but the central knot had untied because only four throws had been used per knot.

INCISIONS FOR OBESE PREGNANT WOMEN

Obesity is a recognized high-risk factor for wound infections. Pitkin (1976) reported a 4 percent wound complication rate in nonobese women undergoing abdominal hysterectomy, compared with 30 percent in obese women. Krebs and Helmkamp (1984) reported a wound infection rate of 25 percent in massively obese women in whom a periumbilical transverse incision was used. Because muscle cutting may be needed for this transverse incision, entry time can be lengthy and the resulting incision relatively bloody. If any transverse incision is chosen for obese wom-en, it should be far removed from the anaerobic moist environment of the subpannicular fold.

Morrow and colleagues (1977) suggested modifications of preoperative care, intraoperative techniques, and postoperative care in obese women undergoing gynecologic surgery and observed a relatively low wound infection rate of 13 percent. Gallup (1984) subsequently modified these techniques and compared retrospectively a group of 97 high-risk obese women with a control group in which the modified protocol was not used. The wound infection rate in protocol-operated obese women was only 3 percent compared with 42 percent in controls.

The technique demonstrated in Figure 4–11 is ideal for massively obese pregnant women when incisions in the lower abdomen are necessary. When time permits, preoperative care should include pHisoHex showers and thorough cleansing of the umbilicus. Clip removal of abdominal hair is preferred. Prophylactic antimicrobials are used for the usual obstetric indications (see Chap. 38). The midline incision is made by first retracting the panniculus caudad, below the superior margins of the symphysis, in order to avoid the anaerobic area. The skin incision is a periumbilical incision, which is usually extended around the umbilicus. When a hysterectomy is necessary, a wound protector is used to improve exposure in the pelvis.

Fascia is closed with a Smead-Jones or running mass closure. Subcutaneous sutures are not used. A Jackson-Pratt or Blake drain is placed anterior to the fascia after irrigating with normal saline. This drain is removed in 72 hours, or when the output is less than 50 mL in 24 hours. The skin is closed with a suture stapler, and these staples are left in place for 2 weeks.

There have been no randomized prospective studies regarding the use of subcutaneous sutures versus subcutaneous drains. Of the women who had wound infections in the series reported by Morrow and colleagues (1977), none had subcutaneous drains. A time-honored surgical principle is to eliminate dead space although subcutaneous areas rarely contain adequate supportive tissues for approximation. If sutures are used, a running tech-

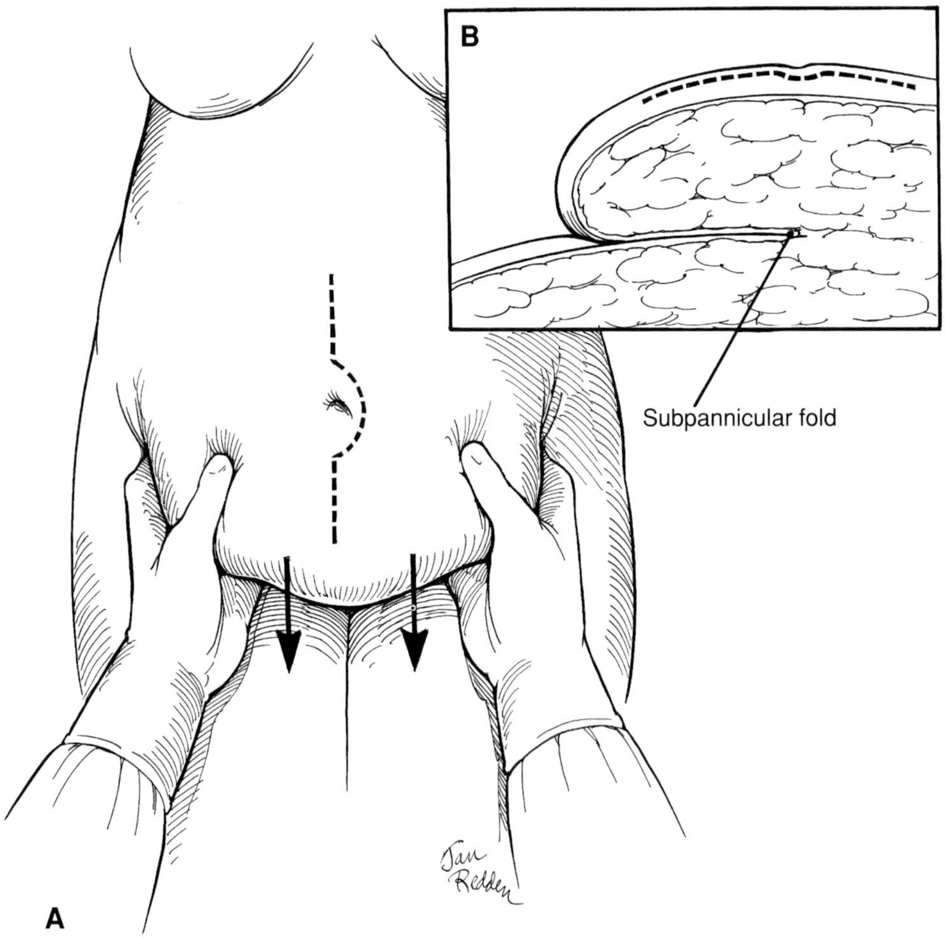

Figure 4–11. A. To perform a periumbilical midline incision in the obese woman, the panniculus is retracted inferiorly so that the incision avoids the most anaerobic environment. **B.** Cross section showing subpannicular fold. An incision in this area is at high risk of infection.

nique using fine, polyglycolic acid suture is performed. The relatively low wound infection rate in obese women in whom this technique was used supports this type of operative management (Gallup and colleagues, 1989, 1990).

DELAYED CLOSURE, SECONDARY CLOSURE

Occasionally clinical situations are encountered when it is best not to perform primary incision closure at the time of cesarean delivery or other celiotomy. These include contaminated wounds such as those with a ruptured appendix, intraabdominal abscess, or injury to unprepared bowel. In these cases, following fascial closure, a bridge consisting of rolls of gauze can be used to support loosely tied, interrupted 3-0 monofilament polypropylene skin sutures (Menendez, 1985). These sutures can be placed about 2 cm apart using a mattress technique. Dressing sponges (4 × 8 in.) are laid in the wound posterior to the sutures and are changed periodically following wound cleansing. In 5–7 days, the dressing gauze is removed, and the previously placed sutures are simply tied to approximate the skin edges. Steri-strips may be used for further support.

If a wound infection develops anterior to the fascia and requires drainage, early secondary closure is preferable to healing by secondary intention (Hermann and associates, 1988; Walters and co-workers, 1990). A study by Dodson and colleagues (1992) has clearly shown that secondary closure can be performed under local anesthesia in a treatment room setting. The infected wound is opened and debrided under local anesthesia. Saline soaked gauzes, with or without hydrogen peroxide, are changed three times a day. Most wounds are ready for closure after 4–5 days of wound care when they appear beefy-red and are free of necrotic tissue. After local anesthesia, No. 1 polypropylene interrupted sutures, placed 3–4 cm from the skin edge, are used to reapproximate the wound and are also reinforced with steri-strips.

SUMMARY

Clinical circumstances often will be the most important determinant of the type of abdominal wall incision made. When speed is of the essence, the midline incision is most advantageous. Excellent visualization of the intraabdominal structures can be obtained with either the midline, the Maylard, or supraumbilical transverse incision. The best cosmetic result is obtained with the Pfannenstiel incision. Transverse incisions result in better healing and greater wound strength than do vertical incisions. In patients at high risk for poor wound healing and dehiscence or evisceration, a Smead-Jones or running mass closure should be considered.

REFERENCES

Alexander HC, Prudden JF. The causes of abdominal wound disruption. Surg Gynecol Obstet 1966; 122:1223.

Archie JP, Feldman RW. Primary wound closure with permanent continuous running monofilament sutures. Surg Gynecol Obstet 1981; 153:721.

Cherney LS. A modified transverse incision for low abdominal operations. Surg Gynecol Obstet 1941; 72:92.

Cruse PJE. Infection surveillance: Identifying the problem in the high-risk patient. South Med J 1977; 70 (Suppl 1):40.

Cruse PJE, Foord R. A five year prospective study of 23,649 surgical wounds. Arch Surg 1973; 107:206.

Daversa B, Landers D. Physiologic advantages of the transverse incision in gynecology. Obstet Gynecol 1961; 17:305.

Dineen P. A critical study of 100 conservative wound infections. Surg Gynecol Obstet 1961; 113:91.

Dodson MK, Magann EF, Meeks GR. A randomized comparison of secondary closure and secondary intention with superficial wound dehiscence. Obstet Gynecol 1992; 80:321.

Fagniez P, Hay JM, Lacaine F, Thomsen C. Abdominal midline incisions closure. A randomized prospective trial of 3135 patients, comparing continuous vs. interrupted polyglycolic acid sutures. Arch Surg 1985; 120:1351.

Farnell MB, Worthington-Self S, Mucha P Jr, Ilstrup DM, McIlrath DC. Closure of abdominal incisions with subcutaneous catheters. Arch Surg 1986; 126:641.

Gallup DG. Modification of celiotomy techniques to decrease morbidity in obese gynecologic patients. Am J Obstet Gynecol 1984; 150:171.

Gallup DG. Opening and closing the abdomen. In: Phelan JP, Clark SL. Cesarean Delivery. New York: Elsevier, 1988.

Gallup DG, Talledo OE, King LA. Primary mass closure of midline incisions with a continuous running monofilament suture in gynecologic patients. Obstet Gynecol 1989; 73:67.

Gallup DG, Nolan TE, Smith RP. Primary mass closure of midline incisions with a continuous polyglyconate monofilament absorbable suture. Obstet Gynecol 1990; 76:872.

Gallup DG, King LA, Messing MJ, Talledo OE. Para-aortic lymph node sampling using an extraperitoneal approach with a supraumbilical transverse "Sunrise" incision. Am J Obstet Gynecol 1993; 169:307.

Greenburg G, Salk RP, Peskin GW. Wound dehiscence. Patho-physiology and prevention. Arch Surg 1979; 114:143.

Guillou PJ, Hall TJ, Donaldson DR, Broughton AC, Brennan TG. Vertical abdominal incisions—a choice? Br J Surg 1980; 67:359.

Helmkamp BF, Krebs HB, Amstey MS. Correct use of surgical drains. Contemp Ob/Gyn 1984; 23:123.

Helmkamp BF. Abdominal wound dehiscence. Am J Obstet Gynecol 1977; 128:803.

Hermann GG, Pagi P, Christofferson I. Early secondary suture versus healing by second intention of incisional abscesses. Surg Gynecol Obstet 1988; 167:16.

Jurkiewicz MJ, Morales L. Wound healing, operative incisions, and skin grafts. In: Harvey JD (ed): Hardy's Textbook of Surgery. Philadelphia: Lippincott, 1983, p. 108.

Knight CD, Griffen FD. Abdominal wound closure with a continuous monofilament polypropylene suture. Arch Surg 1983; 118:1305.

Krebs HB, Helmkamp F. Transverse periumbilical incision in the massively obese patient. Obstet Gynecol 1984; 63:241.

Maylard AE. Direction of abdominal incision. Br Med J 1907; 2:895.

Menendez MA. The contaminated closure. In: O'Leary JP, Woltering EA (eds), Techniques for Surgeons. New York, John Wiley & Sons, 1985, pp 36–37.

Morrow CP, Hernandez WL, Townsend DE, DiSaia PJ. Pelvic celiotomy in the obese patient. Am J Obstet Gynecol 1977; 127:335.

Mowat J, Bonnar J. Abdominal wound dehiscence after cesarean section. Br Med J 1971; 2:256.

Murray DH, Blaisdell FW. Use of synthetic absorbable sutures for abdominal and chest closures. Arch Surg 1978; 113:477.

Parson L, Ulfelder H. Atlas of Pelvic Surgery, 2nd ed. Philadelphia: Saunders, 1968, p. 156.

Pitkin RM. Abdominal hysterectomy in obese women. Surg Gynecol Obstet 1976; 142:532.

Pratt JH. Wound healing—evisceration. Clin Obstet Gynecol 1973; 16:126.

Rees VL, Coller FA. Anatomic and clinical study of the transverse abdominal incision. Arch Surg 1943; 47:136.

Richards PC, Balch CM, Aldrete JS. Abdominal wound closure. Ann Surg 1983; 197:238.

Shepherd JH, Cavanagh D, Riggs D, et al. Abdominal wound closure using a nonabsorbable single-layer technique. Obstet Gynecol 1983; 61:248.

Sutton G, Morgan S. Abdominal wound closure using a running, looped monofilament polybutester suture: Comparison to Smead-Jones closure in historic controls. Obstet Gynecol 1992; 80:650.

Tollefson DG, Russell KP. The transverse incision in pelvic surgery. Am J Obstet Gynecol 1954; 68:410.

Thompson JB, Maclean KF, Collier FA. Role of the transverse abdominal incision and early ambulation in the reduction of postoperative complications. Arch Surg 1949; 59:1267.

Wallace D, Hernandez W, Schlaerth JB, Nalick RN, Morrow CP. Prevention of abdominal wound disruption utilizing the Smead-Jones closure technique. Obstet Gynecol 1980; 56:226.

Walters MD, Dombroski RA, Davidson SA, Mandez PC, Gibbs RS. Reclosure of disrupted abdominal incisions. Obstet Gynecol 1990; 76:597.

CHAPTER 5

Pelvimetry

Pelvimetry, once used widely, now is employed primarily to evaluate the feasibility of vaginal delivery of the fetus in breech presentation. This chapter examines the development of pelvimetry, describes the major techniques now employed, and considers the role that newer techniques might play in expanding indications for its use.

HISTORY

Concern over the bony pelvis and its adequacy to allow any vaginal delivery predates the invention of the x-ray; the concept of the bony pelvis as an obstruction to labor appears in the literature as early as the eighteenth century. As cesarean section became a safe way to bypass pelvic obstruction, earlier determination of surgical necessity received increased emphasis. During the first half of this century, before availability of blood products and antibiotics, by far the safest time to perform a cesarean delivery was before the onset of labor or rupture of membranes. The high morbidity and mortality of operative delivery in the presence of infection highlighted the importance of defining the limits of pelvic dimensions at which abdominal delivery was indicated.

After the invention and refinement of the x-ray, numerous investigators developed techniques intended to describe normal and abnormal pelvic architecture and dimensions. They also attempted to devise algorithms to accurately predict the ease or difficulty of vaginal birth.

DEVELOPMENT OF PELVIMETRY

Modern pelvimetry can be said to have originated in 1939 with the publication of a now classic three-part article by Caldwell, Moloy, and Swenson (1939a, b, c). The authors outlined a standard method of x-ray pelvimetry, stereo pelvioroentgenography, and demonstrated the accuracy and reproducibility of their method. They divided the pelvis into planes and determined average measurements. Their classification, still the most commonly used today, was based on the shape of the anterior and posterior segments of the pelvic inlet (Fig. 5–1). Both pelvic size and shape were integrated with the mechanisms of labor for specific fetal presentations in the hope that this could lead to more intelligent management in the event of arrest of the fetal head (Caldwell and Moloy, 1939a, b, c). Management often included manual and instrumental maneuvers to accomplish delivery.

Caldwell, Moloy, and Swenson's use of stereoscopic views was one attempt to overcome divergent distortion, a common problem encountered with all types of conventional pelvimetric measurement. Divergent distortion is the magnification that results when a point source (x-ray) is at a varying distance to the object imaged and the objects (different pelvic bones, fetal head) are at a varying distance from the film.

Realizing both the importance and difficulty of obtaining accurate measurements, especially of the fetal head, in establishing a fetal head–pelvic diameter ratio, Ball (1936)

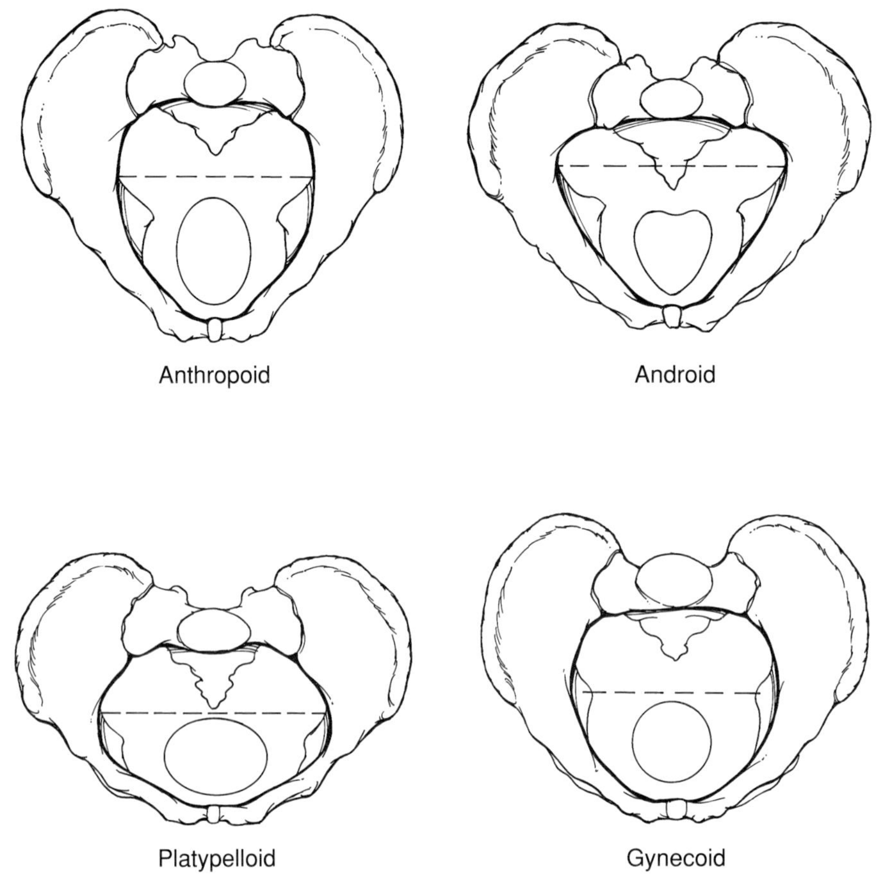

Figure 5–1. The four parent pelvic types as classified by Caldwell et al. (1939a,b,c). Frequencies for pure pelvic types are from Steer (1958). (Adapted from Cunningham and associates, 1993, with permission.)

proposed a technique that compared the fetal cranial volume and the volume capacity of two pelvic planes: the inlet (true conjugate) and the midplane (ischial spines). The fetal cranium was assumed to be spherical and was averaged between the two films (anteroposterior [AP] and lateral views). The distance from bone to film on one film was used to correct for magnification on the other. Critical values for these volumes were later computed and delivery outcomes were predicted from those values (Friedman and Taylor, 1969) (Table 5–1).

Both Thoms (1941) and later Colcher and Sussman (1944) sought to further simplify the technique of pelvimetry. In the Thoms' method (Fig. 5–2), the patient is positioned (AP), the x-ray film shot, a perforated lead ruler positioned at the level of the inlet as measured on

TABLE 5–1. BALL PELVIMETRY AND CRITICAL PELVIC CAPACITIES

	Pelvic Volumes vs Fetal Head Volume		C.S. Rate
	Inlet	*Midplane*	
No disproportion	≥ Fetal head vol.	0 to −150 mL	1%
Borderline	0 to −50 mL	−150 to −200 mL	33%
High disproportion	> −50 mL	> −200 mL	80%

After Friedman and Taylor (1969).

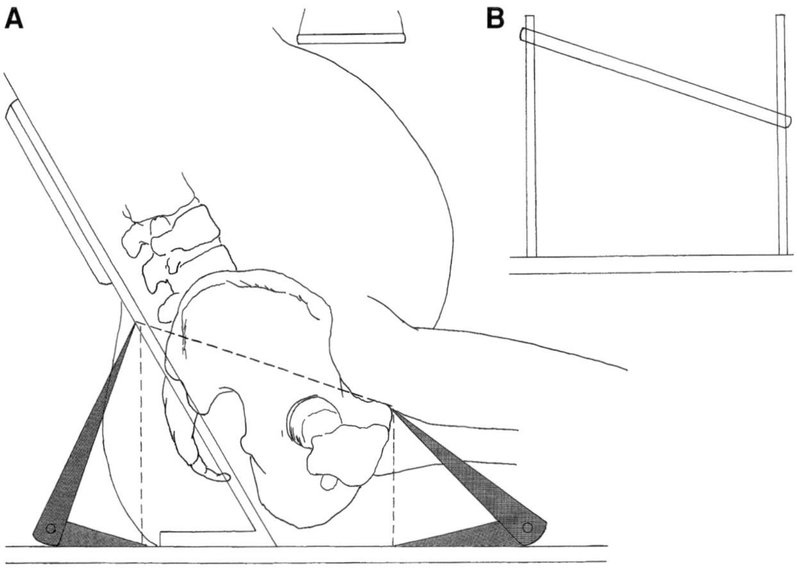

Figure 5–2. Use of centimeter grid markers and patient positioning for AP pelvic x-ray by Thoms' method.

the patient, and a flash exposure made over the same film. On the lateral view, the ruler is placed at the midpelvic level and the process is repeated.

In the Colcher-Sussman method, by careful patient positioning, a single ruler is placed (Figs. 5–3, 5–4) at a point where the transverse diameters of the pelvic inlet, the midplane, and outlet are in the same plane. Although positioning of either patient or scale may result in error, the simplicity of this method led to its wide use; the Colcher-Sussman is employed even today when plain film x-ray pelvimetry is performed.

Both the Thoms and Colcher-Sussman methods emphasized pelvic measurements as criteria for establishing adequacy of the bony pelvis. While the need for cesarean section could not be ascertained with certainty, a table of critical measurements was developed (Hellman and Pritchard, 1971). Values below these levels indicated a contracted pelvis (Table 5–2).

Other yardsticks based on the values obtained by x-ray pelvimetry were created in an attempt to predict the outcome of labor and the likelihood of a difficult forceps or cesarean delivery. Mengert (1948) determined that the area of the inlet and midpelvis assisted his prediction of outcome. A normal (100%) inlet was 145 cm^2 (AP × TV), with the borderline lower limit (85%) being 123.25 cm^2. The midplane values (BI × AP midplane) were 126 cm^2 (100%) and 106 cm^2 (85%), respectively. Kaltneider (1951, 1952) used Mengert's areas in a large series of patients to review the expected levels of difficulty, defined as cesarean section after a trial of labor or difficult forceps with intracranial injury to the fetus. Using percentages of "normal" as defined by Mengert, the midplane was more important as a cause of disproportion (Fig. 5–5). Importantly, while 100 percent of normal in both pelvic planes was highly predictive of vaginal delivery (97%), still the overwhelming majority of infants delivered vaginally even when pelvic dimensions were at the 80–85 percent levels.

Other techniques that have been employed to predict pelvic contraction include:

1. **Mengert's Drawings** (1946). Graphic drawings from pelvimetry measurements that correspond to Caldwell and Moloy's planes. An overlay of a small, medium, and large head is used to predict passage.
2. **Allen's Areas** (1947). Inlet and midplane are considered to be an ellipse and areas are calculated using the ellipse formula.
3. **Moir's Method** (1946, 1947). Biparietal diameter is measured antenatally and correlated with various diameters of the inlet and midplane using a graph.

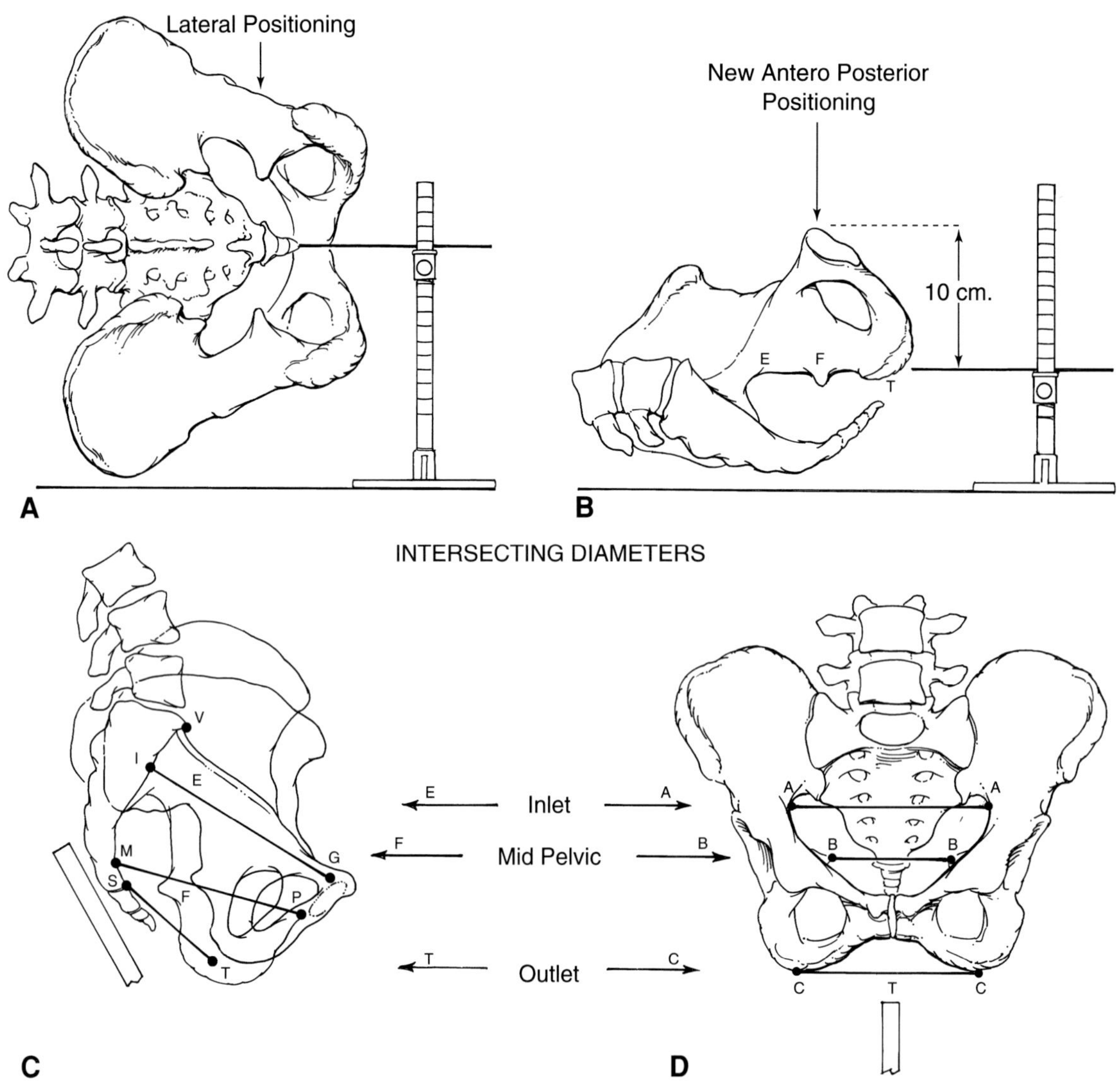

Figure 5–3. **A** and **B.** Diagrams showing lateral and anteroposterior positions with ruler. **C** and **D.** Diagrams of the three pelvic levels with intersecting diameters. Inlet: Actual anteroposterior diameter of inlet line G-I crosses through inlet transverse diameter A-A′. Midpelvis: Anteroposterior diameter P-M crosses transverse diameter B-B′. Outlet: Anteroposterior diameter of outlet T-S bisects midpoint of transverse diameter line C-C′. (Adapted from Colcher and Sussman, 1944, with permission.)

TABLE 5–2. MEASUREMENTS INDICATING A CONTRACTED PELVIS

	Diameters (cm)		
Planes	*Anterior Posterior*	*Transverse*	*Posterior Sagittal*
Inlet	10.0	12.0	—
Midplane	11.5	9.5	4.0
Outlet	11.5	10.0	7.5

From Helman and Pritchard, 1971, with permission.

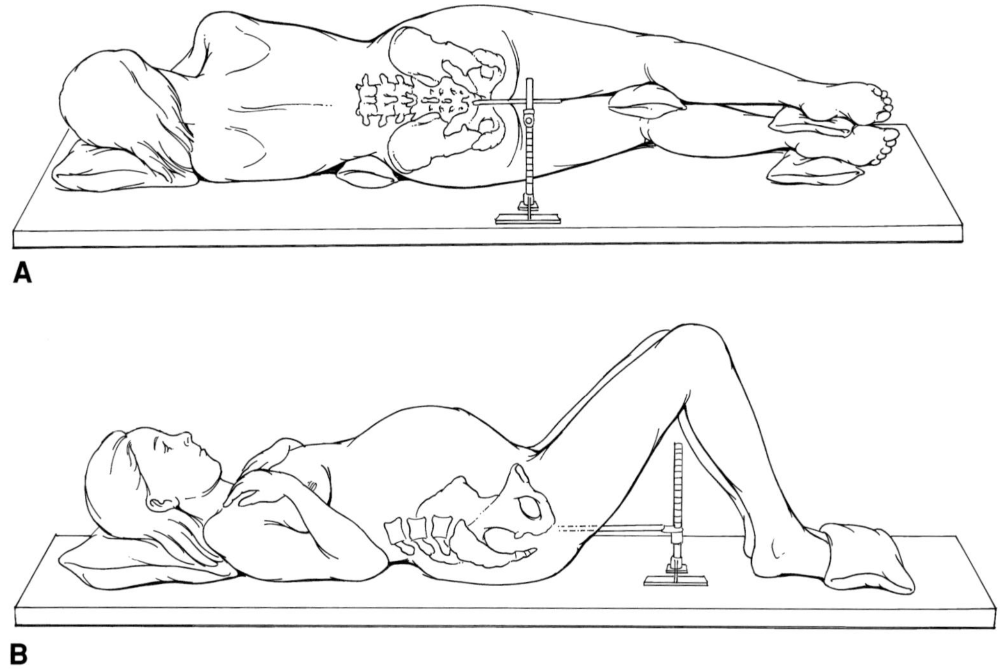

Figure 5–4. A. Lateral positioning. Patient on side; knee and thighs semiflexed. Ruler is at level of midsacral spine; the central ray is directed through the greater trochanter of the femur at any distance. **B.** Anteroposterior positioning. Patient flat on back; knees and thighs semiflexed and slightly separated. Ruler is placed at the level of the tuberosities of the ischium. Central ray is directed above the symphysis at any distance. (Adapted from Colcher and Sussman, 1944, with permission.)

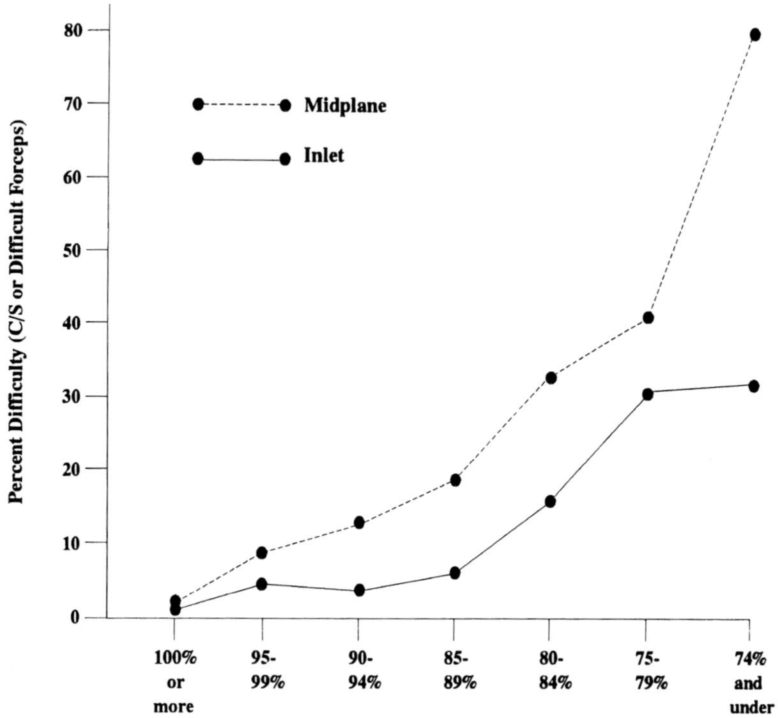

Figure 5–5. Kaltneider's data from 1169 pelvimetries (1951–52) plotted vs. percent difficult deliveries (cesareans and forceps with fetal injury). Note that even below the borderline limits (85%) of pelvic capacity (Mengert, 1948) most patients delivered normally. The midplane, however, did seem to be the more important predictor. (Adapted from Kaltneider, 1951, 1952, with permission.)

CHALLENGES TO THE USE OF PELVIMETRY

By the 1950s when the use of x-ray pelvimetry was at its peak, advances in medicine already marked its decline. In particular, the availability of effective antibiotics and safe blood products had transformed cesarean section into a much safer and acceptable procedure. Consequently, the role of x-ray pelvimetry in the conduct of labor was reappraised.

As a by-product of his assessment of pelvic inlet and midplane contracture, Kaltneider (1951, 1952) concluded that establishing exact criteria for a contracted pelvis could not be based on purely analytic scientific data. This was especially true with the fetus in vertex presentation, where considerable molding of the fetal head might allow it to conform to and pass through even a significantly contracted pelvis. Kaltneider accordingly recommended that a trial of labor was indicated in all patients who had a suspect pelvis or vertex presentation and who had not had prior cesarean sections. He did recommend x-ray pelvimetry for breech presentations because of insufficient time for molding of the fetal head to occur. He also suggested that lateral pelvimetry might be useful in cases where caput and molding were confusing the interpretation of station.

In a classic article, Steer (1958) reviewed x-ray pelvimetry and the outcome of labor in a large series of patients. He emphasized three distinct aspects to the passage of the baby through the birth canal:

1. The relation of the size and shape of the bony pelvis to the size and position of the baby itself;
2. The efficacy of uterine activity; and
3. The moldability of the fetal head.

Steer identified the failure to measure the baby as the greatest error in pelvimetry interpretation, and lamented the inability of x-ray to evaluate labor efficacy. Important observations from this study further limited the indications for pelvimetry:

1. Because x-rays alone would give an accurate prognosis only in the presence of gross pelvic distortion or possibly when the difference at the inlet (circle fitting inlet minus circle fitting head) was less than 1.0 cm, all other women should be given a trial of labor.
2. Because the probability of arrest of labor was only 49 percent when the biparietal diameter was larger than the interspinous diameter, clinical suspicion of this disparity was not a strong indication for pelvimetry, and even when this disparity was found it was not an indication for cesarean delivery.
3. The absence of fetopelvic disproportion allowed a long trial of labor and, if necessary, the use of drugs to stimulate labor. Succinctly stated, except for a grossly distorted or deformed pelvis, disproportion would not be proven by pelvimetry.

Also contributing to the decline of x-ray pelvimetry were retrospective studies suggesting an increase in childhood malignancy rates from in-utero x-ray exposure. Stewart and associates (1956, 1958) reported an association between irradiation in utero and a greater risk of childhood leukemia and other malignancy. With this potential radiation risk as a backdrop, Hannah (1965) reported that at least 95 percent of all x-ray pelvimetry was not helpful. Moreover, he pointed out that most fetopelvic disproportion was relative and could be overcome by careful administration of oxytocin to correct hypotonic uterine inertia. Conceptually the decision to perform a cesarean section should be based on cessation of progress in labor despite adequate uterine contractile and/or maternal expulsive efforts, but not on pelvimetry. Kelly and associates (1975) reiterated this recommendation, noting that normal pelvimetry gave little confidence that a cesarean would not be necessary. Additionally, the duration of labor in those women needing a cesarean delivery was not altered by pelvimetry (Fig. 5–6).

As the electronic fetal monitoring era began and active management of labor with amniotomy and oxytocin was established, Joyce and associates (1975) concluded that pelvimetry was warranted only in breech presentation. Jagani and associates (1981) reported that pelvimetry did not influence vaginal or cesarean delivery rates among women who received oxytocin, and again noted that 95 percent of pelvimetries were unnecessary. They proposed that an accurate estimate of fetal weight by ultrasound was more important.

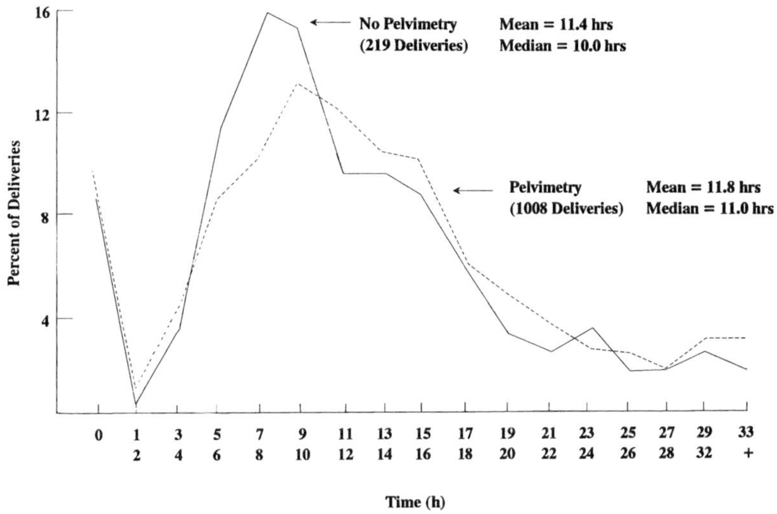

Figure 5–6. Demonstration of lack of difference in lengths of labor experienced by patients managed with and without the use of pelvimetry, who ultimately had a cesarean delivery for "cephalopelvic disproportion" (Kelly and associates, 1975, with permission.)

Finally, in two prospective studies, Laube (1981) and Parsons (1985) and their colleagues showed that pelvimetry did not alter management, that clinical judgment was usually more accurate than pelvimetry, and that in fact the cesarean rate increased in borderline cases when pelvimetry was performed. By the end of the 1980s, the list of indications for pelvimetry (Table 5–3) was small; the only compelling indication was anticipated vaginal delivery of the fetus in breech presentation.

PELVIMETRY FOR SELECTED VAGINAL BREECH DELIVERY

Vaginal delivery was preferred for most breech fetuses until the late 1950s. Routine cesarean delivery to reduce excessive perinatal morbidity and mortality was first suggested by Hall and Kohl (1956). As others (Morgan and Kane, 1964) reported more than a fivefold increase in the perinatal morbidity rate (PNMR) for breech versus cephalic delivery, the cesarean delivery rate for breeches increased from below 5 percent to over 90 percent.

TABLE 5–3. INDICATIONS FOR PELVIMETRY

1. Breech presentation when vaginal delivery anticipated:
   - Frank or complete breech
   - Flexed or military head
   - EFW approximately 2000–3800 g
   - Noncephalic second twin >2500 g
2. Previous injury or disease resulting in contracted or deformed pelvis
3. Use in predicting CPD in fetuses >4500 g or success rates in VBAC trials (fetal-pelvic index)

Todd and Steer (1963) reviewed the results of 364 pelvimetry studies among 1,006 breech deliveries. On the one hand, the authors noted the hazards of breech delivery: In the 52 women with a contracted pelvic inlet who delivered vaginally, the perinatal mortality rate was 6 percent. In comparison, 85 percent of women with an adequate pelvic inlet delivered vaginally with a perinatal mortality rate of 0.5 percent. Beischer (1966) also advised against a trial of labor in breech presentation if significant pelvic contraction existed because neither abnormal uterine activity nor failure to progress in labor was a reliable indicator of cephalopelvic disproportion. In women with a contracted pelvis who delivered vaginally, the perinatal mortality rate was 12 percent (4/32). The high perinatal mortality resulted from the inability of the pelvis to accommodate the unmolded fetal head—not tested until delivery and heralded by entrapment of the fetal head and a traumatic delivery. A strong correlation between the obstetric conjugate and pelvic capacity was shown by Joyce and associates (1975), who additionally noted that larger pelvic diameters were needed for any given size breech delivery when compared to cephalic presentations. He emphasized that fetal size needed to be taken into account with more precise measurements of the fetus in order to have safe vaginal breech delivery protocols.

Protocols for Selected Breech Delivery

In theory, cesarean section could lead to a corrected perinatal mortality rate of 0 in breech presentations. Universal abdominal delivery is not, however, without a price in terms of maternal morbidity and mortality. Moreover, fetal and perinatal outcome and morbidity in the breech presentation is not related solely to the method of delivery, that is, vaginal versus cesarean section. For example, it is well-known that the incidence of cerebral palsy is greater in fetuses that present as a breech regardless of whether delivery is abdominal or vaginal. Clearly many breeches can be delivered vaginally with optimal outcome for both mother and infant; the question is, "Which ones?"

By 1965, Hall and colleagues had recommended cesarean delivery in the following circumstances: borderline or contracted pelvis, poor obstetric history, elderly primigravida, and with uterine dysfunction or prolonged rupture of membranes. In vaginal breech delivery, the need for both reliable estimated fetal weight and pelvimetric measurements was again underscored in the early 1970s. Russell and Richards (1971), however, found no difference in pelvic measurements between women with difficult and easy breech births, and Kauppila (1975) reported that the size of the maternal pelvis alone did not correlate with the incidence of difficult breech deliveries.

Many authors have explored selected vaginal breech delivery and reported excellent outcomes (Benson, 1972; Collea, 1978, 1980; Gimovsky, 1983; Watson, 1984; Kopelman, 1986; Christian 1990; and their colleagues). Table 5–4 summarizes the pelvimetric and fetal weight criteria used by these investigators. Of note, these protocols address only the normal-sized term or near-term breech. Main and colleagues (1983) emphasized that premature infants weighing less than 1500 g had better outcomes when delivered by cesarean section. Experience also has shown that the excessively large breech is more likely to sustain significant birth trauma than is the normal-sized fetus.

Benson (1972) and Watson (1984) and their colleagues believed that a large posterior sagittal diameter indicated additional room in the posterior pelvis, which could compensate for a smaller interspinous measurement. They used a combination of interspinous and poste-

TABLE 5–4. BREECH PELVIMETRY PROTOCOLS

	Series (Type)			
	Benson (1972)[a] Watson (1984) (X-ray)	*Collea (1980) (X-ray)*	*Gimovsky (1983)[c] (X-ray)*	*Kopelman (1986) Christian (1990) (CT)*
EFW (g)	> 2500[b] –(3630)	2500–3800	2000–4000	2000–4000
AP inlet (cm)	≥ 10 cm[b] (< 9.5)	≥ 10.5	≥ 11.0	≥ 10.0
Inlet Mengert (%)	≥ 90%	—	—	—
Transverse inlet	—	≥ 11.5	≥ 12.0	≥ 11.5
Interspinous (T.V. Mid) (cm)	≥ 9.5 cm[b] (< 9.0)	≥ 10.0	≥ 10.0	≥ 9.5
AP midplane (cm)	—	≥ 11.5	—	—
Posterior sagittal (cm)	—	—	—	≥ 4.0
Interspinous plus post sagit (cm)	> 13.5 cm (<13)	—	—	—

[a]Primagravida breeches only
[b]Pelvis categorized as adequate, borderline or contracted ( ) with > 8 lb = oversize infant = no oxytocin with any borderline measurement
[c]Non-frank breeches

rior sagittal diameters of the midplane to define midplane contracture. They also defined a borderline group in which oxytocin should not be given and the oversized fetus, defined by them as greater than 8 lb, was excluded from consideration for vaginal birth. The computed tomogram (CT) protocols of Kopelman (1986) and Christian (1990) and their associates defined absolute lower limits for the interspinous and posterior sagittal dimensions. The University of Southern California protocols (Collea, 1978, 1980; Gimovsky, 1983, and their colleagues) used traditional AP and transverse measurements obtained with the standard Colcher-Sussman technique. Capeless and Mann (1985) used Ball pelvimetry and gave a trial of a vaginal delivery if head volume was less than both the inlet and midplane volumes and no other anomalies of the bony pelvis were noted.

Reasons for exclusion from a trial of labor based on pelvimetry films are outlined in Table 5–5. It is assumed that the fetus meets the weight criteria for inclusion as estimated either clinically or by ultrasound evaluation. The variance in the number of women otherwise considered candidates for vaginal birth but excluded for an extended fetal head may be explained by subjective interpretation of head extension. The most infrequent exclusion criteria was the interspinous distance.

The success of the vaginal delivery protocols is reviewed in Table 5–6. The wide variance in overall cesarean delivery rates depends upon the restrictiveness of the protocol in terms of pelvimetric measurements, estimated fetal weight, and other restrictions. Once the patient has been determined to be a candidate for a trial of labor, the success of vaginal delivery is fairly uniform (76–85%). The exceptions are in studies by Capeless and Mann (1985) in which no oxytocin was used and by Gimovsky and colleagues (1983) which included non-frank breeches. Importantly, even when the most liberal or least restrictive pelvimetric criteria were used, the neonatal outcome was excellent with careful obstetric management.

Method of CT-Pelvimetry

While protocols for selected vaginal delivery of the breech resulted in lower cesarean section rates and maternal morbidity, the potential morbidity from the radiation dose to mother and fetus remained an important concern even in the 1980s. Because obstetric patients often present during "off hours," the quality of x-ray pelvimetry was at times less than optimal. In addition, because pelvimetry had become an infrequently performed procedure, the need to repeat the study would increase the radiation dose to the fetus from the normal 1.1 rads with plain film to nearly 4 rads. In 1982, Federle and colleagues described a technique using digital radiographs obtained with a CT scanner. The technique was easy to perform, required no corrections for magnification, and delivered only 3 percent of the standard dose of radiation. Gimovsky and colleagues (1985) used both laboring patients

TABLE 5–5. REASONS FOR EXCLUSION FROM TRIAL OF LABOR IN BREECH PRESENTATION USING PELVIMETRY

	Series (Type)					
	Christian (1990) (CT)		*Watson (1984) (X-ray)*		*Collea (1980) (X-ray)*	
No. with pelvimetry	122		111		112	
Inadequate measurement	37	(30.3%)	20	(18%)	52	(46.4%)
Extended fetal head	20	(16.3%)	5	(4.5%)	excluded prior	
Transverse inlet	8	(6.6%)	—		3	(2.7%)
AP inlet	—		0		0	
Interspinous	4	(3.3%)	5	(4.5%)	21	(18.8%)
AP midplane	—		—		7	(6.3%)
Posterior sagittal midplane	5	(4.1%)	3	(2.7%)	—	
Multiple factors	—		7	(6.3%)	21	(18.8%)

TABLE 5–6. BREECH VAGINAL DELIVERY EXPERIENCE USING PELVIMETRY PROTOCOLS

	Series						
	Benson (1972)	*Collea (1978)*	*Gimovsky (1983)*	*Watson (1984)*	*Capeless (1985)*	*Kopelman (1986)*	*Christian (1990)*
No. of patients	107	122	70 TOL	151	107	32	122
Initial C/S	3.7%	Randomized (5 elective) 71.3%	Randomized	39.7%	20%	46.9%	30.3%
Type breech	All	Frank	Non-frank	Frank	Frank/ complete	Term breech	Frank
Oxytocin use	Yes	Yes	Yes	Yes	Yes	Yes	Yes
Overall C/S	21.6%	75.5%	56%[a]	36%	52%	56.2%	43.4%
Vag del in labored group	84.4%	85.7%	44%[a]	76%	59%	82.4%	81.2%
Perinatal deaths[b]	0	0	1	0	0	0	0

[a] TOL group
[b] Corrected (multiple congenital anomalies)

TABLE 5–7. CT VS. CONVENTIONAL X-RAY PELVIMETRY

	CT	X-ray
Expense	Same	
Radiation	60–82 millirad	900 ± 100 millirad
Accuracy	+1–2%	Consistently larger
Technical difficulty	Easier (read directly with electronic cursor/can remeasure easily)	Harder (measurements estimated using rulers/often extra exposures needed)
Outcome predictability	Good	Good

and a model of the pelvis to compare CT with standard x-ray pelvimetry (Table 5–7). The results not only suggested that CT was more accurate than conventional x-ray pelvimetry, but that conventional techniques yielded consistently larger measurements than those obtained by CT.

Subsequent studies of CT pelvimetry to prospectively evaluate selected vaginal breech deliveries (Kopelman, 1986; Christian, 1990; and their associates) defined CT as the current benchmark for pelvimetry. The technique is as follows:

1. Ultrasound is used to confirm a living fetus with a normal anatomic survey in frank or complete breech position with a flexed head. Ideal estimated fetal weight is between 2000 and 4000 g. If the fetal head is extended, it should be determined that it can be placed into flexion by transabdominal manipulations.
2. The patient is maintained in the dorsal supine position and centered in the gantry.
3. The anteroposterior digital radiograph (22 mrad) serves as a fetogram and allows clear visualization of the attitude of the fetal head and position of the limbs (Fig. 5–7). The transverse diameter of the pelvic inlet is measured from this film and the level of the foveae capitalis is obtained to be used to determine the level of the axial section.
4. The lateral digital radiograph (22 mrad) is used to measure the anteroposterior diameter of the pelvic inlet (Fig. 5–8) and the posterior sagittal diameter of the midplane (Fig. 5–9). The lateral view permits visualization of the sacral contour and a measurement of the A-P of the midplane if desired.
5. The axial section (38 mrad) at the level of the fovea capitalis is employed to accurately measure the bispinous diameter (Fig. 5–10).
6. Measurements are evaluated. If a question arises, electronic calipers can be repositioned and measurements recalculated without additional exposures. (For measurement criteria see Table 5–4).

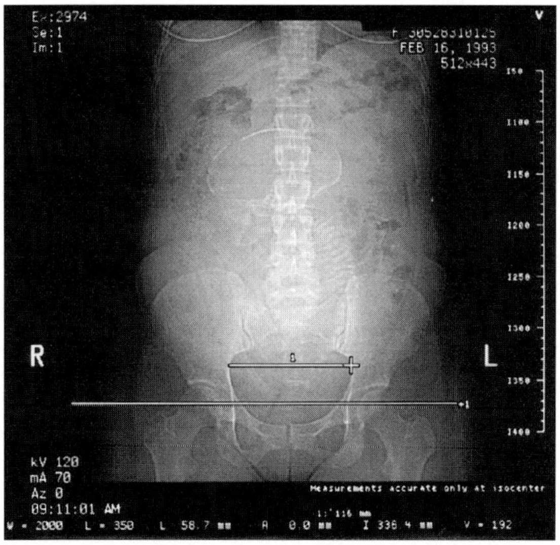

Figure 5–7. Anteroposterior digital radiograph used to obtain fetogram (Frank Breech, head military), transverse diameter of the inlet, and level (foveae) for the axial section.

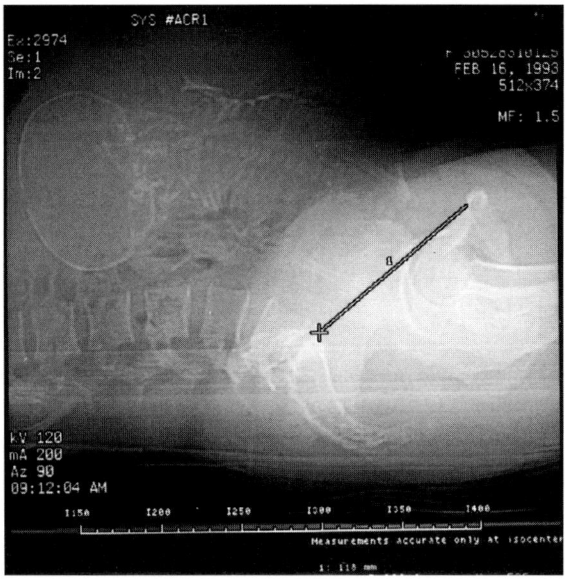

Figure 5–8. Lateral digital radiograph demonstrating the anteroposterior diameter of the pelvic inlet.

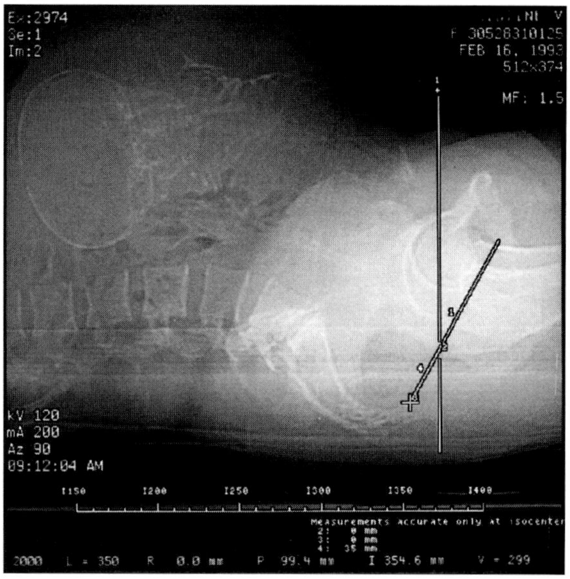

Figure 5–9. Lateral digital radiograph demonstrating measurement of the posterior sagittal diameter.

In general, CT pelvimetry is easier to perform, read, and interpret than conventional pelvimetry. CT pelvimetry can be performed in about 10 minutes and the total fetal radiation dose is approximately 82 mrad. Occasionally, if positioning of the patient results in the foveae capitalis not being on the same plane with each other, an error in measurement may result. Aronson and Kier (1991) have questioned the use of the fovea as a landmark for measurement of the ischial spines. They found no cases in which the spines were above the foveae whereas 15 of 25 (65%) pregnant women had the spines below the foveae. This may result in up to a 1-cm overestimation of the interspinous distance. The ischial spines can often be found on the lateral or AP digital radiograph and the correct level for the axial section determined. Alternatively, an extra axial scan can be performed; otherwise the single axial section should always be obtained slightly below the foveae. Thus far this potential error of measurement has had no clinically adverse consequences in any published series (Kopelman, 1986; Christian, 1990; and their associates).

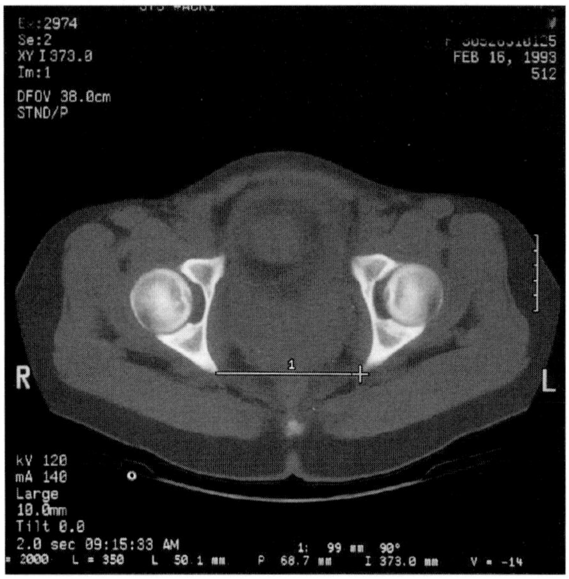

Figure 5–10. Axial section at level of foveae capitalis demonstrating the bispinous diameter.

Use of Fetal and Pelvic Index Measurements for Vertex Presentations

Mengert (1948) described five components of cephalopelvic disproportion: (1) size and shape of the bony pelvis, (2) size of the fetal head, (3) force exerted by the uterus, (4) moldability of the fetal head, and (5) fetal presentation and position.

In 1948 only the first of these five components could be measured accurately. However, with the introduction of intrauterine pressure monitoring and bedside ultrasonography in the 1970s and 1980s, components 2, 3, and 5 could be determined. Steer (1958) previously provided information on fetal head moldability, especially as pertains to the BPD and the interspinous diameter. It was hypothesized that with accurate knowledge of Mengert's other four components, adjustments could be calculated that would minimize the impact of moldability. The cephalopelvic index and fetal-pelvic index both represent such an effort.

Cephalopelvic Index

Yamazaki and Uchida (1983) proposed a cephalopelvic index (CPI) using 10 different x-ray pelvimetric measurements of the pelvis and fetal head. The measurements dealt with the inlet and pelvic aperture angles using elaborate mathematical modeling. The low end of the CPI (< 69) was 100 percent predictive of vaginal delivery and the high end (> 110) correctly predicted cesarean delivery in all cases. A CPI of > 95 was predictive of a cesarean delivery in 92 percent (277/300) of cases.

Fetal-Pelvic Index

Beginning in 1986, Morgan and Thurnau and their co-workers developed the concept of the fetal-pelvic index (FPI) (Morgan, 1986; Morgan, 1988; Thurnau, 1988; Thurnau, 1991; Morgan, 1992; and their colleagues). This index utilized real-time ultrasound measurements of head circumference (HC) and abdominal circumference (AC) in combination with Colcher-Sussman x-ray pelvimetry. The method for calculation of the FPI is presented in Table 5–8. The simplicity of this index is in the methods used and the ease of interpretation: a positive number equals disproportion (the fetus is larger than the pelvis); a negative number means that there is no disproportion (the fetus is smaller than the pelvis). Fetal measurements that show the best correlation with size and weight, the HC and AC, are used along with determination of both important pelvic planes, the inlet and midplane. The accurate interpretation of the data and high predictive ability (Table 5–9) depend upon the patient's being in active labor as defined by a cervical dilatation of ≥ 5 cm.

Within the limitations noted, the fetal-pelvic index provides valuable information. First, it is highly predictive of delivery route in a number of pregnancies that are at high risk for fetopelvic disproportion. Second, a high percentage of false negative values have been associated with persistent occiput posterior presentations. Third, vaginal delivery is highly likely in the presence of a negative index value and absence of fetal malposition. Fourth, the presence or absence of fetal abdominal-pelvic disproportion is the most important single variable, especially in the macrosomic fetus. Fifth, all shoulder dystocias occurred in vaginal deliveries with a positive value for the fetal-pelvic index.

While the FPI looks promising in various groups of high-risk patients, there are still a number of concerns that must be addressed before the FPI can be applied generally. First is the radiation exposure risk. Even if the risk is dismissed as suspect, the method would still be more acceptable if CT or MRI replaced conventional x-ray pelvimetry. Second, CT or MRI methods have not been validated for the index

TABLE 5–8. CALCULATION OF FETAL-PELVIC INDEX

Ultrasound Measurements (outer to outer)
TD_h Transverse-Diameter of head
APD_h Anterior-Posterior Diameter of head (OFD)
APD_a Anterior-Posterior Diameter of abdomen
TD_a Transverse-Diameter of abdomen
Calculate:

(HC) Head Circumference = $(TD_h + APD_h) \times 1.57$
(AC) Abdomen Circumference = $(APD_a + TD_a) \times 1.57$

Pelvimetry Measurements (Colcher-Sussman Technique)

Inlet:	Transverse (TD_I)	
	Anteroposterior (AP_I)	
Midplane:	Transverse (TD_m)	
	Anteroposterior (AP_m)	

Calculate:

Inlet Circumference (IC) = $(TD_I + AD_I) \times 1.57$
Midplane Circumference (MC) = $(TD_m + APD_m) \times 1.57$

Index Calculation
HC – IC =
HC – MC =
AC – IC =
AC – MC =
Add sum of 2 most positive numbers:

_____ + _____ = _____

Interpretation
positive number = total pelvic disproportion
negative number = no fetal-pelvic disproportion

TABLE 5–9. THE USE OF MORGAN AND THURNAU'S FETAL-PELVIC INDEX

	Initial Study		> 4000 g		Labor Induction		Augmentation		VBAC		Nulliparas	
	1986	$N = 75$	*1988*	$N = 34$	1988	$N = 49$	1988	$N = 46$	1988	$N = 65$	1992	$N = 137$
Delivery outcome: FPI	+	–	+	–	+	–	+	–	+	–	+	–
Operative[a]			17	1	12	2	17	7			55	18
Cesarean	23	4	12	1	10	2	14	5	13	5	50	15
Vaginal			5	0	2	0	3	2			5	3
SVD	4	44	1	15	0	35	1	21	0	47	2	0
Shoulder dystocia	1		3	0	2	0	1	0			2	0
Statistical analysis:												
Sensitivity %[b]	85		94		86		71		72		75	
Specitivity %	92		94		100		95		100		97	
Overall predictability %	89		94		96		83		92		85	
p value	<0.001		<0.001		<0.001		<0.001		<0.00001			

Note: All results assume an adequate trial of labor (≥ 5 cm over 2 hr with 3 contractions in 10 min, > 60 sec, > 40 mm Hg).
[a]Operative delivery defined as a cesarean section, midplane vaginal delivery (forceps or vacuum extractor), or a maneuver to reduce shoulder dystocia.
[b]Operative vs. spontaneous vaginal deliveries.

computations, and validation would be required prior to clinical implementation.

At present the best application for the fetal-pelvic index might be in vaginal birth after cesarean delivery (VBAC) situations in which a high likelihood of success is important to the patient and obstetrician. Another potential application is the macrosomic fetus (> 4500 g), where the likelihood of success of achieving vaginal delivery and the risk of shoulder dystocia are both important issues. Pelvimetry could be performed after any primary cesarean section for cephalopelvic disproportion and used to calculate the FPI. The data would then be available in any subsequent pregnancy without any radiation exposure to the fetus.

Abitbol and colleagues (1991) reported a simpler Cephalopelvic Disproportion Index in which the smallest diameters of the inlet and/or midplane are compared with the biparietal diameter (BPD) obtained on ultrasound. Vaginal delivery is "impossible" if the smallest bony diameter minus the BPD is less than 9 mm. While this index is specific (100%), it lacks sensitivity (51%) and does not indicate if a vaginal delivery is possible with a high index. The primary value of this index, like many of its predecessors, is in cases of obvious disproportion. If prior maternal disease or a clinically contracted pelvis indicates pelvimetry (Table 5–3), and cesarean delivery prior to labor is under consideration, the use of the FPI or CPI may be considered.

Magnetic Resonance Imaging Pelvimetry

The two major reasons for not obtaining pelvimetry are its lack of value in the decision-making process and the fact that it delivers ionizing radiation to the fetus. If further research verifies the value of the FPI (Morgan and associates, 1986) or some modification thereof, pelvimetry may be seen as an aid to decision making. With MRI, which uses no ionizing radiation, high-power magnets temporarily alter the state of the hydrogen proton, which spins from low to high energy (nuclear magnetic moments). Using a resonant radiofrequency pulse, which is dependent on the strength of the magnet, the system is perturbed, moving macroscopic magnetic moments within the sample, which are measurable and form the MR spectrum or image (Mattison and associates, 1988). To date there have been no reports indicating that exposure to the various fields used in clinical MR scanners is harmful to the fetus.

Stark and associates (1985) reported that MRI pelvimetry not only was accurate, but provided good images of soft tissue as well as bony structures. In fact, MRI has several advantages over both conventional and CT pelvimetry. Because tissue contrast is high and landmarks are easily recognized, MRI pelvimetry is highly accurate even in obese patients (Wright and associates, 1992a, b). In addition, patient position is not critical with MRI pelvimetry. The scanner can obtain information in axial, sagittal, and coronal planes, and any scan plane can be transformed into an oblique view if the patient is not straight. MRI provides high-quality images of both fetal tissue and maternal pelvic soft tissue; the latter, a potential source for dystocia, can also be evaluated (Table 5–10). The placenta also can be localized precisely by MRI.

The disadvantages of MRI are expense, equipment availability, and the time required for the examination. Cost, originally several times that of CT, should decrease as more machines come on line and as techniques to shorten exam time are devised. Wright and associates (1992a, b) have described a technique of MR pelvimetry that uses T1-weighted gradient echo sequences. This technique enables the operator to perform a full pelvimetry examination in fewer than 5 minutes of scanning time. Urhahn and colleagues (1991) have described a snapshot flash MRI technique in 20 pregnant women, which results in an acquisition time for pelvimetry of only a few seconds. This technique avoids motion

TABLE 5-10. PELVIMETRY USING MAGNETIC RESONANCE IMAGING

Advantages:	1. No ionizing radiation
	2. Accurate measurements
	3. Fetal imaging
	4. Soft tissue evaluation
Disadvantages:	1. Expensive
	2. Limited equipment availability
	3. Time required for imaging studies
Contraindications:	1. Metallic heart valve or surgical clips/other metal within patient
	2. Claustrophobia

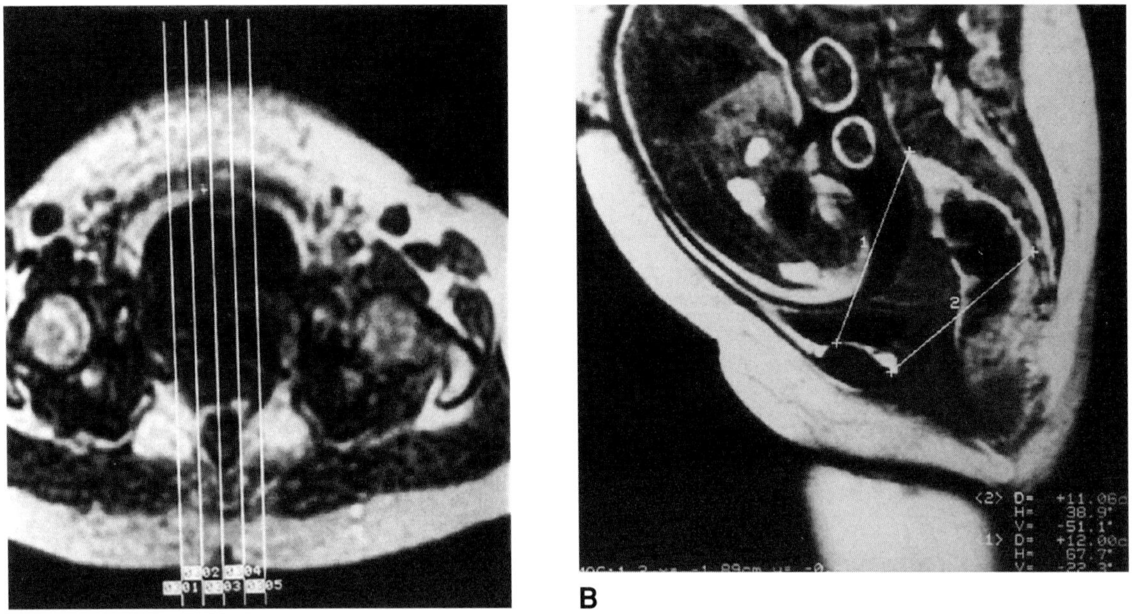

Figure 5–11. Gradient echo pelvimetry scans. **A.** An axial pilot scan is used to prescribe a set of sagittal scans. From these, the median sagittal image **(B)** is used to measure the sagittal inlet and outlet. Fetal and maternal anatomy are also well displayed. (From Wright and associates, 1992, with permission.)

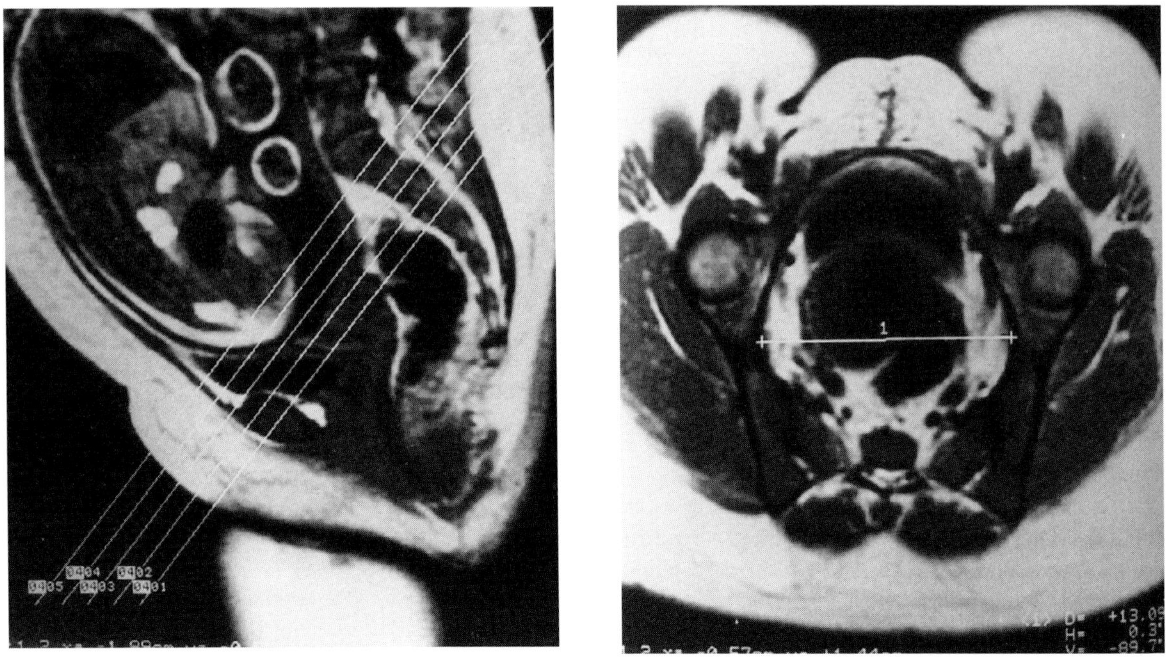

Figure 5–12. The median sagittal image is used to prescribe a set of scans in a plane parallel to the pelvic inlet **(A).** These scans allow measurement of the transverse inlet and assessment of the overall shape of the inlet **(B).** (From Wright and associates, 1992, with permission.)

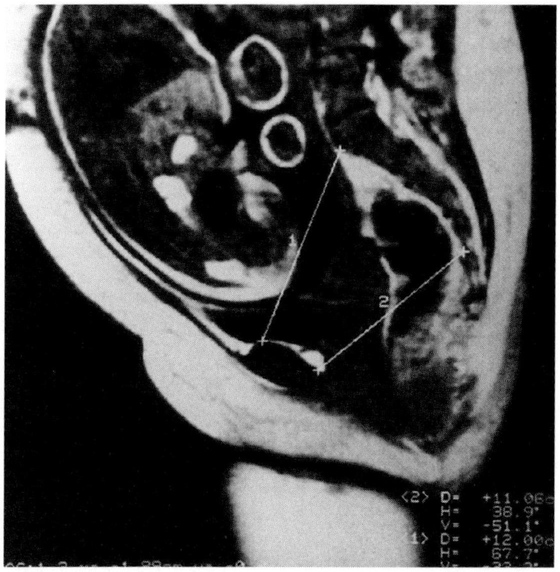

A

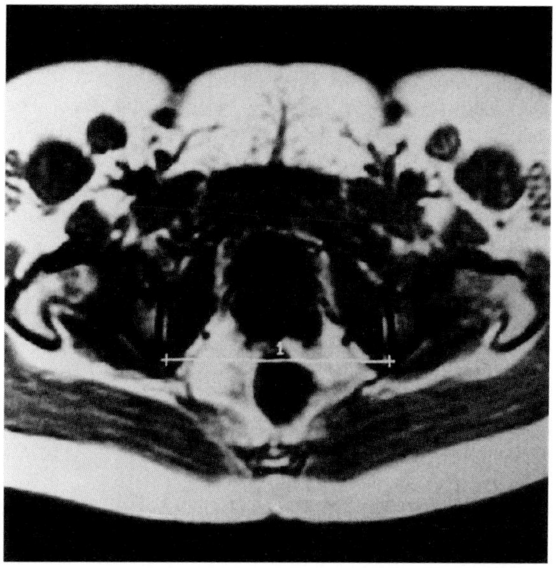

B

Figure 5–13. The median sagittal image is again used to prescribe a set of axial oblique images in the plane shown **(A)**. Measurement of the bispinous distance is made from one of these **(B)**. (From Wright and associates, 1992, with permission.)

artifact but maintains good contrast of bone and soft tissues. The reduced total exam time also results in greater patient comfort.

With the barriers to MRI use for pelvimetry rapidly declining, research will be needed to validate the measurements for the FPI and for various management algorithms such as that for planned vaginal breech delivery. MRI pelvimetry allows unlimited axial slices in different planes, thereby enabling one to obtain linear measurements as well as map the pelvic architecture (Figs. 5–11, 5–12, 5–13). In series by Wright and associates (1992a, b) and VanLoon and associates (1990), the transverse diameters (bispinous and transverse of the inlet) were found to be larger by MRI than by conventional pelvimetry. Because of the high quality of the MR images, the difference (ie, interspinous mean is 1.1 cm greater) is thought to be due to underestimation on conventional pelvimetry (Wright and associates, 1992a, b). Certainly further investigation and clinical validation are needed.

SUMMARY

The techniques, interpretation, and use of pelvic imaging have changed dramatically over the years. The pendulum has swung from extensive use to almost no use. As technology improves, costs decrease, and radiation exposure is potentially eliminated, perhaps pelvimetry may again be used widely in the development of critical clinical pathway protocols.

REFERENCES

Abitbol MM, Taylor UB, Castillo I, Rochelson GL. The cephalopelvic disproportion index. Combined fetal sonography and x-ray pelvimetry for early detection of cephalopelvic disproportion. J Reprod Med 1991; 36:369–73.

Allen EP. Standardised radiological pelvimetry: interpretation of pelvimetry. Br J Radiol 1947; 20:205–18.

Aronson D, Kier R. CT pelvimetry: the foveae are not an accurate landmark for the level of the ischial spines. Am J Roentgen 1991; 156:527–30.

Ball RP. Roentgen pelvimetry and fetal cephalometry. Surg Gynecol Obstet 1936; 62:798–810.

Beischer NA. Pelvic contracture in breech presentation. J Obstet Gynecol Br Commun 1966; 73:421–27.

Benson WL, Boyce DC, Vaughn DL. Breech delivery in the primagravida. Obstet Gynecol 1972; 40:417–28.

Caldwell WE, Moloy HC, Swenson PC. The use of the roentgen ray in obstetrics. Part I. Roentgen pelvimetry and cephalometry; technique of pelvioroentenography. Am J Roentgenol Rad Ther 1939a; 41:305–16.

Caldwell WE, Moloy HC, Swenson PC. The use of the roentgen ray in obstetrics. Part II. Anatomical variations in the female pelvis and their classification according to morphology. Am J Roentgenol Rad Ther 1939b; 41:505–26.

Caldwell WE, Moloy HC, Swenson PC. The use of the roentgen ray in obstetrics. Part III. The mechanism of labor. Am J Roentgenol Rad Ther 1939c; 41:719–41.

Capeless EL, Mann LI. A vaginal delivery protocol for the term breech infant utilizing Ball pelvimetry. J Reprod Med 1985; 30:545–48.

Christian SS, Brady K, Read JA, Kopleman JN. Vaginal breech delivery: A five-year prospective evaluation of a protocol using computed tomographic pelvimetry. Am J Obstet Gynecol 1990; 163:848–55.

Colcher AE, Sussman W. A practical technique for roentgen pelvimetry with a new positioning. Am J Roentgenol 1944; 51:207–14.

Collea JV, Chein C, Quilligan EJ. The randomized management of term frank breech presentation: a study of 208 cases. Am J Obstet Gynecol 1980; 137:235–44.

Collea JV, Rabin SC, Weghorst GR, Quilligan EJ. The randomized management of term frank breech presentation: vaginal delivery vs. cesarean section. Am J Obstet Gynecol 1978; 131:186–95.

Cunningham FG, MacDonald PC, Grant NF, et al., eds. Williams Obstetrics, 19th ed. Norwalk, CT: Appleton & Lange, 1993.

Federle MP, Cohen HA, Rosenwein MF, Brant-Zawadzki MN, Cann CE. Pelvimetry by digital radiography: a low dose examination. Radiology 1982; 143:733–35.

Friedman EA, Taylor MB. A modified normographic aid for x-ray cephalopelvimetry. Am J Obstet Gynecol 1969; 105:1110–15.

Gimovsky ML, Willard K, Neglio M, Howard T, Zeme S. X-ray pelvimetry in a breech protocol: a comparison of digital radiography and conventional methods. Am J Obstet Gynecol 1985; 153:887–88.

Gimovsky ML, Wallace RL, Schifrin BS, Paul RH. Randomized management of the non-frank breech presentation at term: a preliminary report. Am J Obstet Gynecol 1983; 146:34–40.

Green JE, McLean F, Smith LP, Usher R. Has the increased cesarean section rate for breech deliveries reduced the incidence of birth asphyxia, trauma and death? Am J Obstet Gynecol 1982; 142:643–48.

Hall JE, Kohl S. Breech presentation: a study of 1456 cases. Am J Obstet Gynecol 1956; 72:977–90.

Hall JE, Kohl S, O'Brien F, et al. Breech presentation and perinatal mortality, a study of 6,044 cases. Am J Obstet Gynecol 1965; 91: 665–83.

Hannah WJ. X-ray pelvimetry—a critical appraisal. Am J Obstet Gynecol 1965; 91:333–41.

Hellman LM, Pritchard JA. Williams Obstetrics, 14th ed. New York: Appleton-Century-Crofts, 1971:313.

Jagani N, Schulman H, Chandra P, Gonzalez R, Fleischer A. The predictability of labor outcome from a comparison of birth weight and x-ray pelvimetry. Am J Obstet Gynecol 1981; 139:507–11.

Joyce DN, Giwa-Osagie F, Stevenson GW. Role of pelvimetry in active management of labor. Br Med J 1975; 4:505–07.

Kaltneider DF. Criteria of inlet contraction. What is their value? Am J Obstet Gynecol 1951; 62:600–06.

Kaltneider DF. Criteria of midplane contraction. What is their value? Am J Obstet Gynecol 1952; 63:392–99.

Kauppila O. The perinatal mortality in breech deliveries and observations on affecting factors. Acta Obstet Gynecol Scand 1975; 39:1.

Kelly KM, Madden DA, Arcarese JS, Barnett M, Brown RF. The utilization and efficiency of pelvimetry. Am J Roentgenol Radium Ther Nucl Med 1975; 125:66–74.

Klapholz H. A computerized aid to Ball pelvimetry. Am J Obstet Gynecol 1975; 121:1067–70.

Kopelman JN, Dutt P, Karl RT, Schipel AH, Read JA. Computed tomographic pelvimetry in the evaluation of breech presentation. Obstet Gynecol 1986; 68:455–58.

Laube DW, Varner MW, Cruikshank DP. A prospective evaluation of x-ray pelvimetry. JAMA 1981; 246:2187–88.

Main DL, Main EK, Maurer MM, et al. Cesarean section versus vaginal delivery for the breech fetus weighing less than 1500 grams. Am J Obstet Gynecol 1983; 146:580–84.

Mattison DR, Kay HH, Miller RK, Angtuaco T. Magnetic resonance imaging: a noninvasive tool for fetal and placental physiology. Biol Reprod 1988; 38:39–49.

Mengert WF, Eller WC. Graphic portrayal of relative pelvic size. Am J Obstet Gynecol 1946; 52:1032–40.

Mengert WF. Estimation of pelvic capacity. JAMA 1948; 138:169.

Moir JC. The use of radiology in predicting difficult labor: I. J Obstet Gynecol Br Empire 1946; 53:487–97.

Moir JC. The use of radiology in predicting difficult labor. Lecture 2: Forcasting the course of labor. J Obstet Gynecol Br Empire 1947; 54:20–33.

Morgan HS, Kane SH. An analysis of 16,327 breech births. JAMA 1964; 187:262–64.

Morgan MA, Thurnau GR. Efficacy of the fetal-pelvic index in nulliparous women at high risk for fetal-pelvic disproportion. Am J Obstet Gynecol 1992; 166:810–14.

Morgan MA, Thurnau GR. Efficacy of the fetal-pelvic index in patients requiring labor induction. Am J Obstet Gynecol 1988b; 159:621–25.

Morgan MA, Thurnau GR. Efficacy of the fetal-pelvic index for delivery of neonates weighing 4000 grams or greater: a preliminary report. Am J Obstet Gynecol 1988a; 158:1133–37.

Morgan MA, Thurnau GR, Fishburne JI. The fetal-pelvic index as an indicator of fetal-pelvic disproportion: a preliminary report. Am J Obstet Gynecol 1986; 155:608–13.

Parsons MT, Spellacy WN. Prospective randomized study of x-ray pelvimetry in the primagravida. Obstet Gynecol 1985; 66:76–79.

Russell JGB, Richards B. A review of pelvimetry data. Br J Radiol 1971; 44:780.

Stark DD, McCarthy SM, Filly RA, Parer JT, Hricak H, Callen PW. Pelvimetry by magnetic resonance imaging. Am J Radiol 1985; 144:947–50.

Steer CM. X-ray pelvimetry and the outcome of labor. Am J Obstet Gynecol 1958; 76:188–231.

Stewart A, Webb J, Giles D, Hewitt D. Malignant disease in childhood and diagnostic irradiation in utero. Lancet 1956; 2:447.

Stewart A, Webb JW, Hewitt D. A survey of childhood malignancies. Br Med J 1958; 1:1495–1508.

Thoms H. The clinical application of roentgen pelvimetry and a study of the results in 1100 white women. Am J Obstet Gynecol 1941; 42:957–75.

Thurnau GR, Morgan MA. Efficacy of the fetal-pelvic index as a predictor of fetal-pelvic disproportion in women with abnormal labor patterns that require labor augmentations. Am J Obstet Gynecol 1988; 159:1168–72.

Thurnau GR, Seates DH, Morgan MA. The fetal-pelvic index: a method of identifying fetal-pelvic disproportion in women attempting vaginal birth after previous cesarean delivery. Am J Obstet Gynecol 1991; 165:353–58.

Todd WD, Steer CM. Term breech: review of 1006 term breech deliveries. Obstet Gynecol 1963; 22:583–95.

Urhahn R, Lehnen H, Drobnitzky M, Klose KC, Gunther RW. Ultrafast pelvimetry using snap-shot-flash-MRI—a comparison with the spin echo and flash techniques [German]. Rofo Fortschr geb Rontgenstr Neuen Bilogeb Verfahr 1991; 155:432–35.

VanLoon AJ, Mantingh A, Thijn CJP, Mooyaart EL. Pelvimetry by magnetic resonance imaging in breech presentation. Am J Obstet Gynecol 1990; 163:1256–60.

Watson WJ, Benson WL. Vaginal delivery for the selected frank breech infant at term. Obstet Gynecol 1984; 64:638–40.

Wright AR, English PT, Cameron HM, Wilson JB. MR pelvimetry—a practical alternative. Acta Radiol 1992a; 33:582–87.

Wright AR, Cameron HM, Lind T. Magnetic resonance imaging pelvimetry: a useful adjunct in the management of the obese patient. Br J Obstet Gynecol 1992b; 99:852–53.

Yamazaki H, Uchida K. A mathematical approach to problems of cephalopelvic proportion at the pelvic inlet. Am J Obstet Gynecol 1983; 147:25–37.

CHAPTER 6

Symphysiotomy

Symphysiotomy, a controversial procedure in modern obstetrics, has a long and interesting history (Gebbie, 1982). Symphysiotomy continues to have a role in the management of cephalopelvic disproportion in Third World countries where pelvic contraction is common, high parity is the rule, patients often live in remote areas, and transportation is poor. In such circumstances, a scarred uterus is a definite and potentially life-threatening handicap.

Between 1957 and 1963, over 1200 symphysiotomies were performed in a single institution in South Africa (Crichton, 1963). Where there is adequate access to prenatal care and facilities to perform cesarean section, symphysiotomy has little role in the management of cephalopelvic disproportion.

Symphysiotomy may be a lifesaving procedure in the management of the arrested aftercoming head of a breech when the problem cannot be resolved by standard maneuvers. We have performed symphysiotomy for this complication on four occasions. All patients arrived unscheduled in the delivery unit in the second stage of labor. In three cases, the breech was on the perineum with the patient bearing down. The fourth case involved unexpected arrest of the aftercoming head during breech delivery of a second twin; the occiput had rotated posteriorly into the hollow of the sacrum, and the recommended maneuvers failed. All babies were delivered without complication and were in satisfactory condition after resuscitation, although long-term follow-up is not available. There were no short-term maternal complications.

Menticoglou (1990) comprehensively reviewed the use of symphysiotomy for entrapment of the breech fetus. Symphysiotomy was performed for the trapped aftercoming head (114 cases) or the trapped upper body or arms (4 cases). Symphysiotomy was usually delayed and performed after other methods had failed; nevertheless, 80 percent of the babies were born alive and undamaged. Symphysiotomy has also been reported in conjunction with maneuvers to relieve shoulder dystocia (Hartfield, 1986).

MATERNAL AND PERINATAL MORBIDITY AND MORTALITY

Properly performed, symphysiotomy has no deleterious effects on the fetus; the condition of the baby at birth is directly related to its condition prior to the procedure.

Maternal mortality also is not increased by symphysiotomy. In fact, when compared with cesarean section performed under similar circumstances, maternal mortality actually may be lower with symphysiotomy (Van Roosmalen, 1990). Lasbrey (1963) studied symptomatic sequelae following symphysiotomy; patients followed for up to 2 years had the same incidence of pelvic symptoms as women who delivered without symphysiotomy.

TECHNIQUE

The symphysis pubis is a secondary cartilaginous joint (Fig. 6–1). The articular sur-

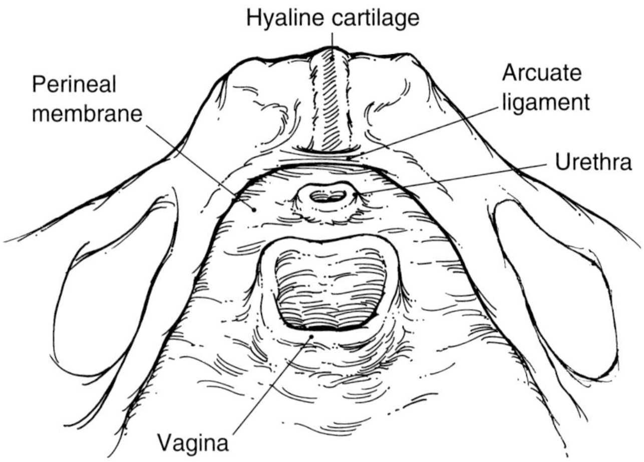

Figure 6–1. Anatomy of the symphysis pubis.

faces are covered with hyaline cartilage. The main uniting medium is a disc of fibrocartilage. Symphysiotomy is the separation of this joint and surrounding ligaments with a scalpel.

With the aid of two assistants supporting the patient's legs, the patient is placed in an exaggerated lithotomy position with the buttocks brought down over the edge of the delivery table. The angle of abduction of the thighs should not exceed 80 degrees. Additional abduction of the thighs to gain further separation of the symphysis pubis is inappropriate because it may result in damage to the sacroiliac joints.

The patient is prepared and draped as for a routine assisted vaginal delivery. If an epidural block is not in place, the skin and soft tissue overlying the symphysis pubis are infiltrated with 0.5 percent or 1 percent lidocaine solution. The inferior aspect of the joint should be liberally infiltrated because it is the most sensitive area. The perineum is also infiltrated in the line of an intended episiotomy.

A catheter is inserted into the urethra to empty the bladder and to identify the urethra. A Foley catheter is adequate although the more rigid No. 6 Jacques catheter is often used. For a right-handed surgeon, the index and middle finger of the left hand are used to displace the urethra laterally. These fingers then will lie directly under the cartilage (Fig. 6–2). The thumb of the same hand can be used to palpate the joint anteriorly.

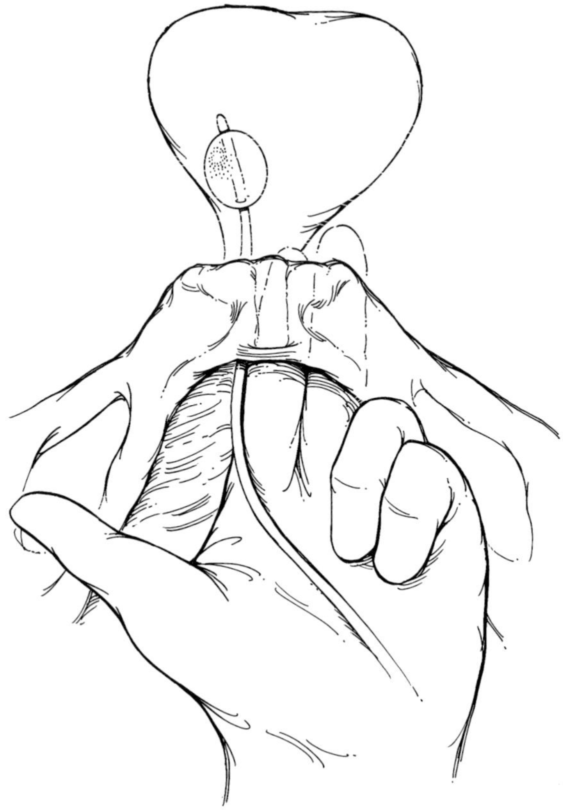

Figure 6–2. The index and middle fingers displace the catheterized urethra laterally and palpate the posterior aspect of the symphysis pubis.

A solid-bladed scalpel is recommended. More readily available detachable scalpels also may be used; however, they are much sharper than solid-bladed scalpels and more liable to injure the operator. The scalpel is inserted vertically into the skin overlying the symphysis pubis. The blade is facing the operator. The joint is entered in the midline at the center of the joint. The scalpel passes through the joint until the tip is palpable by the vaginal finger; the vaginal tissues separate the tip of the scalpel from the operator's finger. The blade should pass through the cartilage easily; if there is any significant resistance, the surgeon probably is not in the midline, and the scalpel should be repositioned. Ease of penetration is probably the best indicator that the scalpel is in the correct position.

The cephalad uncut portion of the joint is used as a fulcrum against which the scalpel is levered to cut the caudad portion of the symphysis pubis and overlying ligaments, including the arcuate ligament. Once this has been achieved, the scalpel is rotated 180 degrees so that it is facing cephalad. The cephalad portion of the symphysis pubis and overlying ligaments then are incised. A separation of 2.5 cm is usually adequate, and this is gauged by the surgeon's being able to insert the thumb of the vaginal hand between the divided joint. If required, greater separation is achieved by further dividing of any uncut ligaments rather than by increasing the abduction of the thighs. An episiotomy is then performed if indicated. Performance of the entire procedure generally requires fewer than 2 minutes.

Following symphysiotomy, delivery is usually rapid. During delivery of the head and shoulder, continual downward traction is applied in order to keep pressure away from the urethra and anterior vaginal wall, which are unsupported and vulnerable to injury at this stage. If delivery is not easy and spontaneous, the degree of fetopelvic disproportion was probably underestimated. If further assistance is required, a vacuum extractor may be used. The use of forceps should be avoided because of the potential for maternal trauma.

Following delivery, the episiotomy is repaired and a detailed inspection for any additional injuries takes place. A Foley catheter is inserted at this time if it was removed for delivery. The small incision over the pubic symphysis may require a single suture.

COMPLICATIONS

Bleeding at the operative site may occur, but is usually easily controlled with local pressure. The lower genital tract should be inspected for lacerations, which should be repaired as after any assisted vaginal delivery. Van Roosmalen (1987) reviewed the literature and found that the rate of serious morbidity after symphysiotomy was 8.1 percent. A total of 1752 cases were reported. Vesico-vaginal fistulas occurred in 30 cases (1.7%); however, 15 of these fistulas were not due to the procedure itself, but were the result of pressure necrosis due to obstructed labor. Vestibular and/or urethral lesions occurred in 33 (1.9%), osteitis pubis or retropubic abscess complicated 10 (0.6%), long-term walking disability or pain occurred in 32 (1.8%), and stress incontinence was present in 36 (2.1%) cases after symphysiotomy.

POSTOPERATIVE CARE

The symphyseal joint heals by dense fibrosis. The patient should remain on her side while in bed for about 5 days. In some institutions, the thighs are gently bound together using a gauze bandage, although such binding is probably unnecessary. The catheter is usually removed after 24–48 hours but should remain until the urine is clear if there is significant hematuria. Prophylactic antibiotics (a first generation cephalosporin) are routinely administered, and analgesics are prescribed as required. If available, a physical therapist should supervise the patient's ambulation. Most patients ambulate well by postoperative day 5 and may be discharged. Patients are advised to perform no strenuous activity for 6 weeks.

The pelvis may remain permanently enlarged after symphysiotomy and thus may provide permanent relief from mild to moderate cephalopelvic disproportion (Van Roosmalen, 1987). In a review of the outcome of labor in 229 women with previous symphysiotomy, Van Roosmalen found that uncomplicated vaginal delivery occurred in 73 percent; assisted vaginal delivery in 14 percent; and cesarean section was required in 11 percent.

SUMMARY

In Third World settings, symphysiotomy will remain a useful technique for allowing vaginal delivery in cases of mild to moderate cephalopelvic disproportion where cesarean section is not available. Such a technique also allows avoidance of a uterine scar in situations where subsequent labors will take place in remote, unsupervised settings. In most developed countries, where the maternal risks associated with cesarean section are minimal (Frigoletto, 1980), abdominal delivery is preferable.

Although a trapped head following vaginal breech delivery is rarely encountered in modern obstetrics, this complication is often devastating for the involved infant. In such situations, symphysiotomy may be a useful and lifesaving technique. The absence of experience with this procedure in most training programs in the United States unfortunately precludes even its occasional use.

REFERENCES

Crichton D, Seedat EK. The technique of symphysiotomy. S Af Med J 1963; 37:227.

Frigoletto FD, Ryan KJ, Phillippe M. Maternal mortality rate associated with cesarean section: an appraisal. Am J Obstet Gynecol 1980; 136:969.

Gebbie D. Symphysiotomy. Clin Obstet Gynecol 1982; 9:663.

Hartfield VJ. Symphysiotomy for shoulder dystocia. Am J Obstet Gynecol 1986; 155:228.

Lasbrey AH. The symptomatic sequelae of symphysiotomy. S Af Med J 1963; 37:231.

Menticoglou SM. Symphysiotomy for the trapped aftercoming parts of the breech: A review of the literature and a plea for its use. Aust NZ J Obstet Gynecol, 1990; 30:1-9.

Van Roosmalen J. Symphysiotomy as an alternative to cesarean section. Int J Gynaecol Obstet 1987; 25:451.

Van Roosmalen J. Safe motherhood: cesarean section or symphysiotomy? Am J Obstet Gynecol 1990; 163:1.

CHAPTER 7

Episiotomy

The precise origin of the episiotomy is difficult to determine; however, one of the first to describe it was a Dublin midwife, Sir Fielding Ould. As early as 1742, in his *Treatise of Midwifery in Three Parts,* he recommended the procedure for some cases in which the external vaginal opening was so tight that labor was dangerously prolonged (Ould, 1742). The first report of episiotomy in the United States is attributed to Taliaferro of Virginia. Almost 110 years after Ould's *Treatise,* in a journal entitled *The Stethoscope and Virginia Medical Gazette,* Taliaferro (1852) published an account of a delivery of a 16-year-old eclamptic woman. After 18 hours of labor and at least a quart of bloodletting, her perineum was sufficiently distended to deliver the infant. Thinking a tear of the rectum was imminent, Taliaferro used a scalpel to cut a 1-inch left mediolateral episiotomy to facilitate delivery. The infant was stillborn, but the convulsions ceased postpartum, and the woman regained consciousness the following evening. Taliaferro wrote, "When this was undertaken by me, I was not aware of its having been done before, and was really afraid that my professional brethren would condemn me."

Indications for using the episiotomy were greatly expanded in the United States when two prominent obstetricians, Pomeroy and DeLee, became champions of the procedure. In *The Prophylactic Forceps Operation,* DeLee (1920) claimed the episiotomy would preserve the integrity of the pelvic floor and introitus, forestall uterine prolapse and rupture of the vesicovaginal septum, and restore virginal conditions. Further, episiotomy combined with forceps delivery would save the fetal brain from injury, reduce the amount of epilepsy and mental retardation, and prevent anoxia. DeLee recommended a forceps delivery with a mediolateral episiotomy for all nulliparas.

In addition to the strong advocacy of episiotomy by the most notable obstetricians of the day, changing practices surrounding the birthing process also contributed to the increasing use of this procedure. In 1900 less than 5 percent of the women in the United States delivered in hospitals; by 1930, about 25 percent; and by 1950, more than 80 percent were in hospitals (Thacker and Banta, 1983). The shift to in-hospital deliveries, while no doubt in large part responsible for improvements in maternal and neonatal morbidity and mortality, also was closely associated with the increased frequency with which episiotomies were performed.

In the United States in the early 1920s and 1930s women frequently were given *twilight sleep,* a powerful combination of drugs that rendered the laboring woman oblivious. Her inability to cooperate actively in the birth process increased the use of forceps, which required extra room for vaginal manipulations. With the move into the hospital, the most common place for giving birth became the delivery room table, and lithotomy the most common position, one believed by many to often unnecessarily place additional stress on the perineal body and lead to tears whether or not an episiotomy is cut (Bromberg, 1986; Thompson, 1987; Yeomans, 1991).

During the back-to-nature movement of the 1970s the emphasis was on decreasing interventions during parturition. Opposition to routine episiotomy surfaced in both the United States and Britain (Arms, 1975; Haire, 1972; Kitzinger, 1981; Thacker and Banta, 1983). Two publications were particularly important in demanding a reassessment of routine episiotomy; the first was published by the National Childbirth Trust in London (Kitzinger, 1981) and the other, by the epidemiologists Thacker and Banta (1983) in the United States. These investigators concluded that the widespread use of episiotomy did not withstand scientific scrutiny, that the risk of episiotomy had been largely ignored, and that if women were fully informed of the risk/benefit ratio, they would be unlikely to consent readily to having a routine episiotomy performed.

INTERPRETATION OF DATA

Influence of Practice Differences

In the United States, the majority of deliveries are performed by medical doctors, and when employed the midline episiotomy is most often preferred (Gass, 1986; Shiono, 1990; Thorp, 1987; and their associates). In contrast, midwives perform the majority of deliveries in Great Britain (Harrison and colleagues, 1984; Reynolds and Yudkin, 1987), Belgium (Buekens and associates, 1985), Sweden (Larsson and co-workers, 1991; Rockner and collaborators, 1988, 1989; Rockner and Olund, 1991), and Denmark (Thranov and colleagues, 1990). Mediolateral episiotomy is performed almost entirely to the exclusion of midline episiotomies in Europe, as well as South Africa (Bex and Hofmeyr, 1987). In Canada mediolateral episiotomies also are more commonly performed than in the United States (Walker and associates, 1991).

Thus there are major differences in practice, which must be considered when evaluating the vast database available concerning episiotomies and their risks and benefits. For example, the complications of the midline episiotomy are largely limited to spontaneous extension involving injury to the anal sphincter and/or rectal mucosa. In the majority of midline episiotomies, a satisfactory repair is easily achieved; however, the incidence of rectovaginal fistulas and breakdown with cloaca formation is higher than with mediolateral episiotomies. On the other hand, mediolateral episiotomies are more often complicated by poor wound healing and long-term pelvic pain and dyspareunia.

To interpret the data correctly, one also must know the definition being employed for each degree of laceration. In Europe, episiotomies commonly are classified only as first-, second-, or third-degree, with the latter encompassing injuries to either the anal sphincter or rectal mucosa. The classification most often employed in the United States, and the one that we use is:

- **First-degree laceration:** Superficial laceration of the vaginal mucosa or perineal body not requiring suturing.
- **Second-degree laceration or episiotomy:** Involving the vaginal mucosa and/or perineal skin and deeper subcutaneous tissue and requiring suturing.
- **Third-degree laceration or episiotomy:** Extension of the laceration to involve any part of the capsule or anal sphincter muscle.
- **Fourth-degree laceration or episiotomy:** Extension to include involvement of the rectal mucosa.

Influence of Study Design

The majority of studies evaluating efficacy and complications of episiotomies have been retrospective. In most of these studies, the indication confounders, that is, the indication for performing the episiotomy alone, also have been found to be indicators of risk for third-degree or fourth-degree tears. Studies based on observational data and not on randomized controlled trials can only provide limited evidence of benefits and hazards of the widespread use of episiotomy (Blondel and Kaminski, 1985). While these observational studies are perhaps a prerequisite to the design of pragmatic randomized trials, they are nonetheless poor substitutes, and it is surprising to find that there are only three prospective randomized trials that have attempted to determine the merits of the routine use of episiotomy (Harrison and associates, 1984; Sleep and colleagues, 1984; Argentine Episiotomy Trial Collaborative Group, 1993). Appropriately designed and randomized prospective trials are both time consuming and costly. For instance, to test the hypothesis that the restricted use of episiotomy would double the incidence of damage to the anal sphincter or rectal mucosa from a rate of 0.6 percent with mediolateral episiotomies to a rate of 1.2 percent, would require a randomized controlled trial including 5000 women in each group (Blondel and Kaminski, 1985).

EPISIOTOMY RATES

Episiotomies are more often performed in nulliparous women, regardless of the background episiotomy rate (Sleep and associates, 1984, 1989). Harrison and co-workers (1984) reported the episiotomy rate in primigravidas delivered at the Rotunda Hospital in Dublin, Ireland, as 90 percent in the 6 months preceding a randomized trial, one arm of which entailed performing episiotomy only if essential. In the latter group, the episiotomy rate fell to 8 percent, with 20 percent delivering over an intact perineum and 25 percent sustaining only a first-degree tear. Although not reported until 1990, Shiono and colleagues reported a 62 percent episiotomy rate among women in the Collaborative Perinatal Project, which accumulated data from 1959 to 1966. McGuiness and colleagues (1991), reporting on a low-income inner-city population, found that almost half the women underwent episiotomy. This rate compares favorably to that reported by Olson and associates (1990) from a three-person family practice group in the rural United States. These physicians reported an overall episiotomy rate of 44 percent, 60 percent in nulliparas and 36 percent in multiparas. This rate is comparable to the 53 percent rate reported by Thranov and colleagues (1990) from Denmark. However, for all of Denmark, the episiotomy rate is 77 percent of nulliparas when cesarean section and instrumental delivery are excluded. Buekens and colleagues (1985) reported a 28 percent rate of episiotomies from 10 Belgium hospitals. The mean incidence of episiotomies in Sweden was 30 percent with a range in individual hospitals of 9 percent to 77 percent (Rockner and Olund, 1991). Among the lowest rates reported are those from Israel, where only 17 percent of women having their first child and 10 percent having a subsequent child will have an episiotomy (Adoni and Anteby, 1991).

The trend observed at the John Radcliffe Hospital, Oxford, has been a steady decline in episiotomy rates for both nulliparous and multiparous women with more intact perineal bodies and no increased significant perineal trauma. These trends, shown in Table 7–1, seem to reflect current trends in industrial-

TABLE 7–1. PERINEAL MANAGEMENT DURING LABOR AMONG 24,439 WOMEN AT JOHN RADCLIFFE HOSPITAL, OXFORD, BETWEEN 1980 AND 1984

Variable	1980	1981	1982	1983	1984
No. of women					
Primiparas (n = 10,412)	2231	2149	1974	2018	2040
Multiparas (n = 14,027)	2903	2856	2755	2747	2766
Episiotomy rate, %					
Primiparas	72.6	69.9	58.7	49.8	44.9
Multiparas	36.8	33.9	24.9	21.3	15.4
Women with intact perineum, %					
Primiparas	7.4	8.5	9.5	11.2	13.7
Multiparas	26.1	26.6	27.7	29.6	33.8
Rate of first-degree tear, %					
Primiparas	6.3	9.0	10.4	18.8	16.4
Multiparas	15.3	15.8	19.6	24.7	24.1
Rate of second-degree tear, %					
Primiparas	6.7	8.6	15.8	16.3	20.3
Multiparas	13.3	20.3	23.9	22.2	24.3
Rate of third- or fourth-degree tear, %					
Primiparas	.44	.46	.35	.55	.49
Multiparas	.21	.21	.25	.11	.18

Modified from Reynolds and Yudkin (1987).

ized nations. The literature does not, however, readily allow direct comparison of identical or even similar time intervals worldwide.

INDICATIONS FOR EPISIOTOMIES

Affecting the final decision regarding the need for and relative merits of episiotomy are a host of factors including training and clinical experience as well as the individual woman's desires. To illustrate this, Graham and colleagues (1990) asked providers in New Mexico if they performed episiotomies in more than three-fourths of their nulliparous patients. The "yes" answers were distributed along a continuum: 100 percent of obstetrical residents, 80 percent of obstetricians, 65 percent of family practitioners, 25 percent of nurse midwives, and less than 5 percent of lay midwives. The rates for episiotomies in multiparous women were lower but distributed along the same continuum.

Most practitioners agree that episiotomy is justified in instances of perceived fetal or maternal distress. Episiotomy also is indicated albeit on an intuitive basis in operative vaginal deliveries requiring additional room to safely accomplish the delivery. Included in this category are delivery of the breech, multifetal gestations, and persistent occiput posterior presentations. Low and midforceps deliveries also are accepted indications, as are vacuum extraction deliveries, which may be facilitated by an episiotomy. The woman who has undergone prior pelvic reconstructive surgery is also a candidate for episiotomy; however, there is no substantial data to support this position. The woman should be educated that in most cases the birth attendant must make a clinical decision for which the majority of the prerequisite information will not be available until the moment that birth is about to occur.

PERFORMANCE OF EPISIOTOMY

Suture Materials and Techniques for Repair of Perineal Trauma

The choice of suture materials as well as technique for repair of perineal trauma have been subjects of debate, but have remained largely the choice of the individual surgeon. Principal materials used for repairs include absorbable and nonabsorbable suture. Absorbable suture materials include chromic catgut, glycerol-impregnated catgut, polyglycolide (Dexon), and polyglactide (Vicryl). For transcutaneous suturing, the absorbables have virtually replaced the previously used nylon and silk sutures.

Grant (1989) reviewed 14 controlled trials that addressed choice of suture material and technique for repair of perineal trauma. The derivatives of polyglycolic acid—Dexon and Vicryl—were the absorbable materials of choice for both deep and skin closure. Compared to catgut, polyglycolic acid sutures were associated with about a 40 percent reduction in short-term pain and need for analgesia. Their early benefit, however, may be more than offset by the frequent need for removal of the polyglycolic acid sutures during the puerperium. Mahomed and colleagues (1989) found that one-third of women required removal of the polyglycolic acid derivatives within the first 10 days after delivery compared with only 12 percent of the chromic group. The finding persisted up to 3 months after delivery with 41 percent of the former and 21 percent of the latter presenting for removal of suture material. The most common reasons given were perineal irritation and tightness. In comparison, the principal drawback to chromic suture is the rapidity with which it loses tensile strength, accelerated even more by infection or inflammation, resulting in the occasional need to resuture perineal wounds closed with catgut (Banninger and colleagues, 1978; Livingstone and co-workers, 1974; Mahomed and associates, 1989).

Spencer and associates (1986) compared glycerol-impregnated chromic catgut with chromic catgut in a randomized comparison for the repair of childbirth perineal trauma. Glycerol-impregnated chromic catgut caused more pain than chromic catgut 10 days after delivery and it was found to be associated with significantly more dyspareunia both at 3 months and 3 years after delivery. The importance of what might seem such a mundane decision, that is, choice of suture material for episiotomy repair, was emphasized by Grant (1986), who estimated that in England and Wales alone, the choice of suture material for perineal repair could make a difference of as many as 30,000 new cases of dyspareunia per year. There is no role for glycerol-impregnated catgut in episiotomy repair.

When compared with nonabsorbable materials (both silk and nylon), polyglycolic acid skin sutures were associated with less short-term perineal pain. However, continuous, subcuticular stitches result in significantly less perineal pain than occurs with transcutaneous sutures. Additionally, there seldom is a need to remove subcuticular sutures postpartum, a common occurrence with polyglycolic acid derivative sutures when used for transcutaneous closure. As an alternative, limited studies using a Histoacryl adhesive for coaption of skin edges with mediolateral episiotomies resulted in virtual abolition of need for postpartum analgesics or sitting aids and appeared far superior to the subcuticular suturing technique (Adoni and Anteby, 1991).

Surgical Technique for Mediolateral Episiotomy

This surgical incision may be quite large and accordingly an adequate pudendal block or conduction analgesia is important. Under emergency conditions the procedure may be carried out with local infiltration of an anesthetic agent. Large straight scissors with enough leverage to incise the tissue with a single cut are used. The procedure is performed when the perineum is bulging and when about 4 cm of fetal scalp is visible during a contraction. The incision is placed at 5 o'clock for a left mediolateral episiotomy and at 7 o'clock for a right mediolateral episiotomy. Regardless of the site, the incision is directed toward the ipsilateral ischial tuberosity. The operator's two fingers in the vagina separate the labia and exert outward pressure on the perineum to flatten it slightly and to protect the presenting fetal part (Fig. 7–1). The incision must be deep enough to remove all perineal resistance to delivery of the infant and should extend at least 3–4 cm onto the perineum. Some clinicians feel that the fat in the

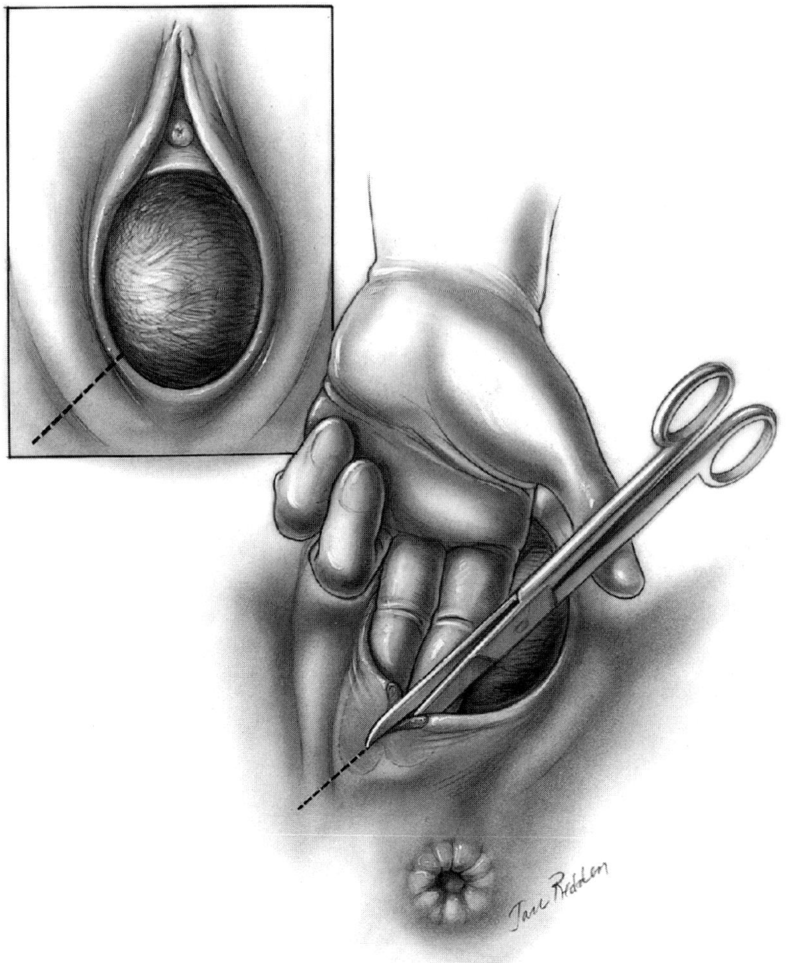

Figure 7–1. The timing of performance of a right mediolateral episiotomy when approximately 3–4 cm of the fetal head is seen distending the perineum during a uterine contraction. Care should be taken that the incision is at 5 or 7 o'clock in order to avoid extension into the rectal sphincter muscle.

ischiorectal fossa is commonly exposed when the episiotomy is of adequate depth (Willson, 1969).

If the episiotomy has been placed too far laterally, it will not provide the desired relaxation of the median portion of the levator plate. When the episiotomy is too small, it usually will not relieve the tensions on the perineal tissues, but rather will provide a weak point from which may arise an associated extension in the form of an uncontrolled laceration. While an episiotomy can be enlarged with several successive cuts, this is not advisable because following the first incision, the wound edges become distorted by the pull of the muscles. Thereafter additional perineal cuts tend to produce a zigzag incision line.

Suture Repair

Prior to suture repair, the birth canal is exposed either manually or with suitable retractors. Retractors should be used cautiously because these instruments themselves may cause additional lacerations. Cervical or vaginal lacerations requiring suturing generally should be repaired prior to the episiotomy because exposure will be maximal if repairs are performed in this sequence (Chap. 14). If necessary, either for removal of the placenta or because of atony and bleeding, manual exploration of the uterus should be performed prior to episiotomy closure if possible.

The surgeon places the second and third fingers of the left hand into the vagina to spread the vaginal and perineal wound margins. This provides access to the uppermost wound angle where suturing begins. Either 00 chromic on a taper CT1 needle or 00 Vicryl on a taper CTX needle are suitable for repair. Placement of the anchor suture approximately 1 cm above the apex of the incision assists in hemostasis at the wound apex (Fig. 7–2). Each

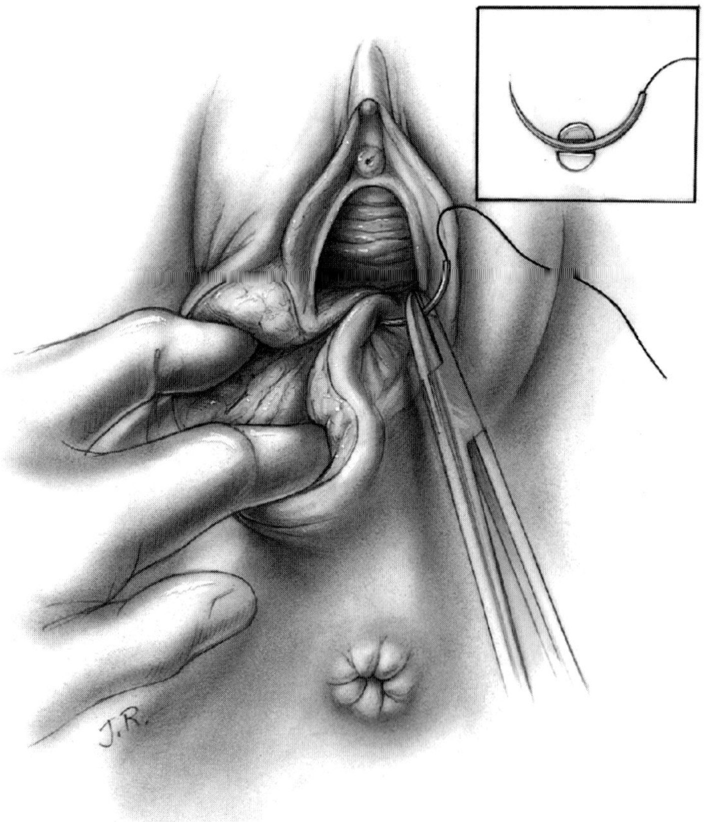

Figure 7–2. Repair of the mediolateral episiotomy. The operator is exposing the full extent of the episiotomy using the left hand. The first suture is placed at the vaginal apex approximately 1 cm cephalad to the most superior margin of the episiotomy or laceration. It is important to place the initial suture above the apex to ensure hemostasis of the repair. Insert shows correct position of the needle at the tip of the needle holder.

bite should include the supporting tissue between the vagina and the rectum as well as the vaginal mucosa to provide strong support. Sutures—either interrupted or continuous locking—of the vaginal mucosa are carried to the level of or slightly past the cut edges of the hymen to the introitus.

Attention is next directed toward the urogenital diaphragm, which is carefully reconstructed using deep interrupted sutures. During this portion of the repair, it must be remembered that the lateral tissues are located at a higher level than the corresponding median structures by virtue of the muscular distortion and retraction. Additionally, the fascia on the medial side usually retracts somewhat toward the midline and beneath the more superficial structures. Medially the tissues lie close to the anterior rectal wall through which a suture can easily be placed inadvertently. The deep sutures should not be placed horizontally, but rather at a diagonal with the median side lower than the lateral (Fig. 7–3). In this way, comparable wound surfaces are united. To minimize discomfort and maximize healing, the operator should place the minimal number of sutures—usually between four and six—required to achieve adequate coadaptation of the tissues and hemostasis. Repair of this portion of the episiotomy is more difficult for the novice and may demand additional time to achieve correct coadaptation of the tissue surfaces. Failure to achieve correct coadaptation of tissue will result in the reconstruction of the pelvic floor being anatomically incorrect. In addition healing and the aesthetic results will be poor.

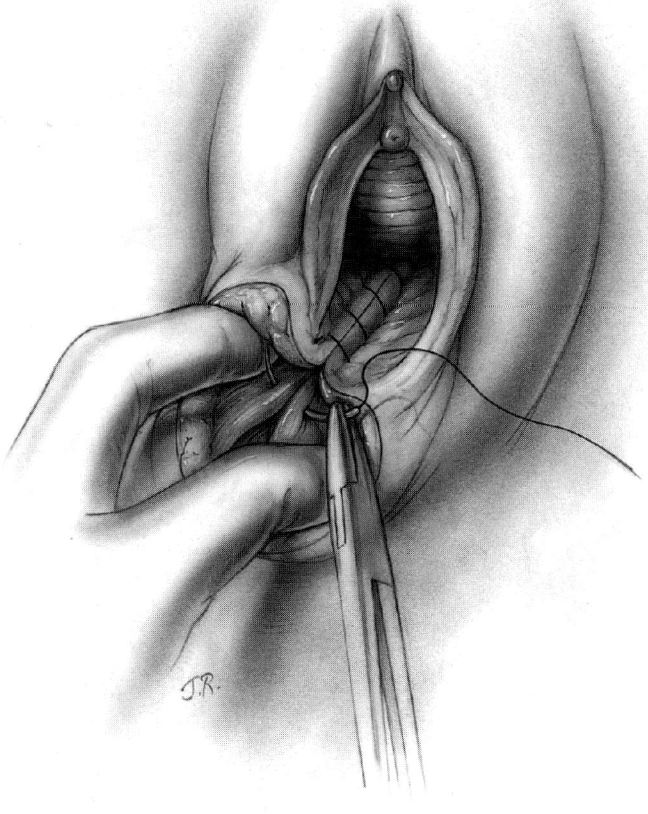

Figure 7–3. Repair of the mediolateral episiotomy. The vaginal mucosa has been approximated not quite to the posterior commissure. The surgeon spreads the perineum widely and unites the deep perineal tissues in order to avoid leaving dead space. Medially, relatively little tissue is taken on the needle for suturing so as to ensure that the rectum will not be punctured. The wound surfaces are not reapproximated in a horizontal plane, but rather at an angle with lower medial tissues joined to higher lateral tissues.

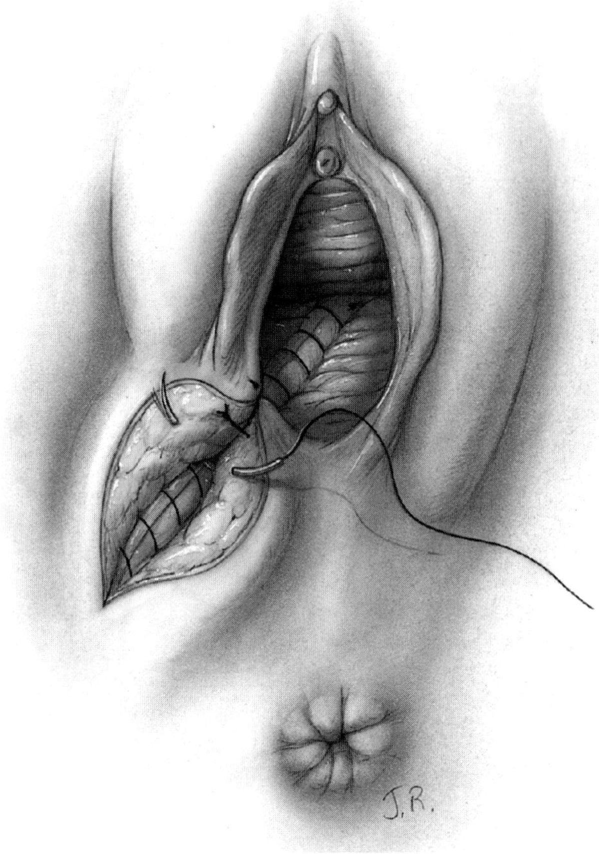

Figure 7–4. Repair of the mediolateral episiotomy. The vaginal wound has been sutured to the approximate level of the posterior commissure. The deep perineal tissues have been joined together by means of interrupted sutures. The operator unites the perineal tissues with additional sutures, again taking care that the sutures join lower medial tissues to higher lateral structures.

The cut ends of the bulbocavernous muscle are approximated as the first step in closing the superficial layer of tissue. Because the muscle ends tend to retract upward, the skin edges must be pulled laterally and superiorly to facilitate visualization, and a deep bite is required to incorporate the necessary structures. This is an important stitch; unless the tissues are properly approximated, the introitus will gape.

Subcutaneous sutures usually will be required to reapproximate the subcutaneous fatty tissue (Fig. 7–4). Again it is important to suture at a diagonal with the lateral side higher than the medial. The repair is completed by placement of either interrupted transcutaneous sutures through the perineal body or, preferably, a subcuticular closure using either the 00 or 000 suture of choice of the surgeon (Fig. 7–5).

Surgical Technique for Midline Episiotomy

The midline episiotomy is the preferred procedure in the United States largely because of the ease of repair and the reduced pain during healing. As emphasized previously, when making the incision, the operator should take care to protect the presenting fetal part by placing at least two fingers between the presenting part and the episiotomy site. Adequate pain control may be achieved with conduction analgesia, pudendal block, or local tissue infiltration with an anesthetic agent. The perineum is incised from the midline of the posterior fourchette toward the anus. Either scissors or scalpel may be used for the incision. The position of the anal sphincter is easily ascertained by visualization and palpation and the episiotomy will be cut while attempting to avoid

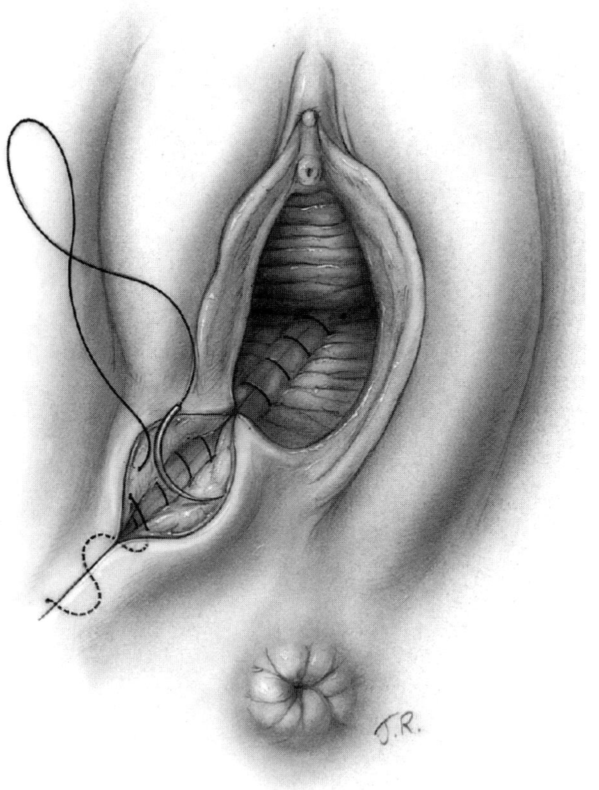

Figure 7–5. Repair of the mediolateral episiotomy. The perineal skin edges are approximated using a subcuticular stitch of reabsorbable suture.

direct injury to the anal sphincter or rectal mucosa. Even when the anal sphincter or rectal mucosa have not been cut as a part of the episiotomy, up to one-fourth of midline episiotomies will extend to involve these structures. Because the midline episiotomy often involves tears of the anal sphincter muscle and/or rectal mucosa, the repair is described sequentially as a fourth-degree repair.

Following delivery, the vagina and cervix are inspected for the presence of any lacerations requiring repair. Lacerations that are not bleeding or that are not deep into the tissues rarely require suture repair. Because exposure is optimal prior to episiotomy repair, any sidewall or cervical lacerations should be sutured before the episiotomy is repaired. Because extension through the rectal mucosa may have contaminated the field with fecal material, it is important to irrigate the wound with copious amounts of fluids. Normal saline, mixtures of normal saline and povodine iodine solution, or mixtures of normal saline and hexachlorophene are all appropriate for irrigation; the choice depends largely upon availability and whether or not the woman has any allergies.

Suture Repair

The full extent of the laceration of the rectal mucosa must be ascertained. Either a 0000 chromic on a taper SH1 needle or a 000 chromic on a T5 needle is appropriate for closing the rectal mucosa. An anchor stitch is placed approximately 0.5–1 cm above the apex of the incision, and the rectal mucosa is closed with a continuous running suture carried approximately 1 cm onto the perineal body (Fig. 7–6). This will build a cradle in which the rectal sphincter can be repaired. Polyglycolic acid derivative suture is appropriate for this closure, as are interrupted submucosal stitches. While there is no conclusive evidence that submucosal stitches are superior to transmucosal stitches, we prefer to avoid placing of stitches into the rectal lumen.

The cut ends of the anal sphincter next must be identified. These muscular structures usually will have retracted laterally and are best visualized when grasped with an Allis clamp incorporating both the muscle and its capsule. The anal sphincter is closed with sutures incorporating both the fascial sheath and small amounts of muscle (Fig. 7–7). Some

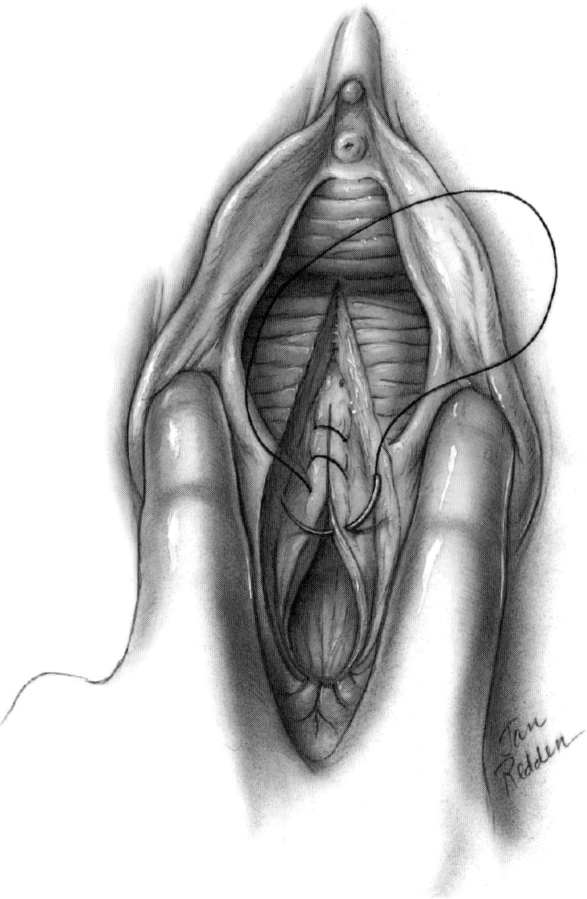

Figure 7–6. Repair of the midline episiotomy. The anchor stitch for closure of the rectal mucosa is placed 0.5–1 cm above the apex of the laceration. The rectal mucosa is then closed using either interrupted or running submucosal sutures of 000 or 0000 chromic or polyglycolic acid derivatives. Exposure can usually adequately be provided without assistance by use of the second and third finger of the operator's nondominant hand placed into the vagina and widely spread to provide exposure of the wound.

prefer to use 00 Vicryl on a taper CTX needle because the polygalactic acid maintains its tensile strength longer than chromic, and thus allows a longer period for healing. It is important to emphasize that the strength of this closure is obtained by incorporating fascia and not muscle. The fascial sheath is easier to close if the posterior capsule (commencing at 6 o'clock) is the first suture placed. The most cephalad stitch is placed next, at the 9 o'clock position of the left half of the sphincter capsule as viewed on cut end. The remainder of the capsule is closed with two or three interrupted stitches, the sequence of which is less important because visualization for these latter stitches is usually easy. It is important that approximately 1 cm of the sphincter capsule should be incorporated on each side and that the suture should be tied snugly but not so tight as to strangulate the tissue. Most caution against the use of a figure-of-eight stitch because it tends to bundle and strangulate tissue.

Next, the depth of the episiotomy is judged by placing two fingers of the left hand into the vagina and visualizing the apex of the episiotomy as the edges are pushed laterally. At this stage, three or four interrupted chromic or Vicryl stitches are placed in the rectovaginal fascia, effectively placing a second layered closure over the rectal mucosa (Fig. 7–8). In placing this stitch, the surgeon's attention is directed toward avoiding entry into the lumen of the rectum. Some individuals prefer to place this layer before repairing the anal sphincter.

The remainder of the episiotomy closure is simply that of a second-degree repair. Visualizing the apex of the incision into the vaginal mucosa, an anchor stitch is placed approximately 1 cm cephalad (Fig. 7–9). The vaginal mucosa then is closed with a running or run-lock 00 chromic or 00 Vicryl suture carried to the level of the hymenal ring. The final vaginal stitch may be either tied at this point or directed from inside the vagina out onto the

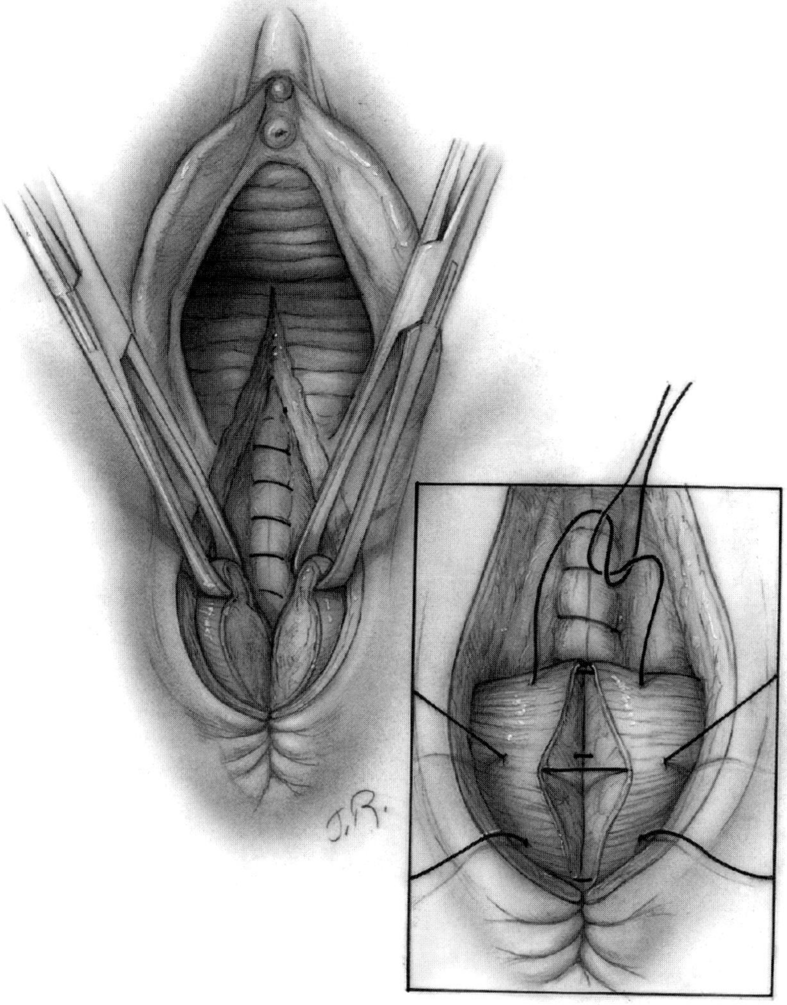

Figure 7–7. Repair of the midline episiotomy. Successful closure of the anal sphincter depends upon reapproximation of the capsule of the sphincter muscle. Approximately 1 cm of capsule should be grasped on each side with closure by interrupted sutures. Avoid figure-of-eight sutures because they may lead to strangulation and compromise the blood supply during the healing phase.

perineal body in the midline (Fig. 7–10). At this point, the depth of the defect on the perineal body must be assessed to determine whether closure can be adequately achieved in one layer or whether deep interrupted sutures will result in a superior closure. Where the cavity depth exceeds 1–1.5 cm, we prefer to place deep interrupted sutures in order to restore the perineum to its predelivery state. The deepest muscle layer that may have been incised or separated is the pubococcygeus. Two or three interrupted stitches usually will close this space.

Attention next is directed to placing the so-called crown stitch. This stitch is important to restore perineal anatomy and accomplishes reapproximation of the bulbocavernosus muscles and the labia. Reapproximation may be accomplished by interrupted sutures, the beginning of a new suture which will be used for a continuous closure, or a continuation of the suture used for the vaginal mucosa. Attention should be directed to ensuring that the reapproximation does not overly restrict the introitus and lead to dyspareunia. Following placement of the crown stitch, a continuous running suture is used to close the subcutaneous fat and the transverse perineal muscles. This stitch is carried to the inferior extension of the episiotomy on the perineal body, or to the end of the rectal mucosal closure, if one has been performed. At this point, a subcuticular suture is used to reapproximate skin edges (Fig. 7–11). At the apex the suture can again be directed from the midline into the vagina, following which the stitch can be placed through both sides of the vaginal mucosa and tied upon itself. The tissues should be snugly reapproximated, but not strangulated by undue tension. Such tension

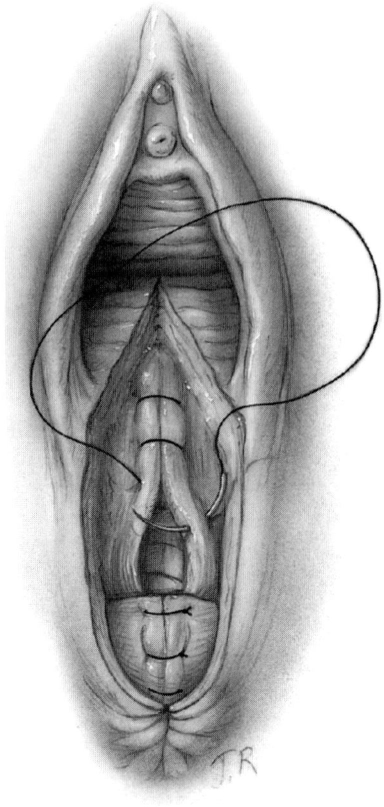

Figure 7–8. Repair of the midline episiotomy. A second layered closure is placed over the rectal mucosa by incorporating the rectovaginal fascia. Care is again exercised to avoid passing the needle and suture material into the lumen of the bowel. This layer is usually effectively closed with three or four interrupted sutures.

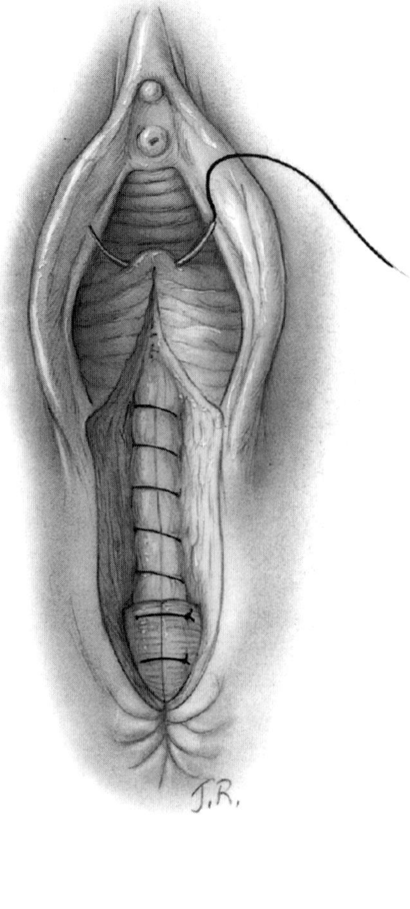

Figure 7–9. Repair of the midline episiotomy. Similar to the principal with the mediolateral episiotomy, an anchor stitch is placed approximately 1 cm beyond the most superior extent of the episiotomy. This is an important stitch to ensure that cut or bleeding vessels are not missed at the apex of the wound.

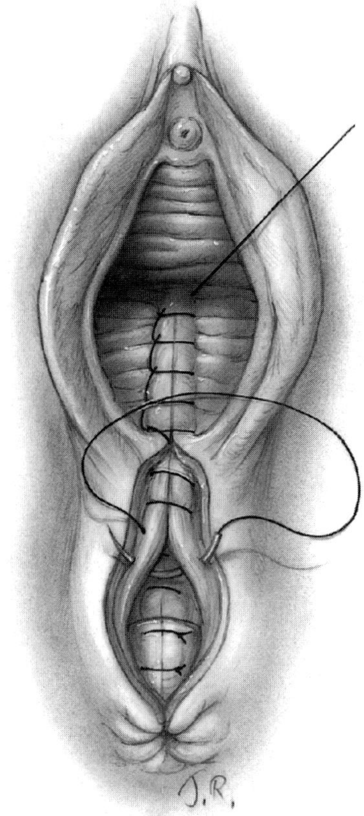

Figure 7–10. Repair of the midline episiotomy. The technique of using one suture for closure of the midline episiotomy is demonstrated. Once the vaginal mucosa has been reapproximated to the hymenal ring, the needle is passed from the midline of the vagina out onto the perineal body. The same suture can now be used for placement of the crown stitch.

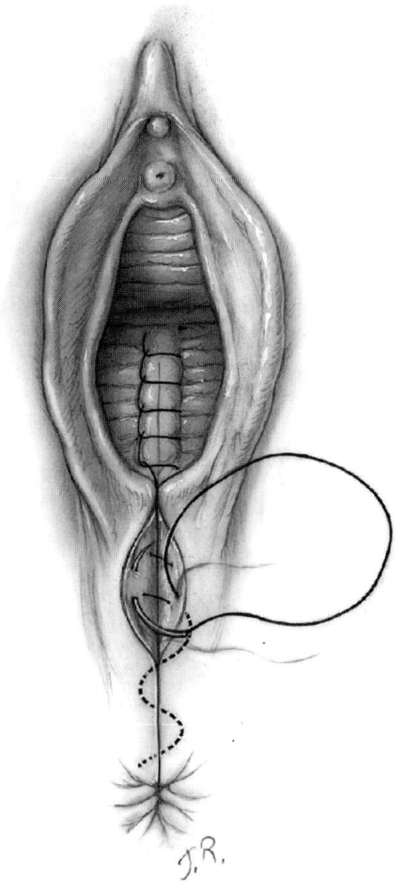

Figure 7–11. Repair of the midline episiotomy. The repair is completed by use of a subcuticular suture carried out from the inferior margin of the episiotomy upwards toward the hymenal ring. The suture is passed back into the vagina, where it is tied upon itself as opposed to leaving a knot on the perineal body.

is certain to increase episiotomy site swelling and subsequent discomfort.

Postpartum Pain Relief

Assuring postpartum comfort entails both local wound care as well as analgesics. Local measures begin immediately post-delivery and include such simple maneuvers as applying perineal ice packs. Efforts should be made to keep the perineal body and any injury sites clean and dry. Twenty-minute sitz baths performed two or three times daily are soothing and help to keep the site clean. A spray bottle or a surgigator device used after each voiding is helpful. Women should be instructed to blot the area dry. Hair dryers can also be used to keep the area dry.

A number of analgesic agents have been evaluated for postpartum pain treatment. Schachtel and colleagues (1989) demonstrated that ibuprofen (400 mg) and acetaminophen (1000 mg) were effective for postpartum pain relief compared with placebo. Ibuprofen was more effective than acetaminophen. Hopkinson (1980) evaluated single-dose ibuprofen (400 mg and 800 mg), propoxyphene hydrochloride (65 mg), and placebo in 322 women. He found both doses of ibuprofen to be significantly more effective than propoxyphene, which was more effective than placebo. In a comparison of single-dose ibuprofen (400 mg), zomepirac (100 mg), aspirin (600 mg), and placebo in 120 postpartum women, Sunshine and colleagues (1983) found ibuprofen to be most effective. As an alternative to oral therapy, indomethacin given as a 200-mg suppository was found to be highly effective in relieving early postpartum pain (Odigie, 1988).

EPISIOTOMY COMPLICATIONS

Postpartum Pain and Dyspareunia

Many studies of postpartum pain have centered upon the episiotomy as the dominant, if not the only cause of pain. With significant stretching of the maternal soft tissues, and to a lesser extent the bony pelvis, it is doubtful that all postpartum pain can be attributed to either an episiotomy or other lacerations. Thranov and colleagues (1990) studied 227 nulliparas delivered from the vertex presentation. They reported that episiotomy failed to account for differences in either magnitude of postpartum perineal symptoms or duration of those symptoms among three cohorts delivered by nurse midwives with episiotomy rates classified as low (20 percent), medium (35 percent), and high (70 percent). There was a significant correlation between postpartum pain and the duration of second-stage labor, viz., only 20 percent had perineal pain postpartum when the second stage was less than 15 minutes, half had pain if the second stage was 15 to 60 minutes, and 70 percent had pain when the second stage was longer than 60 minutes.

In the West Berkshire Perineal Management trial, Sleep and associates (1984) found that women managed with restrictive episiotomy had comparable pain at 10 days and 3 months postpartum when compared with women who underwent more liberal episiotomy. Harrison and co-workers (1984) made similar observations among women undergoing episiotomy in comparison with those who sustained a spontaneous second-degree tear at delivery. There were no differences in pain scores in the morning or afternoon on postpartum days 1–4 (Fig. 7–12). Larsson and associates (1991), however, reported pain at the 8-week postpartum examination in 4.6 percent of women who had undergone mediolateral episiotomies and in 2.9 percent of those who sustained spontaneous lacerations. At 8 weeks 16 percent with episiotomies and 11 percent with spontaneous lacerations reported dyspareunia. These results are similar to those in the West Berkshire trial, in which 22 percent of women in the restrictive group and 18 percent in the liberal group experienced dyspareunia at 3 months postpartum.

Identification of the precise etiology of postpartum perineal pain would appear important in assessing risk of episiotomy as well as treating pain effectively. Unfortunately, these issues are seldom addressed. One study reported that while up to a third of women had some perineal complaint—the dominant being dyspareunia—in only 25 percent of these, or less than 10 percent of the total study population, was the complaint directly referable to the episiotomy. In three-fourths of the cases, the source of the complaint was elsewhere, most often related to tenderness of the levator muscles (Isager-Sally and colleagues, 1986). When the study by Sleep and associates (1984), was followed up 3 years later, 15 percent of the women in both the restrictive and liberal episiotomy groups experienced at least occasional dyspareunia.

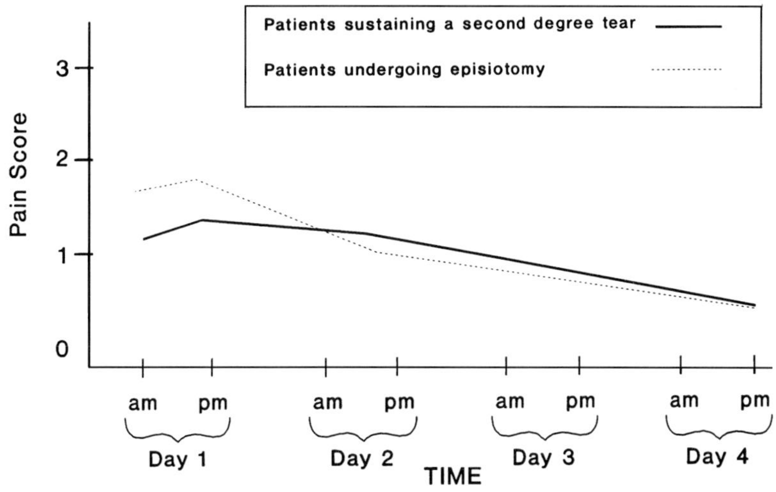

Figure 7–12. Mean pain score plotted against time for 40 women who underwent episiotomy and 37 who sustained a second-degree tear. All patients had unassisted deliveries. (From Harrison and associates, 1984.)

In a retrospective postal questionnaire, Bex and Hofmeyr (1987) attempted to address the incidence of dyspareunia 1–2 years following delivery. Surprisingly, almost 20 percent of women who were delivered by cesarean section, and who had never delivered vaginally, had dyspareunia. This was similar to the rate in women delivering vaginally with an intact perineum. No woman having a spontaneous tear at delivery experienced or reported dyspareunia, but almost 40 percent of the women undergoing episiotomy complained of dyspareunia. These authors noted a high rate of relationship difficulties—almost half—among women with pain and dyspareunia. Unfortunately, the data were insufficient to ascertain whether dyspareunia caused the dysfunctional relationship or vice versa.

In all of the above-referenced studies, mediolateral episiotomies were performed. In many, transcutaneous sutures were used to repair the perineal body, and in a significant number permanent sutures, which required subsequent removal. These factors may have contributed to increased perineal discomfort when compared with techniques using subcuticular closure (Grant, 1989). Studies of short- or long-term postpartum pain and dyspareunia involving midline episiotomies are notably scarce (Shiono and colleagues, 1990). In a direct comparison of 116 women with midline episiotomies and 192 with mediolateral episiotomies, Coats and associates (1980) found that 18 percent of the former and only 6 percent of the latter had resumed intercourse by the end of the first postpartum month. Thereafter, the percentages were roughly comparable, with the exception that 8 percent of women with mediolateral episiotomies and 4 percent with midline episiotomies had not resumed sexual intercourse by the end of the third month.

Endometriosis and the Episiotomy Scar

There are approximately 100 reported cases of endometriosis developing in episiotomy sites (Salamalekis and colleagues, 1990; Sayfan and associates, 1991). The latent period between the last episiotomy and symptoms ranges from a few months to several years. Cyclical pain during menses at the episiotomy site or a palpable mass are among the first symptoms. Some may manifest bloody discharge from the episiotomy scar either into the vagina or onto the perineal body during menstruation. Rare presentations include involvement of the anal sphincter, delayed infection, and abscess formation. Pathophysiologically it appears that decidual cells and endometrial glands become incorporated in the surgical repair site. Supporting this are observations of Paul and Tedeschi (1972), who reported 15 cases of endometriosis developing in the episiotomy scar site among 2028 consecutive deliveries who underwent uterine curettage at delivery prior to episiotomy repair. In comparison, none of 13,800 deliveries without curettage developed endometriosis. They found that lochia from curettage contained a much higher number of decidual and endometrial cells and glands than did lochia collected after delivery but without uterine curettage. Among all the cases reported, none followed a

TABLE 7–2. COMPARISON OF LACERATIONS INVOLVING THE ANAL SPHINCTER AND/OR RECTAL MUCOSA WITH SPONTANEOUS DELIVERIES WITHOUT EPISIOTOMY COMPARED TO THOSE WITH MIDLINE AND MEDIOLATERAL EPISIOTOMIES

Investigator (First Author)	Year	Country	No. of Patients	Episiotomy	Third Degree and/or Fourth Degree (%)
Kaltreider	1948	USA	15,167	Midline	4.5
			799	Mediolateral	5.0
			23,643	None	0.25
Sieber	1962	USA	1774	Midline	23.1*
			121	Mediolateral	0
			150	None	0
Harris	1970	USA	7477	Midline	13
Coates	1980	Great Britian	163	Midline	23.9
			244	Mediolateral	9.0
Harrison	1984	Great Britain	89	Mediolateral	6
			92	None	0
Sleep	1984	Great Britian	502	Mediolateral	0.2
			498	None	0.8
Beukins	1985	Belgium	6041	Mediolateral	1.4
			15,237	None	0.9
Thorp	1987	USA	265	Midline	13.2
			113	None	1.8
Borgatta	1989	USA	111	Midline	22.5
			130	None	2.3
Shiono	1990	USA	7264	Midline	9.7
			8508	Mediolateral	1.8
			7398	None	0.2
McGuiness	1991	USA	180	Midline	15
			187	None	2
Larsson	1991	Sweden	410	Mediolateral	3.9
			1479	None	2.6
Rockner	1991	Sweden	244	Mediolateral	.95
			556	None	.64
Walker	1991	Canada	3816	Midline	3
			1640	Mediolateral	4
			3538	None	1

*136 were intentional third degree.

spontaneous laceration. Treatment consists of simple surgical excision of all involved areas. Long-term results with this approach have been excellent, and there have been no reported recurrences.

Severe Posterior Perineal Trauma

Table 7–2 shows the incidences of injuries to the anal sphincter and/or rectal mucosa in women delivering without an episiotomy, as well as those undergoing mediolateral and midline episiotomies. Data presented are absolute rates, and the three groups were not controlled for confounding variables such as parity, indications for expedited delivery, maternal size, fetal size, or other factors. The risk of these injuries varies from 0 to 2.3 percent in women who do not require an episiotomy, from 0.2 to 9 percent in those with a mediolateral episiotomy, and from 3 to almost 24 percent in those undergoing a midline episiotomy.

The liberal use of midline episiotomy has not been compared with its restricted use in any randomized controlled trials. As discussed, three such studies have been conducted concerning mediolateral episiotomies (Harrison and associates, 1984; Sleep and colleagues, 1984; Argentine Episiotomy Trial Collaborative Group, 1993). Three other studies of mediolateral episiotomies appear to have adequate randomization without bias such that the effect of episiotomy on perineal trauma can be evaluated. In the West Brookshire trials (Sleep and associates, 1984), women were allocated to one of two groups. In the first, the midwife was asked to try to prevent a perineal laceration by performing an episiotomy if considered necessary to prevent imminent lacerations; the goal was delivery without any trauma if possible. In the second, the midwife was asked to try to avoid an episiotomy; its use was restricted to the indication of fetal or maternal distress. The resulting episiotomy rates in the two groups were 50 and 10 percent, respectively. In the trial by Harrison and associates (1984), women were allocated either to routine episiotomy in all cases or to restricted episiotomy performed only as indicated. The more stringent indications for episiotomy resulted in a rate of 8 percent.

The Argentine Episiotomy Trial Collaborative Group in a randomized prospective study compared selective episiotomy, limited to specified maternal or fetal indications, to routine episiotomy following the participating hospital's usual practice. The ratios of episiotomy were 30.1 percent in the selective group and 82.6 percent in the routine group: 39.5 percent and 90.7 percent, respectively among nulliparous women and 16.3 percent and 70.5 percent, respectively, among primiparous women. As expected, the need for surgical repair of any posterior perineal trauma was greater in the routine versus the selective episiotomy group (Table 7–3). However, severe perineal trauma, defined as the extension through the anal sphincter and/or the anal or rectal mucosa, was 1.2 percent in the selective group and 1.5 percent in the routine group, yielding a relative risk of 1.28 (95 percent CI 0.65–2.5).

In three other trials conducted similarly, the episiotomy rates were 43 percent in the routine group versus 20 percent in the restrictive group (Stewart and colleagues, 1983), 42 versus 34 percent (Flint and Poulengeris, 1987), and 55 versus 22 percent (Henrikson and associates, 1992). Liberal or routine use of episiotomy was associated with higher overall rates of posterior perineal trauma (Table 7–3). Further, there was no evidence that a policy of liberal episiotomy use reduced the risk of serious perineal or vaginal trauma. Borgatta and associates (1989) emphasized that the risk of a third- or fourth-degree episiotomy extension is increased by use of a delivery table and stirrups. In comparison to women whose legs were unrestrained and in either a modified supine, semisitting, lateral, chair, or squat position, women delivered in stirrups were 14 times more likely to sustain a third- or fourth-degree laceration. Similarly, the odds ratio for third- or fourth-degree lacerations was 22 if an episiotomy was required. In data from the Collaborative Perinatal Project, Shiono and collaborators (1990) found that women undergoing a midline episiotomy were 50 times more likely to sustain a third- or fourth-degree injury compared with those without an episiotomy. Women undergoing a mediolateral episiotomy were eight times more likely to sustain a third- or fourth-degree laceration compared with those who did not undergo episiotomy. The peripartum factors associated with the occurrence of third- or fourth-degree lacerations are shown in Table 7–4.

The dramatic effect of changing the mode of practice from exclusive use of mediolateral episiotomies to near exclusive use of midline episiotomies is demonstrated in Figure 7–13. During the period from 1935 to 1965 when mediolateral episiotomies were used almost exclusively, less than 1 percent of women sustained third- or fourth-degree tears. Beginning in 1965 when midline episiotomies virtually replaced mediolateral episiotomies, the rate of third- and fourth-degree injuries increased to a plateau level of 11 percent for third-degree and 6.4 percent for fourth-degree lacerations.

Anterior Perineal Trauma

A consistent finding in women delivered without episiotomy has been a higher frequency of anterior tears involving the clitoris and the labial folds. In the West Berkshire randomized prospective study, such tears complicated 26 percent of those in the restrictive group compared with 17 percent in those for whom episiotomy was more liberally used. The Argentine group reported similar results; anterior perineal trauma occurred in 19 percent of the selective episiotomy group and in 8 percent of the routine episiotomy group. Most investigators report that only about a third of all women will successfully negotiate childbirth without sustaining either an episiotomy or a spontaneous laceration that requires suturing (Harrison, 1984; Larsson, 1991; Rockner, 1991; Sleep, 1984; Wilkerson, 1984 and their many colleagues).

TABLE 7–3. EFFECT OF LIBERAL USE OF MEDIOLATERAL EPISIOTOMY IN SPONTANEOUS VAGINAL DELIVERY ON ANY POSTERIOR PERINEAL TRAUMA

Study	Liberal Use		Restrictive Use		Odds Ratio	Graph of Odds Ratios and Confidence Intervals
	n	*(%)*	*n*	*(%)*	*(95% CI)*	*0.01 0.1 0.5 1 2 10 100*
Sleep et al. (1984)	380/502	(75.70)	329/498	(66.06)	1.59 (1.21–2.09)	
Stewart et al. (1983)	76/90	(84.44)	68/94	(72.34)	2.03 (1.01–4.08)	
Flint and Poulengeris (1987)	334/438	(76.26)	336/443	(75.85)	1.02 (0.75–1.39)	
Harrison et al. (1984)	89/89	(100.0)	73/92	(79.35)	8.90 (3.45–22.97)	
Henriksen et al. (1992)	440/597	(73.7)	502/808	(62.13)	1.8 (1.4–2.2)	
Argentine Collaborative (1993)	1138/1291	(88.1)	817/1296	(63.1)	1.39 (1.33–1.47)	
Typical odds ratio (95% confidence interval)					1.47 (1.21–1.78)	

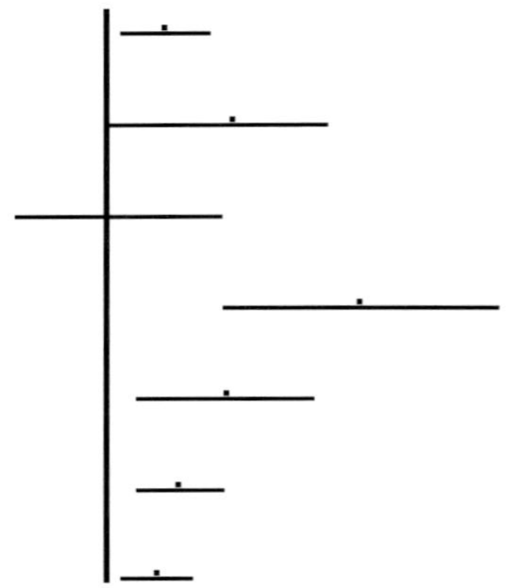

TABLE 7–4. FACTORS ASSOCIATED WITH THIRD- AND FOURTH-DEGREE LACERATIONS

Factor	Laceration		Odds Ratio	95% CI	*P* Value for Differences
	None–2°	*3–4°*			
Episiotomy					
None	7398	16 (0.2%)	1.0		
Mediolateral	8502	153 (1.8%)	8.3	5.0, 13.9	
Midline	7264	781 (9.7%)	49.7	30.3, 81.6	
Forceps					
None	12,357	123 (1.0%)	1.0		
Outlet	3701	287 (7.2%)	7.8	6.3, 9.7	
Low	4077	322 (7.3%)	7.9	6.4, 9.8	
Mid + high	2516	189 (7.0%)	7.5	6.0, 9.5	
Parity					
0	7850	711 (8.3%)	5.8	5.0, 6.8	
1+	15,282	237 (1.5%)	1.0		
Race					
Black	12,009	301 (2.5%)	1.0		
White	11,155	649 (5.5%)	2.3	2.0, 2.7	
Presentation					
Occiput anterior	20,188	787 (3.8%)	1.0		
Occiput transverse	1000	75 (7.0%)	1.9	1.5, 2.4	
Occiput posterior	1532	80 (5.0%)	1.3	1.1, 1.7	
Vertex unspecified	375	7 (1.8%)	0.5	0.2, 1.0	
Other, non-breech	69	1 (1.4%)	0.4	0.1, 2.7	
Birth weight (g)[a]	3148	3310			< .0001
Maternal age (yr)[a]	24.0	21.7			< .0001
Maternal height (cm)[a]	161.5	161.0			.06
Prepregnant weight (kg)[a]	59.4	55.7			< .0001

CI = confidence interval
[a]Data are presented as means
Modified from Shino and associates (1990).

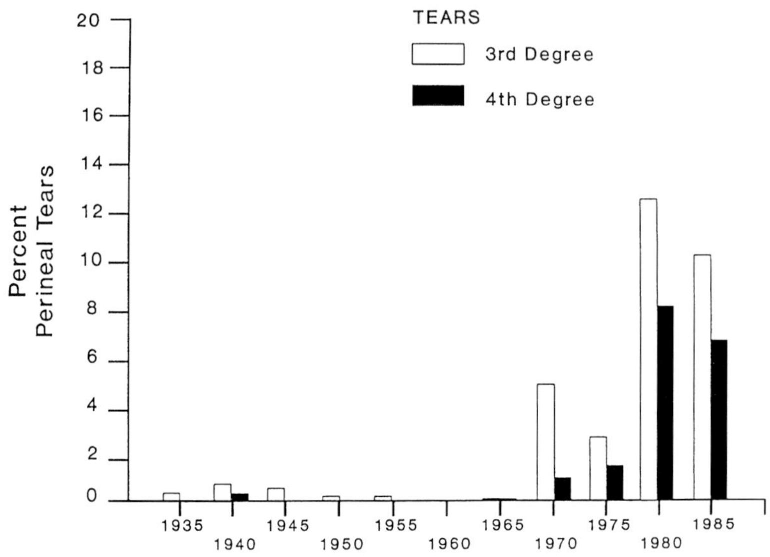

Figure 7–13. Percentage of third- and fourth-degree perineal tears for vaginal deliveries between 1935 and 1985. (From Legino and associates, 1988.)

Injury to the Pelvic Floor and Urinary and Fecal Incontinence

The question of whether stress incontinence is caused or aggravated by vaginal delivery remains controversial. A long-held belief is that injury to the pelvic muscles or to their nerve supply or interconnecting fascia is an inevitable consequence of vaginal delivery, particularly if the delivery is difficult. Before onset of labor, the vaginal diameter is approximately 4–5 cm, and the cervix is closed. Both organs must dilate to a diameter of 10 cm during childbirth, causing the connective tissue of the cervix to undergo more dilation because of its initially smaller size. Nevertheless, cervical connective tissue almost always recovers to the point that dilation before any subsequent curettage requires considerable effort. Additionally, cervical incompetence is a rare phenomenon relative to the number of deliveries. Because the vagina undergoes less dilation and distension than the cervix, it is questionable that damage to the endopelvic fascia would be any greater than that to the cervix. Also questionable is the concept that the cardinal ligaments are damaged during labor due to tension as the fetus descends. The cardinal ligaments may come under progressively *less* tension as the cervix dilates and they are actually pushed toward their points of attachment. Additionally, as the cervix does not descend markedly within the pelvis with progression of labor, and even though it can at times be pulled all the way through the vaginal introitus while being inspected for lacerations after the fetus has been delivered, examination at 6-weeks and 1-year postpartum usually discloses a normally supported cervix. It therefore seems unlikely that the cardinal and uterosacral ligaments are irreparably stretched and more likely that the response to traction occasionally noted immediately after delivery reflects connective tissue softening as opposed to actual tissue damage and destruction.

The levator ani muscles may be injured by one of two mechanisms during parturition: first, direct injury either by mechanical disruption or overelongation; second, damage to the nerve supply to the muscle. Obstetricians performing forceps delivery occasionally have reported feeling something snap or the sudden loss of resistance, suggesting tearing of the levator ani muscles from a purely mechanical injury. When stretched more than 50 percent of its total length, striated muscle may suffer major damage. Portions of the levator ani muscles must elongate by at least 50 percent in order to surround the fetal head (Fig. 7–14). Superimposed upon the potential muscle damage accompanying vaginal birth are the effects of aging. Striated muscle function normally decreases by 1 percent annually after peaking in midlife. This cumulative decrease will be added to whatever connective tissue damage is also present. Neurologic injury to these muscles is also well documented (Smith and colleagues, 1989; Snooks and Swash, 1984; Snooks and associates, 1984, 1985). As the small nerves are torn away from their muscle fibers, contractile ability is diminished and normal function is lost.

Maternal pelvic birth-related trauma includes both reversible and irreversible injuries, even in the context of what is usually considered an uncomplicated delivery. Because the opening in the pelvic floor through which the fetal head must pass is relatively small, the head pushes the floor downward until it has dilated the opening sufficiently to pass through (Fig. 7–14). Descent not only causes potentially damaging elongation of the levator ani muscles, but also stretches their attached nerves, causing possible neuromuscular injury. Because the nerve begins at the ischial spine and runs on the inner surface of the muscle, damage can occur from direct elongation (Fig. 7–15). The more the floor must descend before the head passes through it, the greater the possible neural injury. In addition, further downward descent would cause more damage to connective tissue supports and attachments.

The question then is not whether vaginal delivery will cause injury to the pelvic diaphragm, but rather the degree of injury and whether episiotomy affords protection. A frequent claim made in support of liberal use of episiotomy is that it prevents pelvic floor relaxation during delivery and thereby prevents urinary incontinence and genital prolapse (Flood, 1982; Willson, 1981). If the intention is to protect the pelvic floor, however, a much more extensive incision than is usual would almost certainly be required and could not be accomplished with a midline episiotomy (Goodlin, 1983). As previously noted, liberal and restricted use of episiotomy are associated with contrasting patterns of trauma: liberal episiotomy is associated with a lower frequency of anterior vaginal and labial tears,

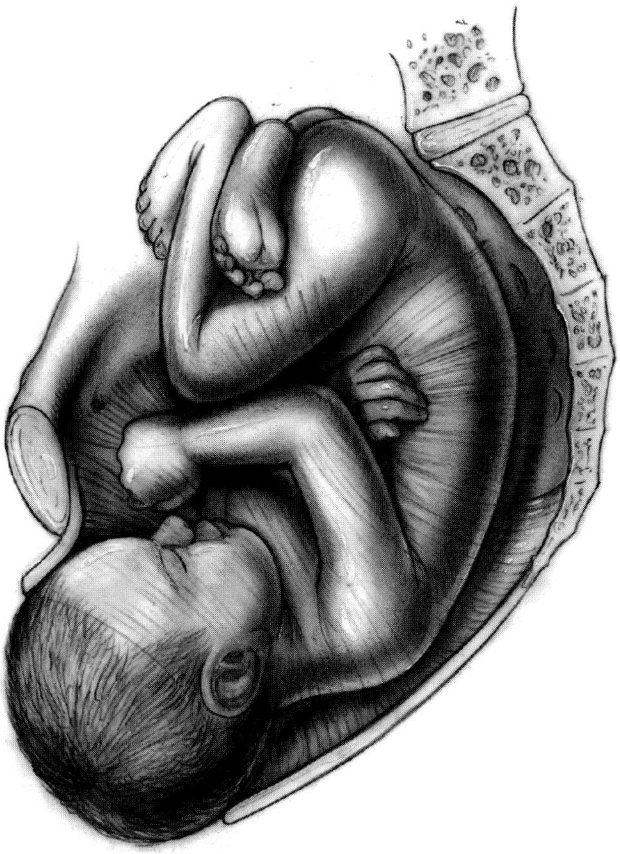

Figure 7–14. As the fetus descends through the birth canal, portions of the levator ani muscles elongate far in excess of 50 percent in order to surround the fetal head. Such elongation may contribute to irreversible damage of the striated muscle.

but with increased posterior trauma. This raises the possibility that episiotomy may have a more specific protective effect on the tissues around the bladder neck. The findings in an observational study of two groups of women that were matched on some prognostic variables, but who had different forms of perineal care, is consistent with this. Women with vaginal tears not only had more labial tears, but also had a higher incidence of cystocele (Brendsel and colleagues, 1981). A small matched pair study, however, found no statistically significant difference in the rates of genital prolapse between women who had and had not had episiotomies, and perineometer readings were similar in the two groups (Brendsel and associates, 1979).

Incontinence

Childbirth itself is often blamed for long-term, persistent stress incontinence, yet many women have stress incontinence for the first time **during pregnancy.** The prevalence of this symptom increases steadily to a rate of 40–70 percent by the end of pregnancy (Francis, 1960a,b; Stanton and associates, 1980). For most women, stress incontinence resolves in the first few weeks after birth, but in an important minority, the symptom persists. According to Stanton and colleagues (1980), about 6 percent of primiparas have stress incontinence at the 6-week postnatal examination; some had had the symptom before pregnancy. About 10 percent of multiparas, most of whom had this symptom prior to pregnancy, also have stress incontinence at 6 weeks postpartum. Francis observed (1960a,b) that only 6 percent of the women who had stress incontinence in pregnancy had persistent incontinence, but the symptoms returned in another 40 percent when they developed a precipitating factor such as a cough. Francis emphasized that in

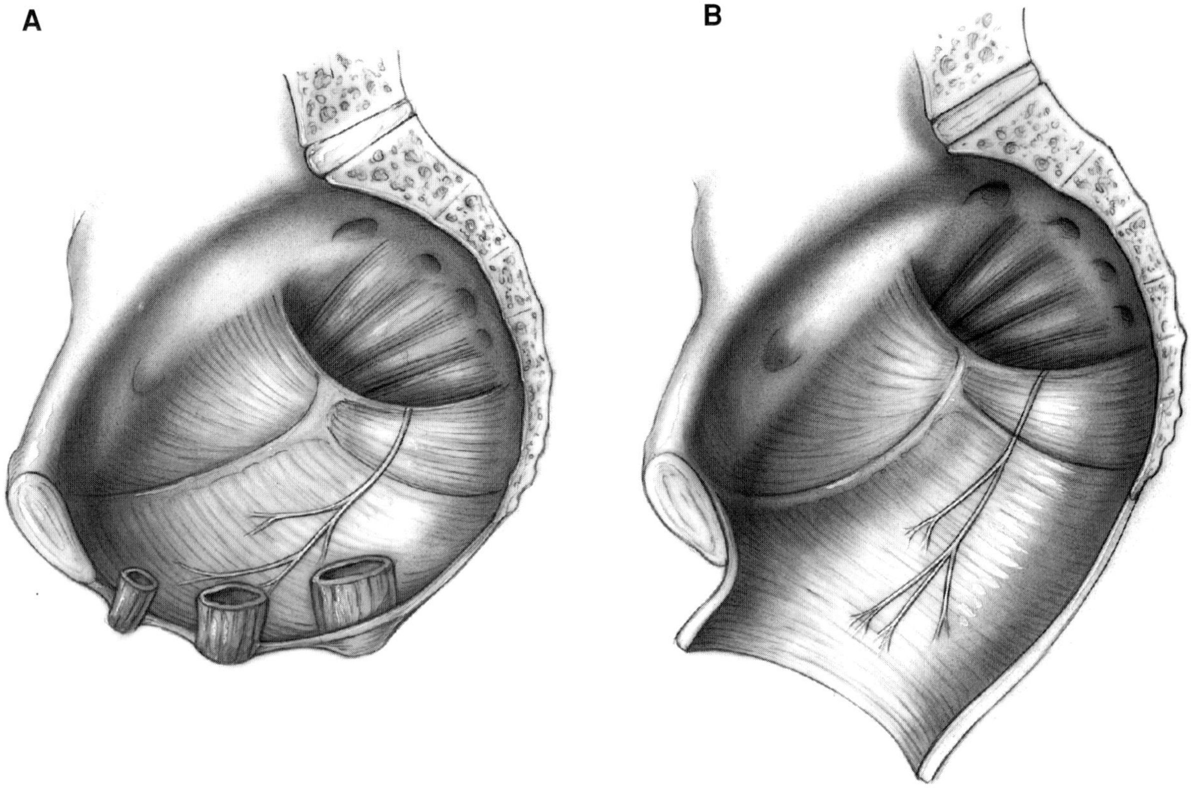

Figure 7–15. A. The normal position of the pelvic floor and the nerve that supplies the levator ani muscles. **B.** Structural changes in the levator ani muscle are shown at the time that the fetus is being expelled. Note the tremendous elongation and stretch of the nerve, which may result in temporary or permanent injury.

none of the women did stress incontinence appear for the first time postnatally. Others, however, have reported that in 4–20 percent of women who have stress incontinence, the symptom first developed in the peripartum period (Beck and Hsu, 1965; Iosif, 1981).

Evidence that both urinary and fecal incontinence result from damage to the nerves of the pelvic floor has come from Snooks and Swash and their colleagues (1984, 1985). They found that in three-fourths of women with fecal incontinence of no clear cause, there is histologic evidence of denervation of pelvic floor muscles, especially the puborectalis and the external anal sphincter. Among women who sustained an injury to the sphincter, Harris (1970) reported that 3 percent had only fair tone, whereas 4 percent had poor tone. His measurements were subjective and based upon the ability of the patient to contract the rectal sphincter around the examiner's finger. When evaluating 20 women with complete third-degree lacerations, Go and Dunselman (1988) performed both anal manometry and single-needle electromyography of the external sphincter. Among these women, mediolateral episiotomy was performed in seven, and median episiotomy in four; in nine, no episiotomy was cut and the tear was spontaneous. Contrary to observations by others, these investigators found an uneventful recovery in all women as confirmed by restoration of the anal pressures of both voluntary and involuntary control to within low to low-normal limits. Notwithstanding, three women complained of incontinence despite normal test of innervation, physiologic function, and appearance of the repair.

Women who have stress urinary incontinence also have slowed conduction of the perineal branch of the pudendal nerve, which innervates the periurethral voluntary sphincter muscle (Snooks and Swash, 1984). Further studies in women with isolated stress urinary incontinence have shown slowed conduction in the perineal branch of the pudendal nerve with normal conduction to the external anal sphincter muscle (Snooks and colleagues, 1985). Slowed conduction of the pudendal nerve is common immediately after vaginal delivery and is usually transitory (Snooks and associates, 1984). As perhaps expected, conduction is unchanged following cesarean delivery. Delay in return to normal conduction is more common following instrumental delivery and in multiparous women. Not all women with stress incontinence show abnormal conduction patterns. Stress incontinence associated with vaginal delivery is still most commonly attributed to stretching or damage to pelvic muscle and fascia, and in particular the perineal body.

Whatever the etiology of postpartum stress incontinence, there is little evidence that more liberal use of episiotomy protects against this sometimes debilitating condition. Early follow-up of women in the West Berkshire trial indicated that 20 percent of women in both groups had involuntary loss of urine at 3 months after delivery and 6 percent reported occasional use of a perineal pad (Sleep and associates, 1984). Using a postal inquiry, investigators followed up 674 of the original 1,000 women 3 years after delivery. In the group undergoing restrictive use of episiotomy (10 percent rate), 22 percent reported incontinence less than once per week compared with 25 percent in the liberal episiotomy group (51 percent rate). In the restrictive episiotomy group, 12 percent reported incontinence once or twice a week compared with 11 percent in the liberal episiotomy group; in both groups more than 2 percent of patients reported leakage of urine more than three times weekly (Sleep and Grant, 1987). The problem was severe enough that 8 and 7 percent of the patients in the restrictive and liberal groups, respectively, used a perineal pad occasionally, 2 percent on at least some occasions, and 1 percent every day. Rockner (1990) reported a similar incidence of stress urinary incontinence among women who had an episiotomy (36 percent) versus a spontaneous tear (36 percent). Incontinence symptoms sufficient to merit wearing a pad developed in 10 percent of women with episiotomy and in 14 percent with a spontaneous tear. Rockner studied women 4 years postpartum. It is possible that differences in the degree of incontinence manifest in each of these groups, based upon perineal management during childbirth, will only emerge over much longer observation times.

That perineal management has little effect on subsequent muscle function is also consistent with the findings of an observational study of perineal muscle function using a perineometer performed 1 year after childbirth (Gordon and Logue, 1985). There was no association between pressure measurements and the degree of perineal trauma. In a study with a significantly different design, Rockner and colleagues (1991a) used vaginal cones weighing from 10 to 100 g to evaluate pelvic floor muscle strength. The experimental design consisted of insertion of cones with increasing weights until the heaviest cone could not be retained for at least 1 minute in the erect standing position or while walking. These investigators observed that at 36 weeks' gestation, all women could maintain a vaginal cone weighing 90 grams or greater. When subsequently measured 8 weeks postpartum, those women who had cesarean deliveries had no decrement in the weight of cone they could support. In contrast, women who had spontaneous vaginal deliveries with intact perineum had a 19-g decrement in weight that they could support, those who sustained a spontaneous laceration also had a 19-g decrement, whereas those who had mediolateral episiotomies had a 30-g decrement. Notably, the episiotomy group did significantly worse than the other women delivering vaginally even though there was no difference between groups in maternal weight, duration of either first- or second-stage labor, Apgar scores, or birthweights.

Only three long-term studies have evaluated the effects of perineal management at 10 years or more following delivery. The studies are impaired because they are retrospective and descriptive. Shown in Figure 7–16 are data from one long-term study, in which 1,000 women in whom forceps deliveries and episiotomies were used were compared with controls without an episiotomy. The investigators concluded that episiotomy limited damage to the pelvic floor. The incidence of urethral detachment, cystoceles, rectoceles, and levator injury were reduced by greater than half relative to controls. Smith and colleagues (1989) indirectly supported these observations; among 105 women studied who had stress urinary incontinence, genital prolapse, or both, only one was nulliparous. Data from a period beginning in the late 1940s indicates that protecting the pelvic floor by the methods cited

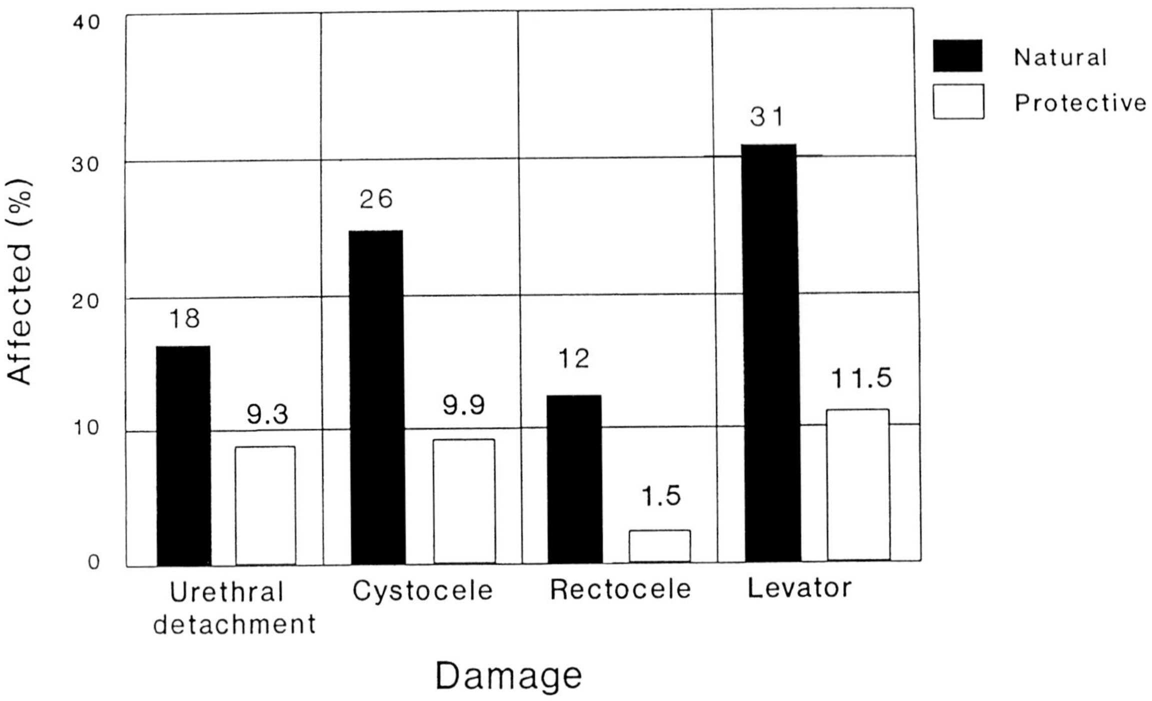

Figure 7–16. Comparative study of 1,000 women delivered without an episiotomy compared with 1,000 women with an episiotomy. The data show the difference in damage to the pelvic floor as manifested by urethral detachment, cystocele, rectocele, and injury to the levator ani muscles. (From Gainey, 1955.)

above effectively reduced the incidence of genital prolapse later in life (Ranney, 1990). One would expect that the prevalence of prolapse might be unaffected during the first 20 years after instituting a program of protecting the pelvic floor because women of an age likely to develop prolapse would have been delivered with older methods. However, once the women studied reached an age at which prolapse might be expected, prevalence of cystocele, rectocele, and enterocele decreased significantly. Analysis showed this result could not be explained simply by changes in demographics or parity.

Wound Healing and Infection

Considering that episiotomies or spontaneous tears take place in an area that is always colonized with bacteria and always subject to at least a degree of mechanical trauma from the birthing process, it is surprising that poor healing and infection are not more common. Generally, wound healing complications occur more often following mediolateral episiotomies than they do following midline operations. The lowest frequency of healing complications, however, are in women with spontaneous lacerations. Some authors report excellent results with mediolateral episiotomies and cite no cases of infection, wound breakdown, or delayed healing (Harrison and colleagues, 1984). In contrast, others have reported that women with mediolateral episiotomies have more complications than those with spontaneous tears (Rockner and associates, 1988). Specifically, 22 percent of those with episiotomies developed wound infections compared with 2 percent of those with spontaneous tears. Hematoma or bruising at the episiotomy site was found in 38 percent of women with episiotomies versus 13 percent of those sustaining spontaneous tears. Local swelling was three times as likely among those with episiotomies, and closure was judged to be insufficient in 40 percent compared with 13 percent who had spontaneous tears. When evaluated on the sixth postpartum day, the wound had not yet healed in half of those with episiotomies compared with 20 percent with spontaneous tears. These poor outcomes were no doubt partially accounted for by use of transcutaneous dexon or ticron stitches, which were removed on the sixth day. In a Swedish study, Rockner and Olund (1991) reported infection in 10 percent of women with mediolateral episiotomies compared with 2 percent of women who sustained spontaneous lacerations. Disturbed healing was noted in 30 percent of the former group and 10 percent of the latter.

McGuinness and colleagues (1991) described primarily midline episiotomies and found that 8 percent of women experienced delayed healing with complications mostly confined to those sustaining damage to the anal sphincter or rectal mucosa. In comparison, delayed healing was noted in 2 percent of women without episiotomies; however, the number increased to 4 percent if spontaneous lacerations had occurred. The reported frequency of midline episiotomy infections ranges from the low of 0.05 percent reported by Owen and Hauth (1990), to 0.1 percent reported by Harris (1970), to 2.5 percent reported by Kaltreider and Dixon (1948), to 3.7 percent reported by Jacobs and Adams (1960). The infection rate is higher when lacerations extend to involve the anal sphincter and/or rectal mucosa. In this select population, O'Leary and O'Leary (1964) reported a 10 percent infection rate.

Perineal abscess, rectovaginal fistula, and complete dehiscence are among the most debilitating complications of episiotomies. A rectovaginal fistula or dehiscence with cloacal formation is far more frequent following midline episiotomy. Sieber and Kroon (1962) observed that 2 percent of cases involving extensions into the rectal mucosa resulted in a perineal abscess and 0.25 percent developed a rectovaginal fistula. This is similar to the 0.3 percent rectovaginal fistula rate in women with fourth-degree episiotomies reported by Harris (1970). Brantley and Burwell (1960) reported that 1.4 percent of women with a fourth-degree perineal laceration developed rectovaginal fistula. The highest incidence of such fistulas was in women in whom an episioproctotomy was performed intentionally (Norris, 1962). Beynon (1974) surveyed the literature and found 18 cases (0.65 percent) of rectovaginal fistula that followed a total of 27,655 midline episiotomies.

Classification and Treatment of Episiotomy Infections

Episiotomy and lower genital tract infections can be classified according to the depth of infection (Table 7–5). An accurate and early diagnosis is important, and the depth of infection must be clinically assessed to guide management (Owen and Hauth, 1990; Shy and Eschenbach, 1979). The more benign infections involve only the skin and subcutaneous tissues (simple) and the edge of the superficial fascia but without necrosis. An intermediate depth consists of necrotizing infection limited to the superficial fascia. Deep infections involve deep fascial layers to potentially include the rectus sheath, inferior fascia of the urogenital diaphragm, or inferior fascia of the levator ani and underlying muscle layers (Fig. 7–17).

Simple Episiotomy Infection. This is a local infection limited to the skin and superficial fascia along the episiotomy incision. In contrast to deeper infection, the associated edema and erythema are adjacent to the episiotomy. Any progression into skin or superficial fascia

TABLE 7–5. CLASSIFICATION OF EPISIOTOMY INFECTIONS

Superficial	Simple—skin and subcutaneous tissues Superficial fascial infection without necrosis
Intermediate	Superficial fascial necrosis (necrotizing fasciitis) 1. Extensive necrosis with widespread undermining of surrounding tissue 2. Moderate-to-severe systemic reaction with altered mental status 3. Absence of muscle involvement 4. Failure to demonstrate clostridia in wound and blood cultures 5. Absence of major vascular occlusion 6. Pathologic examination of debrided tissue showing intense leukocytic infiltration, focal necrosis of fascia and surrounding tissues, and thrombosis of microvasculature
Deep	Myonecrosis

Modified from Fisher and colleagues (1979).

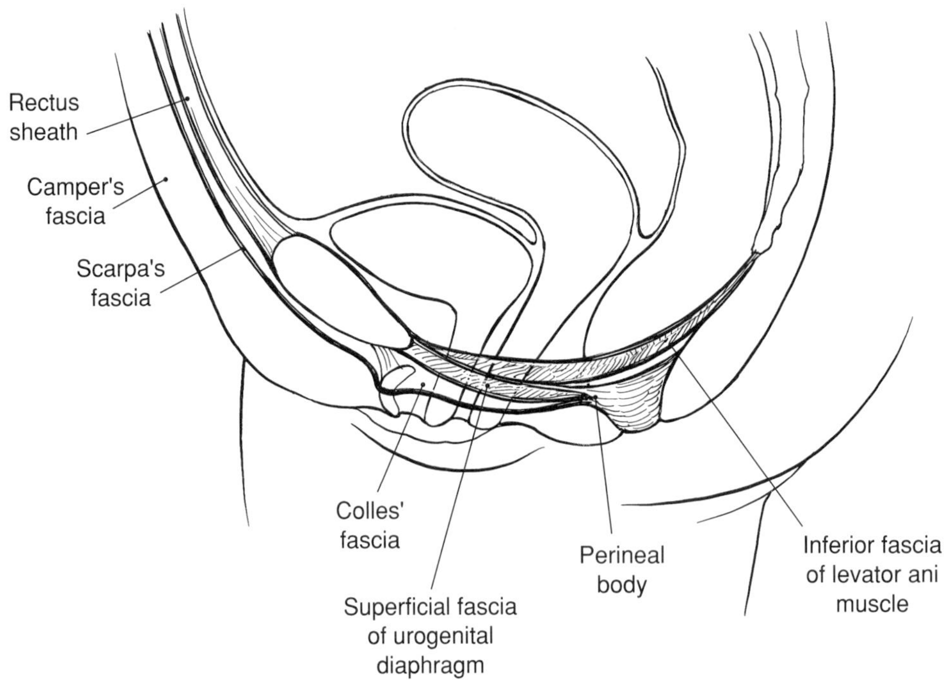

Figure 7–17. Sagittal section of the perineum and lower abdominal wall showing the significant muscle groups and superficial fascial layers.

of the thigh, buttock, or abdominal wall is presumptive evidence of a substantially more severe infection. Bullae formation, skin necrosis, and systemic manifestation are not characteristic of simple episiotomy infection.

Management includes exploration and debridement under adequate anesthesia. Associated hematomas are drained. An acutely infected episiotomy should not be resutured. If the superficial fascial layer is extensively infected, antimicrobials are given. Coverage should be targeted to streptococcal organisms including Group A, Group D, and anaerobic species; staphylococci; aerobic enterobacteriaceae; and anaerobes, including *Bacteroides* species and *Fusobacterium necrophorum* (Fisher and colleagues, 1979; Shy and Eschenbach, 1979).

Superficial Fascial Infection. Infection involving Colles fascia on the perineum or Camper and Scarpa fascia on the lower abdominal wall, constituting the superficial fascia, is an infection of intermediate depth. It is important to distinguish these infections from simple episiotomy infections and from the more severe and deeper fascial infections. There are two infections of the superficial fascia: the more common is infection of the superficial fascia without necrosis, and less common but more severe is infection with associated necrosis.

Signs and symptoms of superficial fascial infection without necrosis are neither striking nor distinctive. Consequently, surgical exploration may be necessary to rule out necrosis. If there is no necrosis, the skin may be erythematous and edematous, but there will be no severe systemic manifestations. Response to antimicrobial therapy should occur within 24–48 hours; however, if there is a poor clinical response, or if the woman's condition worsens during therapy, then the episiotomy should be surgically explored. In these instances, debridement is the hallmark of therapy and should be carried laterally until vital tissues are encountered.

Necrotizing Fasciitis. The first description of rapidly progressive fascial necrosis caused by superficial bacterial infections was in 1871 by Joseph Jones, a Confederate Army surgeon. The term "necrotizing fasciitis" is attributed to Wilson (1952), who introduced it to describe an uncommon, severe superficial infection associated with fascial necrosis. This infection has an acute onset and a rapid course with prominent systemic manifestations and a high fatality rate, variously reported from 20 to 80 percent. Necrotizing fasciitis has been known by a host of terms, including gangrenous erysipelas, hospital gangrene, acute dermal gangrene, and necrotizing erysipelas.

Both layers of the superficial perineal fascia become necrotic as infection spreads along fascial planes (Fig. 7–17). The superficial layer of the superficial fascia (Camper's fascia) is fibroadipose tissue and comprises most of the labia majora. On the anterior abdominal wall, this fascia is recognized as subcutaneous fat. The deep layer of the superficial fascia on the perineum (Colles' fascia) is membranous and without adipose tissue. The deep layer of the superficial fascia in the abdominal wall (Scarpa fascia) is simply a continuation of the deep layer of superficial fascia from the perineum (Colles' fascia).

While the deep layer of the superficial fascia may prevent infection from reaching deeper structures, infection may spread along this fascial plane from the perineum to the anterior abdominal wall. Characteristically, only the superficial fascia is involved, and deep fascia such as the inferior fascia of the urogenital diaphragm and the inferior fascia of the levator ani are relatively spared. Fisher and colleagues (1979) have proposed six criteria that allow exclusion of closely allied soft tissue infections that may mimic necrotizing fasciitis from actual necrotizing fasciitis (Table 7–5).

Because the skin is not the primary site of infection in necrotizing fasciitis, superficial manifestations are variable, and diagnosis by inspection alone is unreliable. Nevertheless, initially there usually is cutaneous edema and erythema with indistinct margins that gradually fade into normal areas. The color of affected skin may become blue or brown as infection progresses. As nutrient vessels to the skin become occluded, vesicles and bullae form, and the skin may become gangrenous. Progressive edema follows. An initial marked local tenderness is frequently seen, but once the cutaneous nerves are affected the lesion may become hypesthetic or even anesthetic. Because of associated bacterial toxin production, there are profound volume shifts, and underlying anemia may be masked by hemoconcentration.

While treatment of these women is multifaceted and includes empirical broad-spectrum antimicrobial coverage and support of cardiovascular and respiratory systems, the hallmark of successful treatment is surgical exploration and debridement. Shown in Table 7–6 are 13 maternal deaths from necrotizing fasciitis arising from an episiotomy wound. Importantly, although antimicrobial and general supportive therapy were instituted in a timely fashion in all of these women, surgical exploration often was delayed or too limited. Surgical exploration should be performed if there is skin edema or erythema beyond the immediate area of the episiotomy, if severe systemic manifestations are present, or if the infection does not resolve after 24–48 hours of intravenous antimicrobial therapy. During exploration, separation of the skin from the underlying deep fascia and a bloodless incision through superficial fascia are strong prognostic signs of necrotizing fasciitis (Fig. 7–18). Often the surgeon finds a serosanguineous exudate rather than grossly purulent accumulations. The necrotic superficial fascia usually forms a dull gray layer with partial liquefaction of subcutaneous fat. Debridement margins are reached when the subcutaneous tissue cannot be separated from the underlying normal deep fascia or from normal skin and when there is free flow of blood at the margins of dissection. A frozen tissue section may clarify the diagnosis when fascial necrosis is uncertain; often, however, it is obvious.

Myonecrosis. Infection beneath the deep fascia may involve the muscles and produce necrosis. Myonecrosis is most commonly caused by *Clostridium perfringens* infection, although it can develop from neglected necrotizing infection of deep fascia. Another cause of myonecrosis of the gluteal or psoas muscles is from bacteria introduced into this deep space by a paracervical or pudendal needle.

Clostridial infections may develop early postpartum, as illustrated in Table 7–6. Typically the severity of the pain is disproportionate to physical findings. Appropriate treatment for both myonecrosis and clostridial infection is a combination of wide surgical debridement and antimicrobial therapy. For clostridial infection, high-dose penicillin is given. Hyperbaric oxygen may be used as an adjunct, but it is not a substitute for extensive surgical debridement. Fisher and associates

TABLE 7–6. MATERNAL DEATHS ASSOCIATED WITH EPISIOTOMY AND PERINEAL TRAUMA

Year	First Author	Age	Delivery	Perineal Trauma	Initial Symptoms (Days)	Presentation	Initial Treatment	Surgery	Delivery to Death	Final Diagnosis	Cultures	Underlying Disease
1986	Soper	24	Forceps	Med[a], 3° tear	4	Perineal discomfort	Antibiotics and steroids	No[b]	4	Myonecrosis	Clostridia, *E. coli*, *Klebsiella*	None
1979	Shy (1)	23	NS	Med. with tear over right ischial spine	2	Pain induration	Explored and opened into ischiorectal fossa; antibiotics, steroids, hyperbaric oxygen	Yes	6	Fascial necrosis Myonecrosis	Clostridia	None
	Shy (2)	21	SVD	Med.	3	Induration	Local incision, antibiotics, steroids	No	8	Fascial necrosis	*E. coli*	None
	Shy (3)	22	Forceps	Med.	5	Perineal, leg, and gluteal pain	Antibiotics, steroids	Yes	9	Myofascial necrosis	*E. coli*, Bacteroides	None
1979	*Scott	23	SVD	Med.	1	Vulvar edema	Antibiotics	No	4	Fascial necrosis	Clostridia	None
1979	*Hibbard (1)	30	NS	Med., 4° tear	2	Left labial edema	Antibiotics, steroids	No	10	Presumed fascial necrosis	None	None
	Hibbard (2)	19	NS	Mediolateral episiotomy	2	Swelling of left labia and buttock	Antibiotics, hyperbaric oxygen	No	3	Presumed myonecrosis	*E. coli*, strep, clostridia	None
1979	Ewing (1)	19	Forceps	Procto-episiotomy	2	Vulvar edema	Antibiotics	Yes[c]	6	Presumed fascial necrosis	Not cultured	None
	Ewing (2)	16	Forceps	Med., 3° tear[d]	2	Vulvar edema	Antibiotics, steroids	No	4	Presumed fascial necrosis	Not cultured	None
	Ewing (3)	24	SVD	Med.	2	Vulvar edema	Antibiotics, steroids	No	4	Presumed fascial necrosis	Streptococci, clostridia, staphylococci	None
1977	Golde (1)	30	SVD	Med., 4° tear	2	Edema of left labia majora	Antibiotics, human serum, local treatment	No	10	Fascial necrosis	Anaerobic, Streptococci, *E. coli*	None
	Golde (2)	23	SVD	Med., 3° tear	3	Perineal pain	Antibiotics, steroids	Yes	4	Fascial necrosis	Staphylococci, clostridia	None
1972	Jewett	23	NS	Med., 3° tear	5	Severe abdominal pain, fever	Antibiotics, heparin[e]	No	24	Retro-peritoneal	*E. coli*	None

[a]Med., median episiotomy [b]Died during preparation for surgery [c]Limited to exploration of ischiorectal fossa [d]Suspected rectal involvement with suture or occult 4° tear
[e]Had concurrent pulmonary embolism SVD = Spontaneous vaginal delivery NS = Not stated—but presumed SVD
**See Ewing, 1979 (Discussion)*

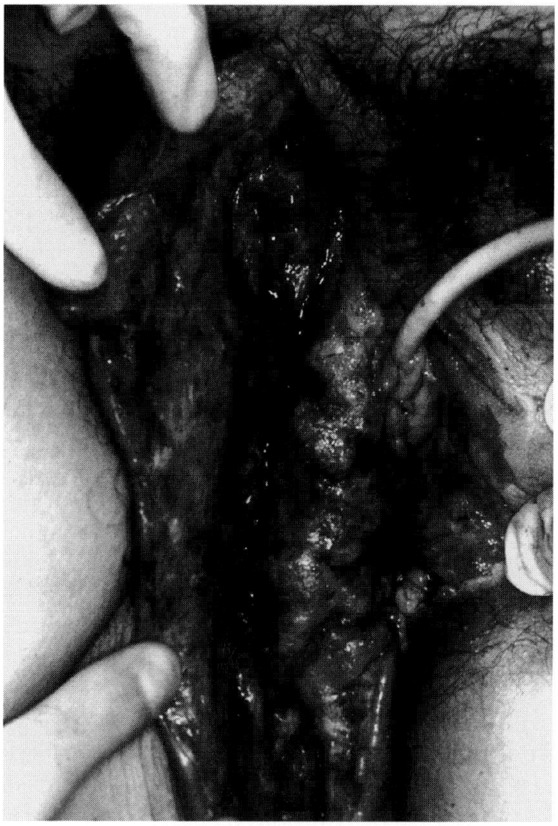

Figure 7–18. Woman 8 days postpartum whose episiotomy became infected and failed to respond to antimicrobial therapy. Surgical exploration and wide local debridement were performed shortly after presentation to the tertiary referral hospital. There is obvious necrosis of the skin and fibroadipose tissue and the majority of blood vessels contained clot.

(1979) emphasized that in each of their 22 patients who underwent radical debridement of all nonviable fascia and tissue, fascial necrosis extended farther than the area of cutaneous involvement. In their series, four of five deaths were women with infections involving the groin area.

Blood Loss and Hematoma Formation. Any practitioner who has ever cut an episiotomy can attest to the fact that women who have episiotomies experience greater blood loss than those who deliver over an intact perineum. Thacker and Banta (1983) estimated that the episiotomy itself accounted for approximately 200 mL of blood loss during vaginal birth. Rockner and associates (1989) reported increased frequency of excessive blood loss—greater than 600 mL—with episiotomy; however, they offered no objective data in support of this observation. Thranov and colleagues (1990) also observed that attendants reported increased blood loss with an episiotomy; however, objective measurements based on postpartum hematocrits failed to show a difference. Nevertheless, the primary factor associated with the development of vulvovaginal hematomas during childbirth is the performance of an episiotomy.

Neonatal Lidocaine Intoxication

While rare, there are convincing cases of neonatal lidocaine intoxication from administration of a pudendal block for vaginal birth and episiotomy (DePraeter and colleagues, 1991; Kim and associates, 1979). The clinical syndrome is characterized by neonatal apnea episodes up to and including respiratory arrest. Frequently, there are hypotonia and seizures at or shortly after birth. Fixed, dilated pupils, loss of the oculocephalic reflex, and either bradycardia or ventricular tachycardia may develop. Toxic effects have been noted with neonatal serum lidocaine levels as low as 3 μg mL (Shnider and Way, 1968). Among cases reported, maximal lidocaine levels in the neonate as high as 22.5 μg/mL have been extrapolated based on measured serum drug concentrations and the half-life of the compound. The delay in onset of symptoms is hypothesized to be secondary to direct injection into the fetus, with a time delay for absorption accounting for the interval until manifestation of symptoms.

Castration at Birth

That even the simplest of surgical procedures may have devastating complications for both mother and baby is illustrated by a report of castration at birth (George, 1988). In a breech delivery of a multiparous woman, a generous right posterolateral episiotomy was performed quickly as the woman was pushing and the breech was distending the perineum. Soon afterwards a pearly, grayish pink, spherical structure measuring about 1.5 cm in diameter fell out of the vagina. The woman kept pushing, and another similar structure was expelled. There was no undue bleeding. Delivery was spontaneous and completed without further assistance. The newborn had profuse bleeding; his scrotum had been almost completely severed except for an anterior tag. The two pearly structures were testicles, and the scrotum had been severed with the episiotomy. This happened despite the obstetrician's 30 years' experience.

EPISIOTOMY DEHISCENCE REPAIR

Prior to the mid-1980s, conventional medical doctrine held that if episiotomy repair at the time of delivery failed, a second attempt at repair should be deferred for a minimum of 3–4 months (Mattingly and Thompson, 1985). This delay was believed necessary to ensure an adequate blood supply to the margins of the defect and the return of optimal viability of perineal tissue. The cost to the woman of delayed repair, a cost which included fecal incontinence with potential inability to function socially or in the workplace, the loss of sexual function, and the prolonged dread and anxiety while awaiting ultimate repair, was judged to be minimal relative to the risk of failure of early repair (Cogan and Harris, 1966). These dicta were especially inviolate when the injury extended to involve the anal sphincter or rectal mucosa.

The first series of women undergoing early repair of an anal sphincter muscle and rectal mucosal dehiscence was reported by Hauth and associates in 1986. These observations were subsequently updated and extended to include 22 women with breakdown of a fourth-degree episiotomy, four with breakdown of a third-degree episiotomy, and five with a mediolateral dehiscence (Hankins and colleagues, 1990). The mean interval from delivery to dehiscence was 6.6 ± 2.6 days for fourth-degree lesions and 5.3 ± 2.2 days for third-degree and mediolateral lesions. On average the time required to prepare the wound for surgical reapproximation was 6 days with a range of from 1 to 11 days.

Technique of Early Repair

In performing early repair of episiotomy dehiscence, there are important specific tenets for preoperative, intraoperative, and postoperative management of these women.

Preoperative

When dehiscence is first recognized, the wound is carefully inspected. Anesthesia required for such inspection will vary from none to general anesthesia, but the majority of women require only intravenous sedation. If infected, the episiotomy is completely taken down and the wound fully exposed. If there is no evidence of infection, gentle lateral traction is applied at the wound margins. In the absence of separation, the remaining intact repair is not disturbed. The wound then is cleaned briskly using surgical gauze and a mixture of equal parts of 10 percent povidone iodine solution, hydrogen peroxide, and normal saline. Any remaining suture is removed from the previous repair. Thereafter, the wound is scrubbed and irrigated two or three times daily. Application of 2 percent lidocaine jelly to the wound 5 minutes before each cleaning decreases patient discomfort. The woman is instructed to use sitz baths after all bowel movements and to keep the perineum as clean and dry as possible.

The day before surgery, women with breakdown involving the rectal mucosa undergo a mechanical bowel preparation with a commercially available electrolyte solution (Golytely). The solution is consumed at the rate of 1 L/hour until clear, colorless diarrhea is produced. Oral antibiotics are not given as a part of the bowel preparation.

Perioperative Management

A broad-spectrum antimicrobial is given intravenously on call to the operating room and continued for 48–72 hours. For women in whom infection is associated with episiotomy breakdown, the duration of preoperative antimicrobial treatment is increased.

The wound is judged ready for surgical repair when its surface is free of exudate and covered by healthy, pink granulation tissue. Operative dissection is performed until all tissue layers have good mobility and can be reapproximated without tension on the suture lines. Extensive retraction of the anal sphincter is a consistent finding, and particular attention is required for its identification to ensure that the fibrous capsule can be mobilized and reapproximated without tension. The rectal mucosa is reapproximated with a running submucosal 000 or 0000 chromic gut suture. This is reinforced with a layer of rectovaginal septal tissue using either a running or interrupted 00 or 000 chromic gut suture. The external anal sphincter is approximated with four or five interrupted 00 chromic gut or polyglactin sutures. The remainder of the repair is the same as a simple second-degree episiotomy.

Postoperative Management
Patients are encouraged to use a sitz bath three times daily, and then to dry the perineum. If the rectal mucosa is repaired, diet is designed to avoid bowel movements during the initial postoperative period. Diarrheal stool during the immediate post-repair period is a substantially greater threat to wound healing than is formed stool. At 48–72 hours postoperatively patients are advanced to a clear liquid diet, which is continued for 3 days, following which a regular diet is resumed. Women with injuries involving the rectal mucosa are not discharged until they have resumption of normal bowel function. They are instructed to avoid placing anything intravaginally for at least 6 weeks. When the repair does not involve the rectal mucosa, the diet is rapidly advanced postoperatively.

Follow-up averaged 2 years for the 22 women with dehiscence of a fourth-degree episiotomy described by Hankins and associates (1990). With the exception of two women who developed a pinpoint rectovaginal fistula, the remainder of the repairs were judged highly successful by both physicians and patients. Both women with pinpoint fistulas were subsequently repaired using an anal flap, one at 6 weeks and the other 6 months from discovery of the fistula. All women were continent of both stool and flatus 1 year following the repair. About 10 percent noted occasional mild dyspareunia.

Among those women with third-degree or mediolateral dehiscence, follow-up averaged 17 months. Early complications were limited to superficial separation of the skin edge on the perineal body; however, these healed spontaneously. All women were continent and reported normal bowel function. Again, about 10 percent had occasional dyspareunia. These results concerning fecal continence and dyspareunia are equivalent to those reported for women undergoing primary episiotomy repair. While a pinpoint fistula is certainly not desirable, this complication rate was not significantly different from that of 10 percent reported with delayed repairs (Given and Browning, 1988).

These earlier reports by Hauth (1986) and Hankins (1990) and their colleagues included a military population of middle to lower-middle class, predominantly white women. Ramin and colleagues (1992) subsequently reported their results with a similar management schema used for an indigent population at Parkland Hospital. Whereas these previous reports described infection as the obvious cause of dehiscence in only a quarter of fourth-degree episiotomies, Ramin and colleagues (1992) found related infection in two-thirds of 41 episiotomy dehiscences. Despite this, an average of 6.4 days (range, 3–13) was required to prepare tissue for resuturing. Questionably infected tissue was not reapproximated. A successful anatomic repair was achieved in 94 percent of patients; the two failures were third-degree episiotomies that again broke down. In both instances, these wounds were allowed to heal by secondary intention.

A somewhat different approach to the separated, and in their experience, often infected, episiotomy was described by Monberg and Hammen (1987). They reported 35 women with dehiscence of a mediolateral episiotomy. These women were randomized to two divergent protocols. In the first group, 20 women underwent immediate repair by primary resuturing. They were given clindamycin 2 hours before suturing and continuously for 5 days thereafter. The second group of 15 women were managed by local wound cleaning with healing by secondary intention. Infection was identified in half of women in both groups. In the early-repair group, women with purulent wounds underwent sharp resection until vital tissue was reached followed by closure with 2-0 Vicryl. They were discharged on average 1 day sooner than women managed conservatively. They also required significantly fewer clinic and home health visits. Dyspareunia at 6-months postpartum was reported in 6 percent of women undergoing early repair and in 14 percent of those with repair by secondary intention.

There is little doubt that complete dehiscence of a mediolateral, third-degree, or fourth-degree episiotomy is associated with significant morbidity. Both anatomic reapproximation and physiologic function following early repair are comparable to those achieved with delayed repair. The general protocols that have been published provide guidelines that individuals can use to address these infrequent, but very morbid events in a more timely fashion.

SUMMARY

Episiotomy, despite being performed for nearly 250 years, is highly controversial. It is increasingly apparent that even *normal* childbirth is associated with trauma to the maternal pelvic soft tissues and nerves, some of which is irreversible and most of which cannot be prevented by an episiotomy. In contrast, it is clear that both third-degree and fourth-degree lacerations are greatly increased when an episiotomy is performed. The routine performance of an episiotomy should be replaced by a more restrictive policy where use of the procedure is based on the specific clinical conditions encountered at the time of delivery.

REFERENCES

Adoni A, Anteby E. The use of Histoacryl for episiotomy repair. Br J Obstet Gynaecol 1991; 98:476.

Argentine Episiotomy Trial Collaborative Group. Routine vs selective episiotomy: a randomised controlled trial. Lancet 1993; 342:1515.

Arms S. Immaculate deception. Boston: Houghton Mifflin, 1975.

Banninger V, Buhrig H, Schreiner We. Vergleichende Studie uber die Verwendung von Polyglykolsaure (Dexon) and Chromicatgut als Nahtmaterial bei der Episiotomeinaht. Geburtsholfe Frauenheilkd 1978; 30:30.

Beck RP, Hsu N. Pregnancy, childbirth and the menopause related to the development of stress incontinence. Am J Obstet Gynecol 1965; 91:821.

Bex PJM, Hofmeyr GJ. Perineal management during childbirth and subsequent dyspareunia. Clin Exp Obstet Gynecol 1987; 14:97.

Beynon CL. Midline episiotomy as a routine procedure. J Obstet Gynaecol Brit Commonw 1974; 81:126.

Blondel B, Pusch D, Schmidt E. Some characteristics of antenatal care in 13 European countries. Br J Obstet Gynaecol 1985; 92:565.

Blondel B, Kaminski M. Episiotomy and third-degree tears. Br J Obstet Gynaecol 1985; 92:1297.

Borgatta L, Piening SL, Cohen WR. Association of episiotomy and delivery position with deep perineal laceration during spontaneous delivery in nulliparous women. Am J Obstet Gynecol 1989; 160:294.

Brantley JT, Burwell JC. A study of fourth-degree perineal lacerations and their sequelae. Am J Obstet Gynecol 1960; 80:711.

Brendsel C, Peterson G, Mehl LE. Episiotomy: facts, fictions, figures, and alternatives. In: Stewart D, Stewart L (eds), Compulsory Hospitalization or Freedom of Choice in Childbirth. National Association of Parents and Professionals for Safe Alternatives in Childbirth (NAPSAC), 1979; pp. 139.

Brendsel C, Peterson G, Miehl C. The role of episiotomy in pelvic symptomatology. In: Kitzinger S (ed), Episiotomy—Physical and Emotional Aspects, London: National Childbirth Trust, 1981; pp. 36.

Bromberg MH. Presumptive maternal benefits of routine episiotomy. A literature review. J Nurs-Midwif 1986; 31:121.

Buekens P, Lagasse R, Dramaix M, Wollast E. Episiotomy and third-degree tears. Br J Obstet Gynaecol 1985; 92:820.

Chalmers I. Evaluating the quality of new procedures. Arch Gynecol Obstet 1987; 241:S101.

Chatterjee SK. Scar endometriosis: a clinicopathologic study of 17 cases. Obstet Gynecol 1980; 56:81.

Coats PM, Chan KK, Wilkins M, Beard RJ. A comparison between midline and mediolateral episiotomies. Br J Obstet Gynaecol 1980; 87:408.

Cogan JE, Harris HW. Rectal complications after perineorrhaphy and episiotomy. Arch Surg 1966; 93:634.

DeLee JB. The prophylactic forceps operation. Am J Obstet Gynecol 1:34, 1920.

DePraeter C, Vanhaesebrouck P, DePraeter N, et al. Episiotomy and neonatal lidocaine intoxication. Eur J Ped 1991; 150:685.

Enkin MW, Hunter DJ, Snell L. Episiotomy: Effects of a research protocol on clinical practice. Birth 1984; 11:145.

Ewing TL, Smale LE, Elliott FA. Maternal deaths associated with postpartum vulvar edema. Am J Obstet Gynecol 1979; 134:173.

Fisher JR, Conway MJ, Takeshita RT, Sandoval MR. Necrotizing fasciitis. Importance of Roentgenographic studies for soft-tissue gas. JAMA 1979; 241:803.

Flint C, Poulengeris P. The "know your midwife" report. London: Heinemann, 1987.

Flood C. The real reasons for performing episiotomies. World Med 1982; 6 Feb:51.

Francis WJA. Disturbances of bladder function in relation to pregnancy. J Obstet Gynaecol Br Empire 1960a; 67:353.

Francis WJA. The onset of stress incontinence. J Obstet Gynaecol Br Empire 1960b; 67:899.

Gass MS, Dunn C, Stys SJ. Effect of episiotomy on the frequency of vaginal outlet lacerations. J Repro Med 1986; 31:240.

Gainey HL. Postpartum observation of pelvic tissue damage: Further studies. Am J Obstet Gynecol 1955; 70:800.

Gainey HL. Postpartum observation of pelvic tissue damage. Am J Obstet Gynecol 1943; 45:457.

George S. Castration at birth. Br Med J 297:1313 1988.

Given FT Jr, Browning G. Repair of old complete perineal lacerations. Am J Obstet Gynecol 1988; 159:779.

Go PMNYH, Dunselman GAJ. Anatomic and functional results of surgical repair after total perineal rupture at delivery. Surg Gynecol Obstet 1988; 166:121.

Golde S, Ledger WJ. Necrotizing fasciitis in postpartum patients: A report of four cases. Obstet Gynecol 1977; 50:670.

Goodlin RC. On protection of the maternal perineum during birth. Am J Obstet Gynecol 1983; 62:393.

Gordan H, Logue M. Perineal muscle function after childbirth. Lancet 1985; 2:123.

Graham SB, Catanzarite V, Bernstein J, Varela-Gittings F. A comparison of attitudes and practices of episiotomy among obstetrical practitioners in New Mexico. Soc Sci Med 1990; 31:191.

Grant A. Repair or episiotomies and perineal tears. Br J Obstet Gynaecol1986; 93:417.

Grant A. The choice of suture materials and techniques for repair of perineal trauma: an overview of the evidence from controlled trials. Br J Obstet Gynaecol 1989; 96:1281.

Haire D. The cultural warping of childbirth, a special report on US obstetrics. Minneapolis: ICEA, 1972.

Hambrick E, Abcarian H, Smith D. Perineal endometrioma in episiotomy incisions. Clinical features and management. Dis Colon Rectum 1979; 22:550.

Hankins GDV, Hauth JC, Gilstrap LC, et al. Early repair of episiotomy dehiscence. Obstet Gynecol 1990; 75:48.

Harris RE. An evaluation of the median episiotomy. Am J Obstet Gynecol 1970; 106:660.

Harrison RF, Brennan M, North PM, et al. Is routine episiotomy necessary? Br Med J 1984; 288:1971.

Hauth JC, Gilstrap LC, Ward SC, Hankins GDV. Early repair of an external sphincter ani muscle and rectal mucosal dehiscence. Obstet Gynecol 1986; 67:806.

Henriksen TB, Bek KM, Hedegaard M, Secher NJ. Episiotomy and perineal lesions in spontaneous vaginal deliveries. Br J Obstet Gynaecol 1992; 99:950.

Hopkinson JH. Ibuprofen versus propoxyphene hydrochloride and placebo in the relief of postepisiotomy pain. Curr Ther Res 1980; 27:55.

Iosif S. Stress incontinence during pregnancy and in the puerperium. Int J Gynaecol Obstet, 1981; 19:13.

Isager-Sally L, Legarth J, Jacobsen B, Bostofte E. Episiotomy repair—immediate and long-term sequelae. A prospective randomized study of three different methods of repair. Br J Obstet Gynecol 1986; 93:420.

Jackson MB, Dunster GD. Episiotomy: Who gets one and why. J R Coll Gen Pract 1984; 34:603.

Jacobs WM, Adams BD. Midline episiotomy and extension through the rectal sphincter. Surg Gynecol Obstet 1960; 111:245.

Jewett JF. Committee on Maternal Welfare: Fatal perineal sepsis. N Engl J Med 1972; 286:1213.

Kaltreider DF, Dixon DM. A study of 710 complete lacerations following central episiotomy. South Med J 1948; 36:814.

Kim WY, Pomerance JJ, Miller AA. Lidocaine intoxication in a newborn following local anesthesia for episiotomy. Pediatrics 1979; 64:643.

Kitzinger S. Episiotomy: Physical and emotional aspects. London, National Childbirth Trust, 1981.

Larsson PG, Platz-Christensen JJ, Bergman B, Wallstersson G. Advantage or disadvantage of episiotomy compared with spontaneous perineal laceration. Gynecol Obstet Invest 1991; 31:213.

Legino LJ, Woods MP, Rayburn WF, McGoogan LS. Third- and fourth-degree perineal tears. 50 years' experience at a university hospital. J Repro Med 1988; 33:423.

Livingstone E, Simpson D, Naismith WCMK. A comparison between catgut and polyglycolic acid suture in episiotomy repair. J Obstet Gynaecol Br Commonw 1974; 81:245.

Mahomed K, Grant A, Ashurst H, James D. The Southmead perineal suture study. A randomized comparison of suture materials and suturing techniques for repair of perineal trauma. Br J Obstet Gynaecol 1989; 96:1272.

Mattingly RF, Thompson JD. Anal incontinence and rectovaginal fistulas. In: TeLinde's Operative Gynecology. 6th ed. Philadelphia: JB Lippincott, 1985; p. 669.

McGuinness M, Norr K, Nacion K. Comparison between different perineal outcomes on tissue healing. J Nurs-Midwif 1991; 36:192.

Monberg J, Hammen S. Ruptured episiotomia resutured primarily. Acta Obstet Gynecol Scand 1987; 66:163.

Norris F. Episioproctotomy. Surg Clin North Am 1962; 42:947.

Odigie EA. Effectiveness of indomethacin (indocid) suppositories as post-episiotomy analgesia. Int J Gynaecol Obstet 1988; 26:57.

O'Leary JL, O'Leary JA. The complete episiotomy. Analysis of 1224 complete lacerations, sphincterotomies, and episioproctotomies. Obstet Gynecol 1964; 25:235.

Olson R, Olson C, Cox NS. Maternal birthing positions and perineal injury. J Fam Pract 1990; 30:553–57.

Ould F. A Treatise of Midwifery. Dublin, 1742.

Owen J, Hauth JC. Episiotomy infection and dehiscence. In: Gilstrap LC, Faro S (eds), Infections in Pregnancy. New York: Alan R. Liss, 1990; p. 61.

Paciornik M. Commentary: Arguments against episiotomy and in favor of squatting for birth. Birth 1990; 17:104.

Paul TH, Tedeschi LG. Perineal endometriosis at the site of episiotomy scar. Obstet Gynecol 1972; 40:28.

Pilkington JW, Cunningham CB, Johnson RC. Median episiotomy and complete perineotomy. South Med J 1963; 56:284.

Pomeroy RH. Shall we cut and reconstruct the perineum for every primipara? Am J Obstet Dis Woman and Child 1918; 78:211.

Ramin SM, Ramul RM, Little BB, Gilstrap LC. Early repair of episiotomy dehiscence associated with infection. Am J Obstet Gynecol 1992; 167:1104.

Ranney B. Decreasing numbers of patients for vaginal hysterectomy and plasty. S D J Med 1990; 43:7.

Reynolds JL, Yudkin PL. Changes in the management of labour: 2. Perineal management. CMAJ 1987; 136:1045.

Rockner G, Henningsson A, Wahlberg V, Olund A. Evaluation of episiotomy and spontaneous tears of perineum during childbirth. Scan J Caring Sci 1988; 2:19.

Rockner G, Wahlberg V, Olund A. Episiotomy and perineal trauma during childbirth. J Adv Nurs 1989; 14:264.

Rockner G. Urinary incontinence after perineal trauma at childbirth. Scan J Caring Sci 1990; 4:169.

Rockner G, Jonasson A, Olund A. The effect of mediolateral episiotomy at delivery on pelvic floor muscle strength evaluated with vaginal cones. Acta Obstet Gynecol Scan 1991; 70:51.

Rockner G, Olund A. The use of episiotomy in primiparas in Sweden. Acta Obstet Gynecol Scan 1991; 70:325.

Salamalekis E, Vasiliadis TX, Kairi P, Zourlas PA. Perineal endometriosis. Int J Gynecol Obstet 1990; 31:75.

Sayfan J, Benosh L, Segal M, Orda R. Endometriosis in episiotomy scar with anal sphincter involvement. Dis Colon Rectum 1991; 34:713.

Schachtel BP, Thoden WR, Baybutt RI. Ibuprofen and acetaminophen in the relief of postpartum episiotomy pain. J Clin Pharmacol 1989; 29:550.

Shiono P, Klebanoff MA, Carey JCC. Midline episiotomies: More harm than good? Obstet Gynecol 1990; 75:765.

Shnider SM, Way EL. Plasma levels of lidocaine (xylocaine) in mother and newborn following obstetrical conduction anaesthesia. Anesthesiology 1968; 29:951.

Shy KK, Eschenbach DA. Fatal perineal cellulitis from an episiotomy site. Obstet Gynecol 1979; 54:292.

Sieber EH, Kroon JD. Morbidity in the third-degree laceration. Obstet Gynecol 1962; 19:677.

Sleep J. Episiotomy in normal delivery. Nursing 1984; 2:614.

Sleep J, Grant A. West Berkshire perineal management trial: three year follow up. Br Med J 1987; 295:749.

Sleep J, Grant A, Garcia J, et al. West Berkshire perineal management trial. Br Med J 1984; 289:587.

Sleep J, Roberts J, Chalmers I. Care during the second stage of labour. In: Effective Care in Pregnancy and Childbirth. Chalmers I, Enkin M, Keirse MJNC (eds), Vol 2. Childbirth. Oxford: Oxford University Press, 1989; p. 1129

Smith ARB, Hosker GL, Warrell DW. The role of partial denervation of the pelvic floor in the aetiology of genitourinary prolapse and stress incontinence of urine: A neurophysiological study. Br J Obstet Gynaecol 1989; 96:24.

Snooks SJ, Swash M. Abnormalities of the innervation of the urethral striated musculature in incontinence. Br J Urol 1984; 56:401.

Snooks SJ, Setchell M, Swash M, Henry MM. Injury to innervation of pelvic floor sphincter musculature in childbirth. Lancet 1984; ii:546.

Snooks SJ, Badenoch DF, Tiptaft RC, Swash M. Perineal nerve damage in genuine stress incontinence—an electrophysiological study. Br J Urol 1985; 57:422.

Soper DE. Clostridial myonecrosis arising from an episiotomy. Obstet Gynecol 1986; 68:26S.

Spencer J, Grant A, Elbourne D, et al. A randomized comparison of glycerol-impregnated catgut with untreated chromic catgut for the repair of perineal trauma. Br J Obstet Gynaecol 1986; 93:426.

Stanton SL, Kerr-Wilson R, Grant Harris V. The incidence of urological symptoms in normal pregnancy. Br J Obstet Gynaecol 1980; 87:897.

Stewart P, Hillan E, Calder AA. A randomised trial to evaluate the use of a birth chair for delivery. Lancet 1983; 1:1296.

Sunshine A, Olson NZ, Laska EM, et al. Ibuprofen, zomepirac, aspirin, and placebo in the relief of post episiotomy pain. Clin Pharmacol Ther 1983; 34:254.

Taliaferro RM. Rigidity of soft parts: Delivery effected by incision in the perineum. Stethoscope Va Med Gazette 1852; 2:383.

Thacker SB, Banta HD. Benefits and risks of episiotomy: An interpretive review of the English language literature, 1860–1980. Obstet Gynecol Surv 1983; 38:322.

Thompson DJ. No episiotomy?! Aust NZ J Obstet Gynaecol 1987; 27:18.

Thorp JM, Bowes WA, Brame RG, Cefalo R. Selected use of midline episiotomy: effect on perineal trauma. Obstet Gynecol 1987; 70:260.

Thranov I, Kringlebach AM, Melchior E, et al. Postpartum symptoms. Episiotomy or tear at vaginal delivery. Acta Obstet Gynecol Scand 1990; 69:11.

Walker MPR, Farine D, Rolbin SH, Ritchie JWK. Epidural anesthesia, episiotomy, and obstetric laceration. Obstet Gynecol 1991; 77:668.

Wilkerson VA. The use of episiotomy in normal delivery. Midwives Chronicle 1984; 97:106.
Willson JR. Obstetrics—gynecology: a time for a change. Am J Obstet Gynecol 1981; 141:857.
Willson JR. Atlas of Obstetric Technique. 2nd ed. C. V. Mosby Company, St. Louis, 1969.
Wilson B. Necrotizing fasciitis. Am Surg 1952; 18:416.
Yeomans ET. Operative vaginal delivery. ACOG Technical Bulletin No. 152, February 1991.

CHAPTER 8

Forceps Delivery

"The art and science of forceps delivery is becoming a thing of the past" (Douglas and Stromme, 1982, 1988). "The status of forceps in modern obstetrics is constantly under discussion (and scrutiny) within the specialty" (Dennen, 1989). Neither of these observations should be surprising when one considers that forceps were invented as an extricating tool to be used in desperation in the most difficult circumstances and usually as a last resort. Indeed, primitive varieties of forceps may have existed for 2500 years before they were ever used for delivery of a viable child. Further contributing to a decline in use of forceps has been the increase in litigation, particularly in America. Overreliance on cesarean section as a remedy for abnormal labor and suspected fetal jeopardy has led to a generation of providers skilled in surgery and midwifery, but lacking proficiency in operative vaginal delivery. The reclassification of the forceps delivery system by the American College of Obstetricians and Gynecologists in 1988 and subsequent studies showing that the new classification accurately stratifies risk for both mother and fetus (Hagadorn-Freathy and associates, 1991) should serve as an impetus for continued or even increased use of forceps under appropriate clinical conditions.

HISTORY

Development of Instrumentation

For centuries, accoucheurs searched for mechanical means to aid women in labor. In 1500 BC, leather straps with handles were used for traction in Persia (Plauche, 1992). A second-century marble bas relief found near Rome depicts a paired instrument (Douglas and Stromme, 1976). The earliest forceps were instruments of destruction, and an instrumental vaginal delivery either followed or resulted in the death of the infant. Albucasis developed a pair of forceps in 1000 AD that might have been used for delivery of a viable child (O'Grady, 1988); however, the most widely recorded and historically accurate use of forceps for extraction of a living child is credited to the Chamberlen family of England. It is believed that Peter Chamberlen "the elder," son of William, designed the first pair in the sixteenth century. The earliest forceps consisted of separate 12-inch branches, each with a cephalic curve and fenestrated blade. These instruments had no pelvic curve or lock and were joined, once applied to the fetus, with a rivet or thong at the handle. This was kept a family secret until the early eighteenth century, when it was sold to an enterprising group of physicians in Amsterdam. Later, the "secret" was made public (Williams, 1903). By 1929 there had been 515 recorded modifications of the original Chamberlen model (Das, 1929).

Around 1740 there was a significant advance in forceps construction: development of the pelvic curve. Credit for this adaptation should be given equally to three practitioners, each working independently and unaware of the other; Smellie of Scotland, Pugh of England, and Levret of France (Shute, 1992). In

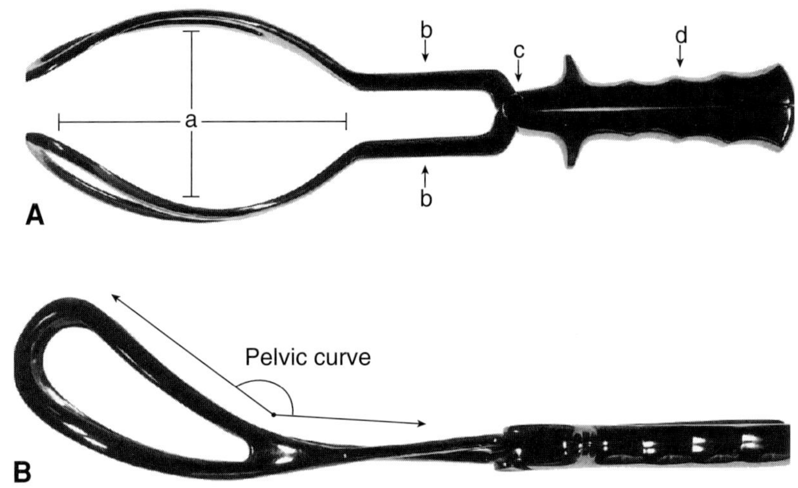

Figure 8–1 A. Simpson forceps as viewed from above demonstrating the cephalic curve of wide radius (a), parallel shanks (b), English lock (c), and corrugated handles (d). **B.** Simpson forceps in lateral view. Note the upward curve of the blade of the forceps from the shank of the forceps such that the anterior tip of the toe of the forceps rests well above the handle of the forceps.

1745, William Smellie also described accurate application and rotation to occiput anterior prior to delivery rather than the previously practiced pelvic application and traction without regard to position of the fetal head (Dennen, 1989). Smellie is also credited with development of the English lock. Levret's forceps also introduced the French lock and were the first forceps constructed entirely of steel. The instrument was multipurpose, designed not only to deliver the living infant, but to serve as an instrument of destruction if necessary. One handle converted to a hook and on the tip of the other handle was a screw cap, which concealed a perforator. Numerous obstetricians designed forceps containing minor variations in the cephalic curve, using closer or more widely separated shanks, and changing the length, shape, and corrugation of the handles. In 1845, Sir James Y. Simpson, the first obstetrician to use chloroform, developed an instrument for delivery, not only the most popular in his time, but in ours as well. The Simpson forceps consisted of a cephalic curve of wide radius, parallel shanks above a loosely fitting English lock, and corrugated handles (Fig. 8–1). The problem of uncontrolled cephalic compression served as impetus for Elliot to insert a set screw between the handles of the forceps that bear his name to counter dangerous approximation of the blades above the scissors lock (Fig. 8–2). Both the Elliot forceps and the Simpson forceps are classified as classical forceps.

Tarnier of France introduced the principle of axis-traction. To encourage smooth cranial descent through the Curve of Carus (pelvic axis), his instrument consisted of a relatively flat cephalic curve, a French lock, and short handles to which the axis-traction device could be attached. The influential obstetrician Pajot enthusiastically endorsed the Tarnier forceps and the principle of axis-traction. The concept of solid blade construction to facilitate ease in pelvic rotation was advocated by Osiander in 1799 and popularized by McLane in the 1880s. Luikart modified the solid blade by thinning its inner portion. Thus, the pseudofenestrated blade combines the assets of external solidity and internal fenestration (Fig. 8–3). Other inventors designed forceps for special applications: the Barton and Kielland (Figure 8–4) for correction of transverse arrest and pelvic rotations, the Piper (Figs. 8–5 and 8–6) for the aftercoming head of the fetus delivered in breech position, and the Laufe divergent forceps (Fig. 8–7) to avoid intracranial damage by undue compression.

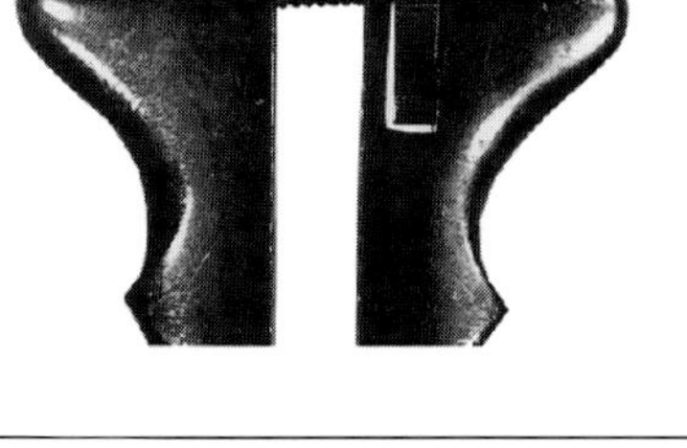

Figure 8–2. A close-up view of the handle of the Elliot forceps demonstrating the set screw between the handles designed to reduce cephalic compression.

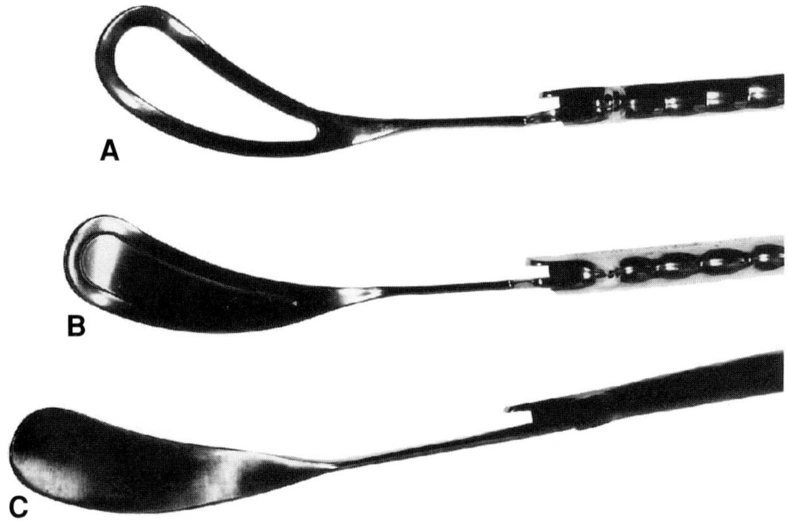

Figure 8–3. Forceps demonstrating **A.** a fenestrated blade (Simpson), **B.** pseudofenestrated blade (Luikart-Simpson), and **C.** solid forceps blade (Tucker-McLane).

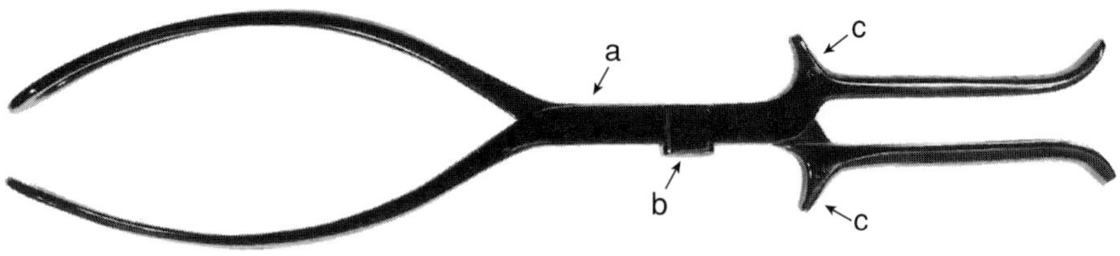

Figure 8–4. The Kielland forceps as viewed from above. The cephalic curve has a wide radius. The shanks overlap (a) and are connected by a sliding lock (b). The two elevations (c) on the handle near the finger guards serve for orientation of the forceps and are usually directed toward the fetal occiput.

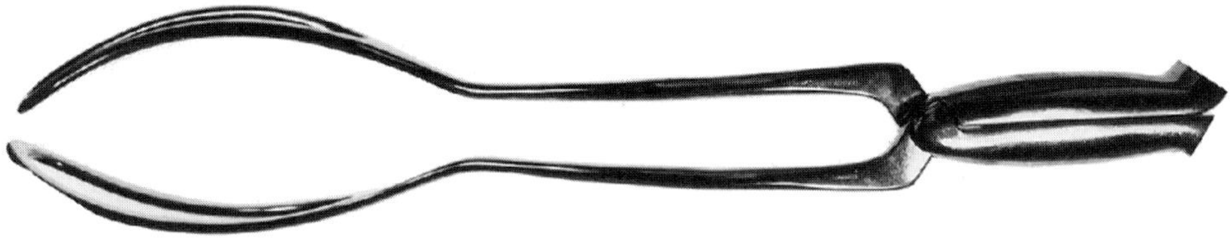

Figure 8–5. Piper forceps as viewed from above. The forceps are notable for the parallel shanks connecting at the handle by an English lock. The shanks of these forceps are much longer than those of most other forceps.

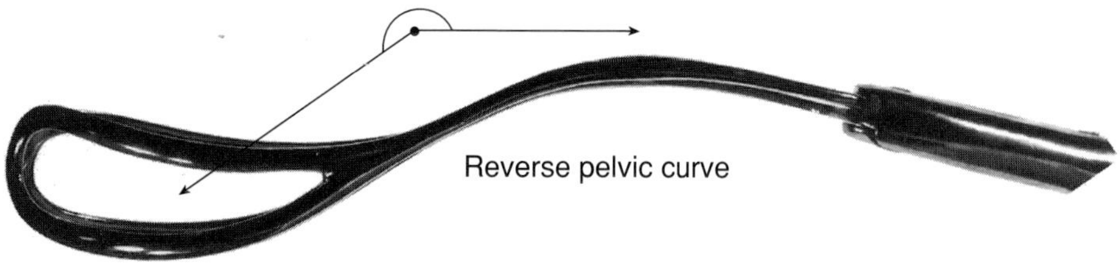

Figure 8–6. Piper forceps in lateral projection. Notable is the reverse pelvic curve of these forceps. Accordingly, axis-traction generally will be in line with and parallel to the handle of the forceps.

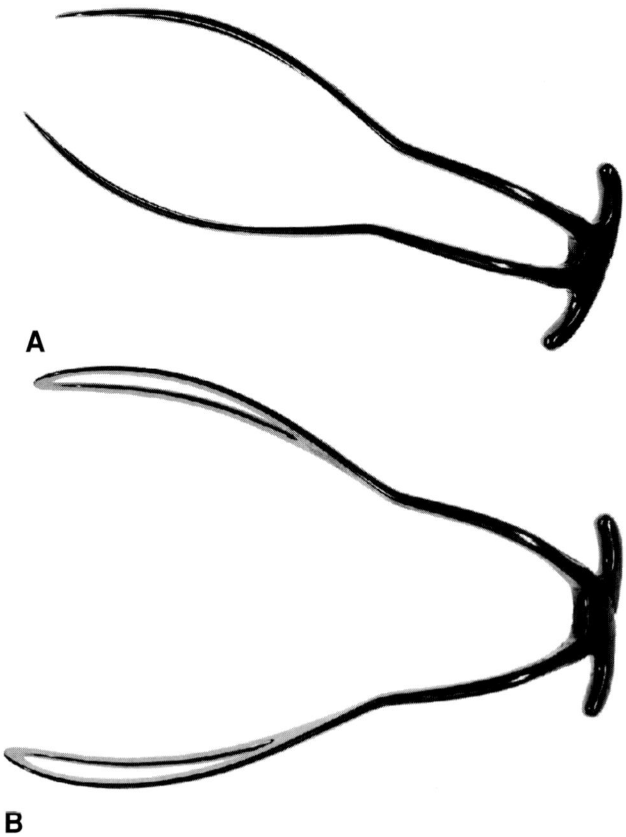

Figure 8–7. A. The Laufe divergent forceps are shown as viewed from above. They are characterized by parallel shanks and by a locking mechanism incorporated into the handle. **B.** When traction is placed upon the finger guards of the forceps, the blades will tend to diverge, minimizing compressive forces on the fetal skull. If viewed in lateral projection, the forceps would be notable for a pronounced reverse pelvic curve.

Practice of Forceps Delivery

Use of obstetric forceps has been controversial since their invention. William Smellie in 1752 recommended using forceps in his "Treatise on the Theory and Practice of Midwifery." The instrument then became widely available and was used by unskilled practitioners, resulting in injury to mother and child. By the early nineteenth century, forceps had been almost abandoned, but the case of Princess Charlotte in 1817 figured in their reemergence (Holland, 1951). The princess had a 24-hour second stage of labor. Her obstetrician, Sir Richard Croft, was the son-in-law of Sir Thomas Denman, one of the most influential physicians in England. One of Denman's maxims was that instrumental delivery not be attempted until the fetal head had rested on the perineum for 6 hours. Ultimately, through delay and questionable advice from a consultant, the never-to-be prince remained on the perineum for 10 hours and was stillborn. The princess died of a postpartum hemorrhage, and the inconsolable Dr. Croft committed suicide 6 weeks later. The consensus was that this "triple obstetric tragedy" could have been avoided by a timely forceps delivery.

This event in part accounted for a resurgence in forceps use that lasted for more than 100 years. The development of obstetric anesthesia in the mid-nineteenth century further increased the popularity of forceps and patient acceptance. The concept of the prophylactic use of forceps, introduced by DeLee (1920), contributed to a nearly 70 percent incidence of forceps deliveries by the late 1940s. Since this record-high incidence, the more difficult forceps deliveries have prudently been eliminated in favor of cesarean section. This trend has continued to the present; but along the way, many not-very-difficult forceps deliveries also were abandoned. Furthermore, the liberal use of cesarean section in the first stage of labor has led to a generation of obstetricians inexperienced and uncomfortable with forceps use. However, the economic cost, the morbidity of cesarean delivery, and the minimal fetal morbidity of properly selected cases have refocused attention on operative vaginal deliveries (Hagadorn-Freathy and associates, 1991).

MODERN FORCEPS INSTRUMENTS

In the last 200 years, the design of the basic instrument has changed only slightly. Although over 600 varieties of forceps have been catalogued, only a few features are important, and these can be obtained with the use of relatively few basic instruments, which are described in this chapter.

Anatomy of the Forceps

Except when used at cesarean delivery, obstetric forceps are a paired instrument. The two members are customarily referred to as the left and right blades. However, because each distal end of the forceps is also referred to as a blade, throughout this chapter, we use the less common terms left branch and right branch. The left branch is grasped by the operator's left hand and applied to the left side of the maternal pelvis, while the right branch is grasped by the right hand and introduced into the right side of the maternal pelvis. Prior to the application of the forceps, they should be examined for symmetry to ensure that they are in good repair. In addition, the operator should ascertain that the blades are a matched set by examining the inside of the handle of the instrument: the arabic numerals on each blade should be identical. Both the right and left branch of the forceps can be further subdivided into four parts: handle, lock, shank, and blade (see Fig. 8–1). Some forceps, such as DeLees, are fitted with an additional device known as an axis-traction bar. As mentioned, while each half of the forceps is customarily referred to as a left or right blade, the "blade" is actually limited to the widened, curved portion that is applied to the head of the fetus. Forceps blades may be either fenestrated (Simpson's), pseudofenestrated (Luikart-Simpson's), or solid (Tucker-McLane) (see Fig. 8–3) (Luikart, 1937). The open blades facilitate traction but are prone to injure maternal soft tissue if significant degrees of rotation are required. In contrast, solid blades are well designed for rotation; they cause less maternal soft tissue injury, but increase the risk of slippage on the fetal head.

Articulated, the forceps present two curves in planes at right angles to each other. The curve that corresponds to the fetal head is known as the cephalic curve (see Fig. 8–1), which varies from one forceps to another. The cephalic curve should be well shaped and measure approximately 7.5 cm in its widest diameter. All forceps can be subdivided into two groups. The first consists of elongated and bayonet-shaped blades with a shallow curve, which is well suited for application to the molded head. The Simpson forceps and the DeLee forceps are examples of instruments ideally suited for delivery of the molded head. The second grouping of forceps has a shorter and more rounded cephalic curve and is ideal for delivery of the fetal head with little or no molding. The Bailey-Williamson forceps are excellent in this clinical setting (Fig. 8–8).

The second curve of the forceps, which corresponds to the curve of the pelvis, is known as the pelvic curve. In conventional for-

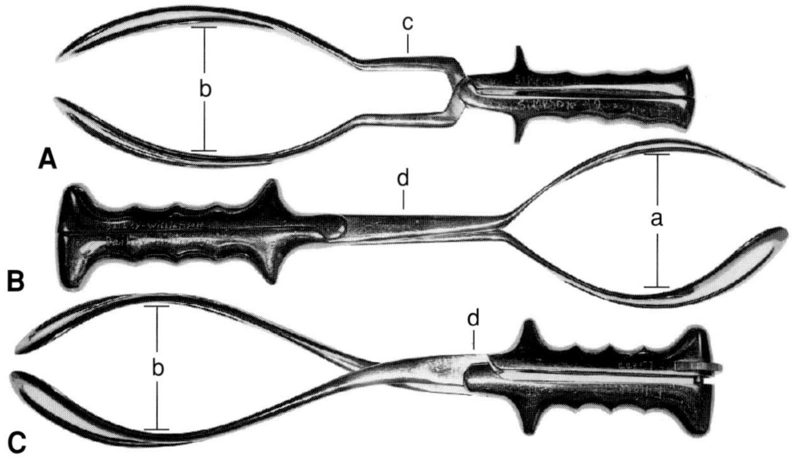

Figure 8–8. Top view of **A.** Simpson, **B.** Bailey-Williamson, and **C.** Elliot forceps. Note the more rounded cephalic curve of the Bailey-Williamson forceps (a) relative to the Simpson (b) or the Elliot forceps (b). Also note the parallel shanks of the Simpson forceps (c) compared to the overlapping shanks of the Bailey-Williamson or Elliot forceps (d).

ceps, the pelvic curve is directed upward so that when the forceps are applied to the fetal head presenting in an occiput anterior position (OA), the curve of the instrument approximates the pelvic Curve of Carus (Fig. 8–9). The tips of the blades of classical instruments, such as the Simpson and Elliot forceps, rise from 2.75 to 3.5 inches above the level of the handles (Fig. 8–10). When the head lies in a transverse position, however, as frequently occurs with midpelvic arrest, the pelvic curve is no longer desirable. The Kielland forceps were designed so that the pelvic curve is almost entirely eliminated. In contrast, Piper forceps (see Fig. 8–6) and the Hawks-Dennen forceps have a reverse pelvic curve.

The handle and blades of the forceps are connected by the intervening shank. The shank is longer in instruments such as the Kielland and Bailey-Williamson forceps, which are designed for midpelvic delivery. The shanks may be parallel (Simpson forceps) or may overlap (Elliot [Fig. 8–8] and Tucker-McLane forceps).

Each forceps has a locking mechanism located either on the shank or where the shank joins the handle. By convention, the lock is built into the left branch. The most commonly used locks are the sliding lock (Kielland forceps) and the English type (Simpson forceps) (Fig. 8–11). The English lock is a groove or slot lock at a fixed point for each member; articulation is rapid and easy. In comparison, the sliding lock of the Kielland forceps is built exclusively into the left branch and accordingly is not fixed when articulated. This lock is of the slot-type flanged design and is particularly useful where ideal application cannot at first be made because one unit must ride higher than its partner (Fig. 8–12), as often occurs with transverse arrest with asynclitism. The Laufe and short Piper forceps both use a pivot lock mechanism. The pivot lock is incorporated into the finger grip han-

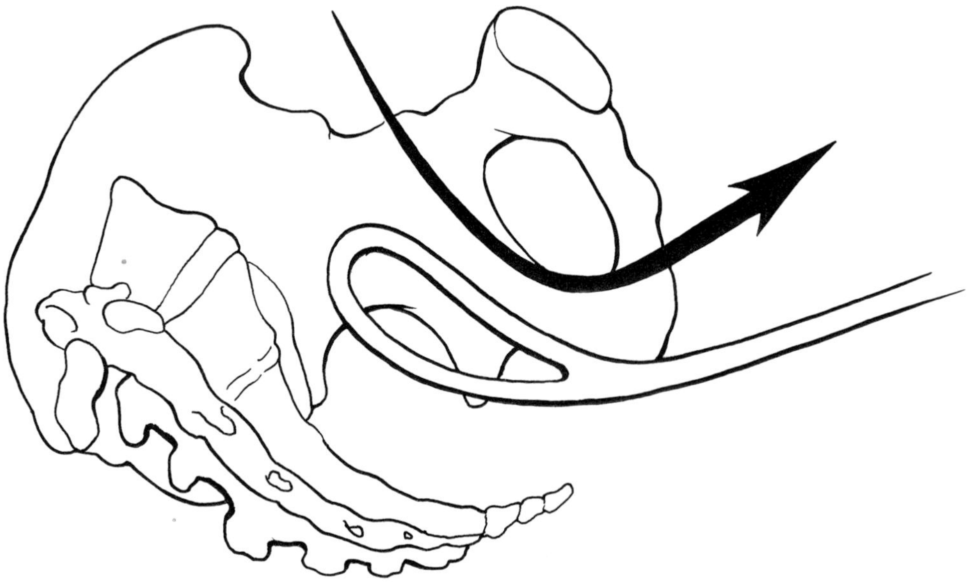

Figure 8–9. The cavity of the true pelvis is comparable to an obliquely truncated, bent cylinder with its greatest height posteriorly. Note the curvature of the pelvic axis, the so-called Curve of Carus.

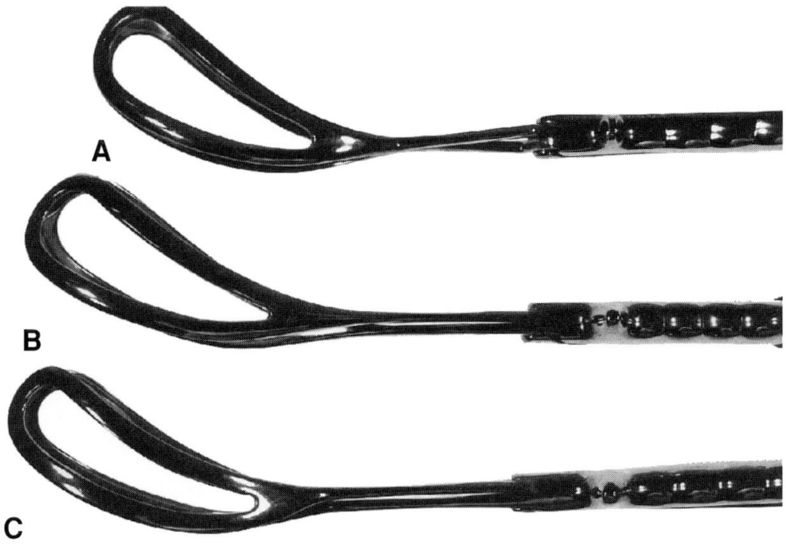

A

B

C

Figure 8–10. Lateral view of the **A.** Simpson, **B.** Bailey-Williamson, and **C.** Elliot forceps demonstrating the pelvic curve.

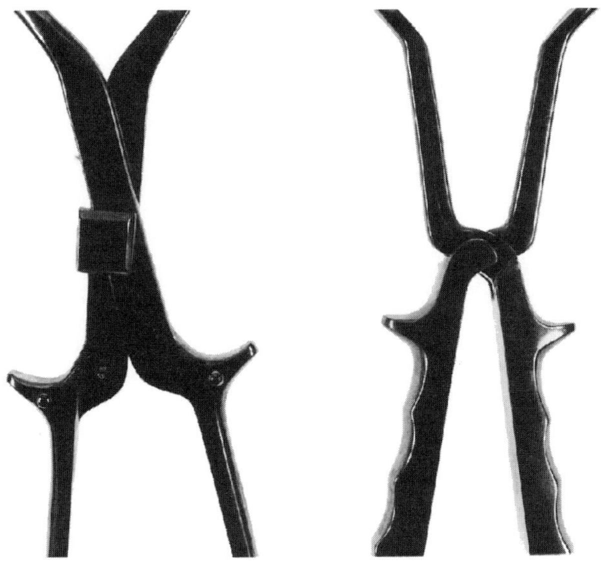

A B

Figure 8–11. Shown is **A.** the sliding locking mechanism of the Kielland forceps and **B.** the fixed English lock of the Simpson forceps.

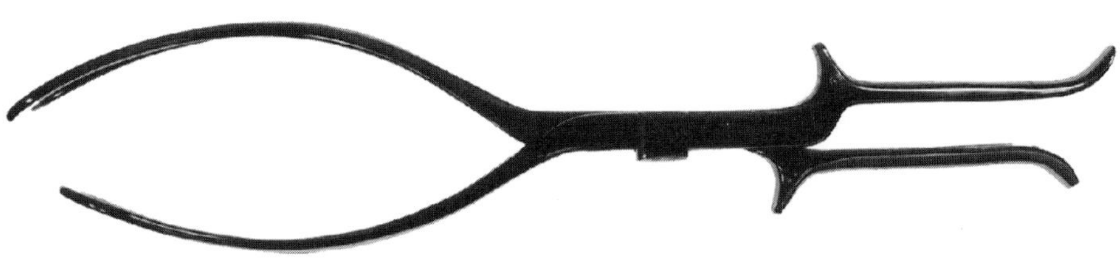

Figure 8–12. The Kielland forceps as viewed from above. This view could easily represent the forceps as applied to a right occiput transverse (ROT) position with asynclitism. In this situation, the anterior blade is inserted higher into the pelvis than the posterior blade. The asynclitism would be corrected by adjusting the shanks of the forceps after the sliding lock had been engaged.

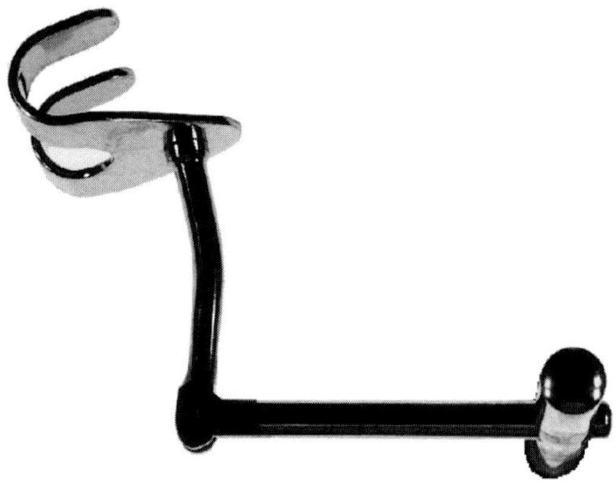

Figure 8–13. A Bill axis-traction device. This device is designed so that it will fit on the handle of many forceps including Simpson, Luikart-Simpson, Elliot, Bailey-Williamson, etc. When properly used, the hinge adjoining the handle to the arm extending to the forceps will be at approximately a 90-degree angle.

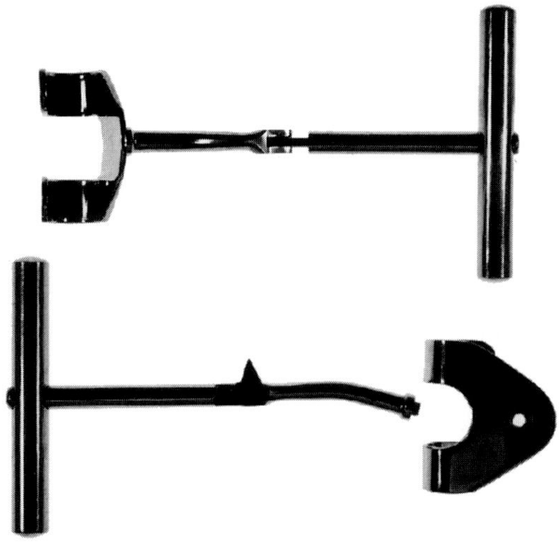

Figure 8–14. An intact and a broken axis-traction device. While breakage could result from mechanical failure and stress from use over a period of many years, it is by no means desirable to break metal instruments during an instrumented pelvic delivery.

dles of the forceps and traction tends to cause the blades to diverge, minimizing compressive forces on the fetal head (see Fig. 8–7).

The final portion of the forceps is the handle. Finger grips or lateral flanges are incorporated into the majority of forceps in contemporary use.

The principle of axis-traction has been incorporated into the design of some instruments such as the Hawks-Dennen forceps and can be obtained with others by use of a traction bar (Fig. 8–13). The Bill axis-traction device can be attached to the handle flange of several forceps instruments. It assists the operator in applying traction in the proper plane by maintaining the vector force in an out and downward direction (Bill, 1925). Figure 8–14 shows a Bill traction handle that was broken during a midpelvic delivery. This breakage suggests that excessive traction forces were being applied. Fortunately the fetus sustained no injury.

Contemporary Instruments

Classical Instruments

The forceps selected depends upon the nature of the procedure and the clinical indications (Table 8–1). The Simpson and Elliot forceps are considered all-purpose or classical instruments. These forceps have English locks, which allow locking only at one point and only when the shank of the right branch overlies the left (Fig. 8–8d). The Simpson forceps have parallel shanks, fenestrated blades, and a long, tapered cephalic curve designed to fit the molded fetal head. Elliot forceps have overlap-

TABLE 8–1. FORCEPS DELIVERY—INSTRUMENT TYPE

Procedure	Instrument
Outlet delivery	Classical forceps: Simpson or Elliot type Laufe divergent forceps
Low forceps delivery	
<45° rotation	Classical forceps
>45° rotation	Classical forceps Kielland Tucker-McLane Bailey-Williamson
Midforceps delivery	Keilland or Tucker-McLane Hawks-Dennen
Breech delivery	Piper Bailey-Williamson
Cesarean section	Vectis Blade—Murless Type Classical Forceps Laufe Forceps

ping shanks and short, fenestrated blades with a shorter and more rounded cephalic curve that is somewhat better suited for application to the unmolded head. A wheel and screw device is built into the handle of the instrument to avoid compression of the fetal head if the handles are squeezed (see Fig. 8–2). The Tucker-McLane forceps, a variant of the Elliot type, have short, solid blades. The overlapping shanks and solid blades make this a popular instrument for rotations.

Specialized Instruments

Specialized forceps have been developed to effect delivery in situations not amenable to solution with the classical instruments. The Kielland forceps, with no pelvic curve and a sliding lock (see Fig. 8–4), originally was designed for use in mid-pelvic arrest, but they have been used since extensively for rotations. The sliding lock is useful to correct asynclitism, a common problem in transverse arrest. Kielland forceps also are occasionally used to effect delivery of the face presentation.

Piper forceps have long shanks with a reverse pelvic curve for ease of application to the aftercoming fetal head in a breech delivery (see Figs. 8–5 and 8–6). The forceps stabilize and protect the fetal head and neck during delivery. When difficulty is encountered in spontaneous delivery of the fetal head, use of Piper forceps may produce lower morbidity than manual maneuvers.

The Laufe outlet forceps incorporate the unique design of a pivot lock and finger grips (see Fig. 8–7). Divergent blades diminish the compressive force on the fetal head, and traction on the finger grips applies no additional force at the toes of the blades. The short length of the instrument makes it easy to apply at cesarean section. The Laufe modification of the Piper forceps is useful for delivery of the aftercoming head of the premature breech fetus.

Other instruments designed during this century include highly specialized forceps and traction devices. The Barton forceps, which consist of a hinged anterior blade, a posterior blade with an acute curvature, and a sliding lock, were developed for high transverse arrest. Although they are used infrequently today, there has been renewed interest in the application of these forceps for delivery of the fetal head at cesarean section (Megison, 1993).

CLASSIFICATION OF FORCEPS OPERATIONS

One reason forceps have remained controversial is the lack of agreement regarding classification of the operation. It is clear that different categories of forceps operations are associated with significantly different morbidity. The forceps operation has classically been described according to the station of the fetal bony head in the pelvis. There was disagreement as to whether station should be determined by the leading bony edge or the biparietal diameter (BPD) as well as whether the pelvis should be divided by centimeters or by thirds.

Titus Classification

In 1949, Titus, Greenhill, McCormick, and Eastman formulated a classification of forceps operations that they felt was simple, practicable with or without x-ray pelvimetry, and safe (Dennen, 1952). The major purpose of their system was to identify instances in which general practitioners could perform an instrumental delivery without consulting a specialist. Their system involved only three levels and resulted in a narrow definition of low forceps, a broad definition of midforceps, and a well-accepted definition of high forceps.

ACOG Classification

Nearly 16 years later, in 1965, the American College of Obstetricians and Gynecologists (ACOG) adopted the Titus scheme for high, mid-, and outlet forceps operations. The term *outlet forceps* was used in preference to *low forceps*, but was defined equivalently. This classification was not well accepted, even at the time, because the definition of outlet forceps was too restrictive and resulted in the classification of many relatively simple operations as midforceps. The midforceps category included all instrumental deliveries commencing from the ischial spines down to the level of the pelvic floor as well as those in which rotation was required. Many clinicians felt that this distance in the pelvis (from the ischial spines to the perineum) was too great to be classified as a single operation.

Dennen Classification

In contrast to Titus and associates, E. H. Dennen proposed an alternative classification system in 1952 based on the four major obstetric planes of the pelvis. He defined high forceps as the BPD in the plane of the inlet and the leading bony edge slightly above the ischial spines. The term *midforceps* described operations with the BPD through the inlet, the leading bony part at or just below the ischial spines, and with the hollow of the sacrum not yet filled. A low-midforceps delivery was one in which the BPD was in the plane of the spines, the leading bony point within a finger breadth of the perineum between contractions, and with the hollow of the sacrum filled. Outlet forceps referred to operations wherein the BPD was below the plane of the spines and the sagittal suture was in the anteroposterior diameter with the head visible during a contraction. The major points of contention with Dennen's scheme were the confusing references to the plane of the BPD and the category of low-midforceps, which was later specifically disapproved in the 1965 ACOG classification scheme.

TABLE 8–2. CLASSIFICATION OF FORCEPS DELIVERIES ACCORDING TO STATION AND ROTATION

Type of Procedure	Classification
Outlet forceps	1. Scalp is visible at the introitus without separating labia. 2. Fetal skull has reached pelvic floor. 3. Sagittal suture is in anteroposterior diameter or right or left occiput anterior or posterior position. 4. Fetal head is at or on perineum. 5. Rotation does not exceed 45°.
Low forceps	Leading point of fetal skull is at station ≥ +2 cm, and not on the pelvic floor. 1. Rotation ≤ 45° (left or right occiput anterior to occiput anterior, or left or right occiput posterior to occiput posterior). 2. Rotation >45°
Midforceps	Station above +2 cm but head engaged
High	Not included in classification

American College of Obstetricians and Gynecologists. Obstetrics forceps. ACOG Committee Opinion 71. Washington, DC: ACOG, 1989.

ACOG Classification

In 1988, ACOG issued a new classification that emphasized two factors. First, the station of the fetal head in the pelvis was estimated in centimeters. Station referred to the level of the leading bony point of the fetal head at or below the level of the maternal ischial spines (Table 8–2). Engagement implied that the BPD had passed through the pelvic inlet, and that the leading bony edge of the fetal head was usually at the level of the ischial spines (0 station). The fetal head was classified as +5 cm when crowning. The category of high forceps was eliminated. Under virtually no circumstance were forceps to be applied to an unengaged presenting part, a fetus with intact membranes, or if the cervix had not dilated completely. The second important factor emphasized in the new classification was the degree of rotation, which was classified as ≤45 degrees and greater than 45 degrees.

The 1988 classification was modeled closely after the Dennen scheme and has led to a clearer stratification of risks among types of operations. Hagadorn-Freathy and associates (1991) reported on 281 midforceps and 76 outlet forceps deliveries as classified by the 1965 ACOG criteria. When reclassified according to the 1988 ACOG criteria, only 22 percent of the original 281 midforceps operations remained as midforceps. One hundred seventy-eight (63%) of the operations that were previously classified as midforceps became low forceps deliveries, and all but 27 involved less than 45 degrees of rotation. As shown in Table 8–3, adverse maternal and fetal outcome correlate both with station and with amount of rotation involved. In evaluating the data shown in Table 8–3 it is important to consider that the maternal injury rate with cesarean delivery is 100% and that maternal infection and transfusion rates are both higher with cesarean section. Further, the fetal injuries were facial nerve palsies (n = 10), brachial plexus palsy (n = 3), clavicular fracture (n = 5), and cephalohematoma (n = 24); most of these injuries resolved within days of delivery with no permanent sequelae, and all of the injuries resolved by 5 months of age.

INDICATIONS

Indications for forceps delivery have changed little since early in this century. Forceps delivery may be indicated on behalf of mother, fetus, or both.

TABLE 8–3. MATERNAL AND FETAL OUTCOME BY FORCEPS OPERATION

	Outlet (%) (*N* = 116)	Low ≤45° (%) (*N* = 151)	Low >45° (%) (*N* = 27)	Mid (%) (*N* = 63)
Maternal				
Episiotomy				
(3° or 4°)	9	14	30	21
Vaginal laceration	5	10	26	22
Blood transfusion	0.9	0.7	—	3.2
Hospital stay >5 d	7	7	19	14
Neonatal				
Apgar score				
1 min <3	2	3	—	6
5 min <7	1	3	—	3
Umbilical arterial				
pH <7.20	17	25	30	37
Fetal injury	5	11	7	19

Maternal Indications

Maternal indications include disease states that impair the ability to push or conditions that may be worsened by prolonged voluntary expulsive effort. Examples of the former include neurologic disorders associated with weakness and certain pulmonary diseases; maternal cardiac disease is the classic example of the latter. Collectively, these diseases are uncommon. More often forceps delivery is indicated by maternal fatigue or by a dense regional block that inhibits motor fibers. The latter was common when saddle block anesthesia was used for vaginal delivery, but a properly dosed epidural block should not interfere with muscular control and expulsive efforts to the same degree. Other anesthetic considerations are discussed in the section that follows.

Fetal Indications

Fetal indications for forceps delivery include non-reassuring fetal heart rate patterns. The degree of heart rate abnormality justifying or necessitating operative intervention is not well quantified whether it is diagnosed in the first or the second stage of labor. In the first stage, provided that the pattern cannot be resolved by intrauterine resuscitative measures, cesarean section is the only management option. In the second stage of labor, the obstetrician must carefully evaluate the clinical situation to determine whether abdominal or operative vaginal delivery will produce the best maternal and perinatal outcome. Forceps delivery may be more expedient than assembling an operating team for cesarean section. Conversely, a traumatic instrumental delivery from the midpelvic cavity may be avoided by judicious selection of cesarean delivery. It is well established that even the uncomplicated second stage of labor is associated with progressive fetal acidosis; safe shortening of this stage may be desirable. These decisions require judgment, skill, and individualization on the part of the operator.

Combined Maternal and Fetal Indications

Two other indications for forceps delivery are probably best classified as combined maternal and fetal indications. The first is termination of a prolonged second stage of labor. The 1991 ACOG Technical Bulletin states that operative delivery should be considered when the second stage of labor has exceeded 3 hours in the nulliparous woman with a regional anesthetic, or 2 hours without a regional anesthetic. Similarly, a multiparous patient should be carefully evaluated after 1 hour without regional anesthesia or after 2 hours with regional anesthesia. These recommendations are intended to serve as guidelines rather than strict rules. The times can be exceeded safely if there is continued, albeit slow progress in descent without evidence of fetal or maternal compromise. Less often, arrest of descent may be diagnosed before these suggested time limits have been reached.

Epidural Anesthesia

In the last 10 years, the use of epidural anesthesia for labor has increased, undoubtedly due to enhanced maternal satisfaction with the pain relief offered by this technique as well as its relative safety for the fetus (ACOG, 1991). However, two important questions have been raised about the use of epidural anesthesia: (1) Does it affect maternal expulsive efforts and duration of the second stage of labor? (2) Does paralysis of the pelvic diaphragm result in fetal malposition? Hoult and colleagues (1977) prospectively studied the frequency of instrumental deliveries and the incidence of malposition, defined as any position requiring assisted rotation, in women with epidural anesthesia. They found that nulliparous women were three times as likely to have malposition of the vertex and to require instrumental delivery. Institution of epidural blockade before cervical dilatation of 5 cm was not responsible for the increased incidence of operative vaginal delivery. However, when the anesthesia level was reduced and the woman's sensation returned, the need for instrumental deliveries declined. The results of this study may have been influenced by the use of 0.5% bupivacaine in contrast to the 0.25% or 0.125% more often used today. Still, Chestnut and colleagues (1987) found that even 0.125% bupivacaine prolonged the second stage of labor and increased operative vaginal deliveries.

Phillipsen and Jensen (1989) prospectively randomized patients to regional anesthesia or intravenous opiates in the first stage of labor. The epidural analgesic effect was allowed to wear off in the second stage, and women were not redosed after reaching 8 cm of dilation. With this protocol, the investigators found that there were an equal number of instrumental and spontaneous deliveries in each group. In contrast, when Thorp (1989) studied laboring women with epidural anesthetics in whom the anesthesia had not been decreased or turned off, he found that 25 percent had been delivered by forceps as opposed to 7 percent of those who had not had epidural anesthesia. Kaminski and co-workers (1987), controlling for fetal size and malposition, reported a twofold increase in instrumental deliveries, as well as an incidence of midforceps deliveries that was three times greater in women with epidural anesthesia. The incidence of malposition, such as persistent occiput posterior, was tripled.

Thus, most of the published evidence suggests that epidural anesthesia prolongs the second stage of labor and increases instrumental deliveries. As previously discussed, many of these studies have involved intermittent bolus doses of local anesthetic agents administered in higher concentrations than currently used. Proponents of epidural anesthesia emphasize reports that low concentrations of anesthetic agents given by continuous infusion do not result in increased instrumental delivery (Wittels, 1991). However, these are controlled situations managed by obstetric anesthesiologists, and the same outcome may not be achievable in other settings.

PREREQUISITES FOR FORCEPS APPLICATION

The decision to perform a forceps operation is at least as important as a decision to perform a cesarean operation. Accordingly, unless a forceps operation is performed under emergency circumstances, the physician should write a thorough and complete preoperative note. Included should be documentation that the operation is to be performed with the patient's knowledge and consent. The following are the minimum prerequisites for an operative forceps delivery:

1. The fetal head is engaged at 0 station or lower.
2. The membranes are ruptured.
3. The cervix is fully dilated and effaced.
4. The exact position of the fetal head is known.
5. The patient's pelvis has been assessed for adequacy and the maternal–fetal size relationship evaluated.
6. Appropriate maternal anesthesia is available.
7. Necessary personnel and support equipment are available.
8. The surgeon is knowledgeable about the instruments and technique and possesses the skills necessary to use them.
9. There is a willingness to abandon attempts if the forceps delivery does not proceed readily.
10. The patient's informed consent has

been obtained orally or preferably in written form.

Far more critical than technical proficiency is the knowledge of when forceps should be used and when they should not.

Anesthesia Requirements for Forceps Delivery

Adequate levels of anesthesia are important to ensure the safest delivery for both the mother and the fetus (ACOG, 1991). Generally, pudendal block anesthesia is sufficient for outlet forceps and for low forceps operations involving rotation ≤45 degrees. For low forceps operations with rotation >45 degrees and for midforcep operations, regional anesthesia is preferred. General anesthetic agents also may be used for forceps deliveries, but their use is unusual.

Training

One of the most important prerequisites for the conduct of a forceps delivery is a skilled operator. The physician must be able to adequately assess the capacity of the bony pelvis and any soft tissue obstruction, determine that the cervix is fully dilated and, that the fetal vertex is engaged, and must know unequivocally the fetal position and station. Also important is the physician's ability to determine flexion, asynclitism, caput, and molding. The forceps must be properly applied to the fetal head (cephalic placement) because incorrect application increases the risk of injury. Finally, the operator must properly apply traction by using the minimum amount of force in the direction of least resistance. Station should be gained with each application of traction; the majority of deliveries should require five or fewer "pulls" (Sjostedt, 1967). These skills are acquired only through experience, and competence is maintained by use. Overreliance on Cesarean section reduces the opportunities for acquiring and maintaining the skills necessary to perform forceps deliveries.

A survey of 144 US and Canadian residency programs was conducted in the early 1980s to determine existing attitudes on the use of forceps (Healy and Laufe, 1985). Of the 73 percent of programs that responded, all still used outlet forceps. Further, all but one program reported that they still performed midforceps procedures. In 1990, Ramin and colleagues repeated this survey to assess the impact of the 1988 classification system on practice patterns. Ninety-nine percent of responding residency programs stated they were aware of the new definitions, and 80 percent were using them. Although all programs continued to use outlet forceps, 14 percent no longer performed midforceps deliveries. The trend was toward fewer operative vaginal deliveries and increased reliance on cesarean section. In one half of all programs, less than 5 percent of all deliveries were performed by outlet or low forceps. The decline in midforceps use probably reflects the more stringent new definitions; less than 1 percent of all deliveries are by midforceps in 75 percent of training programs; the rate is probably lower in private practice (Ramin and associates, 1993).

The decrease in the actual number of forceps deliveries in part reflects the attitude of the residency program directors. In 1990, 75 percent believed that outlet forceps operations were "important" or "extremely important" and 40 percent believed midforceps were "important" or "very important." Twenty percent thought midforceps training was of no importance. Lack of training in forceps deliveries is a major reason for their decline (Seiler, 1990). Training should occur at the podium and in the delivery room. Application of forceps by trainees should be supervised by experienced operators to guard against bad outcomes and to avoid the acquisition of bad habits.

Fetopelvic Relationship

One of the most important prerequisites for forceps deliveries is an accurate assessment of fetopelvic relationships (see Chap. 5, Pelvimetry). An essential component of training for instrumental vaginal deliveries is clinical evaluation of the pelvis—regrettably ill, if not a dying art. The frequent and quick retreat to cesarean section to solve a wide variety of obstetrical problems has diminished the emphasis on knowledge of the mechanical aspects of obstetrics during residency training and in clinical practice.

The Fetus

The exact position of the fetal head can be diagnosed by careful vaginal examination. It is, however, not always an easy feat. Caput and molding, redundant maternal soft tissue, and reliance on palpation of the fontanelles all contribute to incorrect diagnosis.

Using a systematic approach, the examiner should first attempt to locate the sagittal suture (Fig. 8–15). This suture should be traced in both directions, the shape of each fontanelle assessed, and the number of lines of intersection counted. At the posterior fontanelle, the two lambdoid sutures and the sagittal suture account for three intersecting lines. At the anterior fontanelle, the right and left halves of the coronal suture intersect with the frontal (metopic) suture and the sagittal suture, producing a total of four intersecting lines (Fig. 8–15). Sometimes the shape of the fontanelle (the posterior is triangular, the anterior is diamond shaped) will suffice for diagnosis; but meticulous counting of sutures

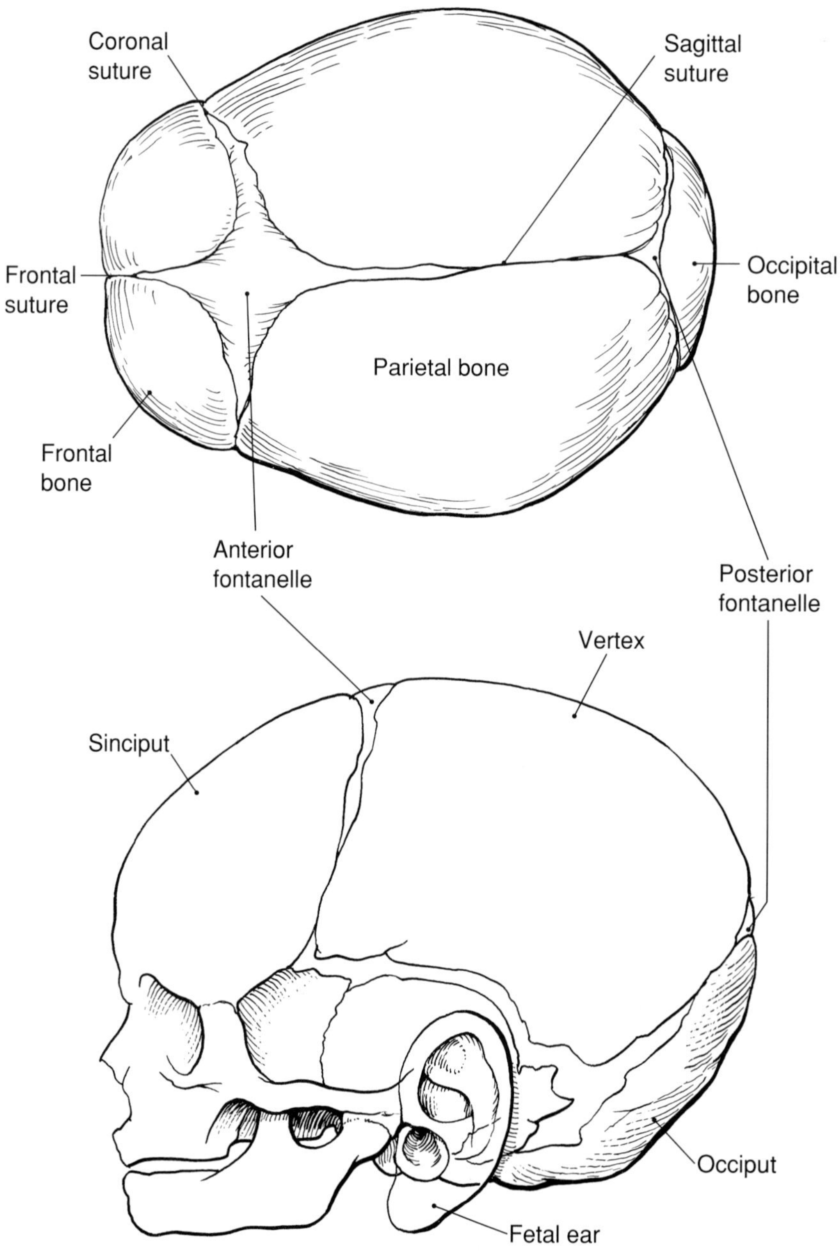

Figure 8–15. The landmarks of the fetal skull necessary for determining fetal position.

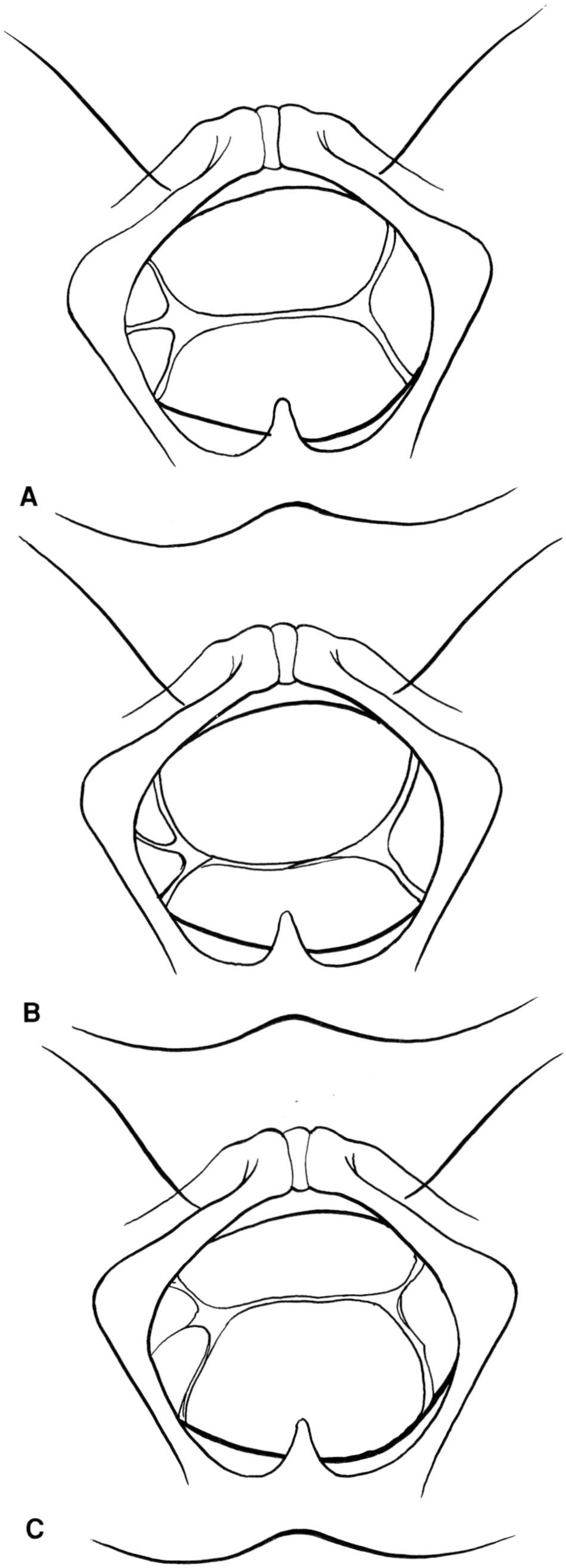

Figure 8–16A. The fetus in LOT position with normal synclitism. **B.** LOT position with anterior parietal presentation due to anterior asynclitism. Note that the sagittal suture has been displaced into the posterior segment of the maternal pelvis. **C.** LOT position with posterior parietal presentation due to posterior asynclitism. The sagittal suture has been displaced into the anterior pelvis.

is preferable. If diagnosis of position remains in doubt, the examiner should locate a fetal ear. The posterior ear is usually more readily accessible, and both the external auditory meatus and the pinna should be sought. Knowing the relative position of these two structures should always lead to a correct assessment of position.

The presence of asynclitism, the tilting of the fetal head toward either the left or right shoulder of the fetus, should be carefully addressed during assessment of the fetus. In the fetus in left occiput transverse position, if the fetal head is tilted down toward the left fetal shoulder, the right parietal bone will be primarily presenting and represent anterior asynclitism. In this instance, the sagittal suture will be displaced toward the posterior aspect of the pelvis (Fig. 8–16B). In contrast, in left occiput transverse position with posterior asynclitism, the fetal head is tilted toward the right shoulder and the sagittal suture displaced into the anterior maternal pelvis (Fig. 8–16C). The obstetrician also should ascertain the degree of flexion or extension of the fetal head. In the occiput anterior position, the posterior fontanelle should be easily palpated in the anterior quadrant of the maternal pelvis. Greater ease in palpating the anterior fontanelle relative to the posterior fontanelle suggests problems with deflexion of the fetal head for anterior positions.

The Pelvis

Intrapartum assessment of the pelvis should begin at the inlet and proceed downward. The diagonal conjugate represents the distance from the inferior margin of the symphysis pubis to the sacral promontory (Fig. 8–17). Subtracting 1.5–2.0 cm from the diagonal conjugate gives an estimate of the obstetric conjugate, the narrowest anteroposterior diameter through which the fetal head must pass. A deeply engaged head precludes determination of the diagonal conjugate, but at the same time renders the determination unimportant because

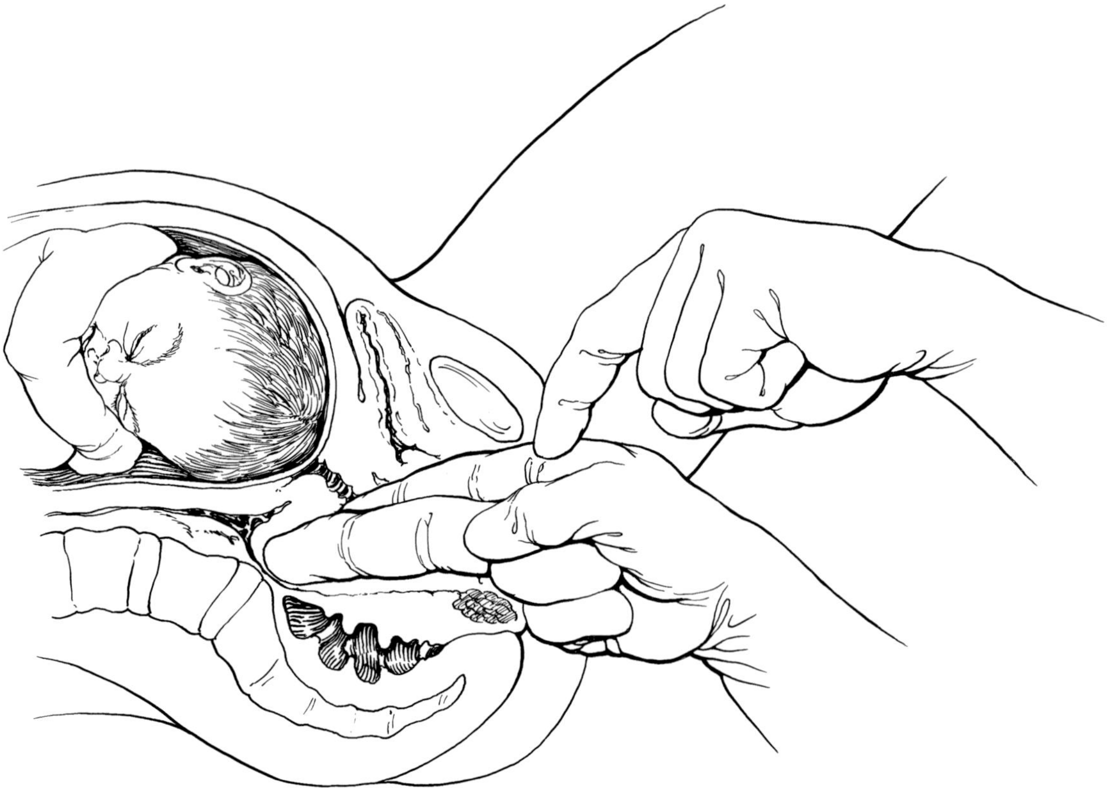

Figure 8–17. Vaginal examination to determine the diagonal conjugate. Subtracting 1.5–2 cm from the diagonal conjugate yields a good approximation of the obstetric conjugate.

the head has already passed through the pelvic inlet. The transverse diameter of the inlet cannot be determined clinically (see Chap. 5).

The important features of the midplane of the pelvis include the shape and position of the sacrum, the prominence of the ischial spines, and the width of the sacrosciatic notch. This last feature is approximated by determining the width in finger breadths of the connecting sacrosciatic ligament (Fig. 8–18). It should be at least two finger breadths wide. Prominent spines and a forward flat sacrum are characteristic of a contracted midpelvis. A midforceps delivery in such a pelvis, wherein the BPD has not yet passed the midplane, would increase the risk of injury to the infant.

In addition, the operator should assess the outlet by estimating with the closed fist the interischial-tuberosity distance (normally >8 cm), palpating the coccyx and lower sacrum, and evaluating the forepelvis. The forepelvis is examined by placing two fingers under the symphysis to determine the shape of the arch. The fingers are then curved superiorly to palpate the retropubic angle, which is rounded in gynecoid, angulated sharply in android, and nearly flat in platypelloid pelvis (Fig. 8–19). The degree of convergence of the pelvic sidewalls should also be noted.

The final step in assessing the pelvis consists of combining and integrating the information gained from both the fetal position assessment and the estimation of maternal pelvic configuration. Is the head asynclitic? Does the head fill or partially fill the hollow of the sacrum? Where is the most usable room in the pelvis? Can the head be rotated if necessary? The answers to these questions will provide the operator with important information as to whether or not to deliver by forceps and if so, how.

Adequate knowledge of the pelvis is critical for maintaining the viability of forceps delivery. In addition, an understanding of clinical pelvimetry not only increases the safety of forceps procedures, but improves decision making regarding induction of labor, use of oxytocin, method of anesthesia, management of prolonged labor, and choice of route of delivery.

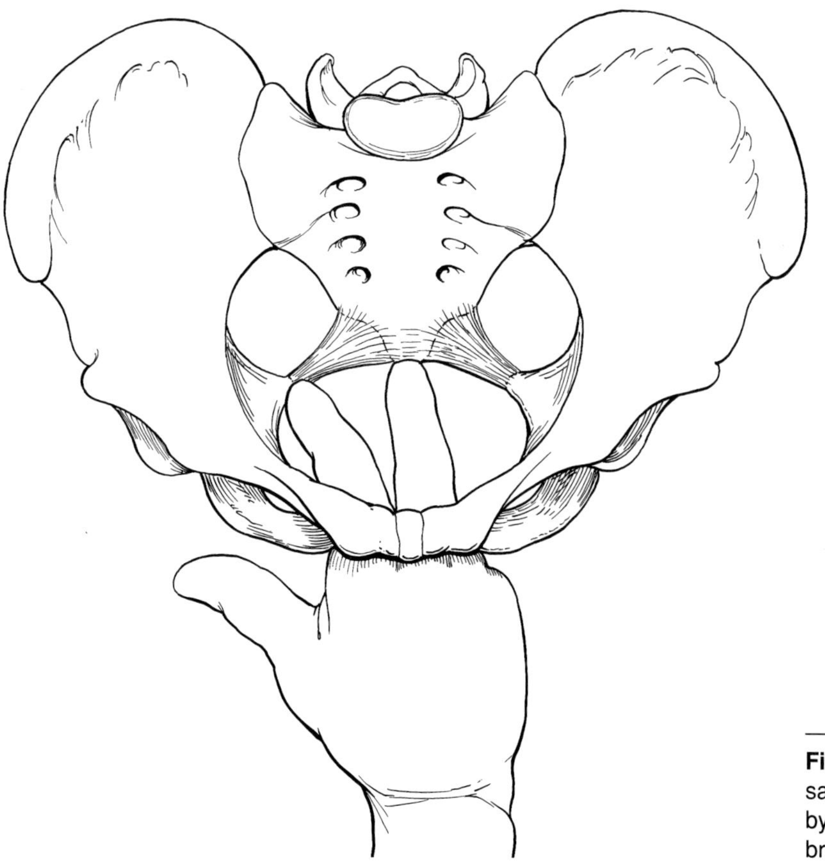

Figure 8–18. The length of the sacrospinous ligament is estimated by determining the width in finger breadths of the sacrosciatic notch.

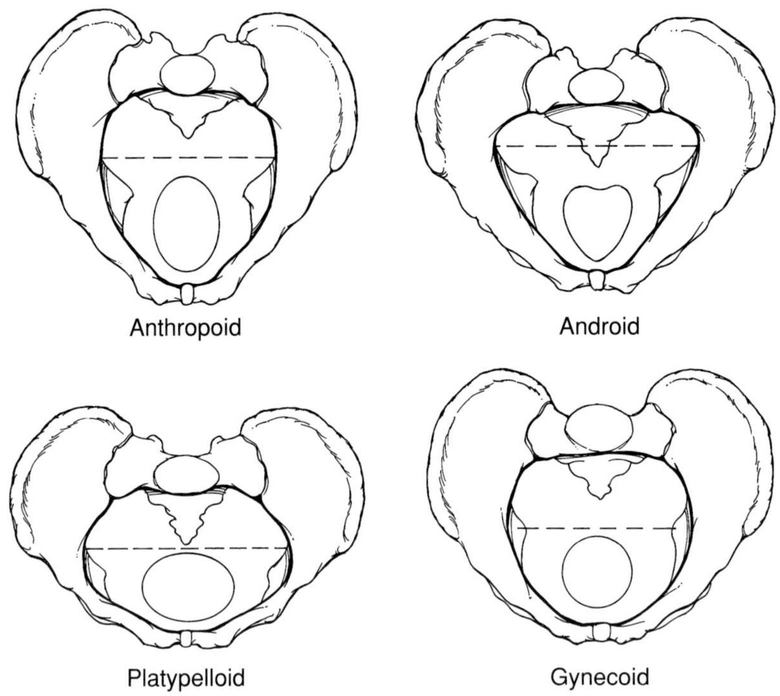

Figure 8–19. The four parent pelvic types of the Caldwell-Moloy classification system.

TECHNIQUE FOR FORCEPS DELIVERY

General

The patient is placed in lithotomy position with the legs suitably supported in flexion and abduction with the buttocks resting at the edge of the table. Care should be taken that the level of abduction is not so great as to put undue stress on the perineal body, which could lead to either spontaneous tears or extension of the episiotomy if performed. If the length of the pubic hair might interfere with the procedure or a repair, it can be clipped with scissors. The vulva and perineum are scrubbed with an appropriate antiseptic solution. Next, the patient is sterilely draped. The bladder should be assessed and if necessary, drained. Careful vaginal examination is performed once again to ensure that all prerequisites for forceps delivery have been met. Finally, adequacy of anesthesia for the operation is ensured before proceeding.

Appropriate and suggested forceps for different operations are listed in Table 8–1. It is good practice to hold the forceps in front of the perineum in an articulated fashion and align them so that they approximate the position once applied to the fetal head. Regardless of the fetal position, we prefer to insert the posterior forceps branch first in order to prevent loss of station of the fetal head. The left forceps branch is held in the left hand while the right hand serves as a guide during introduction. To position the right branch, the operator holds it in the right hand and uses the left hand as a guide during introduction. When the sagittal suture is in the anterior-posterior diameter, the left blade is inserted first. This facilitates locking the handles after application of the right blade because the lock is on the left blade. If the forceps are inserted in reverse order, they must be crossed on the perineum in order to articulate them. During insertion, the obstetrician should be careful that the toe of the forceps blade does not injure the fetal face.

The goal of cephalic application is for the forceps blades to fit the head as evenly and as symmetrically as possible. The blades should lie evenly against the side of the head and reach to and beyond the malar eminences, symmetrically covering the space between the orbits and the ears (Fig. 8–20). The correct application prevents soft tissue and nerve injury as well as bony injuries of the fetal head. Pressure is evenly distributed and applied to the least vulnerable areas, the malar eminences. Correct application depends upon the operator's knowledge of the attitude

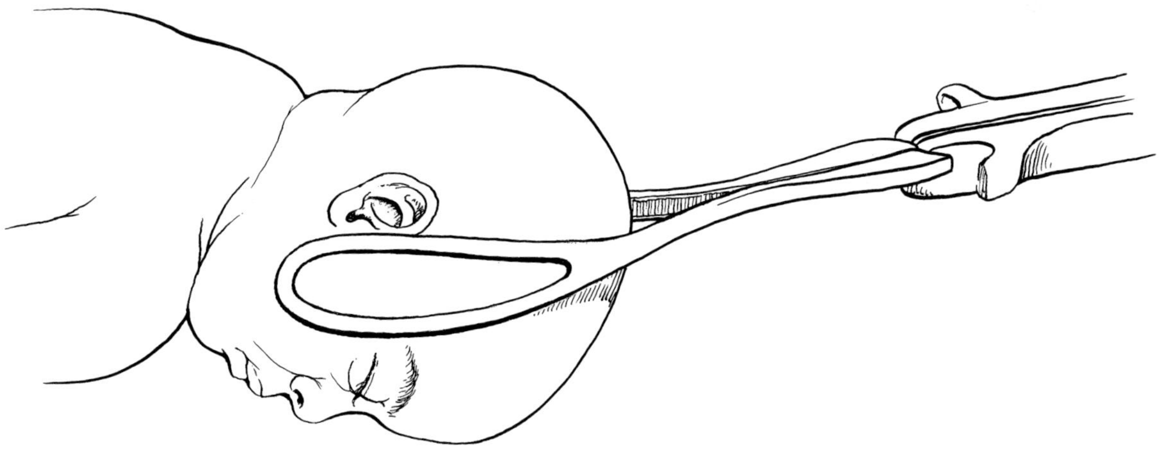

Figure 8-20. Cephalic application of forceps. This application is also referred to as the biparietal or bimalar application. The blade should lie evenly against the sides of the head, reaching to and beyond the malar eminences, symmetrically covering the space between the orbits and the ears.

of the fetal head. This knowledge allows the operator to facilitate descent in the proper attitude of flexion. The tractive force necessary to achieve delivery is thereby minimized, and trauma to maternal and fetal tissue is decreased. As shown in Figure 8–9, the cavity of the true pelvis is comparable to an obliquely truncated bent cylinder with its greatest height posteriorly. The descent of the fetus through the pelvis must follow the pelvic axis.

After the forceps are introduced and locked, they should be checked to ensure that the branches are appropriately applied before they are used for rotation or retraction. Three checks for proper application to the head in occiput anterior or oblique positions are (1) the sagittal suture throughout its length is perpendicular to the plane of the shanks, (2) the posterior fontanelle is one finger breadth away from the plane of the shanks and equidistant from the sides of the blades, directly in front of the locked point of the articulated forceps, and (3) if fenestrated blades are used, the amount of fenestration in front of the fetal head should not admit more than the tip of one finger (Fig. 8–21). The purpose of these checks is to prevent asymmetric compression of the fetal head, a notable risk with brow mastoid application. The perfectly symmetric grip on the fetal head ensured by these checks also reduces the amount of traction necessary and is less likely to result in forceps marks on the newborn.

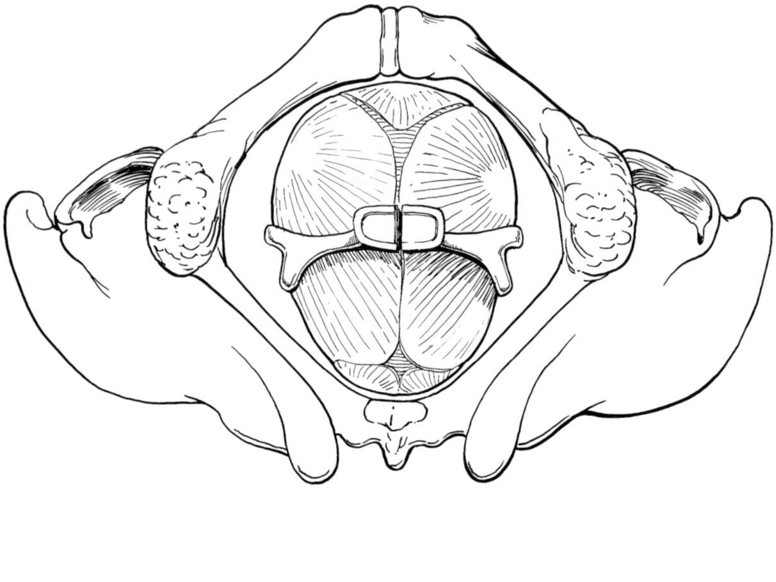

Figure 8–21. Proper application of the forceps to the fetal head in occiput anterior position is ascertained by checking that (1) the sagittal suture throughout its length is perpendicular to the plane of the shanks, (2) the posterior fontanelle is one finger breadth away from the plane of the shanks equidistance from the sides of the blades, directly in front of the locked point of the articulated forceps and, (3) if fenestrated blades are used, the amount of fenestration in front of the fetal head will admit no more than the tip of one finger.

Occiput Anterior (OA)

The forceps are locked and held in front of the bulging perineum in the same position they will assume on the fetal head. For application in the direct occiput anterior position, the left instrument is held delicately between the thumb and first and second fingers in much the same way as a pencil. The left blade is introduced first, with the fingers of the right hand placed between the labia and the fetal head to serve as a guide. The left branch is carried in a sweeping arch across the perineum from above such that the handle begins in an almost vertical position (Fig. 8–22A). The blade is guided into position by the first two fingers of the right hand. As the blade is inserted, the handle is dropped into a horizontal position. Great gentleness is important; this is a procedure of finesse, not force. The instrument should be guided into place with relative ease. Sometimes lubrication of the forceps with an antiseptic solution facilitates

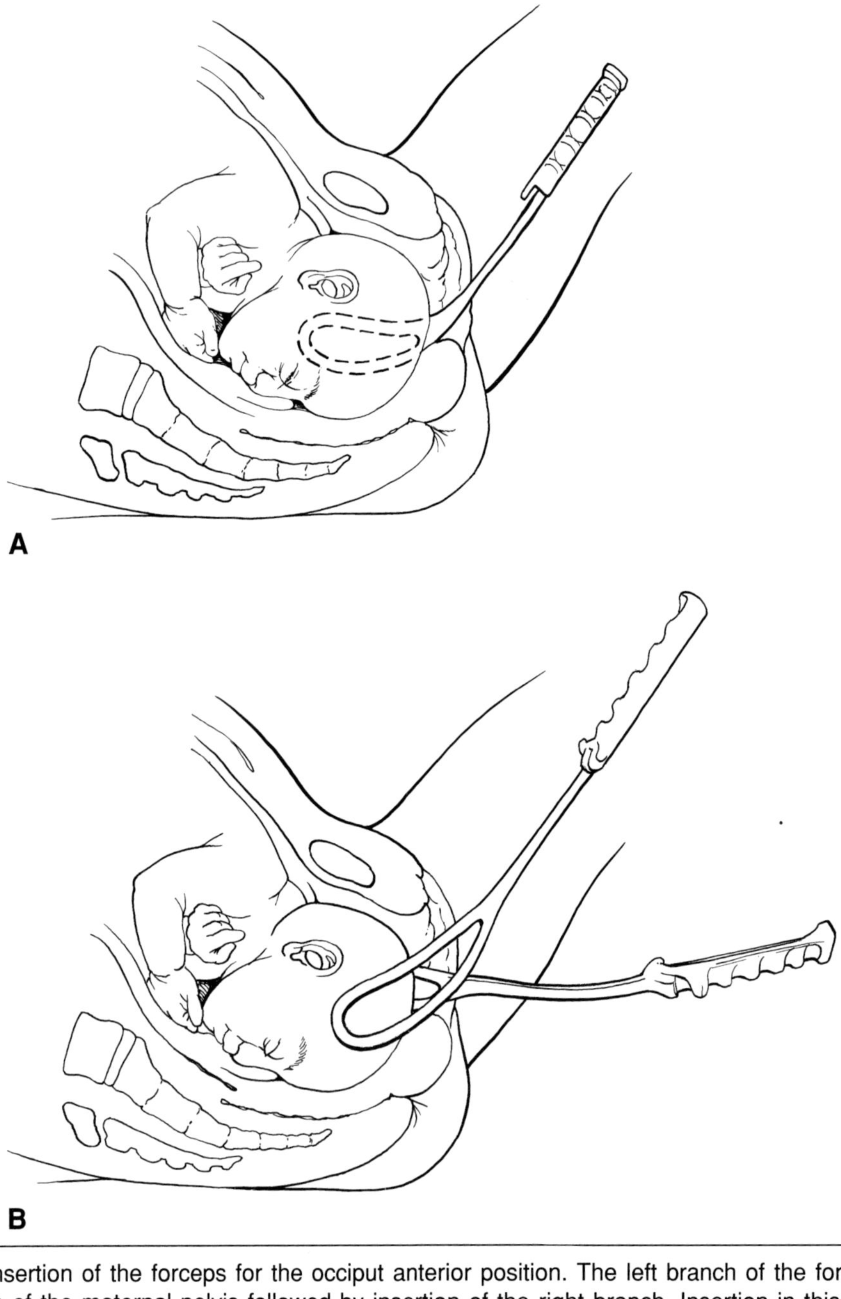

A

B

Figure 8–22. Insertion of the forceps for the occiput anterior position. The left branch of the forceps is inserted into the left side of the maternal pelvis followed by insertion of the right branch. Insertion in this order facilitates locking of the branches without crossing the handles of the instruments. **A.** Insertion of the left branch. **B.** Insertion of the right branch.

placement. The blade then can be held in position by an assistant or alternatively held in position by compressive forces of the maternal soft tissues. The opposite branch is then grasped in a similar manner with the right hand and inserted into the right side of the pelvis, the left hand serving as a guide (Fig. 8–22B). Either branch can be further positioned to achieve best placement by gentle wandering of the branch after the initial insertion. For the left branch this is performed using the fingers of the right hand against the blade of the forceps while the left hand gently supports the handle and shank of the forceps. The reverse procedure is performed for wandering of the right forceps branch. The branches are then locked and the application is checked by vaginal examination as previously described. If difficulty is encountered in articulating the forceps branches, position should be rechecked and correct position ascertained before additional attempts to articulate the branches.

Left Occiput Anterior (LOA)

When the fetus is in LOA position, the left ear is posterior. Dennen's four cardinal points emphasize that for LOA the left branch should be held in the left hand and inserted into the left side of the pelvis in front of the left ear of the fetus. Application is similar to that for a direct occiput anterior (OA) except that the curve of the blade is directed in a more downward position with the cephalic curve inward toward the vulva. The plane of the shank initially is oriented vertically relative to the floor. The blade is directed along the curved plane of the fetal head and the left posterior side of the pelvis to its position in front of the left ear and over the malar eminence. The middle and index fingers of the right hand are inserted into the vagina opposite the left parietal bone to guide the toe of the blade along the side of the head. The right thumb is placed against the heel of the blade as the cephalic curve of the blade is positioned against the curve of the fetal skull (Fig. 8–23). The force necessary to

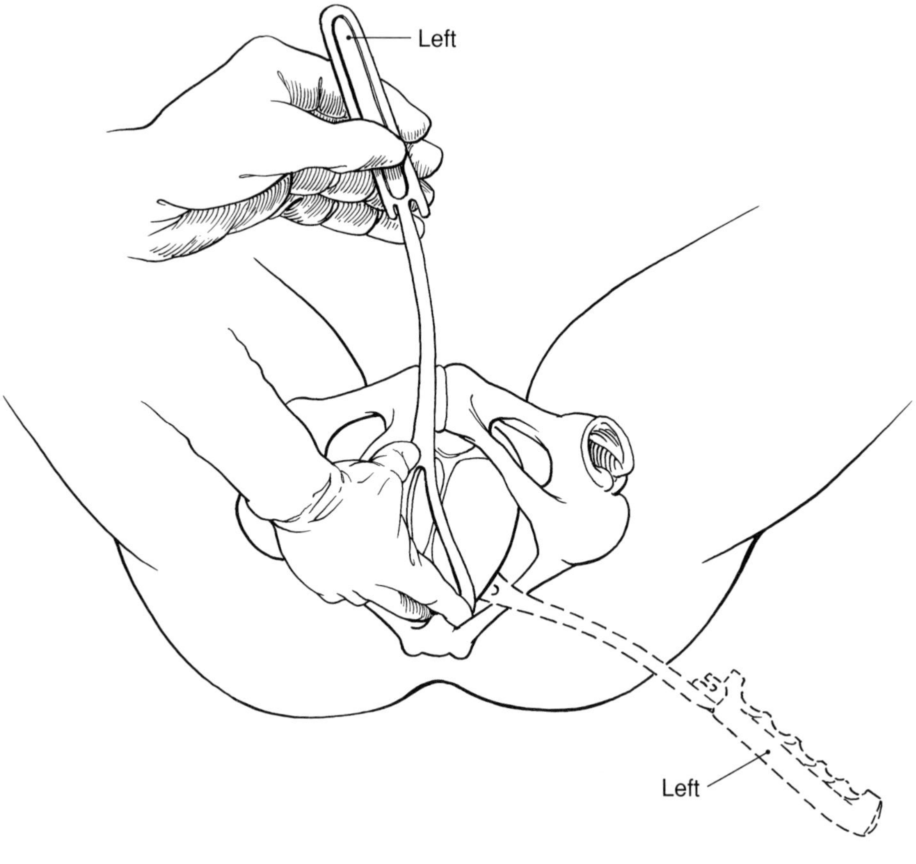

Figure 8–23. The left forceps branch is held in the left hand. The middle and index fingers of the right hand are inserted into the vagina opposite the left parietal bone to guide the toe of the blade along the side of the fetal head.

position the blade in the vagina is applied mainly with the thumb on the heel of the blade as opposed to the left hand at the handle. The left hand serves to guide the handle downward over an arc, first outward toward the right thigh, then inward toward the midline as the blade enters the vagina. In the LOA position, the plane of the handle should be parallel to the left oblique diameter of the pelvis, at right angles to the sagittal suture, approximating a line connecting the 10 and 4 o'clock positions. Next, the right branch is inserted by holding it in the right hand and using the left hand both to guide the toe of the blade and to introduce the necessary force for insertion with the thumb on the heel of the blade. The right branch should be inserted posteriorly in a fashion similar to that used to insert the left branch (Fig. 8–24). With the middle and index fingers positioned at the heel of the blade, the operator then guides the right branch around the brow to the proper position. The arc described by the handle of the right branch is longer in its downward component in order to carry the toe of the blade into the anterior quadrant and over the right malar eminence. Once both branches are in place, the handles are locked. The left branch is more apt to be in the correct position than the right. If articulating the branches is difficult, the position of the right blade should be adjusted first. If the handles do not lock easily, or if they diverge widely when locked, the application is incorrect. Usually this is due to incomplete rotation of the anterior blade beyond the brow onto the cheek and a short application. This can be overcome by lowering the handle after unlocking it and elevating the blade by exerting upward pressure on the heel of the right blade with the middle and index fingers of the left hand. This will carry the right blade farther up into the pelvis and around to the side of the head. If this maneuver is not successful, the forceps should be removed and the position of the head rechecked prior to reapplication.

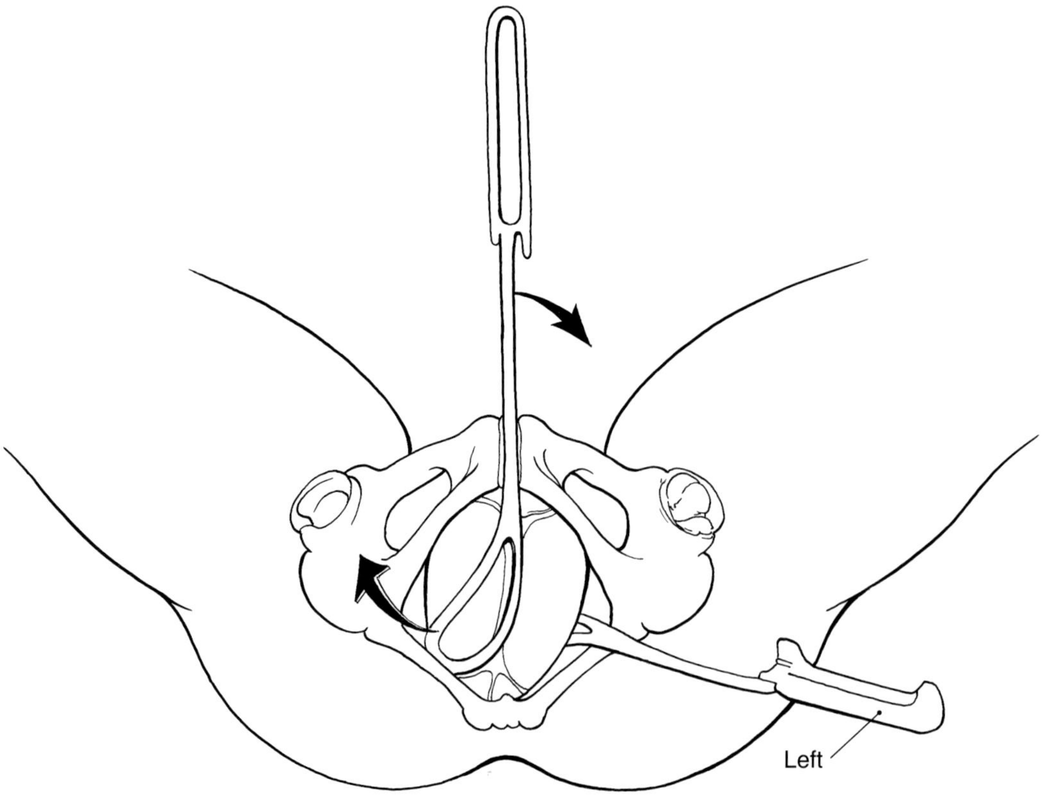

Figure 8–24. Introduction of the right or anterior branch for the LOA position. The right branch is inserted posteriorly in a fashion similar to that used for insertion of the left branch.

Simpson Forceps

The proper application of Simpson forceps is illustrated in Figure 8–25. In performing the cardinal checks for forceps placement, the operator may find that specific readjustments of the forceps are required. For instance, if the posterior fontanelle is more than one finger's breadth above the plane of the shanks, traction will result in attempts at delivery of a deflexed head. Because the pivot point of the head is above the center of the blades, traction would cause further extension of the head and necessitate far greater tractive force for the delivery. This misapplication can be corrected easily by unlocking the handles, elevating the branches one at a time to the required level, and then relocking them. Similarly, if the posterior fontanelle is less than a finger's breadth above the plane of the shanks, the pivot point of the head will be below the center of the blades. The toes of the blades are too far forward on the cheeks in this overflexed attitude, and traction causes further deflexion of the head. The forceps should again be unlocked and each branch lowered one at a time toward the perineum until the desired level below the posterior fontanelle is achieved, at which point they are relocked. If the sagittal suture is found to be running obliquely to the plane of the shanks, a brow–mastoid application has occurred. Milder degrees of this misapplication may not be recognized unless the examining finger is passed along the entire length of the sagittal suture. Adjustments should be made by unlocking the blades and repositioning them. Just as the posterior blade is usually applied first, it is also usually repositioned first. The handle should be moved slightly off midline so that the toe of the blade is carried away from the fetal head, thereby avoiding soft tissue trauma to the fetus. The index and middle fingers are used to apply pressure to the heel of the blade with counterpressure on the handle in order to shift the branch until the plane of the shank is perpendicular to the sagittal suture. The opposite branch is adjusted similarly until its shank is also perpendicular to the sagittal suture. If more than one finger can pass between the fetal head and the fenestration of the forceps blade, it signifies a short application, with the toe of the blade potentially on the malar eminence or higher on the fetal face. This misapplication poses significant risk for fetal soft tissue trauma, including the forceps slipping completely off the fetal head. The branches should again be unlocked and repositioned one at a time. This is usually best accomplished by using the index and middle fingers of the right hand for positioning the left blade with gentle

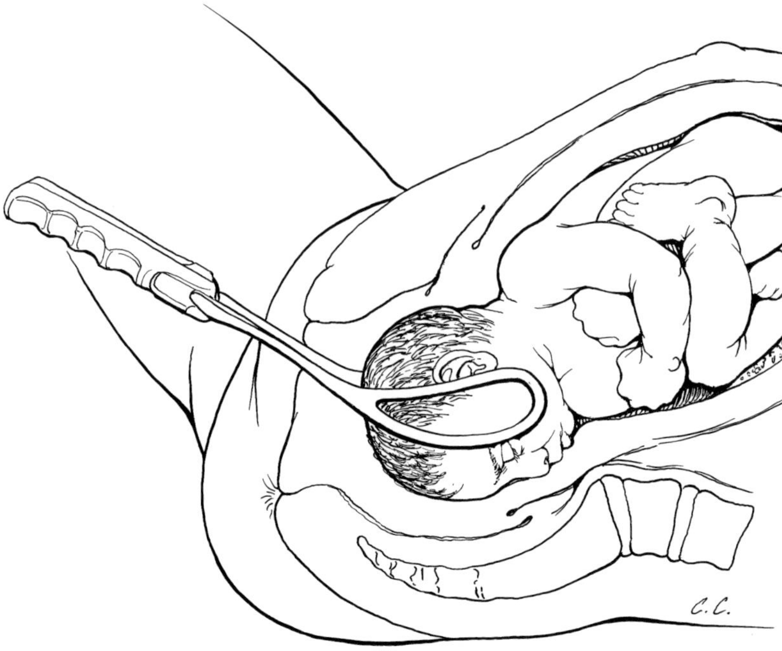

Figure 8–25. Proper application of Simpson forceps illustrating blade position on fetal head.

upward force. The handle and shank of the branch are supported with the left hand during this maneuver. The procedure is reversed for advancement of the left blade. The branches are again articulated and locked, and a final check of the application is made prior to rotation or traction.

Right Occiput Anterior (ROA)

The application for right occiput anterior (ROA) is similar to that for the LOA position except that the order of applying the branches is reversed. In the ROA position, the right or posterior branch is inserted first. Again, insertion of the posterior branch first will prevent loss of station and minimize the chances of rotation of the occiput into the transverse position. Following positioning of the right branch, the left branch is inserted. It is again emphasized that the right blade will rest in the right lower quadrant of the maternal pelvis. The left branch, held in the left hand, is applied anteriorly to the left side of the pelvis in front of the left ear. This blade, after initial application, usually requires some amount of wandering to achieve the correct position. It is necessary to separate the handles and cross them prior to locking, and attention should be directed to ensuring that the toe of the forceps blade does not traumatize fetal soft tissue during this procedure. The branches of the forceps are then articulated and the application is checked prior to rotation.

Rotation

Rotation from LOA or ROA to OA is usually easily accomplished. For all rotations we prefer to place the index and middle fingers of the right hand on either the anterior or posterior fontanelle and corresponding suture lines and rest the palm of the hand on the heel of the forceps blades and shanks while using the opposite hand and handles to perform the rotation. Rotations from LOA and ROA to OA virtually never require any loss of station and often can be accomplished during application of traction.

Traction

Two important elements of traction are direction and amount. The relationship of the station of the fetal head at which the forceps are applied to the plane of the pelvis at that level is critically important (see Fig. 8–9). The direction of the pull at any given level should be perpendicular to the plane of that level. Some have compared the pelvic curve to a stovepipe with an elbow at its lower end (Dennen, 1989). The BPD should serve as the reference point in maintaining traction forces perpendicular to the axis of the pelvis. Accordingly, the higher the forceps application, the greater the direction of the initial downward pull. It was precisely for this reason that axis-traction devices were developed. With descent of the head, the line of traction moves forward following the curve of the sacrum; the direction then turns upward through the outlet. Because of the pelvic curve of the classical instruments, the handles lie in a plane anterior to the plane of the pelvis in which the head is stationed. Traction in the direction of the handles thus would result in prematurely pulling the fetal head into the symphysis pubis.

Regardless of station, traction forces should be applied in the plane of least resistance, that is, in the axis of the pelvis (axis-traction) (see Fig. 8–9). Application of manual axis-traction should be sufficient for all outlet and low forceps deliveries. Manual axis-traction is obtained by using one hand to grasp the shanks and the other to grasp the handles at the finger guards. The hand on the shanks exerts force downward, the hand on the handles, outward. Exerting downward force from above with the palm of the hand on the forceps shanks is the Pajot maneuver. The Saxtorph maneuver is performed from the seated position using the fingers of the hand on the shanks to pull downward perpendicular to the shanks. The sum of the forces exerted by both hands results in a vector determined by the relative strengths of the outward and downward forces. If Simpson type forceps are used, insertion of the middle finger in the space

TABLE 8–4. NUMBER OF TRACTION EFFORTS REQUIRED TO ACHIEVE VAGINAL DELIVERY

Traction Efforts	Forceps	Malmstrom Vacuum Extractor
1–2	213 (38.4%)	296 (68.4%)
3–4	270 (48.6%)	108 (24.9%)
≥ 5	72 (12.9%)	29 (6.7%)
Total	555 (100%)	433 (100%)

Modified from Sjostedt (1967).

between the shanks during traction will result in the force at the time of traction being exerted at the lock rather than from the handles, decreasing compressive forces. Interrupted traction coordinated with uterine contractions is preferable to continuous traction because the latter may result in increased intracranial pressure and stimulation of a vagal response by the fetus with resultant bradycardia. The fetal heart should be monitored carefully throughout the operative delivery. Often the fetal scalp electrode is disconnected to facilitate forceps application. In these instances, a scalp electrode either can be reconnected or the heart rate can be monitored with a Doppler device.

When true axis-traction is being exerted, the maximum forces should not exceed 45 pounds in a primipara and 30 pounds in a multipara. An axis-traction pull will be in a direct line with the anterior toe of the forceps blade (Fig. 8–26). It is important to recognize that some instruments, such as the Hawks-Dennen forceps, are designed to provide axis-traction when the pull is applied directly to the handles. These instruments have either a reverse pelvic curve or no pelvic curve. Their handles should not be elevated higher than 45 degrees above the horizontal in order to avoid sulcus tears.

Once the fetal head produces bulging of the introitus, the forceps handles of the classic instruments are elevated, again approaching a position perpendicular to the floor with crowning and expulsion of the fetal head. The need for episiotomy is assessed during the terminal phases of the delivery. The fetal head can be delivered with the forceps still attached. Alternatively, the forceps can be disarticulated once the fetal head is in a position to be controlled using the modified Ritgen maneuver. Disengagement of the forceps branches is performed in reverse order to that of application. Each forceps branch is swept backward and up across the opposite groin for removal (Fig. 8–27).

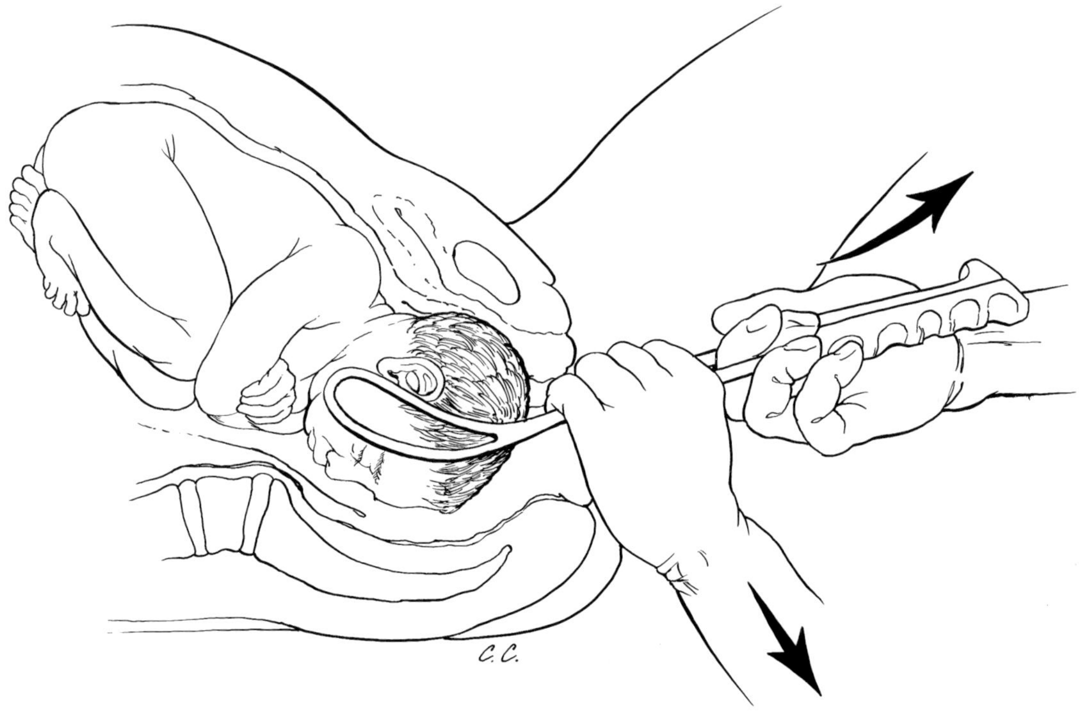

Figure 8–26. Application of axis-traction is by virtue of the vectors exerted by downward displacement on the shank of the forceps combined with outward forces exerted upon the handle of the forceps.

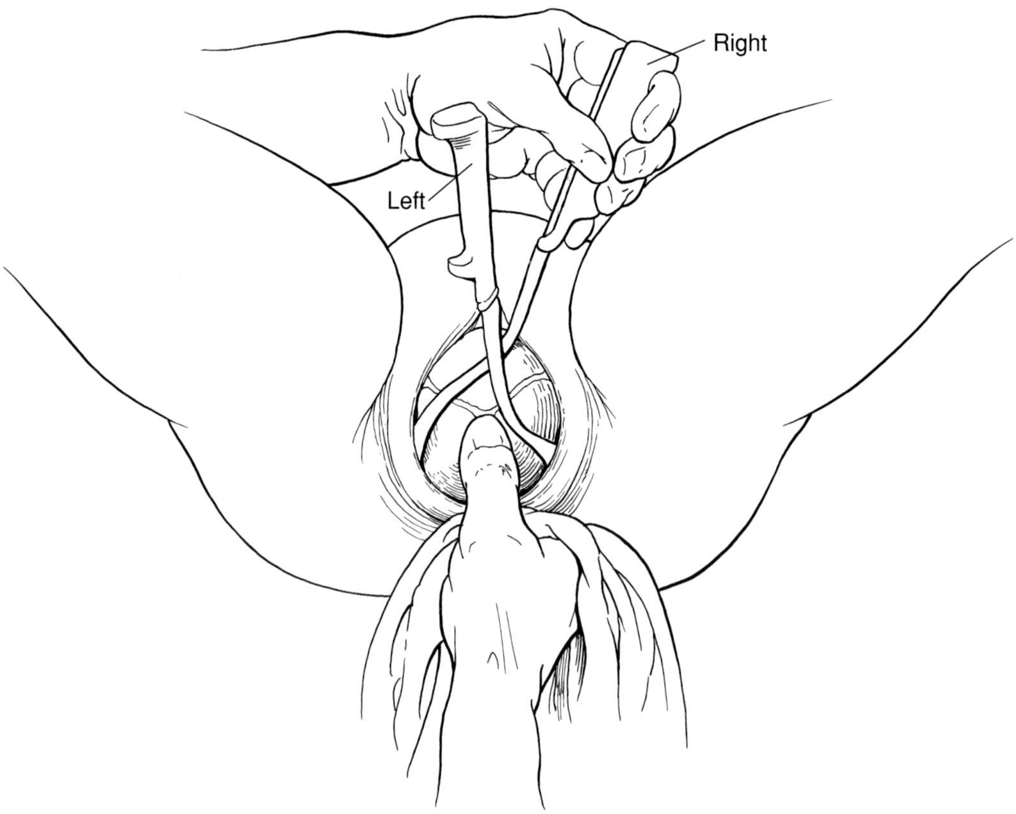

Figure 8–27. The forceps blades are removed while the head is controlled with a modified Ritgen maneuver. The forceps are removed in a sequence opposite to that in which they were inserted, with the right or anterior blade removed first.

Occiput Transverse Positions (OT)

Malpositions of the fetal head such as occiput transverse predispose to failure of spontaneous delivery. Not all malpositioned fetuses need to be rotated prior to delivery; with a platypelloid pelvis, the fetus may deliver as an occiput transverse. In some cases, however, rotation may represent the only means to achieve vaginal delivery. The obstetrician should carefully evaluate each available option for achieving delivery, including manual rotation, autorotation using a vacuum extractor, forceps rotation, and cesarean delivery. Unless the operator has experience with instrumental rotation, cesarean section often is the safer alternative.

Digital Rotation—Left Occiput Transverse (LOT)

Digital rotation is unlikely to produce any fetal or maternal injury and may be used without anesthesia. In the LOT position, the tips of the index and middle fingers of the right hand are placed in the anterior segment of the lambdoidal suture near the posterior fontanelle and the thumb is positioned on the anterior parietal bone. Upward pressure is exerted with the index and middle fingers on the parietal suture line while the thumb provides a counterclockwise downward motion. If this maneuver is successful in rotating the head into the LOA or OA position, the fingers of the right hand are left in the left lower quadrant of the maternal pelvis to prevent backward rotation and to act as a guide for introducing the left forceps blade.

Manual Rotation—LOT

If digital rotation is unsuccessful, the manual maneuver can be attempted with the LOT position. The operator uses the right hand, introducing four fingers into the vagina behind the posterior parietal bone with the palm up and the thumb over the anterior parietal bone. During this maneuver, care should be taken to minimize the amount of station lost, as it can further complicate instrumental delivery as well as result in a prolapsed umbilical cord. The head should be simultaneously flexed and rotated counterclockwise to the anterior or oblique position. The maneuver may be facilitated by using the left hand abdominally to move the fetal back toward the right side of the mother and into the midline. If successful, the fingers should be left against the parietal bone and the mother encouraged to push in order to gain descent of the fetus into the birth canal. Following manual rotation the forceps can be applied as previously described for the LOA or OA positions. For the fetus in right occiput transverse position, the identical procedures will be performed by using the left hand for both the digital and manual rotations. Similarly, the right forceps blade would be placed first in order to prevent rotation back to the transverse position.

Classical Forceps Application—LOT

Application of forceps to the fetal head in the transverse position is the most difficult forceps operation to master and carries the highest risk for both mother and fetus. We describe only the wandering application because we regard the classical application of the Kielland forceps as a far greater risk for maternal trauma.

Either classical instruments (Simpson or Elliot types) or special instruments (Kielland) can be used for this operation. If a classical instrument is chosen for the wandering technique, the maneuver may be more easily accomplished with the Elliot or Tucker-McLane instruments. The more rounded cephalic curve of both instruments tends to offer less resistance than the Simpson forceps to passage beneath the symphysis. The overlapping shanks also offer less resistance to rotation than the parallel shanks of the Simpson forceps. Additionally, a solid bladed instrument (Tucker-McLane) produces less tissue trauma than a fenestrated blade (Elliot and Simpson).

In the LOT position, the posterior or left branch is introduced first. The forceps are held in front of the perineum in the position desired after application to the fetal head (Fig. 8–28). The blade is introduced directly posterior with the shank running oblique to the horizontal to allow for the pelvic curve of the blade. The toe of the blade is positioned directly posterior and runs parallel to the plane of the sacrum with the shank following obliquely along the plane of the sacrum. The index and middle fingers of the right hand are

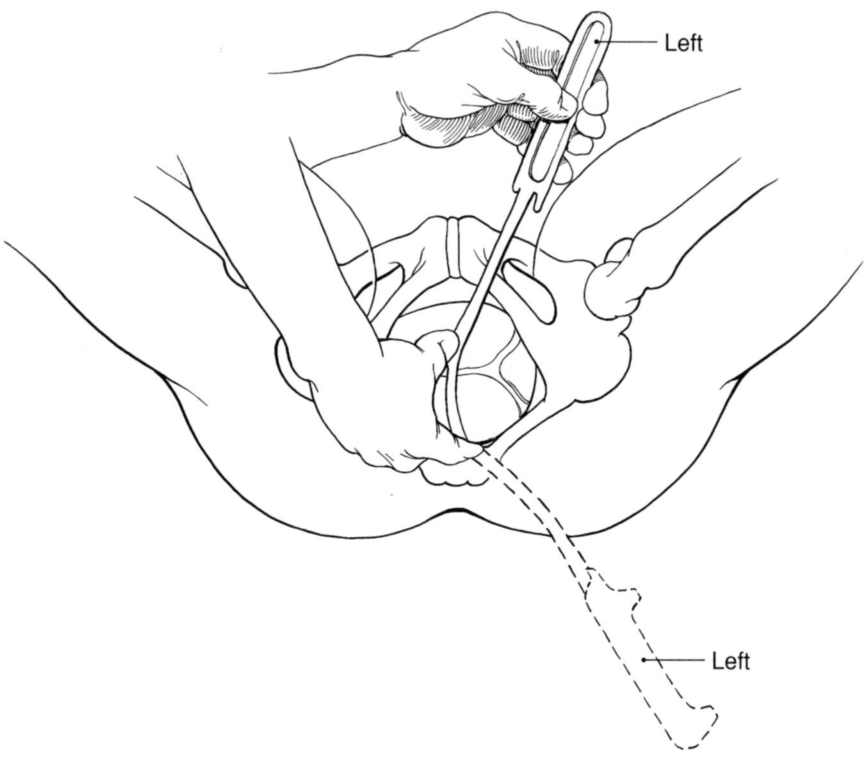

Figure 8–28. Insertion of the Elliot forceps in the LOT position. The left or posterior blade is inserted first.

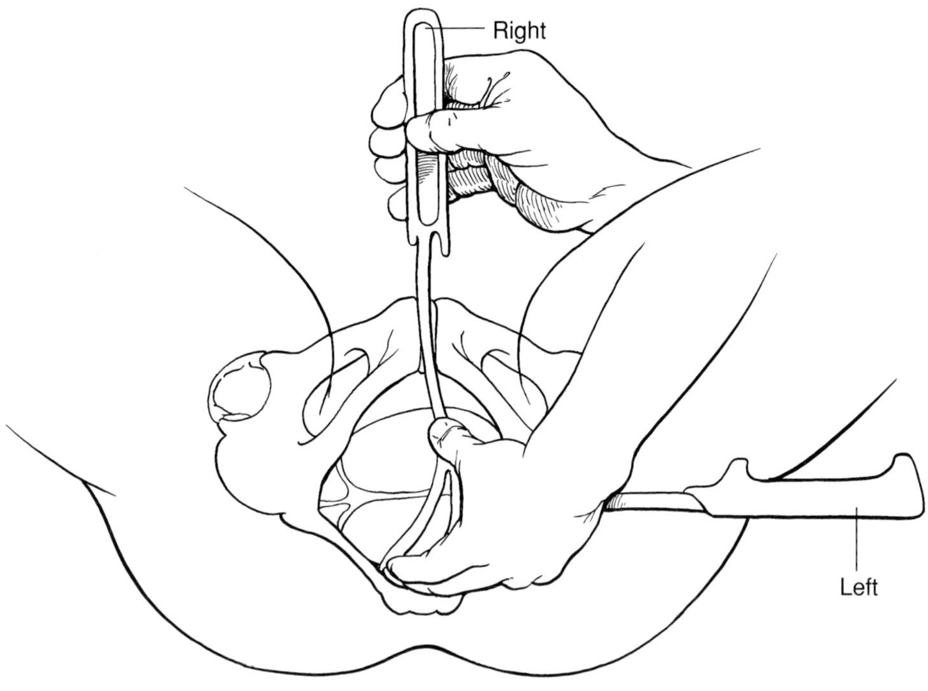

Figure 8–29. The right or anterior blade is introduced into the right lower quadrant of the maternal pelvis. The blade is then wandered around the brow and face of the fetus and positioned on the right parietal bone and malar eminence beneath the symphysis pubis.

used to keep the blade in close apposition to the fetal head in order to minimize obstructions to insertion. As the toe of the forceps is advanced, the handle is lowered until it reaches a point just below the horizontal with the fenestration barely felt below the head. The angle of the handle with the horizontal is dependent upon the station of the fetal head. The angle is closer to horizontal with low stations and points more directly toward the floor at higher stations. The right branch, held with the right hand and guided with the thumb and forefinger of the left hand, is introduced into the right maternal pelvis (Fig. 8–29). After the blade has been inserted, gentle upward pressure is exerted with the index and middle fingers of the left hand while the handle of the left branch descends over an arc close to the left thigh. This maneuver should remove the toe of the blade from the anterior frontal eminence of the fetus, allowing the blade to be wandered around the head and into place in front of the anterior ear. The handle of the wandering or anterior branch will usually be in a lower plane than the posterior branch. To lock the forceps, the handle of the right branch must be elevated.

This maneuver causes the right blade to slide further up into the pelvis behind the symphysis until the handles meet. The plane of the shanks will be directed toward the side on which the occiput lies, obliquely away from the midline of the long axis of the patient at an angle approaching 50 degrees. Locked, the handles will lie in a plane obliquely to the left of the midline of the patient with the shanks one finger breadth medial to the posterior fontanelle.

Classical Forceps—Rotation of LOT

When classical forceps are used for rotation, the handles must describe a relatively wide arc in order to reduce the arc of rotation of the toe of the blades (Fig. 8–30). Controlling the size of the arc described by the blade reduces the danger of tearing vaginal and paravaginal soft tissue. Additionally, if this technique is used, the rotation is more readily accomplished because of the limited field of movement of the head within the confines of the bony pelvis. Conceptually the operator should visualize that the toes of the forceps blade remain at the same point; only the handles should describe the arc of the rotation. Although it is generally easier

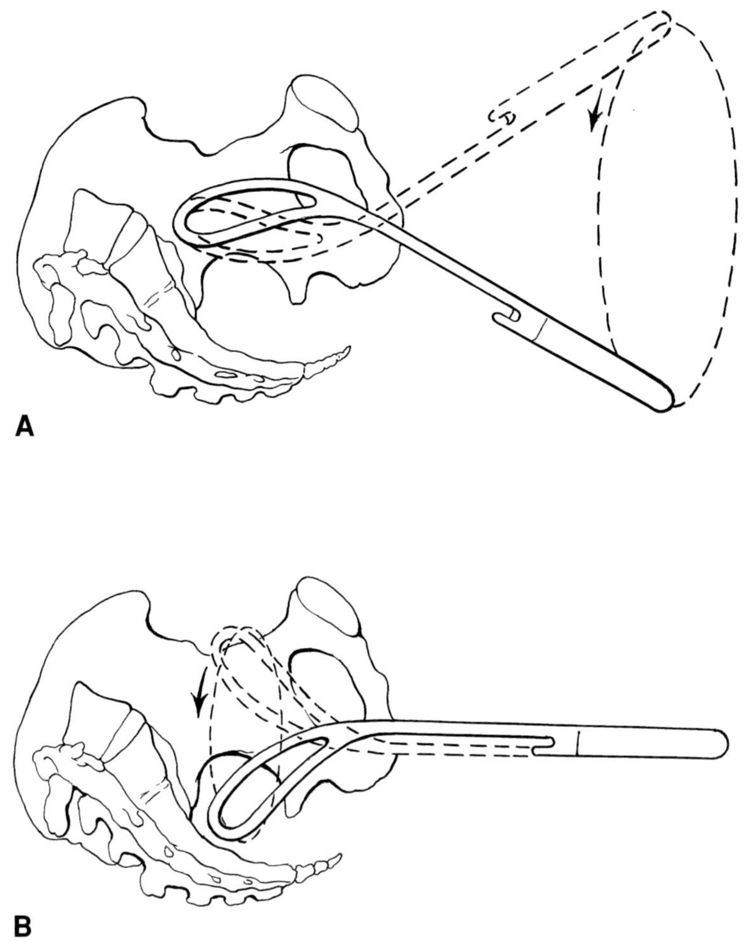

Figure 8–30. Rotation technique. **A.** Correct technique. When a classical instrument is used to perform a rotation, the handle must describe a large arc so that the toe will remain relatively stationary within the maternal pelvis. **B.** Incorrect technique. Failure to describe a large arc with the handles of the forceps will result in the toe of the blade circling in a wide arc, which can cause significant trauma to the maternal pelvis. The rotation will also be prone to failure for lack of sufficient room to describe this larger turning radius when performed incorrectly.

to accomplished rotation at the midpelvic level if rotation is required, it should be attempted initially at whatever station the forceps have been applied. If resistance is met, slight destationing toward the midpelvis may be attempted. As previously noted, the authors prefer to place one hand on the handle of the forceps with the palm of the opposite hand resting upon the shank of the forceps and the index and middle fingers positioned on suture lines. This allows not only some assistance in the rotation digitally but also detection of any slippage of the forceps on the fetal head. Difficulty in rotating the head is usually secondary either to extension or to failure to move the forceps handles in a sufficiently wide arc. As the approximate 90 degree rotation is completed, the occiput will come to rest beneath the symphysis (Fig. 8–31). At this point the handles are depressed to further improve flexion. The application is again checked and any necessary adjustments made prior to application of traction.

Kielland Forceps—Rotation of LOT

The Kielland forceps, characterized by a slight to reverse pelvic curve, overlapping shanks, and a sliding lock, is shown in Figure 8–4. The inner surfaces of the blades are beveled to prevent injury to the fetal head; injury can be further reduced by using a modification incorporating pseudofenestrated blades. Knobs are

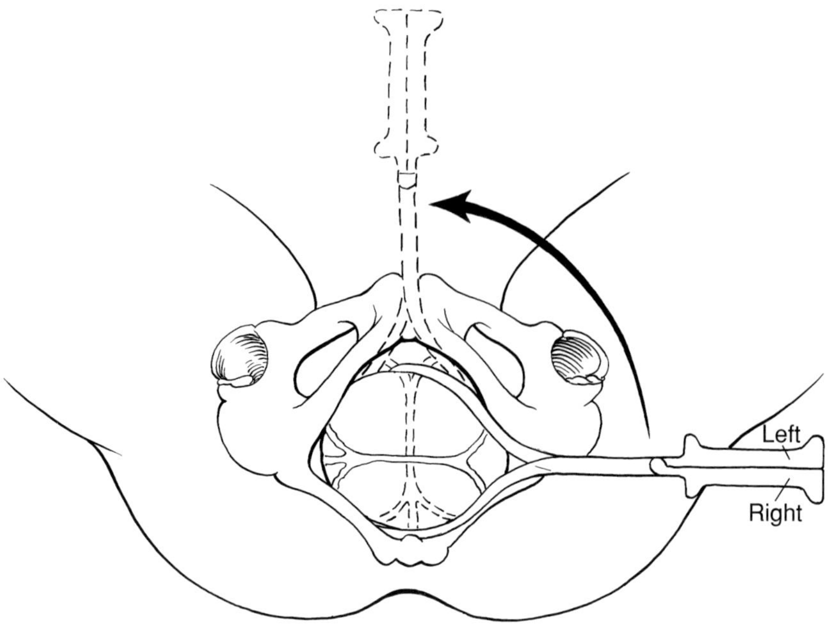

Figure 8–31. The forceps have been applied correctly and rotation will be accomplished in a counterclockwise fashion. Attention is directed to describing a large arc with the handle of the forceps. The handle should be moved laterally toward the maternal left thigh. Movement should continue in an arc that carries the handle to the midline and above the symphysis pubis. Conceptually, the operator should visualize the toe of the forceps blades remaining at the same level in the pelvis.

located on the finger guards to identify the anterior surfaces of the instrument and assist during forceps application. Kielland forceps are excellent for rotation as well as for traction. They are superior to all other forceps for correction of asynclitism by virtue of the sliding lock mechanism, which allows locking of the handles at any level of the shank (see Fig. 8–11). Because of the reverse pelvic curve, Kielland forceps also exert axis-traction when forces are directed in a straight line with the handle. Finally, their straight design allows the shanks and handles to lie on the same axis as the fetal head; the toes describe a very small circle during rotation and the handles basically remain in the midline. It is important to note that the Kielland forceps is not a "classical" instrument. If used in a fashion similar to that employed with the classical instruments, the reverse pelvic curve is prone to cause sulcus tears and third- and fourth-degree lacerations.

Wandering Application—LOT. As is the procedure with all forceps applications, the instruments should be positioned near the perineum outside the woman's body in the approximate position that they will occupy once inserted. In applying the Keilland forceps, the operator may place either the anterior or the posterior blade first. If the posterior blade is to be placed first, the branch is gently held in the left hand between the thumb and middle finger with the index finger resting on the hand guard. The buttons on the handle should face toward the occiput. The middle and index fingers of the right hand are placed into the posterior vagina, and the forceps are gently guided into position. Lubricating the forceps with Betadine soap solution may decrease resistance and facilitate placement. The right hand advances the toe of the blade into the vagina. The position of the handle and shank will move in a virtual straight line from their initial vertical position to rest in a horizontal position relative to the floor at completion of application. The operator then grasps the right or anterior branch with the right hand, using the middle and index fingers of the left hand to guide the toe of the blade into the right lower quadrant of the maternal pelvis. As the anterior blade is inserted, the handle will describe an arc close to the woman's left leg. Gentle pressure is exerted on the heel of the blade with the left hand, with simultaneous counterpressure on the shank and handle serving to wander the blade across the fetal brow and into position beneath the symphysis. If resistance is met during the wandering of this blade, moving the handle toward the woman's left leg should remove the toe of the forceps from the fetal face. Further efforts to guide the forceps into place should be made at this point. If these efforts are unsuccessful, there may be obstruction by maternal soft tissue, and slight movement of the forceps toward the midline may facilitate further positioning. Alternatively, if neither of these maneuvers overcomes resistance to wandering the blade around the side of the fetal face, the blade can be inserted into the left side of the maternal pelvis in an upside-down position and then wandered around the occiput and into position. Once both blades have been brought into position, their position relative to the suture lines again should be checked. Asynclitism is corrected by placing traction on the finger guard that is near the perineum while simultaneously applying pressure in the opposite direction to the other finger guard until the handles are aligned.

Direct Application—LOT. If the head is so low in the pelvis that a wandering application of the anterior blade is precluded, direct application can be attempted. In this situation the head is near the outlet in a transverse position with an anterior parietal presentation. The asynclitism combined with the low station will place the anterior ear just behind the symphysis. In the direct application, the anterior or right blade is applied directly under the symphysis to the anterior ear. The approach is from below upward with the handle pointing toward the floor and initially held below the edge of the delivery table. Placement may be facilitated either by elevation of the delivery table or by the operator kneeling on the floor. The toe of the forceps is directed under the symphysis toward the anterior ear with the concave beveled surface of the blade kept in close apposition to the anterior parietal bone. Often gentle upward pressure results in the blade sliding into the desired location over the malar eminence of the anterior cheek. Although previous authors (Dennen, 1989; Douglas and Stromme, 1988) taught that the anterior blade always should be applied first with the Kielland's instrument, they also stated their preference for the classical application technique with Kielland forceps. We, like Kielland, prefer the wandering technique that we have described.

Classical Application—LOT. The classical or inversion method of application is associated with a higher incidence of trauma involving the lower uterine segment and maternal bladder. The anterior or right branch of the forceps is applied first. The right branch is held in an inverted manner, with the inner surface of the cephalic curve facing upward and the shank 45 degrees above the horizontal (Fig. 8–32A). The operator places the left hand into the vagina with the tips of the middle and index fingers inserted under the symphysis, anterior to the fetal head. The blade is advanced under the symphysis anterior to the operator's left hand as the handle is simultaneously lowered toward the midline level to the horizontal. Excessive force should not be used during this maneuver. If there is resistance, this method of application should be abandoned. As the blade passes under the symphysis, the handle is gently depressed to an angle 45 degrees below the horizontal. The toe of the blade may now be seen elevating the lower abdominal wall through the lower uterine segment (Fig. 8–32B).

The right branch now must be rotated so that the cephalic curve will align with the fetal head. The operator's right hand grasps the handle and rotates the branch counterclockwise with a twist of the wrist. The rotation is complete when the knob of the branch points toward 3 o'clock (Fig. 8–33). As the rotation is completed, the handle is depressed slightly. As stated previously, we prefer not to use the classical application in an effort to avoid rupturing the bladder and lower uterine segment.

Kielland Rotation—LOT. The reverse pelvic curve of the Kielland forceps, as previously mentioned, allows almost direct rotation on the axis of the shanks. When the rotation has been completed, the handles should be dropped to maximize flexion. At higher stations, the handles of the forceps must be low-

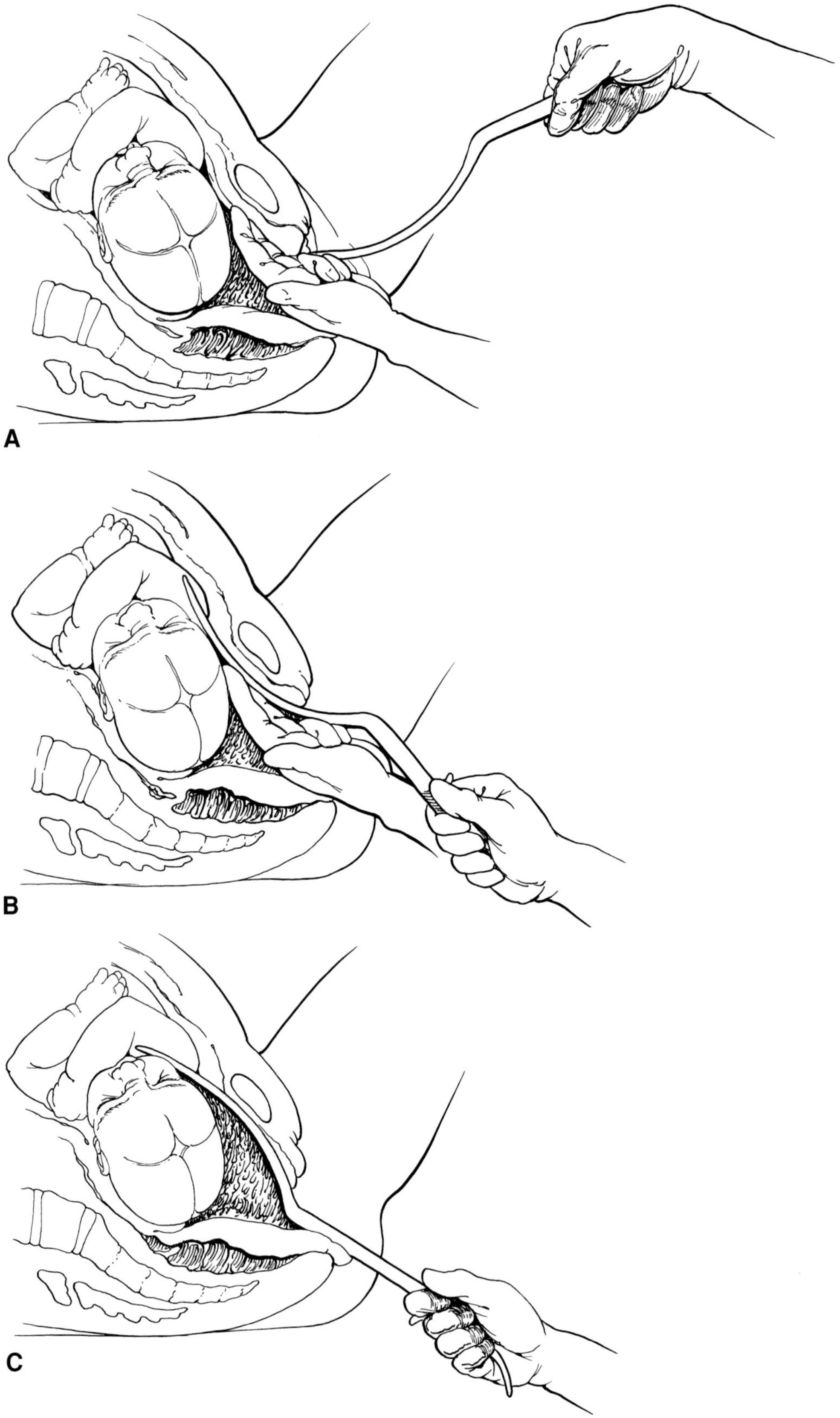

Figure 8–32. **A.** The left hand is placed in the vagina between the fetal head and the symphysis. **B.** The right branch is advanced in an upside-down position as the operator simultaneously lowers the handle toward the floor. **C.** The branch is rotated 180 degrees, the application is rechecked, and adjustments are made as required.

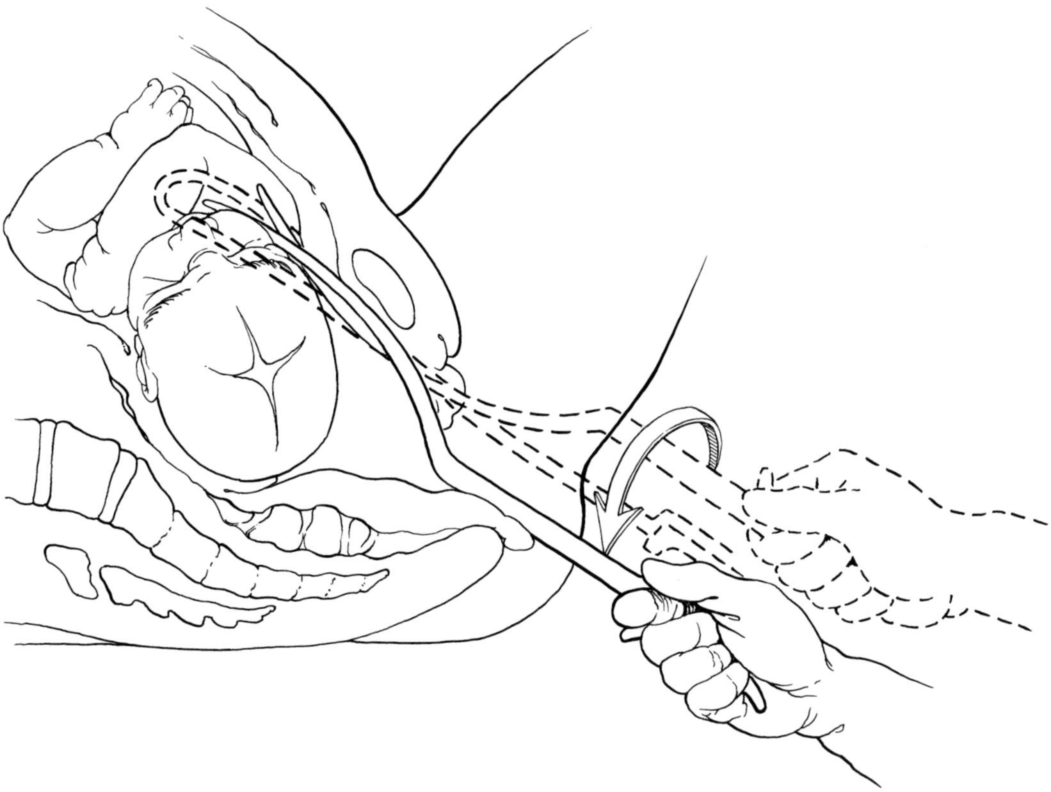

Figure 8–33. Rotation of the right branch of the Kielland forceps counterclockwise after classical insertion will align the cephalic curve with the fetal head.

ered in order to achieve successful rotation. After flexing the head, the operator should check the forceps to see if a readjustment is needed so that the shanks are positioned within a finger's breadth anterior to the posterior fontanelle. If rotation at the level of application proves difficult, efforts should be made to gain station at which time rotation can be attempted again. If rotation again is unsuccessful, the head should be displaced approximately 1 cm above its original station. Rotation then should be attempted again. As with all attempts at forceps delivery, the operator should be willing to abandon the procedure if difficulty is encountered.

Right Occiput Transverse (ROT)

Delivery with either classical or specialized instruments for the right occiput transverse is similar to that described for the fetus in left occiput transverse position. The posterior or right forceps blade is generally inserted first, with the left or anterior blade wandered into position. Rotation and traction are as described for the left occiput transverse.

Occiput Posteriors (OP)

The occiput posterior may be managed by manual rotation, instrument rotation, or a combination of these methods. Alternatively, some occiput posterior presentations are easily delivered in that presentation.

Manual Rotation

Manual rotation is similar to that described from the occiput transverse presentation with the exception that the arc of the rotation is greater. If the fetus is in the LOP position, the fingers of the operator's right hand should be inserted into the posterior vagina along the posterior parietal bone with the thumb positioned on the anterior parietal bone (Fig. 8–34). If rotation to the anterior quadrant of the pelvis is successful, the fingers of the right

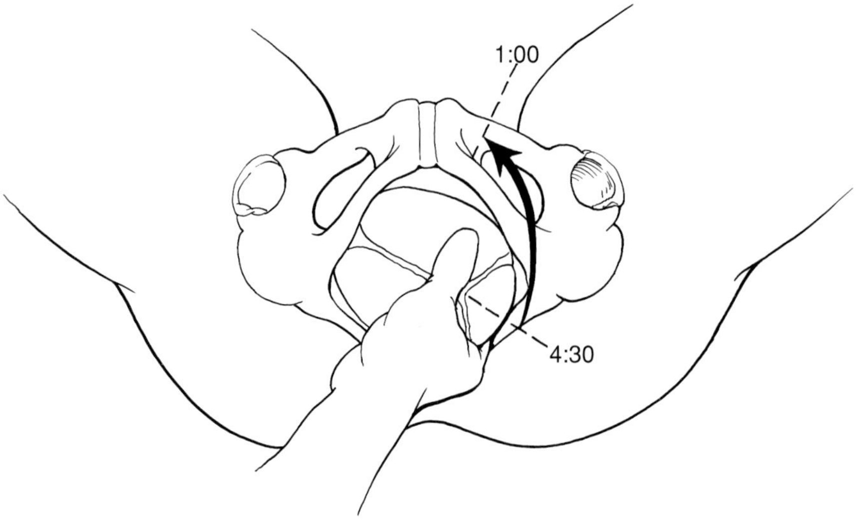

Figure 8–34. Manual rotation of LOP to LOA. The fingers of the right hand are inserted into the posterior vagina, where they rest largely upon the left parietal bone. The thumb will rest on the right parietal bone. The rotation is performed in a counterclockwise direction with the abdominal hand used to assist in moving the right shoulder of the fetus into the midline and toward the right side of the maternal abdomen.

hand are kept in the vagina to splint the parietal bone while the left forceps blade is applied. Using the abdominal hand to assist in rotating the fetal body during this maneuver may facilitate success. When rotation has been successful in conversion to the LOA or OA position, forceps can be applied as previously described.

Classical Forceps Application—LOP

If the fetus is in the LOP position, the forceps are applied as if the fetus were in the right occiput anterior position. The right blade is introduced into the right lower quadrant of the maternal pelvis as previously described (Fig. 8–35). The right blade then lies in close juxtaposition to the left parietal bone and left malar eminence. The left blade of the forceps is then introduced into the left lower quadrant of the maternal pelvis and wandered into an anterior position (Fig. 8–36). The handles then are crossed and the shanks locked. A preliminary check should reveal the posterior fontanelle lying just below the plane of the shanks with the sagittal suture perpendicular to the plane of the shanks. The head is then rotated counterclockwise to the anterior position (Fig. 8–37). Because of the pelvic curve of classical instruments, the handles must describe a wide arc in order to keep the toe of the blades in the center of the pelvis. If rotation is difficult, flexion should be performed and the attempted rotation repeated. Following rotation, the head should be fixed in the new position by slight downward traction. At this point, the forceps are in an upside-down position with the toes pointing posteriorly, and they should be removed, inverted, and reapplied. The posterior or right blade (residing in the anterior position) is the easiest to remove initially. We favor having a second pair of forceps available so that the right or anterior blade can be inserted in the correct position prior to withdrawing the remaining blade, which is in the upside-down position. After the removal of the left or posterior blade, it should be replaced. Alternatively, the anterior blade can be removed first. Because it is the left blade, it can be reinserted between the head and the blade that is still in place opposite the left ear as in the LOA position. The right blade is then removed in a downward direction and reapplied over the right or anterior ear. When this operation was first described, both forceps blades were removed following the rotation and then reapplied. Unfortunately, this frequently led to spontaneous rotation to the original position before reapplica-

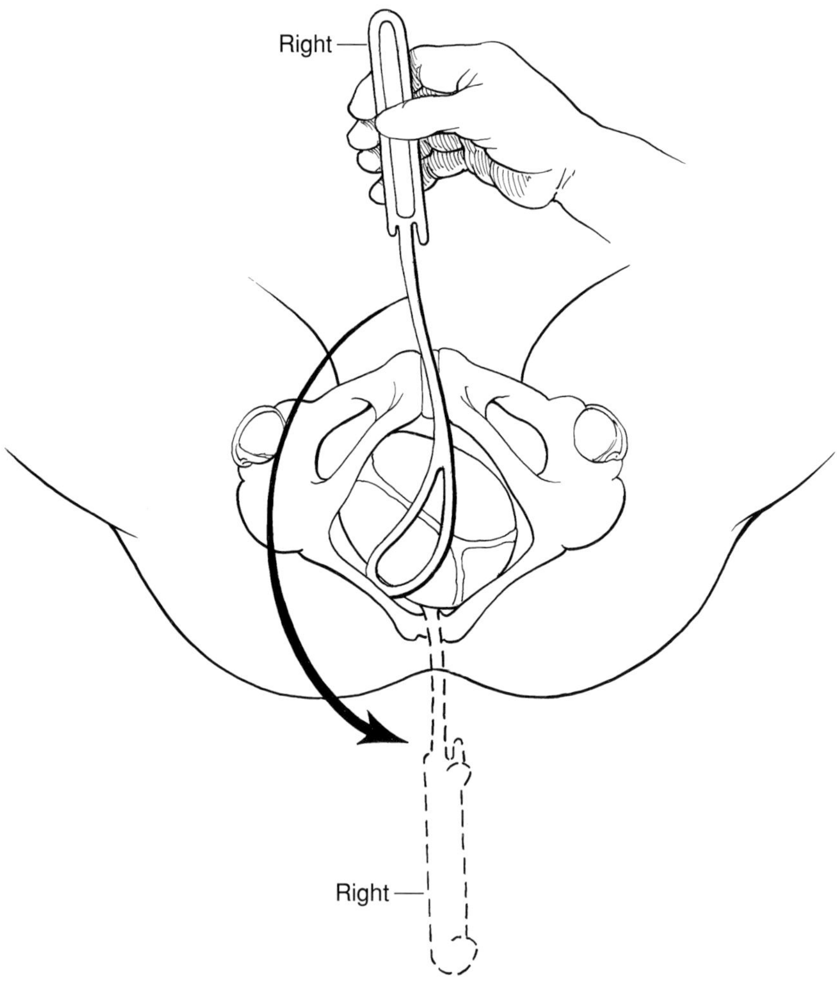

Figure 8–35. Using classical instruments, the fetus in the LOP position will have the forceps applied in a fashion identical to that used for the fetus in the right occiput anterior position. The right or posterior blade will be applied first.

tion could be accomplished. The previously mentioned advantages of overlapping shanks and solid or pseudofenestrated blades, such as found on Tucker-McLane or Elliot forceps with a Luikart modification, are even more advantageous with occiput posterior presentations than in transverse presentations because the arc of the rotation is even greater.

Scanzoni Maneuver—ROP

The right occiput posterior position is treated as if it were an LOA position for application of the forceps blades. Rotation is clockwise to the anterior quadrant, following which removal and reapplication are performed in a manner similar to that for LOP.

Direct Occiput Posterior

For the direct OP, classical instruments are inserted as if the fetus were in the OA presentation. Whether the initial attempt to rotate is clockwise or counterclockwise should be determined based on the location of the fetal back. The occiput should always rotate through the side on which the back lies: with the back to the left, the rotation is counterclockwise; with the back to the right, clockwise.

Kielland Forceps—OP

That the knobs on the handle of the Kielland forceps should always be directed toward the occiput is standard teaching. However, the authors have found that when applied in a manner similar to the classical instruments,

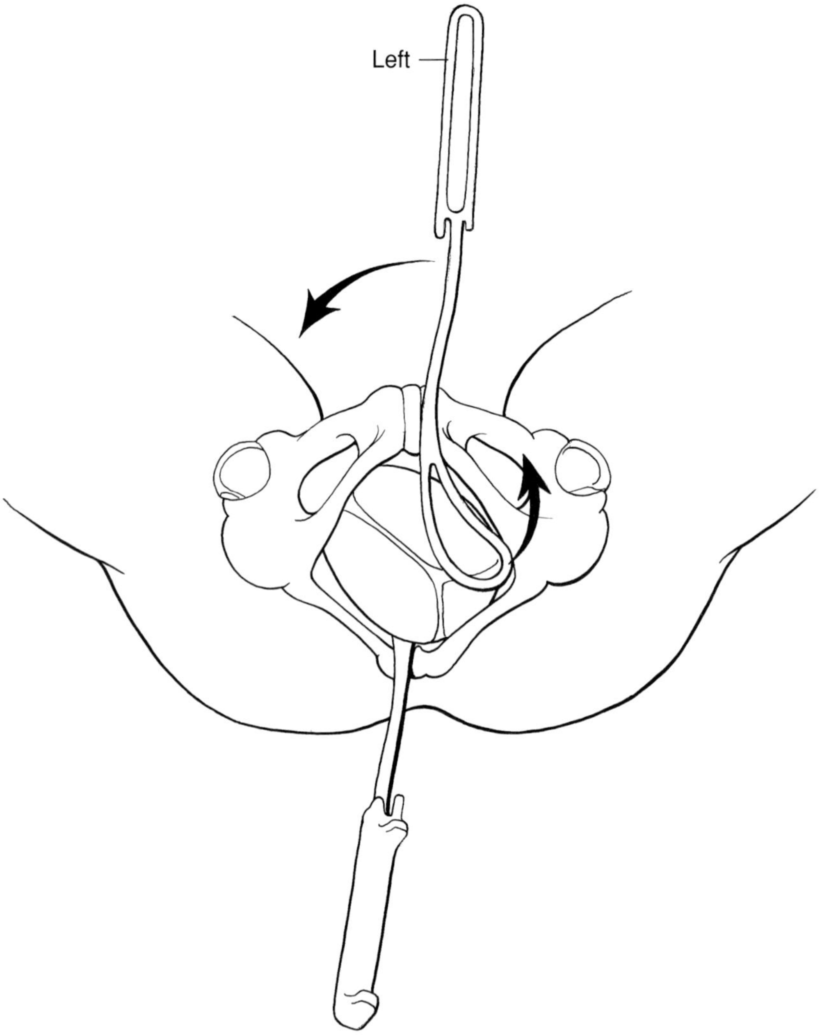

Figure 8–36. The left or anterior blade of the classical instrument is introduced into the left lower quadrant of the maternal pelvis, following which it is wandered into position around the fetal occiput.

that is, an initial upside-down application, Kielland forceps are satisfactory for rotation of OP, LOP, and ROP. Positioning of the forceps is similar to that previously described. Because of the absence of a pelvic curve and the alignment of the toe of the forceps with the handle, the rotation can be performed in the midline without the wide arcing of the handles required with classical instruments. Following the rotation, traction is exerted to gain station. The forceps blades then can be removed and replaced one at a time. It is important not to remove both blades simultaneously because this may result in reversion to the original position. Alternatively, the forceps can be applied to the OP positions as more classically taught with the buttons on the handles pointing toward the occiput.

Kielland Application—LOP

The Kielland forceps should be positioned near the perineal body in the position intended after placement about the fetal head. The right branch is held in the right hand and the left hand serves as a guide to introduce the blade into the right lower quadrant of the maternal pelvis. The index and middle fingers of the left hand are then used to wander the blade across the brow and into position over the right parietal bone, beneath the sym-

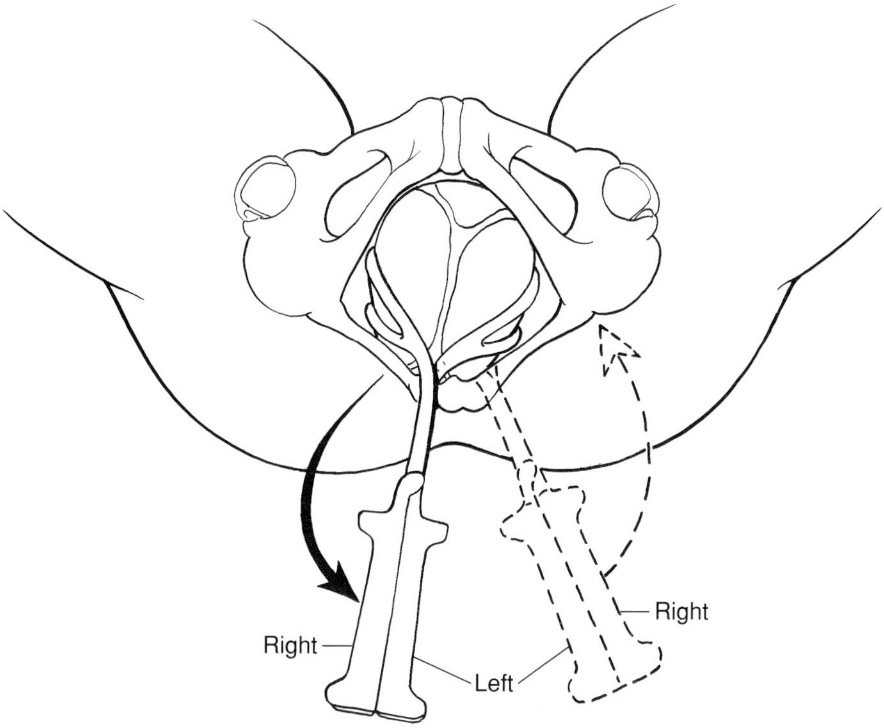

Figure 8–37. Following articulation of the branches of the classical instrument, the rotation is performed in a counterclockwise direction. It is emphasized that the handles must describe a wide arc that begins at the left maternal thigh, describing a wide arc up toward the pubic symphysis and then continued to completion at the level of the right maternal thigh. This represents the modified Scanzoni maneuver.

physis pubis at approximately 2 o'clock. In this instance, the rotation of the blade will be in a clockwise fashion and will traverse approximately 180 degrees. The posterior blade then can be inserted in a more direct application with little wandering of the blade required to achieve the correct application. It is held in the right hand with the button facing the maternal left thigh. The left hand assists in introducing the toe of the blade between the vaginal tissues and the left fetal parietal bone. If difficulty is encountered in positioning the forceps, efforts can be made to reinsert it either more in the midline at the 6 o'clock position or closer to the 9 o'clock position, thereafter wandering it into the 7–8 o'clock position. After the handles are locked, the asynclitism is corrected by pulling down on the finger guard nearest the perineal body and by exerting upward pressure on the opposite finger guard. The head is then flexed and rotated counterclockwise over approximately 135 degrees to the anterior position. Application and flexion are rechecked and, if appropriate, traction is applied.

Right Occiput Posterior—ROP

For the right occiput posterior position, the left forceps branch is grasped with the left hand and the right hand is used to guide it into the right lower quadrant of the maternal pelvis. The forceps is then wandered around the brow over approximately 180 degrees, beneath the symphysis and into the right upper quadrant of the maternal pelvis in juxtaposition to the left fetal parietal bone. The right forceps branch is then grasped with the left hand and guided into the left lower quadrant of the maternal pelvis using the right index and middle fingers to guide the toe of the forceps with the thumb exerting pressure at the heel of the blade. The handle of the forceps will again proceed from a near vertical orientation toward the horizontal as the toe is advanced into the pelvis. Fine adjustments then can be made by exerting gentle pressure at the heel of the blade. The branches are then articulated, and position is checked. Asynclitism can be corrected, following which rotation will proceed in a clockwise fashion.

Kielland—Direct OP

As previously noted, we prefer the inversion method of application for the direct OP. Alternatively, a reverse or upside-down direct application can be employed. In the upside-down direct application the forceps are again positioned outside the maternal body in the position intended following application. The right branch is taken in the left hand and introduced from below the patient's right thigh upward at a 45 degree angle. The toe of the blade passes directly to the right side of the fetal head in the left maternal pelvis (Fig. 8–38). The left branch, held by the right hand, is inserted from below the patient's left thigh to the left side of the fetal head. The forceps are locked, the application is checked, and need for flexion is assessed. Rotation will require turning the fetus through 180 degrees. The position of the handles relative to the horizontal will depend upon the station of the fetal head: the higher the fetal head, the lower the forceps will point below the horizontal; the lower the fetal head is in the pelvis, the closer the forceps will approach being parallel to the floor (Fig. 8–39). The direct application technique is best suited to the fetal head that is low in the pelvis. At higher stations, the reverse pelvic curve of the Kielland forceps interferes with application.

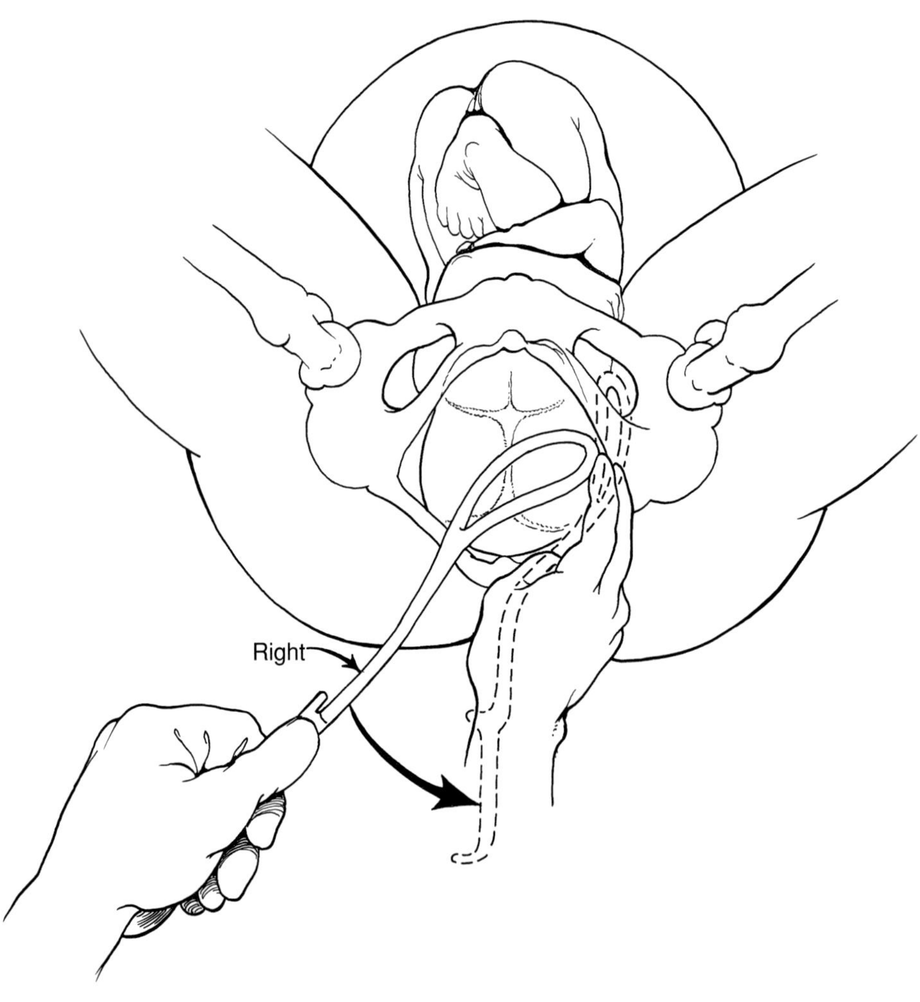

Figure 8–38. In the upside-down direct application of the Kielland forceps for the OP presentation, the right blade, with the anterior surface of the shank pointing downward, is held in the left hand and introduced to the left side of the patient's pelvis. The application is often facilitated by performing it from below upward.

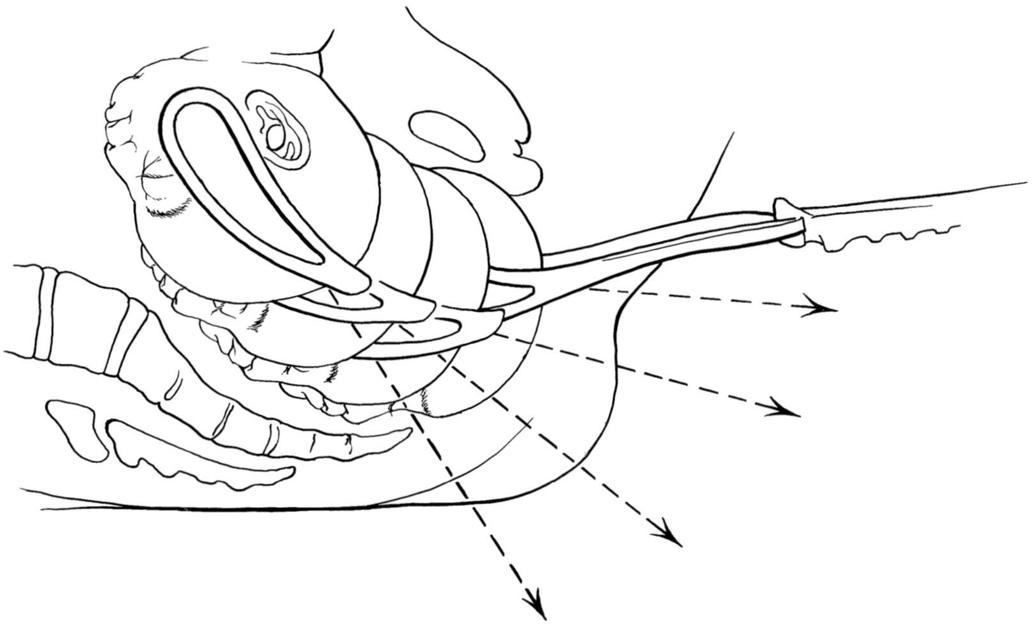

Figure 8–39. The position of the Kielland forceps depends upon the station of the fetal head. At higher stations, the handles point well below the horizontal, whereas at lower stations, they approach the horizontal.

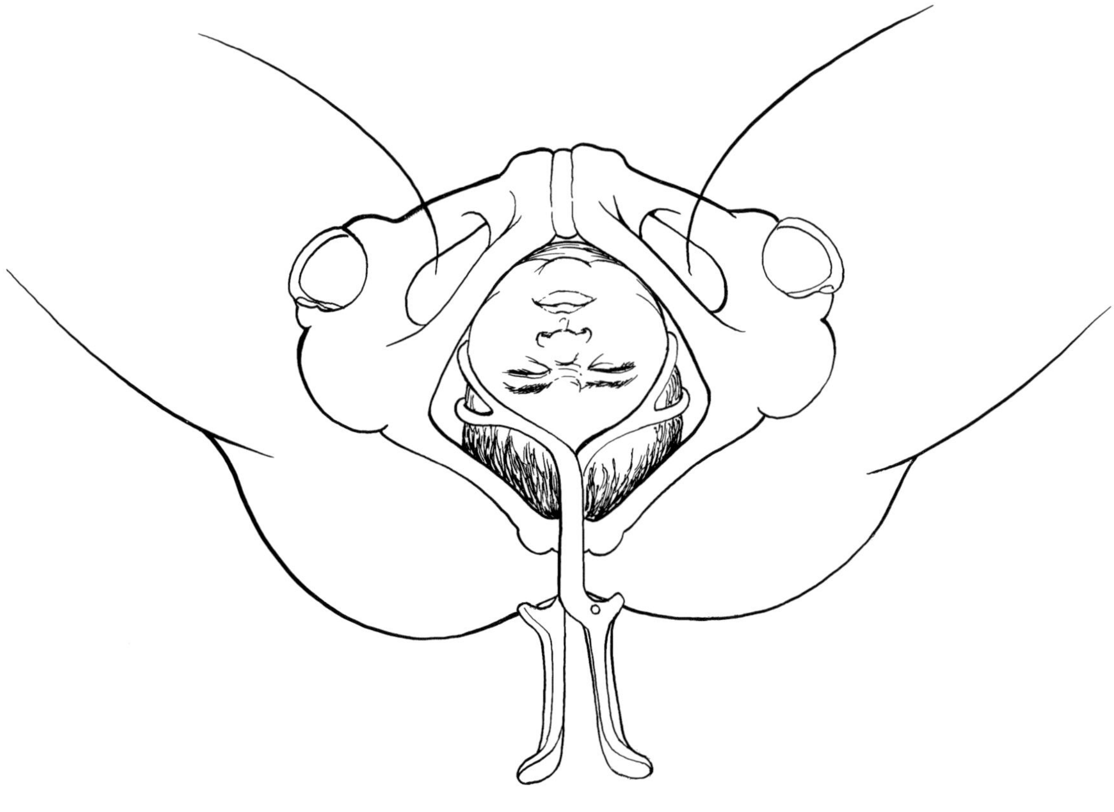

Figure 8–40. Application of Kielland forceps to a face presentation, mentum anterior. The forceps are applied as if dealing with a direct OA position.

Face Presentation

Face presentations are rare, and any given physician is apt to have limited experience with them. The only face presentation in which we would consider use of forceps is the mentum anterior. In this presentation, either Kielland or a classical instrument can be used. Regardless of the instrument selected, the forceps are applied as if dealing with a direct occiput anterior position. Landmarks are different. The chin substitutes for the occiput, and the mouth substitutes for the posterior fontanelle as the reference point. Traction should be downward in an effort to preserve complete extension until the chin passes under the symphysis. Great care must be taken to avoid hyperextension. The handles are then elevated gradually to the horizontal with traction so that the occiput is delivered over the perineum and the head is delivered by flexion (Fig. 8–40).

TRIAL OF FORCEPS/ FAILED FORCEPS

A trial of forceps applies to only a small number of deliveries; the literature contains few reports, none of which describe a large group of women. All of the reports are descriptive as opposed to randomized trials. The spectrum of opinion concerning the procedure is broad. Dyer (1965) believed that "failure to be successful in the use of forceps should occur extremely rarely, if ever, in the lifetime of a well-trained obstetrician." At the time, training in forceps delivery was readily available, and the overall cesarean section rate was less than 5 percent. More recently, Dennen (1989) expressed the belief that the trial of forceps is an available and an eminently acceptable procedure. This opinion was rendered at a time when training in forceps delivery was much less readily available and when the overall cesarean section rate was 25 percent, and significantly higher in some centers. It appears that both Dyer and Dennen may have been right in relation to the prevailing mode of practice in their respective times.

The distinction between trial of forceps and failed forceps is based on more than semantics. A trial of forceps is one in which the operator has anticipated the possibility of failure and has made advance preparations for cesarean delivery. The forceps attempt occurs in a fully equipped operating suite with appropriate support personnel including an anesthesiologist. Failed forceps implies failure to anticipate failure. The delivery takes place in a setting not amenable to immediate cesarean delivery. Sometimes the woman must be moved to another room, and other times the operating team must be hurriedly assembled. Although reports of such cases are sparse, the outcomes appear to be worse than those in which a trial of forceps fails.

Usually, a failed trial of forceps (cumbersome but accurate terminology) occurs when the operator cannot achieve satisfactory application of the forceps to the fetal head. The procedure can also fail when moderate traction does not produce descent. With proper training and experience, the frequency of failure drops precipitously. Using a Bill axis-traction handle to optimize the direction of force may increase the success rate in some cases. Sometimes, delivery may be accomplished by changing instruments after an initial attempt fails.

There is no evidence in the literature that perinatal or maternal outcome is worsened by a properly conducted trial of forceps. Boyd and colleagues (1986) found that among 53 cases of failed trial of forceps in 6,524 otherwise uncomplicated primiparous deliveries, birth depression and encephalopathy occurred with a frequency similar to that which occurred when cesarean section was done for failure to progress in the second stage of labor. Further, birth trauma was no more common than with successful midforceps delivery. The incentive to try is best stated in risk-benefit terms: avoiding an unnecessary cesarean section with its increased maternal morbidity without assuming substantive risk to the infant.

MORBIDITY

Lacerations of the vagina and cervix, pelvic hematomas, episiotomy extension, and the hemorrhage resulting from these events are the most common maternal complications associated with instrumental deliveries. Episiotomies and lacerations disrupting the sphincter are associated with sphincter weakness, incontinence, and rarely rectovaginal fistula formation (Coombs and colleagues, 1990). Periurethral and anterior vaginal vault lacerations are associated with hemorrhage and possible damage to the urethra and/or bladder. Urinary retention can result from edema or hematoma formation at the urethra. Very infrequently uterine rupture occurs secondary to instrumental delivery. Uterine rupture is most likely due to perforation occurring during attempted insertion of the forceps blade.

Cesarean Section versus Forceps Delivery

Because cesarean section is often the only alternative to forceps deliveries, it is worthwhile to compare the morbidity of these two operations. The laceration rate in cesarean section is 100 percent. There is always a uterine scar, which carries at least a 1 percent risk of uterine rupture with a subsequent pregnancy (Cowan, 1994; Miller, 1994; Rosen, 1991; Videla, 1994; and their colleagues). Maternal morbidity is more frequent and likely to be more severe following a cesarean than following a vaginal delivery. Following a cesarean, nearly 3 percent of women may have serious complications, including uterine rupture, placenta accreta, placenta previa, and hemorrhage (Cowan, 1994; Cunningham, 1993; Miller, 1994; Rosen, 1991; Videla, 1994; and their associates). Women who have had cesarean sections also are at risk of having all subsequent deliveries by cesarean section because vaginal birth after cesarean is not uniformly promoted and practiced in spite of the ACOG position that a "woman with one previous cesarean delivery with a low transverse incision should be counseled and encouraged to attempt labor in her current pregnancy." Furthermore, a woman with more than one low transverse cesarean section "should not be discouraged" from attempting a vaginal birth after cesarean (ACOG, 1988).

One of the most prominent causes of postcesarean morbidity is infection. Bashore and colleagues (1990) reported a sixfold increase in febrile morbidity in women undergoing cesarean as opposed to midforceps delivery. Hemorrhage is greater and transfusion much more common with cesarean section than with operative vaginal deliveries (Gilstrap, 1987). Robertson and colleagues (1990) determined that for all operative vaginal deliveries, there was a "significant" decrease in maternal morbidity, blood loss, and length of hospital stay when compared with cesarean section." However, they found a 5 percent increase in fetal morbidity with all operative vaginal deliveries compared to matched cesarean sections. Fetal morbidity included serious complications such as skull fractures, brachial plexus injuries, facial nerve injuries, and clavicular fractures. Furthermore, deep vein thrombosis and pulmonary embolism are significantly increased with cesarean delivery (Bashore and colleagues, 1990). Two other reports documented an increased rate of maternal morbidity with rotations greater than 45 degrees and midforceps (Hagadorn-Freathy, 1991; Robertson, 1990; and their coworkers). However, none of these injuries was clinically serious. Fetal injuries occurred in 7 percent of the deliveries.

Gilstrap and Hauth surveyed 700 infants delivered by indicated low (293), indicated mid (234), and elective forceps (177) with regard to fetal acidosis, trauma, and neurologic deficit. They compared 303 spontaneous deliveries and 111 cesarean sections to these groups. They noted that there was no significant difference in outcome between the spontaneous vaginal delivery and the low-forceps delivery groups. The midforceps group had increased vaginal lacerations and lower hematocrits at discharge than did the low-forceps group, but neonatal outcome was similar. A comparison of cesarean delivery for cephalopelvic disproportion and indicated forceps for arrest of descent failed to show a significant difference in neonatal acidoses. When forceps delivery for fetal distress was compared with cesarean sections for the same indication, no significant difference was found.

Fetal Injury

Concern for fetal injury is one of the major reasons for the decline in operative vaginal delivery. Fear of litigation certainly contributes; however, most obstetricians deny this as a large factor. Most cite concern for fetal morbidity, which can include minor lacerations, forceps marks, facial and brachial plexus palsies, cephalhematoma, skull fracture, intracranial hemorrhage, antenatal depression, and seizures. Friedman and colleagues (1984) examined long-term development sequelae; this widely quoted work is from a collaborative study of 55,908 pregnancies of which only 1,194 infants were followed until age seven. He found a statistically significant lower IQ in the midforceps group compared to the spontaneously delivered group. Many have criticized this study because it was conducted during the 1960s with limited intrapartum fetal monitoring, has almost no comparative cesarean delivery data, and does not address socioeconomic status or educational level of the mother. Also, the significant IQ difference found at both 3–4 and 7 years of age was not seen at 18 months of age. In 1993, Wesley studied infants born between 1964 and 1967 in California. This retrospective analysis was designed to address the deficiencies of Friedman's work. It evaluated 1,951 children with respect to spontaneous vaginal, forceps, and cesarean section delivery relative to IQ at 5 years of age. These infants had no fetal heart rate abnormalities in labor. When maternal educational level and socioeconomic status were taken into account, no difference in IQ was found, regardless of route of delivery (Wesley and associates, 1993). Seidman and colleagues (1991) retrospectively evaluated more than 52,000 infants born between 1964 and 1972 by an IQ test given at age 17. They too found no evidence of cognitive impairment. McBride and colleagues (1979) also found no difference in IQ relative to route of delivery. Over 770 infants born between 1970 and 1974 were examined by a battery of tests at age five, and no evidence of cognitive impairment could be related to route of delivery.

ILLUSTRATIVE CASE

A 22-year-old nullipara at 40 weeks' gestation has been in labor for 12 hours and has pushed for just over 2 hours. A functioning epidural catheter is in place. The fetal head is at +2 station, left occiput transverse. Both anterior and posterior fontanelles are at the same level in the pelvis and located in the posterior quadrants. The sagittal suture connecting the two fontanelles is deviated toward the sacral promontory. There is no appreciable molding of the fetal head, and only minimal caput succedaneum. The same examiner has detected no progress in descent over the last hour despite adequate uterine activity and maternal pushing efforts. The pelvis clinically is gynecoid with normal capacity throughout. The estimated fetal weight is 8 pounds (3600 g). The fetal heart rate is 150 beats per minute with normal beat-to-beat variability and moderate variable decelerations with each pushing effort. The maternal temperature is 37°C and there is no evidence of dehydration.

Discussion

The case represents a deep transverse arrest with associated anterior asynclitism and a military attitude (slight deflexion) of the fetal head. Although the time elapsed in the second stage is less than the 3-hour limit suggested by ACOG guidelines, there has been no progress in descent for 1 hour, indicating a true arrest disorder. Importantly, this case emphasizes one of the most controversial aspects of the new classification scheme: it depends critically on clinical estimation of station of the fetal head. As described, this case represents a low forceps with greater than 45 degrees rotation. However, if the fetal head were a millimeter or two higher, the proper designation would be a midforceps delivery. There are no studies of interobserver or intraobserver differences in the estimation of station, and such estimation is known to be affected by factors such as caput formation and asynclitism.

The case is well-suited to operative vaginal delivery; an acceptable indication is present (arrest of descent), fetopelvic relationships have been adequately assessed, and other prerequisites for forceps delivery have been satisfied. The delivery should be conducted in the manner outlined in the trial of forceps section above. One choice would be to apply the anterior (right) blade of the Kielland forceps first by wandering it over the face, and then positioning the blade between the symphysis pubis and the fetal head. Given the presence of anterior asynclitism, another acceptable approach to the application of this blade would be the direct application. The application of the posterior blade should present no problem, although occasionally it may have to be repositioned posterolaterally if the toe of the blade cannot be positioned beyond the sacral promontory. Once the forceps have been successfully applied and articulated, the operator will note that the handles are not at equal depth. The sliding lock feature of the Kiellands allows for correction of asynclitism by equalizing the depth of insertion. Assuming that the application has been checked and is proper, the next move should be a slight deviation of the handles toward the maternal right leg, thereby enhancing fiexion. Using only the left hand, rotation should be easily accomplished. Two fingers of the right hand should be placed on the lambdoid sutures to monitor the progress of the rotation. Some operators prefer to complete the delivery using the Kielland forceps, mindful of the fact that the handles should rarely be raised above the horizontal plane. Others choose to replace the Kielland instrument with a classical forceps such as Simpson-Luikart. The latter instrument has a pelvic curve and may be less likely to cause vaginal lacerations or extension of an episiotomy. With regard to episiotomy, we recommend individualized management according to size of perineal body and anticipated space requirements. If the operator does elect to change forceps, care should be taken to ensure that the head does not spontaneously rotate back to the original transverse position. Forceps delivery in the situation outlined above should not involve a high degree of difficulty. It does require training, experience, and incisive clinical judgment. Properly executed, this delivery method should produce excellent maternal and perinatal outcome.

SUMMARY

For over 50 years, there has been a heated debate about the role of midforceps in obstetrical practice. E. S. Taylor (1953) posed the question, "Can midforceps operations be eliminated?" Ten years later, Danforth lamented that the use of forceps was a vanishing art. Friedman and associates (1984) implicated forceps delivery as the cause of the decreased IQ among infants so delivered. Fortunately, recent information has greatly clarified issues surrounding forceps deliveries ((ACOG, 1988, 1991; Hagadorn-Freathy, 1991; Robertson, 1990; Wesley, 1993; Seidman, 1991; and their associates). The new classification system advanced by the American College of Obstetricians and Gynecologists in 1988 for the first time allows a reasonable stratification of risk based on the operation performed. It has become obvious that the greatest risk of both maternal and fetal injury is associated with deliveries performed at 0 and +1 station and with high degrees of rotation. By the same token, it is also obvious that the outlet forceps delivery carries little risk to mother or fetus and often represents the best option available for the birthing process. Risk of maternal and fetal injury increase somewhat with outlet forceps and with increasing degrees of rotation. In this chapter we have concentrated on the use of classical instruments and one special instrument, the Kielland forceps. Critical criteria for use of forceps have been outlined and detailed information has been provided concerning application, rotation, and traction. Forceps deliveries, when properly executed by trained providers, can avoid the maternal morbidity associated with cesarean section while imposing no additional short- or long-term neonatal risk.

REFERENCES

American College of Obstetricians and Gynecologists, Committee on Obstetrics, Maternal and Fetal Medicine. Obstetric Forceps. Technical Bulletin No. 59, February 1988.

American College of Obstetricians and Gynecologists. Operative vaginal delivery. Technical Bulletin No. 152, February 1991.

American College of Obstetricians and Gynecologists. Manual of Standards of Obstetric-Gynecologic Practice: American College of Obstetricians and Gynecologists, 2nd ed. Washington, DC: ACOG, 1965.

Bashore RA, Phillips WH, Brinkman CR III. A comparison of the morbidity of midforceps and cesarean delivery. Am J Obstet Gynecol 1990; 162:1428.

Bill AH. A new axis traction handle for solid blade forceps. Am J Obstet Gynecol 1925; 9:606.

Boyd ME, Usher RH, McLean FH, Norman BE. Failed forceps. Obstet Gynecol 1986; 68:779.

Chestnut DH, Vandewalker GE, Owen CL. The influence of continuous epidural bupivacaine analgesia on the second stage of labor and method of delivery in nulliparous women. Anesthes 1987; 66:774.

Coombs CA, Robertson PA, Laros RK Jr. Risk factors for third-degree and fourth-degree perineal lacerations in forceps and vacuum deliveries. Am J Obstet Gynecol 1990; 163:100.

Cowan RK, Kinch RAH, Ellis B, Anderson R. Trial of labor following cesarean delivery. Obstet Gynecol 1994; 83:933.

Cunningham FG, MacDonald PC, Gant NF. Williams Obstetrics. 19th ed. Norwalk, CT: Appleton & Lange, 1993.

Danforth DN, Ellis AH. Midforceps delivery: a vanishing art? Am J Obstet Gynecol 1963; 86:29.

Das K. Obstetric forceps. Its history and evolution. Calcutta: The Art Press, 1929.

DeLee JB. The prophylactic forceps operation. Am J Obstet Gynecol 1920; 1:34.

Dennen EH. A classification of forceps operations according to station of head in pelvis. Am J Obstet Gynecol 1952; 63:272.

Dennen PC. Dennen's Forceps Deliveries. 3rd ed. Philadelphia: Avis, 1989.

Douglas RB, Stromme WB. Operative Obstetrics. 3rd ed., New York: Appleton-Century-Crofts, 1976.

Douglas RB, Stromme WB. Operative Obstetrics. 4th ed. New York: Appleton-Century-Crofts, 1982.

Douglas RB, Stromme WB. Operative Obstetrics. 5th ed. Norwalk, CT: Appleton & Lange, 1988.

Dyer I. Trial and failed forceps. Clin Obstet Gynecol 1965; 8:914.

Friedman EA, Sachtleben-Murray Mr, Dahrouge D, Neff RK. Long-term effects of labor and delivery on offspring: a matched-pair analysis. Am J Obstet Gynecol 1984; 150:941.

Gilstrap LC, Hauth JC, Hankins GDV, Patterson AR. Effect of type of anesthesia on blood loss at cesarean section. Obstet Gynecol 1987; 69:328.

Hagadorn-Freathy AS, Yeomans ER, Hankins GDV. Validation of the 1988 ACOG forceps classification system. Obstet Gynecol 1991; 77:356.

Healy DL, Laufe LE. Survey of obstetric forceps training in North America in 1981. Am J Obstet Gynecol 1985; 151:54.

Holland E. The Princess Charlotte of Wales. A triple obstetric tragedy. Obstet Gynecol 1951; 58:905.

Hoult IJ, MacLennan AH, Carrie LES. Lumbar epidural analgesia in labor: relation to fetal malposition and instrumental delivery. Br Med J 1977; 1:14.

Kaminski HM, Stafl A, Aiman J. The effect of epidural analgesia on the frequency of instrumental obstetric delivery. Obstet Gynecol 1987; 69:770.

Luikart R. A modification of the Kielland, Simpson, and Tucker-McLane forceps to simplify their use and improve function and safety. Am J Obstet Gynecol 1937; 34:686.

McBride WG, Black BP, Brown CJ, et al. Method of delivery and developmental outcome at five years of age. Med J Aust 1979; 1:301.

Megison JW. Save the Barton forceps. Obstet Gynecol 1993; 82:313.

Miller DA, Diaz F, Paul RH. Vaginal birth after cesarean: a 10-year experience. Obstet Gynecol 1994; 84:255.

O'Grady JP. Modern Instrumental Delivery. Baltimore: Williams & Wilkins, 1988.

Philipsen T, Jensen NH. Epidural block or parenteral pethidine as analgesic in labor: a randomized study concerning progress in labour and instrumental deliveries. Eur J Obstet Gynecol Reprod Biol 1989; 30:27.

Plauche WC. Surgical Obstetrics. Philadelphia: Sanders, 1992.

Ramin SM, Little BB, Gilstrap LC. Survey of forceps delivery in North America in 1990. Obstet Gynecol 1993; 81:307.

Robertson PA, Laros RK Jr, Ahao RL. Neonatal and maternal outcome in low-pelvic and midpelvic operative deliveries. Am J Obstet Gynecol 1990; 162:1436.

Rosen MG, Dickinson JC, Westhoff CL. Vaginal birth after cesarean: a meta-analysis of morbidity and mortality. Obstet Gynecol 1991; 77:465.

Seidman DS, Laor A, Gale R, et al. Long-term effects of vacuum and forceps deliveries. Lancet 1991; 337:1583.

Seiler JS. The demise of vaginal operative obstetrics: a suggested plan for its revival. Obstet Gynecol 1990; 75:710.

Shute WB. History of obstetrical forceps from 1750 to the present era. Acta Belg Hist Med 1992; 5:65.

Sjostedt JE. The vacuum extractor and forceps in obstetrics: a clinical study. Acta Obstet Gynecol Scand 1967; 46:3.

Taylor ES. Can midforceps operations be eliminated? Obstet Gynecol 1953; 2:302.

Thorp JA. The effect of epidural analgesia on instrumental vaginal delivery: a multivariate analysis. Society of Perinatal Obstetricians, 9th Annual Meeting, New Orleans, LA, February 1989.

Videla FL, Satin AJ, Barth WH Jr, Hankins GDV. Trial of labor: a disciplined approach to labor management resulting in a high rate of vaginal delivery. Am J Perinatol (in press).

Wesley BD, van den Berg BJ, Reece EA. The effect of forceps delivery on cognitive development. Am J Obstet Gynecol 1993; 169:1091.

Williams JW. Obstetrics: A Textbook for the Use of Students and Practitioners. New York: D. Appleton and Company, 1903.

Wittels B. Does epidural anesthesia affect the course of labor and delivery? Sem Perinatol 1991; 15:358.

CHAPTER 9

Vacuum Delivery

The earliest recordings of the use of vacuum or suction to hasten the delivery of a fetus was by Younge in 1706 in Europe. In his treatise, he stated, "I could neither fasten or crochet nor draw it out by a copping-glass fixt to the scalp with an air pump." Saemann (1797) advanced the concept of an instrument that could be attached by suction to the fetal head and by traction decrease the diameter of the head and facilitate its delivery (MacCahey, 1890). Approximately 50 years later Simpson (1848), in Edinburgh, designed the first instrumental vacuum cup. It consisted of a slender, short brass syringe with a double-valve piston attached to an inner metal cup which was covered by an outer, flexible, vulcanized rubber cup (Laufe and Berkus, 1992). He suggested that his "air tractor" could substitute for forceps in difficult labors (Fig. 9–1).

In 1890, MacCahey presented the second design of a vacuum cup, which he called the "atmospheric tractor." The cup was made of elastic material that could mould to the shape of the fetal head. A firm handle attached to the base of the soft cup allowed the cup to be pressed against the head and vacuum would be formed by traction (much like a rubber commode plunger). None of these devices reached any level of popularity until Malmstrom introduced his metal cup modification, which he called the vacuum-extractor (Malmstrom, 1954). It differed from the "suction cups" that preceded it in that it also functioned as a tractor cup. While in principle this instrument was designed merely as an aid to maternal uterine contraction and expulsive efforts, it now for the first time served as a usable suction forceps (Malmstrom, 1954).

The Malmstrom vacuum-extractor consists of a bell-shaped steel cup with a smooth slightly turned in lip with the outside diameter 60 mm (Fig. 9–2). The dome of the cup is attached to a rubber suction tube through which is passed a traction chain that is anchored in the cup and has a traction handle at the other end of the tubing. The interior of the cup contains a mesh that prevents the scalp from being drawn into the vacuum port. Beyond the traction handle, the tubing is attached to a wide-mouthed bottle with a 3-holed stopper. The other two connections are for a vacuum gauge and a bicycle air pump with a backward valve to create negative pressure in the bottle and cup system (Fig. 9–3). By gradual increments of negative pressure, the fetal scalp tissue is sucked into the hollow of the shallow cup to create a caput succedaneum called a "chignon." This chignon acts as a traction area for the cup. Traction is exerted in conjunction with uterine contractions and voluntary maternal pushing. If properly placed on the fetal scalp, traction on the cup will flex the fetal head. By maintaining the traction axis parallel to the axis of the birth canal through which the head is traversing, the head will usually rotate to an occiput anterior position as it encounters the muscular levator ani sling posteriorly. This same movement occurs in unassisted spontaneous delivery and is called "autorotation."

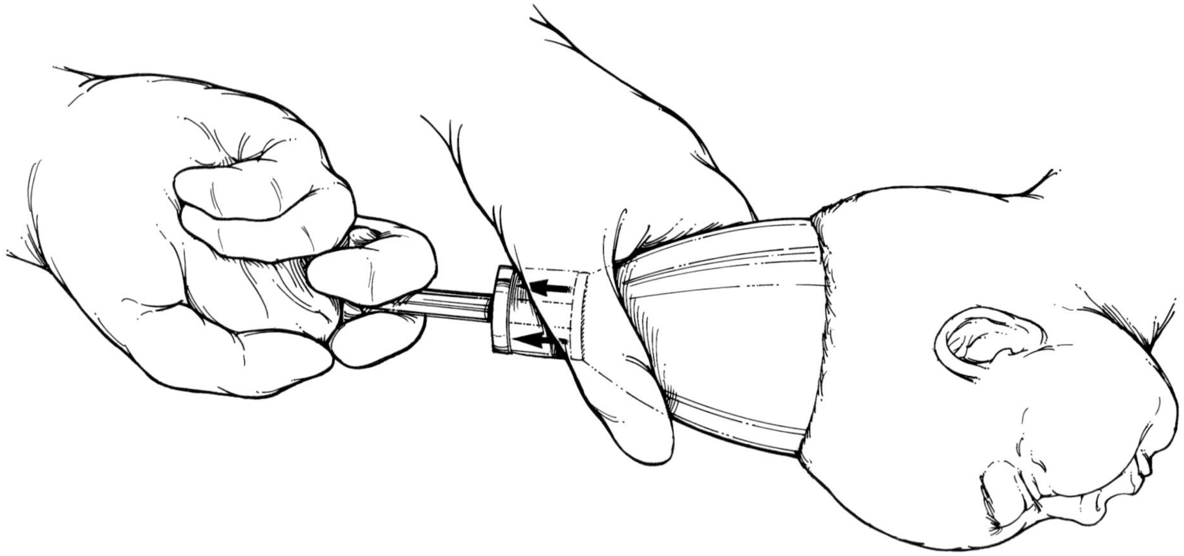

Figure 9–1. Early vacuum extractor described by Simpson. Vacuum is created by pulling back on the plunger. *(Adapted from Laufe and Berkus, 1992, with permission.)*

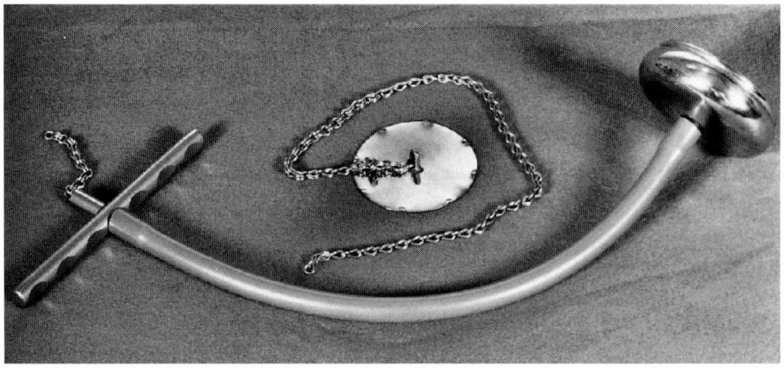

Figure 9–2. Photograph of Malmstrom device showing the metal cup, handle, and chain. The metalic disk with attached chain fits inside the metal cup and prevents the fetal scalp from being sucked into the vacuum tubing.

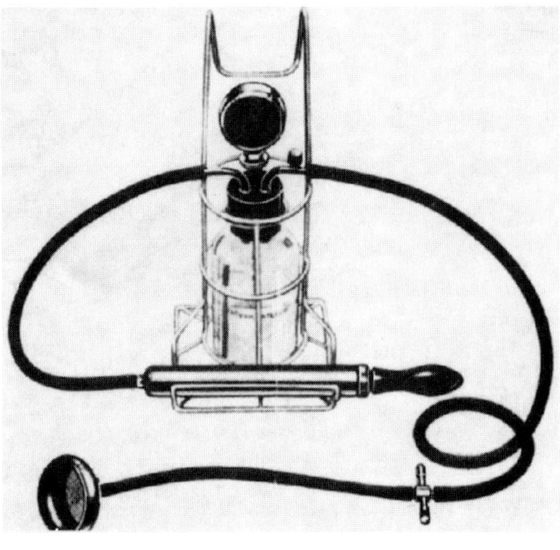

Figure 9–3. An original Malmstrom vacuum extractor system.

Instrument Modifications

Malmstrom Metal Cup Devices

Modifications to the Malmstrom vacuum-extractor were introduced by Bird (1976). He moved the vacuum hose away from the center of the cup and attached the traction chain to the center of the dome of the cup (Fig. 9–4). Touted advantages were easier cup placement and traction at an acute angle to the plane of the cup with less tendency to elevate one edge of the cup and "pop off." He modified another cup for easier placement on the occiput posterior head, moving the vacuum hose attachment to one side of the cup.

The vacuum-extractor became increasingly popular in Europe: used not only in place

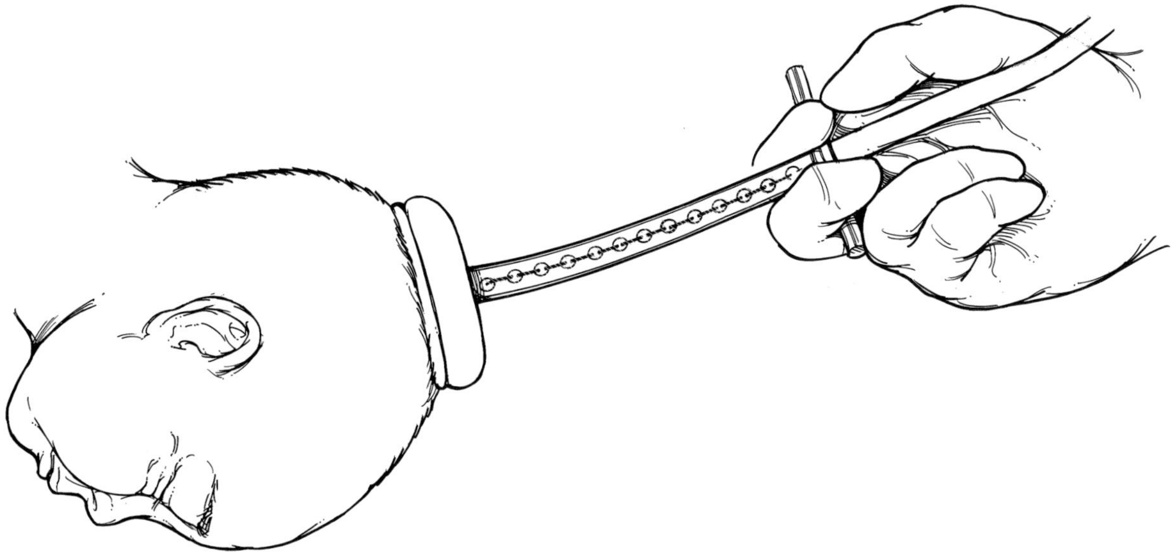

Figure 9–4. The short traction chain attached to the center of the cup avoids angle traction of the vacuum extractor.

of obstetrical forceps, but also to stimulate or enhance the first stage of labor by application to the fetal scalp before full dilatation of the cervix. Smaller diameter cups were designed for this latter purpose. Since use of the vacuum-extractor was felt to be simpler and require less anesthesia than obstetrical forceps, its use had particular appeal in Third World countries (Lasbrey and colleagues, 1964; Chukwudebelu, 1977).

Earn (1967), in reviewing the literature comparing the Malmstrom vacuum-extractor to forceps, found approximately 150 articles. All but one study (Lasbrey and colleagues, 1964) were either retrospective or descriptive. Earn concluded the following: (1) maternal morbidity and perinatal deaths were lower with vacuum delivery than with forceps, (2) there was a higher incidence of non-serious scalp trauma with vacuum-extractors than with forceps, (3) considerable skill was required when using the vacuum extractor if the cervix was not fully dilated, (4) the vacuum extractor is efficacious in select cases of prolapsed umbilical cord when the cervix is almost or fully dilated, (5) the vacuum extractor is efficacious on a second twin in a transverse or oblique lie to convert it to a vertex. Subsequently three randomized controlled trials that compared the Malmstrom vacuum-extractor to forceps have validated Earn's finding (Ehlers, 1974; Fall, 1986; Vacca, 1983, and their colleagues). Use of the vacuum extractor for the second twin has also more recently been discussed by O'Brien and Shaver (1993).

Malmstrom's instrument was widely introduced into American obstetrical practice in the early 1960s (Tricomi, 1961; Kelly and Mishell, 1962; McCullough and Pisani 1963; Pauly, 1963; Nyirgesy, 1963; Barth, 1965; and their colleagues). Results in America with the device were just as favorable as had been reported from Europe. For instance, Matheson and associates (1968) reported on 168 deliveries with no significant maternal complications, a fetal cephalhematoma rate of 2 percent, and a corrected perinatal mortality of 18/1000.

Despite the above encouraging reports, vacuum delivery did not become popular in America, mainly because of reports of associated fetal complications. Not only were scalp abrasions and the caput succedaneum caused by the metal cup aesthetically unpleasant; life-threatening complications of intracranial bleeding and subaponeurotic or subgaleal hemorrhages were also reported (Aguero,

1962; Ahuja, 1969; and their colleagues). That Ott (1975) noted the infants in one report (Ahuja and colleagues, 1969) to have been poorly selected for delivery by vacuum extraction due to greatly prolonged labors was of little consequence; the popularity of this device had been greatly reduced nonetheless.

Three comparisons of the Malmstrom vacuum extractor with forceps are particularly notable inasmuch as they altered the practice in America relative to than in Europe (Ott, 1975). First, Wider and colleagues (1967) discouraged use of the vacuum extractor in the first stage of labor, as well as its prolonged use (over 15 minutes), as both were found to increase perinatal mortality. Using a plexiglass replica of the metal cup they also demonstrated that a delay in excess of 2 minutes to allow chignon formation before exerting traction is unnecessary once the desired level of vacuum is produced. In a second study Greis and colleagues (1981) compared the Bird modification of the Malmstrom vacuum extractor to either a forceps or cesarean delivery. Neither perinatal mortality nor serious traumatic complications were attributable to vacuum extraction when the operation was limited to approximately 15 minutes and/or two "pop-offs." Finally, Baerthlein and colleagues (1986) evaluated instrumental delivery from the midpelvis when the indication was limited to prolonged second stage of labor, uterine inertia, or maternal exhaustion. Similar to prior studies, they confirmed a higher maternal morbidity with the use of forceps. There was, however, no significant difference in neonatal morbidity except for a higher incidence of inconsequential cephalhematomas in the mid-vacuum group.

Significant changes in vacuum delivery technique evolved as a result of the aforementioned studies. The vacuum-extractor, like forceps, was limited to use in the second stage of labor with full cervical dilation (Tricomi and co-workers, 1961). This practice prevailed throughout America, supported by reports from other countries whose collective experience also suggested that the high rate of perinatal mortality and morbidity in cases of failed trial of vacuum extraction was likely due to improper case selection (Fahmy, 1968). Other refinements in technique included time (15 min) and "pop-off" (two) limits as criteria for abandonment of the procedure (Greis and colleagues, 1981; Schenker and Serr, 1967).

Soft Cup Devices

The next advance in vacuum extraction delivery involved improved instrumentation; in 1973 soft vacuum extraction cups made of pliable plastic material were introduced. The Kobayashi Silastic cup with a stainless steel valve on the stem allowed release of a significant amount of the suction force between contractions without loss of cup application to the fetal head. The Silastic cup diameter (65 mm) is the largest of any of today's instruments. It fits over the fetal occiput similar to a skull cap, offering the advantage of less scalp trauma as it better adapts to the fetal head, requires no chignon, and has no rigid metal edge.

Paul and associates (1973) reported favorable results with a three-component plastic vacuum extractor system composed of a disposable plastic replica of the Malmstrom metal cup with a flexible handle stem, disposable plastic tubing, and reusable hand pump. The cup diameter was 50 mm and required the development of a chignon. The advantage over the Malmstrom system was the simplicity of assembly and few parts. The diameter of the plastic cup was subsequently increased to 60 mm and the cup reconfigured by making the dome deeper to remove the necessity of forming a chignon. This device is now called the Mityvac (Fig. 9–5).

The soft cup device resulted in a reawakening of interest in the vacuum extractor. In one report of 432 vacuum extraction deliveries using the Kobayashi Silastic cup (Maryniak and Frank, 1984), much less scalp trauma occurred than had been cited in several series using the metal cup. Five randomized studies comparing the Silastic cup to the metal cup (Kuit, 1993; Hofmeyer, 1990; Chenoy, 1992; Cohn, 1989; Hammarstrom, 1986; and their colleagues) verified this observation. The Silastic cup extractor was also found to effect delivery in a shorter time period; however, they did have a higher failure rate than occurred with metal cups. Hammarstrom and associates (1986) found the metal cup to be clearly superior with occiput posterior presentations, a presentation acknowledged to present larger fetal head diameters relative to the occiput anterior presentations. Kuit and

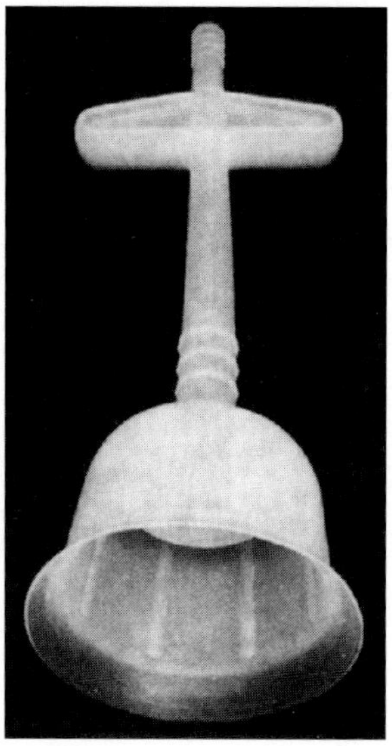

Figure 9–5. Mityvac vacuum extractor.

colleagues (1993) found no significant differences in cord pH, Apgar scores, or retinal hemorrhage between infants delivered with a Silastic or with a metal cup.

In one randomized and four retrospective studies comparing Silastic vacuum delivery to forceps delivery, the Silastic vacuum delivery was associated with less maternal soft tissue trauma. While delivery with the Silastic vacuum caused no increase in major neonatal morbidity, there were more minor scalp changes than occurred with forceps delivery (Berkus, 1985; Meyer, 1987; Svigos, 1990; Hastie, 1986; Johanson, 1989; and their colleagues). Berkus and colleagues (1986) suggest that a judicious trial of Silastic vacuum extractors adds no significant morbidity to mother or infant and may avoid a difficult midforceps or cesarean delivery. However, in a randomized study Johanson and coworkers (1989) reported a higher success rate with forceps (90%) than with the Silastic vacuum extractor (73%).

There is a paucity of studies evaluating the Mityvac cup. In a prospective randomized study the CMI Soft Touch disposable polyethylene cup (formerly called Mityvac) used with a CMI hand vacuum pump was compared to forceps for midpelvic and outlet applications in 99 patients (Williams and associates, 1991). There were no difference in either safety or efficacy between the two groups; however, there were a limited number of midpelvic applications. Delivery by sequential application of instruments occurred in 15 percent of patients with no apparent impact as regards whether vacuum or forceps was tried (and failed) first. Dell and colleagues (1985) randomly assigned 118 nulliparous women who met standard criteria for low forceps delivery to delivery with forceps (Tucker-McLane), Silastic cup, or Mityvac vacuum extraction. All three instruments were effective in achieving outlet delivery. Because of its smaller size, the Mityvac instrument was easier to place into the vagina and failed less often from loss of suction than did the Silastic cup. If the Silastic cup lost suction, successful delivery was achieved in only 30 percent of women, whereas after loss of suction with the Mityvac, delivery was still accomplished in 70 percent of women. Silastic cup failure secondary to a less than perfect seal was most likely to occur in the setting of asynclitism, irregular or excessive moulding of the fetal head, or extensive caput formation (Chenoy and Johanson, 1992). Dell and colleagues (1985) emphasized that with the soft vacuum instruments "the dramatic usefulness of these instruments to quickly deliver multiparas whose infants experienced fetal distress in late labor was far more impressive than their performance as outlet instruments in nulliparas." This no doubt relates to the requirement for less tractive force to deliver the multiparous relative to the nulliparous woman.

There was more maternal trauma in the forceps group and more neonatal trauma in the vacuum group with all injuries involving minor soft tissue trauma. Caput and scalp discoloration were more apparent with the Mityvac than with the Silastic instrument. While loss of suction with the soft cups occurs more often than with the metal cups (about 30% of the time); it is much more innocuous. Loss of suction of the metal vacuum cup was closely correlated with both scalp injuries and instrumental failures (Plauche, 1979).

In current practice in the United States the soft cup vacuum extractors have almost completely replaced the rigid cup devices. The most common instrument now used is the Silastic cup. The American College of Obstetricians and Gynecologists (1991) has published a description of and suggested guidelines for use of vacuum extractors.

VACUUM PRESSURE AND TRACTION FORCES

A number of systems have been used to create the vacuum. Negative or vacuum pressures were initially generated using a bicycle hand pump with the valve reversed. The Mityvac system uses a pistol grip hand pump that connects directly to the cup via a collection filter. Most labor and delivery units have portable electric pumps specifically designed for vacuum extractors such as the Ameda-Egnell suction pump with attached foot pedal control (Fig. 9–6). Many general purpose suction pumps or wall vacuum regulated through a pressure controlling valve are satisfactory alternatives. There must be a gauge, however, to constantly read the negative pressure generated in order to ensure that it is maintained within both effective and safe limits. The recommended operating vacuum pressures for the majority of cups are between −0.6 kg/cm^2 and −0.8 kg/cm^2. The equivalent vacuum pressure reading are summarized in Table 9–1.

An average tractive force of 16 kg in nulliparous women and 12 kg in multiparous women is needed to effect forceps delivery (Wylie, 1935; Laufe, 1971; Moolgaoker and colleagues, 1979). Some have suggested that 22.7 kg (50 lb) of traction force may be the upper limit for fetal safety; however, many apparently normal neonates have been delivered by forceps using greater traction forces (Moolgaoker, 1979; McIntire, 1964; and their colleagues). Mishell and Kelly (1962) were the first to demonstrate quantitatively that 40 percent less traction is exerted by the Malmstrom vacuum extractor (38 lb) as compared with a Simpson forceps delivery (67.5 lb). Duchon and associates (1988) evaluated the traction forces of rigid and soft cup vacuum extractors using a laboratory model. At the commonly recommended vacuum pump settings (550–600 mm Hg), the traction force required for each type of cup before detachment were as follows: the Malmstrom 60 mm cup was 19 kg, the Silastic cup was 20 kg, and the Mityvac 60 mm cup was 18 kg. In terms of force per unit area, they demonstrated that within the working range of 550–600 mm Hg, the Malmstrom has the greatest tractive force (0.79 kg/cm^2), whereas the Mityvac is intermediate (0.68 kg/cm^2) and the Silastic cup has the least (0.63 kg/cm^2). This group observed that on occasion a portion of the soft lip of the Silastic cup would tend to buckle or roll under causing erratic performance and detachment at lower traction forces. In a subsequent laboratory model study, these investigators examined the effect of off-axis traction on the performance of modern vacuum extractors (Muise and colleagues, 1992). By measuring the maximal tractive force (pop-off) for each device at 10-degree increments from the vertical, they found that the rigid cups allowed higher traction force at more acute angles than did the soft cups. The single mold design of most of the soft cups resulted in a tendency for the

TABLE 9-1 VACUUM PRESSURES PRESENTED IN EQUIVALENT UNITS

kg/cm^2	kPa	mm Hg	in. Hg	cm H_2O	lb/in^2
0.23	13	100	3.9	134	I.9
0.27	27	200	7.9	268	3.9
0.41	40	300	11.8	402	5.8
0.54	53	400	15.7	536	7.7
0.68	67	500	19.7	670	9.7
0.82	80	600	23.6	804	11.6
0.95	93	700	27.0	938	13.5
1.03	101	760	29.9	1018	14.7

From Vacca, 1990, with permission.

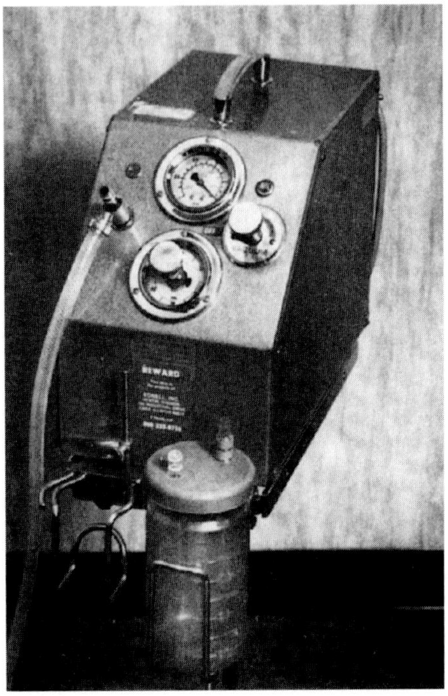

Figure 9–6. Ameda-Egnell suction pump.

cup to tilt, deform, and subsequently detach with off-axis traction at lower traction forces. These investigators felt that an ideal vacuum extractor has yet to be designed; "it should have a large contact area to distribute the tractive force as much as possible. It should be rigid enough to prevent it from collapsing against the fetal head, decreasing its effective diameter, yet flexible enough so that adherence and sealing are achieved with the device and not the scalp." In the quest for a better device, Elliot and associates (1992) have evaluated an obstetric scalp bonnet using models with encouraging preliminary results.

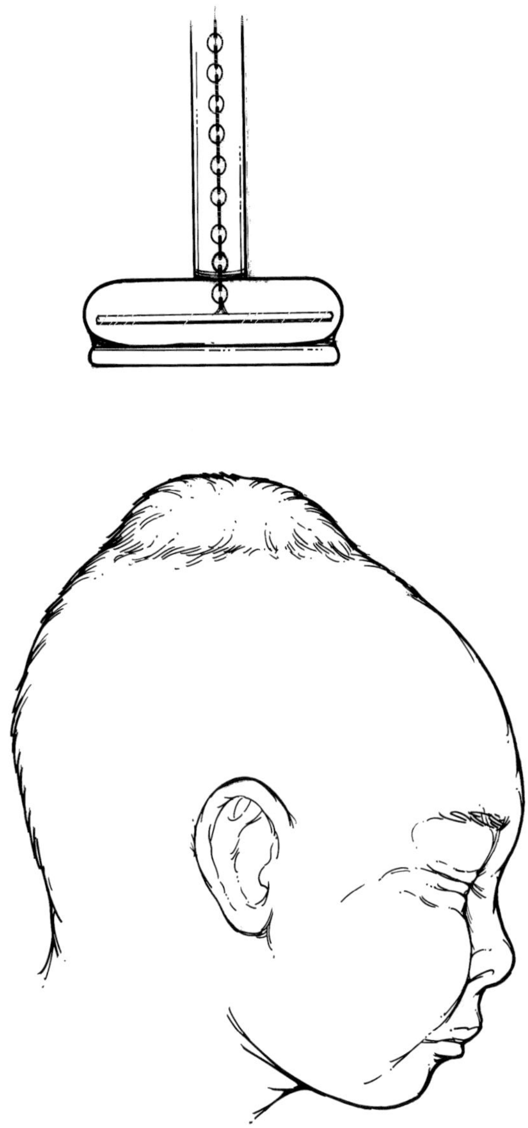

Figure 9–7. Caput succedaneum (chignon).

NEONATAL COMPLICATIONS

Superficial Scalp Markings

Marking of the scalp is always present after vacuum extractor delivery using rigid devices, but disappears after a few days. The caput succedaneum required for delivery with metal cups is the cause of most of this trauma (Fig. 9–7). Plauche (1979) reported an incidence of abrasions or lacerations of the fetal scalp that ranged from 0.8 to 37.6 percent with a mean incidence of 12.6 percent in 12 studies. The Silastic cup and, to a lesser extent, other plastic cups mold to the scalp and create less caput and therefore less injury. Berkus and co-workers (1985) found no increase in scalp abrasions and lacerations with the use of the Silastic cup when compared to forceps.

Cephalhematomas

A more serious but transient form of scalp trauma is development of a cephalhematoma (Fig. 9–8), caused by bleeding due to rupture of a diploic or emissary vein beneath the periosteum. Since bleeding is subperiosteal, it is limited to a single cranial bone, usually one of the parietal bones. The incidence of cephalhematoma in 19 studies involving vacuum delivery ranged from 1 to 25 percent with a mean incidence of 6 percent (Plauche, 1979). Fahmy (1971) examined 116 cases of Malmstrom vacuum extraction deliveries with cephalhematoma and compared them to 116 cases of randomly selected Malmstrom vacuum extraction deliveries without a cephalhematoma. Factors significantly related to cephalhematoma formation included high station of the fetal head, traction for more than 10 minutes, more than one cup detachment, and fetal weight greater than 3.6 kg. The incidence of cephalhematoma with the Silastic cup is increased over that of forceps and spontaneous birth; however, it is well below that of the metal cup. Cephalhematomas usually resolve in 7–10 days.

Subgaleal Hematomas

A more serious and potentially fatal complication of vacuum delivery is the subgaleal or subaponeurotic hematoma, caused by rupture of the diploic vessels in the loose subaponeurotic tissues of the scalp (Fig. 9–9). The subaponeurotic or subgaleal space extends from the

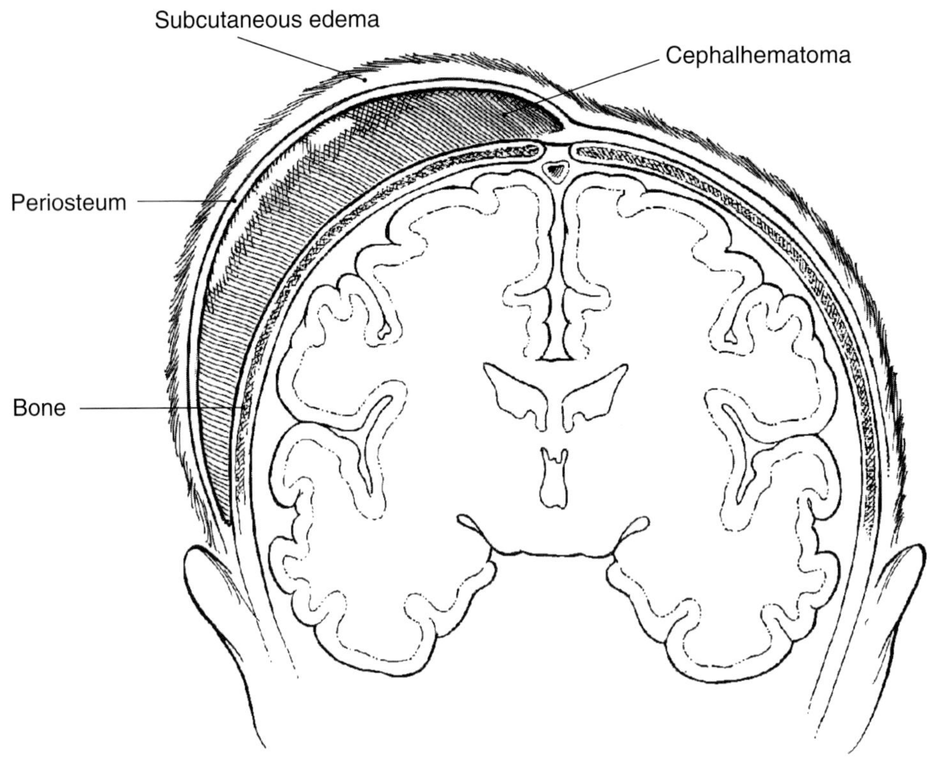

Figure 9–8. Cephalhematoma formation.

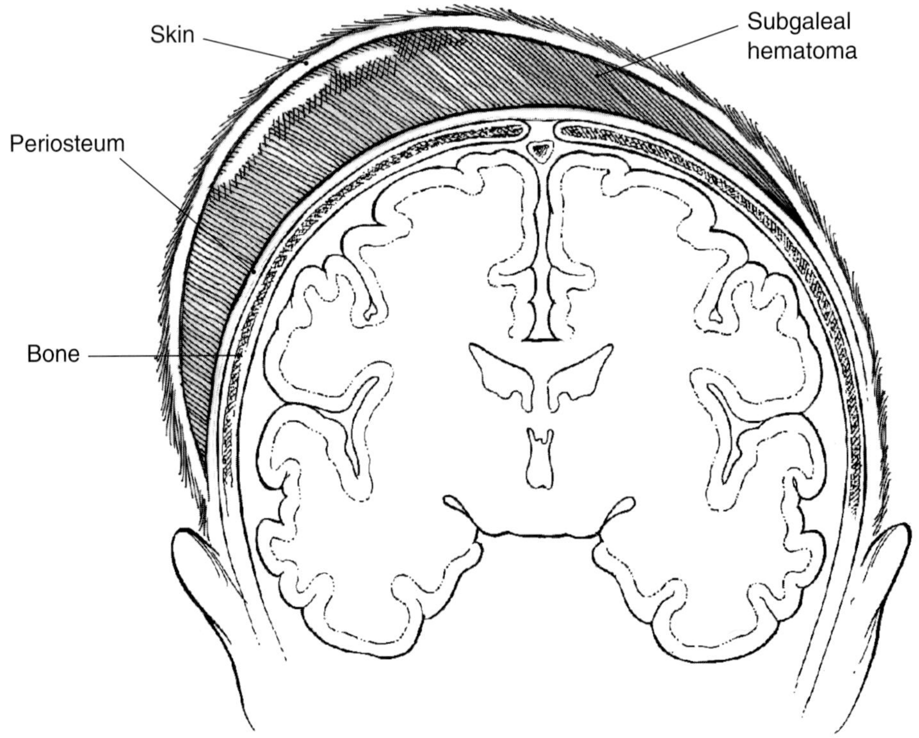

Figure 9–9. Subgaleal hematoma formation.

orbital ridges to the nape of the neck and would hold the entire blood volume of a newborn if filled to a depth of only 1 cm. Thus, this type of bleed can simultaneously be significant yet easily missed as it tends to manifest late in the nursery course, many hours or even days after delivery (Ahuja and associates, 1969). Boo (1990) reported that 101 of 64,424 Malaysian neonates (1.6/1,000 live births) were found to have subaponeurotic hemorrhage after delivery. The occurrence was highest in neonates weighing over 4.0 kg, with only 5 percent of affected neonates demonstrating hypoprothrombinemia. Two-thirds of affected neonates had a history of a trial of vacuum extraction and the remainder had either a prolonged labor or difficult delivery. In one series of subgaleal hematomas, 49 percent followed vacuum extraction, 28 percent followed spontaneous delivery, 14 percent followed a midforceps delivery, and 9 percent followed a cesarean delivery (Plauche, 1980). The incidence of subgaleal hematomas in the general obstetric population is 5/10,000 compared to 50/10,000 Silastic vacuum extractor deliveries and 160/10,000 Malmstrom vacuum deliveries (Benaron, 1993). Subgaleal hematomas have been associated with asphyxia of the newborn, with difficult deliveries from high stations, and with application during the first stage of labor. The only subgaleal hematomas reported in association with the soft cup extractors that have resulted in serious injury to the infant involved a concomitant clotting abnormality as well (Laufe and Berkus, 1992). The neonate's head should be carefully examined after all vacuum extraction applications with periodic reexaminations if the extraction attempt proves difficult. Prompt recognition of subgaleal bleeding, use of a pressure bandage, and blood transfusion will greatly reduce mortality and morbidity (Plauche, 1980).

Fetal Hemorrhage

Fetal hemorrhage in association with vacuum extraction following fetal scalp blood sampling has been reported, but is a rare event (Roberts and Stone, 1978). In one prospective study of 63 cases of vacuum extraction following fetal scalp blood sampling, Lee (1970) found no cases of this complication.

Intracranial Hemorrhage

Intracranial hemorrhage presents a much more serious threat to the newborn than does scalp injury. Plauche (1979) found 51 intracranial hemorrhages in 15 reports involving 7,124 vacuum extractor deliveries for an incidence of 0.35 percent. Hannigan and colleagues (1990) reported on three neonates with tentorial hemorrhages that were associated with soft cup vacuum extractor deliveries. These authors emphasize that vacuum extraction may produce vertical stress in the occipitofrontal diameter of the fetal cranium, causing tentorial venous hemorrhage. Intracerebral hemorrhage occurs so rarely in term infants that it is reasonable to assume an anatomic or developmental abnormality of the vascular system as a predisposing factor. Since intracranial bleeding is much more common in preterm infants, vacuum extraction is relatively contraindicated in these cases.

Retinal Hemorrhages

Retinal hemorrhages are found fairly frequently in the newborn; the incidence following spontaneous delivery is 28 percent, following forceps delivery is 38 percent, and following Malmstrom vacuum extractor delivery is 64 percent (Ehlers and associates, 1974). The more severe retinal hemorrhages have often been associated with vacuum deliveries. One study has reported a similar incidence of retinal hemorrhages with successful delivery whether by Silastic vacuum extractor, forceps, or spontaneous vaginal delivery (Berkus and colleagues, 1985). However, retinal hemorrhage was increased from 28% with a successful delivery to 56% after an unsuccessful trial of Silastic vacuum extraction (Berkus and colleagues, 1986). While it has been suggested that retinal hemorrhage may relate to subclinical cerebral trauma, Svenningsen and associates (1987) found no correlation between retinal hemorrhages, neurobehavior of infants, or the tractive forces required to achieve delivery.

Long-term Infant Follow-up

In a prospective study of 40 infants delivered by Malmstrom vacuum extractor and examined in the newborn period and again at 14 months of age, neurobehavioral testing revealed no risk for serious cerebral sequelae (Blennow and co-workers, 1977). Another study of 121 children delivered via instrumental vaginal delivery (101 by vacuum-extractor) showed no difference in neurobehavioral sequelae compared to infants who delivered spontaneously (Bjerre and Dahlin, 1974). Carmody and associates (1986) in a randomized controlled comparison of vacuum extraction (152) and forceps delivery (152) found no significant differences between groups with regard to growth parameters when assessed at 9 months of age. One child in each group exhibited developmental delay. In another study of 295 children delivered by vacuum extractor, there was no difference in incidence of neurologic abnormalities when compared to 302 controls (Nagan and colleagues, 1990). The longest follow-up study to date included draft board intelligence testing results and medical examinations done at 17 years of age. Analyzed were 1,747 individuals delivered by vacuum-extraction, 937 by forceps, 47,500 by spontaneous vaginal delivery, and 2,098 by cesarean section. These data indicate that infants delivered by vacuum extraction are not at risk of either physical or cognitive impairment when evaluated at 17 years of age (Seidman and associates, 1991).

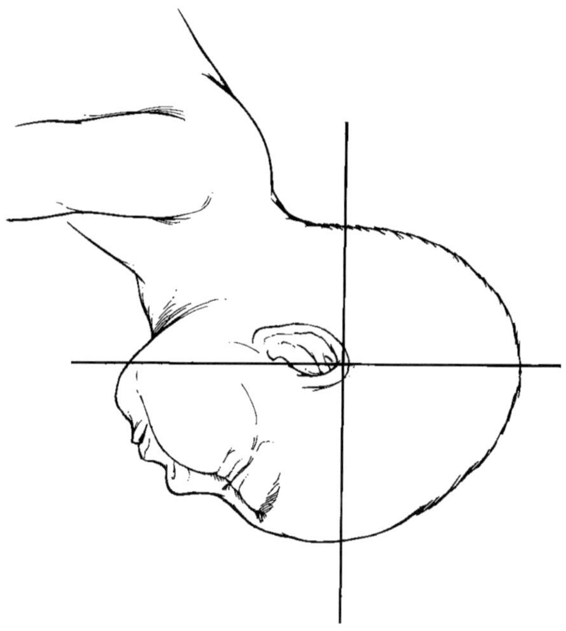

Figure 9–10. The flexing point located on the sagittal suture 3 cm in front of the posterior fontanelle.

APPLICATION TECHNIQUE

The obstetrician must abide by four major principles when performing a vacuum extraction delivery. The first is that flexion of the fetal head must be maintained. The fetal head is completely flexed when the mentovertical diameter points in the direction of descent and this diameter emerges on the sagittal suture 3 cm in front of the posterior fontanelle (Ryberg, 1954) (Fig. 9–10). Vacca (1990) has termed this the flexing point, an important landmark on the fetal head for vacuum extraction. If the vacuum cup is attached to the fetal head so that the center of the cup is over the flexing point, then traction in the axis of descent will maintain the flexion attitude and synclitism of the fetal head. When the vacuum cup is placed too far toward the anterior fontanelle traction will deflex the head. If the vacuum cup is displaced from the center of the sagittal suture, traction can cause or exaggerate asynclitism (Fig. 9–11). Since the sagittal suture is approximately 9 cm in length, a properly placed 60 mm cup will have one edge 3 cm from the anterior fontanelle and the other edge will encroach upon the posterior fontanelle; the sagittal suture will bisect the cup at the posterior fontanelle. Bird (1976) noted that the Malmstrom vacuum cup was usually applied to the most accessible part of the fetal scalp because of limited maneuverability secondary to the centrally placed suction tube. He redesigned the cup to place the vacuum tubing eccentrically but kept the traction chain centrally, allowing proper cup placement over the flexing point. For occiput posterior positions he used a modified cup with the vacuum tubing coming off the edge of the cup. These redesigned vacuum extractor cups reduced his failed vacuum extraction rates. By comparison, the Silastic vacuum cup and the Mityvac have even less maneuverability because of their traction stems, limiting their proper application to fetal heads that are deflexed or asynclitic. Improper application of these instruments results in higher failure rates. While the ideal situation for their use is a flexed and synclitic fetal head, if such conditions existed instrumented delivery would seldom be indicated anyway.

Another important principle for vacuum extraction delivery is the requirement for adequate uterine contractions and maternal expulsive effort. If the mother is under epidural anesthesia or has been overly sedated, time should be allowed for these effects to dissipate and maternal expulsive efforts encouraged. Decreases in traction force and in the number

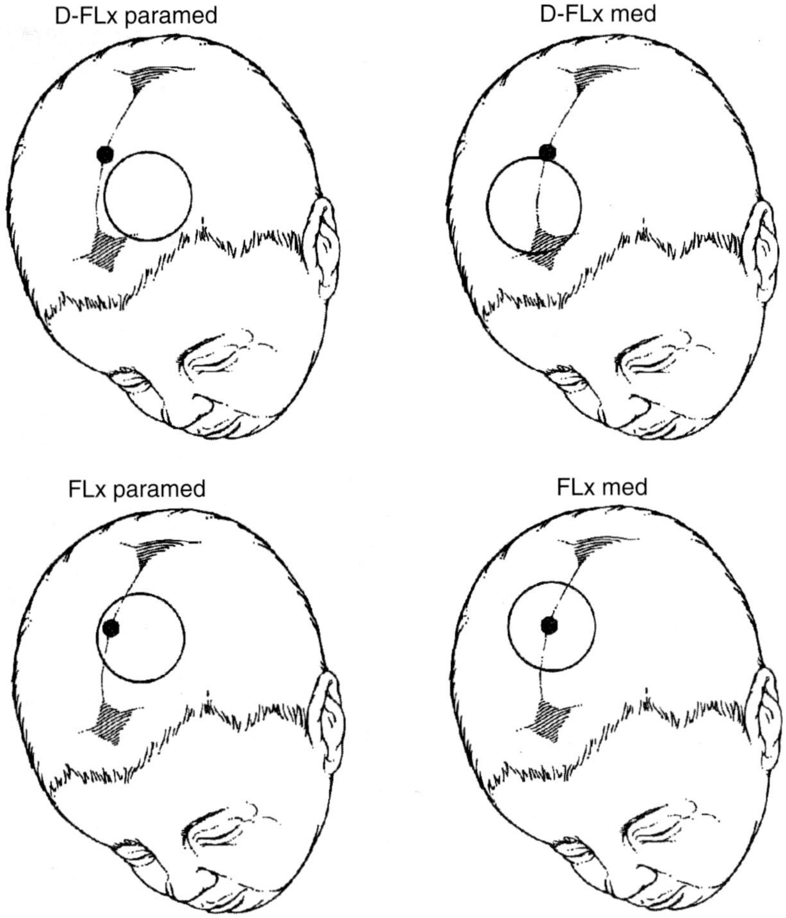

Figure 9–11. Application of the vacuum cup, demonstrating how misapplication can lead to deflexion, asynclitism, or combinations thereof.

of traction episodes will lessen the risk for scalp trauma.

The third principle is that the least resistance to fetal head descent occurs when the direction of traction is parallel with the axis of the birth canal through which the widest part of the flexed fetal head (biparietal diameter) is traveling. Attachment of the cup to the scalp is also most secure, and pop-offs are fewer, when the direction of traction is perpendicular to the cup. This principle can usually be adhered to for low vacuum extractions; however, for midpelvic rotations or for asynclitism, oblique traction will often be necessary. Oblique axis pulls are likely to dislodge the cup as they tend to depress one side of the cup while elevating the opposite side. Compensation for this can be attempted by using the thumb, index, or middle finger of the nontraction hand to apply counterpressure on the side of the cup that is tending to elevate. This maneuver is not, however, possible with the soft cups, thus relegating these cups to low pelvic applications or "easy" rotational procedures.

The fourth and perhaps most important principle of vacuum extraction is the willingness of the obstetrician to abandon the procedure if progress with each traction is not obtained or after two detachments (pop-offs) occur. The vast majority of the literature suggests that delivery of the fetal head should occur after three to five traction events and total application time of 15 minutes or less. Cup detachment should not be regarded as a safety mechanism of the vacuum extractor, but as a warning sign of possible cephalopelvic disproportion.

Appropriate patient selection for vacuum delivery requires considerable judgment and careful evaluation of a number of clinical variables: dilation of the cervix, station, position, moulding, and the condition of the fetus and mother. Vacuum extraction should be limited to a second-stage procedure done by a delivery team led by an experienced attendant familiar with the type of equipment used. In order not to overestimate descent of the fetal head, some have advocated estimating the proportion of the fetal head, expressed in fifths, that is palpable abdominally. Engagement is confirmed when no more than one fifth of the head is palpable. A severe degree of moulding of the fetal head suggests the possibility of cephalopelvic disproportion. A method for assessing moulding has been proposed by Stewart (1980). According to this method, if the parietal bones are not overlapping at the sagittal suture line, moulding is slight (+); if one parietal bone is overlapping the other, but can be reduced by finger pressure, moulding is moderate (++); and if the overlapping cannot easily be reduced, moulding is severe (+++) (Fig. 9–12). Fetal condition should allow the expected time and stress of vacuum extraction delivery; otherwise it should not be attempted.

Few indications for vacuum extraction are absolute. Indications may be divided into standard (low risk) and special (high risk) categories according to the judgment and operative skills required (Vacca, 1990). Standard indications include a non-reassuring fetal heart rate pattern, prolonged second stage of labor, and indicated shortening of the second stage of labor for fetal or maternal reasons. Special uses of vacuum extraction include delay in the second stage of labor associated with malposition of the fetal head where relative cephalopelvic disproportion is suspected or prolapse of the umbilical cord when the cervix is fully dilated and the head engaged. These special uses have been described using the Malmstrom vacuum extractor only.

Initially, the operator should assemble the vacuum extractor system and check to ensure that there are no leaks in the system. Perineal infiltration with local anesthesia will usually be all that is necessary, but some attendants may prefer a pudendal nerve block. The first step in the application of the vacuum extractor is the insertion of the cup into the vagina. The bell and the vaginal opening are prelubricated using surgical soap. The pliable Silastic cup is then collapsed into the smallest possible

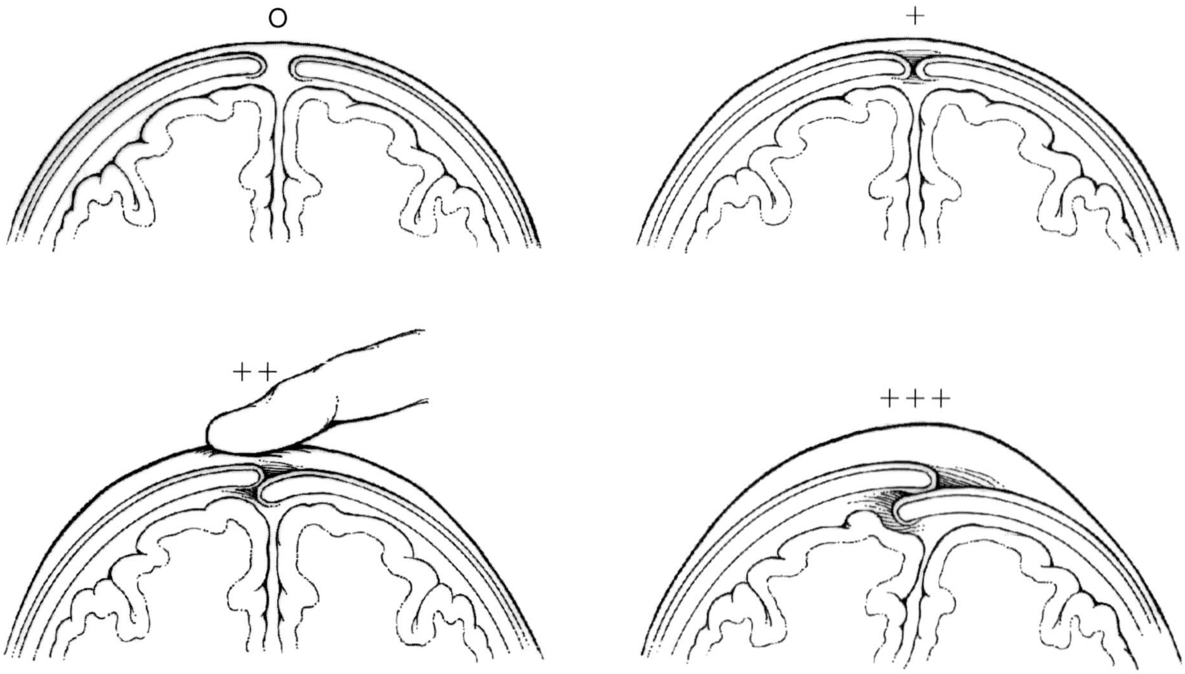

Figure 9–12. Degrees of moulding according to Stewart (1980); 0 is applied when the suture line is open, + when the parietal bones merge and obscure space in the suture line, ++ when the parietal bones overlap but can be reduced with digital pressure, and +++ when the parietal bones overlap and cannot be reduced. *(Adapted from Vacca, 1990, with permission.)*

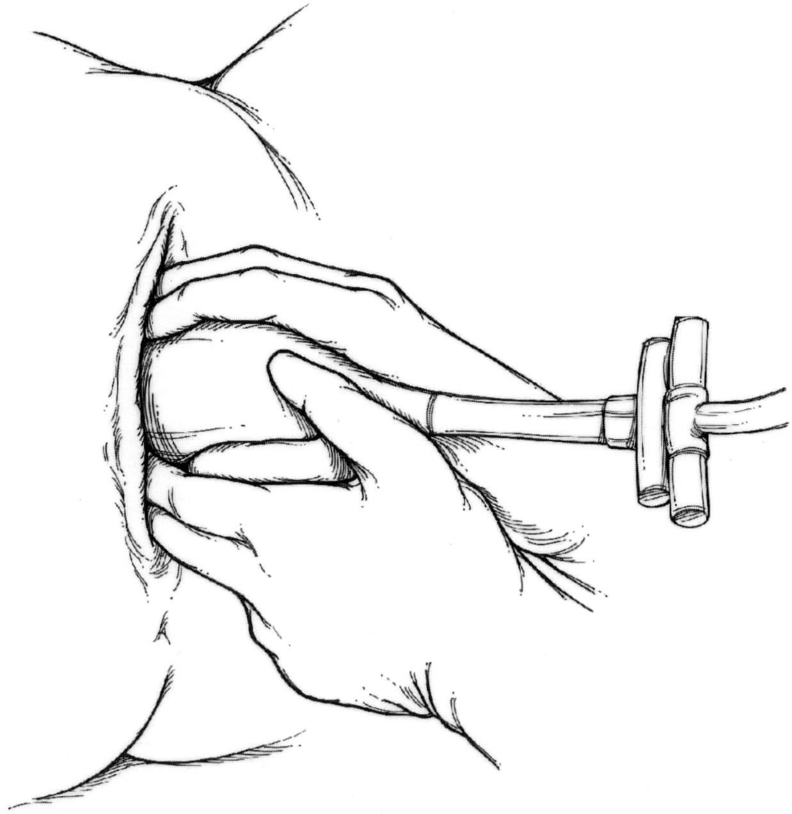

Figure 9–13. When the vacuum cup is inserted, attention is directed to application on the flexing point.

diameter and carefully inserted avoiding the urethral opening by directing pressure toward the posterior vagina (Fig. 9–13). Even the edges of this soft cup can lacerate labial and vaginal tissues. The cup is placed on the scalp as far back toward the occiput and over the flexing point as possible. The blue direction line on the Silastic cup should be directed toward the posterior fontanelle. Simple rotation unfolds the cup edges, which are then palpated to ensure that no cervical or vaginal tissues are trapped (Fig. 9–14). Suction of about

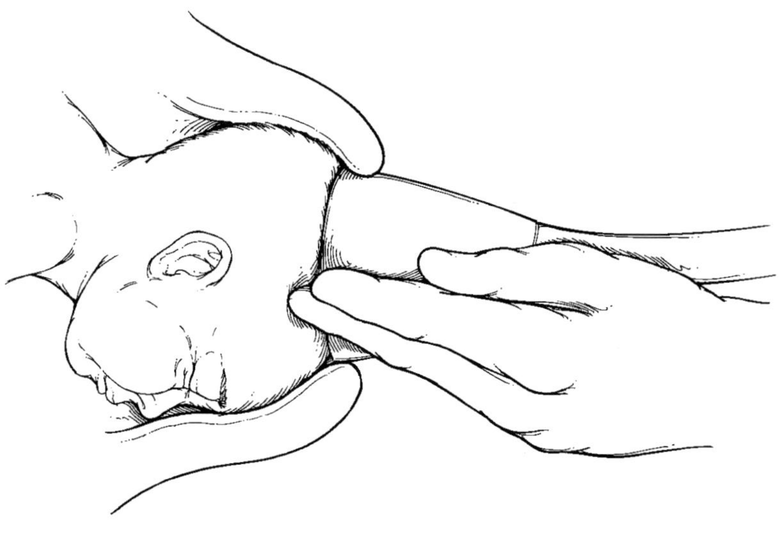

Figure 9–14. When checking the application of the vacuum cup, the physician should ensure that no maternal tissues have been trapped in the vacuum cup.

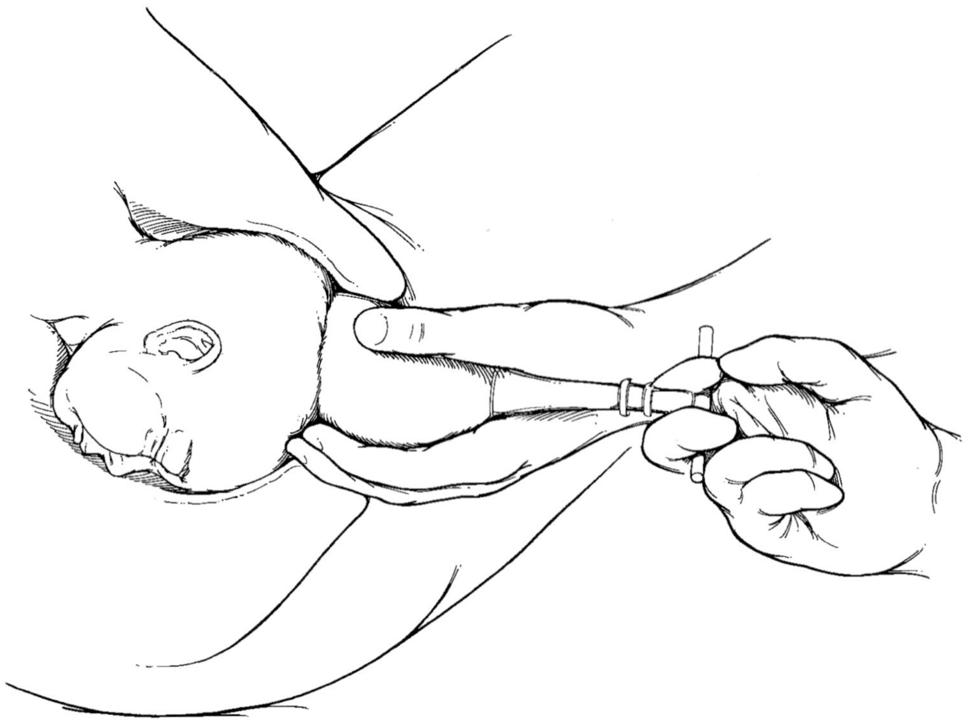

Figure 9–15. Traction is applied along the pelvic axis as the mother pushes, the fingers of the nontraction hand palpating the edges of the cup.

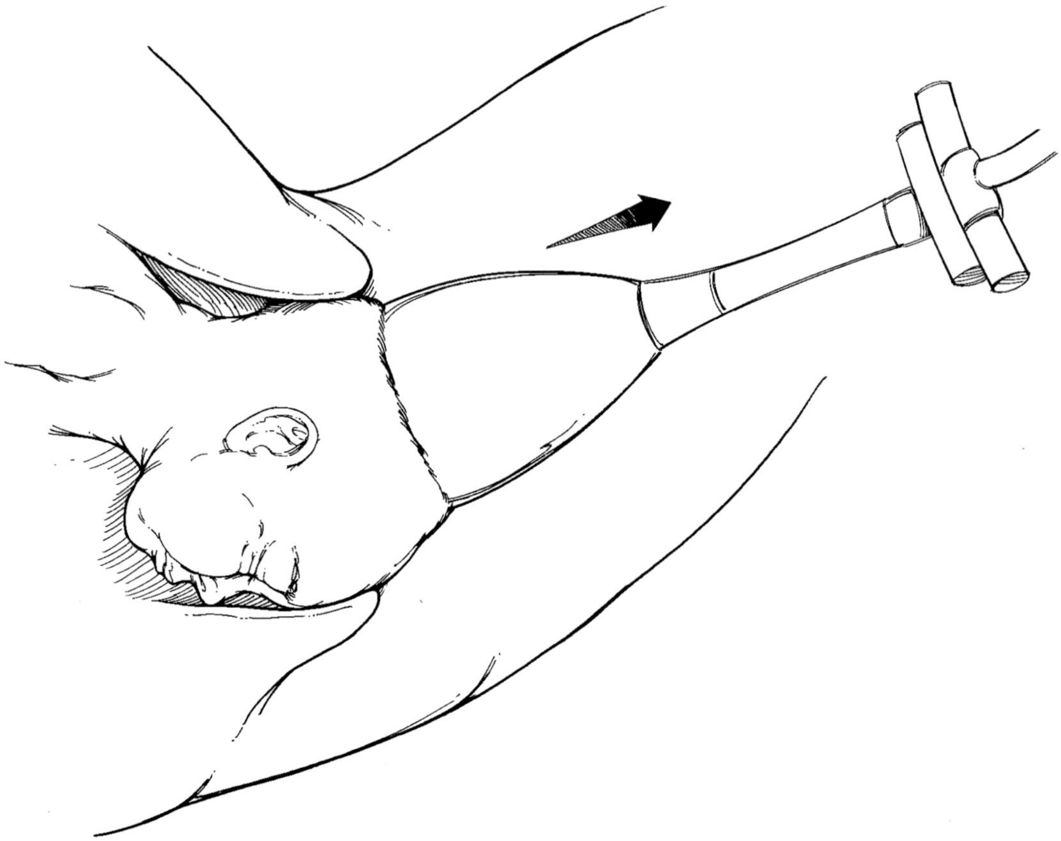

Figure 9–16. As the vertex is delivered, the cup assumes a 90-degree orientation to the horizontal as the head is extended over the perineal body.

200 mm Hg is applied and the cup edges reexamined. This is most easily accomplished by obtaining a full vacuum with the pump to 600 mm Hg, then depressing the trumpet valve above the handle, which is calibrated to release the vacuum pressure down to a baseline of 200 mm Hg. The same control of pressures can be achieved with a foot pedal and the Ameda-Egnell electric vacuum pump system. It is again emphasized that positioning the center of the cup over the flexing point is the key to a successful vacuum delivery. For this reason, the Silastic cup is not well suited for delivery of an infant in the occiput posterior position.

At the beginning of a uterine contraction, the vacuum is increased to 600 mm Hg by releasing the trumpet valve. Traction is applied along the pelvic axis as the mother pushes. The fingers of the non-traction hand should be palpating the edges of the cup (Fig. 9–15). This finger-thumb technique can monitor fetal head movement and descent, the direction of traction adjusted accordingly. One can also detect early on if detachment of the cup is occurring by feeling an edge as it begins to roll under. If detected, the operator should reduce the amount of traction force. The vacuum pressure is released to low levels between contractions. The operator must keep the traction axis parallel to the pelvic axis at that point where the fetal biparietal diameter lies. As the vertex is delivered, the cup should assume a 90-degree orientation to the horizontal as the head is extended over the perineal body (Fig. 9–16). The edges of the cup should be palpated before each traction event. Failure rates of vacuum extraction are between 10 and 13 percent and are usually due to either cephalopelvic disproportion or inappropriate cup positioning.

SUMMARY

Controlled trials comparing vacuum extraction and forceps delivery have shown that serious injury to the fetus directly attributable to the vacuum extractor are rare when it is used in appropriately selected cases. Injuries attributable to the vacuum extractor for the most part are cosmetic and temporary and use of the Silastic vacuum extractor has virtually eliminated these injuries. Long-term follow-up studies have shown no neurobehavioral sequelae to be associated with the use of the vacuum extractor. When using the vacuum extractor it is important to adhere to the basic principles of flexion of the fetal head, efficient maternal uterine contractile and expulsive efforts, maintaining the traction axis parallel to the pelvic axis, and most importantly, a willingness to abandon the technique if progress is not obtained.

REFERENCES

Aguero O, Alvarez H. Fetal injuries due to the vacuum extractor. Obstet Gynecol; 1962; 19:212,.

Ahuja GL, Willoughby MLN, Kerr MM, Hutchison JH. Massive subaponeurotic haemorrhage in infants born by vacuum extraction. Br Med J 1969; 3:743.

American College of Obstetricians and Gynecologists. Operative vaginal delivery. ACOG Technical Bulletin 152. Washington, DC: ACOG, 1991.

Baerthlein WC, Moodley S, Stinson SK. Comparison of maternal and neonatal morbidity in midforceps delivery and midpelvis vacuum extraction. Obstet Gynecol 1986; 67:594.

Barth W, Newton M. The use of the vacuum extractor. Am J Obstet Gynecol 1965; 91:403.

Benaron DA. Sugaleal hematoma causing hypovolemic shock during delivery after failed vacuum extraction: A case report. J Perinatol 1993; 13:228.

Berkus MD, Ramamurthy RS, O'Connor PS, et al. Cohort study of Silastic obstetric vacuum cup deliveries: I. Safety of the instrument. Obstet Gynecol 1985; 66:503.

Berkus MD, Ramamurthy RS, O'Connor PS, et al. Cohort study of Silastic obstetric vacuum cup deliveries: II. Unsuccessful vacuum extraction. Obstet Gynecol 1986; 68:662.

Bird GC. The importance of flexion in vacuum extractor delivery. Br J Obstet Gynaecol 1976; 83:194.

Bjerre I, Dahlin K. The long-term development of children delivered by vacuum extraction. Dev Med Child Neurol 1974; 16:378.

Blennow G, Svenningsen NW, Gustafson B, et al. Neonatal and prospective follow-up study of infants delivered by vacuum extraction. Acta Obstet Gynecol Scand 1977; 56:189.

Boo N. Subaponeurotic hemorrhage in Malaysian neonates. Singapore Med J 1990; 31:207.

Carmody F, Grant A, Mutch L, et al. Follow up of babies delivered in a randomized controlled comparison of vacuum extraction and forceps delivery. Acta Obstet Gynecol, Scand 1986; 65(7):763.

Chenoy R, Johanson R. A randomized prospective study comparing delivery with metal and silicone rubber vacuum extractor cups. Br J Obstet Gynaecol 1992; 99:360.

Chukwudebelu WO. The vacuum extractor in difficult labor. Int Surg 1977; 62:89.

Cohn M, Barclay C, Fraser R, et al. A multicentre randomized trial comparing delivery with a silicone rubber cup and rigid metal vacuum extractor cups. Br J Obstet Gynaecol 1989; 96:545.

Dell DL, Sightler SE, Plauche WC. Soft cup vacuum extraction: a comparison of outlet delivery. Obstet Gynecol 1985; 66:624.

Duchon MA, DeMund MA, Brow RH. Laboratory comparison of modern vacuum extractors. Obstet Gynecol 1988; 71:155.

Earn AA. An appraisal of Malmstrom's vacuum tractor (vacuum extractor): Obstetric and pediatric results. Am J Obstet Gynecol 1967; 99:732.

Ehlers N, Jensen IK, Hansen KB. Retinal haemorrhage in the new forceps and by vacuum extractor. Acta Ophthalmol 1974; 52:73.

Elliott BD, Ridgeway LE, Berkus MD, et al. The development and testing of new instruments for operative vaginal delivery. Am J Obstet Gynecol 1992; 167:1121.

Fahmy K. Failed trial vacuum extraction followed by cesarean section. Int Surg 1968; 49:262.

Fahmy K. Cephalhematoma following vacuum extraction. J Obstet Gynaecol Br Commonw 1971; 78:369.

Fall O, Ryden G, et al. Forceps or vacuum extraction? A comparison of effects on the newborn infant. Acta Obstet Gynecol Scand 1986; 65:75.

Greis JB, Bieniarz J, Scommegna A. Comparison of maternal and fetal effects of vacuum extraction with forceps or cesarean section. Obstet Gynecol 1981; 57:571.

Hammarstrom M, Csemiczky G, Belfrage P. Comparison between the conventional Malmstrom extractor and a new extractor with Silastic cup. Acta Obstet Gynecol Scand 1986; 65:791.

Hannigan W, Morgan A, Kokinski L, et al. Teutorial hemorrhage associated with vacuum extraction. Pediatrics 1990; 85:534.

Hastie SJ, MacLean AB. Comparison of the use of the Silastic obstetric vacuum extractor to Kielland's forceps. Asia-Oceania J Obstet Gynaecol 1986; 12:63.

Hofmeyr GJ, Gobetz L, Sonnendecker EW, Turner MJ. New design rigid and soft vacuum extractor cups: a preliminary comparison of traction forces. Br J Obstet Gynecol 1990; 97:681.

Johanson R, Pusey J, Livera N, Jones P. North Staffordshire/Wigan assisted delivery trial. Br J Obstet Gynaecol 1989; 96:537.

Kelly JV, Mishell D Jr. Experience with the vacuum extractor. Surg Gynecol Obstet 1962; 114:609.

Kuit JA, Eppinga HG, Wallenburg HC, Huikeshoven FJ. A randomized comparison of vacuum extraction delivery with a rigid and a pliable cup. Obstet Gynecol 1993; 82:280.

Lasbrey AH, Orchard CD, Crichton D. A study of the relative merits and scope for vacuum extraction as opposed to forceps delivery. South Afr J Obstet Gynaecol 1964; 2:1.

Laufe LE. Divergent and crossed obstetric forceps: Comparative study of compression and traction forces. Obstet Gynecol 1971; 38:885.

Laufe LE, Berkus MD. Assisted Vaginal Delivery: Obstetric Forceps and Vacuum Delivery Techniques. New York: McGraw-Hill, 1992.

Lee KH. Vacuum extraction after fetal blood sampling. Aust NZ J Obstet Gynecol 1970; 10:205.

MacCahey P. Med Surg Reporter 1890; 63:619.

Malmstrom T. Vacuum extractor—an obstetrical instrument. Acta Obstet Gynaecol Scand 1954; 33(S4):4.

Maryniak G, Frank J. Clinical assessment of the Kobayashi vacuum extractor. Obstet Gynecol 1984; 64:431.

Matheson GW, Davajan V, Mishell DR. The use of the vacuum extractor: A reappraisal. Acta Obstet Gynecol Scand 1968; 47:155.

McIntire MS, Pearse WH. Follow-up evaluation of infants delivered by electronically recorded forceps delivery. Am J Obstet Gynecol 1964; 89:540.

McCullough CD, Pisani BJ. Preliminary report of use of vacuum extractor with caudal anesthesia. New York J Med 1963; 63:2649.

Meyer L, Mailloux J, Marcoux S, et al. Maternal and neonatal morbidity in instrumental deliveries with the Kobayashi vacuum extractor and low forceps. Acta Obstet Gynecol Scand 1987; 66:643.

Mishell D Jr, Kelly JV. The obstetrical forcep and the vacuum extractor: An assessment of their compressive forces. Obstet Gynecol 1962; 19:204.

Moolgaoker AS, Ahamed SOS, Payne PR. A comparison of different methods of instrumental delivery based on electronic measurements of compression and traction. Obstet Gynecol 1979; 54:299.

Muise KL, Duchon MA, Brown RH. Effects of angular traction on the performance of modern vacuum extractors. Am J Obstet Gynecol 167:1125, 1992.

Ngan H, Miu P, Ko L, Ma H. Long term neurological sequelae following vacuum extractor delivery. Aust NZ J Obstet Gynecol 1990; 30:111.

Nyirgesy I, Hawk BL, Falls HC, et al. A comparative clinic study of the vacuum extractor: reassessment of their compressive forces. Am J Obstet Gynecol 1963; 85:1071.

O'Brien JM, Shaver DC. Vaginal delivery of a second, nonvertex twin by high vacuum after failed breech extraction and successful external version. J Mat Fet Med 1993; 2:243.

Ott WJ. Vacuum extraction. Obstet Gynecol Surv 1975; 30:643.

Paul R, Staisch K, Pine S. The "new" vacuum extractor. Obstet Gynecol 1973; 41:800.

Pauly J, Bepko F, Olson. Experience with the negative pressure extractor. South Med J 1963; 56:1219.

Plauche WC: Fetal cranial injuries related to delivery with the Malmstrom vacuum extractor. Obstet Gynecol 1979; 53:750.

Plauche WC. Subgaleal hematoma: a complication of instrumental delivery. JAMA 1980; 244:1597.

Roberts IF, Stone M. Fetal hemorrhage: complication of vacuum extractor after fetal blood sampling. Am J Obstet Gynecol 1978; 132:109.

Rydberg E (ed). The Mechanisms of Labour. Springfield: Charles C Thomas 1954; p 3.

Schenker JG, Serr DM. Comparative study of delivery by vacuum extraction and forceps. Am J Obstet Gynecol 1967; 98:32.

Seidman DS, Laor A, Gale R, et al: The long-term effects of vacuum and forceps deliveries. Lancet 1991; 337:1583.

Simpson JV. On a suction-tractor or new mechanical power as a substitute for forceps in tedious labours. Edinburgh Mon J Med Sci 1848; 32:556.

Stewart KS. In Myerscough PR (ed), Munro Kerr's Operative Obstetrics. 10th ed. London: Bailliere Tindall, 1980; p 32.

Svenningsen L, Lindfemann R, Eidal K, Jensen O. Neonatal retinal hemorrhages and neurobehavior related to tractive force in vacuum extraction. Acta Obstet Gynaecol Scand 1987; 66:165.

Svigos JM, Cave DG, Vigneswaran R, et al. Silastic cup vacuum extractor or forceps: a comparative study. Asia Oceanic J Obstet Gynecol 1990; 16:323.

Tricomi V, Amorosi L, Gottschalk W. A preliminary report on the use of Malmstrom's vacuum-extractor. Am J Obstet Gynecol 1961; 81:681.

Vacca A. The place of the vacuum extractor in modern obstetric practice. Fet Med Rev 1990; 2:103.

Vacca A, Grant A, Wyatt G, Chalmers I. Portsmouth operative delivery trial: A comparison of vacuum extraction and forcep delivery. Br J Obstet Gynaecol 1983; 90:1107.

Vacca A, Keirse MJNC. Instrumental vaginal delivery. In Chalmers I, Enkin M, Keirse MJNC (eds), Effective Care in Pregnancy and Childbirth. Oxford: Oxford University Press, 1989; p 1216.

Wider JA, Erez S, Steer CM. An evaluation of the vacuum extractor in a series of 201 cases. Am J Obstet Gynecol 1967; 98:24.

Williams MC, Knuppel RA, O'Brien WF, et al. A randomized comparison of assisted vaginal delivery by obstetric forceps and polyethylene vacuum cup. Obstet Gynecol 1991; 78:789.

Wylie B. Traction in forceps deliveries. Am J Obstet Gynecol 1935; 2:425.

Younge, J. An account of the balls of hair taken from the uterus and ovaria of several women. Phil Trans 1706; 25:2387.

CHAPTER 10

Breech Delivery

The prevalence of breech presentation varies according to gestational age. Scheer and Nubar (1976) reported that breech presentation occurred in approximately one-third of pregnancies at 21–24 weeks and 14 percent of those at 29–32 weeks, but by term only 3–4 percent of all singleton deliveries are associated with a breech presentation. Table 10–1 summarizes factors associated with breech presentation; gestational age is the single most important factor.

There are three basic types of breech presentation. With the frank breech presentation, the fetal legs are flexed at the hips and extended at the knees (Fig. 10–1). With the complete breech, the legs are flexed at the hips and one or both knees are also flexed (Fig. 10–2). With the incomplete or footling breech presentation, one or both feet or knees lie below the fetal buttocks as the main presenting part (Fig. 10–3). This latter presentation is especially at risk for prolapse of the umbilical cord.

COMPLICATIONS

Both mother and fetus are at greater risk for complications with breech presentation compared to cephalic presentation. These risks include an increase in perinatal morbidity and mortality, prolapsed umbilical cord, placenta previa, congenital anomalies, and cesarean delivery.

Fetal Risks

There is little question that the prognosis for the fetus presenting as a breech either in labor or at delivery is worse than that for a fetus in cephalic presentation. Perinatal mortality and morbidity in these fetuses is most commonly secondary to either prematurity, congenital anomalies, or birth trauma. Congenital anomalies are two to three times greater for the fetus in breech presentation compared to those in cephalic presentation (Brenner and colleagues, 1974). Perinatal mortality is also three to four times greater in breech compared to cephalic presentations. Gimovsky and Paul (1982) reported a mortality rate of 8.5 percent for the fetus in breech presentation and 2.2 percent for those in cephalic presentation. The increased mortality rate for the fetus presenting as a breech was seen despite a 75 percent cesarean delivery rate.

With the exception of the frank breech, cord prolapse increases significantly with breech presentation compared to cephalic presentation (Collea and co-workers, 1978; Barrett, 1991). The risk of cord prolapse according to presentation is summarized in Table 10–2.

Persistent breech presentation also may be a predictor of a neurologically abnormal fetus. In an analysis of over 57,000 pregnancies, Schutte and associates (1985) concluded "it is possible that breech presentation is not coincidental but is a consequence of poor fetal quality, in which case medical intervention is unlikely to reduce the perinatal mortality

TABLE 10–1. FACTORS ASSOCIATED WITH BREECH PRESENTATION

Gestational age
Great parity
Multiple fetuses
Hydramnios
Oligohydramnios
Uterine anomalies
Pelvic tumors
Anomalous fetus
Previous breech presentation

associated with breech presentation to the level associated with vertex presentation." This concept is further supported by the findings of Hytten (1982) and Susuki (1985). Nelson and Ellenberg (1986), as well as Torfs and associates (1990), found breech presentation to be a risk factor for cerebral palsy regardless of delivery route.

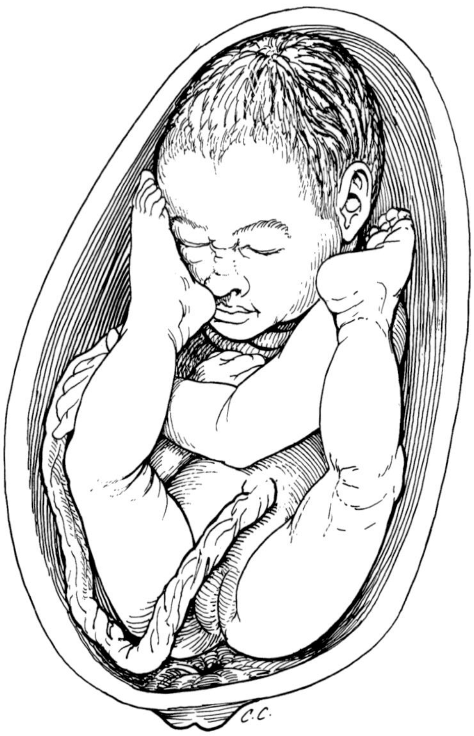

Figure 10–1. Frank breech. The hips are flexed and the knees are extended with the feet lying near the infant's face.

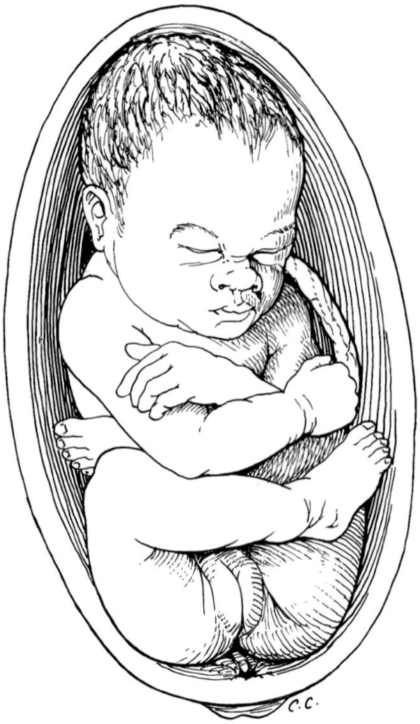

Figure 10–2. Longitudinal lie. Complete breech presentation: both the hips and the knees are flexed and the feet present with the buttocks. This attitude is easily recognized by vaginal examination once the cervix has dilated to 4–5 cm.

Maternal Risks

The major maternal complications associated with breech presentation are those coincident with cesarean delivery. Although maternal mortality is rare, death is significantly more common with cesarean section than following vaginal delivery. Maternal morbidity is also significantly increased with operative delivery. Weiner (1992) has estimated that routine cesarean delivery for all breech presentations in 1990 cost society almost $1.5 billion. Delivery of only 50 percent of breech presentation vaginally would save more than $700 million annually.

VAGINAL DELIVERY VERSUS CESAREAN SECTION

Over the last 35 years or so, the equivalent of one professional life span for an obstetrician, there has been a dramatic change in opinion

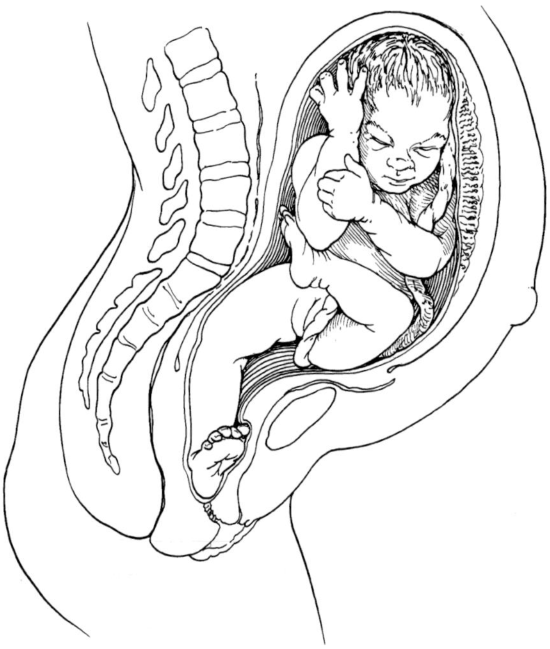

Figure 10–3. Single-footling breech presentation in labor with membranes intact. Note possibility of umbilical cord accident at any instant, especially after rupture of membranes.

regarding the most appropriate route of delivery for the persistent breech presentation. In contemporary obstetric practice, the vast majority of fetuses presenting as breeches are delivered via cesarean section (ACOG, 1986). Green and associates (1982) reported that the cesarean section rate for breech presentation had increased from 22 percent in the decade 1963 through 1973 to 94 percent by 1979. Breech presentations now account for approximately 15 percent of all cesarean sections (Weiner, 1992). The major reason for the high cesarean section rate for breech presentation is the belief that both perinatal mortality and morbidity can be reduced by avoiding vaginal delivery. A second factor is the inadequate

TABLE 10–2. FREQUENCY OF CORD PROLAPSE

Presentation	Frequency (%)
Cephalic	0.4
Frank breech	0.5
Complete breech	4–6
Footling breech	15–18

instruction and training in vaginal breech delivery received by the majority of residents in obstetrics and gynecology. Furthermore, even obstetricians proficient at vaginal breech delivery at the completion of residency are unlikely to encounter enough breeches in practice to remain proficient. For example, Moore (1988) has estimated that the "average" practitioner of 240 deliveries per year will encounter only 10 breeches per year and of these only 2 would be candidates for a trial of labor.

Has the increase in cesarean delivery rate for breech presentation resulted in an improvement in fetal outcome? In select cases such as birth weights of 500–1,000 g, who are at highest risk for entrapment of the fetal head, the answer appears to be yes. A more clinically relevant question is whether cesarean section improves outcome for all breech presentations (ie, footling v. frank presentation) at all gestational ages (ie, term v. preterm). Additionally, most busy delivery services occasionally will have patients who present with a partially or mostly delivered fetus in breech presentation at a stage when it is too late to proceed with an abdominal delivery.

The Term Breech Fetus

Collea and co-workers (1980) and Gimovsky and associates (1983) reported the results of prospective studies regarding the method of delivery for the term breech presentation. In the 1980 report, 115 of 208 infants in the frank breech presentation were randomized to a trial of labor. Following x-ray pelvimetry, only 60 women were judged to be candidates for vaginal delivery and of these 49 (82%) delivered vaginally. There were two transient brachial plexus injuries in the vaginal delivery group. Maternal morbidity was significantly higher in the 148 women who underwent cesarean section. In 105 women at term with a non-frank breech presentation, Gimovsky and colleagues (1983) reported 31 of 70 (44%) patients randomized to a trial of labor following x-ray pelvimetry delivered vaginally. Neonatal morbidity in the vaginal and cesarean groups was similar. The one neonatal death occurred in the cesarean group.

In a review of the literature regarding vaginal breech delivery at term, Weiner (1992) found that in 13 retrospective studies of 3,729 breeches, 2,133 (57%) delivered vaginally. The corrected perinatal mortality was 3.1/1,000 for those delivered via cesarean section compared to 3.7/1,000 for neonates delivered vaginally (Table 10–3). In a review of 1,240 singleton breech infants (term and preterm) from the California Kaiser Permanente Program (term and preterm), Crough-Minihane and associates (1990) found that 75 percent were delivered by cesarean section and 25 percent vaginally. There was no significant association between route of delivery and frequency of head trauma, newborn seizures, mental retardation, or cerebral palsy.

In contrast, Thorpe-Beeston and colleagues (1992) reported a significant increase in intrapartum and neonatal deaths in term breeches without congenital anomalies when they compared vaginal delivery to cesarean section [8 of 961 (0.83%) v. 1 of 2,486 (0.03%)]. Moreover, Cheng and Hannah (1993) reviewed 24 studies regarding planned vaginal versus elective cesarean delivery for the singleton term breech. Both perinatal mortality (odds ratio 3.86; 95% CI 2.2–6.7) and neonatal morbidity (odds ratio 3.96; 95% CI 2.76–5.67) were higher for the planned vaginal delivery groups. However, as the authors pointed out "because of selection bias in the majority of studies, differences in outcome may be due to factors other than the planned method of delivery."

The Preterm Breech Fetus

There may be significant disparity between the size of the fetal head and buttocks in the premature infant. In such cases, the body of the fetus may pass through the cervix easily while the head may become trapped. There are no large randomized prospective studies addressing delivery of the premature breech. However, several retrospective studies have suggested improved neonatal outcome, as measured by perinatal mortality, developmental abnormalities, and intracranial hemorrhage with cesarean delivery of preterm breech fetuses weighing less than 1,500–2,000 g (Ingemarsson, 1978; Westgren, 1985a,b; Morales, 1986; Bodmer, 1986). Although preterm fetuses in this weight range most commonly undergo cesarean section in the United States, the value of operative delivery for these infants is not universally accepted (Cox, 1982; Effer, 1983).

PELVIMETRY

X-ray pelvimetry has been recommended by some for the management of breech presentation (see Chapter 5). For example, Ridley and associates (1982) reported that the cesarean section rates were 40 percent, 61 percent, and 89 percent when the pelvis was adequate, marginal, or inadequate, respectively. Because of the relatively high-dose exposure from conventional x-ray pelvimetry (1–5 rads), computed tomography (CT) is now recommended. With CT pelvimetry, exposure may be as low as 250 mrad (Moore and Shearer, 1989). An adequate pelvic inlet by plain film pelvimetry was defined by Collea and associates (1980) as a transverse diameter of 11.5 cm and an anterior-posterior diameter of 10.5 cm. For the midpelvis the bispinous diameter would be 10.5 cm and the anterior-posterior diameter should be 11 cm or greater.

EXTERNAL CEPHALIC VERSION

When a breech presentation is detected in the third trimester, external cephalic version may be attempted. Van Dorsten and colleagues (1981) reported 70 percent success with this procedure. This procedure is discussed in detail in Chapter 12.

CESAREAN SECTION

Cesarean section is used for the delivery of the majority of breech presentations. Cesarean delivery is recommended for (1) a known or suspected large fetus (> 4000 g), (2) a contracted pelvis, (3) fixed hyperextension of the fetal head as occurs with a neck mass, (4) prematurity at 24–30 weeks, gestation or birthweight 500–1,500 g, (5) inadequate skills to perform the delivery, and (6) inadequate support services, that is, anesthesia, pediatrics, surgery team. Induction of labor is a reasonable approach under appropriate circumstances. Cesarean section is preferred to oxytocin augmentation in cases of active phase or second stage arrest of labor.

The choice of uterine incision should be dictated by the degree of development of the lower uterine segment and the relative size of the fetus. In the vast majority of breeches, a low transverse uterine incision can be used.

TABLE 10–3. VAGINAL BREECH DELIVERIES ≥ 2000 g ≤ 3900 g (OR GREATER THAN 35W) RETROSPECTIVE

Author	(y)	Number of Candidates for Vaginal Delivery	Breech Types Included	Management Protocol	Used Oxytocin	Vaginal Delivery (%)	Abnormal X-ray (%)	Corrected[a] PNM/1000		Perinatal[b] Morbidity (%)	
								Vaginal	*Cesarean*	*Vaginal*	*Cesarean*
Bowes	(79)	353	all	Y	?	265 (75)	—	7.5	22.7	—	—
Mann	(79)	334	all	N	?	209 (63)	—	0	8	—	—
O'Leary	(79)	81	frank	Y	N	48 (59)	—	0	0	0	0
Jaffa	(81)	321	all	Y	Y	260 (81)	10.2	0	0	.3[d]	0
Gimovsky	(82)	153	frank	N	Y	54 (35)	—	0	0	3.2[d]	1.3[d]
Rosen	(84)	325	x footling	?	?	68 (21)	—	14.7[c]	0	11.8[d]	9.7[d]
Watson	(84)	147	frank	Y	Y	69 (47)	23	0	0	?	?
Tatum	(85)	397	x footling	Y	Y	155 (38)	43	0	0	1.5[d]	.50[d]
Flanagan	(87)	369	variable	?	Y	175 (47)	?	0	10	0	0
Songane	(87)	571	all	±Y	Y	453 (79)	?	11[e]	0	1.7[d]	.7[d]
Bingham	(87)	149	frank	Y	?	90 (60)	?	0	0	1	.5
Mahomed	(88)	213	x footling	±Y	?	88 (41)	?	0	0	0	0
Weiner	(90)	316	all	±Y	Y	199 (63)	—	0	0	2.1[d]	3.3[d]
Total		3729				2133 (57)		3.7[f]	3.1		

[a]Lethal anomalies excluded.
[b]Many studies included bruising.
[c]RDS
[d]No permanent nerve palsies.
[e]Includes 2 intrapartum deaths (hypoxia, 2nd stage) and 3 neonatal deaths (meconium aspiration, hypoxia, trapped head).
[f]PNM 1.4/100 excluding Songane.
x is an abbreviation for "except."
From Weiner CP (1992), with permission

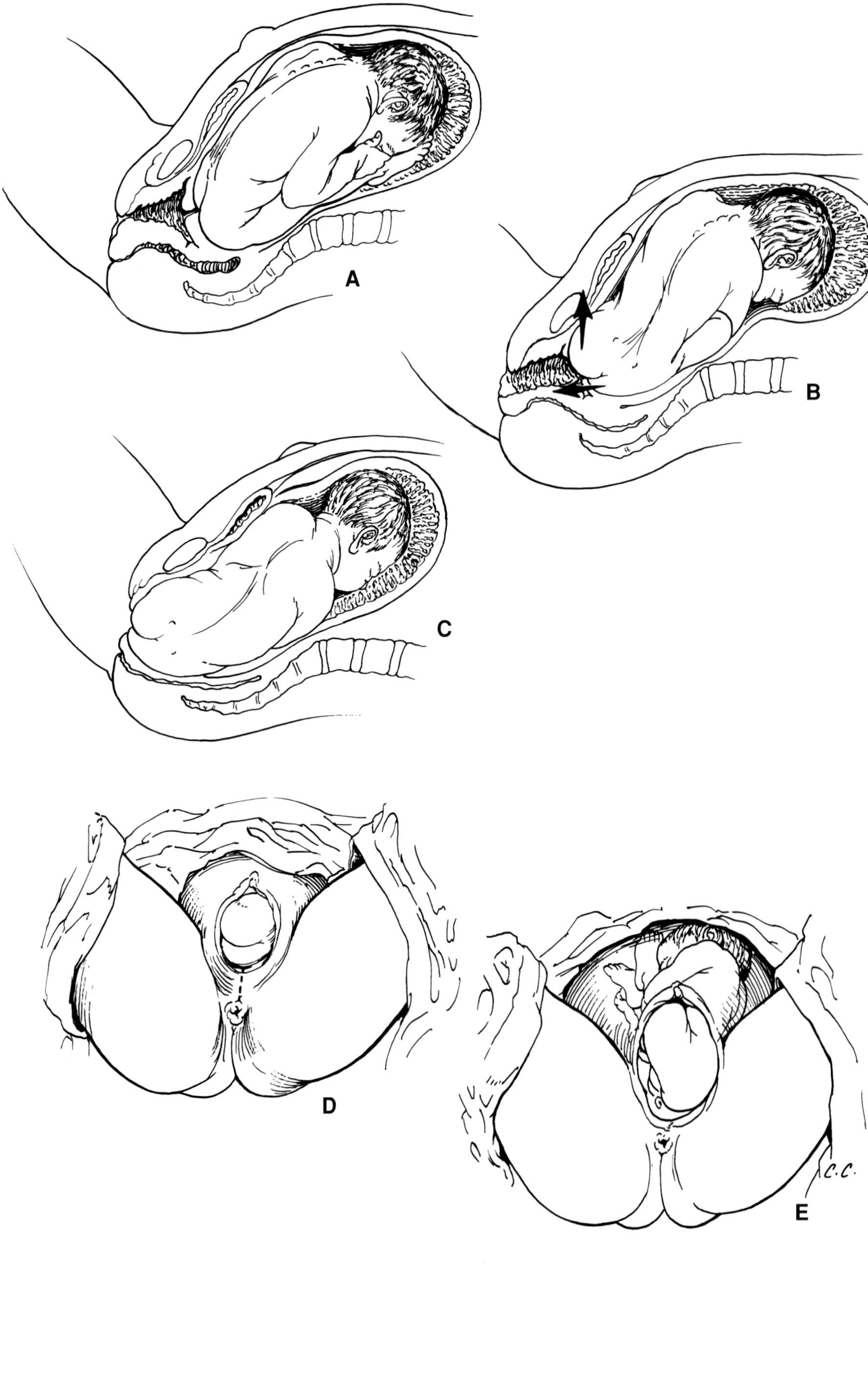
A
B
C
D
E
C.C.

← **Figure 10–4.** Mechanism of labor in frank breech presentation. **A.** At commencement of labor the presenting part usually lies above the level of the ischial spines, with the infant's back directed in an oblique anterior position. **B.** The presenting part may remain high until the cervix is completely dilated. In breech labors, most descent occurs during the second stage. As the buttocks descend, the anterior hip slides up the levator on one side until the bi-ischial diameter lies in the anterior-posterior diameter of the maternal pelvis. **C.** The anterior hip has descended to a position beneath the pubic arch. Next the posterior hip will be forced upward over the perineum while the fetal spine bends laterally to accommodate to the curve of the birth canal. **D.** Episiotomy is performed when the genital crease becomes visible through the distended introitus. **E.** With further descent of the presenting part the posterior hip is pushed completely through the introitus.

In some cases, especially when dealing with a thick, poorly developed lower uterine segment and a preterm breech fetus, a low vertical or classical uterine incision may be necessary in order to avoid fetal trauma. It must be emphasized however, that cesarean section does not guarantee an atraumatic delivery, especially if improper technique is used. The technique of breech extraction at the time of cesarean section is the same as for vaginal delivery.

VAGINAL DELIVERY OF THE BREECH FETUS

Moore (1988) summarized several key steps that should be taken before delivering the breech fetus (Table 10–4). The experience and skill of the obstetrician should be considered when choosing the route of delivery. An anesthesiologist and pediatric attendant should be present at delivery. An operating room and team should also be readily available should emergency abdominal delivery be required.

Technique of Vaginal Breech Delivery

The mechanism of labor in frank breech presentation is detailed in Figure 10–4. A major potential problem with vaginal breech delivery is the possibility that the smaller feet and body may deliver through a partially dilated cervix, leaving the fetal head trapped in the pelvis by the cervix. For this reason, it is imperative to avoid premature traction on the lower fetal body or feet. The cardinal rule of vaginal breech delivery is to avoid touching the fetus before delivery has occurred to the level of the umbilicus. The scenario depicted in Figure 10–5 is *not* an obstetrical emergency as long as the fetal heart rate is normal; even with both feet presenting, spontaneous delivery to the level of the umbilicus is awaited unless fetal heart rate abnormalities merit earlier assistance with delivery.

TABLE 10–4. KEY STEPS BEFORE DELIVERING THE BREECH FETUS

Obtain informed consent
Estimate gestational age
Determine type of breech
Evaluate for presence of hyperextension of fetal head
Perform pelvimetry
Estimate fetal weight
Evaluate delivery team

Adapted from Moore (1988).

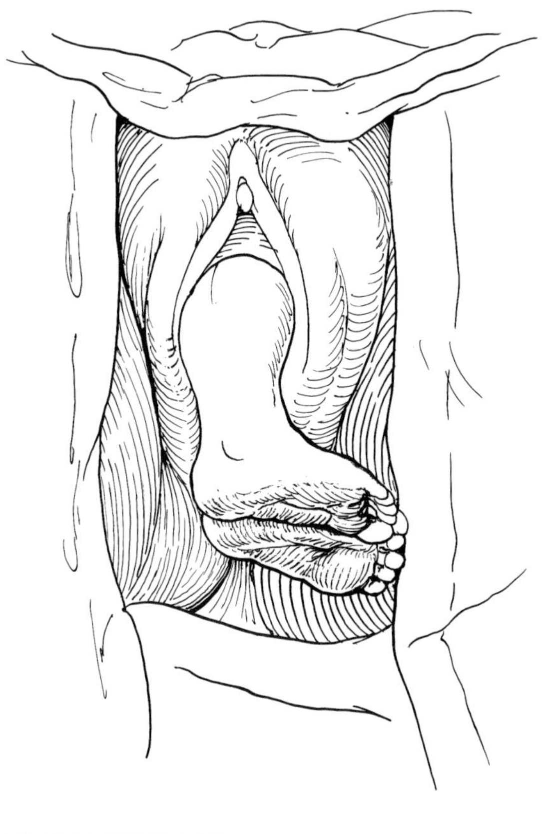

Figure 10–5. This is not an obstetric emergency! In performing a vaginal breech delivery, do not grasp the feet until the body has delivered to the umbilicus if the fetal heart rate is normal.

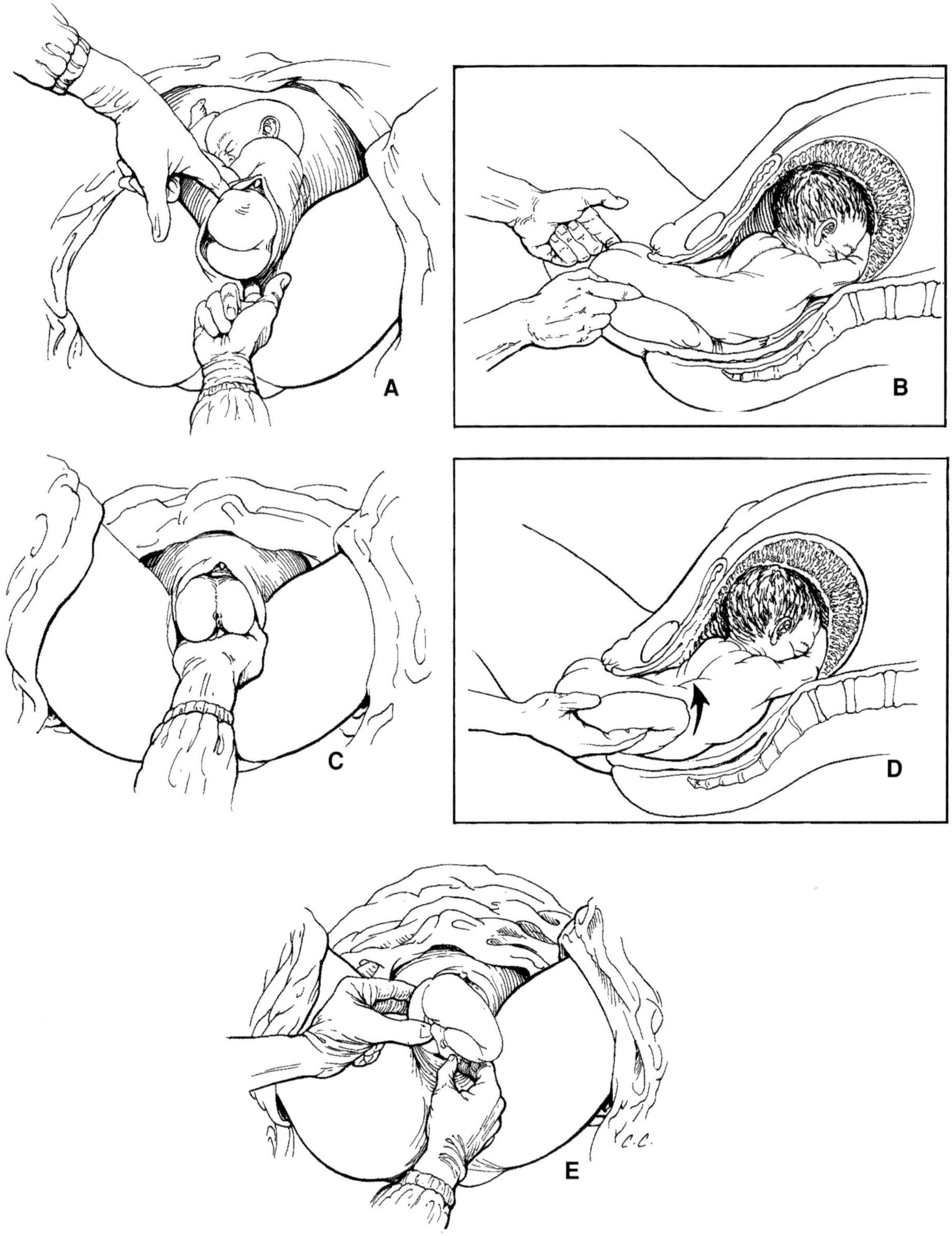

Figure 10–6. A, B. Downward traction is made with the operator's index fingers in the groin of the fetus. **C, D, E, F.** When the knees of the fetus reach the perineum, the knee is flexed by pressure on the thigh, allowing the foot to be delivered. (**G, H**). The procedure is then repeated with the other leg.

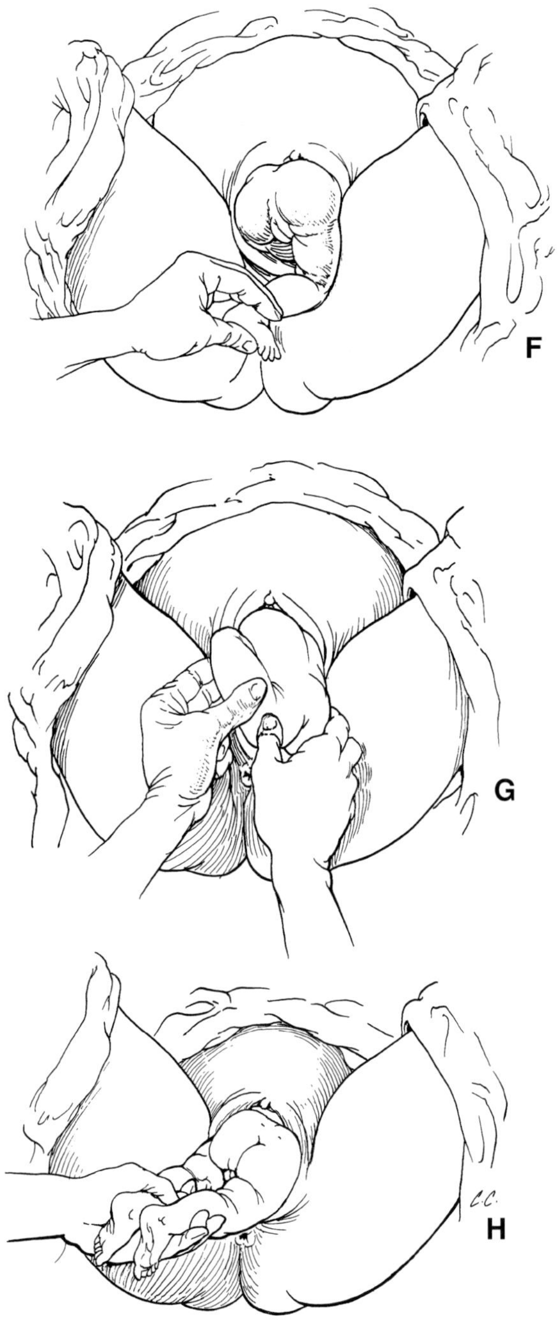

Figure 10–6. (continued).

Only after spontaneous delivery to the level of the fetal umbilicus should active delivery of the fetus begin. A finger is placed in each groin and gentle downward traction is used (Fig. 10–6). A breech decomposition is then performed by converting the fetus to a footling breech (Fig. 10–6). The Pinard maneuver is especially useful for atraumatically obtaining the feet of the fetus and deserves special emphasis on technique when performed at higher stations (Fig. 10–7). With this procedure, two fingers are placed along one fetal thigh to the level of the knee, which is then pushed away from the midline to effect flexion of the leg. The obstetrician's fingers are kept parallel to the femur and serve as a splint as the upper leg is swept laterally. With flexion, the foot then can usually be easily grasped and brought down and out. These same maneuvers may be employed in the technique of total breech extraction. During this procedure, the feet of the fetus are grasped and held by the ankles. Then with gentle traction the feet are brought down into the vagina and through the vulva. If both feet cannot be grasped at once, one foot at a time should be brought down into the vagina. These procedures are sometimes appropriately employed by applying traction to the fetus *prior* to delivery to the umbilicus when delivering the second twin or in emergencies when rapid cesarean delivery is not possible. An episiotomy should be used in most such cases; an exception is the multiparous patient with marked relaxation of the vaginal perineum.

Following delivery of the legs, they may be wrapped with a moist towel for a better grasp; gentle traction is continued until the buttocks emerge (Fig. 10–8). The thumbs of the obstetrician should be placed over the sacrum and the fingers over the anterior illiac crests of the fetus. Along with continued downward traction, gentle and slight rotation from side to side should be applied until the scapulas become visible (Fig. 10–9). This *slight* rotation or "corkscrew" motion will decrease the incidence of nuchal or trapped arms. The mother should be encouraged to aid in delivery by bearing down and pushing if possible. If too much downward traction is applied, the arms may become trapped behind the occiput.

Once the axilla become visible, the shoulders and arms can be delivered. With the scapulas visible, the trunk is rotated so that one arm is in an anterior position. The anterior arm then may be freed by placing one or two fingers parallel to the humerus until the elbow is reached and the arm is swept downward and through the vulva (Fig. 10–10). The body is then rotated in the reverse direction to deliver the other shoulder.

If trunk rotation is difficult, it may be best (or necessary) to deliver the posterior shoulder first. With this technique, the feet

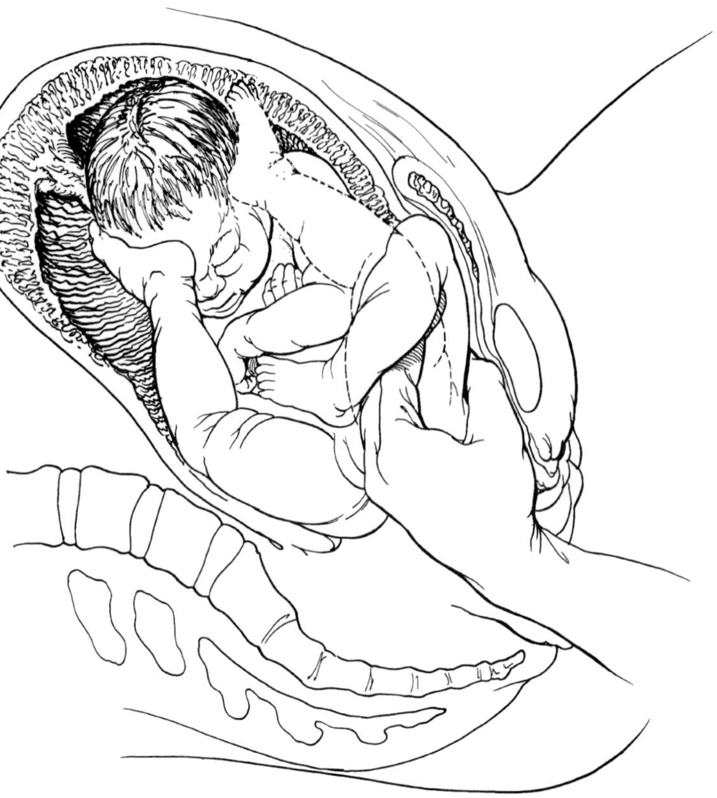

Figure 10–7. Details of the Pinard maneuver, which is sometimes used in a case of a frank breech presentation to deliver a foot into the vagina. The obstetrician's fingers are kept parallel to the femur. Pressure in the popliteal fossae results in flexion at the fetal knee.

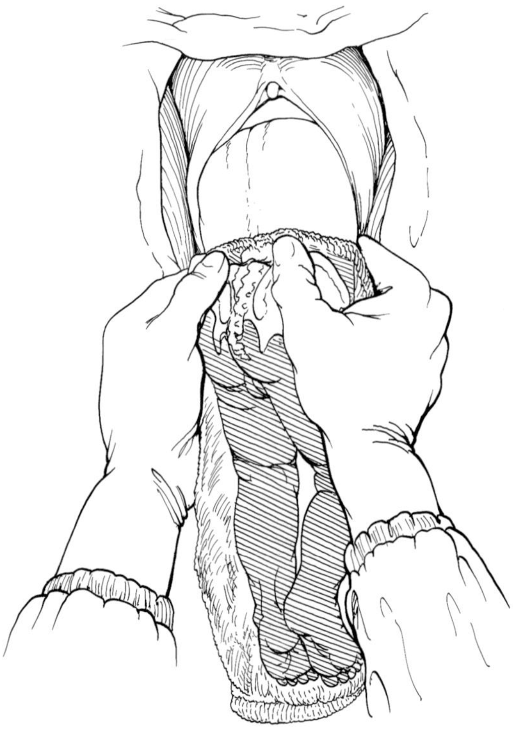

Figure 10–8. Breech extraction. The hands are applied over, but not above, the infant's pelvis, with the thumbs resting on the sacrum and the fingers on the anterior illiac crests.

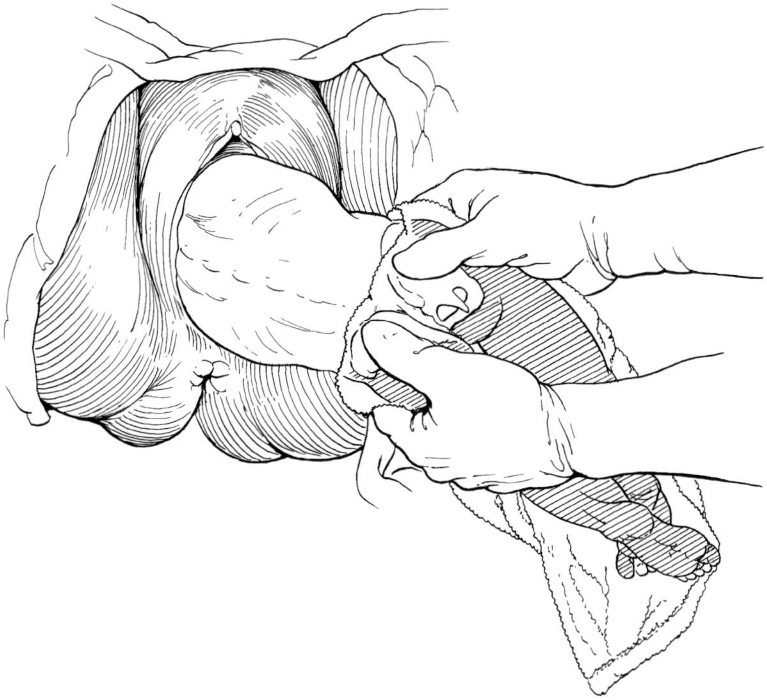

Figure 10–9. The thumbs of the obstetrician should be placed over the sacrum and the fingers over the anterior illiac crests of the fetus. Along with continued downward traction, gentle and slight rotation from side to side should be applied until the scapulas become visible.

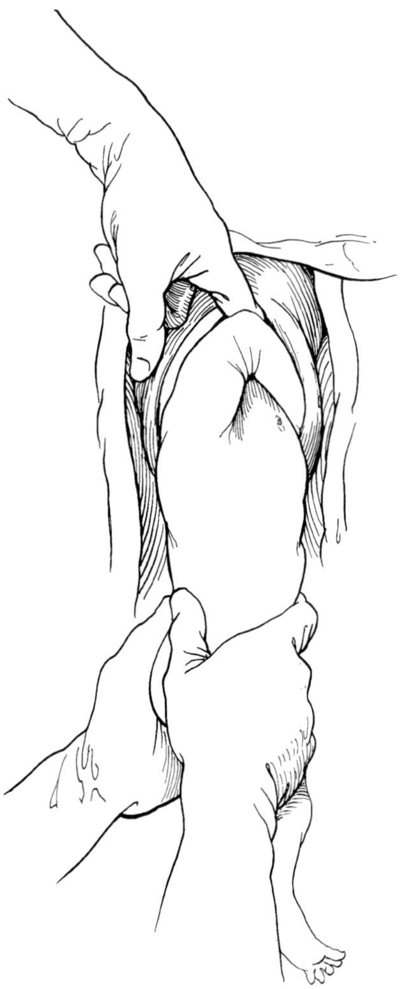

Figure 10–10. Breech extraction. Delivery of the anterior shoulder by downward traction. The anterior arm may be freed by splinting the humerus with the fingers and sweeping it down and out.

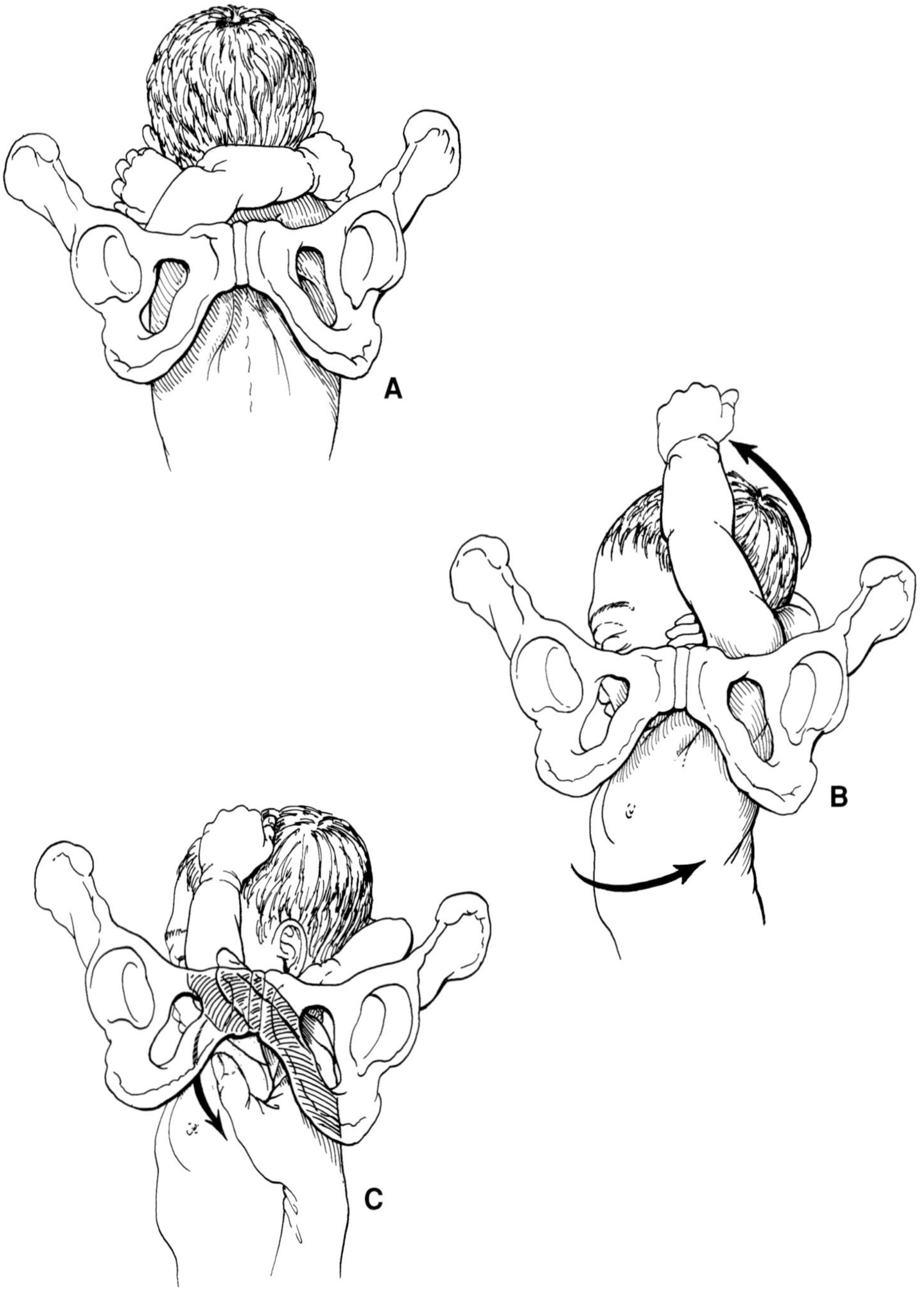

Figure 10–11. Nuchal arms. **A.** The back is directed anteriorly and the operator can feel the left arm crossed over the right arm below the occipital area of the head. **B.** The head and shoulders are pushed upward slightly to free them from the pelvic inlet. The body is rotated at least 90 degrees until the back is directed toward the left side of the pelvis. During the rotation, the left arm will usually be forced into a position of extension behind the pubic symphysis and lateral to the head by the pressure from the brim of the pelvis. **C.** The arm is swept downward over the face and chest and through the cervix with the index and second finger of the obstetrician's hand. The left arm is free, but the right remains in the nuchal position, thereby preventing delivery of the head.

should be grasped and the fetus should be elevated over the inner thigh of the mother until the posterior arm is visible and the arm freed. Subsequent head entrapment can be avoided by having an assistant maintain flexion of the fetal head by applying trans-abdominal pressure to the fetal occiput as the body is being delivered.

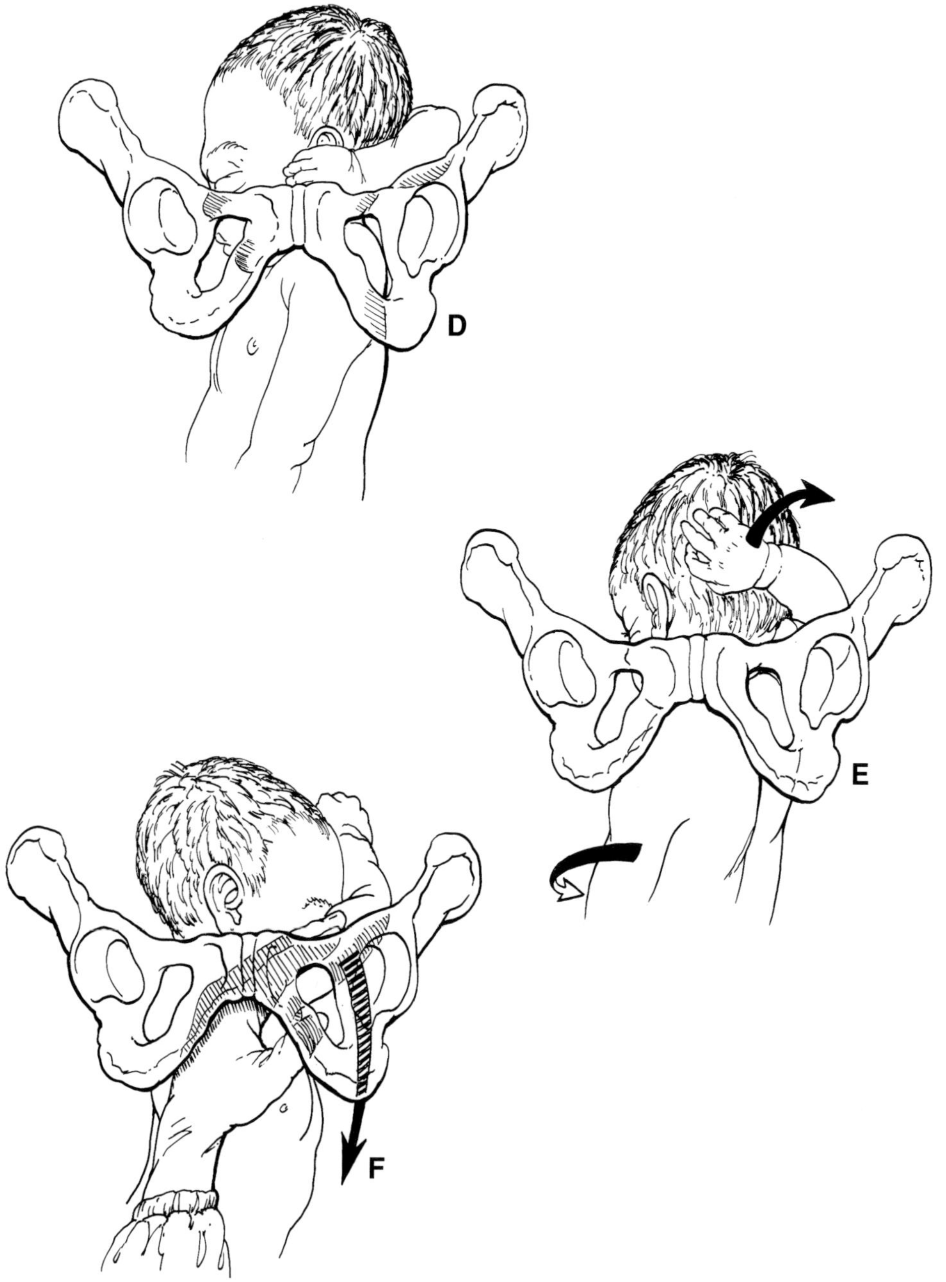

Figure 10–11 (continued). D and **E.** As the infant's body is rotated from left to right the remaining nuchal arm will be forced over the occiput to an extended position. This is the mirror image of the initial maneuver. **F.** The body and head have been rotated 180 degrees until the back is directed toward the right side of the maternal pelvis. The right arm now lies in front of the face, from which it can be swept over the chest and delivered with the index and second fingers of the obstetrician's right hand. The head is then delivered in the usual fashion.

Nuchal Arms

Nuchal arms occur when one or both fetal arms are trapped around the back of the neck (Fig. 10–11). If the nuchal arms are not freed by rotating the fetus to deliver either the anterior or posterior shoulder, extraction may be accomplished by rotating the fetus through 180 degrees so that friction exerted by the vagina will cause the arm to be released. Occasionally, it may be necessary to rotate the fetus 360 degrees. If the nuchal arms cannot be freed with such rotation, an attempt should

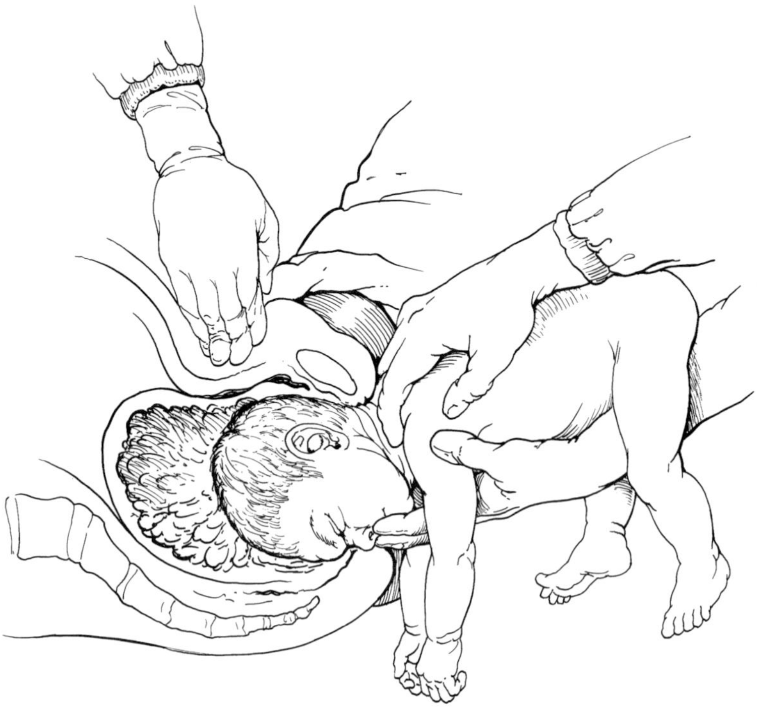

Figure 10–12. Delivery of aftercoming head using the Mauriceau maneuver. Note that as the fetal head is being delivered, flexion of the head is maintained by suprapubic pressure provided by an assistant, and simultaneously by pressure on the maxilla by the operator as traction is applied.

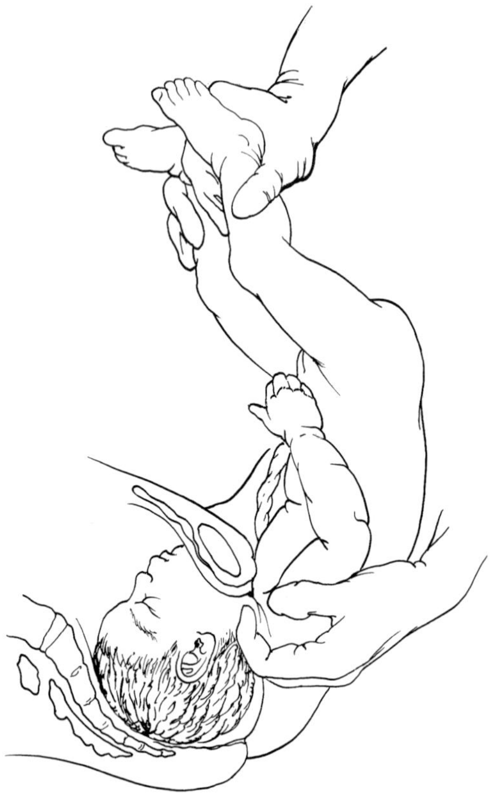

Figure 10–13. Delivery of the aftercoming head using the modified Prague maneuver necessitated by failure of the fetal trunk to rotate anteriorly.

be made to push the fetus upward with rotation to release the arms. If this attempt is unsuccessful, the fetal arms can be extracted forcibly by the obstetrician's hooking a finger over one or both of them. It is usually easier to release a second trapped arm once the first arm has been released. Releasing one or both arms by force may result in fracture of the humerus. Sherer and colleagues (1989) have recommended cesarean section if nuchal arms are suspected or detected on imaging studies.

Mauriceau-Smellie-Viet Maneuver

This maneuver is used for controlled delivery of the breech fetal head. The obstetrician applies the index and middle fingers of one hand over the maxilla while two fingers of the other hand are hooked over the fetal neck and grasp the fetal shoulders. Gentle downward traction usually results in delivery of the fetal head (Fig. 10–12). This maneuver is especially useful for guiding the head in the presence of rapid labor and delivery.

Modified Prague Maneuver

This maneuver is used for vaginal delivery of the breech in whom the back remains in a posterior position. With this maneuver, two fingers of one hand are used to grasp the

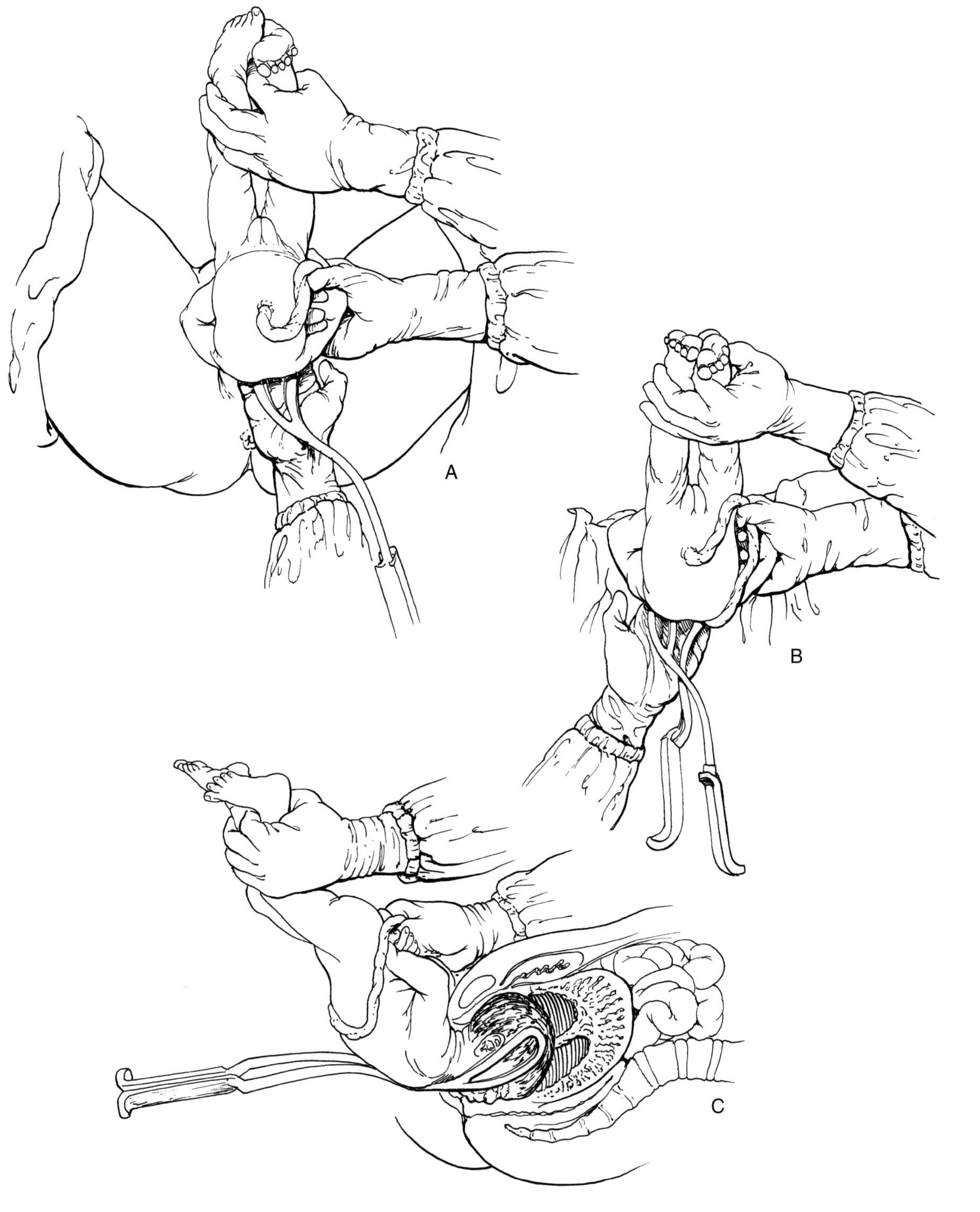

Figure 10–14. Application of Piper forceps. **A.** An assistant elevates the infant's body to expose the face and the introitus. It is important that the assistant elevate the cord and upper extremities out of the operative field while the operator applies the Piper forceps. The arch in the shanks and the absence of the pelvic curve permits the application of the blades beneath the body of the baby directly to the side of the head. The fingers of the operator's right hand are inserted into the left side of the vagina and the tip of the forceps blade is passed through the introitus against the palmar surface of the fingers with the operator in the kneeling position. The handle is held in the left hand below the medial surface of the patient's right thigh. The blade is inserted in pelvic application by sighting its cephalic curve around the side of the infant's face. **B.** The right blade is applied similar to the left blade, which has previously been applied. **C.** After locking the forceps, the handles are elevated to flex the head slightly. The infant's body is lowered against the shanks of the forceps. The head is extracted by pulling outward and raising the handle simultaneously; thereby rolling the face and forehead over the perineum while the suboccipital area remains fixed beneath the pubic ramis.

shoulders while the other hand draws the feet up over the abdomen of the mother (Fig. 10–13). The original Prague maneuver, which was used when the fetal back was directed upward, is no longer recommended.

Piper Forceps

Application of Piper forceps to the aftercoming head may prove especially useful in the primigravida, but also may be used electively in the multiparous patient in lieu of the Mauriceau-Smellie-Veit maneuver. Prophylactic use of Piper forceps ensures that the main force of traction is directed to the fetal head instead of the neck. With adequate anesthesia, the forceps can be applied to the head once it has reached the pelvis. While kneeling, the operator applies the forceps from beneath the breech, which is elevated (Fig. 10–14). The left blade is usually placed first followed by the right blade. After proper application, traction is applied outward and upward.

Analgesia and Anesthesia

Although continuous epidural analgesia is commonly used for labor and delivery in the woman with a breech presentation, an increase in the need for oxytocin augmentation has been reported in such patients (Confino and colleagues, 1985; Chadha and colleagues, 1992). In 643 women with a singleton breech presentation, Chadha and colleagues (1992) reported that continuous epidural analgesia was associated with longer labors, increased use of oxytocin for augmentation, and a higher cesarean rate in the second stage of labor. Narcotic analgesia may be used effectively for the first stage of labor and to allow spontaneous delivery to the level of the fetal umbilicus. A pudendal block is generally satisfactory for episiotomy and repair and for application of forceps to the aftercoming head. If additional anesthesia is required for breech delivery, general anesthesia may be helpful; halogenated agents are especially useful for entrapment of the aftercoming head or if intrauterine manipulation is necessary.

Entrapment of the Fetal Head

Very few situations are as anxiety-provoking for the obstetrician or as dangerous for the fetus as entrapment of the aftercoming head with a breech delivery. This is seen more often with the premature than the term breech infant. As mentioned above, a halogenated agent will often provide sufficient uterine and cervical relaxation to allow for delivery.

If the cervix cannot be successfully reduced over the fetal head, it may be necessary to perform Dührssen incisions in the cervix. With this technique, two or three incisions are made into the cervix at 2, 6, or 10 o'clock. This technique should not be used unless the cervix is dilated at least 7 cm. If Dührssen incisions are employed, it is essential to avoid incision at 3 to 4 or 8 to 9 o'clock, in order to avoid possible incision of the uterine vessels and serious hemorrhage.

ROLE OF VAGINAL BREECH DELIVERY IN MODERN OBSTETRICS

Unfortunately, discussions of the role of vaginal breech delivery in modern obstetrics are often clouded by emotion and rhetoric, with some individuals claiming that any vaginal breech delivery is "unsafe," while others maintain that in select cases, vaginal breech delivery is "safe." A critical assessment of the available evidence suggests that labels such as "safe" or "unsafe" are misleading and tend to confuse the real issues. The prospective randomized studies discussed earlier demonstrate increased neurologic injury or death in carefully selected fetuses delivered vaginally, compared to the cesarean delivery groups (Collea, 1980; Gimovsky, 1983; and their associates). Because of small sample sizes, however, these differences are not statistically significant. The metanalysis of Cheng and Hannah (1993) discussed before confirmed a higher fetal risk with vaginal breech delivery. Clinical experience also suggests that despite careful selection, cord prolapse and trapped head or nuchal arms will occasionally be encountered. Although these complications often can be successfully managed by an alert and experienced clinician, unless a selection process is devised to eliminate the possibility of these complications, they will still occur—albeit rarely—and lead to adverse outcomes. Thus, the issue is not whether vaginal breech delivery is absolutely safe; even in carefully selected cases, it is clearly less safe for the fetus than cesarean section. Rather, the real issue involves whether the small risk to the fetus incurred with planned vaginal delivery of carefully selected patients is justified by the major reduction in maternal morbidity and cost associated with vaginal birth. There is no uniformly correct answer to this question; it appears that after appropriate informed consent, either delivery route might be justified in select cases. However, it is inappropriate to tell a patient that vaginal breech delivery is as safe as cesarean section for the fetus, and equally inappropriate to imply that cesarean section is the safest option without a discussion of the increased maternal risks of cesarean delivery. Such an approach takes on special significance in residency training programs, where those women electing vaginal breech delivery will contribute to the ability of future obstetricians to deal with unplanned precipitous breech deliveries and to be comfortable in managing entrapped heads or nuchal arms.

SUMMARY

In appropriately selected candidates, planned vaginal breech delivery is the safest and most cost efficient choice for the mother. However, there is a slight increase in the risk of birth trauma and injury to the fetus. It is important that all obstetricians be trained in the technique of vaginal breech delivery because this knowledge undoubtedly will be required at some point in their career when they encounter the woman who presents with the breech fetus already spontaneously delivering to the level of the umbilicus.

REFERENCES

American College of Obstetricians and Gynecologists. Management of the breech presentation. ACOG Technical Bulletin 95. Washington, DC: ACOG, 1986.

Barrett JM. Funic reduction for the management of umbilical cord prolapse. Am J Obstet Gynecol 1991; 165:654.

Beck AC, Rosenthal AH. Obstetric Practice. 6th ed. London: Balliere, Tindal and Cassel, 1955, p. 499.

Bingham P, Lilford RJ. Management of the selected term breech presentation: assessment of the risks of selected vaginal delivery versus cesarean section for all cases. Obstet Gynecol 1990; 76:750.

Bodmer B, Benjamin A, McClean FH, Usher RH. Has use of cesarean section reduced the risks of delivery in the preterm breech presentation? Am J Obstet Gynecol 1986; 154:144.

Bowes WA, Taylor ES, O'Brien M, Bowes C. Breech delivery: evaluation of the method of delivery on perinatal results and maternal morbidity. Am J Obstet Gynecol 1979; 135:965.

Brenner WE, Bruce RD, Hendricks CH. The characteristics and perils of breech presentation. Am J Obstet Gynecol 1974; 188:700.

Chadha YC, Mahmood TA, Dick MJ, et al. Breech delivery and epidural analgesia. Br J Obstet Gynaecol 1992; 99:96.

Cheng M, Hannah M. Breech delivery at term: a critical review of the literature. Obstet Gynecol 1993; 82:605.

Collea JV, Chein C, Quilligan EJ. The randomized management of term frank breech presentation: a study of 208 cases. Am J Obstet Gynecol 1980; 137:235.

Collea JV, Rabin SC, Weghorst GR, Quilligan EJ. The randomized management of term frank breech presentation: vaginal delivery vs cesarean section. Am J Obstet Gynecol 1978; 131:186.

Confino E, Ismajovich B, Rudick V, David MP. Extradural analgesia in the management of singleton breech delivery. Br J Anaesth 1985; 57:892.

Cox C, Kendall AC, Hommers M. Changed prognosis of breech-presenting low birthweight infants. Br J Obstet Gynaecol 1982; 89:881.

Croughan-Minihane MS, Petitti DB, Gordis L, Golditch I. Morbidity among breech infants according to method of delivery. Obstet Gynecol 1990; 75:821.

Effer SB, Saigal S, Rand C, et al. Effect of delivery method on outcomes in the very low-birth weight breech infant: Is the improved survival related to cesarean section or other perinatal care maneuvers? Am J Obstet Gynecol 1983; 145:123.

Flanagan TA, Mulchahey KM, Korenbrot CC, et al. Management of term breech presentation. Am J Obstet Gynecol 1987; 156:1492.

Gimovsky ML, Paul RH. Singleton breech presentation in labor: experience in 1980. Am J Obstet Gynecol 1982; 142:733.

Gimovsky MI, Wallace RL, Schifrin BS, Paul RH. Randomized management of the nonfrank breech presentation at term: a preliminary report. Am J Obstet Gynecol 1983; 146:34.

Green JE, McLean F, Smith LP, Usher R. Has an increased cesarean section rate for term breech delivery reduced the incidence of birth asphyxia, trauma, and death? Am J Obstet Gynecol 1982; 142:643.

Hytten FE. Breech presentation: Is it a bad omen? Br J Obstet Gynecol 1982; 89(11):879.

Ingemarsson I, Westgren M, Svenningsen NW. Long-term follow-up of preterm infants in breech presentation delivered by caesarean section. A prosective study. Lancet 1978; 2(8082):172.

Jaffa AJ, Peyser MR, Ballas S, Toaff R. Management of term breech presentation in primigravidae. Br J Obstet Gynaecol 1981; 88:721.

Mahomed K. Breech delivery: a critical evaluation of the mode of delivery and outcome of labour. Int J Gynaecol Obstet 1988; 27:17.

Mann LI, Gallant JM. Modern management of the breech delivery. Am J Obstet Gynecol 1979; 134:611.

Moore MM, Shearer DR. Fetal dose estimates for CT pelvimetry. Radiology 1989; 171:265.

Moore TR. Malpresentation: breech and transverse lie. In: Phelan JP, Clark SL (eds), Cesarean Delivery. New York: Elsevier, 1988.

Morales WJ, Koerten J. Obstetric management and intraventricular hemorrhage in very-low-birth-weight infants. Obstet Gynecol 1986; 68:35.

Nelson KB, Ellenberg JH. Antecedents of cerebral palsy: multivariate analysis of risk. N Engl J Med 1986; 315:81.

O'Leary JA. Vaginal delivery of the term breech: a preliminary report. Obstet Gynecol 1979; 53:341.

Ridley WT, Jackson P, Stewart JA, et al. Role of antenatal radiography in the management of breech deliveries. Br J Obstet Gynaecol 1982; 89:342.

Rosen MG, Chik L. The association between Cesarean birth and outcome in vertex presentation. Am J Obstet Gynecol 1984; 150:775.

Scheer K, Nubar J. Variation of fetal presentation with gestational age. Am J Obstet Gynecol 1976; 125:269.

Schutte MF, van Hemel OJ, van de Berg C, van de Pol A. Perinatal mortality in breech presentations as compared to vertex presentations in singleton pregnancies: an analysis based upon 57819 computer-registered pregnancies in The Netherlands. Eur J Obstet Gynecol Reprod Biol 1985; 19:391.

Sherer DM, Menashe M, Palti Z, et al. Radiologic evidence of a nuchal arm in the breech-presenting fetus at the onset of labor: an indication for abdominal delivery. Am J Perinatol 1989; 6:353.

Songane FF, Thobani S, Malik H, et al. Balancing the risks of planned cesarean section and trial of vaginal delivery for the mature, selected, singleton breech presentation. J Perinat Med 1987; 15:531.

Suzuki S, Yamamuro T. Fetal movement and fetal presentation. Early Human Dev 1985; 11:255.

Tatum RK, Orr JW, Soong SJ, Huddleston JF. Vaginal breech delivery of selected infants weighing more than 2000 grams. Am J Obstet Gynecol 1987; 156:1492.

Thorpe-Beeston JG, Banfield PJ, Saunders NJ St G. Outcome of breech delivery at term. Br Med J 1992; 305:746–7.

Torfs CP, van den Berg BJ, Oechsli FW, Cummins S. Prenatal and perinatal factors in the etiology of cerebral palsy. J Pediatr 1990; 116:615–9.

Van Dorsten JP, Schifrin BS, Wallace RL. Randomized control trial of external cephalic version with tocolysis in late pregnancy. Am J Obstet Gynecol 1981; 141:417.

Watson WJ, Benson WL. Vaginal delivery for the selected frank breech at term. Obstet Gynecol 1984; 64:638.

Weiner CP. Vaginal breech delivery in the 1990's. Clin Obstet Gynecol 1992; 35:559–69.

Westgren LMR, Songster G, Paul RH. Preterm breech delivery: Another retrospective study. Obstet Gynecol 1985a; 66:481.

Westgren M, Paul RH. Delivery of the low birth weight infant by cesarean section. Clin Obstet Gynecol 1985b; 28:752.

CHAPTER 11

Multifetal Gestation

Although the diagnosis of multiple gestation, especially twins, is often a time of joy and excitement for the patient and her family, it may be a time of anxiety and guarded optimism for the obstetrician. There is little question that multifetal gestations are at increased risk of maternal complications and fetal/neonatal morbidity and mortality.

Twins may be either dizygotic or monozygotic. The former results from the release and fertilization of two separate ova and the latter from a single fertilized ovum that subsequently divides (ie, identical twins). Monozygotic twins occur approximately one-third as often as dizygotic twins.

MATERNAL COMPLICATIONS

One of the most common complications associated with multiple fetuses is pregnancy-induced hypertension, which occurs more frequently and develops earlier in multifetal gestation compared to singleton pregnancies. Moreover, parity does not appear to play a significant role; hypertension occurs at least as often in multiparous as in nulliparous women. In a review of 341 twin pregnancies, Thompson and colleagues (1987) reported an 18 percent incidence of pregnancy-induced hypertension while Long and Oats (1987) reported a 26 percent incidence of hypertension in 642 twin gestations. In the latter report, almost three-fourths of the cases of preeclampsia occurred prior to 37 weeks gestational age.

Anemia is also much more common with multifetal gestations, especially in women who do not consume a diet adequate in folic acid. There is an increased demand for iron due to the marked expansion in blood volume. The mother is also at an increased risk for postpartum hemorrhage, usually secondary to uterine atony, which is associated with an overdistended uterus.

FETAL/NEONATAL MORBIDITY AND MORTALITY

That perinatal mortality is higher with multifetal gestations than with singletons is well documented. For example, Spellacy and associates (1990) in a review of 1253 twin gestations reported a perinatal mortality rate of 54/1000 live births for twins compared to 10.4/1000 live births for singletons. Perinatal mortality was higher for twin B compared to twin A (64 v. 49/1000 births). Much of the perinatal mortality with twins can be directly attributed to prematurity. Unfortunately, there has been little, if any, significant progress in the prevention and treatment of premature birth in twins (Gilstrap and Brown, 1988). The perinatal mortality is even higher for monozygotic twins—2.5 times that for dizygotic twins in one report (Kovacs and associates, 1989). An even higher mortality rate has been reported when monozygotic twins occupy the same amniotic sac (ie, monoamniotic twins). Fortunately, this latter complication is rare, occurring in approximately 1 percent of monozygotic twins (Tessen and Zlatnik, 1991). Much of the mortality is no doubt due to the intertwining of umbilical cords, which has been reported to occur in 50 percent or more of cases (Benirschke, personal communication, 1983) (Fig. 11–1). Interestingly, Carr and associates (1990) reported that the survival of monoamniotic twins does not decrease after 30 weeks' gestation. In a review of 24 sets of monoamniotic twins, 17 sets reached 30 weeks' gestation with at least one fetus alive. There were no subsequent fetal deaths.

Another cause for the increased perinatal mortality associated with twin gestations is the increased frequency of congenital anomalies (Neal and Hankins, 1992). Twice as many malformations occur in twins as do in singletons and malformations occur more often in monozygotic than dizygotic twins (Fig. 11–2A,B). Vascular communication also may occur between monozygotic fetuses and be associated with significant morbidity and mortality. These anastomoses, frequent in monochorionic placentas (rarely in dichorionic placentas), may be artery to artery, artery to vein, or vein to vein and may result in hypoperfusion, intrauterine malnutrition, growth retardation, and death in one of the twin pair. Bejar and associates (1990) reported that monochorionic twins were frequently complicated by antenatal necrosis of cerebral white matter.

Other factors reported to be associated with increased morbidity and mortality include intrauterine growth retardation, prolapsed umbilical cord, and premature placental separation (Table 11–1). Twins also may have less than optimal subsequent physical and intellectual development (Nilsen and colleagues, 1984) and a greater frequency of cerebral palsy; the latter is seen especially in premature twins (Rydhstrom, 1990).

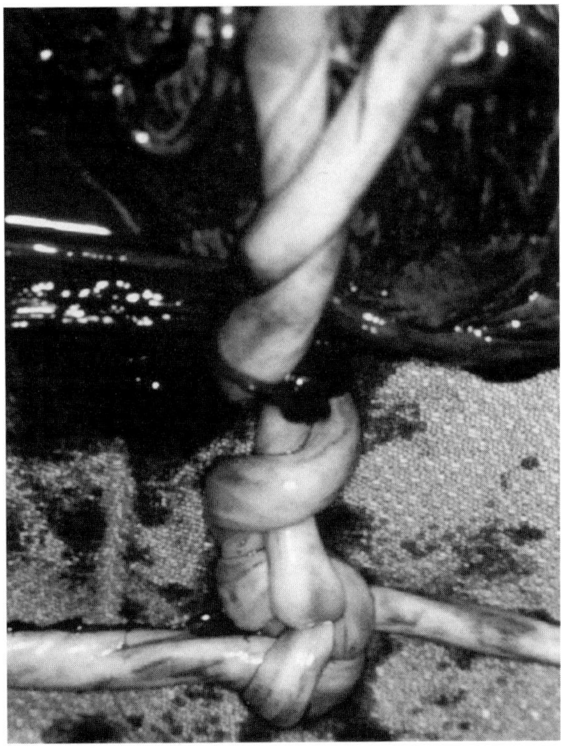

Figure 11–1. Massive cord entanglement of monoamniotic twins as seen at cesarean delivery at 30 weeks and 6 days EGA. Delivery was prompted by one fetus showing significant variable decelerations on NST. (Photo courtesy Dr. Andrew J. Satin.)

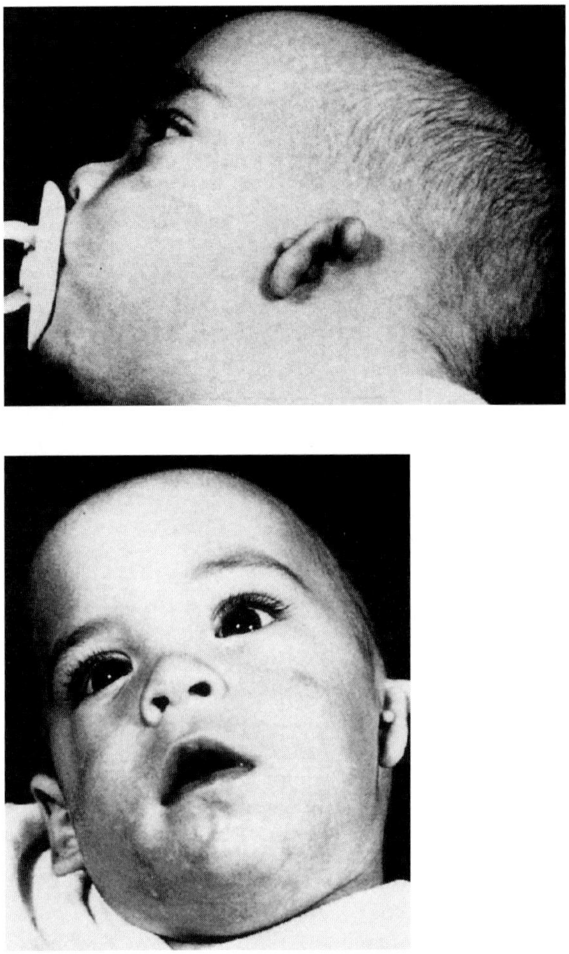

Figure 11–2. Ear deformity, microtia, in one of monozygotic twins. This twin also had a single umbilical artery. (Photo courtesy of Dr. Greg Neal.)

TABLE 11–1. FACTORS ASSOCIATED WITH AN INCREASE IN PERINATAL MORTALITY AND MORBIDITY IN MULTIFETAL GESTATION

Prematurity
Monoamniotic twins
Congenital anomalies
Vascular communication between fetuses
Intrauterine growth retardation
Prolapsed umbilical cord
Premature separation of placenta

INCIDENCE AND DIAGNOSIS

Incidence

The incidence of twin gestation in the United States is approximately 12/1000 births (Hrubec and Robinette, 1984); the incidence of triplets, approximately 1/10,000. The frequency of twinning is related to the type of twins, that is, monozygotic versus dizygotic. The incidence of monozygotic twins is approximately 1/250 births and is independent of age, race, parity, and heredity. The incidence of dizygotic twins, on the other hand, is related to age, race, parity, heredity, and the use of fertility drugs (Callahan, 1994; Neumann, 1994; and their colleagues). For example, dizygotic twinning is more common in blacks than whites and even less common in Asians. Advancing age and parity increase twinning. With regard to heredity, it is the genotype of the mother that is important.

Diagnosis

With the development of technically advanced ultrasonographic equipment, the majority of twins are diagnosed prior to labor, with fewer than 5 percent undiagnosed (Chervenak and associates, 1985). In a review of over 250 multifetal gestations, Persson and Kullander (1983) reported that 98 percent were detected antenatally.

Monoamniotic Twins

The diagnosis of monoamniotic twins can be made accurately when entanglement of the umbilical cords of the two fetuses can be demonstrated. For example, Townsend and Filly (1988) correctly diagnosed five nonconjoined monoamniotic twins by identifying cord entanglement sonographically. One case without cord entanglement was not recognized antenatally. With modern equipment, the diagnosis can often be suspected sonographically even without obvious cord entanglement. However, failure to see a dividing membrane does not confirm the diagnosis of monoamniotic twins.

Lavery and Gadwood (1990) reported the successful diagnosis of monoamniotic twins by using amniography. Carlan (1990) and Sargent (1991) and their associates reported the use of computed tomographic imaging to diagnose monoamniotic twins.

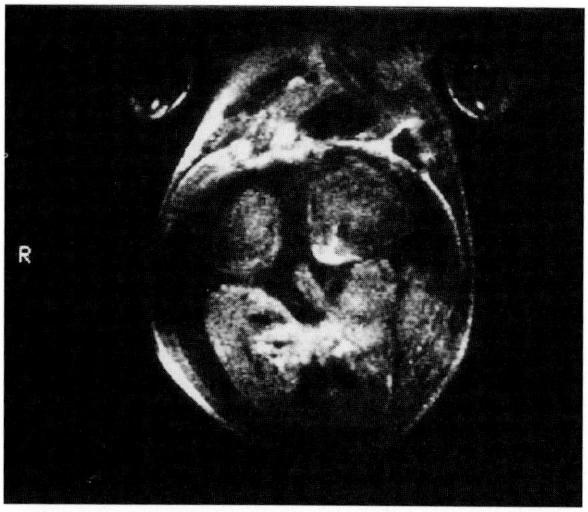

Figure 11–3. Magnetic resonance imaging study showing a liver bridge and body wall communication. The twins were successfully separated following cesarean birth.

Conjoined Twins

Conjoined twins most often can be diagnosed sonographically. The four major types include (1) thoracopagus (anterior), (2) pygopagus (posterior), (3) craniopagus (cephalic), and (4) ischiopagus (caudal). Thoracopagus is the most common variety. Magnetic resonance imaging and sonography are both useful in defining the extent of organ involvement and sharing in these cases (Fig. 11–3) (Turner and associates, 1986).

INTRAPARTUM MANAGEMENT OF MULTIPLE GESTATIONS

Labor

There are several complications of labor that may be associated with multifetal gestations, including premature labor, hypotonic uterine dysfunction, abnormal presentations, prolapse of the umbilical cord, premature separation of the placenta (especially after the birth of the first twin), and postpartum hemorrhage. Once labor is confirmed, several key prerequisites should be adhered to as outlined in Table 11–2. It is also of paramount importance to determine the presentation and position of both fetuses prior to delivery. Oxytocin for labor induction or augmentation should be used judiciously in twin gestations, as is the case any time there is uterine overdistention.

Analgesia and Anesthesia

Conduction analgesia, such as continuous epidural analgesia, is advocated by some for both labor and delivery and in many cases will prove satisfactory. Crawford (1987), in a series of 130 women with twins who delivered vaginally, reported that the 105 women who received epidural anesthesia had a significantly longer second stage of labor compared to those who did not (90 minutes v. 30 minutes). If the patient has not received conduction anesthesia, a pudendal block with supplemental nitrous oxide may prove satisfactory. If intrauterine manipulation or internal podalic version is required, it may be necessary to use general anesthesia with a halogenated agent in order to achieve adequate uterine relaxation. Either conduction or general anesthesia is acceptable in most cases of multifetal gestation requiring cesarean delivery.

Vaginal Delivery

The decision to perform vaginal delivery should be based on gestational age, estimated fetal weight, experience of the obstetrician, presence of complications, and presentation and position of both fetuses. The most common presentation for twin gestation is the vertex–vertex followed by vertex–breech presentation.

TABLE 11–2. PREPARATION FOR DELIVERY OF TWIN GESTATIONS

Skilled obstetric attendant throughout labor
Immediate availability of blood
Well-functioning intravenous system
Availability of two obstetricians at delivery
Availability of anesthesiologist at delivery
Skilled personnel and ability for resuscitation and care of both newborns
Ability to perform emergency cesarean section

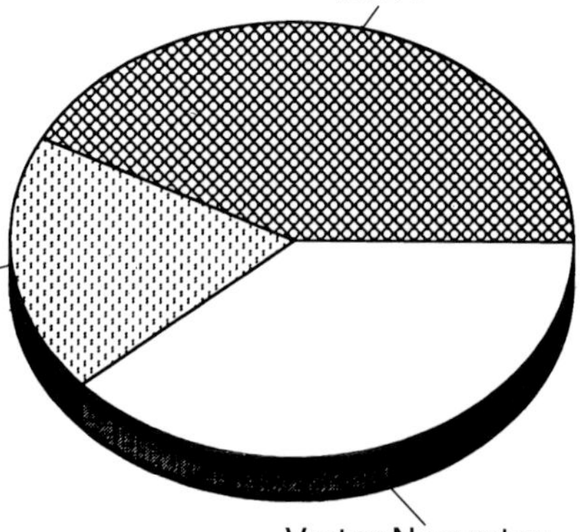

Figure 11–4. Presentation of 362 consecutive twin pairs at delivery. (Modified from Chervenak and colleagues, 1985.)

Together these account for almost two-thirds of all presentations (Fig. 11–4).

Vertex–Vertex

Approximately 40 percent of the time, both twins A and B present in the vertex position (Chervenak and co-workers, 1985). Vaginal delivery can be anticipated for the vast majority of such presentations. Following delivery of the first twin, the presenting part of the second twin should be ascertained immediately. Intrapartum real-time sonography is a valuable aid for confirming the presenting part of the second twin as well as monitoring the fetal heart rate. When the vertex of the second twin is fixed in the pelvis, moderate fundal pressure should be applied and the membranes ruptured.

Prevailing wisdom once held that the interval between delivery of the first and second twin should be less than 30 minutes. However, in a review of 115 twin pairs by Rayburn and associates (1984), the mean interval between delivery of twins was 21 minutes with a range of 1–134 minutes. In almost two-thirds of cases, the interval was 15 minutes or less. Although the cesarean section rate increased when the interval was greater than 15 minutes, there was no excess trauma or fetal depression.

If contractions do not resume within 10 minutes after delivery of the first twin, dilute oxytocin should be used to stimulate labor and delivery of the vertex twin B. With reestablishment of labor, there is no urgent need to hasten delivery unless significant bleeding or a nonreassuring fetal heart rate pattern develops.

Vertex–Nonvertex Twin Presentation

There is no unanimity of opinion or standard of care regarding the most appropriate route of delivery when twin A is in the vertex position and twin B is in the nonvertex position, that is, breech or transverse. Almost 40 percent of twin gestations will present as vertex for twin A and either breech or transverse for twin B (Chervenak and associates, 1985). If vaginal delivery is planned for the vertex–nonvertex presentation, an experienced operator skilled in intrauterine manipulation is required (Table 11–2).

There are numerous reports attesting to the safety of vaginal delivery for the nonvertex second twin (Acker, 1982; Chervenak, 1984; Rabinovici, 1987; Laros, 1988; Bergland, 1989; Gocke, 1989; Wells, 1991; Fishman, 1993; and their colleagues). For example, Acker and colleagues (1982) in a review of 150 nonvertex second twins reported a corrected neonatal mortality of 0 for 74 twins delivered by cesarean section and 0 for 76 second twins extracted vaginally. There was also no significant difference in Apgar scores between the two groups (Table 11–3).

Chervenak and associates (1984) reviewed the management of 93 vertex–breech and 42 vertex–transverse twin gestations. Seventy-eight percent of the former and 53 percent of the latter were delivered vaginally. There were no cases of neonatal death or intraventricular hemorrhage in newborns weighing more than 1500 g who were delivered vaginally. More recently, Fishman and colleagues (1993) in a review of 390 vaginally delivered second twins (183 delivered as breech) reported no significant differences in neonatal outcome between vaginal breech (95% as breech extractions) and vaginal vertex deliveries. Moreover, there was no increase in either morbidity or mortality regardless of whether twin A or twin B was larger or whether there was a 20 percent or greater difference in birthweight (ie, discordance).

The technique for vaginal breech delivery is the same for the breech second twin as for the single breech presentation as outlined in Chapter 10. Briefly, after delivery of the first twin, vaginal examination should be performed immediately to ascertain the type of breech, that is, frank or footling. If the breech is a frank presentation and is fixed in the birth canal, fundal pressure should be applied and the membranes ruptured. A partial breech extraction then can be performed after spontaneous delivery to the umbilicus. A total breech extraction should be performed if emergency delivery is required or if a footling breech is encountered. Membranes should not be ruptured purposefully until the feet are brought down into the vagina.

TABLE 11–3. COMPARISON OF INCIDENCE OF 5-MINUTE APGAR SCORE ≤ 7 IN ASYMPTOMATIC TWINS (FIRST- OR SECOND-BORN) IN NONVERTEX PRESENTATION DELIVERED BY CESAREAN SECTION AND TWINS DELIVERED BY BREECH EXTRACTION (SECOND TWIN ONLY)

Birthweight (g)	No. of liveborn infants with Apgar score ≤ 7/total no. of liveborn infants			Significance
	Cesarean section	*Breech extraction*	*t*	
1,500–1,999	1/7	5/13	1.28	NS
2,000–2,499	6/22	4/23	0.80	NS
2,500+	0/45	2/40	1.45	NS
Total	7/74 (9.5%)	11/76 (14.5%)	0.95	NS
Corrected total[a]	6/67 (8.9%)	6/63 (9.5%)	0.11	NS

NS = not significant
[a]Corrected for birth weight less than 1,999 g
From Acker and colleagues (1982), with permission.

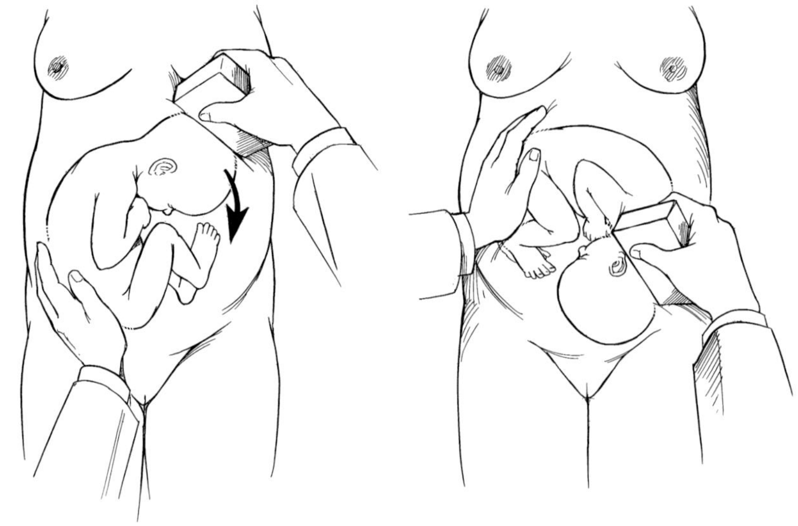

Figure 11–5. Method of using ultrasound transducer to guide vertex into pelvis. (From Chervenak and associates, 1983, with permission.)

If an experienced operator is not present, a cesarean section should be performed. A relatively common scenario is vaginal delivery of the first twin followed by cesarean delivery of twin B. In a review of 510 twin pregnancies Samra and colleagues (1990) reported that 36 percent were delivered by cesarean section. Of the 184 twin gestations delivered by cesarean section, 22 (12%) were combined vaginal/abdominal deliveries. The major reasons for this combined approach were persistent transverse lie or high breech presentation, and the hour of delivery "when experienced obstetricians may not be immediately available." In the absence of an operator experienced in vaginal delivery of vertex–nonvertex twins, we believe that it would be prudent to perform a cesarean section for both twins at the outset in order to avoid the frequent emergency situations that can arise for twin B following the vaginal delivery of twin A.

Intrapartum External Version

The subject of external cephalic version is discussed in detail in Chapter 12. External cephalic version also has been utilized for the intrapartum management of the nonvertex second twin (Fig. 11–5). For example, Chervenak and associates (1983) reported on the results of attempted intrapartum cephalic version on 11 breech and 14 transverse twin B presentations. Version was successful and resulted in subsequent vaginal delivery in approximately three-fourths of all patients

TABLE 11–4. MODE OF DELIVERY OF TWIN B AFTER ATTEMPTED EXTERNAL VERSION ACCORDING TO METHOD OF ANESTHESIA

Method of anesthesia	Successful version		Unsuccessful version		Total
	Subsequent vaginal delivery	*Subsequent cesarean delivery*	*Subsequent vaginal delivery*	*Subsequent cesarean delivery*	
Peridural	8	0	0	0	8
Pudendal and/ or local	10	2	2	3	17
Total	18	2	2	3	25

From Chervenak and colleagues (1983), with permission.

(Table 11–4). Moreover, successful version was not influenced by either gestational age or birthweight. Version was successful in 75 percent of primiparas and 71 percent of multiparas. As shown in Table 11–4, all 8 attempted versions under peridural analgesia were successful compared to 10 (59%) of 17 attempts under pudendal and/or local anesthesia. Successful version was also related to disparity in twin size; there were no successful versions when twin B's birthweight was 500 g or greater than twin A's.

In another review of 136 vertex–nonvertex twins, 41 patients underwent attempted external version, 55 underwent attempted breech extraction, and 40 patients had a primary cesarean section (Gocke and co-workers, 1989). There were no significant differences in either neonatal mortality or morbidity among the three groups (Table 11–5). Of note in this study was that external version was associated with an increase in fetal complications such as "fetal distress," cord prolapse, and compound presentations. In this report, successful version was not related to type of anesthesia (20 of 27 with an epidural v. 6 of 14 without; $p > .10$).

Wells and associates (1991) in a comparison of primary abdominal delivery, breech extraction, and external version for the nonvertex second twin, reported that there were no differences in neonatal outcome relative to delivery routes. However, patients in the external version group were more likely to undergo abdominal delivery of the second twin and required more emergency anesthesia than the breech extraction group. Chervenak and associates (1983) have proposed a protocol for the intrapartum management of twin gestations (Fig. 11–6).

Internal Podalic Version

In cases in which neither the breech nor the occiput is over the pelvic inlet or when emergency delivery is mandated (ie, nonreassuring fetal heart rate pattern, excessive bleeding, or prolapse of the umbilical cord), it may be necessary to perform internal podalic version. This procedure, which requires a skilled obstetrician and an anesthesiologist, ideally involves the obstetrician's use of both hands, one transvaginally and one transabdominally. The procedure varies somewhat depending upon whether the fetus is in the ventral presentation (Fig. 11–7), scapula presentation (Fig. 11–8), or vertex presentation (Fig. 11–9). This procedure is performed most easily when

TABLE 11–5. NEONATAL OUTCOME VERSUS ATTEMPTED ROUTE OF DELIVERY

	External Version (n=41)	Breech Extraction (n=55)	1° C-S (n=40)	P
Birthweight of first twin (g)	2399	2544	2356	NS
Birthweight of second twin (g)	2365	2569	2347	NS
1 min Apgar score < 4	5	5	1	NS
5 min Apgar score < 7	0	1	0	NS
Neonatal intensive care unit admission (%)	18	13	18	NS
Respiratory distress syndrome	0	2	1	NS
Birth trauma	0	0	0	NS
Intraventricular hemorrhage	0	0	0	NS
Neonatal death	0	0	0	NS
Postpartum infant length of hospital stay (days)	10.1	5.0	10.2	<0.05
Postpartum infant length of hospital stay minus maternal stay (days)	6.4	2.6	5.8	NS

From Gocke and associates (1989), with permission.

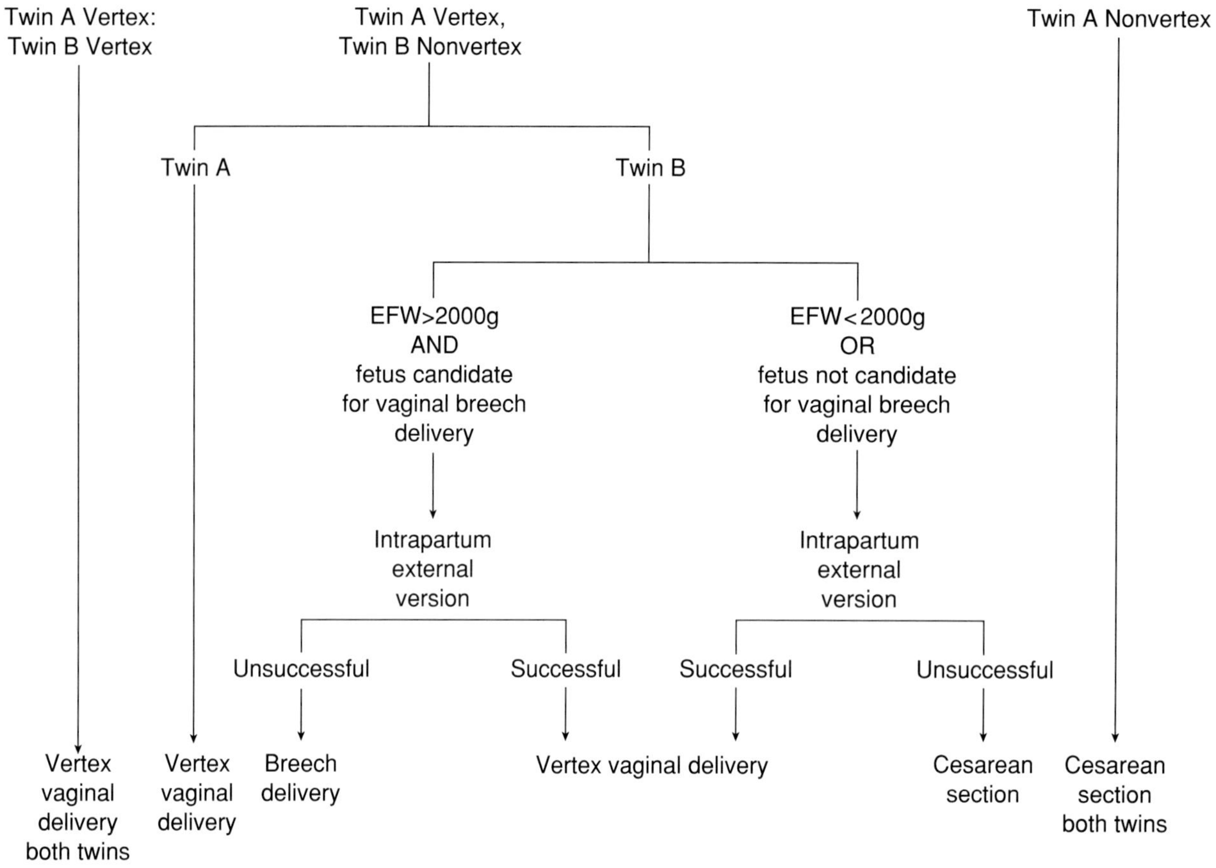

Figure 11–6. Protocol for intrapartum management of twin gestation. (From Chervenak and associates, 1983, with permission.)

the fetus is in the ventral position and requires the greatest degree of skill when internal version and breech extraction are performed on the vertex presentation that has failed to descend into the pelvis. If the fetal head is obstructing the lower uterine segment or pelvic inlet, it should be displaced with the vaginal hand to the point that the abdominal hand can sweep it into the upper uterus. The next step with this procedure is to identify and grasp both feet of the fetus. Intrapartum ultrasound examination often is helpful in identifying the exact position of the fetus. Both feet should be brought down into the vagina prior to rupture of the membranes if possible; if not, a single foot can be delivered first and the second located as the fetus descends through the birth canal. As men-

Figure 11–7. Internal version from the ventral presentation. **A.** This version is usually uncomplicated as the ventral surface of the infant is directed toward the pelvic inlet with the feet in easy position to be grasped with little additional intrauterine manipulation. The obstetrician's hand and forearm are introduced through the vagina and the cervix into the uterus and the exact position and attitude of the infant determined. The feet are grasped and positively identified as such, following which they are pulled through the cervix. **B.** Once the feet have been brought out through the introitus, the membranes are ruptured if they have not previously spontaneously ruptured. The buttocks will follow, and the head will automatically assume a position in the fundus of the uterus. Although it usually is not necessary to apply external pressure in an attempt to push the head upward, this is a reasonable practice to institute with every internal version. The version is now complete and if extraction is to follow, it is performed as for the primary breech positions. (See illustration on opposite page.)

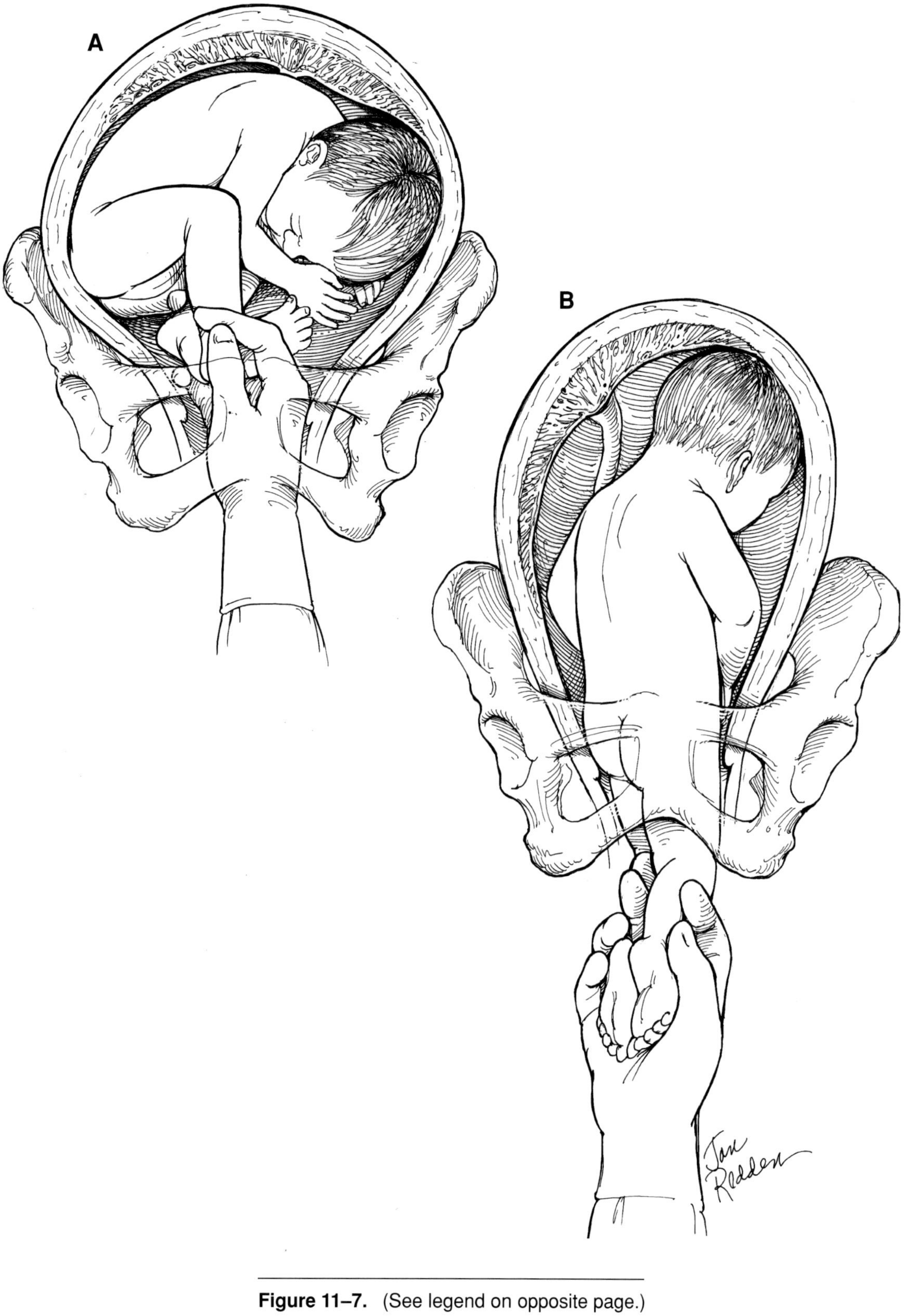

Figure 11–7. (See legend on opposite page.)

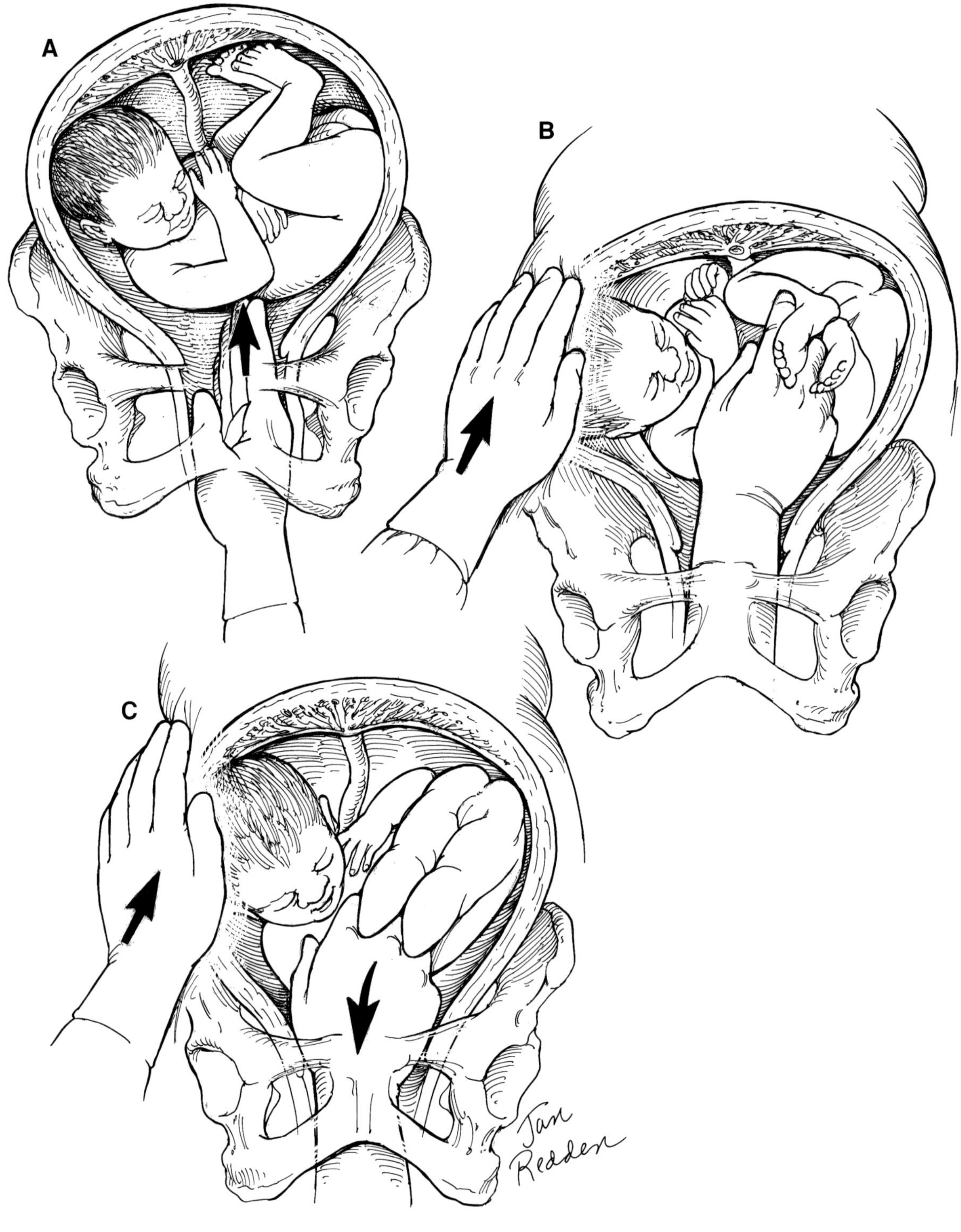

Figure 11–8. Internal podalic version is more difficult and requires a greater degree of skill when the infant is in either the left or right scapular anterior position. The obstetrician's hand must be introduced deeper into the uterus to reach the feet, and far more manipulation is required to rotate the back upward and simultaneously to correct the transverse lie. In addition, the arm may be prolapsed and the uterine wall thin. Uterine relaxation may be required in order to effect this delivery. **A.** The presenting shoulder is pushed upward well out of the pelvis. **B.** The vaginal hand and the abdominal hand simultaneously assist with elevating the presenting part. Either hand may be used as the vaginal hand and will depend upon operator preference and the position of the fetus. **C.** Both feet are identified and grasped with the vaginal hand. In the scapular left anterior position, the feet are shown being pulled anteriorly and downward. Simultaneously the baby's head and shoulder are lifted out of the pelvis. The delivery is completed by sweeping the head and shoulders into the fundus with the abdominal hand as the feet are drawn down into the lower birth canal with the vaginal hand. The procedure is greatly facilitated by uterine relaxation and intact membranes.

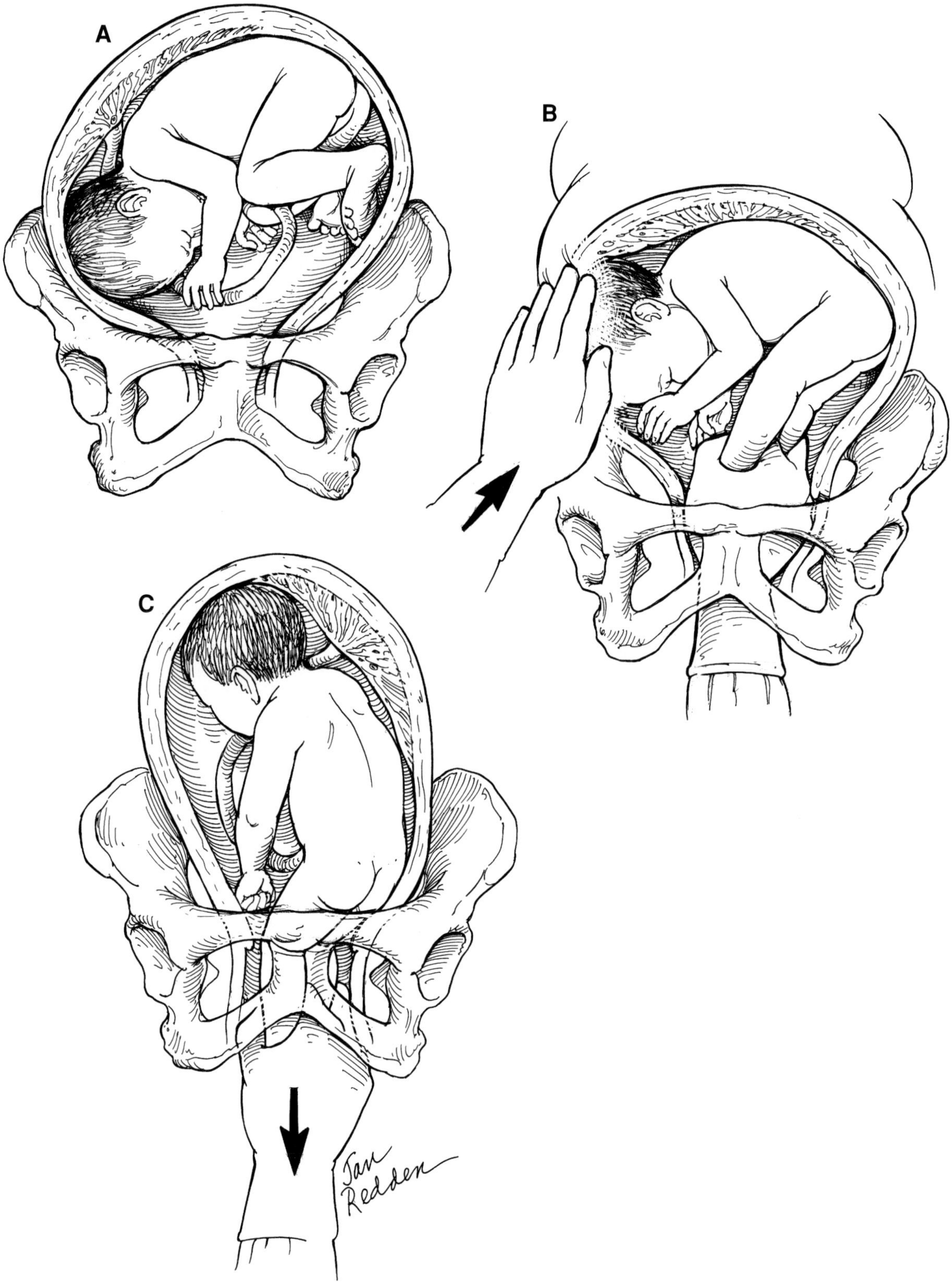

Figure 11-9. A. For a version in the vertex position, the abdominal and vaginal hands are used simultaneously and in coordination. The head often is at the level of or slightly lower than the feet. The vaginal hand is used to elevate the head to the abdominal hand, which then sweeps it up into the fundus. **B.** Simultaneously the vaginal hand locates the feet. **C.** Once the feet have been grasped, they are brought down into the lower birth canal, the membranes ruptured, and the remainder of the breech extraction performed as for a primary breech delivery.

tioned above, the vertex can be elevated with the operator's abdominal hand or by an assistant using the ultrasound transducer. Once the feet have been successfully brought down into the birth canal, the membranes can be ruptured and a total breech extraction can be carried out. Often the membranes have ruptured prior to grasping the fetal feet; occasionally it is necessary to rupture the membranes in order to correctly identify the fetal feet. Great care must be taken to avoid grasping one foot and one arm of the fetus. In the absence of a skilled operator, prompt delivery by cesarean section is a reasonable and prudent choice.

Premature Twins

As they would with term twins, most obstetricians will allow vaginal delivery for preterm twins presenting as vertex–vertex and perform cesarean section when the presenting twin is nonvertex. However, there is no consensus of opinion regarding the most appropriate route of delivery for preterm twins when twin A is vertex and twin B non vertex. In a review of 862 twin gestations less than 1500 g, Rydhstrom (1990) reported that although the cesarean section rate had increased from 7.7 percent in 1973–1976 to almost 70 percent in 1981–1983, "analysis failed to reveal any significant impact of abdominal birth on the fetal outcome for low-birth-weight twins, even when fetal presentation was taken into account."

Davison and associates (1992) reviewed the outcomes of 54 breech extracted second twins that weighed 750–2000 g. While confirming better outcome for the first delivered twin, regardless of route, these investigators found no significant differences in perinatal outcome when they compared breech extracted second twins to those delivered by cesarean section. Adam and colleagues (1991) reported outcomes of 578 sets of twins delivered between 1980 and 1987. The only perinatal death occurred in a vaginally delivered infant weighing less than 1500 g. Grieg and associates (1992) examined perinatal outcomes in 457 sets of twins delivered between 1985 and 1990. The authors found no support for routine cesarean delivery of twins of any birthweight. However, their series contained only 9 nonvertex fetuses under 1500 g who were delivered vaginally. Conclusive data documenting improved outcome of small nonvertex presenting second twins delivered by cesarean section is currently lacking; thus route of delivery for vertex–nonvertex preterm twins cannot be considered an issue of standard of care. One conservative approach to this problem is the recommendation by the American College of Obstetricians and Gynecologists that nonvertex second twins weighing less than 1500–2000 g be delivered by cesarean section. Chauhan and associates (1993) suggested that to avoid vaginal delivery of a nonvertex second twin with a birthweight of less than 1500 g, an estimate of 1700 g or greater via ultrasound is appropriate.

Nonvertex First Twin

Most clinicians choose cesarean section when twin A presents as a breech (Chervenak and associates, 1985). Of particular concern have been "interlocking" twins, when the first twin presents in the breech position and the second twin is vertex. However, Cohen and colleagues (1965) reported that interlocking occurred only once in 817 twin gestations. More recently, Oettinger and associates (1993) compared the outcome of 82 twins in which the first twin presented as a breech. The patients were divided into two time periods for analysis. Although the cesarean section rate increased approximately 21 percent to almost 95 percent over the two time periods, neither neonatal morbidity nor mortality was related to method of delivery. There were no cases of interlocking twins among the 36 twin pairs delivered vaginally. However, maternal morbidity was higher in the group delivered via cesarean section.

Cesarean Section

Many clinicians choose cesarean section to deliver twins with at least one twin in a nonvertex presentation. No doubt some clinicians prefer to deliver all twins via cesarean section. There is little question that the former position can be justified if the attendant is an obstetrician with little or no experience in intrauterine manipulation; however, there is little if any data to support routine cesarean section when both twins are vertex.

The type of uterine incision should be based on the size and weight of the twins, the skill of the operator, and the degree of development of the lower uterine segment. The low segment transverse incision probably can be used in the majority of cases, but a high level of skill is required for the extraction of the second twin. Vertical incisions should be considered in cases where the lower uterine segment is thick. Vertical incisions are also easily and quickly extended if more space is required to effect an atraumatic delivery. Either conduction or general anesthesia may be used for cesarean section for twin gestations. However, anesthesia personnel should be prepared to provide uterine relaxation for extraction of the second twin—even at cesarean section!

TRIPLETS AND HIGHER ORDER BIRTHS

Maternal and fetal/neonatal morbidity with three or more fetuses is similar to that of twins but occurs even more frequently. Because of the degree of manipulation required with three or more fetuses, most clinicians (including the authors) prefer to deliver such pregnancies by cesarean section. However, there is little data to support a specific route of delivery. If vaginal delivery is chosen for triplets, it is imperative to be well prepared as outlined in Table 11–2 for twins. In a report by Lipitz and associates (1989) of 76 triplet pregnancies, all fetuses were delivered vaginally in 16 (21%) and by cesarean section in 60 (79%) patients. Recent data suggests that fetal survival for triplets now approaches 95% (Creinin, 1988; Lipitz, 1990; Newman, 1989; Sasson, 1990; and their colleagues).

SUMMARY

Multifetal gestations represent a substantial obstetric challenge. Successful vaginal delivery requires considerable skill; mastery of intrauterine manipulations is especially important. The ability to quickly perform a cesarean section with adequate operating room personnel, anesthesia, and pediatric support are important prerequisites for attempted vaginal delivery of twins.

REFERENCES

Acker D, Lieberman M, Holbrook H, et al. Delivery of the second twin. Obstet Gynecol 1982; 59:710.

Adam C, Allen AC, Baskett TF. Twin delivery: influence of the presentation and method of delivery on the second twin. Am J Obstet Gynecol 1991; 165:23–7.

Beck AC, Rosenthal AH. Obstetrical Practice. 6th ed. Baltimore: Williams & Wilkins, 1955, p. 915.

Bejar R, Vigliocco G, Gramajo H, et al. Antenatal origin of neurological damage in newborn infants. II. Multiple gestations. Am J Obstet Gynecol 1990; 162:1230.

Berglund L, Axelsson O. Breech extraction versus cesarean section for the remaining second twin. Acta Obstet Gynecol Scand 1989; 68:435.

Callahan TL, Hall JE, Ettner SL, et al. The economic impact of multiple-gestation pregnancies and the contribution of assisted-reproduction techniques to their incidence. N Engl J Med 1994; 331:244.

Carlan SJ, Angel JL, Sawai SK, Vaughn V. Late diagnosis of nonconjoined monoamniotic twins using computed tomographic imaging: a case report. Obstet Gynecol 1990; 76:504.

Carr SR, Aronson MP, Coustan DR. Survival rates of monoamniotic twins do not decrease after 30 weeks' gestation. Am J Obstet Gynecol 1990; 163:719.

Chauhan SP, Washburne JF, Martin JN, et al. Intrapartum assessment by house staff of birth weight among twins. Obstet Gynecol 1993; 82:523.

Chervenak FA, Johnson RE, Berkowitz RL, Hobbins JC. Intrapartum external version of the second twin. Obstet Gynecol 1983; 62:160.

Chervenak FA, Johnson RE, Berkowitz RL, et al. Is routine cesarean section necessary for vertex-breech and vertex-transverse twin gestations? Am J Obstet Gynecol 1984; 148:1.

Chervenak FA, Johnson RE, Youcha S, et al. Intrapartum management of twin gestation. Obstet Gynecol 1985; 65:119.

Cohen M, Kohl SG, Rosenthal AH. Fetal interlocking complicating twin gestation. Am J Obstet Gynecol 1965; 91:407.

Crawford JS. A prospective study of 200 consecutive twin deliveries. Anaesthesia 1987; 42:33.

Creinin M, MacGregor S, Socol M, et al. The Northwestern triplet study. Am J Obstet Gynecol 1988; 159:1140.

Davison L, Easterling TR, Jackson JC, Benedetti TJ. Breech extraction of low-birth-weight second twins: can cesarean section be justified? Am J Obstet Gynecol 1992; 166:497.

Fishman A, Grubb DK, Kovacs BW. Vaginal delivery of the nonvertex second twin. Am J Obstet Gynecol 1993; 168:861.

Gilstrap LC, Brown CEL. Prevention and treatment of preterm labor in twins. Clin Perinatol 1988; 15:71.

Gocke SE, Nageotte MP, Garite TJ, et al. Management of the nonvertex second twin: primary

cesarean section, external version, or primary breech extraction. Am J Obstet Gynecol 1989; 161:111.
Grieg PC, Veille JC, Morgan T, Henderson L. The effect of presentation and mode of delivery on neonatal outcome in the second twin. Am J Obstet Gynecol 1992; 167:901.
Hrubec Z, Robinette D. The study of human twins in medical research. N Engl J Med 1984; 310:435.
Kovacs BW, Kirschbaum TH, Paul RH. Twin gestations. I. Antenatal care and complications. Obstet Gynecol 1989; 74:313.
Laros RK, Dattel BJ. Management of twin pregnancy: the vaginal route is still safe. Am J Obstet Gynecol 1988; 158:1330.
Lavery JP, Gadwood KA. Amniography for confirming the diagnosis of monoamniotic twinning: a case report. J Reprod Med 1990; 35:911.
Lipitz S, Frenkel Y, Watts C, et al. High-order multifetal gestation—management and outcome. Obstet Gynecol 1990; 76:215.
Long PA, Oats JN. Preeclampsia in twin pregnancy—severity and pathogenesis. Aust NZ J Obstet Gynaecol 1987; 27:1.
Neal GS, Hankins GDV: Left microtia in one monozygotic twin. J Reprod Med 1992; 37:375–7.
Neumann PJ, Gharib SD, Weinstein MC. The cost of a successful delivery with in vitro fertilization. N Engl J Med 1994; 331:239.
Newman RB, Harner C, Miller MC. Outpatient triplet management: a contemporary review. Am J Obstet Gynecol 1989; 161:547.
Nilsen ST, Bergsjo P, Nome S. Male twins at birth and 18 years later. Br J Obstet Gynaecol 1984; 91:122.
Oettinger M, Ophir E, Markovitz J, et al. Is cesarean section necessary for delivery of a breech first twin? Gynecol Obstet Invest 1993; 35:38.
Persson PH, Kullander S. Long term experience of general ultrasound screening in pregnancy. Am J Obstet Gynecol 1983; 146:942.
Rabinovici J, Barkai G, Reichman B, et al. Randomized management of the second nonvertex twin: vaginal delivery or cesarean section. Am J Obstet Gynecol 1987; 156:52.
Rayburn WF, Lavin JP Jr, Miodovnik M, Varner MW. Multiple gestation: time interval between delivery of the first and second twins. Obstet Gynecol 1984; 63:502.
Rydhstrom H. Prognosis for twins with birth weight < 1500 gm: the impact of cesarean section in relation to fetal presentation. Am J Obstet Gynecol 1990; 63:528.
Samra JS, Spillane H, Mukoyoko J, et al. Caesarean section for the birth of the second twin. Br J Obstet Gynaecol 1990; 97:234.
Sargent SK, Young W, Crow P, Simpson W. CT amniography: value in detecting a monoamniotic pair in a triplet pregnancy. AJR 1991; 156:559.
Sasson DS, Castro LC, Davis JL, Hobel CJ. Perinatal outcome in triplet versus twin gestations. Obstet Gynecol 1990; 75:817.
Spellacy WN, Hondler A, Fene CD. A case-control study of 1,253 twin pregnancies from a 1982–1987 perinatal data base. Obstet Gynecol 1990; 75:168.
Sutter J, Arab H, Manning FA. Monoamniotic twins: antenatal diagnosis and management. Am J Obstet Gynecol 1986; 155:836.
Tessen JA, Zlatnik FJ. Monoamniotic twins: a retrospective controlled study. Obstet Gynecol 1991; 77:832.
Thompson SA, Lyons TI, Makowski EL. Outcomes of twin gestations at the University of Colorado Health Sciences Center, 1973–1983. J Reprod Med 1987; 32:328.
Townsend RR, Filly RA. Sonography of nonconjoined monoamniotic twin pregnancies. J Ultrasound Med 1988; 7:665.
Turner RJ, Hankins GDV, Ziaya PR, et al. Magnetic resonance imaging and ultrasonography in the antenatal evaluation of conjoined twins. Am J Obstet Gynecol l55:645, l986.
Wells SR, Thorp JM Jr, Bowes WA Jr. Management of the nonvertex second twin. Surg Gynecol Obstet 1991; 72:383.

CHAPTER 12

External Cephalic Version

External cephalic version, described in the medical literature since the writings of Hippocrates, was a commonly performed procedure earlier in this century (Friedlander, 1966; Hibbard and Schumann, 1973; Ranney, 1973; Stevenson, 1951). However, in the 1960s and '70s, external cephalic version fell out of favor because of increasing reports of maternal and fetal complications, high rates of spontaneous conversion to cephalic presentation, and spontaneous reversion to breech after successful external cephalic version (Brosset, 1956). Further, external cephalic version was being contrasted with vaginal breech delivery, which at the time was considered a totally acceptable approach to the breech presentation. Data then emerged that suggested that vaginal breech delivery was associated with excess perinatal morbidity and mortality even when congenital anomalies associated with breech presentation were excluded (Morgan, 1964; Smith, 1970; Tank, 1971; Rovinsky, 1973; Brenner, 1974; Mayer, 1978; and their colleagues). Long-term follow-up of the vaginally delivered breech also revealed evidence of neurologic damage that had been undetected in the perinatal period (Berendes, 1965; Muller, 1971; Manzaki, 1978; and their co-workers), and analysis suggested that the poorer outcome resulted from the type of delivery rather than breech presentation itself (Rovinsky and associates, 1973).

The obstetric community, not surprisingly, responded with almost universal cesarean delivery for intrapartum breech presentation, irrespective of gestational age (Taffel and associates, 1991), and breech presentation became a major component of a significantly increasing cesarean rate (Shiono and colleagues, 1987). Some physicians continued to embrace the concept of vaginal breech delivery but, even when various protocols for "safe" vaginal delivery were applied, most cases of breech presentation ultimately defaulted to cesarean delivery (Zatuchni, 1965; Bird, 1975; Collea, 1978; Gimovsky, 1980; and their associates). By 1989, 84 percent of all intrapartum breeches were managed by cesarean delivery (Taffel and colleagues, 1991).

If there were not excess maternal morbidity/mortality and excess expense with cesarean delivery (Petitti, 1982; Zhang, 1993; and their co-workers), alternative approaches to the breech presentation would probably never have been sought. Because the problem seemed to be the breech presentation itself, strategies to convert the presentation to the safer cephalic one seemed logical. External cephalic version was thus resurrected in the past decade. Successful version rates from various institutions of 60–70 percent resulted in parallel reductions in intrapartum breech presentation and subsequent cesarean delivery (Van Dorsten, 1981; Stine, 1985; Morrison, 1986; Savona-Ventura, 1986; Robertson, 1987; and their colleagues).

HISTORY OF EXTERNAL CEPHALIC VERSION

In the mid 1960s, the state of external cephalic version was best characterized by

MacArthur: "There are those who enthusiastically recommend it, others who violently oppose it, and still others who express a rather elegant distaste for it" (MacArthur, 1964). Skepticism was grounded in the following:

1. Fetal risk in the form of placental separation or cord accident (Bradley-Watson, 1975; Berg and Kunze, 1977).
2. Suspected high rate of spontaneous conversion from breech to cephalic presentation if external cephalic version were not attempted (Brosset, 1956).
3. Suspected high rate of spontaneous reversion to breech presentation after successful external cephalic version (Brosset, 1956).
4. Poor success rates if attempted later in pregnancy (Ranney, 1973).

To circumvent some of these problems and rekindle interest in external cephalic version, Saling and Muller-Holve (1975) reported a series of patients who had undergone external cephalic version under tocolysis near term. They selected term patients so that in the unlikely event of fetal distress, the fetus would be mature enough for immediate delivery. Aware of others' poor success late in pregnancy, they employed the beta-sympathomimetic fenoterol to relax the uterus and minimize the amount of force required. Saling and Muller-Holve succeeded in 75 percent of version attempts without apparent maternal, fetal, or neonatal ill-effects and reduced term intrapartum breech presentations 1.6 percent during the study period as compared to 3.8 percent in the era immediately preceding. Investigators from Finland and Sweden corroborated these findings (Fall and Nilsson, 1979; Ylikorkala and Hertiakinen-Sorri, 1977); still, skeptics questioned the role of external cephalic version and cited the lack of randomized prospective trials.

Beginning with Van Dorsten and associates (1981), four randomized prospective trials worldwide, including a total of 570 patients, have tested the role of external cephalic version at term (Hofmeyr, 1983; Brocks, 1984; Mahomed, 1991; and their colleagues). All studies were of similar design and all have shown a significant reduction in both intrapartum breech presentation and cesarean delivery rate (Tables 12–1 and 12–2). The higher the institutional cesarean rate for breech presentation, the greater will be the impact of external cephalic version. For example, Morrison and colleagues (1986) employed external cephalic version routinely in term breech presentation. External cephalic version was performed on 2.3 percent of all patients between 1982 and 1984. Vaginal breech deliveries decreased from 1.8 percent to 1.1 percent and cesarean delivery for breech presentation fell from 2.8 percent to 1.6 percent compared to the three preceding years when external cephalic version was not employed. Using the most conservative estimates from the North American and European randomized trials, Hofmeyr (1991a) has estimated that in the United Kingdom, "every 100 external cephalic versions at term should prevent 34 breech births and 14 cesarean sections. If external cephalic version at term were attempted in

TABLE 12–1. EXTERNAL CEPHALIC VERSION: RANDOMIZED PROSPECTIVE TRIALS

First Author	Location	Patients	Para 0 (%)	Reactive NST[a]	Tocolytic	Operator	Technique
Van Dorsten (1981)	S. California	48	?	Yes	Yes	Two	Lateral tilt: backward and forward
Hofmeyr (1983)	S. Africa	60	?	Yes	Only with 7 failures	One	Steep lateral: backward and forward
Brocks (1984)	Copenhagen	65	68%	Yes	Yes	?	Single attempt, left lateral, tilt
Mahomed (1991)	Zimbabwe	208	26%	Yes	Yes	One	Single attempt with lateral tilt: forward or backward

[a]NST = non-stress test

TABLE 12–2. EXTERNAL CEPHALIC VERSION: RANDOMIZED PROSPECTIVE TRIALS

First Author	Success Rate (%)	Cesarean Rate		Intrapartum Cephalic Presentation		Failure Factors	Morbidity	Spontaneous Conversion to Vertex	
		Study (%)	*Control (%)*	*Study (%)*	*Control (%)*			*Study (%)*	*Control (%)*
Van Dorsten (1981)	68	28	14	18	18	Obesity Nulliparity	None	0	17
Hofmeyr (1983)	97	20	43	67	3	None	None	0	33
Brocks (1984)	41	23	35	55	85	Obesitiy Nulliparity Ant. Placenta	None	9	14

only 2% of the 750,000 pregnancies in the United Kingdom each year, these 15,000 external cephalic version attempts should reduce the number of breech births by 5100 and the number of cesarean sections by 2100." With higher cesarean delivery rates in the United States, the effect of a program of successful external cephalic version should be even more dramatic.

Zhang and co-workers (1993) reviewed 25 studies published in the last 12 years, 13 of which were conducted in the United States. Based on the 1,339 patients from U.S. studies and a 64.5 percent success rate with version, they hypothesized that for every 100 normal pregnant women with a breech presentation in a program of external cephalic version, 63.3 percent (95% CI 60.7–65.9) would deliver vaginally and 36.7 percent (95% CI 34.1–39.3) would delivery by cesarean. Among controls the overall cesarean delivery rate was 83.2 percent (95 percent CI 79.8–86.6), which is in agreement with the current cesarean birth rate for breech presentation in the United States.

The same review article included a cost analysis on a hypothetical 100 normal pregnant women with breech presentation at term. Based on costs of uncomplicated deliveries at the North Carolina Memorial Hospital, a program of external cephalic version would save $583 per birth (12.3% of the total cost). This analysis did not account for any extension of hospitalization from a complicated delivery.

These authors further speculated on the ultimate impact of external cephalic version on the national cesarean rate. Using data from US studies, they concluded that a reduction in the cesarean rate among patients with term breech presentation from 83.2 percent to 36.7 percent would reduce the overall cesarean birth rate by only 1.9/100 deliveries.

The safety of external cephalic version at term is established. The risk to the fetus is quite small. In a review of 979 cases of external cephalic version at term, Hofmeyr (1991b) reported no fetal losses in cases where anesthesia had not been used. Whatever risks external cephalic version might pose, they must be weighed against the risk of persistent breech presentation. There is probably inherent risk to vaginal breech delivery (Brenner, 1974; Rovinsky, 1973; Morgan, 1964; Tank, 1971; Smith, 1970; Mayer, 1978; and their colleagues). There is also the risk of precipitate delivery before arrival in the hospital and the increased risk of prolapsed cord. There is also a risk of birth trauma at cesarean and possibly increased risk of pulmonary hypertension (Tatum, 1985; Heritage, 1985; and their coworkers).

For the mother, the savings are more easily quantifiable. Cesarean delivery poses excess morbidity, mortality, and cost (Petitti, 1982; Zhang, 1993; and their associates). There is the likely possibility of a future repeat cesarean and potential negative psychologic effects. However, this latter effect must be weighed against the disappointment of a failed external cephalic version.

PROTOCOL

Most investigators have used uniform inclusion and exclusion criteria for external cephalic version at term (Van Dorsten, 1981; Morrison, 1986; Stine, 1985; Hofmeyr, 1983; Brocks, 1984; Mahomed, 1991; Flanagan, 1987; Dyson, 1986; Fortunato, 1988; Marchik, 1988; Flamm, 1991; Donald, 1990; Hanss, 1990; O'Grady, 1986; and their co-workers). Absolute contraindications include third trimester bleeding, placenta previa, fetal anomalies that put the fetus at risk for injury, oligohydramnios, premature rupture of membranes (PROM), and presenting fetus with multiple gestations. The relative contraindications to external cephalic version are listed in Table 12–3.

Prerequisites for elective external cephalic version include an established gestational age of 37 weeks or beyond, normal ultrasound evaluation, reactive non-stress test (NST), informed consent, and availability of an operating room and anesthetic support. Intravenous access should be established and the maternal bladder should be empty. Because of the uniformly poor rate of success of external cephalic version at term, most investigators have employed a beta-sympathomimetic to relax the uterus and facilitate manipulation. Acceptable and similar success rates have been reported with a number of different agents, whether administered subcutaneously or intravenously. One randomized trial found no difference in successful version between tocolytic and placebo groups (Robertson and colleagues, 1987). Despite this one study, most clinicians still favor adjunctive tocolysis. In cases of diabetes, magnesium sulfate has been used as a safe and satisfactory tocolytic.

TABLE 12–3 RELATIVE CONTRAINDICATIONS

- Hypertension/preeclampsia
- Diabetes (beta sympathomimetics are contraindicated)
- Morbid obesity
- Previous uterine scar
- Various positions of the fetal back (depending on the author)
- Various locations of the placenta other than previa (depending on the author)
- Engagement of the breech
- Macrosomia
- Maternal congenital or acquired heart disease (if beta sympathomimetics are employed)
- Maternal thyroid dysfunction (if beta sympathomimetics are employed)

TECHNIQUE

Both one- and two-person version techniques have been described. Maternal flexion at the knees and hips relaxes abdominal musculature and lateral uterine displacement prevents supine hypotension. Some authors use powder on the maternal abdomen to facilitate a better purchase on the fetal poles; other authors use a lubricant gel or olive or mineral oil so the hands can slide over the maternal abdomen as the fetus is turned. Some favor the steep lateral position, while most use a lateral tilt. The direction of tilt often varies with the direction of the version attempt. The critical first step is elevation of the fetal breech from the maternal pelvis. If this step cannot be accomplished, success is doubtful and is not facilitated by concurrent vaginal elevation by an assistant. Success is reported with both a forward roll and back-flip. If one direction is not successful, the other is usually tried. After elevation of the breech, a to-and-fro movement on appropriate poles of the fetus facilitates external cephalic version (Fig. 12–1). The patient's pain threshold dictates how much pressure can be exerted. Anesthesia, analgesia, or sedation are not recommended as they might allow excess force to be used, causing abruption, cord accident, or uterine rupture (Bradley-Watson, 1975; Berg and Kunze, 1977). The operator(s) should desist with occurrence of excess pain or prolonged fetal heart rate decelerations. Transient heart rate deceleration (from cord compression or head compression) is not uncommon and invariably recovers when the maneuvers are halted. Experience has shown that manipulation beyond 5 minutes is rarely productive. With proper patient counseling and a willingness to stop for a minute or two during the procedure, most patients do not report a painful experience.

The fetal heart rate is monitored either continuously or intermittently by Doppler or real-time ultrasound throughout the version attempt. After external cephalic version, a reactive NST or negative contraction stress test confirms fetal well-being. Generally the fetus is monitored for at least 30 minutes after version. Follow-up antepartum fetal testing is not recommended unless other ongoing indications exist. The patient is asked to report vaginal bleeding, rupture of the membranes, regular uterine contractions, or decreased fetal movement following the version.

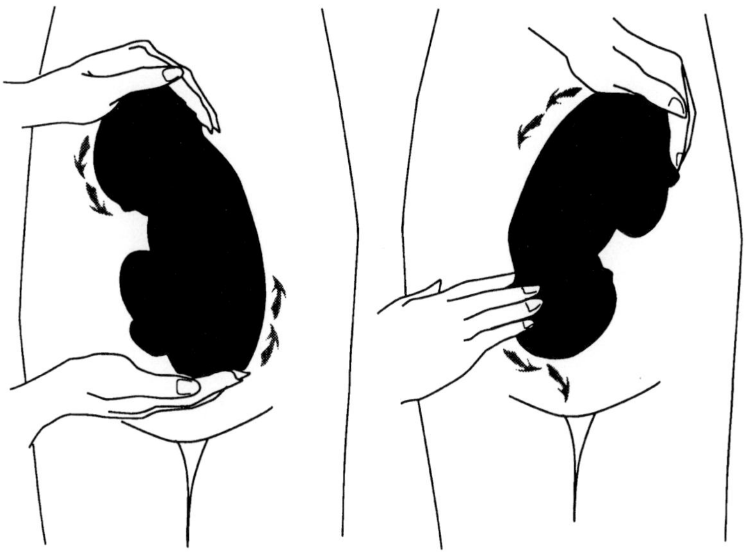

Figure 12–1. After elevation of the breech, a to-and-fro movement on appropriate poles of the fetus facilitates external cephalic version.

Rh-negative patients should receive Rh immune globulin (300 μg), as fetomaternal bleeding, measured by the Kleihauer Betke technique, has been reported in up to 28 percent of cases (Gjode and co-workers, 1980).

EXPANDED INDICATIONS

As clinicians have gained experience and comfort with external cephalic version at term, expanded indications have been tested under stringent protocols: (1) intrapartum breech presentation, (2) antepartum and intrapartum transverse lie, (3) intrapartum management of the breech second twin, (4) breech presentation in patients with a previous cesarean delivery approved for a trial of labor, and (5) preterm breech presentation.

Intrapartum External Cephalic Version

Using virtually the same protocol as with antepartum external cephalic version, Ferguson and Dyson (1985) reported a 73 percent success rate in 15 patients at term in early labor with intact membranes. Ten of 11 successes delivered vaginally for an overall vaginal delivery rate of 67 percent. There were no untoward outcomes. As part of a larger prospective study on external cephalic version at term with tocolysis, Fortunato and associates (1988) included 13 patients in active labor defined as contractions at least every 5 minutes with demonstrated cervical change. Among women in labor, 54 percent underwent successful external cephalic version compared with 61 percent of those at term but not in labor, a nonsignificant difference. A lower intrapartum success rate might be expected because of increased uterine tone and a lower fetal station. No randomized prospective trial has yet tested the efficacy and safety of intrapartum external cephalic version.

Transverse Lie

Phelan and colleagues (1985) reported on a series of 12 patients with intrapartum transverse lie. Inclusion criteria for attempted version included estimated fetal weight > 2000 g, reactive non-stress test, intact membranes, and normal amniotic fluid volume. External cephalic version was performed in the delivery room after ritodrine tocolysis (100 μg/min × 10–15 minutes). Version was successful in 10 of which 6 ultimately delivered vaginally. With the exception of an undiagnosed meningomyelocele, neonatal outcome was good. These results suggested that external cephalic version could avoid 50 percent of cesarean deliveries in patients with intrapartum transverse lie. Though there have been no randomized trials with intrapartum transverse lie, the alternative of cesarean delivery seems obvious.

Phelan and associates (1986) subsequently followed 29 patients with antepartum transverse lie at term expectantly. Though 83 percent had spontaneously converted to a longitudinal lie (vertex or breech) prior to labor, the cesarean delivery rate was 45 percent and there were 4 cases of serious morbidity/mortality including 2 cord prolapses, a neonatal death, and a spontaneous uterine rupture. As a result, these authors recommend external cephalic version with persistent transverse lie at 39 weeks; with failure, prophylactic cesarean should be strongly considered because of the high cesarean rate and major morbidities associated with expectant management.

Preterm External Cephalic Version

There is temptation to employ external cephalic version in the preterm setting where there is abundant amniotic fluid, generally a floating breech, and a soft uterus. The only randomized prospective trial of preterm version was performed at the University of Zimbabwe (Kasule and colleagues, 1985) and involved 310 patients who underwent version between 33 and 36 weeks. With initial failure, the procedure was subsequently repeated up to three times. Three hundred and thirty patients were also randomized to a control group, with no intervention. Two hundred and twenty patients (71%) had a successful version between 33 and 36 weeks. The success rate was 78 percent in multiparas and 46 percent in nulliparas. An additional 30 patients had a follow-up successful external cephalic version between 36 and 40 weeks. Of 250 successful antepartum external cephalic versions, only 134 were still cephalic intrapartum, for a final success rate of 43% (as opposed to an initial 80% overall procedure success rate). Overall, the spontaneous reversion rate after successful external cephalic version was 46 percent, and significantly greater among multiparas. Of the 60 patients where external cephalic version failed completely, 14 (23%) spontaneously converted to a cephalic presentation prior to labor. Ultimately, the incidence of breech presentation at delivery was 52 percent in the study group and 51 percent in the control group as 49 percent of patients in the control group spontaneously converted to vertex prior to labor. The cesarean delivery rate was similar in the two groups (16% vs. 15%). More importantly, there were three major complications: two multiparas had an abruption and fetal death within 6 hours of external cephalic version performed at 36 weeks. Another patient went into preterm labor soon after external cephalic version at 33 weeks and delivered a neonate who died of respiratory distress syndrome. The authors concluded that there is no place for antepartum external cephalic version prior to term due to the increased perinatal mortality rate. It is unclear from this study whether fetal surveillance by ultrasound and/or electronic fetal monitoring was performed before, during, or after the procedure. Furthermore, tocolytics were apparently not used.

It is not surprising that the spontaneous conversion rate was so high in the control group. Westgren and colleagues (1985) followed patients with a breech presentation identified at 32 weeks. Spontaneous version occurred in 57 percent of patients prior to term. By 37 weeks, the nulliparas had only a 5 percent chance of subsequent spontaneous conversion, whereas the multiparas still had a 20 percent chance. The four randomized prospective trials of external cephalic version at term corroborates these data.

Though Ranney (1973) demonstrated the safety and efficacy of antepartum preterm external cephalic version (even with repeated attempts), the high spontaneous conversion rate, coupled with the potential risk of iatrogenic prematurity with the procedure, would seem to preclude the routine use of antepartum external cephalic version in the preterm setting. Still unanswered, however, is the intrapartum application of external cephalic version with breech presentation in preterm labor with intact membranes, where tocolysis has failed and where cesarean delivery is the likely alternative. Such a program, if safe and successful, could have a significant impact in the preterm setting, where breech presentation is so prevalent and where cesarean is the rule in most institutions (Malloy and associates, 1991). Perhaps external cephalic version could even be performed at the time of initial tocolysis rather than after tocolysis has failed. It must be emphasized that these expanded applications should be tested in a randomized prospective fashion.

External Cephalic Version in Patients with Previous Cesarean Delivery

Flamm and associates (1991) tested external cephalic version in 56 patients who had undergone one or more previous cesarean deliveries (Flamm and co-workers, 1991). Fifty-six consecutive external cephalic version patients (without uterine scars) who met all inclusion/exclusion criteria served as controls. Using an otherwise standard protocol, external cephalic version was successful in 82 percent of patients with a previous cesarean as compared with 61 percent in controls. Sixty-five percent of the successful external cephalic version patients subsequently delivered vaginally. There were no untoward outcomes, although the limitations of the small sample size must be appreciated. The authors concluded that there is now another option for properly selected patients with breech presentation at term who have had a previous cesarean delivery.

EXTERNAL CEPHALIC VERSION IN TWINS

Interest in external cephalic version for the second twin with either a breech or transverse lie following successful vaginal delivery of the first twin was rekindled by Chervenak and coworkers (1983). Previously, there had been only anecdotal reports regarding external cephalic version in twins. Malpresentation of the second twin is common, with the incidence of cephalic-breech presentation reported to be 27.7–42.8 percent and cephalic-transverse lie, 4.9–7.2 percent (Farooqui, 1971; Guttmacher, 1958; Kohl, 1975; Kurtz, 1955; and their associates). Chervenak and associates (1983) reported retrospectively on 14 transverse lies and 11 breech presentations. External cephalic version was successful and resulted in subsequent vaginal delivery in 71 percent of transverse lies and 73 percent of breech presentations. Successful version was associated with cases where (1) the second twin was not significantly heavier than the first twin and (2) epidural anesthesia had been used. Success was not related to parity, gestational age, or birthweight. One neonatal death from necrotizing enterocolitis followed a successful external cephalic version and vaginal delivery at 28 weeks. There were no other untoward outcomes. In their study, gestational age ranged from 28 to 41 weeks. Chervenak and associates (1983) made the following recommendations:

1. Twin A vertex/twin B vertex: vertex vaginal delivery of both twins
2. Twin A vertex/twin B nonvertex:
    - Twin A: vertex vaginal delivery
    - Twin B:
        - Estimated fetal weight greater than 2000 g and fetus a candidate for a vaginal breech delivery: intrapartum external cephalic version
            - Unsuccessful: vaginal breech delivery
            - Successful: vaginal vertex delivery
        - Estimated fetal weight less than 2000 g or fetus not a candidate for a vaginal breech delivery: intrapartum external cephalic version
            - Successful: vaginal vertex delivery
            - Unsuccessful: cesarean delivery
3. Twin A nonvertex: cesarean delivery for both twins

In this algorithm ultrasound is the cornerstone of diagnosis and therapy. Not only does it assess the configuration and rule out anomalies, but it also estimates fetal weight.

Initial enthusiasm regarding Chervenak's recommendations was tempered by a retrospective review of 136 vertex–nonvertex twins with birthweight greater than 1500 g (Gocke and colleagues, 1989). By physician preference, 41 cases were primarily managed by external cephalic version, 55 primarily by attempted breech extraction, and 40 by outright cesarean delivery. There were no differences in neonatal morbidity/mortality among the three groups. External cephalic version was significantly less likely than breech extraction to result in a vaginal delivery (46% vs. 96%). External cephalic version was associated with fetal distress, cord prolapse, and compound presentation complications not seen in the other two groups. The cesarean rate was also significantly higher in the external cephalic version group (39% vs. 47%). These authors concluded that primary breech extraction of the second twin was a better alternative than either external cephalic version or primary cesarean.

To the contrary, Tchabo and Tomai (1992) reported on a series of 30 malpositioned second twins, all greater than 35 weeks, diamniotic, with normal amniotic fluid volume, intact membranes, and no anomalies. Version succeeded and resulted in vaginal delivery in 11 of 12 transverse lies and 16 of 18 breech presentations. Patients without epidural anesthesia (25%) received terbutaline 0.25 mg subcutaneously to relax the uterus. Two cesarean deliveries were performed, one for a prolapsed cord and the other for a prolapsed arm. There was no significant fetal/neonatal morbidity. There were two maternal complications: a postpartum hemorrhage secondary to uterine atony and a uterine inversion during delivery of the placenta.

In conclusion, external cephalic version would seem to be an acceptable alternative in the malpositioned second twin; however, its advantage over other management schemes is not yet clear.

REPEATED ATTEMPTS

In cases where immediate labor induction does not follow successful external cephalic version, there is a 6–7 percent risk of spontaneous reversion (Stine and colleagues, 1985). Rosen and associates (1992) reported on a multipara who underwent successful external cephalic version at 38 weeks. After prompt reversion to breech, the patient underwent a second successful version the next day. Following a failed induction, the patient requested expectant management. There was again spontaneous reversion to breech at 41 weeks. The patient requested a third external cephalic version, which was successful at 42 weeks. This time, the patient underwent successful induction and uneventful vaginal delivery. The authors concluded that induction of labor would seem reasonable after reversion and a second successful external cephalic version.

PREDICTING SUCCESS OF EXTERNAL CEPHALIC VERSION

Many authors (Fortunato, 1988; Ferguson, 1987; and their colleagues) have identified prognostic factors for success of external cephalic version, but there has not been an attempt to integrate these factors into a simple, quantitative scoring system for predicting success, nor have any prognostic factors been prospectively tested. Newman and associates (1993) examined the clinical characteristics of 108 consecutive external cephalic versions performed between 1984 and 1986. Five factors explained the majority of variability in outcome: parity, placental location, cervical dilatation, station of the presenting part, and estimated fetal weight. This retrospective analysis was used to develop a prognostic scoring system similar to that of Bishop (Table 12–4). The scoring system was then tested on 286 consecutive external cephalic version patients between 1986 and 1992. There was a positive relationship between a rising score and the likelihood of success (Fig. 12–2). No external cephalic versions were successful with a score less than or equal to 2, and all external cephalic versions were successful with a score of 9 or 10. The results of the score may have significantly altered physician recommendation in more than one-third of cases. The authors suggested that women with scores of 4 or less might simply not be candidates for external cephalic version, thus avoiding a costly and probably futile version attempt. Alternatively, those patients with scores of 8 or greater would seem to be opti-

TABLE 12–4 PROPOSED EXTERNAL CEPHALIC VERSION SCORING SYSTEM FOR ESTIMATING LIKELIHOOD OF SUCCESSFUL BREECH VERSION

	0	1	2
Parity	0	1	≥ 2
Dilatation	≥ 3 cm	1–2 cm	0 cm
Estimated weight	< 2500 g	2500–3500 g	> 3500 g
Placenta	Anterior	Posterior	Lateral/fundal
Station	≥ –1	–2	≤ –3

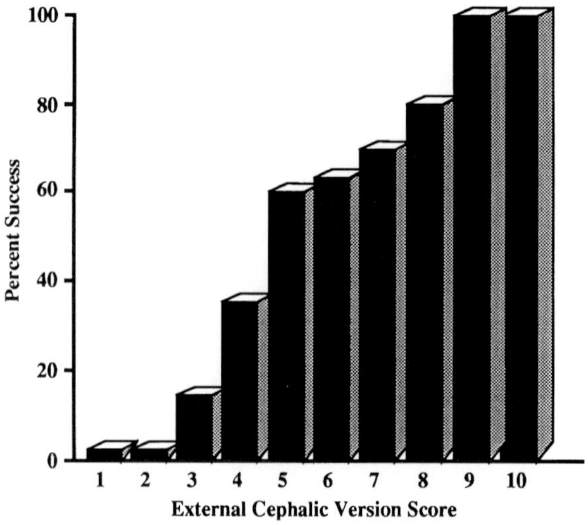

Figure 12–2. External cephalic version score.

mal candidates, with success rates greater than those typically quoted.

SUMMARY

The role of external cephalic version has expanded. In this era of cost containment, a program of external cephalic version can effectively lower the institutional cesarean delivery rate without sacrificing safety. New refinements in technique and new applications, always tested under strict protocol, may make the impact of external cephalic version even greater in the future.

REFERENCES

Berendes HW, Weiss W, Deutschberger J, Jackson E. Factors associated with breech delivery. Am J Public Health 1965; 55:708.

Berg D, Kunze U. Critical remarks on external cephalic version under tocolysis. Report on a case of antepartum fetal death. J Perinat Med 1977; 5:32.

Bird CC, McElin TW. A six-year prospective study of term breech deliveries utilizing the Zatuchni-Andros prognostic scoring index. Am J Obstet Gynecol 1975; 121:551.

Bradley-Watson PJ. The decreasing value of external cephalic version in modern obstetric practice. Am J Obstet Gynecol 1975; 123:237.

Brenner WE, Bruce RD, Hendricks CH. The characteristics and perils of breech presentation. Am J Obstet Gynecol 1974; 118:700.

Brocks V, Philipsen T, Secher NJ. A randomized trial of external cephalic version with tocolysis in late pregnancy. Br J Obstet Gynaecol 1984; 91:653.

Brosset A. The value of prophylactic external version in cases of breech presentation. Acta Obstet Gynecol Scand 1956; 35:555.

Chervenak FA, Johnson RE, Berkowitz RL, Hobbins JC. Intrapartum external version of the second twin. Obstet Gynecol 1983; 62:160.

Collea JV, Rabin SC, Weghorst GR, Quilligan EH. The randomized management of term frank breech presentation: vaginal delivery versus cesarean section. Am J Obstet Gynecol 1978; 131:186.

Donald WL, Barton JJ. Ultrasonography and external cephalic version at term. Am J Obstet Gynecol 1990; 162:1542.

Dyson DC, Ferguson JE, Hensleigh P. Antepartum external cephalic version under tocolysis. Obstet Gynecol 1986; 67:63.

Fall O, Nilsson BA. External cephalic version in breech presentation under tocolysis. Obstet Gynecol 1979; 53:712.

Farooqui MO, Grossman JH, Shannon RA. A review of twin pregnancy and perinatal mortality. Obstet Gynecol Surv 1973; 28:144.

Ferguson JE, Armstrong MA, Dyson DC. Maternal and fetal factors affecting success of antepartum external cephalic version. Obstet Gynecol 1987; 70:722.

Ferguson JE, Dyson DC. Intrapartum external cephalic version. Am J Obstet Gynecol 1985; 152:297.

Flamm BL, Fried MW, Lonky NM, Giles WS. External cephalic version after previous cesarean section. Am J Obstet Gynecol 1991; 165:370.

Flanagan TA, Mulchahey KM, Korenbrott CC, et al. Management of term breech presentation. Am J Obstet Gynecol 1987; 156:1492.

Fortunato S, Mercer LJ, Guzick DS. External cephalic version with tocolysis: factors associated with success. Obstet Gynecol 1988; 72:59.

Friedlander D. External cephalic version in the management of breech presentation. Am J Obstet Gynecol 1966; 95:906.

Gimovsky ML, Petrie RH, Todd WD. Neonatal performance of the selected term vaginal breech delivery. Obstet Gynecol 1980; 56:687.

Gjode P, Ramussen TB, Jorgensen J. Fetomaternal bleeding during attempts at external version. Br J Obstet Gynaecol 1980; 87:571.

Gocke SE, Nageotte MP, Garite T, et al. Management of the nonvertex second twin: primary cesarean section, external version, or primary breech extraction. Am J Obstet Gynecol 1989; 161:111.

Guttmacher AF, Kohl SG. The fetus of multiple gestations. Obstet Gynecol 1958; 12:528.

Hanss JW. The efficacy of external cephalic version and its impact on the breech experience. Am J Obstet Gynecol 1990; 162:1459.

Heritage CK, Cunningham MD. Association of elective repeat caesarean delivery and persistent pulmonary hypertension of the newborn. Am J Obstet Gynecol 1985; 152:627.

Hibbard LT, Schumann WR. Prophylactic external cephalic version in an obstetric practice. Am J Obstet Gynecol 1973; 116:511.

Hofmeyr GJ. Effect of external cephalic version in late pregnancy on breech presentation and caesarean section rate: A controlled trial. Br J Obstet Gynaecol 1983; 90:392.

Hofmeyr GJ. External cephalic version at term: how high are the stakes? Br J Obstet Gynaecol 1991a; 98:1.

Hofmeyr GJ. Breech presentation and abnormal lie in late pregnancy. In Chalmers I, Enkin MW, Keirse MJNC (eds), Effective Care in Pregnancy and Childbirth. Oxford: Oxford University Press, 1991b, pp 653-665.

Kasule J, Chimbira THK, Brown IMcL. Controlled trial of external cephalic version. Br J Obstet Gynaecol 1985; 92:14.

Kohl SG, Casey G. Twin gestation. Mt Sinai J Med 1975; 42:523.

Kurtz GR, Keating WJ, Loftus JB. Twin pregnancy and delivery. Obstet Gynecol 1955; 6:370.

MacArthur JL. Reduction of the hazards of breech presentation by external cephalic version. Am J Obstet Gynecol 1964; 88:302.

Mahomed K, Seeras R, Coulson R. External cephalic version at term. A randomized controlled trial using tocolysis. Br J Obstet Gynaecol 1991; 98:8.

Malloy MH, Onstad L, Wright E, National Institute of Child Health and Human Development Neonatal Research Network. The effect of cesarean delivery on birth outcome in very low birth weight infants. Obstet Gynecol 1991; 77:498.

Manzaki H. Morbidity among infants born in breech presentation. J Perinat Med 1978; 6:127.

Marchik R. Antepartum external cephalic version with tocolysis: A study of term singleton breech presentations. Am J Obstet Gynecol 1988; 158:1339.

Mayer PS, Wingate MC. Obstetrics factors in cerebral palsy. Obstet Gynecol 1978; 51:399.

Morgan HS, Kane SH. An analysis of 16,327 breech births, JAMA 1964; 187:108.

Morrison JC, Myatt RE, Martin JN Jr, et al. External cephalic version of the breech presentation under tocolysis. Am J Obstet Gynecol 1986; 154:900.

Muller PF, Campbell HE, Graham WE, et al. Perinatal factors and their relationship to mental retardation and other parameters of development. Am J Obstet Gynecol 1971; 109:1205.

Newman RB, Peacock BS, Van Dorsten JP, Hunt HH. Predicting success of external cephalic version. Am J Obstet Gynecol 1993; 169:245.

O'Grady JP, Veille JC, Holland RL, Burry KA. External cephalic version: a clinical experience. J Perinat Med 1986; 14:189.

Petitti DB, Cefalo RC, Shapiro S, Whalley P. In-hospital maternal mortality in the United States: time trends and relation to method of delivery. Obstet Gynecol 1982; 59:6.

Phelan JP, Stine LE, Edwards NB, et al. The role of external version in the intrapartum management of the transverse lie presentation. Am J Obstet Gynecol 1985; 151:724.

Phelan JP, Boucher M, Mueller E, et al. The nonlaboring transverse lie: a management dilemma. J Reprod Med 1986; 31:184.

Ranney B. The gentle art of external cephalic version. Am J Obstet Gynecol 1973; 116:239.

Robertson AW, Kopelman JN, Read JA, et al. External cephalic version at term: is a tocolytic necessary? Obstet Gynecol 1987; 70:896.

Rosen DJD, Illeck JS, Greenspoon JS. Repeated external cephalic version at term. Am J Obstet Gynecol 1992; 167:508.

Rovinsky JJ, Miller JA, Kaplan S. Management of breech presentation at term. Am J Obstet Gynecol 1973; 115:497.

Saling E, Muller-Holve W. External cephalic version under tocolysis. J Perinat Med 1975; 3:115.

Savona-Ventura C. The role of external cephalic version in modern obstetrics. Obstet Gynecol Surv 1986; 41:393.

Shiono PH, McNellis D, Rhoads GR. Reasons for the rising cesarean delivery rates: 1978–1984. Obstet Gynecol 1987; 69:696.

Smith RS, Oldham RR. Breech delivery. Obstet Gynecol 1970; 36:151.

Stevenson CS. Certain concepts in the handling of breech and transverse presentation in late pregnancy. Am J Obstet Gynecol 1951; 62:488.

Stine LE, Phelan JP, Wallace R, et al. Update on external cephalic version performed at term. Obstet Gynecol 1985; 65:642.

Taffel SM, Placek PJ, Moien M, Kosary CL. U.S. cesarean section rate steadies — VBAC rises to nearly one in five. Birth 1991; 18:73.

Tank ES, Davis R, Holt JF, Morley GW. Mechanisms of trauma during breech delivery. Obstet Gynecol 1971; 38:761.

Tatum RK, Orr JW, Soong S, Huddleston JF. Vaginal breech delivery of selected infants weighing more than 2000 grams: a retrospective analysis of seven years experience. Am J Obstet Gynecol 1985; 152:145.

Tchabo J-G, Tomai T. Selected intrapartum external cephalic version of the second twin. Obstet Gynecol 1992; 79:421.

Van Dorsten JP, Schifrin BS, Wallace RL. Randomized control trial of external cephalic version with tocolysis in late pregnancy. Am J Obstet Gynecol 1981; 141:417.

Westgren M, Edvall H, Nordstrom L, Svalenius E. Spontaneous cephalic version of breech presentation in the last trimester. Br J Obstet Gynaecol 1985; 92:19.

Ylikorkala O, Hertiakinen-Sorri A. Value of external version in fetal malpresentation in combination with use of ultrasound. Acta Obstet Gynecol Scand 1977; 56:63.

Zatuchni GI, Andros GJ. Prognostic index for vaginal delivery in breech presentation at term. Am J Obstet Gynecol 1965; 93:237.

Zhang J, Bowes WA, Fortney JA. Efficacy of external cephalic version: a review. Obstet Gynecol 1993; 82:306–12.

CHAPTER 13

Shoulder Dystocia

Shoulder dystocia is one of the most dreaded and dramatic complications encountered in obstetrics. When this condition occurs it can result in high rates of maternal morbidity as well as neonatal morbidity and mortality. Resnik (1980) defines shoulder dystocia as a condition requiring special maneuvers in order to deliver the shoulders following an unsuccessful attempt to apply downward traction; Benedetti (1989) more specifically defines this condition as arrest of spontaneous delivery due to impaction of the anterior shoulder against the symphysis pubis (Fig. 13–1). Proper management of shoulder dystocia requires prior consideration of risk factors, a well-conceived plan of action, and rapid execution (Dignam, 1976). The basic clinical tenets of shoulder dystocia management are prompt recognition, specific maneuvers to deliver the impacted shoulders, and avoidance of excessive forces to the fetal and maternal tissues, all during a relatively brief time.

HISTORY

Shoulder dystocia has been described in the medical literature for at least two centuries. Swartz (1960) quoted Smellie, in 1730: "A sudden call to a gentlewoman in labor. The child's head delivered for a long time—but even with hard pulling from the midwife, the remarkably large shoulder prevented delivery. I have been called by midwives to many cases of this kind, in which the child was frequently lost." Even as late as 1966 shoulder dystocia received relatively little attention; in the 13th edition of *Williams Obstetrics* (Eastman and Hellman, 1966), only one page is devoted to the subject.

Morris (1955) described the clinical phenomenon of "broad shoulder dystocia" graphically:

> The delivery of the head with or without forceps may have been quite easy, but more commonly there has been a little difficulty in completing the extension of the head. The hairy scalp slides out with reluctance. When the forehead has appeared it is necessary to press back the perineum to deliver the face. Fat cheeks eventually emerge. A double chin has to be hooked over the posterior vulval commissure, to which it remains tightly opposed. Restitution seldom occurs spontaneously, for the head seems incapable of movement as a result of friction with the girdle of contact at the vulva. On the other hand, gentle manipulation of the head sometimes results in a sudden 90 degree restitution as the head adjusts itself without descent to the antero-posterior position of the shoulders. Time passes. The child's face becomes suffused. It endeavors unsuccessfully to breathe. Abdominal efforts by the mother or by her attendants produce no advance, gentle head traction is equally unavailing. Usually equanimity forsakes the attendants. They push, they pull. Alarm increases. Eventually 'by greater strength of muscle or by some infernal juggle' the difficulty appears to be overcome, and the shoul-

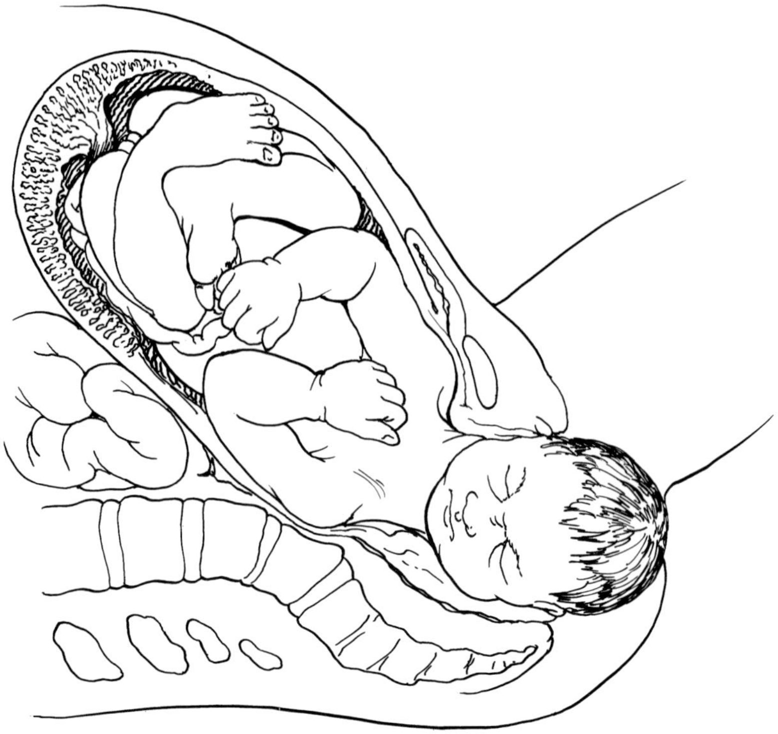

Figure 13–1. Shoulder dystocia. The shoulders are in an anteroposterior diameter, with the anterior shoulder impacted behind the symphysis pubis, and the posterior shoulder behind the sacral promontory.

> ders and trunk of a goodly child are delivered. The pallor of its body contrasts with the plum coloured cyanosis of the face, and the small quantity of freshly expelled meconium about the buttocks. It dawns upon the attendants that their anxiety was not ill-founded, the baby lies limp and voiceless, and only too often remains so despite all efforts at resuscitation.

INCIDENCE

The incidence of shoulder dystocia is difficult to determine because of variations in definition and methods of reporting. Sandmire and O'Halloin (1988) report an overall incidence of approximately 0.2–0.5 percent of deliveries. The incidence has been reported by others as higher, lower, or similar. Hopwood (1982) described an increasing incidence of shoulder dystocia, which was reported to have occurred in 0.2 percent of deliveries between 1966 and 1976, but increased in 1.1 percent between 1976 and 1981. He attributed this increase to the general trend toward larger birthweight, a finding confirmed by Modanlou and co-workers in 1982. It is possible that other factors such as heightened recognition and improved reporting of shoulder dystocia also may play a role in the reported incidence. On the other hand, Sandmire and O'Halloin (1988) reviewed the literature and concluded that there was no evidence of an increased incidence in shoulder dystocia reported during this century. Sack (1969) evaluated infants weighing 10 pounds (4545 g) or more at delivery. Between 1947 and 1956, the incidence of shoulder dystocia was 10 percent; in 1966, the incidence was reduced to 6 percent, possibly due to changes in the clinical management of diabetes and labor. Table 13–1 demonstrates the incidence of shoulder dystocia with respect to birthweight in several series. The incidence of this complication will vary depending upon the methods of reporting, the specific patient population, and the subgroups of patients reported (total population, versus diabetics, versus nondiabetics). Virtually all of these studies also are limited by the retrospective methodology employed. Gonik and associates (1991) hypothesize that shoulder dystocia is underreported in the literature and that unrecognized cases of shoulder dystocia are associated with increased risk of neonatal injury, presumably secondary to excessive traction forces.

TABLE 13–1. BIRTHWEIGHT AND SHOULDER DYSTOCIA

Study	Incidence by Birthweight			Comments
	≤ 4000 g	*> 4000 g*	*> 4500 g*	
Benedetti and Gabbe (1978)	12/8196 0.15%	21/694 3%		8890 vertex vaginal deliveries.
Golditch and Kirkman (1978)		20/667 3%	11/134 8%	801 deliveries with birthweight ≥ 4100 g. Denominator includes cesarean sections.
Modanlou et al. (1980)	1/284 0.4%		22/287 8%	Retrospective study of 287 macrosomic infants and controls. Denominator includes caesareans.
Acker et al. (1985)	144/13,403 1%	113/1100 10%	52/218 24%	14,721 vaginal deliveries with birthweight ≥ 2500 g. Includes diabetics and nondiabetics.
Gross TL et al. (1987)	67/6729 1%[a]	29/338 9%	20/56 36%	Study of 7123 deliveries, including birthweight < 2500 g, diabetics and nondiabetics.
Sandmire and O'Halloin (1988)	26/13,051 0.2%	25/1232 2%	22/523 4%	Denominator is total deliveries.
Keller et al. (1991)	7/75 9%	5/37 14%	3/8 38%	173 gestational diabetics underwent trial of labor, 120 delivered vaginally.
Delpapa and Mueller-Heubach (1991)	1/60 2%	3/52 6%	1/8 13%	242 nondiabetics with EFW by U/S ≥ 4000 g or 90th percentile.

[a]2.9% (39/1,368) at 3,500–3,999 g

DIFFERENTIAL DIAGNOSIS

Swartz (1960) has listed the differential diagnosis of difficulty in completing vaginal delivery of the fetus (Table 13–2). When the fetal shoulders fail to spontaneously follow delivery of the head, and other rare causes of such delay are ruled out by examination, shoulder dystocia is most likely the underlying problem.

TABLE 13–2. DIFFERENTIAL DIAGNOSIS OF DIFFICULTY IN COMPLETING DELIVERY

Short umbilical cord (absolute or relative)
Thoracic or abdominal enlargement of the infant (tumor, anasarca, anomaly)
Locked twins
Conjoined twins
Contraction ring
Shoulder dystocia

From Swartz (1960).

RISK FACTORS

Risk factors for shoulder dystocia may be identified during the antepartum period or during the intrapartum period (Table 13–3). Unfortunately, such risk factors are so com-

TABLE 13–3. SOME RISK FACTORS FOR SHOULDER DYSTOCIA

Antepartum	Intrapartum
Fetal macrosomia	First stage labor abnormalities
Maternal obesity	Protraction disorders
Diabetes mellitus	Arrest disorders
Post-term pregnancy	Prolonged second stage of labor
Male gender	Oxytocin augmentation of labor
Advanced maternal age	Mid-forceps and mid-vacuum extraction
Excessive weight gain	
Prior shoulder dystocia	
Platypelloid pelvis and contracted pelvis	
Prior macrosomic infant	

mon that they lack both sensitivity and specificity and are of limited clinical utility (American College of Obstetricians and Gynecologists, 1989b).

Antepartum Risk Factors

Fetal Macrosomia

Fetal macrosomia has been established as one of the major risks for shoulder dystocia. The degree of risk is dependent upon the weight used to define macrosomia. The incidence of macrosomia in reported series of shoulder dystocia is listed in Tables 13–1 and 13–4. Nathanson (1950) reported on 44,286 full-term deliveries between 1932 and 1947; 756 infants weighed 4500 g or more. Among this group, 720 were delivered vaginally. There were 76 cases of shoulder dystocia, for an overall incidence of 10.6 percent. Twenty-five of the 716 (3.5%) living infants who underwent vaginal delivery suffered "serious infantile injuries." Acker and colleagues (1985) demonstrated that the incidence of shoulder dystocia increased as birthweight increased both for nondiabetics and diabetics (Fig. 13–2). They described a 10 percent incidence of shoulder dystocia in nondiabetic women delivering babies between 4000 and 4499 g, compared to a 22.6 percent incidence in nondiabetic women delivering babies weighing above 4500 g.

In an attempt to further clarify the management of suspected macrosomia, SJ Gross and co-workers (1987) used multiple discriminant analysis to find a model that could predict three outcome categories: no shoulder dystocia, shoulder dystocia without trauma, and shoulder dystocia with trauma. In pregnancies with an infant weighing ≥ 4000 g, the occurrence of shoulder dystocia could not be consistently predicted from clinical characteristics of pregnancy or labor abnormalities. These investigators calculated that if cesarean section were performed on all infants weighing 4000 g or more, 6 cesarean sections would be required to prevent one case of shoulder dystocia. Delpapa and Mueller-Heubach (1991) reached similar conclusions in their study of 242 nondiabetic women at or beyond 36 weeks of gestation with an estimated fetal weight by ultrasound of ≥ 4000 g or the 90th percentile for gestational age. They found an increasing risk of shoulder dystocia with increased birthweight (Table 13–1); however, 5 cases of shoulder dystocia occurred, all without birth trauma. They did not endorse cesarean section or induction to prevent infant morbidity when fetal macrosomia was diagnosed by ultrasound.

An alternative strategy to cesarean delivery for management of macrosomia is labor induction. Combs and co-investigators (1993) retrospectively evaluated induction versus expectant management for pregnancies identified with fetal macrosomia, defined as estimated fetal weight greater than the 90th

TABLE 13–4. INCIDENCE OF MACROSOMIA (≥ 4000 G) IN REPORTED SERIES OF SHOULDER DYSTOCIA

Study	Number of Shoulder Dystocias ≥ 4000 g/ Total Number of Shoulder Dystocias	Percent ≥ 4000 g
Swartz (1960), Baltimore, MD	24/31	77
Seigworth (1966), Baltimore, MD	39/51	77
Benedetti and Gabbe (1978), Los Angeles, CA	21/33	64
Johnstone (1979), Melbourne, Australia	33/47	70
Acker et al. (1985), Boston, MA	165/309	53
Gross TL et al. (1987), Peoria, IL	49/116	42
Sandmire and O'Halloin (1988), Green Bay, WI	47/73	64
Hassan (1988), Amman, Jordan	38/41	93
Al-Najashi et al. (1989), Saudi Arabia	33/56	59
Langer et al. (1991), San Antonio, TX	280/456	61
Morrison et al. (1992), Jackson, MS	26/254	11
Total	755/1467	52

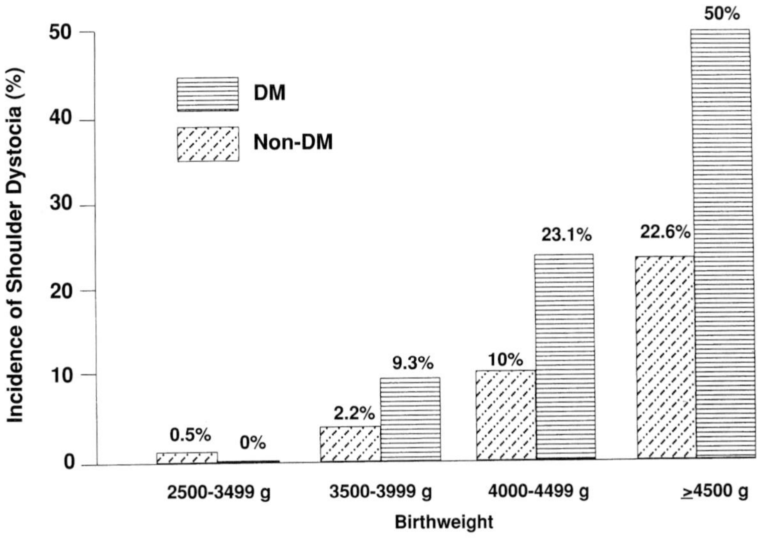

Figure 13–2. The incidence of shoulder dystocia among 14,721 vaginal deliveries with birthweight ≥2500 g, according to birthweight and diabetic status. (Data from: Acker and associates, 1985.)

percentile for gestational age. Unfortunately, they found a significantly higher cesarean section rate with elective induction (57%) versus expectant management (31%), without a significant reduction in shoulder dystocia.

In another retrospective study, Lazer and colleagues (1986) compared 525 macrosomic infants (defined as > 4500 g) with 520 controls (2500 to 4000 g). A significantly increased incidence of shoulder dystocia, Erb's palsy, and clavicular fracture was noted among the macrosomic group. They also studied a subgroup who had had a previous macrosomic child and compared these to the group of women who delivered only one macrosomic infant. Among the subgroup of women who delivered a macrosomic child in a previous pregnancy, there appeared to be a relative decrease in shoulder dystocia, Erb's palsy, and clavicular fracture when compared to the subgroup who delivered only one macrosomic infant. These authors recommended delivery by cesarean section for estimated fetal weight > 4500 g, except for the subgroup of women who have already delivered a macrosomic infant, who they suggested should be allowed a trial of labor. This recommendation is in accord with that of SJ Gross and associates (1987). Although there were relatively fewer complications in this subgroup, it should be recognized that there was still an 8.3 percent incidence of shoulder dystocia, 2.4 percent incidence of Erb's palsy, and 1.2 percent incidence of clavicular fracture in the subgroup with a previous macrosomic infant.

Rydhstrom and Ingemarsson (1989) reviewed the Swedish National Medical Birth Registry for cases of birthweight exceeding 5700 g (12.5 lb) between 1973 and 1984. There were 110 newborns identified, of which 78 underwent vaginal delivery, and 40 percent (31/78) had shoulder dystocia. Four out of the 8 deaths in this group were secondary to shoulder dystocia, and there were 11 brachial plexus injuries. It would be most unusual not to consider the merits of cesarean delivery when the expected birth weight is 5700 g.

In 1991 the American College of Obstetricians and Gynecologists attempted to refine the definition of macrosomia (1991b). It was recognized that while the large-for-gestational-age baby is defined in relation to gestational age, macrosomia refers to an absolute birthweight without regard to gestational age or other demographics. Additionally, different populations manifest different prevalences of macrosomia. Based on the available data on Erb's palsy (Acker, 1985; Lazer, 1986; McFarland, 1986; and their associates) and the vagaries of antepartum estimation of fetal weight, the College defined as macrosomic any fetus with an estimated weight greater than or equal to 4500 g in utero. Adoption of a lower estimated weight would result in the identification of many infants as "at risk" despite only a relatively small increase in the risk of morbidity as a consequence of their size.

Maternal Obesity

Johnson and associates (1987) reported a 5.1 percent incidence of shoulder dystocia if the maternal weight was over 250 pounds versus a 0.6 percent incidence in women who weighed less than 200 pounds at delivery. Spellacy and co-workers (1985) found that obesity was a risk factor for macrosomia, which was in turn a risk factor for shoulder dystocia. Schwartz and Dixon (1958) showed that the overall incidence of shoulder dystocia was 0.2 percent in the general population but 1.5 percent in women weighing over 180 pounds; 32 percent of all cases of shoulder dystocia occurred in women who weighed over 180 pounds. It is not clear whether obesity is an independent risk factor or is related to the common co-occurrence of diabetes mellitus.

Diabetes Mellitus

Neonates of diabetics have increased shoulder-to-head and chest-to-head size differences relative to comparable-weight neonates of nondiabetic mothers (Modanlou and colleagues, 1982). Acker and co-workers (1985) found a relative risk of 5.2 for shoulder dystocia in diabetics when compared to nondiabetics. Cousins and associates (1985) reported that maternal carbohydrate intolerance was associated with increased birthweight, depressed 5 minute Apgar scores, increased incidence of shoulder dystocia, and increased perinatal mortality. Figure 13–2 illustrates the relationship between birthweight, maternal diabetes, and shoulder dystocia. One study of gestational diabetics found a 9 percent incidence of shoulder dystocia with birthweight between 3500 and 3999 g, an incidence that increased to 14 percent with birthweight of 4000–4499 g, and 38 percent with birthweight greater than 4500 g (Keller and co-workers, 1991). Langer and co-investigators (1991) found that birthweight and diabetes ranked highest as risk factors for shoulder dystocia in their population (Table 13–5). These investigators recommended a cesarean section for diabetic women with an estimated fetal weight greater than 4250 g.

Pederson (1954) found a trend in lower birthweight of infants of those diabetics receiving long-term insulin therapy as compared to those undergoing short-term therapy. Coustan and Imarah (1984) also found that insulin therapy decreased the incidence of macrosomia, operative delivery, and birth trauma in gestational diabetics. Berne and associates (1985) confirmed these observations and proposed the use of insulin for this purpose, a practice widely employed today.

Post-term Pregnancy

Post-term pregnancies also have been associated with shoulder dystocia (Johnson, 1987; Eden, 1987; and their colleagues). Several studies have found that nearly half of shoulder dystocia cases were associated with a pregnancy extending beyond 41 weeks of gestation (Johnstone, 1979; Hopwood, 1982).

TABLE 13–5. SHOULDER DYSTOCIA AS RELATED TO BIRTHWEIGHT IN DIABETIC AND NONDIABETIC PREGNANT WOMEN

Weight Category (g)	Diabetic			Nondiabetic			*P* Value
	No.	*Shoulder Dystocia*	*%*	*No.*	*Shoulder Dystocia*	*%*	
2500–3749	1002	5	0.5	61,569	97	0.2	0.0001
3750–3999	251	3	1.2	6979	71	1.0	NS
4000–4249	128	4	3.0	3231	86	2.6	NS
4250–4499	81	6	6.9	1399	73	5.0	0.03
4500–4749	43	12	21.8	528	43	7.5	0.0001
4750–4999	18	10	35.7	176	26	12.9	0.0001
≥ 5000	16	10	38.5	102	10	8.9	0.0001
Total	1539	50		73,984	406		

NS, not significant

Spellacy and associates (1985) suggested that post-term pregnancy is a risk factor for macrosomia, itself a risk for shoulder dystocia. Excluding post-term pregnancies with birthweight greater than 4000 g, Acker and colleagues (1985) found that the overwhelming majority of post-term pregnancies were not associated with shoulder dystocia. Thus, the post-term pregnancy does not appear to be an independent risk factor for shoulder dystocia; rather the risk is macrosomia. Induction of all post-term pregnancies to avoid shoulder dystocia is unwarranted.

Male Gender

Several studies have associated male gender with shoulder dystocia. Parks and Ziel (1978) found that 72 percent of 110 macrosomic (≥ 4500 g) neonates were males. Spellacy and associates (1985) found that 67 percent of 574 macrosomic (> 4500 g) infants were males. In a series of 41 cases of shoulder dystocia reported by Hassan (1988), 28 (68%) were male.

Advanced Maternal Age

Advanced maternal age as a risk factor for shoulder dystocia depends upon the co-existence of diabetes mellitus and obesity, and is not therefore an independent risk factor for shoulder dystocia. Using logistic regression analysis, Langer and co-workers (1991) found that maternal age did not contribute to the risk of shoulder dystocia.

Excessive Maternal Weight Gain

Schwartz and Dixon (1958) studied 50 cases of shoulder dystocia; 14 percent of the mothers gained over 30 pounds, and 32 percent of shoulder dystocia cases occurred in women weighing more than 180 pounds. In 80 percent of these cases, the fetus weighed more than 4000 g. Nathanson (1950) found that of patients who delivered babies weighing 4500 g or more, 27 percent had gained at least 33 pounds. A positive linear association exists between maternal weight gain during pregnancy and birthweight (Niswander and associates, 1969).

Prior Shoulder Dystocia

Shoulder dystocia in a previous pregnancy is thought by some to be a risk factor in subsequent pregnancies; this has been mentioned in the literature but has not been substantiated (Hernandez and Wendel, 1990).

Contracted Pelvis and Platypelloid Pelvis

In one study, a contracted pelvis did not contribute to shoulder dystocia except in cases where birthweight was less than 4000 g; among 10 cases of shoulder dystocia with birthweight under 4000 g, 5 were noted to have borderline maternal pelvic measurements (Schwartz and Dixon, 1958). Seigworth (1966) reported a series of 51 cases of shoulder dystocia; x-ray pelvimetry was available in 9 cases. A platypelloid pelvis was found in 2 cases, and reduced anteroposterior and posterior sagittal diameters of the outlet were evident in a third case. Six cases showed no evidence of contraction of the bony pelvis by x-ray. Clinical pelvimetry indicated that 47 cases were normal and 4 were contracted; a J-shaped coccyx with forward projection was suggested in 10 cases. Although these retrospective observations are interesting, this data is of limited clinical utility because a contracted pelvis cannot be clinically diagnosed with precision.

Prior Macrosomic Infant

From the previous discussion of macrosomia, it is apparent that interpretation of data is made difficult by varying definitions of the weight that defines "macrosomia." Some studies have suggested that delivery of a prior macrosomic infant increases the risk of shoulder dystocia; 8 of 31 women who experienced shoulder dystocia in one series had delivered 4082 g (9 lb) or larger infants in previous pregnancies without difficulty (Swartz, 1960). Schwartz and Dixon (1958) found that 44 percent of women who had shoulder dystocia had previously given birth to infants weighing more than 4000 g. Seigworth (1966) noted that 35 percent of women experiencing a shoulder dystocia had given birth previously to an infant weighing at least 4000 g. In a retrospective analysis of 185 shoulder dystocia patients, one of 79 with birthweight < 4,000 g and 31 of 106 with birthweight > 4000 g had had a previous infant weighing > 4000 g (Nocon and associates, 1993). In contrast, Lazer and colleagues (1986) found a relative decrease in shoulder dystocia, Erb's palsy, and clavicular fracture in women who had previously given birth to an infant weighing > 4500 g. These data would, in composite, seem to best justify an approach of individualized management.

Intrapartum Risk Factors

Prolonged Second Stage of Labor

Prolonged second stage of labor has been associated with increased risk of shoulder dystocia (Benedetti and Gabbe, 1978; Acker, 1985, 1986; SJ Gross, 1987; TL Gross, 1987; and their co-workers). Benedetti and Gabbe (1978) noted that the overall incidence of shoulder dystocia was 0.37 percent of 8890 vertex vaginal deliveries in contrast to 0.16 percent in the absence of a prolonged second stage and midpelvic delivery. However, with a prolonged second stage and midpelvic delivery, the incidence of shoulder dystocia was 4.6 percent. If the birthweight exceeded 4000 g, the second stage was prolonged, and midpelvic delivery was performed, the incidence of shoulder dystocia was 23 percent. TL Gross and associates (1987) reported midforceps delivery in 50 percent and prolonged second stage in 25 percent of their cases of shoulder dystocia, with a combination of prolonged second stage and midforceps delivery in 21 percent of cases of shoulder dystocia. Acker and co-workers (1985) found that 22 percent of patients with a shoulder dystocia had protraction disorders and 8 percent had arrest disorders; however, 70 percent of patients with shoulder dystocia had a normal labor pattern.

Oxytocin Administration

The association of oxytocin administration may be a secondary factor in the development of shoulder dystocia, but there is no evidence of a direct causal link. The apparent connection between shoulder dystocia and oxytocin administration may be related to the compounds used to augment or induce labor in cases of labor disorders or fetal macrosomia.

Mid-forceps and Mid-vacuum Extraction

Operative vaginal deliveries have been associated with shoulder dystocia. Benedetti and Gabbe (1978) found a nonstatistically significant trend toward a higher incidence of shoulder dystocia with vacuum extraction compared to delivery with Kielland forceps. Since the tractive forces that can be achieved with forceps greatly exceed those with a vacuum, these observations may reflect an erroneous assumption by the physician that shoulder dystocias are less likely to occur with vacuum than with forceps. Moreover, Broekhuizen and associates (1987) reported a 3.1 percent incidence of shoulder dystocia in women delivered by vacuum extraction compared to a 0.3 percent incidence in a group delivered by forceps. However, the vacuum group had a higher incidence of midpelvic delivery, an increase in mean birthweight, and an increase in birthweights greater than 4000 g. McFarland (1986) also found a higher incidence of Erb's palsy with midforceps delivery and vacuum extraction compared to deliveries accomplished with low forceps, spontaneous vaginal delivery, and cesarean section.

PREDICTING SHOULDER DYSTOCIA: ULTRASOUND EVALUATION OF THE MACROSOMIC FETUS

Various sonographic parameters such as biparietal diameter, abdominal area, femur length to abdominal circumference ratio, and estimated fetal weight have been studied to predict birthweight and neonatal complications. Seigworth (1966) found that the neonatal chest circumference was greater than or equal to the head circumference in 33 of 41 cases (80%) of shoulder dystocia. Kitzmiller and associates (1987) measured fetal shoulder width by computed tomography in diabetic women. A shoulder measurement exceeding 14 cm predicted a birthweight over 4200 g with a sensitivity of 100 percent, specificity of 87 percent, positive predictive value of 78 percent, and negative predictive value of 100 percent. This technique was limited by factors such as non-longitudinal lie, extreme maternal obesity, fetal motion, and maternal movement.

Elliot and co-workers (1982) defined the "macrosomia index" as the chest diameter minus the biparietal diameter. A macrosomia index of 1.4 cm was proposed as a critical value to avoid hazardous vaginal deliveries and birth injuries. Yarkoni and co-workers (1985) studied fetal clavicular measurements by ultrasound and found a close linear correlation with gestational age, but in this study did not report results with respect to birthweight or the occurrence of shoulder dystocia.

Bochner and colleagues (1987) evaluated the utility of ultrasound measurements of abdominal circumference at 30–33 weeks in gestational diabetics in the prediction of macrosomia. An abdominal circumference at or below the 90th percentile for gestational age accurately predicted the absence of macrosomia, dystocia, and birth trauma. Fetal abdominal circumference greater than the 90th percentile between 30 and 33 weeks was not an accurate predictor of macrosomia at term, but was associated with an increase in labor dystocia, shoulder dystocia, and birth trauma. Four out of 43 infants (9.3%) with an abdominal circumference greater than the 90th percentile at 30–33 weeks had shoulder dystocia, whereas one of 121 (0.8%) with an abdominal circumference less than or equal to the 90th percentile at 30–33 weeks had shoulder dystocia.

Morgan and co-investigators (1986) developed the "fetal–pelvic index" as an indicator of fetal–pelvic disproportion. Ultrasound was used to measure fetal head circumference, and maternal x-ray pelvimetry measured the inlet circumference and the midpelvis circumference. This method had a sensitivity of 85 percent and a specificity of 92 percent in predicting shoulder dystocia. These authors found that the false negatives tended to be occiput posterior at delivery. Even the false positives all had a difficult vaginal delivery.

Accurate prediction of birthweight has been attempted; unfortunately, there is a 15 percent error for estimated fetal weight even by experienced sonographers (Deter and Hadlock, 1985). Benacerraf and co-authors (1988) found the sensitivity of ultrasound for identifying a fetus with macrosomia, defined as a birthweight > 4000 g, to be 65 percent. We agree with Sandmire (1993) that current ultrasound fetal weight estimates are not accurate in detecting fetal macrosomia.

MANAGEMENT OF SHOULDER DYSTOCIA

Since shoulder dystocia is a rare and unpredictable event, prospective clinical trials to determine optimal methods of management have not been and are not likely to be performed. Nocon and co-workers (1993), in an analysis of risk in obstetric maneuvers for shoulder dystocia, felt that no single delivery method for shoulder dystocia was superior to another with respect to neonatal injury. Thus, they felt that no protocol should serve to substitute for clinical judgment and that any reasonable methods were appropriate. Guidelines have been published for the management of shoulder dystocia, primarily to educate the clinician about the importance of implementing a planned series of maneuvers in order to reduce delay and fetal risk. One such protocol is proposed by the American College of Obstetricians and Gynecologists (Table 13–6). The authors recommend that every delivery immediately proceed uninterrupted until the anterior shoulder clears the symphysis pubis before either suctioning the fetus or checking for a nuchal cord. In theory the shoulders should be prevented from going into full extension as they enter the mid-pelvis if rapid delivery of the anterior shoulder is accomplished.

TABLE 13–6. MANAGEMENT OF SHOULDER DYSTOCIA

Additional help is summoned, including anesthesia and pediatrics
Initial gentle attempt at traction, assisted by maternal expulsive forces
Suprapubic pressure
Generous episiotomy
McRoberts maneuver
Rotation of anterior shoulder
Transabdominal: suprapubic pressure
Transvaginal: back of anterior scapula
Woods screw maneuver
Posterior arm extraction
Clavicular fracture
Other Methods to Consider:
Intentional fracture of clavicle
Zavanelli maneuver
Abdominal rescue
Controversial Methods:
Fundal pressure
Symphysiotomy
Cleidotomy

Modified from American College of Obstetricians and Gynecologists (1991a).

Downward Traction

Initial management should include gentle downward traction with maternal expulsive efforts. Swartz (1960) recommended rapid examination of the infant as far within the birth canal as the hand can be inserted, and avoidance of excessive angulation of the fetal neck. Morris (1955) studied the brachial

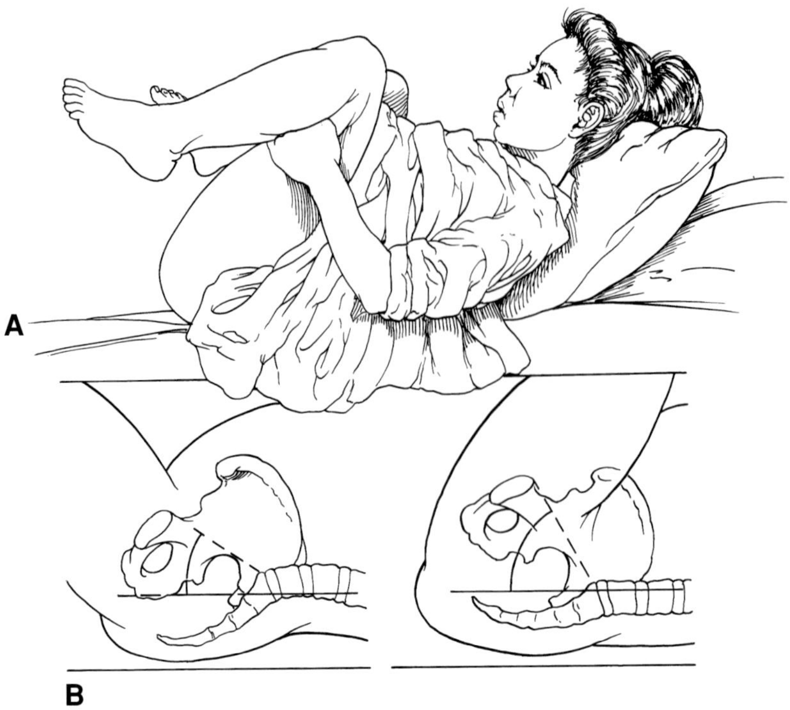

Figure 13–3. McRoberts maneuver. The legs are removed from the stirrups **(A),** and sharply flexed upon the abdomen, thus straightening the sacrum relative to the lumbar spine, with consequent rotation of the symphysis pubis cephalad and a decrease in the angle of inclination **(B).** (Modified from Gabbe, 1986, with permission.)

plexus of babies at autopsy; he concluded that traction is least likely to injure the brachial plexus when the cervical and thoracic spine are in a straight line, and that flexion, torsion, and jerking of the neck should be avoided. Using tactile sensing gloves to measure traction forces, Gonik and co-workers (Sorab, 1988; Gonik, 1989; and their co-workers) studied the clinician-applied forces with varying degrees of difficulty during delivery. The peak force significantly increased from routine delivery (< 60 Newtons), to difficult delivery (60–90 Newtons), and delivery complicated by shoulder dystocia (> 90 Newtons). Gonik's group recommended that the clinician be alert to the degree of force (traction) applied. Coincident with gentle downward traction, a request should be made for delivery assistance, an anesthesiologist, and a pediatric attendant.

Episiotomy

An episiotomy may be cut or extended in order to provide more room for manipulation posteriorly and to avoid other lacerations of the birth canal. The episiotomy may be extended laterally (mediolateral) or medially (episioproctotomy). Resnik (1980) and Hibbard (1969, 1982) favored an episioproctotomy in order to maximize space, reduce blood loss, facilitate repair, and provide more comfortable wound healing. Harris (1984) recommended a mediolateral episiotomy for more room if necessary, and Hopwood (1982) reported the use of bilateral mediolateral episiotomies in certain cases.

McRoberts Maneuver

Many contemporary reviews promote the McRoberts maneuver (Fig. 13–3) as a primary technique to resolve shoulder dystocia. The McRoberts maneuver as described originally by Gonik and co-workers (1983) involves exaggerated flexion of the patient's legs, similar to a knee–chest position. This results in straightening of the sacrum relative to the lumbar spine and consequent rotation of the symphysis pubis cephalad, with a decrease in the angle of inclination. This maneuver is not reported to change the dimensions of the true pelvis, but rather rotates the symphysis superiorly, thus freeing the impacted anterior shoulder without manipulation of the fetus. In a laboratory model, the McRoberts maneuver decreased shoulder extraction forces, brachial plexus stretching, and the incidence of clavicular fracture (Gonik and associates, 1989).

Woods Maneuver

Woods (1943) described a technique to release the impacted shoulder, "based on a well-known law of physics applicable to the screw.

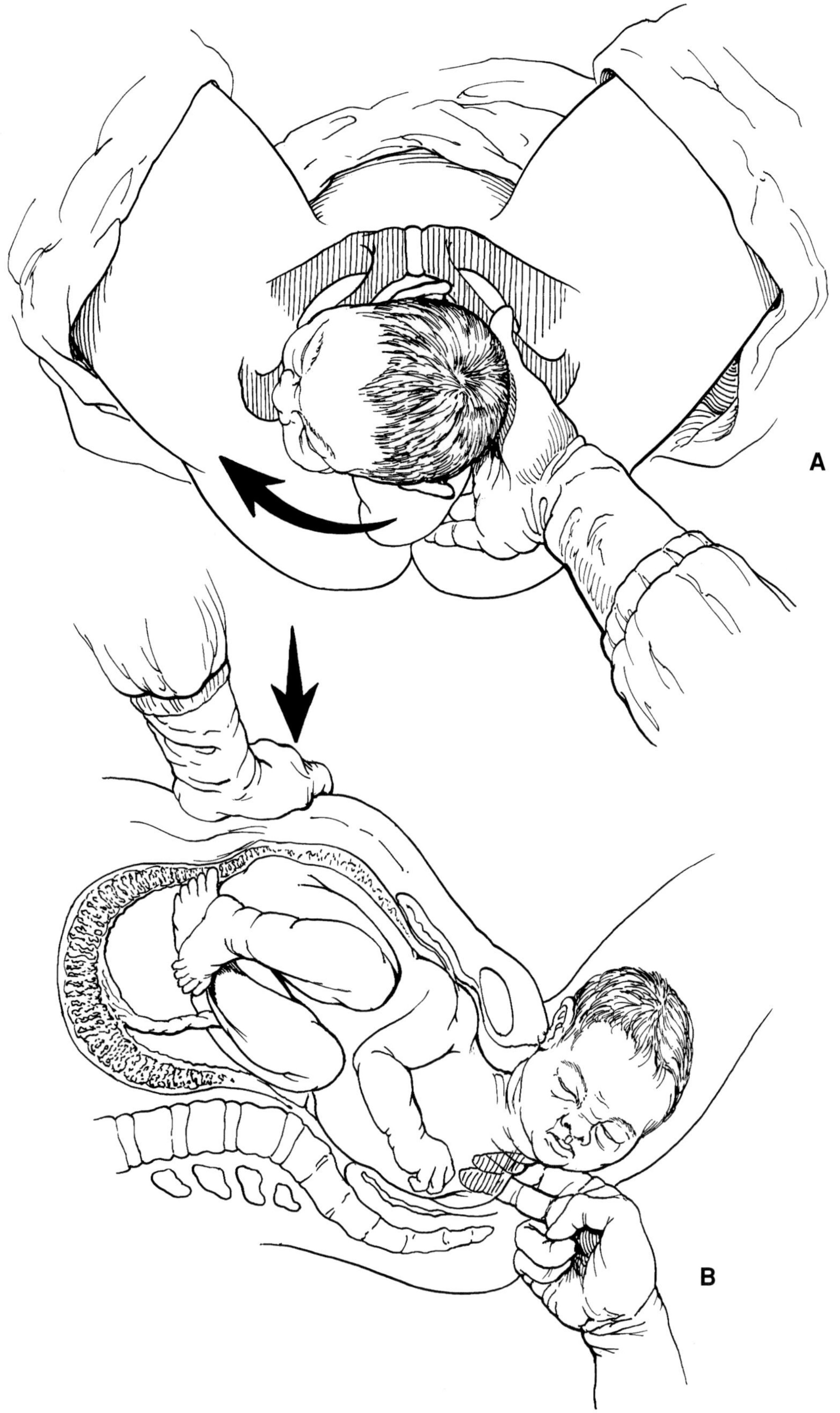

Figure 13–4. Modified Woods maneuver. **A.** The operator's hand is placed on the posterior aspect of the posterior shoulder, which is rotated like a screw in a clockwise fashion, thus releasing the anterior shoulder. **B.** Longitudinal view of Woods maneuver demonstrating rotation of the posterior shoulder. Depicted as originally described with simultaneous fundal pressure.

A screw is a continuous spiral incline plane, which when engaged in suitable threads is used where we wish to create the greatest resistance to its release by a direct pull. It follows, then, that a direct pull is the most difficult way to release a screw." He further described the anterior and posterior fetal shoulder passing through three threads, the symphysis pubis, the sacral promontory, and the coccyx. In the vertex presentation, Woods recommended "a downward thrust . . . with the left hand on the buttocks of the baby. At the same time two fingers of the right hand, on the anterior aspect of the posterior shoulder, make gentle clockwise pressure upward around the circumference of the arc to, and past, twelve o'clock." This maneuver should deliver the posterior shoulder. Woods stated that the pressure on the fetal buttocks should be applied from above by the operator, not by the assistant, in order to synchronize the pressure of the two hands. Figure 13–4 shows the modified Woods maneuver with pressure extended on the posterior aspect of the shoulder.

Posterior Arm Extraction

If delivery of the fetus is unsuccessful at this stage, Hernandez and Wendel (1990) recommend induction of general anesthesia for subsequent maneuvers unless adequate regional anesthesia are already in effect. Many operators at this stage prefer extraction of the posterior arm (Fig. 13–5). The hand is gently inserted along the curvature of the sacrum. If the fetal back is toward the right, the right hand is used, and if the back of the fetus is toward the left, then the left hand is used. The fingers of the operator follow along the humerus to the antecubital fossa, and with the forefinger pressure is made in a maneuver similar to the Pinard maneuver in breech extraction. As the arm flexes, the index finger grabs the forearm of the infant and gently sweeps it across the chest and face of the fetus and out of the vagina. In up to 18 percent of cases in older series it was necessary to deliberately fracture the humerus to accomplish this maneuver. It is then usually possible to complete delivery of the anterior shoulder with traction and pressure. When the baby is excessively large, it may be necessary to rotate the extracted posterior arm and shoulder anteriorly and to repeat the above maneuver on the posterior arm and shoulder. Schwartz and Dixon (1958) noted that traction and fundal pressure resulted in a 16 percent neonatal death rate, whereas all 17 infants delivered by posterior arm extraction survived.

Suprapubic Pressure

Suprapubic pressure also may be used (Fig. 13–6), and the maneuver is simple to perform. Many authors suggest suprapubic pressure as one of the initial measures to overcome shoulder dystocia (ACOG, 1991b; Benedetti, 1989; Carlan and associates, 1991; Harris, 1984; Hernandez and Wendel, 1990; Morrison and associates, 1992; O'Leary and Leonetti, 1990; Resnick, 1980; Rubin, 1964). Lee (1987) reported 6 cases of brachial plexus injury in 1983, with 5 of the 6 cases associated with the use of suprapubic pressure. After implementation of the McRoberts maneuver at their institution in 1984, there was only one case of brachial plexus injury during a similar time interval; thus he recommended avoidance of excessive suprapubic pressure. However, there is no evidence that suprapubic pressure contributes to brachial plexus injury, and it remains a mainstay in shoulder dystocia management.

Rubin's Maneuver

At the University of Pennsylvania, Rubin (1964) described two maneuvers for managing shoulder dystocia. The first uses transabdominal rocking of the fetal shoulders to disimpact the anterior shoulder and permit the shoulders to find a more favorable diameter through the pelvis for descent (Fig. 13–7A). The second maneuver is performed vaginally and uses adduction of the most accessible shoulder to reduce the circumference and transverse diameter of the shoulders (Figs. 13–7B, C). Rubin pointed out that the Woods maneuver abducts the posterior shoulder by placing the operator's fingers on the anterior aspect of the posterior shoulder and pushing the shoulder toward the fetus's back. He states that this results in a larger shoulder circumference and transverse diameter compared to abducting the accessible shoulder. Measuring shoulder dimensions of newborns, Rubin showed that the adducted shoulder has a smaller transverse diameter than the abducted shoulder, which is smaller than the straightened shoulder.

Cephalic Replacement

If the foregoing maneuvers are unsuccessful, other techniques can be used to deliver the baby. The Zavanelli maneuver (cephalic replacement) was originally described by Sand-

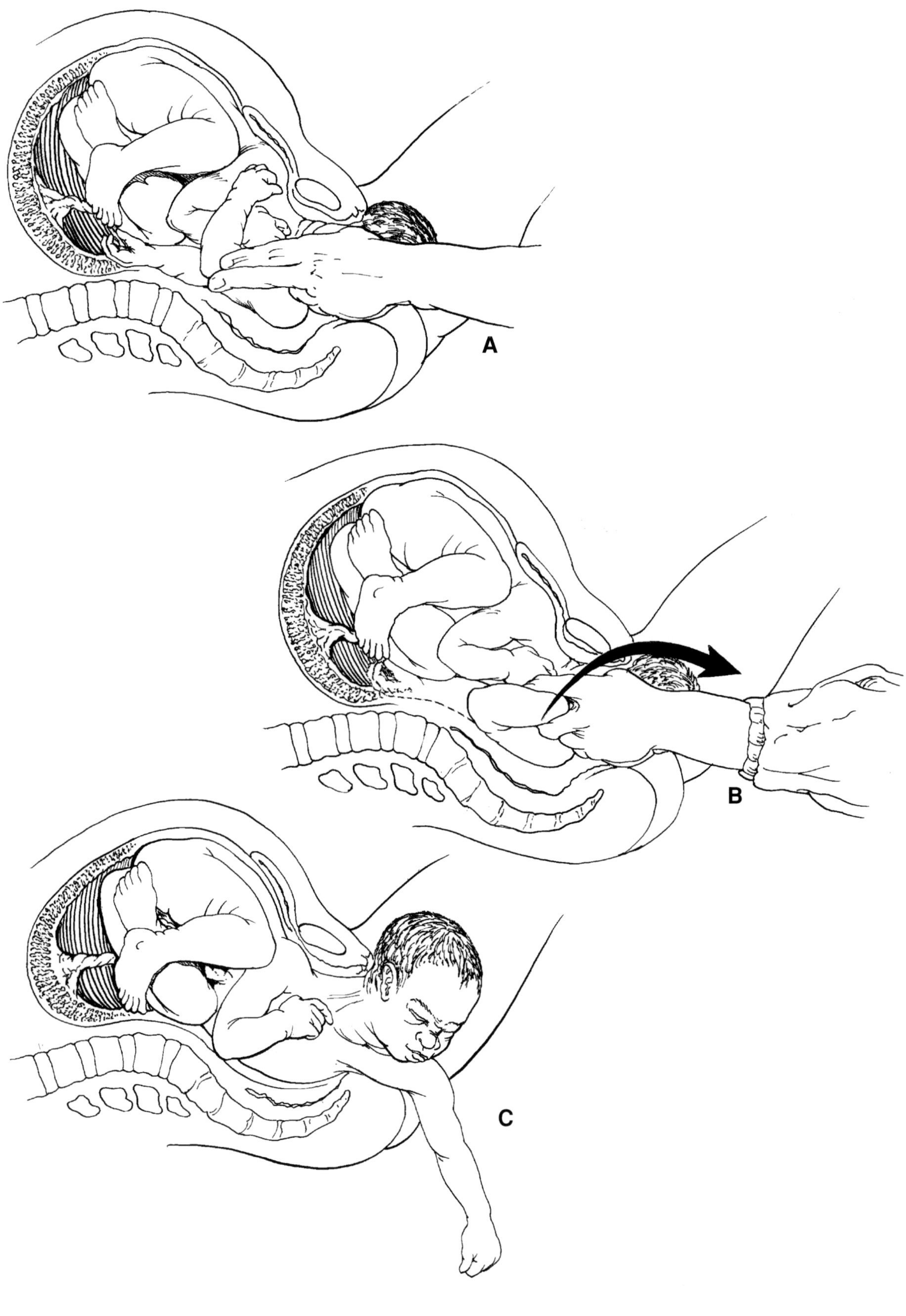

Figure 13–5. Delivery of posterior arm. **A.** The operator's hand is introduced into the vagina and the fetal humerus is located and pressure is applied in the antecubital fossa. **B.** The fetal arm is swept across the chest. **C.** The fetal hand is then grasped and extended along the chest and face, thus delivering the posterior arm from the vagina.

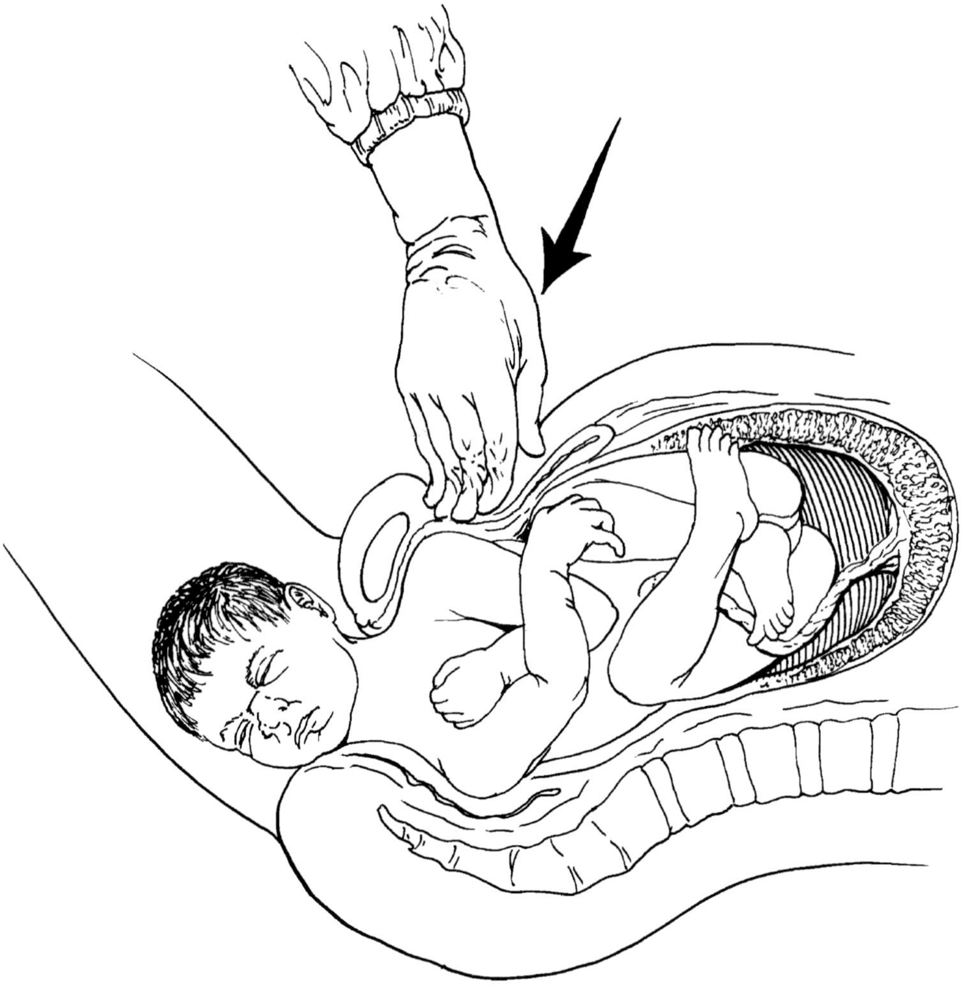

Figure 13–6. Suprapubic pressure. An assistant applies oblique suprapubic pressure to free the anterior shoulder. The force should be directed at about a 45-degree angle off of vertical to move the fetal shoulder not only down, but also laterally toward the fetal chest.

berg (1985), who attributed the first case to Dr. William Zavanelli, performed in 1978. The fetal head is returned to its previous intravaginal location and the fetus is extracted by cesarean section as soon as practical (Fig. 13–8). O'Leary and Gunn (1985) reported four cases that occurred between 1976 and 1985; they recommended placement of a fetal scalp electrode for continuous fetal monitoring and subcutaneous terbutaline for uterine relaxation at delivery. Sandberg (1988) presented 15 additional cases; three of the dystocia cases were secondary to sacrococcygeal teratoma, rather than shoulder dystocia obstruction of delivery. Others have described experience with this maneuver (Gallaspy, 1991; Graham, 1992; and their colleagues). Recently O'Leary (1993) reported 59 cases from a registry; in two cases, hysterectomy was required secondary to uterine rupture.

Abdominal Rescue

O'Leary and Cuva (1992) also have described "abdominal rescue" after failed cephalic replacement as a final effort in delivery of the fetus, whereby low transverse hysterotomy is performed and the fetal shoulder is assisted below the symphysis pubis, followed by vaginal delivery of the infant (Figs. 13–9A, B). The abdominal rescue had previously been

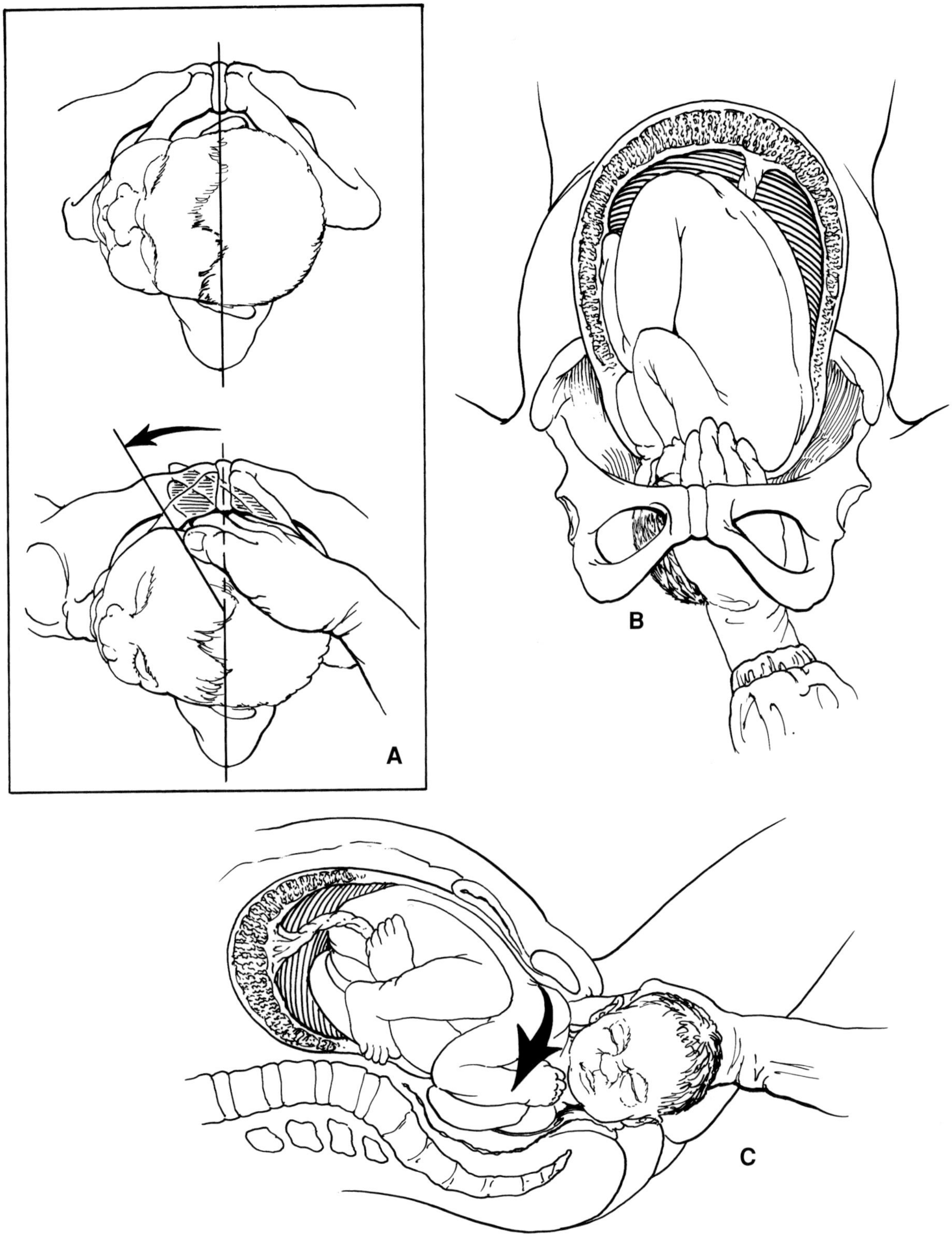

Figure 13–7. Rubin's maneuver. Rubin's first maneuver: The anterior shoulder is transabdominally disimpacted by rocking it from side to side. **A, B.** Rubin's second maneuver: The most accessible shoulder is abducted, thus reducing the shoulder circumference and transverse diameter. **C.** It is abducted by counterclockwise pressure on the anterior shoulder for the fetus in LOT position.

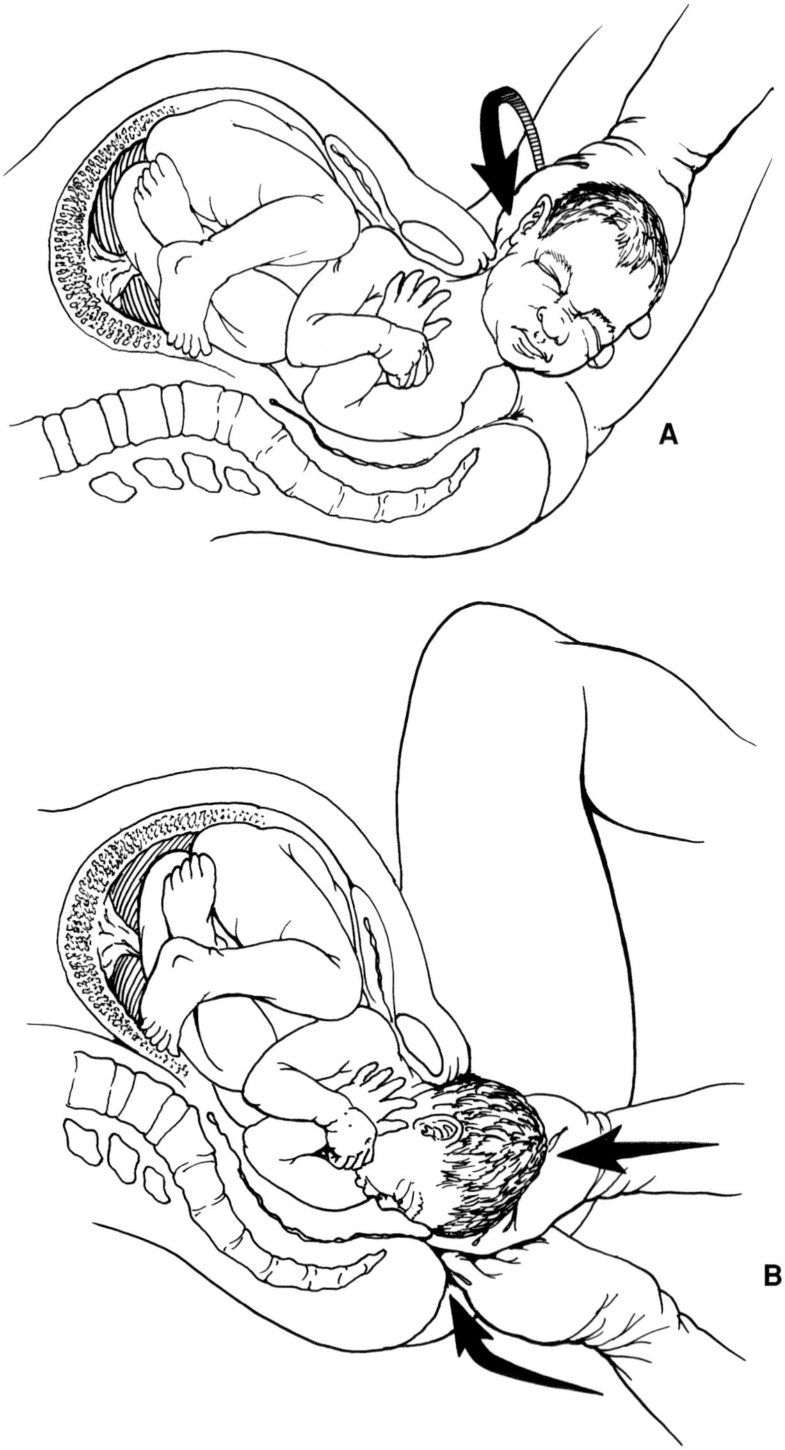

Figure 13–8. Zavanelli maneuver. **A.** If restitution has occurred, the head is manually rotated to the pre-restitution position, full extension, and occiput anterior. **B.** The head is manually flexed recapitulating, in reverse, delivery of the head, with gentle upward pressure.

described in the context of breech delivery with entrapment of the aftercoming fetal head (Iffy and co-workers, 1986).

Symphysiotomy

Subcutaneous symphysiotomy (Chap. 6) has been described as a technique to overcome moderate cephalopelvic disproportion and avoid cesarean section in developing countries (Hartfield, 1973a, 1986). It can be performed with a urethral catheter and a scalpel in just 5 minutes (Hartfield, 1973a, 1986). Although this technique is described primarily to overcome cephalopelvic disproportion, some

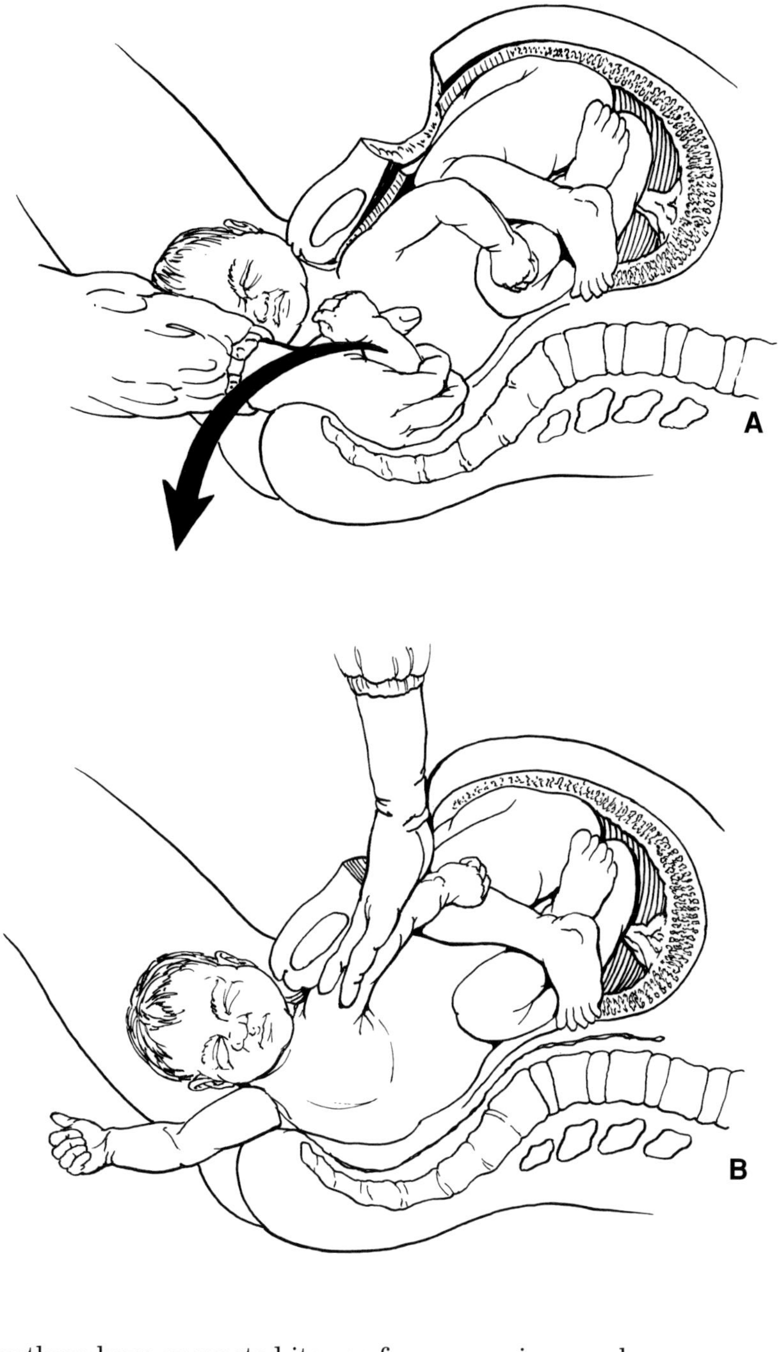

Figure 13–9. Abdominal rescue **A.** As the anterior shoulder is abducted and slightly rotated, the infant descends, allowing the posterior arm to be grasped and delivered. **B.** Abdominally applied direct downward pressure on the anterior shoulder allows the infant's body to be delivered.

authors have suggested its use for overcoming shoulder dystocia (Schramm, 1983; Sandberg, 1985; Hartfield, 1986).

Clavicular Fracture

Deliberate fracture of the clavicle can be performed in order to reduce the diameter of the fetal shoulders. To avoid subclavian vascular injury, the clavicle is broken most safely by upward pressure against its midportion (Rubin, 1964). Cleidotomy, or cutting of the clavicle with scissors, is usually reserved for a dead fetus (Schwartz and Dixon, 1958; McCall, 1962), because compound fracture often results in trauma to the pleural cavity (Seigworth, 1966).

Fundal Pressure

Fundal pressure is highly controversial. Schwartz and Dixon (1958) noted a significantly higher neonatal death rate with traction and fundal pressure compared to posterior arm extraction. TL Gross and colleagues (1987) found that when used to treat shoulder dystocia, fundal pressure resulted in a 77 percent complication rate and a high incidence of orthopedic and neurologic damage. Fundal pressure may result in further impaction of the shoulder against the symphysis pubis and uterine rupture; in addition, it is associated with the highest rate of neonatal injury of any method to manage shoulder dystocia (ACOG, 1991b). Perhaps the only place for fundal pressure is in concert with either external (suprapubic pressure) or internal rotational procedures such as the Woods or Rubin's maneuvers. Clearly, simultaneous fundal pressure and traction on the fetal head should be used only when brain damage or death of the fetus are likely unless delivery is immediately accomplished.

Other Maneuvers

Birthing centers have proposed other positional maneuvers to correct shoulder dystocia. The "all-fours maneuver" places the patient on her hands and knees (Meenan and associates, 1991). Squatting has been suggested in order to increase the capacity of the pelvic outlet (Kurokawa and Zilkoski, 1985; Carter, 1986). Shute (1962) has reported rotation (but not extraction) of the fetal shoulders with the Shute parallel forceps. A stainless steel instrument called "the shoulder horn" was reported by Chavis (1978–79) for shoulder dystocia management.

ROLE OF CESAREAN DELIVERY

Although O'Leary and Leonetti (1990) recommend a "liberal policy for cesarean section" for risk factors such as diabetes, obesity, postterm pregnancy, excessive fetal weight, or excessive maternal weight gain, Gimbel (1990) points out that it is only the rare obstetric patient that does not have at least one or several of these risk factors. Nagey (1990) concluded that shoulder dystocia is not preventable without an increase in cesarean-related maternal morbidity and mortality. Indeed, while there are occasional opinions to the contrary, no data exist to show that a prospective management scheme involving cesarean section for *any* combination of risk factors actually reduces the risk of shoulder dystocia without an unacceptable increase in maternal morbidity.

The majority opinion is that shoulder dystocia is not preventable without excessive use of cesarean section. Delpapa and Mueller-Heubach (1991) concluded that neither cesarean section nor labor induction would be helpful in nondiabetic women with macrosomic infants weighing more than 4000 g. SJ Gross and associates (1987) felt that cesarean section should be considered in cases with estimated fetal weight in excess of 4500 g. In a study of macrosomic infants weighing over 4500 g, Spellacy and co-workers (1985) found a significantly increased risk of birth injury for vaginal delivery (9.3%) compared to those infants delivered by cesarean section (2.6%). In consideration of a 10 percent error in estimated fetal weight, they recommended cesarean section for an estimated fetal weight over 5000 g to reduce fetal trauma.

Acker and co-workers (1985, 1988) advocate cesarean section for diabetic women with an estimated fetal weight exceeding 4000 g in order to reduce the incidence of shoulder dystocia and Erb-Duchenne palsy. Keller and co-investigators (1991), for their population of gestational diabetics, estimated that a perfectly executed protocol designed to deliver all fetuses weighing over 4000 g by cesarean section would increase the total number of non-elective cesarean sections from 53 to 98. These additional 45 cesarean sections would have prevented 8 of 15 shoulder dystocias and one permanent brachial plexus injury. Emphasizing the limitations of fetal weight estimations, they concluded that a policy of cesarean section for all fetuses thought to weigh more than 4000 g would considerably increase the cesarean rate with minimal fetal/neonatal benefit. In contrast, Langer and colleagues (1991) recommended cesarean delivery for diabetic women with an estimated fetal weight > 4250 g. They estimated that 76 percent of shoulder dystocias could be prevented in the diabetic group with an increase of only 0.26 percent in their institutional cesarean section rate. Calculated another way, 158 cesarean sections would be performed to prevent 38 cases of shoulder dystocia.

Sandmire and O'Halloin (1988) found that only 2 of 73 infants with shoulder dystocia had persistent injuries, specifically mild arm weakness. Both babies in their series had estimated fetal weights below 4000 g. Nocon and co-workers (1993) retrospectively studied 185 cases of shoulder dystocia that occurred between 1986 and 1990. They commented that if newborns weighing > 4000 g could have been accurately predicted, routine cesarean section would have prevented 106 cases of shoulder dystocia, but not permanent injury.

Boyd and associates (1983) showed that increasing the cesarean section rate for macrosomic infants from 8 percent in the 1960s to 21 percent between 1978 and 1980 did not improve perinatal outcome. There was a higher incidence of birth trauma in the latter period, suggesting that decreased experience with difficult vaginal delivery may have reduced the skills of the accoucheur as cesarean delivery became more frequent.

Benedetti (1989) estimated the risk of permanent brachial plexus injury following shoulder dystocia to be 3/100 occurrences; thus the chance of permanent fetal injury reaches 1 percent only when the incidence of shoulder dystocia exceeds 33 percent, which is rare. When the risk of shoulder dystocia is approximately 25 percent (diabetic with fetal weight 4000–4500 g or nondiabetic with fetal weight > 4500 g), the risk for permanent brachial plexus injury is 8/1000. Given the known degree of inaccuracy with current methods to estimate fetal weight, he states there are relatively few indications for performing elective cesarean section to avoid fetal injury.

Hofmeyr (1992) correctly states that decisions regarding mode of delivery should be based upon prevention of birth trauma, as many cases of shoulder dystocia are associated with no adverse sequelae. Furthermore, he believes that more would be achieved in reducing the morbidity associated with shoulder dystocia by assuring that all birth attendants are proficient in shoulder dystocia management, rather than by trying to eliminate shoulder dystocia by abdominal delivery. In summary, while some authors recommend consideration of cesarean section for infants of known diabetic mothers when estimated fetal weight exceeds 4000–4250 g, and abdominal delivery for nondiabetic patients when estimated weight exceeds 4500–5000 g, no data exist to document that such policies actually prevent sufficient neurologic injury to justify the required increase in cesarean section rate. Thus, standard of care cannot be said to mandate cesarean section for fetal macrosomia at any specific estimated weight.

COMPLICATIONS

Neonatal Complications

Neonatal complications of shoulder dystocia include death, asphyxia, brachial plexus injuries, and bone fractures. Fractures of the clavicle are more common than those of the humerus. In a review of the literature, Sandmire and O'Halloin (1988) calculated an 11.8 percent incidence of brachial plexus palsy, 7.9 percent incidence of stillbirth, 4.3 percent incidence of severe asphyxia, 2.9 percent incidence of neonatal death, and 2.9 percent incidence of meconium aspiration associated with shoulder dystocia. Perinatal mortality of shoulder dystocia is reported to range between 19 and 289 per 1000 (Hernandez and Wendel, 1990).

Buschmann and Sager (1987) found that Erb-Duchenne palsy is the most frequent brachial plexus injury. Erb-Duchenne palsy involves C-5 through C-6 nerve roots, Klumpke palsy involves C-8 and T-1 nerve roots, and combined brachial plexus palsies involve C-5 through T-1. Right brachial plexus injuries were more common than left brachial plexus injuries, possibly secondary to the more common left occiput anterior fetal position. McFarland (1986) estimated that one case in six of shoulder dystocia resulted in Erb's palsy. Acker and associates (1988) reported Erb-Duchenne palsy was more common in diabetics (10.5/1000 deliveries) than in nondiabetics (0.56/1000 deliveries).

Curran (1981) defines birth injuries as those associated with mechanical forces producing hemorrhage, edema, tissue disruption, or alteration in organ function, occurring during the intrapartum period. In a review of birth associated injury, Curran reported that 80 percent of Erb's palsies recovered by 3–6 months but only 40 percent of Klumpke palsies recovered by 1 year. The combination of Erb-Duchenne-Klumpke palsy resulted in a poor prognosis for recovery.

In a study of 48 cases of brachial plexus palsy in Sweden, Sjoberg and co-workers (1988) found that most cases recovered within the first 6 months, and all cases that were to recover (73%) did so by 18 months. Data from the Collaborative Perinatal Study identified 52 cases of brachial paralysis: at 4 months of age 88 percent were recovered, and at 12 months 92 percent were recovered (Gordon and colleagues, 1973). Hardy (1981) studied 36 infants in New Zealand with brachial plexus injuries, with shoulder dystocia noted in only 10 cases. Two cases of brachial plexus injuries occurred following cesarean section; 80 percent of brachial plexus injuries were noted to have full recovery by 13 months of age.

Benedetti and Gabbe (1978) reported five humeral or clavicular fractures, three Erb's palsies, and one abnormal neurologic examination among 19 neonates with shoulder dystocia associated with prolonged second stage and midpelvic delivery. In a study of 573 macrosomic (> 4500 g) infants, Spellacy and co-workers (1985) noted a statistically significant increase of birth injury in the vaginal delivery group (9.3%, n = 378) versus the cesarean group (2.6%, n = 195).

Prompt recognition, management, and resolution of shoulder dystocia is necessary to avoid permanent neonatal injury. Following delivery of the fetal head, compression of the umbilical cord in the birth canal occurs with concomitant inability of the fetus to spontaneously breath. Wood and co-investigators (1973) demonstrated a drop in pH of 0.04 units/minute following delivery of the fetal head.

Boyd and associates (1983) reported an incidence of severe birth asphyxia of 14/1000 spontaneous macrosomic deliveries, and 143/1000 macrosomic deliveries complicated by shoulder dystocia. In a case control study of term neonates with early neonatal seizures, Patterson and associates (1989) found shoulder dystocia to be strongly associated with the development of early neonatal seizures.

Maternal Complications

Postpartum hemorrhage can occur secondary to uterine atony and lower genital tract lacerations of the cervix, vagina, and fourth-degree perineal tears. Nathanson (1950) reported increased hemorrhage secondary to uterine atony and lacerations of the birth canal. Hernandez and Wendel (1990) also mention infection, bladder atony, and uterine rupture as complications of shoulder dystocia. Benedetti and Gabbe (1978) reported an estimated blood loss greater than 1000 mL in 68 percent of cases of shoulder dystocia with prolonged second stage of labor.

In a study of 98 cases of shoulder dystocia, El Madany and co-workers (1991) found a 19.3 percent incidence of vaginal tears requiring repair, 14.2 percent incidence of postpartum hemorrhage, and a 1 percent incidence of ruptured uterus, compared to rates of 0.54 percent, 0.38 percent, and 0.06 percent, respectively, for the total hospital population. Goldaber and associates (1993) reviewed 390 cases of fourth-degree perineal tears at Parkland Memorial Hospital; shoulder dystocia was the only intrapartum characteristic that occurred more frequently in women with perineal morbidity than in women without perineal morbidity.

Physician Complications

A case of physical trauma to the physician is described (Schramm, 1983) during a difficult delivery, where a "crack" was heard in the delivery room by the attendants. It was thought that the fetal neck had been broken, but upon delivery of the fetus, the obstetrician noted pain and swelling of the left hand, believed to have been rupture of interosseous ligaments between the third and fourth fingers. The baby's Erb's palsy resolved in 72 hours, whereas the pain and edema of the obstetrician's hand was reported to resolve in 3 weeks. Unfortunately, medical/legal issues rather than physical injury are of more peril to the obstetrician. TL Gross and colleagues (1987) reported that 7 percent of 103 obstetrics and gynecology-related lawsuits filed at an affiliated hospital were related to shoulder dystocia. O'Leary and Leonetti (1990) stated "it is highly probable that in the future all shoulder impaction dystocias with a bad outcome will be litigated." Sandmire (1989) appropriately points out that the occurrence of shoulder dystocia and neonatal injury should not subsume negligence on the part of the physician. Nevertheless, it is incumbent upon all clinicians who deliver babies to be fully prepared for the event of shoulder dystocia, so that the issue can be rapidly and appropriately managed.

In the event of shoulder dystocia, it is important to provide a detailed written or dictated note of events, maneuvers, estimation of traction forces, timing of events, and neonatal evaluation for future review (Benedetti, 1989; Hernandez and Wendel, 1990; Acker, 1991). Acker (1991) has proposed a "shoulder dystocia intervention form." Table 13–7 summarizes pertinent information to be documented in the medical record. Best estimates of time on the perineum are obtained if a "cardiac arrest" or "event" clock is activated or a timekeeper is designated. Awareness of the duration of the shoulder dystocia should be integrated into the vigor of maneuvers being performed. Full discussion of the events should be disclosed to the patient in an honest manner (Benedetti, 1989).

TABLE 13–7. MEDICAL RECORD DOCUMENTATION OF SHOULDER DYSTOCIA

Delivery Note
Spontaneous or operative delivery
Indication for forceps or vacuum
Technique of delivery
Fetal station
Fetal position
Shoulder Dystocia Maneuvers
Estimation of traction forces
Specific maneuvers employed
Time interval from delivery of head to completion of delivery
Neonatal Condition
Estimated fetal weight
Actual fetal weight
Apgar scores
Umbilical cord gases
Moro reflex
Evidence of brachial plexus injury
Evidence of fracture, clavicle or humerus

Not all cases of brachial plexus palsy occur during the intrapartum period, but may be secondary to antepartum intrauterine events (Koenigsberger, 1980; Dunn and Engle, 1985; Jennett and co-workers, 1992; Hankins and Clark, 1995). Brachial plexus injury may also occur following cesarean section for cephalopelvic disproportion (Morrison and associates, 1992).

SUMMARY

Since shoulder dystocia is a rare, unpredictable, and catastrophic complication of obstetrics, a "shoulder dystocia drill" should be taught to all personnel involved in the delivery of babies (Mazzanti, 1959; Hernandez and Wendel, 1990). This practice should not be limited to obstetric residents, but should also include nurse midwives (Mashburn, 1988) and delivery nurses.

Most cases of shoulder dystocia are not preventable and fetal injury cannot always be avoided. The 19th edition of *Williams Obstetrics* (Cunningham and associates, 1993) states "While there are clearly several risk factors statistically associated with shoulder dystocia, actual identification of individual instances of shoulder dystocia before the fact has proven to be extremely difficult, if not impossible." As stated in the ACOG Technical Bulletin No. 159 (1991b), "It is not always possible to deliver an undamaged infant after shoulder dystocia has been encountered. Even when shoulder dystocia is managed optimally, brachial plexus injuries occur. Some of these injuries may be associated with the process of impaction at the symphysis or during descent of the shoulders into the pelvis."

REFERENCES

Acker DB. A shoulder dystocia intervention form. Obstet Gynecol 1991; 78:150–1.

Acker DB, Gregory KD, Sachs BP, Friedman EA. Risk factors for Erb-Duchenne palsy. Obstet Gynecol 1988; 71:389–92.

Acker DB, Sachs BP, Friedman EA. Risk factors for shoulder dystocia. Obstet Gynecol 1985; 66:762–8.

Acker DB, Sachs BP, Friedman EA. Risk factors for shoulder dystocia in the average-weight infant. Obstet Gynecol 1986; 67:614–8.

Al-Najashi S, al-Suleiman SA, el-Yahia A, et al. Shoulder dystocia—a clinical study of 56 cases. Aust NZ J Obstet Gynaecol 1989; 29:129–32.

Allen R, Sorab J, Gonik B. Risk factors for shoulder dystocia: an engineering study of clinician-applied forces. Obstet Gynecol 1991; 77:352–5.

American College of Obstetricians and Gynecologists. Diagnosis and management of postterm pregnancy. Technical Bulletin 130. Washington, DC: ACOG, 1989a.

American College of Obstetricians and Gynecologists. Dystocia. Technical Bulletin 137. Washington, DC: ACOG, 1989b.

American College of Obstetricians and Gynecologists. Operative vaginal delivery. Technical Bulletin 152. Washington, DC: ACOG, 1991a.

American College of Obstetricians and Gynecologists. Fetal macrosomia. Technical Bulletin 159. Washington, DC: ACOG, 1991b.

Benacerraf BR, Gelman R, Frigoletto FD. Sonographically estimated fetal weights: accuracy and limitation. Am J Obstet Gynecol 1988; 159: 1118–21.

Benedetti TJ. Added complications of shoulder dystocia. Contemp Obstet Gynecol 1989; 33:150–61.

Benedetti TJ, Gabbe SG. Shoulder dystocia. A complication of fetal macrosomia and prolonged second stage of labor with midpelvic delivery. Obstet Gynecol 1978; 52:526–9.

Berne C, Wibell L, Lindmark G. Ten-year experience of insulin treatment in gestational diabetes. Acta Paediatr Scand Suppl 1985; 320:85–93.

Bochner CJ, Medearis AL, Williams J, et al. Early third-trimester ultrasound screening in gestational diabetes to determine the risk of macroso-

mia and labor dystocia at term. Am J Obstet Gynecol 1987; 157:703–8.
Boyd ME, Usher RH, McLean FH. Fetal macrosomia: prediction, risks, proposed management. Obstet Gynecol 1983; 61:715–22.
Broekhuizen FF, Washington JM, Johnson F, Hamilton PR. Vacuum extraction versus forceps delivery: indications and complications, 1979 to 1984. Obstet Gynecol 1987; 69:338–42.
Buschmann WR, Sager G. Orthopaedic considerations in obstetric brachial plexus palsy. Orthop Rev 1987; 16:290–2.
Carlan SJ, Angel JL, Knuppel RA. Shoulder dystocia. Am Fam Physician 1991; 43:1307–11.
Carter V. Another technique for resolution of shoulder dystocia (letter). Am J Obstet Gynecol 1986; 154:964.
Chavis WM. A new instrument for the management of shoulder dystocia. Int J Gynaecol Obstet 1978–79; 16:331–2.
Clark SL. Macrosomic fetuses should not routinely be delivered by C/S. Contemp Obstet/Gynecol 1991; 36 (Special Issue): 56–60.
Combs CA, Singh NB, Khoury JC. Elective induction versus spontaneous labor after sonographic diagnosis of fetal macrosomia. Obstet Gynecol 1993; 81:492–6.
Cousins L, Dattel B, Hollingsworth D, et al. Screening for carbohydrate intolerance in pregnancy: a comparison of two tests and reassessment of a common approach. Am J Obstet Gynecol 1985; 153:381–5.
Coustan DR, Imarah J. Prophylactic insulin treatment of gestational diabetes reduces the incidence of macrosomia, operative delivery, and birth trauma. Am J Obstet Gynecol 1984; 150:836–42.
Cunningham FG, MacDonald PC, Gant NF, et al. Williams Obstetrics, 19th ed. Norwalk, CT: Appleton & Lange, 1993.
Curran, JS. Birth-associated injury. Clin Perinatol 1981; 8:111–29.
Delpapa EH, Mueller-Heubach E. Pregnancy outcome following ultrasound diagnosis of macrosomia. Obstet Gynecol 1991; 78:340–3.
Deter RL, Hadlock FP. Use of ultrasound in the detection of macrosomia: a review. J Clin Ultrasound 1985; 13:519–24.
Dignam WJ. Difficulties in delivery, including shoulder dystocia and malpresentations of the fetus. Clin Obstet Gynecol 1976; 19:577–85.
Dunn DW, Engle WA. Brachial plexus palsy: intrauterine onset. Pediatr Neurol 1985; 1:367–9.
Eastman NJ, Hellman LM (ed). Williams Obstetrics, 13th ed. New York: Appleton-Century-Crofts, 1966.
Eden RD, Seifert LS, Winegar A, Spellacy WN. Perinatal characteristics of uncomplicated postdate pregnancies. Obstet Gynecol 1987; 69: 296–9.
el-Madany AA, Jallad KB, Radi FA, et al. Shoulder dystocia: anticipation and outcome. Int J Gynaecol Obstet 1991; 34:7–12.
Elliott JP, Garite TJ, Freeman RK, et al. Ultrasonic prediction of fetal macrosomia in diabetic patients. Obstet Gynecol 1982; 60:159–62.
Gabbe S, Neibyl J, Simpson J. Obstetrics: normal and problem pregnancies. New York: Churchill Livingstone, 1986.
Gallaspy JW, Dunnihoo DR, DeGueurce JC, et al. Cephalic replacement in severe shoulder dystocia. South Med J 1991; 84:1373–4.
Gimbel GL. Can shoulder dystocia be predicted? (letter). Am J Obstet Gynecol 1990; 163:680.
Goldaber KG, Wendel PJ, McIntire DD, Wendel GD. Postpartum perineal morbidity after fourth-degree perineal repair. Am J Obstet Gynecol 1993; 168:489–93.
Golditch IM, Kirkman K. The large fetus. Management and outcome. Obstet Gynecol 1978; 52:26–30.
Gonik B, Allen R, Sorab J. Objective evaluation of the shoulder dystocia phenomenon: effect of maternal pelvic orientation on force reduction. Obstet Gynecol 1989; 74:44–8.
Gonik B, Hollyer VL, Allen R. Shoulder dystocia recognition: differences in neonatal risks for injury. Am J Perinatol 1991; 8:31–4.
Gonik B, Stringer CA, Held B. An alternate maneuver for management of shoulder dystocia. Am J Obstet Gynecol 1983; 145:882–4.
Gordon M, Rich H, Deutschberger J, Green M. The immediate and long-term outcome of obstetric birth trauma. Am J Obstet Gynecol 1973; 142:117–51.
Graham JM, Blanco JD, Wen T, Magee KP. The Zavanelli maneuver: a different perspective. Obstet Gynecol 1992; 79:883–4.
Gross SJ, Shime J, Farine D. Shoulder dystocia: predictors and outcome. A five-year review. Am J Obstet Gynecol 1987; 156:334–6.
Gross TL, Sokol RJ, Williams T, Thompson K. Shoulder dystocia: a fetal–physician risk. Am J Obstet Gynecol 1987; 156:1408–18.
Hankins GDV, Clark SL. Brachial plexus palsy involving the posterior shoulder at spontaneous vaginal delivery. Am J Perinatol (in press) 1995.
Hardy AE. Birth injuries of the brachial plexus. Incidence and prognosis. J Bone Joint Surg 1981; 63:98–101.
Harris BA. Shoulder dystocia. Clin Obstet Gynecol 1984; 27:106–11.
Hartfield VJ. A comparison of the early and late effects of subcutaneous symphysiotomy and of lower segment cesarean section. Aust NZ J Obstet Gynaecol 1973a; 13:147–52.
Hartfield VJ. Subcutaneous symphysiotomy—time for a reappraisal? J Obstet Gynecol Br Commonw 1973b; 80:508–14.
Hartfield VJ. Symphysiotomy for shoulder dystocia (letter). Am J Obstet Gynecol 1986; 155:228.

Hassan AA. Shoulder dystocia: risk factors and prevention. Aust NZ J Obstet Gynaecol 1988; 28:107–9.

Hernandez C, Wendel GD. Shoulder dystocia. Clin Obstet Gynecol 1990; 33:526–34.

Hibbard LT. Coping with shoulder dystocia. Contemp Obstet Gynecol 1982; 20:229–37.

Hibbard LT. Shoulder dystocia. Obstet Gynecol 1969; 34:424–9.

Hofmeyr GJ. Breech presentation and shoulder dystocia in childbirth. Curr Opin Obstet Gynecol 1992; 4:807–12.

Hopwood HG. Shoulder dystocia: fifteen years' experience in a community hospital. Am J Obstet Gynecol 1982; 144:162–6.

Iffy L. Macrosomia (letter). Obstet Gynecol 68:140, 1985.

Iffy L, Apuzzio JJ, Cohen-Addad N, et al. Abdominal rescue after entrapment of the aftercoming head. Am J Obstet Gynecol 1986; 154:623.

Jennett RJ, Tarby TJ, Kreinick CJ. Brachial plexus palsy: an old problem revisited. Am J Obstet Gynecol 1992; 166:1673–6.

Johnson SR, Kolberg BH, Varner MW, Railsback LD. Maternal obesity and pregnancy. Surg Gynecol Obstet 1987; 164:431–7.

Johnstone NR. Shoulder dystocia: a study of 47 cases. Aust NZ J Obstet Gynaecol 1979; 19:28–31.

Keller JD, Lopez-Zeno JA, Dooley SL, Socol ML. Shoulder dystocia and birth trauma in gestational diabetes: a five-year experience. Am J Obstet Gynecol 1991; 165:928–30.

Khatree MH, Gamsu HR, Rudd P, Studd JW. Features predictive of brachial plexus injury during labour. South Afr Med J 1982; 61:232–3.

Kitzmiller JL, Mall JC, Gin GD, et al. Measurement of fetal shoulder width with computed tomography in diabetic women. Obstet Gynecol 1987; 70:941–5.

Klebe JG, Espersen T, Allen J. Diabetes mellitus and pregnancy. A seven-year material of pregnant diabetics, where control during pregnancy was based on a centralized ambulant regime. Acta Obstet Gynecol Scand 1986; 65:235–40.

Koenigsberger MR. Brachial plexus palsy at birth: intrauterine or due to delivery trauma? Ann Neurol 1980; 8:228.

Kurokawa J, Zilkoski MW. Adapting hospital obstetrics to birth in the squatting position. Birth 1985; 12(2):87–90.

Langer O, Berkus MD, Huff RW, Samueloff A. Shoulder dystocia: should the fetus weighing greater than or equal to 4000 grams be delivered by cesarean section? Am J Obstet Gynecol 1991; 165:831–7.

Lazer S, Biale Y, Mazor M, et al. Complications associated with the macrosomic fetus. J Reprod Med 1986; 31:501–5.

Lee CY. Shoulder dystocia. Clin Obstet Gynecol 1987; 30:77–82.

Levine MG, Holroyde J, Woods JR, et al. Birth trauma: incidence and predisposing factors. Obstet Gynecol 1984; 63:792–5.

Lindsay MK, Graves W, Klein L. The relationship of one abnormal glucose tolerance test value and pregnancy complications. Obstet Gynecol 1989; 73:103–6.

Mashburn J. Identification and management of shoulder dystocia. J Nurse Midwifery 1988; 33:225–31.

Mazzanti GA. Delivery of the anterior shoulder: a neglected art. Obstet Gynecol 1959; 13:603–7.

McCall JO. Shoulder dystocia: a study of aftereffects. Am J Obstet 1962; 83:1486–90.

McFarland LV. Erb/Duchenne's palsy: a consequence of fetal macrosomia and method of delivery. Obstet Gynecol 1986; 68:784–8.

Meenan AL, Gaskin IM, Hunt P, Ball CA. A new (old) maneuver for the management of shoulder dystocia. J Fam Pract 1991; 32:625–9.

Meghdari A, Davoodi R, Mesbah F. Engineering analysis of shoulder dystocia in the human birth process by the finite element method. Proc Inst Mech Eng 1992; 206:243–50.

Modanlou HD, Dorchester WL, Thorosian A, Freeman RK. Macrosomia—maternal, fetal, and neonatal implications. Obstet Gynecol 1980; 55:420–4.

Modanlou HD, Komatsu G, Dorchester W, et al. Large-for-gestational-age neonates: anthropometric reasons for shoulder dystocia. Obstet Gynecol 1982; 60:417–23.

Morgan MA, Thurnau GR, Fishburne JI. The fetal-pelvic index as an indicator of fetal-pelvic disproportion: a preliminary report. Am J Obstet Gynecol 1986; 155:608–13.

Morris WIC. Shoulder dystocia. J Obstet Gynaecol Br Empire 1955; 62:302–6.

Morrison JC, Sanders JR, Magann EF, Wiser WL. The diagnosis and management of dystocia of the shoulder. Surg Gynecol Obstet 1992; 175:515–22.

Nagey DA. Can shoulder dystocia be prevented? (letter). Am J Obstet Gynecol 1990; 163:1095–6.

Nathanson JN. The excessively large fetus as an obstetric problem. Am J Obstet Gynecol 1950; 60:54–63.

Niswander KR, Singer J, Westphal M, Weiss W. Weight gain during pregnancy and prepregnancy weight: association with birth weight of term gestation. Obstet Gynecol 1969; 33:482–91.

Nocon JJ, McKenzie DK, Thomas LJ, Hansell RS. Shoulder dystocia: an analysis of risks and obstetric maneuvers. Am J Obstet Gynecol 1993; 168:1732–7.

O'Leary JA. Cephalic replacement for shoulder dystocia: present status and future role of the Zavanelli maneuver. Obstet Gynecol 1993; 82:847–50.

O'Leary JA, Cuva A. Abdominal rescue after failed

cephalic replacement. Obstet Gynecol 1992; 80:514–6.

O'Leary JA, Gunn D. Cephalic replacement for shoulder dystocia (letter). Am J Obstet Gynecol 1985; 153:592–3.

O'Leary JA, Leonetti HB. Shoulder dystocia: prevention and treatment. Am J Obstet Gynecol 1990; 162:5–9.

O'Leary JA, Pollack NB. McRoberts maneuver for shoulder dystocia: a survey. Int J Gynaecol Obstet 1991; 35:129–31.

Parks DG, Ziel HK. Macrosomia. A proposed indication for primary cesarean section. Obstet Gynecol 1978; 52:407–9.

Patterson CA, Graves WL, Bugg G, Sasso SC, Brann AW. Antenatal and intrapartum factors associated with the occurrence of seizures in term infant. Obstet Gynecol 1989; 74:361–5.

Pecorari D. Shoulder dystocia: revisited. Clin Exp Obstet Gynecol 1992; 19:272–3.

Pedersen J. Weight and length at birth of infants of diabetic mothers. Acta Endocrinol 1954; 16: 330–42.

Penney DS, Perlis DW. Shoulder dystocia: when to use suprapubic or fundal pressure. Am J Matern Child Nurs 1992; 17:34–6.

Resnik R. Management of shoulder girdle dystocia. Clin Obstet Gynecol 1980; 23:559–64.

Rogo KO, Okeyo SO, Ojwang SB. Management of shoulder dystocia. East Afr Med J 1992; 69:391–3.

Rooks JP, Weatherby NL, Ernst EK, et al. Outcomes of care in birth centers. The National Birth Center Study. N Engl J Med 1989; 321:1804–11.

Rubin A. Management of shoulder dystocia. JAMA 1964; 189:835–7.

Rubinstein TH, Schifrin BS. Shoulder dystocia. J Perinatol 1992; 12:74–7.

Rydhstrom H, Ingemarsson I. The extremely large fetus—antenatal identification, risks, and proposed management. Acta Obstet Gynecol Scand 1989; 68:59–63.

Sack RA. The large infant: a study of maternal, obstetric, fetal, and newborn characteristics; including a long-term pediatric follow-up. Obstet Gynecol 1969; 104:195–204.

Sandberg EC. The Zavanelli maneuver: a potentially revolutionary method for the resolution of shoulder dystocia. Am J Obstet Gynecol 1985; 152:479–84.

Sandberg EC. The Zavanelli maneuver extended: progression of a revolutionary concept. Am J Obstet Gynecol 1988; 158:1347–53.

Sandmire HF. Case report: brachial plexus injury with shoulder dystocia. Wis Med J 1989; 88:36, 38.

Sandmire HF. Whither ultrasonic prediction of fetal macrosomia? Obstet Gynecol 1993; 82:860–2.

Sandmire HF, O'Halloin TJ. Shoulder dystocia: its incidence and associated risk factors. Int J Gynaecol Obstet 1988; 26:65–73.

Schramm M. Impacted shoulders—a personal experience. Aust NZ J Obstet Gynaecol 1983; 23:28–31.

Schwartz BC, Dixon DM. Shoulder dystocia. Obstet Gynecol 1958; 11:468–71.

Seigworth GR. Shoulder dystocia. Review of 5 years' experience. Obstet Gynecol 1966; 28:764–7.

Shute WB. Management of shoulder dystocia with the Shute/parallel dystocia forceps. Am J Obstet Gynecol 1962; 84:936–9.

Sjoberg I, Erichs K, Bjerre I. Cause and effect of obstetric (neonatal) brachial plexus palsy. Acta Paediatr Scand 1988; 77:357–64.

Smeltzer JS. Prevention and management of shoulder dystocia. Clin Obstet Gynecol 1986; 29: 299–308.

Sorab J, Allen RH, Gonik B. Tactile sensory monitoring of clinician-applied forces during delivery of newborns. IEEE Trans Biomed Eng 1988; 10:1285–6.

Spellacy WN, Miller S, Winegar A, Peterson PQ. Macrosomia—maternal characteristics and infant complications. Obstet Gynecol 1985; 66:158–61.

Swartz DP. Shoulder girdle dystocia in vertex delivery. Obstet Gynecol 1960; 15:194–206.

Turnpenny PD, Nimmo A. Fractured clavicle of the newborn in a population with a high prevalence of grand-multiparity: analysis of 78 consecutive cases. Br J Obstet Gynaecol 1993; 100:338–41.

Wolfe HM, Zador IE, Gross TL, et al. The clinical utility of maternal body mass index in pregnancy. Am J Obstet Gynecol 1991; 164:1306–10.

Wood C, Ng KH, Dounslow D, Benning H. Time—an important variable in normal delivery. J Obstet Gynecol Br Commonw 1973; 80:295–300.

Woods CE. A principle of physics as applicable to shoulder delivery. Am J Obstet Gynecol 1943; 45:796–804.

Yarkoni S, Schmidt W, Jeanty P, et al. Clavicular measurement: a new biometric parameter for fetal evaluation. J Ultrasound Med 1985; 4: 467–70.

Zuspan FP, Quilligan EJ (eds). Douglas-Stromme Operative Obstetrics, fifth ed. Norwalk, CT: Appleton & Lange, 1988.

CHAPTER 14

Puerperal Hematomas and Lower Genital Tract Lacerations

The first reported case of vulvovaginal hematoma is attributed to Rueff in 1554. When Lyons (1949) surveyed the literature some 400 years later, he found 188 cases, and only 12 years later Pedowitz and associates (1961) reported that 770 cases of vulvovaginal hematoma had been described.

FREQUENCY

The reported frequency with which hematomas complicate delivery varies widely. For example, Table 14–1 lists seven reports from the last 45 years in which the reported frequency of vulvovaginal hematomas varied from approximately 1 in 1000 to 1 in 300 deliveries. Criteria used to define a hematoma varied widely. For example, Sotto and Collins (1958) described any hematoma greater than 1.5 inches in diameter, while Benrubi and colleagues (1987) multiplied cross-sectional diameters and reported those greater than 2.5 cm. Others used subjective criteria, including "those instances in our own practice wherein the hematomas were sufficiently troublesome or large enough to be dignified by diagnosis" (McElin and associates, 1954) and those "judged of a size sufficient to require surgical intervention" (Sheikh, 1971; Zahn and Yeomans, 1990). Accordingly, any interpretation of these data will be limited by the lack of a standardized definition and reporting system for vulvovaginal hematomas.

CLASSIFICATION

The most commonly used classification systems for genital tract hematomas are presented in Table 14–2. The simplest, and most frequently used, consists of classifying the hematomas as vulvar, vulvovaginal, paravaginal, and subperitoneal. In this system, a combination of visual inspection and palpation is used to localize the predominant position of the hematoma.

Vulvar Hematomas

Vulvar hematomas are subdivided into those located in the anterior and posterior triangles. The central tendon of the perineum prevents these hematomas from spreading across the midline (Figure 14–1). Using an alternate classification system based on the levator muscle, vulvar hematomas are infralevator in location. Their extension is limited superiorly by the levator ani muscle and they are limited from spread onto the thigh by Colles fascia and the fascia lata. Vulvar hematomas involving the posterior triangle may dissect into the ischiorectal fossa, where considerable blood can accumulate quickly (Figure 14–2). Shown in Figures 14–3A and 14–3B are sagittal and coronal representations of such a hematoma demonstrating both the fascial limitations to spread of the hematoma and the large potential space of the ischiorectal fossa and buttock within which the hematoma can accumulate.

TABLE 14–1. FREQUENCY OF VULVOVAGINAL AND SUPRAVAGINAL HEMATOMAS

Source	Deliveries	Hematomas	Frequency
Cheung and Chang (1991) Hong Kong[a]	31,628	52	1:608
Zahn and Yeomans (1990) USA	5786	11	1:526
Sheikh (1971) UK[b]	37,042	40	1:926
Sotto and Collins (1958) USA	14,548	47	1:310
Pieri (1958) USA	70,543	95	1:742
McElin and associates (1954) USA[c]	40,932	73	1:561
Lyons (1949) USA	1250	3	1:417

[a]Reported only those of a size requiring surgical intervention
[b]Includes any >1.5 inch diameter
[c]Hematomas "sufficiently troublesome or large enough to be dignified by the diagnosis"

Vulvovaginal Hematomas

Vulvovaginal hematomas involve the vulva and the lower portion of the vagina. This type of hematoma most commonly is associated with either a mediolateral episiotomy or a spontaneous lateral vaginal wall tear with extension onto the perineal body. Vulvovaginal hematomas also may complicate midline episiotomies. On visual inspection, it is not always possible to determine whether there has been supralevator extension of the hematoma from a cut or tear of the levator plate or whether there is simply displacement of the levator plate by the most cephalad extension of the hematoma. In contrast, the paravaginal hematoma is clearly a supralevator hematoma that occupies the middle to upper portion of the vagina (Fig. 14–4).

Subperitoneal Hematomas

Subperitoneal hematomas also are known as supravaginal or retroperitoneal hematomas. These hematomas are above the cardinal ligaments and may extensively involve the broad ligament with continued retroperitoneal dissection to the level of the kidneys or even higher. These hematomas can result in significant hemorrhage and may also rupture into the abdominal cavity. While the current outlook for subperitoneal hematomas is much better than the 75 percent mortality rate Lyons (1949) reported, maternal deaths continue from these complications (Jewett, 1972).

TABLE 14–2. COMMONLY EMPLOYED CLASSIFICATION SYSTEMS FOR GENITAL TRACT HEMATOMAS

Soft Tissue Based	Fascia Based
Vulvar Anterior triangle Posterior triangle	Infralevator
Vulvovaginal	Infra- or supralevator
Paravaginal	Supralevator
Subperitoneal	Broad ligament/ retroperitoneal

ETIOLOGY AND RISK FACTORS

The development of puerperal hematomas is associated with several factors that can be divided into broad categories of maternal trauma or maternal disease processes that may predispose to hematoma formation (Table 14–3). The most common risk factor is performance of episiotomy. McElin and colleagues (1954) reported performance of episiotomy, predominantly left mediolateral, in 93 percent of women who subsequently developed hematomas. Similarly, an episiotomy—usually midline—was performed in all women with hematomas reported by Zahn and Yeomans (1990). These authors also described frequent use of forceps and concurrent vaginal sidewall lacerations in a third of their patients. While Sheikh (1971) reported associated episiotomies in only half of women developing hematomas, another third sustained a spontaneous laceration without an episiotomy. Almost 20 percent of his patients developed a significant hematoma despite delivery over an intact perineum. It is also important to remember that 40–65 percent of women who

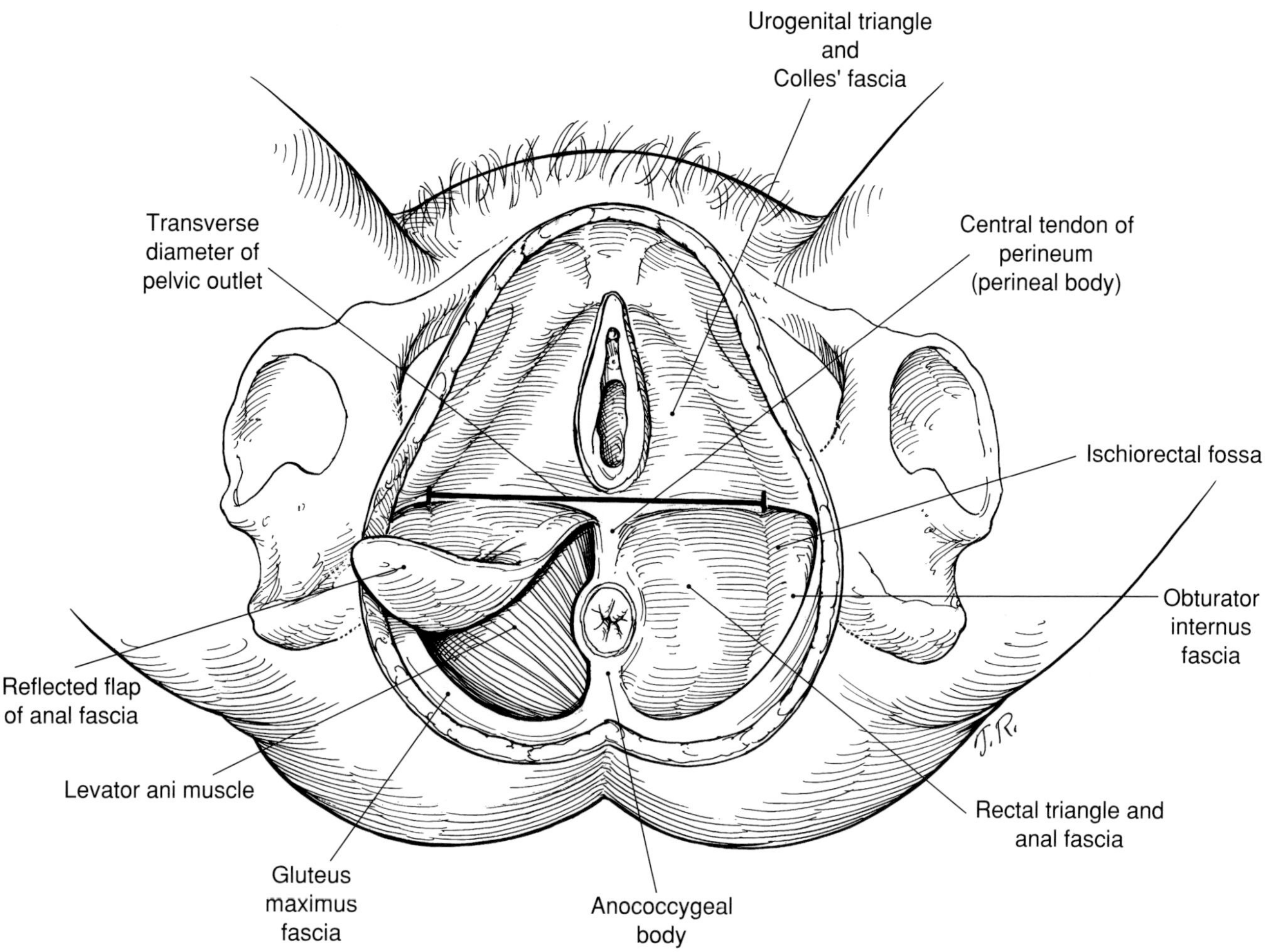

Figure 14–1. Dissection of the female perineum with the integument and superficial fascia removed. The fat has also been removed from the ischiorectal fossae in this diagram.

develop a genital hematoma do so following spontaneous vaginal delivery (Pedowitz and colleagues, 1961; Sheikh, 1971; Benrubi and associates, 1987). Other reported risk factors for puerperal hematomas include primiparity (50–73 percent), preeclampsia (30 percent), multifetal pregnancies (15 percent), instrumented delivery (20–50 percent), and breech delivery (10–17 percent).

VESSEL INJURY

Inured vessels that most commonly cause vulvar hematomas are branches of the pudendal artery: inferior rectal, transverse perineal, and posterior labial arteries (Fig. 14–5). Some vaginal hematomas involve the descending branch of the uterine artery. Subperitoneal hematomas may be associated with the uterine artery and its branches as well as other vessels in the broad ligament (Walsh and Ganser, 1948).

CLINICAL PRESENTATION

Diagnosis and classification of vulvar and vaginal hematomas involves inspection and palpation. Attention is usually first called to the hematoma by the woman herself when she complains of severe perineal pain that is not relieved by analgesics. Unfortunately, the pain is too often attributed to the episiotomy and a hematoma is missed early in its course. Blood loss almost always is underestimated with

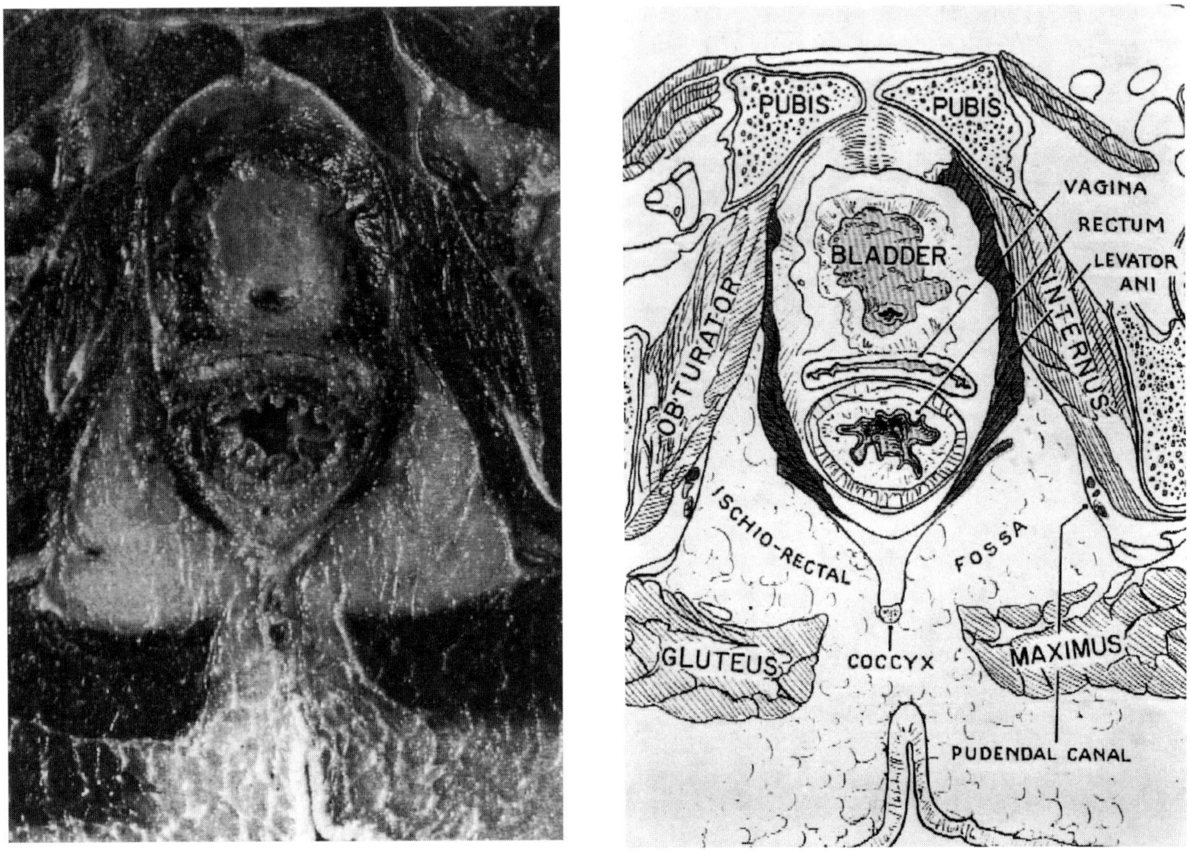

Fig. 14–2. Female pelvis on horizontal section showing muscle groups, bone, and potential spaces and accompanying diagram. (Courtesy of *Grant's Anatomy,* with permission.)

puerperal hematomas (Sheikh, 1971; Scudamore, 1964). The severity of associated anemia depends on the magnitude and rapidity of hemorrhage and volume replacement.

The vulvar or vulvovaginal hematoma will present obvious deformity of the external genitalia with the presence of a mass and associated edema and/or discoloration (Fig. 14–6). There is tenderness to palpation of the mass. The diameter of the hematoma can vary from only a few centimeters to 10 cm or greater with the corresponding degree of tenseness dependent upon both its size and the degree of distention of the surrounding tissue. If an episiotomy was performed, there may be extrusion of fresh blood or clot from the operative site.

Women with a paravaginal or supralevator hematoma often complain of rectal pain and pressure. In these cases, the mass will not be appreciated by external visualization, but rather will require speculum and/or manual rectovaginal examination for assessment.

The subperitoneal hematoma is the most difficult to diagnose. Like patients with other hematomas, these women may present with varying degrees of anemia, although hypovolemic shock is more likely due to the potential for significant retroperitoneal hemorrhage. In many cases, women are asymptomatic until shock develops. Symptoms depend upon the size and the rate of hematoma formation. Pain is more likely to be in the lower abdomen, and the uterine fundus may be displaced cephalad to a greater extent than expected. In many cases, the uterus also is displaced to the side opposite the hematoma. A unilateral fluctuant mass may be felt. These women are at greater risk for developing adynamic ileus and fever than women in whom the hematoma is confined to the lower genital tract.

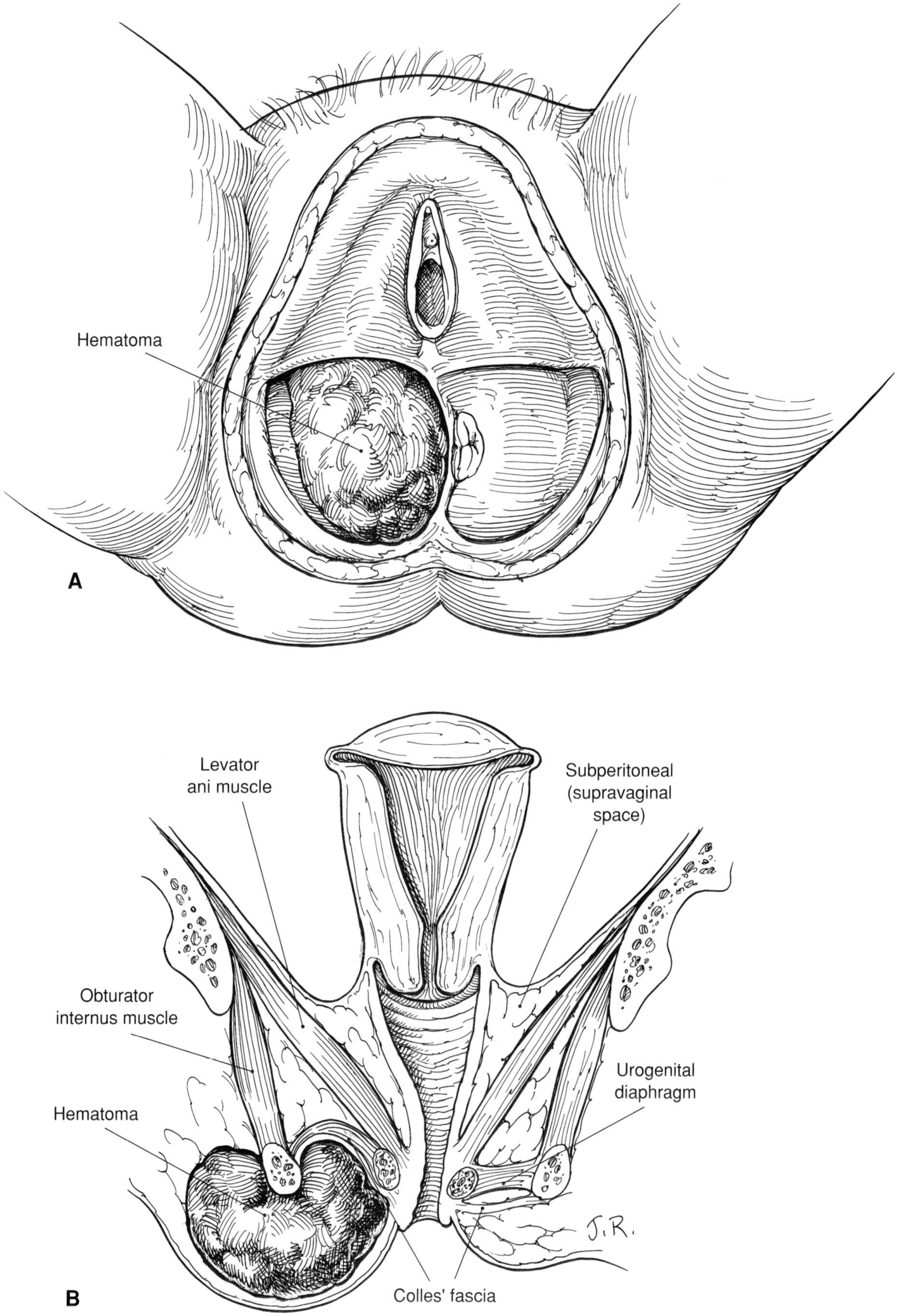

Figure 14–3. **A.** Infrafascial hematoma in rectal triangle. **B.** Coronal section through infrafascial pelvic hematoma illustrating its relationship to adjacent structures .

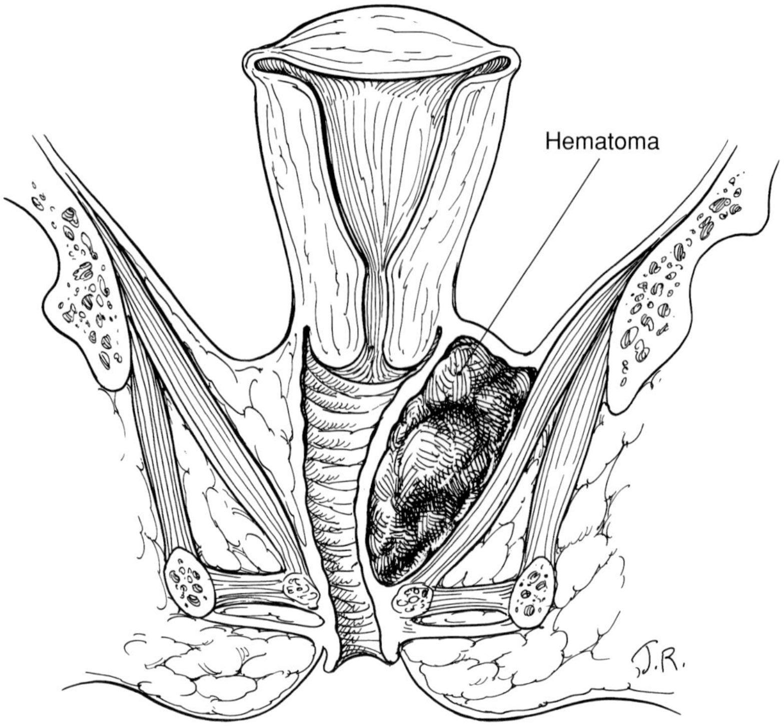

Figure 14–4. Coronal section through a paravaginal or supralevator hematoma.

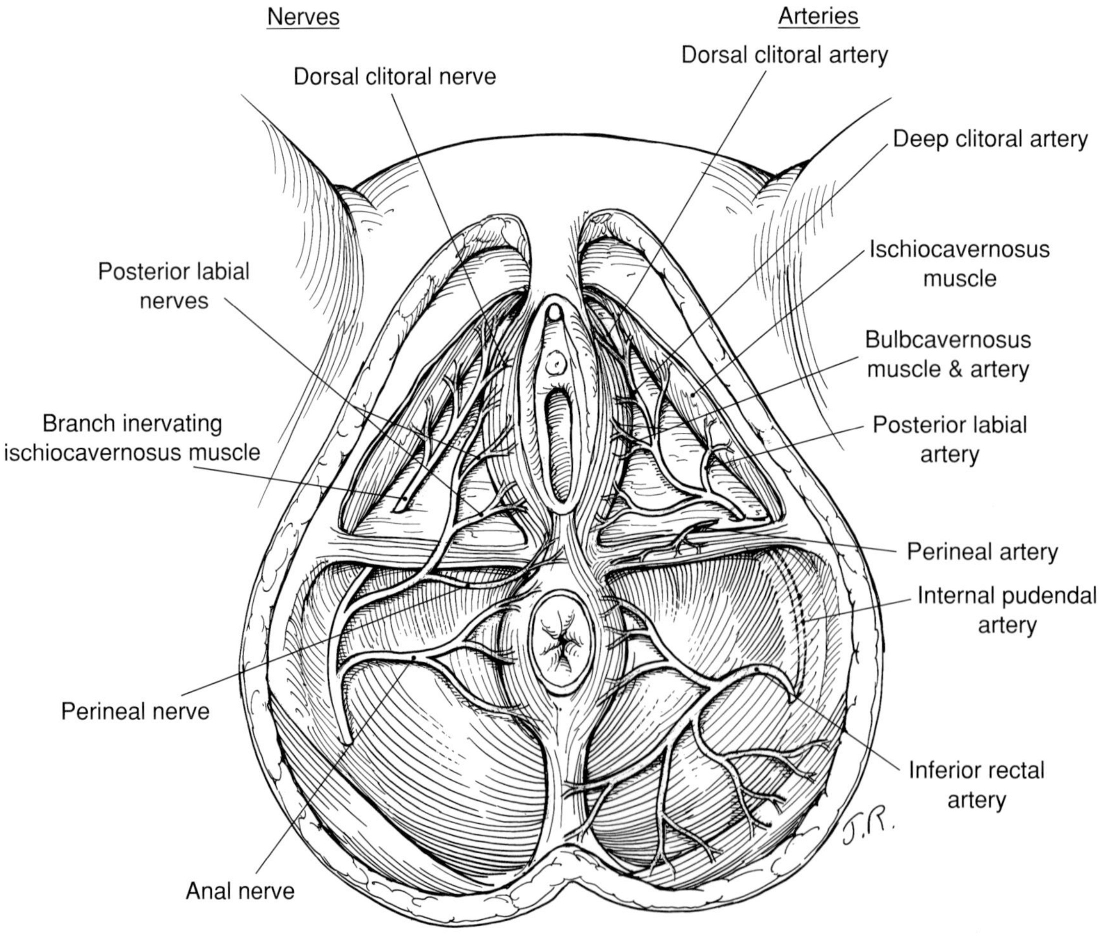

Figure 14–5. The arteries and nerves of the pelvic floor as seen from below demonstrating the branching of the internal pudendal artery and the pudendal nerve. (After Batke).

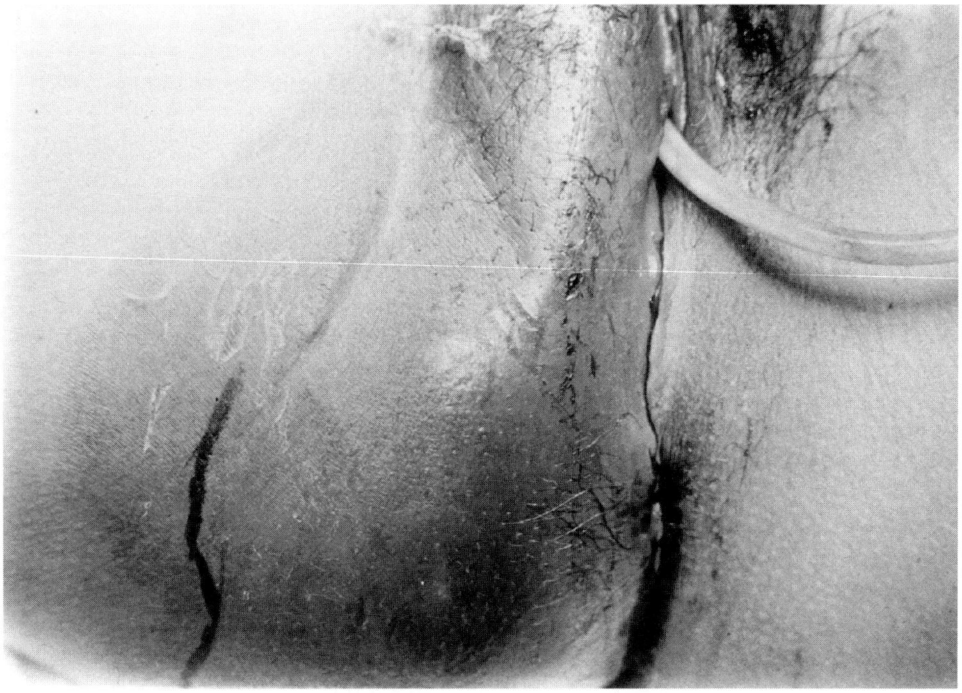

Figure 14–6. A posterior triangle vulvar hematoma, which presented on the 8th postpartum day after an uneventful labor and delivery. There is obviously a mass effect and discoloration of the posterior labia and buttock. The extent of the hematoma has been demarcated with a marking pen, and it can be noted that the hematoma is now expanded beyond the margins that were marked upon admission.

TABLE14–3. RISK FACTORS ASSOCIATED WITH PUERPERAL HEMATOMAS

Trauma	Maternal Disease
Nulliparous	Clotting Abnormalities
Episiotomy	Acquired
Spontaneous laceration	Inherited
Longer labor	
	Pre-eclampsia/Eclampsia
	Varicosities
Improper surgical repair	Infection
Macrosomic infant	
Iatrogenic	
Too vigorous massage	
Retractors	
Pudendal block	
Operative delivery/manipulations	
Forceps, especially rotations	
Vacuum extraction	
Breech delivery	

MANAGEMENT

Management of some puerperal hematomas is controversial and evolving. Historically, the treatment of perineal hematomas was expectant (Walsh and Ganser, 1948). If infection occurred, the hematoma was drained surgically. Such management led to many deaths from sepsis because antimicrobials were not in use. Indeed, the maternal mortality rate was as high as 20 percent for paravaginal and vulvar hematomas (McElin and colleagues, 1954) and 73 percent for subperitoneal hematomas. As a result of such prohibitive mortality, expectant treatment was replaced by evacuation of the blood as soon as thrombosis was complete, generally in about 48 hours. The goal was to prevent sepsis while waiting long enough to reduce the possibility of secondary hemorrhage. With the advent of antimicrobials and modern suture materials, as well as availability of blood transfusion, operative intervention has become more frequent for lower genital tract hematomas with expectant management preferred for subperitoneal hematomas (Fliegner, 1971; Sheikh, 1971).

When the hematoma is small, that is, less than 5 cm, and not expanding, most authors recommend observation (Lyons, 1949; Zahn and Yeomans, 1990). Ice packs and pressure dressings may limit the hematoma expansion. Sufficient analgesics should be given to alleviate pain. The hematoma size should be documented carefully with measurements in centimeters made in at least two dimensions and the peripheral margins of the mass outlined with a marking pen to the greatest extent possible. Such markings allow easy detection of further expansion (Fig. 14–6).

For hematomas greater than 5 cm in diameter or those rapidly expanding, the general consensus has favored surgical intervention (Walsh and Ganser, 1948; Sheikh, 1971). Experience from the past 30 years indicates that surgical intervention has been used in from 70 to 100 percent (Sotto and Collins, 1958; Pedowitz and colleagues, 1961; Sheikh, 1971; Zahn and Yeomans, 1990). Benrubi and associates (1987) reported the only comparison of conservative versus operative management of hematomas. Among 29 obstetric patients with hematomas, 19 were managed expectantly and 10 underwent prompt operative exploration. Of those followed conservatively, 21 percent subsequently required evacuation of the hematoma because of complications, 25 percent were treated with intravenous antibiotics, 15 percent were given blood transfusions, and 10 percent required readmission. None of the women treated surgically had complications. Hospital stays for women managed conservatively averaged 4.7 days compared with 3.8 days for those managed surgically. Importantly, among women managed conservatively, the greatest number of complications developed when the product of the longitudinal and transverse diameter of the hematoma was 15 cm or greater.

PREOPERATIVE ASSESSMENT

Hemodynamic status and cardiovascular stability must be determined prior to surgical intervention. An indwelling bladder catheter allows continuous assessment of urinary output and thus renal perfusion, and ensures adequate bladder drainage should pressure dressings or vaginal packing be used at the conclusion of the surgery. Hemodynamic stability, assessed by pulse, blood pressure, and urine output, should be assured prior to hematoma evacuation because incision and decompression may result in brisk bleeding. Adequate venous access should be established to allow rapid infusion of crystalloid and blood if necessary.

From 10 to 75 percent of women undergoing surgical treatment of lower genital tract hematomas require blood transfusion (Sotto and Collins, 1958; Pedowitz and associates, 1961; Benrubi and colleagues, 1987; Sheikh, 1971; Zahn and Yeomans, 1990). These reports suggest that approximately half of the patients who undergo operative intervention will require blood transfusion. Sheikh (1971) reported the mean transfusion volume was 1125 mL with a maximum of 4 L. McElin and colleagues (1954) reported similar transfusion volumes with a mean of approximately 1000 mL and a maximum of 2500 mL. If an inherited or acquired coagulopathy is suspected, appropriate coagulation studies should be performed and consideration given to correcting any deficiencies prior to surgery.

INTRAOPERATIVE MANAGEMENT

Hematomas should be managed surgically in a fully equipped and staffed operating room. Adequate exposure and pain relief usually necessitate either general or conduction anesthesia. If the woman is hemodynamically unstable, caution is advised with conduction anesthesia because of resultant loss of vascular tone with worsening of hypotension and perfusion pressure.

An incision of at least 3–5 cm usually is required in opening the hematoma. The incision is made over the area of greatest distention. When possible, the incision is made through the vaginal mucosa to minimize scar formation (Hamilton, 1940; Zahn and Yeomans, 1990). Although the clot begins to extrude spontaneously from the hematoma following the surgical incision, complete evacuation often requires the use of a suction catheter, instruments to grasp and remove the clot, and copious irrigation. If distinct bleeding sites are seen after clot evacuation, these areas may be clamped and secured by using either a free tie or suture ligature with 00 to 000 chromic. In many cases, bleeding sites are not distinct; rather, inspection of the hematoma bed reveals multiple oozing areas. Five percent dextrose in water may aid visualization of small arteriolar or venous bleeding sites. In these cases, multiple hemostatic simple or figure-of-eight suture ligatures are used to achieve hemostasis. When there is a continued small ooze and complete hemostasis of the hematoma cavity cannot be achieved, a Jackson-Pratt or similar drain may be placed at the base of the hematoma and brought out through a stab wound onto the perineal body (Fig. 14–7). When the hematoma cavity is extensive multiple drains are used.

Once hemostasis is adequate and hemodynamic stability assured, the hematoma cavity is closed. Depending upon its depth, either a multiple or single layer closure is employed. Attempts are made to begin all closures by placement of the initial suture as far cephalad as possible. Running-locking or interrupted sutures of 00 chromic are used for deep closure. The mucosal closure is begun at least 1 cm above the most cephalad extent of the hematoma and a running-locking suture is used for closure of the vaginal mucosa. At completion of the closure, the vagina is tightly packed with saline- or povidone-iodine moistened gauze, which is removed within 24 hours.

Packing

As an alternative to suture closure, some authors recommend packing. This has been described variously as either selective or routine packing of the hematoma cavity and the

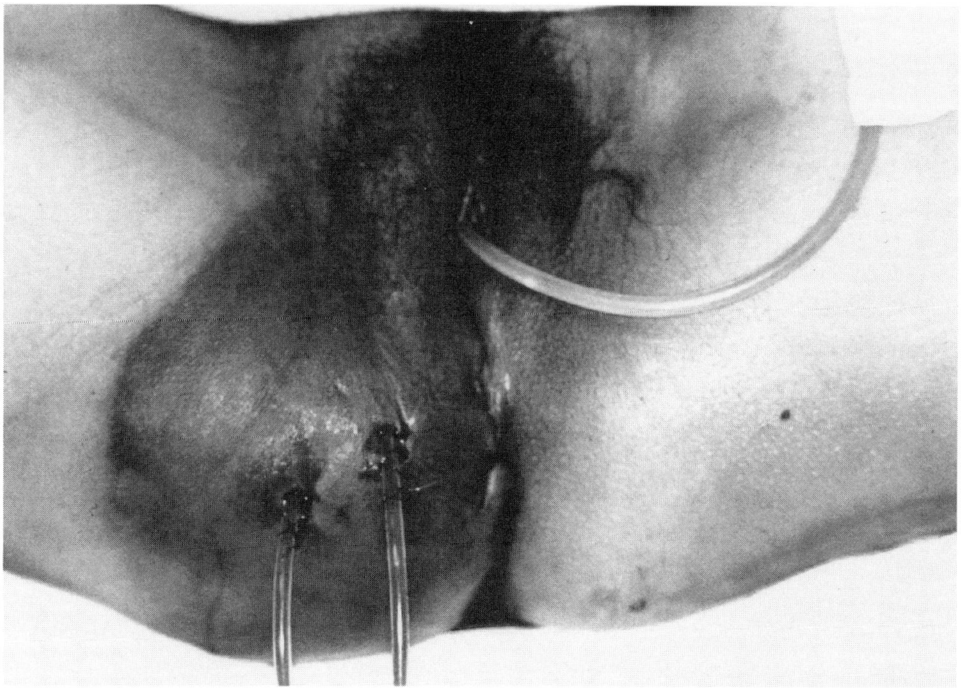

Figure 14–7. A very large vulvo-vaginal hematoma extending into the ischiorectal fossae has required placement of two Jackson-Pratt drains for adequate drainage. Note that these are brought out through a separate stab wound onto the buttock and in a dependent position.

vagina, or alternatively, the vagina alone. Pieri (1958) advised against packing the hematoma cavity because the result might be further tissue dissection and trauma. In contrast, both Hamilton (1940) and Scudamore (1964) advised packing the hematoma cavity loosely and following with a tight pack applied in the vagina. In addition, Hamilton recommended using a tightly applied T-binder for compression.

Drains

Using drains as an adjunct to surgical treatment of puerperal hematomas also is controversial and is predicated on operator preference rather than actual data. Sotto and Collins (1958) used a rubber drain in 7 of 47 cases, but did not mention location or length of time used. Hudock and associates (1955) suggested that if a drain were used, it should be a small Penrose drain left in the incision for fewer than 24 hours. McElin and associates (1954) used drains in approximately 15 percent of their cases, usually if infection were suspected. Zahn and Yeomans (1990) described a closed drainage system using Jackson-Pratt drains that exited through a separate perineal incision (Fig. 14–7). Using the technique of separate stab wounds to bring the drains out through the perineal body results in satisfactory healing (Fig. 14–8). Drainage may help to eliminate dead space and thereby reduce pressure and possible necrosis as well as help to evacuate necrotic material and secretions that might otherwise serve as a nidus of infection. When using the closed system, drains are removed once output is less than 30 mL per day.

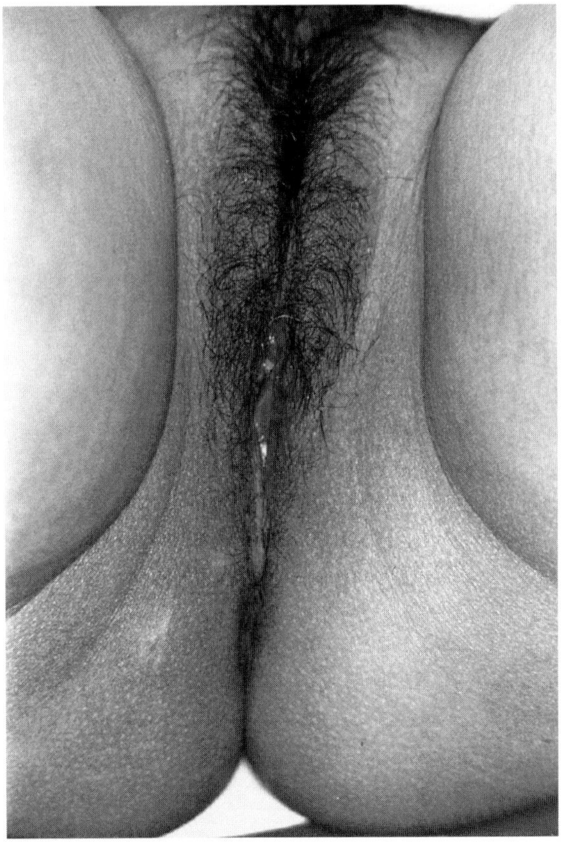

Figure 14–8. Same patient as Figure 14–7 6 weeks later showing healing of incisional site and drain stab wounds.

SUBPERITONEAL HEMATOMAS

Fortunately, subperitoneal hematomas occur far less frequently than other forms of puerperal hematomas; the incidence ranges from 1 in 3500 (Fliegner, 1971) to 1 in 20,000 (Sheikh, 1971). As previously noted, mortality with subperitoneal hematomas once exceeded 70 percent, but maternal deaths now are rare. In the largest series reported, 65 percent were multiparas. About a third each followed spontaneous vaginal delivery, cesarean delivery, and forceps operations (Fliegner, 1971). Two-thirds of the cases associated with forceps operations followed difficult rotations from occiput transverse or occiput posterior positions.

One half of all subperitoneal hematomas are discovered virtually immediately, whereas in the other half presentation is delayed in excess of 24 hours (Table 14–4). An obvious deep cervical laceration, frequently extending into the upper vagina, was apparent in two-thirds of these women. Others reports also emphasize the role of occult uterine rupture in the development of subperitoneal hematomas (McElin and colleagues, 1954; Sheikh, 1971).

Although Pieri (1958) recommended abdominal exploration and evacuation of these hematomas upon discovery, most investigators recommend a more conservative approach of expectant management (McElin and colleagues, 1954; Shiekh, 1971; Fliegner, 1971; Cheung and Chang, 1991). With either approach, blood transfusion usually is indicated. Fliegner (1971) found that 98 percent of women required a blood transfusion and the mean volume transfused was 4000 mL. One woman in this series of 39 was transfused 16,500 mL! Other treatment includes clotting factor replacement, analgesics, and broad-spectrum antimicrobials. Some have recommended a tight abdominal binder, and while not previously reported, the use of military anti-shock trousers (MAST) or pneumatic anti-shock trousers (PAST) may be ideal for this condition.

If the woman is stabilized with these conservative measures, continued expectant management is warranted. Inability to adequately replace blood loss or achieve hemodynamic stability mandates prompt surgical exploration. Generally, the operation of choice is the quickest and least invasive procedure necessary to achieve hemostasis. This is especially important for the woman with a coagulopathy, who is particularly susceptible to complications of an extensive surgical procedure. Hysterectomy as described in Chapter 19 is often necessary to allow adequate exposure to achieve hemostasis. Bilateral hypogastric artery ligation (Chapter 26) has frequently been employed under these circumstances.

In the combined series totaling 48 patients (Fliegner, 1971; Sheikh, 1971; McElin and associates, 1954) conservative nonoperative management was successful in 40 (83 percent). Combined packing of the uterus and vagina served as a successful adjunct in several women.

ANTIMICROBIAL THERAPY

Antimicrobial treatment has almost universally been employed for the treatment of subperitoneal hematomas. Broad-spectrum coverage is recommended when the hematoma has been surgically drained, or if there is evidence of clinical infection.

ANGIOGRAPHY AND EMBOLIZATION

Angiographic localization of bleeding sites and Gelfoam embolization have been described to obtain hemostasis in postpartum hematomas refractory to surgical management. Brown and associates (1979) reported the first success of this technique in a woman in whom multiple surgical attempts failed to obtain hemostasis. Others have described this technique since (Chin and colleagues, 1989; Yamashita and colleagues, 1991). Angiographic embolization offers a number of advantages over surgical approaches. First, angiographic identification of specific bleeding sites, often impossible to find at surgery, is relatively easy. Second, surgical complications such as ureteral and bladder injury as well as fistula formation are minimized or avoided if hemorrhage is controlled by embolization. Third, angiography and embolization is employed in situations that might otherwise require hysterectomy to achieve hemostasis. Heffner and colleagues (1985) described excellent results in three women in whom hemorrhage was refractory to more conservative measures including incision and drainage, ligation of the bleeding sites, vaginal packing, and replacement of volume and coagulation factors. All of these women were found to have an undiagnosed coagulation disorder when

TABLE 14–4. CLINICAL FEATURES IN 39 WOMEN WITH LARGE SUBPERITONEAL HEMATOMAS

Clinical Finding	Immediate (n = 18) (%)	Delayed >24 h (n = 21) (%)
Abdominal pain	100	67
Shock	67	24
Suprapubic mass	100	100
Deep cervical laceration	72	71
Ileus	39	24
Anemia	72	81
Fever	78	86
Urinary symptoms[a]	22	19

[a]Hematuria or urinary retention

studied at 6 weeks postpartum. Similar excellent results have been reported in women with von Willebrand disease and refractory postabortal hemorrhage (Haseltine and colleagues, 1984) as well as in abdominal pregnancy (Pais and associates, 1980).

A well-trained angiographer usually can perform an embolization procedure within 1–2 hours. Angiography is easier when performed prior to internal iliac hypogastric artery ligation. While severe complications of embolization are rare, they include bladder gangrene, sciatica, and femoral neuropathy occasionally resulting in lower limb paresis. Additionally, inadvertent embolization of branches of the femoral artery have occurred. Gluteal pain is reported in up to one-third of women, but both the pain and transient buttock claudication can usually be avoided if only the anterior division of the internal iliac artery is embolized and the superior gluteal artery is spared. Other complications include arterial thrombosis or spasm, arteriovenous fistula, and pseudoaneurysm. Despite these formidable complications, internal iliac artery embolization may prove lifesaving when surgical therapy fails. As additional experience accumulates, embolization may merit consideration even prior to surgical exploration.

CERVICAL LACERATIONS

"Slight degrees of cervical laceration must be regarded as an inevitable accompaniment of childbirth. Such tears, however, heal rapidly and rarely give rise to symptoms. In healing they cause a material change in the shape of the external os, thereby affording us a means of determining whether a woman has borne children or not" (Williams, 1911). In the 83 years since these observations, little has been published on cervical lacerations during childbirth. Indeed, while virtually every obstetric textbook includes a discussion of cervical lacerations, there is no referenced work reporting the incidence of even those lesions associated with hemorrhage sufficient to require surgical repair. Fahmy and associates (1991) recently reported on a series of colposcopic examinations performed in 189 successive parturients within 6–48 hours of delivery with attention directed toward evidence of type, site, and extent of cervical trauma and its relation to various obstetric factors. In 66 percent of the cases these investigators found trauma that presented as an erosion in 79 percent, as lacerations in 56 percent, as bruising in 30 percent, and as a "yellow area" in 17 percent. In approximately two-thirds of the cases, the diameter of the cervical erosion or the length of the laceration did not exceed 5 mm, and 81 percent of the lacerations were first degree. Injury was more frequent in primiparae, in the anterior cervical lip, with occipital-posterior positions, and with premature rupture of membranes. Residual cervical damage was reported in 8 percent of the 117 of these women in whom follow-up colposcopic examination was performed at 6–8 weeks.

Inspecting the lower birth canal and cervix during the third stage of labor is routine. Visualization of the full circumference of the cervix is often facilitated by the surgeon's applying suprapubic pressure, which elevates the uterus out of the pelvis and concurrently causes the cervix to balloon into full vision. Commonly, lacerations of the cervix at both 3 and 9 o'clock will be noted. If there is no evidence of bleeding, repair of such lacerations generally is not warranted. Exposure may be facilitated by a surgical assistant and the use of right angle vaginal retractors. Further visualization of the cervix is aided by the use of ring forceps to grasp the anterior and posterior lips of the cervix and bring any lacerations into full view. Significant lacerations are most prone to occur in association with an instrumental delivery, including midforcep or midvacumn delivery, intrauterine manipulation such as occurs with the delivery of a second twin, or with the delivery of a breech infant. Other clinical settings in which cervical injury is prone to occur include tumultuous and precipitous labors. Cervical and/or vaginal lacerations and even uterine rupture should be suspected when bright red bleeding persists in the face of apparent good uterine tone.

On rare occasions, an edematous anterior cervical lip is caught between the fetal head and the symphysis pubis. If this is undetected, and the edematous lip cannot be manually reduced, lowered perfusion of the tissues in combination with repetitive pressure results in ischemia sufficiently severe that the cervical lip undergoes necrosis and separation. Even more rarely, an angular or circular detachment of the entire cervix may occur. Remarkably, in such instances the blood supply has usually been compromised to the degree that significant bleeding does not occur.

SURGICAL REPAIR

When bleeding does occur and surgical repair is necessary, adequate anesthesia and exposure of the surgical field are key. In the absence of bleeding, cervical lacerations usually are not repaired. The extent of the laceration must be identified and extension to involve the vaginal fornices, either laterally or inferiorly, should be sought.

Important factors to consider in performing the repair include the possibility of extension with involvement of the descending branch of the uterine artery when lacerations extend above the vaginal fornix at either the 3 or 9 o'clock positions. Further assessment of the extent of the laceration may be obtained on bimanual examination. The possibility of injury to the uterine artery with development of a broad ligament hematoma should be considered and the patient observed for this development. Additionally, the proximity of the ureter to the area of surgical repair must be considered. The suture repair should be confined to the proximity of the cervix and not be swept laterally into the broad ligament. If lacerations extending above the vaginal fornix are bleeding and need extensive repair, laparotomy may be required to achieve adequate exposure and ensure that the ureter is not damaged. Insertion of a Foley catheter and monitoring of urinary output, while reassuring, are not conclusive evidence that the ureter has not been incorporated into a repair. If the surgeon has any question about the possibility of ureteral damage, cystoscopy should be performed and drainage of urine into the bladder from the involved ureter should be visualized and/or a stint passed up into the ureter.

For the surgical repair, right angle retractors are inserted anteriorly, ring forceps are used to grasp the cervix posteriorly, and its entire circumference is inspected. A knowledgeable surgical assistant may be indispensable for adequate visualization. The vault of the vagina posteriorly and the lateral fornices are exposed by manipulating the cervix with ring forceps. Lacerations that are hidden behind the redundant cervix would accordingly be exposed (Fig. 14–9). The raw edges of the laceration can be approximated with interrupted absorbable sutures; each stitch is placed through the entire thickness of the cervix (Fig. 14–10). A 00 suture of either chromic catgut, Dexon, or Vicryl is appropriate for such repairs. The apex of a deep laceration may not be obvious if it lies above the vaginal vault. In such cases, visualization may be facilitated by beginning the closure of the laceration at the most distal portion and using each successive suture as a means of traction (Figure 14–11). Unless the higher sutures can confidently be placed accurately and safely above the upper end of the tear, a laparotomy should be considered because extensive bleeding can occur from an unligated vessel. If the

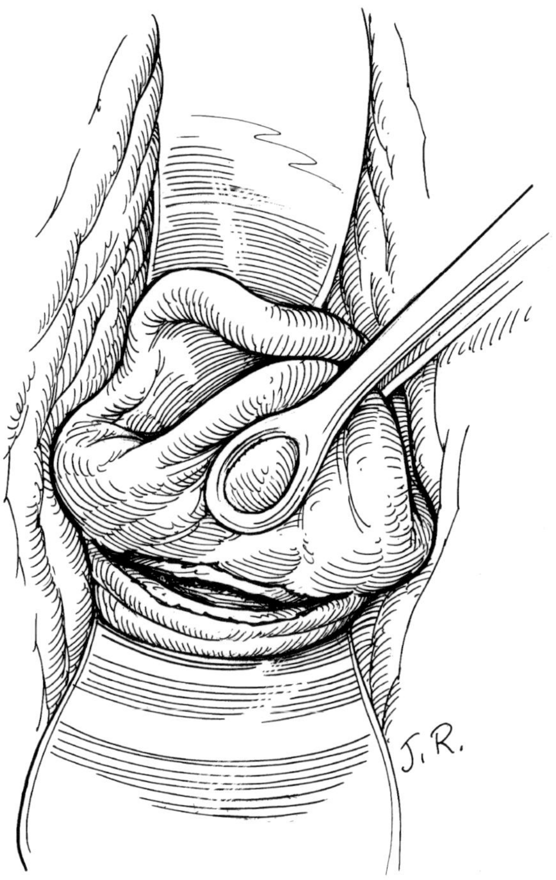

Figure 14–9. Right angle retractor and ring forceps are being used to visualize a cervical laceration in the posterior fornix of the vagina. This laceration can be closed with either a running-locking suture or with interrupted sutures.

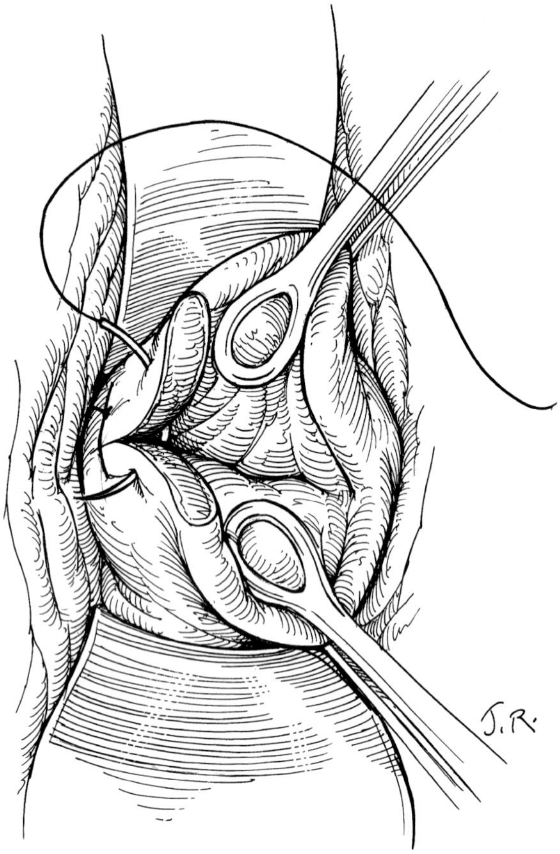

Figure 14–10. A laceration involving the 9 o'clock position of the cervix is shown. The anterior and posterior edges of the wound are well demonstrated with the use of ring or ovum forceps. Interrupted sutures are used for closure with the suture incorporating the full thickness of the laceration.

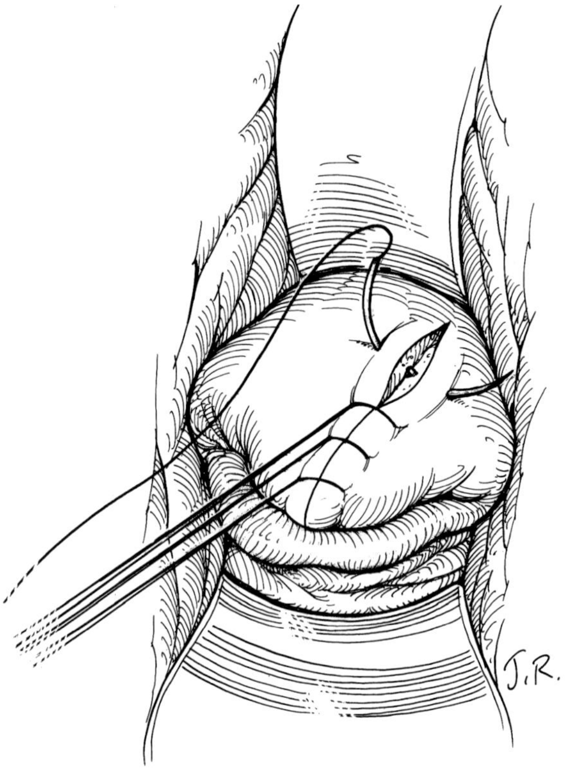

Figure 14–11. An extensive cervical laceration has occurred extending well into the lateral vaginal fornix. Successive interrupted sutures have been placed with traction placed on these sutures, progressively bringing more of the laceration into the surgical field so that it can be repaired.

decision is to observe the patient, close attention to vital signs and urinary output is necessary. When the cervical laceration also extends onto the vagina, the vaginal laceration should be repaired in a similar fashion. Either interrupted sutures or a running-locking suture are appropriate for this closure.

VAGINAL LACERATIONS

The most frequent vaginal lacerations are spontaneous tears involving the midline and occurring posteriorly or in the anterior periurethral areas. Posterior lacerations of the perineal body or vagina should be repaired if they involve more than the vaginal mucosa. Repair of such posterior injuries is described in Chapter 7. Anterior tears involving the labia minora and periurethral area are inspected; if they are not bleeding, they generally do not require repair. If the lacerations are close to the urethra and require repair, it is prudent to insert a Foley catheter. This not only facilitates the repair with the knowledge that the urethra is not being compromised, but also guards against the development of edema, which may make it difficult for the patient to void. Placement of a Foley catheter following repair also may be extremely painful. Repair of these lacerations is generally performed with a fine suture, such as 000 or 0000 chromic catgut, Dexon, or Vicryl.

Occasionally there may be deep sidewall lacerations so extensive that they dissect into the ischiorectal fossae. This is heralded by the appearance of the yellow fibroadipose tissue characteristic of this space. While such injuries are indeed impressive on visualization, they usually are readily repaired with the help of a capable surgical assistant in order to achieve exposure. The fibroadipose tissue itself cannot be sutured as the suture material simply will pull or cut through this tissue. Inspection should be carried out and any isolated bleeding blood vessels ligated with either a clamp and free tie or a suture ligature. Following this the vaginal mucosa can be closed with either a running-locking suture or with interrupted sutures. (The authors prefer the use of a running-locking suture as it is more hemostatic.) A large needle and 00 chromic suture are used for this closure with the successive bites incorporating substantial amounts of tissue. Remarkably, at the postpartum examination there usually is little residual evidence that these injuries ever occurred.

SUMMARY

Puerperal hematomas and lower genital tract lacerations will be encountered in every busy obstetric practice and usually are easily managed. The large and rapidly expanding hematoma will often require surgical intervention. Assessment of the patient's coagulation status and hemodynamic stability preoperatively are key management concepts. Evacuation of the clot with ligation of obvious areas of bleeding is followed by either a layered closure or packing. With the layered closure the authors prefer use of a closed drainage system and prophylactic antibiotics.

REFERENCES

Benrubi G, Neuman C, Nuss RC, Thompson RJ. Vulvar and vaginal hematomas: A retrospective study of conservative versus operative management. South Med J 1987; 80:991.

Brown BJ, Heaston DK, Poulson AM, et al. Uncontrollable postpartum bleeding: a new approach to hemostasis through angiographic arterial embolization. Obstet Gynecol 1979; 54:361.

Cheung TH, Chang A. Puerperal haematomas. Asia-Oceania J Obstet Gynaecol 1991; 17:119.

Chin HC, Scott DR, Resnik R, et al. Angiographic embolization of intractable puerperal hematomas. Am J Obstet Gynecol 1989; 160:434.

Fahmy K, el-Gazar A, Sammour M, et al. Postpartum colposcopy of the cervix: injury and healing. Int J Gynaecol Obstet 1991; 34:133.

Fliegner JRH. Postpartum broad ligament haematomas. J Obstet Gynaecol Br Commonw 1971; 78:184.

Hamilton HG. Post-partum labial or paravaginal hematomas. Am J Obstet Gynecol 1940; 39:642.

Haseltine FP, Glickman MG, Marchesi S, et al. Uterine embolization in a patient with postabortal hemorrhage. Obstet Gynecol 1984; 63:78S.

Heffner LJ, Mennuti MT, Rudoff JC, McLean GK. Primary management of postpartum vulvovaginal hematomas by angiographic embolization. Am J Perinatol 1985; 2:204.

Hudock JJ, Dupayne N, McGeary JA. Traumatic vulvar hematomas. Am J Obstet Gynecol 1955; 70:1064.

Jewett JF. Fatal laceration from normal birth. N Engl J Med 1972; 287:44.

Lyons AW. Post-partum hematoma. N Engl J Med 1949; 240:461.

McElin TW, Bowers VM, Paalman RJ. Puerperal hematomas. Am J Obstet Gynecol 1954; 67:356.

Pais OS, Glickman M, Schwartz P, et al. Embolization of pelvic arteries for control of postpartum hemorrhage. Obstet Gynecol 1980; 55:754.

Pedowitz P, Pozner S, Adler NH. Puerperal hematomas. Am J Obstet Gynecol 1961; 81:350.

Pieri RJ. Pelvic hematomas associated with pregnancy. Obstet Gynecol 1958; 12:249.

Scudamore JH. Vulval and vaginal haematomata. Br Med J 1964; 1:1357.

Sheikh GN. Perinatal genital hematomas. Am J Obstet Gynecol 1971; 38:571.

Sotto LS, Collins RJ. Perigenital hematomas. Obstet Gynecol 1958; 12:259.

Trehan AK. Non-puerperal vulval haematoma. Clin Exp Obstet Gynecol 1991; 18:61.

Walsh FJ, Ganser HI. Puerperal perigenital and perineal hematomas. Am J Obstet Gynecol 1948; 56:869.

Williams JW. Obstetrics. 2nd ed. New York, London: D. Appleton and Company, 1911.

Yamashita Y, Takahashi M, Ito M, Okamura H. Transcatheter arterial embolization in the management of postpartum hemorrhage due to genital tract injury. Obstet Gynecol 1991; 77:160.

Zahn CM, Yeomans ER. Postpartum hemorrhage: placenta accreta, uterine inversion, and puerperal hematomas. Clin Obstet Gynecol 1990; 33:422.

CHAPTER 15

Diagnosis and Management of Uterine Inversion

Uterine inversion is a rare but potentially life-threatening complication of the third stage of labor. The cardinal signs and symptoms of acute inversion are hemorrhage and shock. When it occurs, prompt recognition and treatment reduce morbidity and mortality.

HISTORICAL PERSPECTIVES

A historical review by Das (1940) states: "In the Ayurvedic literature, the Hindu system of medicine (2500–600 BC), there are passages which suggest the condition of inversion of the uterus was known to the Hindus." Hippocrates (460–370 BC) is credited as the first to recognize the inverted uterus. Das suggests, however, that it was Soranus who clearly defined uterine inversion and attributed its cause to traction on the umbilical cord. Subsequently, Aretius (second century AD), Aetius, and Paulus Aegineta (AD 625–699) were acquainted with uterine inversion. Avicenna, an Arabian physician (AD 980–1037), gave the first clear description of the differential diagnosis between inversion of the uterus and prolapse. Since Ambroise Paré (sixteenth century), inversion of the uterus has been recognized as a pathologic entity (Das, 1940).

CLASSIFICATION

A number of classification systems for uterine inversion exist. Most are related to duration or severity of inversion. The following is an example of one system of classification by duration:

1. **Acute inversion.** An inversion diagnosed within 24 hours of delivery; cervical contraction may or may not be present.
2. **Subacute inversion.** An interval between delivery and diagnosis of greater than 24 hours but less than 4 weeks; cervical contraction is always present.
3. **Chronic inversion.** The presence of inversion for 4 weeks or more.

A classification by severity is as follows:

1. **First degree.** Incomplete inversion in which the corpus extends to the cervix but not beyond the cervical ring.
2. **Second degree.** Protrusion through the cervical ring but not to the perineum.
3. **Third degree.** Complete inversion in which the inverted fundus extends to the perineum.
4. **Total.** Inversion of the vagina.

From 1977 to 1986, the Los Angeles County University of Southern California (LAC/USC) Medical Center (Brar and associates, 1989) reported 139,771 births and 56 patients with uterine inversion, for an incidence of 1 in 2495 deliveries. Second-degree inversion occurred in 41 women (73.2%) and third-degree inversion in 15 (26.8%); none had first-degree or total inversion. Fifty-four patients (96.4%) had acute uterine inversion; two had subacute inversion requiring readmission 4–6 days following delivery. An earlier study by Platt and Druzin (1981) reported 68 percent second-degree inversions, 21 percent third-degree inversions, and 11 percent first-degree inversions.

INCIDENCE

The reported incidence of puerperal inversion of the uterus varies widely in the literature, but recent series indicate an incidence of approximately 1 in 2000 (range 1/500 to 1/20,000) (Watson and associates, 1980). In Bunke and Hofmeister's survey (1965) of Milwaukee hospitals between 1940 and 1962, puerperal inversion occurred in 1/4000 and 1/47,000 for an overall incidence of 1/20,000.

Many authors attribute a significant number of uterine inversions to mismanagement of the third stage of labor, by either excessive cord traction, fundal pressure, or both (Jones, 1913, 1914; Gordon, 1936). Jones suggests that traction on a placenta adherent to the fundus with its relatively weakened underlying musculature or pressure on the fundus by the hand of an attendant could produce a dimpled fundus to be gripped by the remaining uterine musculature and expelled through the cervix like a foreign body. In contrast, at the University of Colorado the Crede maneuver was not routinely used and they strongly discouraged vigorous cord traction. Oxytocin and methergine were delayed until after placental separation. When this form of third stage management was used, the authors rejected the association of uterine inversion with mismanagement (Watson and associates, 1980).

In 1925 McCullagh suggested a link between prolonged or precipitous labor and uterine inversion, although no association was confirmed by others (Watson and associates, 1980). After a number of authors (Das, 1940; Gordon, 1936; McCullagh, 1925; Henderson and Alles, 1948) noted the prevalence of primigravidas in large studies, some suggested that inversion is related to the number of primiparas in each patient population rather than to a cause-and-effect relationship. In Watson and co-workers' series (1980), 7 of 18 patients (39%) in the treatment group and 8 of 18 (44%) in the control group were primiparas. In Brar and colleagues' study (1989) 32/56 patients (57%) were primiparas compared to 37% primiparas for the institution as a whole for the same time period. These authors and others (Shah-Hosseini and Errard, 1989; Rachagan and co-workers, 1988) also identified another significant factor; that fundal implantation of the placenta is more common in primiparas. In Brar's study fundal implantation of the placenta occurred in 52 percent of patients. Delivery of a macrosomic fetus was also associated with uterine inversion (Brar, 1989).

Brar also concluded that the use of oxytocin with or without magnesium sulfate placed women at higher risk for inversion; however, magnesium sulfate when used alone did not appear to be a risk factor. In contrast, Platt and Druzin (1981) found an association between the use of magnesium sulfate and uterine inversion and concluded that this was independent of the concomitant use of oxytocin. In their series, 7 of 15 (46%) primigravid women and two multigravid women received magnesium sulfate for the treatment of preeclampsia. Six of these nine women also received oxytocin. Three other patients received only oxytocin. Thus, 9 of 28 women with uterine inversion received magnesium sulfate and 9 of 28 received oxytocin while 6 received both drugs. The authors did not state the overall use of oxytocin or magnesium sulfate in their population.

In one woman puerperal uterine inversion occurred in subsequent pregnancies. Steffen (1957) identified a patient who sustained a uterine inversion and spontaneous rupture of the uterus in her first pregnancy and a uterine inversion in her second. Heyl and colleagues (1984) reported a case of recurrent uterine inversion following the successful reduction of a uterine inversion occurring at the time of delivery. In this patient, a complete uterine inversion was recognized and manually reduced immediately after delivery. Fifteen minutes later, the inversion recurred and was again reduced. Two hours later, the uterus was again inverted. The inversion was corrected under general anesthesia, and 15-methyl prostaglandin $F_{2\alpha}$ and uterine packing were used to prevent a recurrence of the inversion. Although uterine inversion may occur in a woman of any parity, it appears that primiparous women with a fundal implantation of the placenta are more likely to encounter this complication of the third stage of labor.

DIAGNOSIS

While the most common presenting sign of uterine inversion is hemorrhage (94%) (Watson, 1980; Jones, 1913; McCullagh, 1925; Bell, 1953; and their associates), shock is the most common complication of uterine inversion (40%) (Watson, 1980). In the past shock out of proportion to blood loss was noted as one of the cardinal signs of uterine inversion (Das, 1940; Bunke and Hofmeister, 1965; McCullagh, 1925), but this has not been substantiated in more recent series (Platt, 1981; Watson, 1980; Kitchin, 1975; and their colleagues). The appearance of shock out of proportion to the amount of blood loss is more readily explained by an underestimation of blood loss than as the result of a neurologic response to the inverted uterus. Prompt recognition and treatment may prevent or minimize the consequences of the shock.

While uterine inversion generally presents with extensive postpartum hemorrhage, it may present predominantly as a pelvic mass, particularly if the fundus is located in the vagina (Fig. 15–1). If the woman receives oxytocin, the mass may become firm and erroneously lead to a misdiagnosis of a uterine leiomyoma. On bimanual examination, however, the fundus cannot be felt abdominally. In cases where the inverted uterus does not protrude through the introitus, uterine inversion may go undetected and result in a subacute or chronic inversion. Although a diagnosis of uterine inversion is generally possible on a clinical basis, magnetic resonance imaging was recently helpful in a case where the clinical evaluation was inconclusive (Lewin and Bryan, 1989).

MANAGEMENT

Successful treatment of uterine inversion is enhanced by prompt recognition. Treatment of hypovolemia and shock should be addressed immediately with a large intravenous line (18 gauge or larger) and fluid replacement. Initial volume replacement is accomplished with a crystalloid solution given over 15–30 minutes. The volume of initial resuscitation is calculated by multiplying the estimated blood loss by 3. Consideration should be given to establishing additional intravenous access and to summoning support personnel should they be

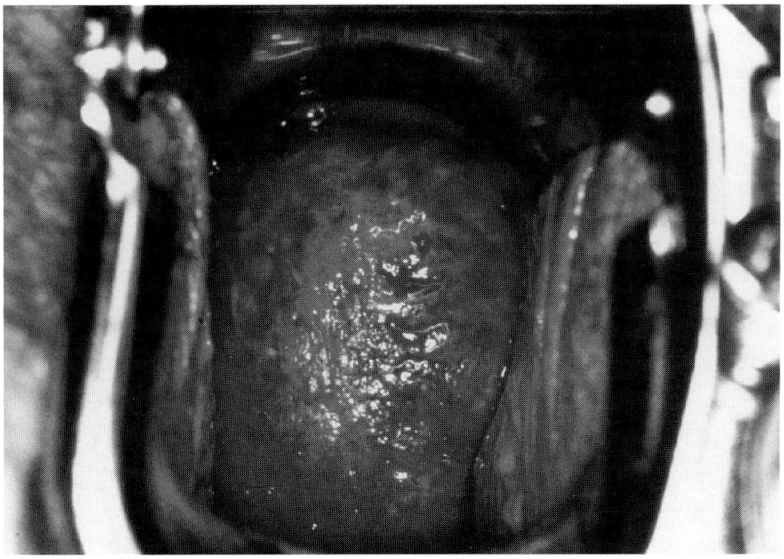

Figure 15–1. Second degree uterine inversion presenting as a vaginal mass and hemorrhage. (Courtesy Dr. Leo Dunn.)

needed. Included would be anesthesia, a full operating room crew, and additional surgical assistants. It is better to err on the side of caution and summon help too early as opposed to too late. Laboratory assessment of the patient's blood count and clotting profile should be obtained, and packed red blood cells and replacement blood products should be made available. Maternal vital signs should be monitored frequently by a designated individual, and as time permits a Foley catheter should be inserted to assess urinary output.

Oxytocic agents should be withheld and an attempt made to reposition the uterus manually via the vagina. The majority of authors recommend a manual attempt at replacement of the uterus prior to removal of the adherent placenta and prior to operative attempts at replacement. If the placenta is removed prior to intrauterine repositioning, the patient is at increased risk for blood loss and shock. After repositioning, the placenta is usually removed easily.

A number of techniques are proposed for the correction of uterine inversion. The Johnson maneuver (1949) (Fig. 15–2) is one of the favored techniques for manual repositioning of the inverted uterus. This method involves grasping the inverted uterus and pushing it through the cervix toward the normal anatomic position. The direction of pressure is toward the umbilicus, and success is enhanced by early efforts at restoration of position. This method minimizes the number of uterine layers required to pass through the cervix at any one time (Watson, 1980; Kitchin, 1975; and their co-workers). Once the uterus is repositioned, the operator's hand should remain in the uterine cavity until a firm contraction occurs and until intravenous oxytocics are administered. Applying ring forceps to the cervical ring for additional countertraction is advocated by some for difficult cases (Henderson and Alles, 1948; Kitchin and associates, 1975). Packing of the uterine cavity is optional and may be of greatest value in those cases where inversion recurs.

In one-third of patients, manual positioning is successful without the use of uterine relaxants (Brar and co-workers, 1989). However, if repositioning of the uterus is not readily accomplished, uterine relaxation may be attempted with 0.125–0.25 mg of intravenous or subcutaneous terbutaline, 0.150 mg of intravenous ritodrine (Clark, 1984), or a 2–4 g bolus of intravenous magnesium sulfate. Drugs generally less familiar to the obstetrician, but which have also been used to assist with uterine repositioning, include intravenous bolus nitroglycerin as well as inhaled amyl nitrate delivered by breaking an ampule beneath the patient's nose. In a substantial number of patients, these drugs effectively relax the traction ring and eliminate the need for general anesthesia. Brar and co-workers (1989) used terbutaline, 0.25 mg intravenously in 18 patients with a success rate of 88.9 percent. Eight patients received 2 g of intravenous $MgSO_4$, of whom seven were successfully repositioned. The three failed cases (two with terbutaline and one with $MgSO_4$) involved third-degree inversion and required the use of general anesthesia for uterine positioning. In patients with significant hypotension and shock, magnesium sulfate should be used rather than vasodilators such as the beta agonist and nitroglycerin. It may be given as a 2–4 g bolus over 5–10 minutes.

When readily available, general anesthesia using halothane at 2 percent or higher concentrations is effective in achieving uterine relaxation and assisting in replacement. Once the uterus is in position, the attendant's hand should remain in the endometrial cavity until a firm contraction occurs and until intravenous oxytocics are administered. Regardless of the method of uterine replacement employed, careful manual exploration afterward is essential to rule out the possibility of uterine rupture, cervical lacerations, and/or lower genital tract trauma.

Another method of treatment for puerperal uterine inversion involving hydrostatic pressure was first suggested by O'Sullivan in 1945. Two liters of warm saline (40°C) are placed on an IV stand and kept approximately 2 m above ground level. The nozzles of two long rubber tubes are placed in the posterior fornix of the vagina. While fluid is allowed to flow quickly, its escape is prevented by blocking the introitus by the operator's hands. The vaginal walls begin to distend, and the fundus of the uterus begins to rise. After correction of the inversion, the fluid in the vagina is allowed to flow out slowly. The uterus is checked for complete replacement, and the patient is given 0.5 mg of ergonovine intramuscularly. An intravenous infusion containing 1,000 mL of 5 percent dextrose with 20 units of oxytocin is begun. Reduction of the

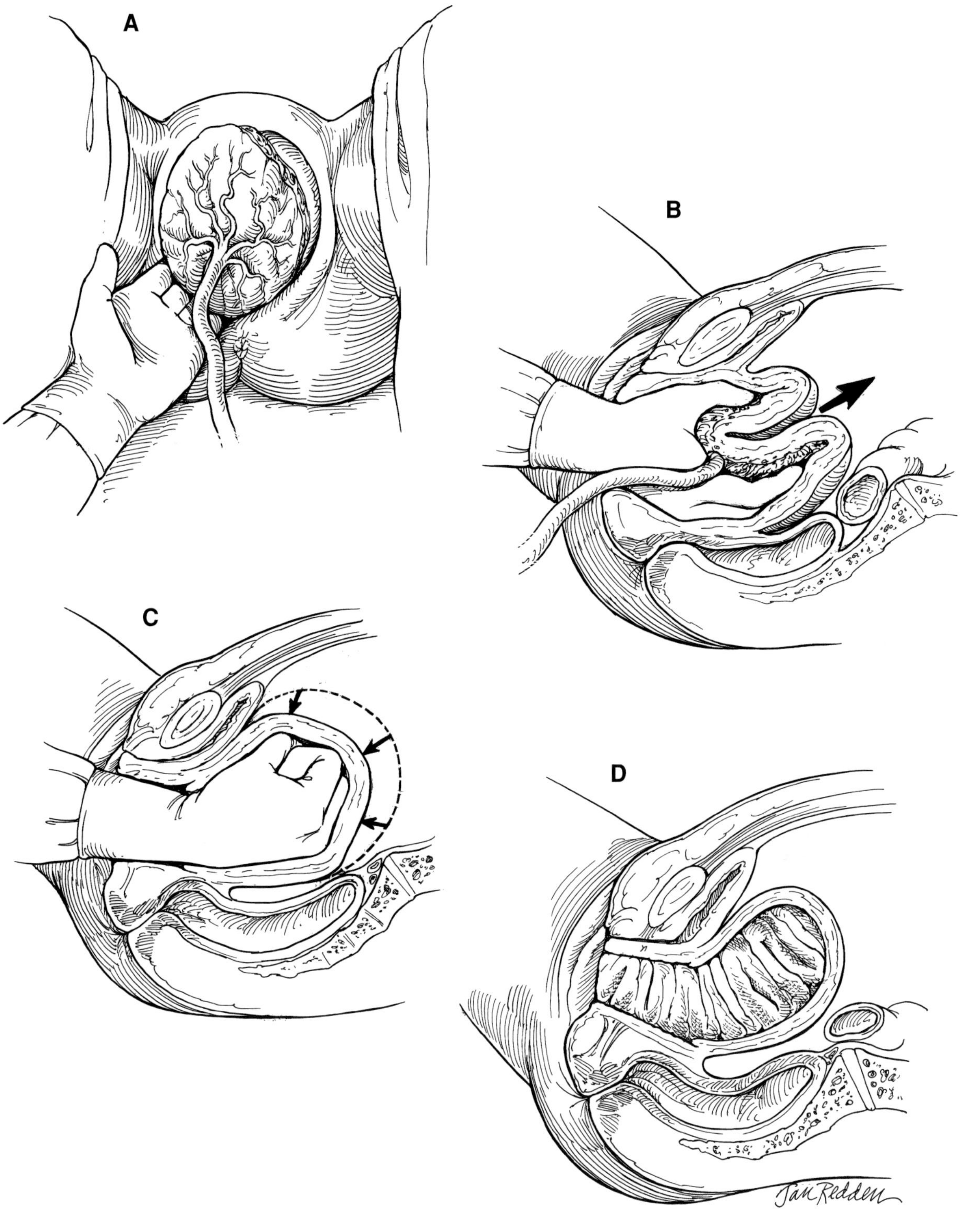

Figure 15–2. The Johnson maneuver. **A.** A third-degree uterine inversion with the uterine fundus delivered through the introitus. The placenta is left attached. **B**. The inverted uterus with the placenta attached is grasped in the operator's entire hand, with the fundus resting on the palmar surface and the finger tips exerting equal pressure around the collar of the uterus within the cervical opening. The fundus is replaced with upward pressure. Replacement usually is not difficult if the inversion is corrected before the uterus contracts firmly. **C**. The repositioned uterus following manual removal of the placenta and uterine exploration. The operator's hand is kept inside the uterus until it begins to contract down around the hand. **D**. Before the hand is removed from the uterine cavity, a tight uterovaginal pack may be inserted. This can be removed after 24 hours.

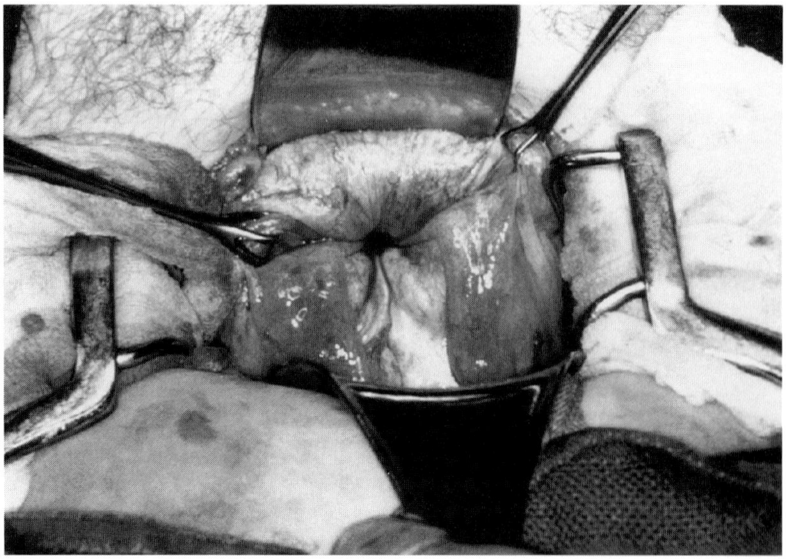

Figure 15–3. Laparotomy was required for replacement of the inverted uterus. The vaginal examination of this patient is shown in Figure 15–1. Note orientation of round ligament and adnexal structures.

inverted uterus is usually achieved in 5–10 minutes after commencement of this technique (Momani and Hassan, 1989).

If conservative attempts at repositioning of the uterus are not successful, an operative approach is indicated (Fig. 15–3). Surgery is more often required for patients with subacute or chronic inversion. The surgical approach of choice is the procedure described by Huntington and colleagues (1928) (Fig. 15–4), which relies on traction of the round ligaments and uterus for restoring normal anatomy. If this is not successful, the procedure described by Haultian (1901) (Fig. 15–5) is recommended; it involves a surgical incision of the cervical ring posteriorly through an abdominal approach, repositioning of the uterus, and subsequent repair of the cervical incision.

The method of repositioning varies with the circumstances. If recognition of the condition is immediate, most patients can undergo manual replacement without uterine relaxants. If unsuccessful, the majority of patients respond successfully to the use of uterine relaxants, which potentially eliminates the need for surgery.

The recent experience of several authors (Brar, 1989; Platt and Druzin, 1981; Watson, 1980) demonstrated only three laparotomies out of a total of 102 uterine inversions. Thirty-eight patients received general anesthesia for manual repositioning. Because a number of these patients did not receive terbutaline or magnesium sulfate, this is probably not a true indication of the need for general anesthesia or surgical intervention. In cases of either subacute or chronic uterine inversion, which may signal the presence of significant tissue necrosis, operative repositioning is almost always required. One case of subacute inversion was diagnosed 5 days after vaginal delivery. Intravenous injection of sodium fluorescein dye identified a clear demarcation between viable and necrotic myometrium (Romo and associates, 1992).

SUMMARY

In all cases of postpartum hemorrhage, uterine inversion should be suspected. If identified, a large bore IV should be started and fluid resuscitation begun. Manual vaginal repositioning of the uterus should be attempted, and an anesthesiologist should be alerted to the possible requirement for general anesthesia. If manual repositioning is successful, the placenta should be removed, the uterus explored, and oxytocic agents begun. If manual repositioning is not immediately successful, terbutaline (0.125–0.25 mg) should be given intravenously or subcutaneously in the absence of hypotension. In the presence of hypotension, magnesium sulfate (2–4 g bolus) should be given intravenously over 5–10 minutes. At this time manual repositioning should again be attempted. If successful, the placenta should be removed, the uterus explored, and

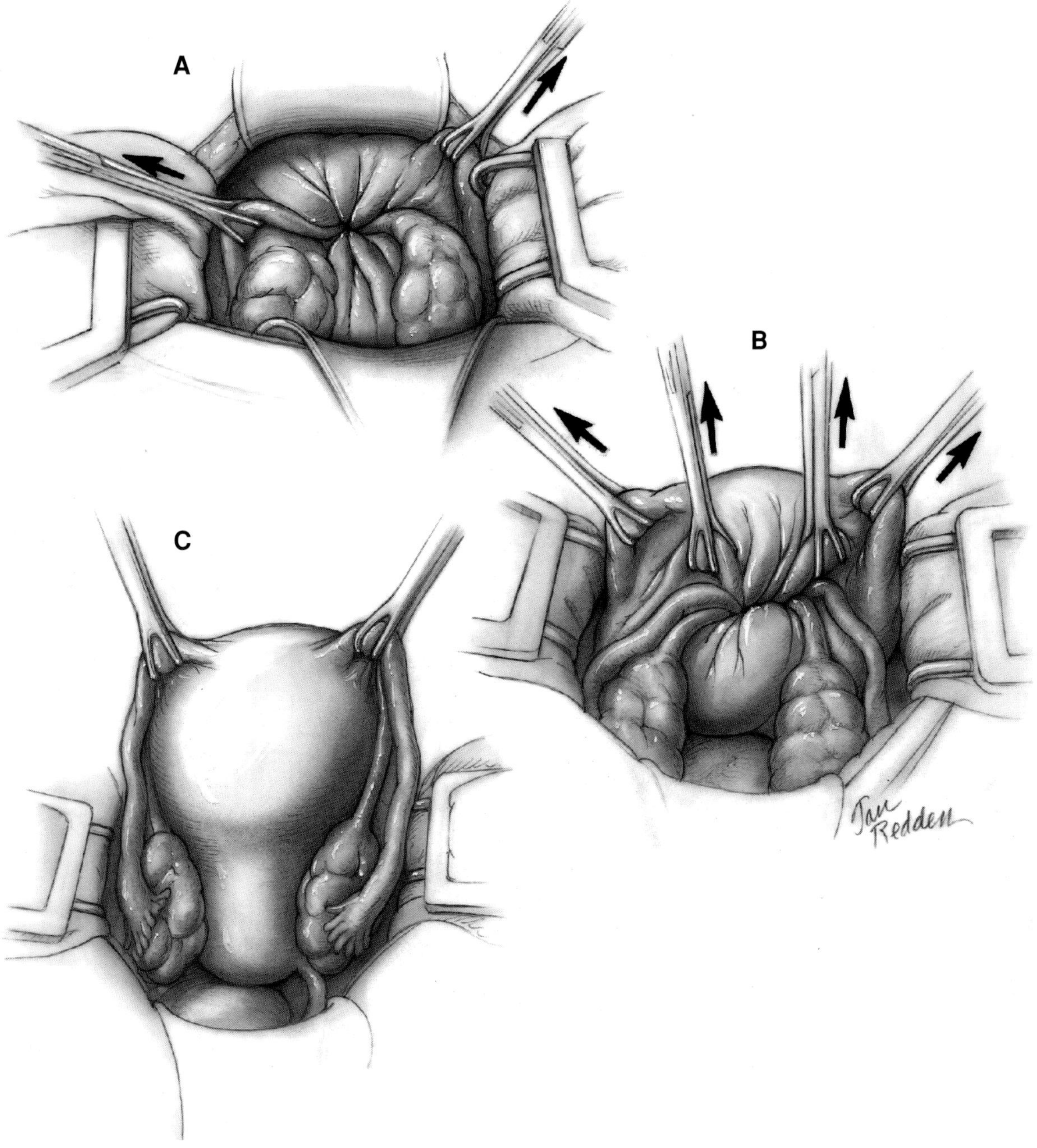

Figure 15–4. The Huntington maneuver. **A**. With an Allis or Babcock forceps, the operator grasps the surface of the uterus in the crater created by the inversion. These are drawn upward, simultaneously pulling a portion of the uterus out of the ring and restoring it to the peritoneal cavity. **B**. Steadying the uterus by the forceps already applied, the surgeon now inserts another Allis clamp into the crater as before and pulls upward. **C**. Thus, by successive bits and upward traction, the uterus is gradually restored to its normal position in the abdominal cavity.

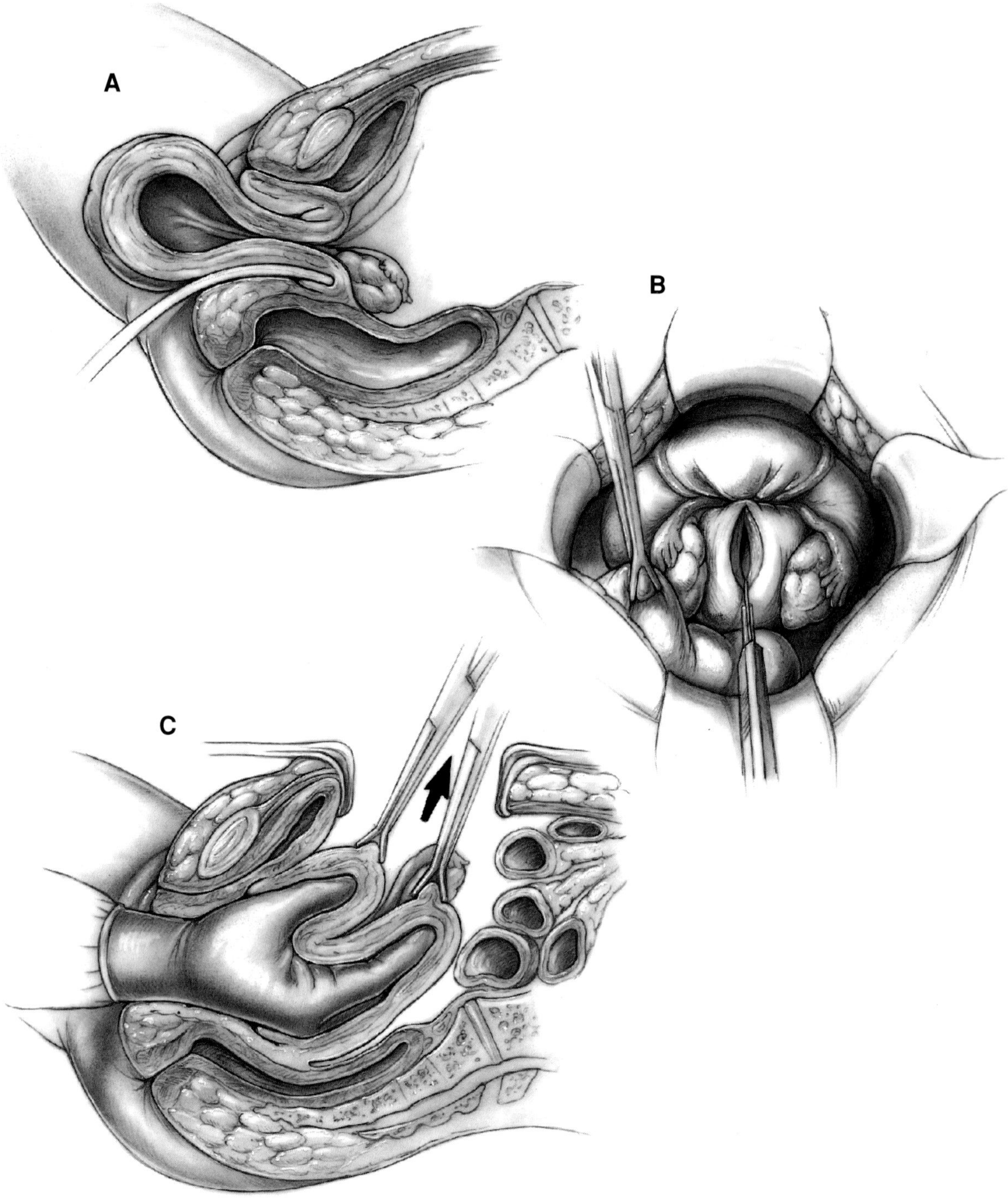

Figure 15–5. A. The uterus is completely inverted, with the fundal portions of the tubes and round ligaments pulled downward through the constricting collar. A malleable retractor is placed in the posterior vagina, with its tip inserted between the posterior lip of the cervix and the inverted uterine wall at the point at which the muscle will be cut. **B**. The rectosigmoid is held out of the way while an incision is made entirely through the uterine wall at the point of greatest constriction. The length of the incision will vary but should be long enough to permit passage of the fundus. If the incision is made over the previously placed malleable retractor, only the uterus will be incised, and the vaginal structures will not be injured. **C**. The fundus is replaced by combined traction on the uterine wall from above by the operator and pressure from below by an assistant. When replacement is complete, the incision is closed with interrupted chromic sutures.

oxytocic agents begun. If unsuccessful, an attempt at repositioning the uterus under general anesthesia should be performed before resorting to abdominal procedures. If an abdominal approach is necessary, the Huntington procedure should be attempted and, if unsuccessful, the Haultin method should be used.

REFERENCES

Bell JE, Wilson F, Wilson LA. Puerperal inversion of the uterus. Am J Obstet Gynecol 1953; 66: 767.

Brar HS, Greenspoon JS, Platt LD, Paul RH. Acute puerperal uterine inversion—new approaches to management. J Reprod Med 1989; 34:173.

Bunke JW, Hofmeister FJ. Uterine inversion—obstetrical entity or oddity. Am J Obstet Gynecol 1965; 91:934.

Clark SL. Use of ritodrine in uterine inversion. Am J Obstet Gynecol 1984; 151:705.

Das P. Inversion of the uterus. J Obstet Gynaecol Br Emp 1940; 47:525.

Gordon OA. A contribution to the etiology and treatment of puerperal inversion of the uterus. Am J Obstet Gynecol 1936; 32:399.

Haultain FWN. The treatment of chronic uterine inversion by abdominal hysterotomy, with a successful case. Br Med J 1901; 2:974.

Henderson H, Alles RW. Puerperal inversion of the uterus. J Obstet Gynecol 1948; 56:133.

Heyl PS, Stubblefield PG, Phillippe M. Recurrent inversion of the puerperal uterus managed with 15(s)-15-methyl prostaglandin $F_{2\alpha}$ and uterine packing. Obstet Gynecol 1984; 63:263.

Huntington JL, Irving FC, Kellogg FS. Abdominal reposition in acute inversion of the puerperal uterus. Am J Obstet Gynecol 1928; 15:34.

Johnson AB. A new concept in the replacement of the inverted uterus and a report of nine cases. Am J Obstet Gynecol 1949; 57:557.

Jones WC. Inversion of the uterus. With report of a case occurring during the puerperium and caused by a fibroid. Surg Gynecol Obstet 1913; 16:632.

Jones WC. Reports of two cases of postpartum inversion of the uterus, with discussion of the pathogenesis of obstetrical inversion. Am J Obstet 1914; 69:982.

Kitchin JD III, Thiagarajah S, May HV, Thornton WN. Puerperal inversion of the uterus. Am J Obstet Gynecol 1975; 123:51.

Lewin JS, Bryan PJ. MR imaging of uterine inversion. Case report. J Comp Assist Tomogr 1989; 13:357.

McCullagh WMH. Inversion of the uterus: a report on three cases and an analysis of 233 recently recorded cases. J Obstet Gynaecol Br Emp 1925; 32:280.

Momani AW, Hassan A. Treatment of puerperal uterine inversion by the hydrostatic method; reports of five cases. Eur J Obstet Gynecol Reprod Biol 1989; 32:281.

O'Sullivan JV. Acute inversion of the uterus. Br Med J 1945; 2:282.

Platt LD, Druzin ML. Acute puerperal inversion of the uterus. Am J Obstet Gynecol 1981; 141:187.

Rachagan SP, Sivanesaratnam V, Kok KP, Raman S. Acute puerperal inversion of the uterus—an obstetric emergency. Aust NZ J Obstet Gynaecol 1988; 28:29.

Romo MS, Grimes DA, Strassle PO. Infarction of the uterus from subacute incomplete inversion. Am J Obstet Gynecol 1992; 166:878.

Shah-Hosseini R, Evrard JR. Puerperal uterine inversion. Obstet Gynecol 1989; 73:567.

Steffen EA. Puerperal inversion of the uterus occurring in consecutive pregnancies in the same patient. Am J Obstet Gynecol 1957; 74:655.

Watson P, Besch N, Bowes WA. Management of acute and subacute puerperal inversion of the uterus. Obstet Gynecol 1980; 55:12.

CHAPTER 16

Uterine Packing for Control of Postpartum Uterine Hemorrhage

Severe postpartum hemorrhage is a potentially life-threatening obstetric complication. Once both upper and lower genital lacerations and retained placenta have been excluded, efforts are directed at increasing uterine muscular tone and maintaining hemodynamic stability. When uterine massage, oxytocin, methergine, and prostaglandin therapies fail to halt blood loss, the physician must resort to other means to control the hemorrhage while simultaneously providing volume and blood and factor replacement to the woman. In this scenario, some sort of invasive procedure is often performed to obstruct the blood supply to the uterus either surgically by vessel ligation or radiologically by embolization of the vessels. The success rates of these procedures are variable, and many times hysterectomy is ultimately required. Time-to-control of the bleeding shows a high correlation with the volume of blood products required, emphasizing the need for both timely and efficacious interventions.

Our forefathers in medicine often employed another therapeutic maneuver, packing the uterine cavity with gauze, which could be performed quickly in the delivery room. Although very effective, uterine packing curiously fell from routine practice during the last 30–50 years. Considering the widespread use of uterine packing in the 1920s, '30s, and '40s, one wonders why the procedure fell into disuse. Was its decline related to poor outcome? Could it be safely used in current medical practice, or have better anesthesia, surgical, and radiologic techniques, and blood and component therapy made it an anachronism?

HISTORICAL PERSPECTIVE

No published data are available regarding the percentage of practicing obstetricians who performed uterine packing in the early to mid 1900s. Textbooks of the time indicate that many prominent obstetricians including Joseph DeLee, J. P. Greenhill, E. Stuart Taylor, and Henricus J. Stander endorsed the practice. In their textbook, *Principles and Practices of Obstetrics*, Doctors DeLee and Greenhill supported uterine packing through all nine editions (1947). *Williams Obstetrics* supported uterine packing until the 10th edition (Eastman, 1950), which corresponded to a change in editors, Nicholas Eastman replacing Henricus J. Stander in 1945. This change from advocating uterine packing for the control of postpartum hemorrhage was not based on specific clinical studies; rather it reflected an endorsement of the views of others (Leff, 1939; Cosgrove, 1936). Since the 11th edition, *Williams Obstetrics* has retained its philosophy of not endorsing uterine packing.

In searching for specific objections to the practice of uterine packing, three can be identified. That the procedure is unphysiologic cannot be denied, but this objection can be set aside for lack of specific scientific relevance. The other two objections were the potential for concealed hemorrhage and infection (Eastman, 1950; Leff, 1939; Cosgrove, 1936). A review of references objecting to uterine packing reveals no instances of either concealed hemorrhage or infection.

Hemorrhage

Concealed hemorrhage is unlikely if uterine packing is performed properly; however, an improperly packed uterus invites continuation of the hemorrhage (Figs. 16–1; 16–2). In 1960 Dr. E. Stuart Taylor cited 15 years of experience and 65,000 deliveries without one example of a postpartum uterus removed purely for atony (Taylor, 1960). Doctors DeLee and Greenhill reported that 398 out of 400 cases treated with uterine packing were successful. The two who failed with the initial packing were successfully treated with a second packing (repacking) of the uterus (DeLee and Greenhill, 1943). In more recent articles, the success of the procedure has been excellent (Cavanagh, 1961; Hester, 1974; Lester and associates, 1965; Pierce and Winkler, 1956; Maier, 1993). All of these reports leave no question that technique is all important, a statement applicable to most areas of surgical practice.

Infection

The potential for infection seems likely when the uterine cavity is filled with a foreign body (gauze). Although literature from the 1930s and 1940s does not indicate occurrence rates or other details, these articles suggest that infection was a problem as the packing instruments used permitted the instillation of a gauze that could be impregnated with an antiseptic (Anderson and co-workers, 1942). More recent articles have mentioned only the use of systemic antibiotics and have used untreated gauze. While earlier articles give few details regarding fever, recent medical reports specifically state that the patients were afebrile when initially packed and generally remained so (Maier, 1993; Druzin, 1989). One example of uterine packing having a favorable outcome in a patient presenting 10 days postpartum with fever and bleeding suggests a favorable outcome may be anticipated even when

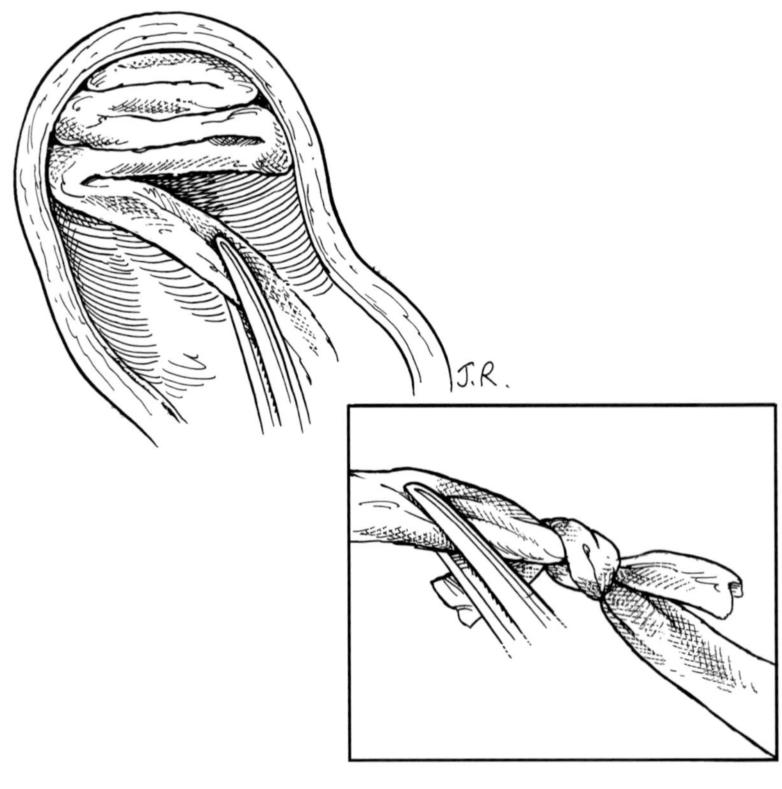

Figure 16–1. Uterine packing is begun in the fundus. More than one roll of gauze is usually required, in which case the ends of the rolls are tied together (inset).

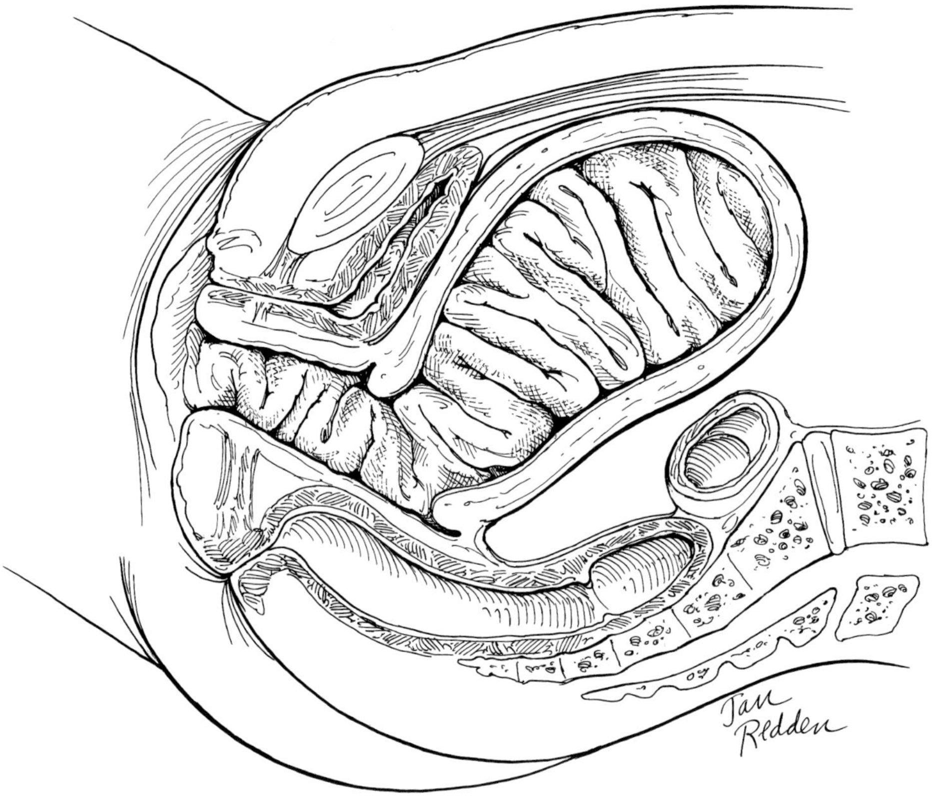

Figure 16–2. Properly packed uterus. The uterine cavity is uniformly packed with pressure uniformly placed on all aspects of the uterine cavity.

used with a coexisting infection. Caution is advised, however, when considering uterine packing in women who appear to be infected. Extended patient observations have reported instances of normal pregnancies and normal pelvic anatomy after uterine packing (Lester and colleagues, 1965; Maier, 1993; Druzin, 1989). The risk of infection seems to be minimal overall and is likely related to antibiotic administration and the removal of the uterine packing material about within 2–3 days of insertion.

Maternal Deaths

To further evaluate the safety of uterine packing for the treatment of postpartum hemorrhage, data regarding maternal deaths related to postpartum hemorrhage or infection during its era of peak use were analyzed. The Maternal Welfare Committee of Philadelphia reviewed 52 deaths from exsanguination occurring in 183,384 deliveries in Philadelphia from 1931 to 1936. In this review, uterine packing was accomplished in 28 of the cases. The author attributed the deaths of the women to neglect and not to the procedure; "rather the picture brought to light by this study was one of steady moderate bleeding over a period of several hours, ending in shock and death because no one became alarmed" (Beecham, 1939). While examples of bleeding through the packing material were cited, the author attributed the lack of any other corrective action by the health care providers as the cause of death. No examples of concealed hemorrhage or infections related to uterine packing were cited. Indeed, the recommended management algorithm was to exclude genital lacerations, give blood transfusions, and perform uterine packing: "In the treatment of postpartum hemorrhage, two procedures stand out above all others; early transfusion and packing" (Beecham, 1939). Hysterectomy was reserved for those patients who failed uterine packing.

PACKING TECHNIQUE

The success of uterine packing is directly related to technique. In uterine atony and postpartum hemorrhage, packing of the uterus must be uniform, tight, and complete. It is not the insertion of a wad of packing material in a single thrust into the uterus. All series that have reported a high level of success have stressed that the packing material is unrolled and evenly placed in all aspects of the uterine cavity through repeated insertion efforts. If more than one roll of material is used, a knot to secure the two rolls is recommended. The gauze is usually supplied in either 5- or 9-yard rolls. Uniform application means side-to-side, front-to-back, top-to-bottom (Fig. 16–1). The entire procedure is accomplished in a very few minutes and involves the obstetrician and an assistant.

The instrument used in the uterine packing is not as important as the technique. DeLee and Greenhill (1947) advocated one hand in the uterus with the second hand advancing the material to the first using uterine packing forceps (Fig. 16–3). Torpin (1941) invented a canister and plunger apparatus (Fig. 16–4); the Holmes Packer and Gomco Packer were other instruments; doubtlessly more existed. The singularly important technical feature was that the material was applied inside the uterus layer by layer and that the upper aspects of the uterus was packed first (Fig. 16–5). The uterus can also be packed successfully without the use of instruments (Fig. 16–6).

After the packing of the uterine cavity is completed, the patient must be observed closely. Bleeding through the packing is the most common failure. When this occurs, the diagnosis is usually made soon after the packing procedure. In successfully packed patients, the gauze will become deeply stained (soaked) with blood, but external bleeding will be less than a menstrual flow or normal lochia. In instances of bleeding through the packing (failure), the blood loss will approximate that seen before the procedure. Broad spectrum

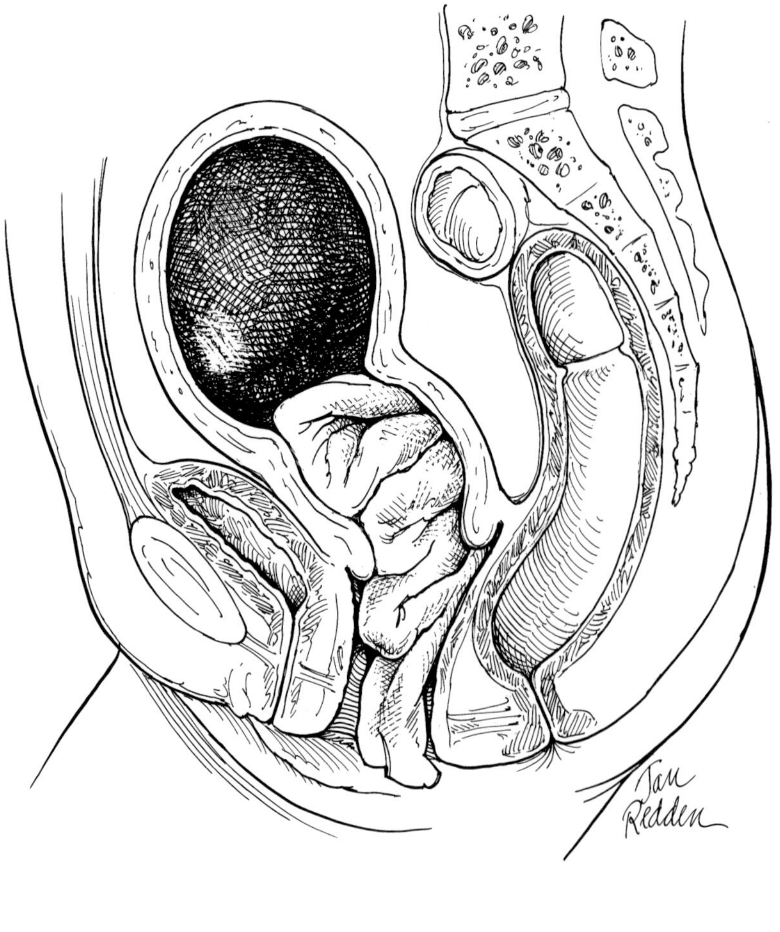

Figure 16–3. Improperly packed uterus. The uterine cavity is not packed properly. Packing material has slipped from the fundal area and the fundal area would continue to bleed due to this improper technique.

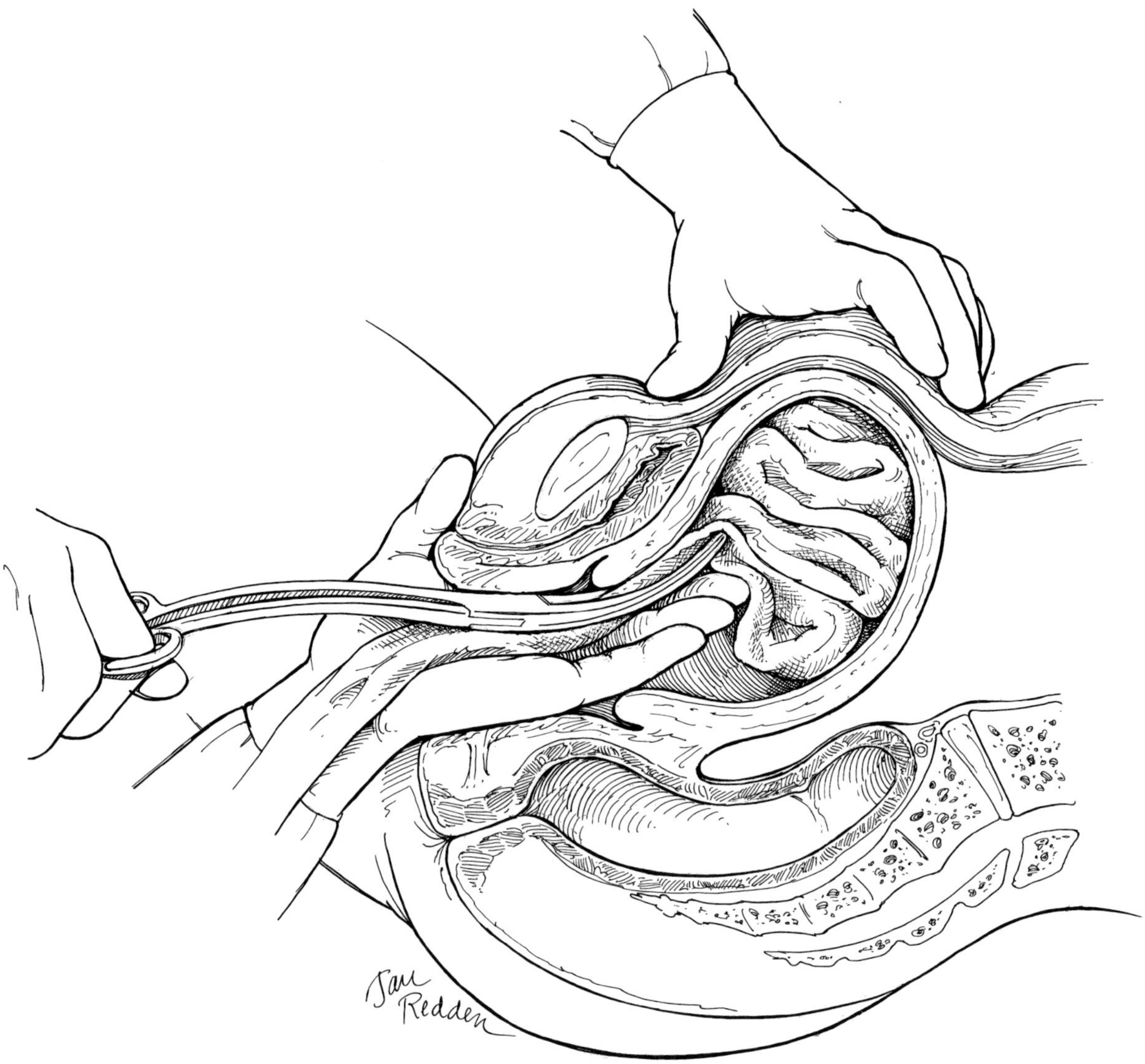

Figure 16–4. The uterus is steadied by an assistant while the operator, using a uterine packing forceps, passes gauze to the hand inside the uterine cavity. The purpose is to advance packing material uniformly and to completely fill the uterine cavity.

systemic antibiotics are given due to intrauterine manipulation and are reasonable as long as the packing material remains in the uterus.

The time for removal of the packing is quite flexible. Early literature suggested 24–36 hours after insertion, but more recent reports vary in their recommendations from 5 to 96 hours. This variation in time primarily reflects the woman's medical condition, as reason would dictate that the patient should be hemodynamically stable before the packing is removed. Removal is generally not associated with unusual degrees of patient pain and no bleeding is to be expected. Rarely are any clots seen; however, the gauze may be soaked with serum and blood. The gauze is withdrawn in a layer-by-layer fashion, identical to the manner in which it was inserted.

INDICATIONS

Uterine packing should be considered in postpartum hemorrhage related to uterine atony and in patients desiring future pregnancies.

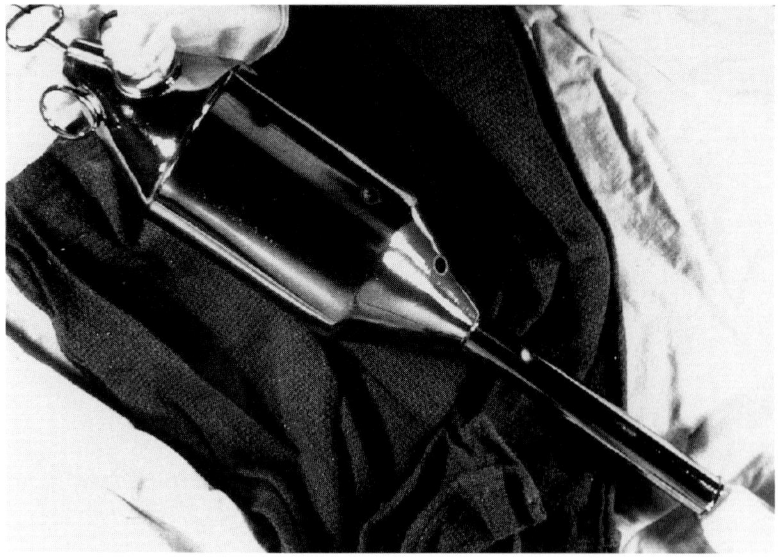

Figure 16–5. The Torpin Packer invented by Robert Torpin. This instrument is shown in its original form. Repeated plunger action (shown in upper left corner) by the operator forces packing material out of nozzle (lower right portion of picture). With side-to-side movement, the uterine cavity will be completely filled.

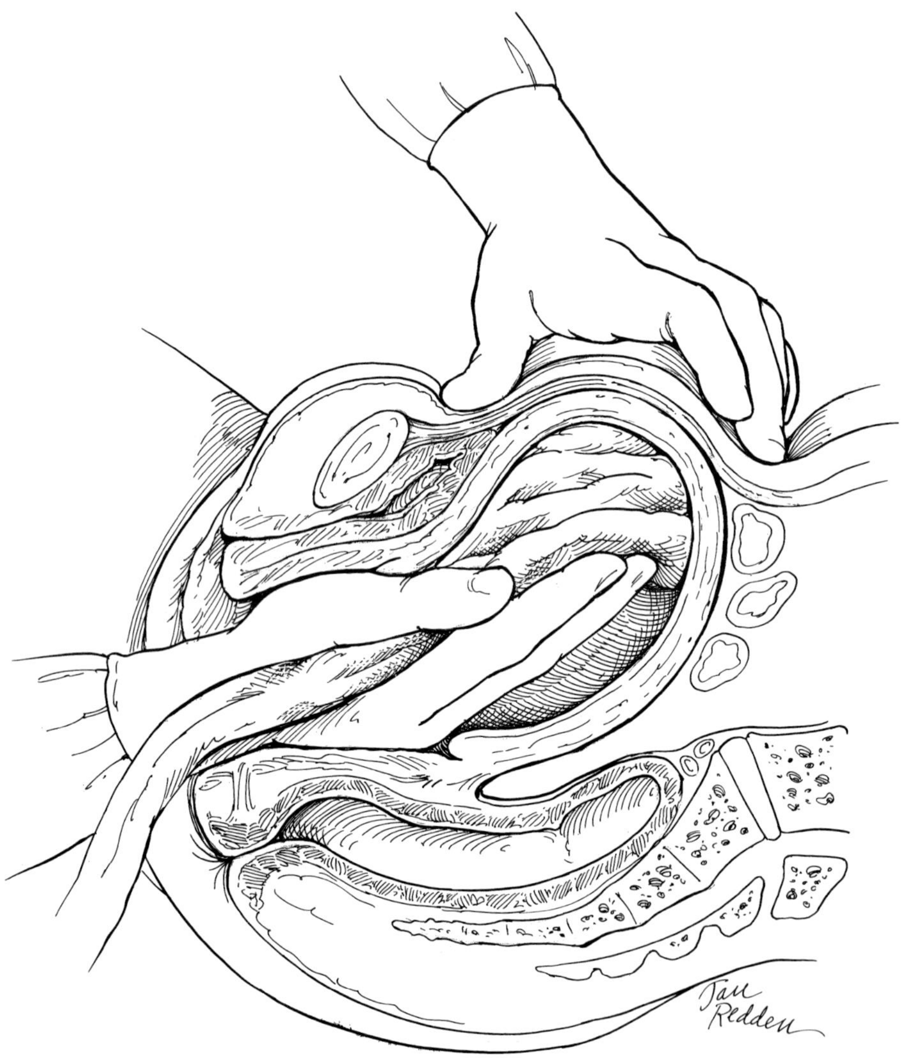

Figure 16–6. Packing of the uterine cavity without the use of any instruments. The operator must assure that the packing material does not become dislodged from the uterine fundus when the intrauterine hand is removed to obtain more packing material.

While the procedure has been used in several different clinical situations including placenta accreta, placenta previa, and uterine atony as well as in women who have delivered either abdominally or vaginally, uterine packing is not for every patient. Distortion of the uterine cavity by leiomyomas or other conditions may make packing of the cavity technically infeasible. Hysterectomy may be preferable when uterine preservation is not desired or when there is other uterine or cervical pathology.

SUMMARY

Using uterine packing to control postpartum hemorrhage due to uterine atony may initially challenge the medical teachings of many physicians. The impact on the young woman whose uterus was removed shortly after her first delivery, or indeed the unexpected and emergency removal of the uterus of any woman, must also be considered. Uterine packing was a time-honored practice in the past and its abandonment cannot be traced to any supportable untoward clinical outcomes. Each practitioner is encouraged to research the issue and to integrate into his or her medical practice those procedures which are deemed appropriate. Gould's 1897 observation is apropos: "We wish to enter a mild protest against the modern egotism that would set aside with a sneer as myth and fancy the testimonies and reports of philosophers and physicians, only because they lived hundreds of years ago." To integrate uterine packing into a plan of corrective procedures for postpartum uterine atony and hemorrhage is reasonable and poses no undue threat to the patient who is given proper medical support.

REFERENCES

Anderson HE, Gardner HL, Gunderson MF, Slack JM. The use of uterine packs impregnated with sulfanilamide. Am J Obstet Gynecol 1942; 43:410.

Beecham CT. Postpartum hemorrhage as a cause of death. Am J Obstet Gynecol 1939; 37:258.

Cavanagh D, ed. Obstetrical emergencies. Springfield, IL: Charles C. Thomas, 1961; 198.

Cosgrove SA. Obstetrical hemorrhage and its management. South Med J 1936; 29:1219.

DeLee JB, Greenhill JP, eds. Pathology of the third stage. In: Principles and Practice of Obstetrics. 8th ed. Philadelphia: WB Saunders, 1943; 813.

DeLee JB, Greenhill JP, eds. Pathology of the third stage. In: Principles and Practice of Obstetrics. 9th ed. Philadelphia, London: WB Saunders, 1947; 723.

Druzin ML. Packing of lower uterine segment for control of postcesarean bleeding in instances of placenta previa. Surg Gynecol Obstet 1989; 169:543.

Eastman NJ, ed. Anomalies of the third stage of labor. In: Williams Obstetrics. 10th ed. New York: Appleton-Century-Crofts, 1950; 917.

Gould GM, Pyle WL, eds. Anomalies and curiosities of medicine. Philadelphia: WB Saunders, 1897; 3.

Hester JD. Postpartum hemorrhage and reevaluation of uterine packing. Obstet Gynecol 1974; 45:501.

Leff M. Management of the third and fourth stages of labor. Surg Gynecol Obstet 1939; 68:224.

Lester WM, Bartholomew RA, Colvin ED, et al. Reconsideration of the uterine pack in postpartum hemorrhage. Am J Obstet Gynecol 1965; 93:321.

Maier RC. Control of postpartum hemorrhage with uterine packing. Am J Obstet Gynecol 1993; 169:317.

Pierce JR, Winkler EG. Why not pack the postpartum uterus? Minn Med 1956; 39:89.

Stander HJ, ed. Textbook of obstetrics. 3rd ed (9th ed., Williams Obstetrics). New York, London: Appleton-Century-Crofts, 1945; 1125.

Taylor ES. Intrapartum and postpartum hemorrhage. Clin Obstet Gynecol 1960; 3:646.

Torpin R. An "automatic" postpartum uterine packer. Am J Obstet Gynecol 1941; 41:334.

CHAPTER 17

Surgical Treatment of Lower Genital Tract Infections

The management of most bacterial and viral lower genital infections in pregnancy is generally accomplished by medical treatment. Many of these infections are caused by sexually transmitted diseases (STDs). Their management is beyond the scope of this chapter but is reviewed in the treatment guidelines of the Centers for Disease Control and Prevention (1993). There is little role for the surgical management of acute bacterial or viral infections, except the surgical drainage of vulvovaginal abscesses. The role of surgery in chronic bacterial or viral infections is also limited and is best deferred until completion of pregnancy unless significant symptoms dictate earlier intervention.

The clinical presentation of vulvovaginal surgical infections is probably affected minimally by pregnancy. However, it may be altered by host factors that should be evaluated prior to decisions regarding medical or surgical treatment. These include, but are not limited to, diabetes mellitus, cancer, human immunodeficiency virus (HIV) infection, and treatment with immunosuppressive drugs. Immunosuppression from human immunodeficiency viral infection and the acquired immunodeficiency syndrome (AIDS) may mask clinical and laboratory signs of local infection and bacteremia due to granulocytopenia and impaired inflammatory response (Berger and associates, 1994). It may also effect the clinical response of chosen therapy, although little is known about this relationship (Macho and Schecter, 1992).

VULVAR ABSCESS

Vulvar or vestibular abscesses occasionally complicate pregnancy. Acute infections may follow pyogenic bacterial folliculitis. Chronic or recurrent vulvar abscesses may occur in women with furunculosis, carbuncles, or hidradenitis suppurativa. Often, small abscesses may be quite debilitating and painful. Most superficial infections become fluctuant and will spontaneously drain. Hot baths or packs may accelerate the temporal course of deeper abscesses to pointing.

It is sometimes difficult to differentiate cellulitis from an abscess; however, needle aspiration of the infected area will generally elucidate the correct diagnosis. Pathogenic bacteria are usually normal skin flora, but mixed aerobic and anaerobic infections are

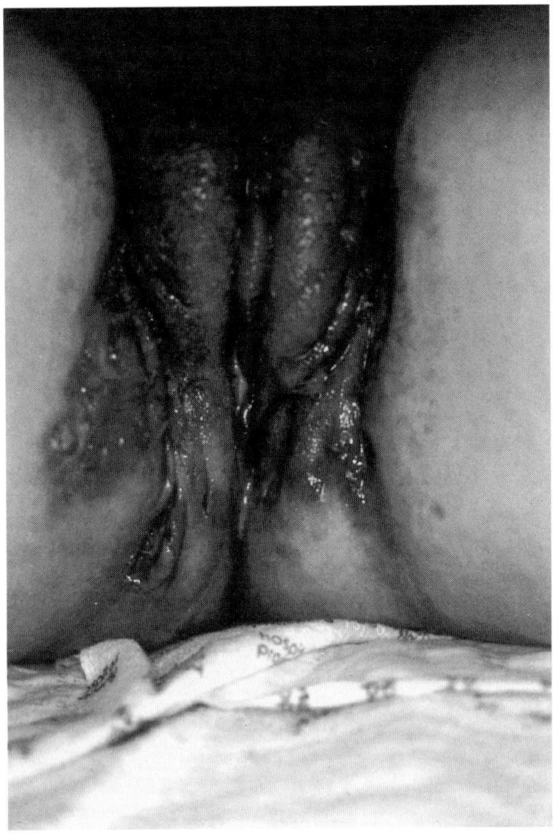

Figure 17–1. Hidradenitis suppurativa showing multiple chronically infected, communicating draining sinus tracts.

common. In immunocompetent patients, Gram stain and bacterial culture add little to the clinical management; however, in complicated infections laboratory identification of the dermatopathogen may be helpful.

Small, superficial vulvar abscesses are best treated by simple incision and drainage. Such minor abscesses may be incised with a No. 11 scalpel blade with a vertical incision following the natural Langer's cleavage lines. Most cases can be performed under local anesthesia and managed as outpatients. Small cavities do not require gauze packing, but local hydrotherapy may assist healing. Many clinicians add broad-spectrum oral antimicrobial treatment after drainage, but this is of uncertain benefit.

Hospitalization for surgical drainage should be considered if there is immunocompromise or significant surrounding cellulitis is present. Overwhelming septicemia and necrotizing fasciitis have been described, complicating surgical treatment in these settings (Cruikshank and McLauchlan, 1987). If the abscess is suspected to be multilocular or deep, surgical exploration may be easier under general anesthesia or spinal analgesia. Broad-spectrum antimicrobials such as cefoxitin or ampicillin with sulbactam are often administered prior to surgery to cover transient bacteremia and treat cellulitis.

There are probably very few indications during pregnancy for definitive surgical therapy for chronic hidradenitis suppurativa (Fig. 17–1). This chronic multifocal vulvar apocrine gland infection during pregnancy may cause recurrent abscesses or a malodorous vulvar exudate. Antepartum isoretinoin and antiandrogen therapy is contraindicated, but prolonged broad-spectrum antimicrobial therapy may improve symptoms. More extensive surgical therapy such as "unroofing" infected pockets and tunnels or wide local excision of involved areas is best postponed until after pregnancy.

BARTHOLIN GLAND ABSCESS

Little is known about the epidemiology of Bartholin gland infection and its complications in adult or pregnant women. In nonpregnant women, it is most commonly associated with age 20–29 years, nulliparity, and lower socioeconomic status. It is not related to ethnicity or marital status (Aghajanian and colleagues, 1994). These women often have prior or concomitant STDs, particularly gonorrhea and chlamydial infection. The demographic characteristics have led to the conclusion that acute Bartholin gland infection is probably an STD. However, recurrent infections or abscesses may be the consequence of scarring of the gland duct damaged by a prior infection.

Microbiology

The microbiology of Bartholin gland infection is similar to that of pelvic inflammatory disease (Brook, 1989; Lee and associates, 1977). Most abscesses have mixed aerobic and anaerobic pathogens, some will be single pathogen infections, and in up to one-third no pathogen is isolated by culture. The predominant organisms are those of the normal vaginal flora, including Gram-negative anaerobic rods, Gram-positive anaerobic rods, *Escherichia coli, Staphylococcus,* and *Streptococcus.* Many investigators have isolated *Neisseria gonorrhoeae* and to some extent *Chlamydia trachomatis* from abscesses (Brook, 1989; Saul and Grossman, 1988). *Mycoplasma hominis* and *Ureaplasma urealyticum* do not appear to be important pathogens in most Bartholin gland abscesses (Lee and colleagues, 1977). While most Bartholin gland cysts are sterile, and most abscesses contain bacteria, there is a spectrum of their clinical presentation and microbiology.

Clinical presentation of a Bartholin gland infection is usually at the abscess stage. Ductal infection alone is unusual. Abscesses are generally unilocular and several centimeters in diameter. Surrounding erythema, induration, and tenderness may obscure actual abscess size. A careful examination for signs of necrotizing fasciitis should precede decisions on the optimal treatment, especially in immunocompromised women, including those with diabetes. Indeed, acute bartholinitis can cause diabetic ketoacidosis. Septic shock and a toxic shock-like syndrome can also complicate Bartholin gland infections (Carson and Smith, 1980; Lopez-Zeno and colleagues, 1990; Shearin and associates, 1989).

Decisions concerning appropriate therapy depend on underlying immune status and severity of infection. In general, immunocompetent women with early, mild infection or a small abscess can be treated with a broad-spectrum oral antimicrobial agent, analgesics, and local heat by packs or Sitz baths. Spontaneous drainage often occurs within 2–3 days during such local therapy. Alternatively, if the abscess is larger and fluctuant, then surgical drainage may be technically easier.

Surgical Therapy

Several surgical techniques have been proposed for management of Bartholin gland abscesses. These include incision and drainage, marsupialization, and catheter drainage. None of these has undergone randomized, prospective evaluation in sufficiently large trials to exclude differences in outcome.

There are four main goals of surgical treatment for Bartholin gland abscesses. First, there must be adequate surgical drainage of the infected gland and abscess. Second, the gland should be preserved, so that it may continue its secretory function. Third, recurrences should be prevented by creation of a new gland ostium or fistula to replace the function of the presumed damaged or occluded duct. Fourth, complications of the infection such as necrotizing fasciitis and sepsis should be prevented.

There is little indication in abscess management for primary excision of the Bartholin gland. Excision may be associated with intraoperative hemorrhage, postoperative hematoma, and subsequent dyspareunia from vulvar scarring and lack of Bartholin gland lubrication (Zuspan and Quilligan, 1988). The purpose of other surgical techniques is to establish immediate drainage and subsequent development of a new gland ostium. The new opening is actually a cutaneous fistula that may take several weeks to fully epithelialize. Patency of this tract allows continued gland secretion without cyst or recurrent abscess formation.

Techniques

The simplest technique is **incision and drainage** that involves creating a 1-cm vertical stab wound with a No. 11 or 15 scalpel blade into the abscess cavity (Fig. 17–2). If the abscess has drained spontaneously, then the opening may be extended further. The cavity is ex-plored with a tissue forceps, evacuated, and irrigated. A self-retaining Word catheter (10 French, 5 cm length, 5 mL balloon tip) is inserted into the cavity, and the proximal bulb is inflated with 2–5 mL of water (Word, 1964). The bulb should be inflated sufficiently to prevent spontaneous catheter expulsion through the gland opening as well as to avoid painful dilation of the gland. Local hydrotherapy or Sitz baths may aid healing, but discomfort from the catheter is common unless the distal end is cephalad from the introitus. The Word catheter may be removed after there has been sufficient epithelialization of the new fistula, usually 1–4 weeks. The recurrence rate with this technique is approximately 10 percent (Heath, 1988).

Marsupialization of the Bartholin gland abscess also can be safely accomplished after drainage (Fig. 17–3). The procedure may require general or regional anesthesia, but usually can be accomplished with local infiltration or pudendal block. The technique has been variously described using fine absorbable suture to exteriorize and reapproximate the abscess lining to the vaginal mucosa or vestibular epithelium. It is important to create an ostium of sufficient diameter to prevent

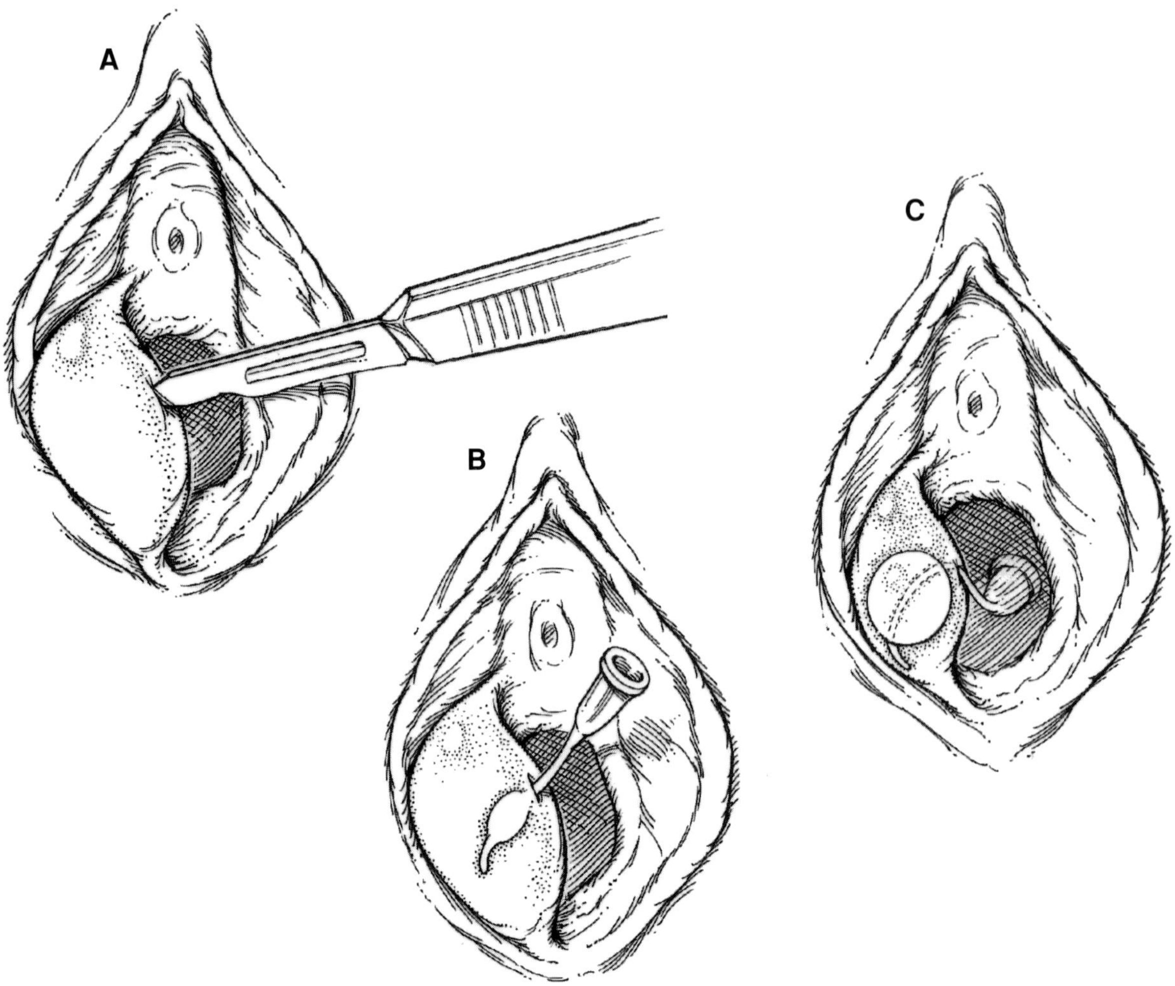

Figure 17–2. Management of a Bartholin gland abscess using the Word catheter. **A.** A stab wound is made into the abscess using a No. 15 scalpel blade. **B.** Insertion of catheter in cavity. **C.** Properly inflated balloon tip with external catheter tip directed into vagina.

secondary closure, for the healed fistula will be of appreciably smaller caliber. The excision of an elliptical or oval specimen of about 1–2 cm is usually adequate (Oliphant and Anderson, 1960). Cho and associates (1990) emphasized the need for excision of a specimen of 2–3 cm in length and 1–1.5 cm in width and renamed the technique the **window operation.** The abscess cavity can be packed loosely with quarter-inch or half-inch plain gauze, which may be removed in 24 hours. Using this method, recurrences have been reported in 5–25 percent of cases.

Three other techniques have limited experience to validate their efficacy, but merit mention. **Carbon dioxide laser** has been used in the management of Bartholin gland cysts, but not abscesses (Davis, 1985; Lashgari and Keene, 1986). This technique creates a neostoma for the gland after vaporization of the cyst roof. Alternatively, it has been used to incise and vaporize the cyst from the inside. Both techniques result in good outcomes, but at significant costs. **Needle aspiration** of infected Bartholin glands along with oral antimicrobial therapy has been described in 21 women (Cheetham, 1985). Failures occurred in 15 percent of cases. Anderson and associates (1992) reported good results with **incision, drainage, gland curettage,** and **suture** with antimicrobial coverage. Two to three vertical mattress sutures under the abscess floor, but not through the cavity, were placed for primary gland closure. Short-term

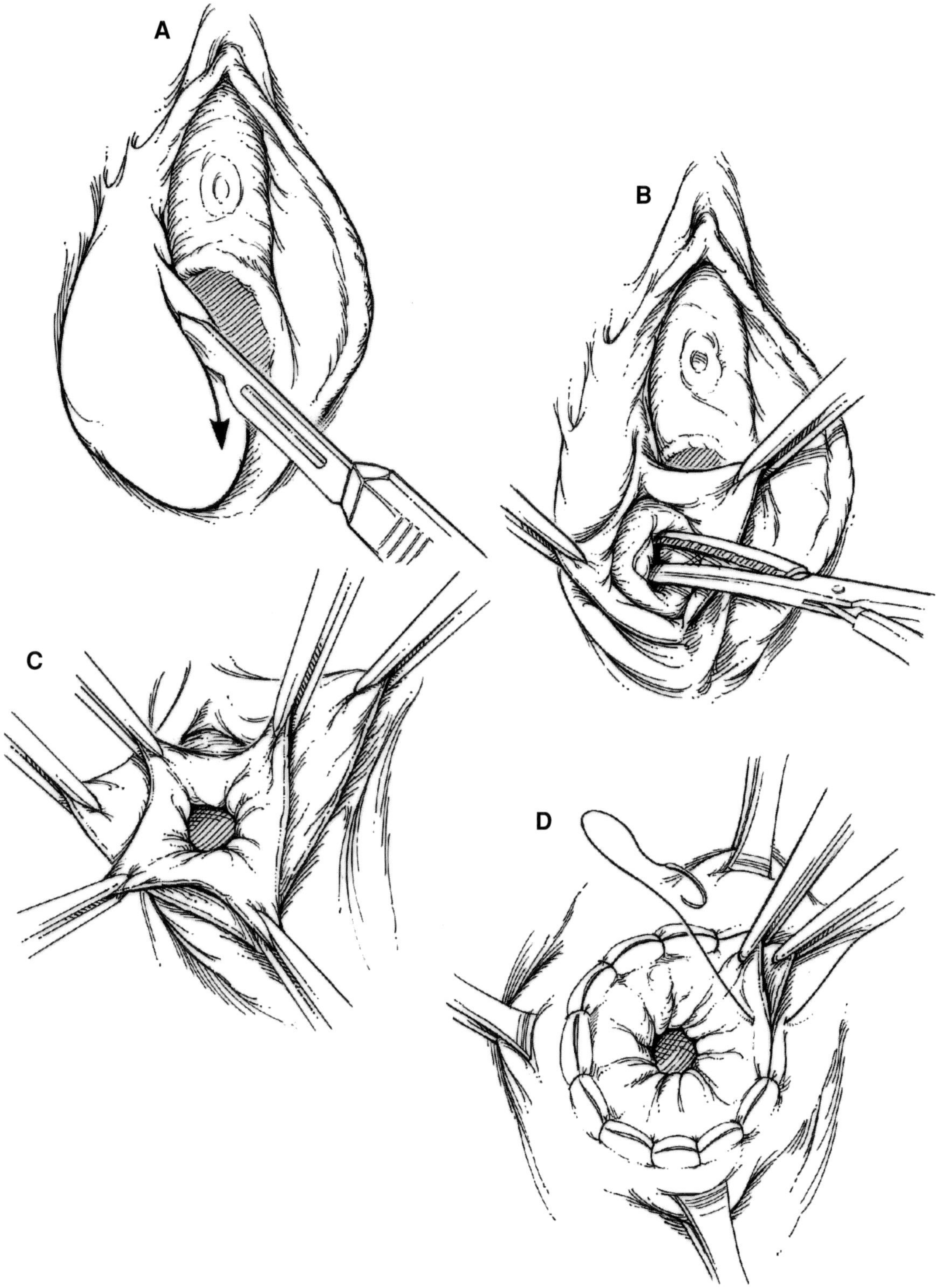

Figure 17–3. Technique of Bartholin gland abscess marsupialization. **A.** Linear incision is made over the abscess as medial and toward the vagina as possible. **B.** Hemostat or similar instrument is used to explore the abscess cavity and break up any loculations. **C.** Abscess cavity lining is identified. **D.** Lining of abscess cavity is sutured to the vaginal mucosa. This may be accomplished with a running-locking stitch or interrupted stitches using absorbable sutures.

outcome and recurrence rates were better than with marsupialization. They did not assess long-term gland function.

VULVAR CONDYLOMATA ACUMINATA

Human papillomavirus (HPV) infection during pregnancy is associated with clinical, subclinical, and latent anogenital infections that have little impact on pregnancy outcome. Papillomavirus types 6 or 11 are most commonly involved, but infection is associated frequently with cervical intraepithelial neoplasia, which also may involve types 16, 18, 31, 33, and 35.

As shown in Figure 17–4, condylomata acuminata or exophytic genital warts frequently increase in number and size during pregnancy, but rarely make vaginal delivery difficult. Accelerated viral replication with advancing pregnancy has been hypothesized to explain the growth of perineal lesions, progression of some to cervical neoplasm, and increased detection of viral DNA from the cervix in pregnant women (Gary and Jones, 1985; Rando and colleagues, 1989). Because these viral infections can be subclinical and multifocal, most women with vulvar lesions also have cervical infection, and vice versa (Spitzer and co-workers, 1989). The management of cervical papillomavirus infection is discussed in Chapter 31.

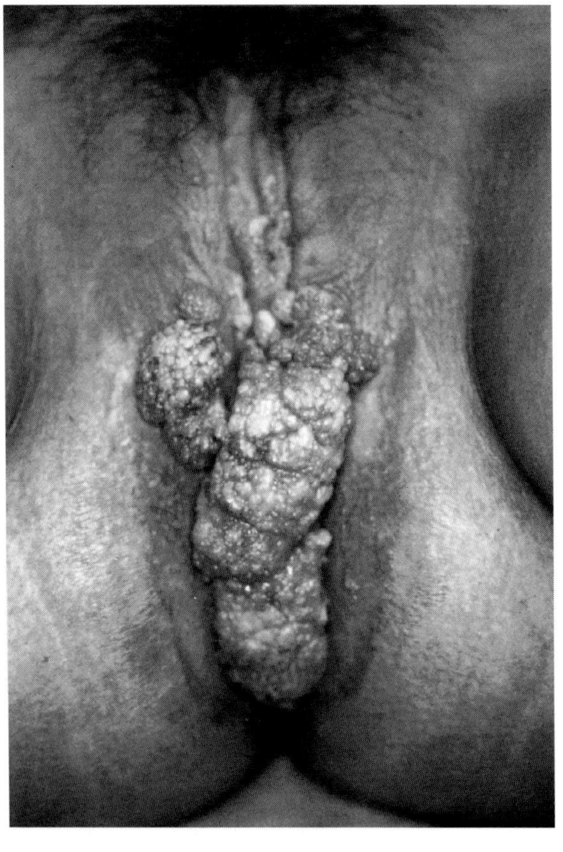

Figure 17–4. Verrucous vulvar condylomata acuminata.

Paradoxically, some vulvar lesions rapidly improve or disappear postpartum without treatment, possibly related to loss of vascularity or of the alleged immunosuppression of pregnancy.

Management

Treatment of HPV in any woman begins with examination, preferably with colposcopy, of the entire lower genital tract. Although condylomata acuminata are generally easily identified, a biopsy for histologic confirmation may be helpful (Felix and Wright, 1994). Without an effective and safe antiviral agent, the goal of treatment is to remove exophytic lesions and ameliorate symptoms of clinical infection (Ferenczy, 1989). No therapy can eradicate the virus completely because it also is present in normal tissue surrounding visible warts. Due to the multifocal and subclinical nature of this genital infection, recurrences are common, particularly in the first 3 months after therapy (Ferenczy and colleagues, 1985; Kirby and Corey, 1987).

Therapy in pregnancy is directed toward minimizing maternal and fetal toxicity and debulking the genital warts in the late second or third trimester to avoid recurrence prior to delivery. Although unproven, it is felt that exophytic warts are more infectious than subclinical or latent infection. Thus, treatment of visible warts by debulking may theoretically decrease the rate of transmission through sexual contact or vaginal birth.

Treatment also should be guided by wart location, size, number; cost; and patient preference. While there have been many clinical trials of treatment of genital warts in adult women, there is less experience with warts during pregnancy. Most methods are effective in cases when vulvar warts are small and have been present less than one year. **Trichloroacetic acid,** either 50 percent or 80–90 percent, applied topically three times weekly or once a week, respectively, is the least expensive mode of therapy (Centers for Disease Control, 1993; Ferenczy, 1989). Mucosal nonkeratinized lesions are moist, soft, and vascular and allow penetration of the topical desiccant acids. **Cryotherapy** and **CO_2 laser ablation** are the preferred modes of therapy in pregnancy for visible lesions in skin and skin appendages—hair follicles and sebaceous glands—especially for extensive keratotic or refractory genital warts (Bergman and associates, 1984; Ferenczy, 1984).

Due to the increased size of lesions and vascularity in pregnancy, **surgical excision** may cause excessive bleeding and tissue denudation. It should be used for large sessile warts with resectable stalks and avoided with extensive genital wart disease. While **loop electrosurgical excision** and **ultrasonic surgical aspiration** have been used effectively for surgical management of vulvar disease, there is limited experience concerning their safety and efficacy in pregnancy (Rader and colleagues, 1991; Wright and associates, 1991).

Unfortunately, failures are identified in about a third of women treated with trichloroacetic acid or laser ablation in the first and early second trimester (Bergman and co-workers, 1984; Ferenczy, 1989; Matsunaga and colleagues, 1987). Most clinical failures or recurrences are thought to be due to reactivation of coexistent latent viral infection rather than reinfection. Podophyllin resin, podophylox (podophyllotoxin) solution, 5-fluorouracil cream, and interferon therapy should not be used in pregnancy due to concerns about maternal and fetal toxicity.

Co-Infection with Human Immunodeficiency Virus

There is increased expression of clinical papillomavirus infection in women with human immunodeficiency viral infection, especially with progressive immunosuppression, low CD_4 lymphocyte counts, or acquired immunodeficiency syndrome (Johnson and associates, 1992; Vermund and colleagues, 1991). Unfortunately, the appropriate treatment and clinical response to therapy are poorly understood in this setting. In women with low CD_4 lymphocyte counts or acquired immunodeficiency syndrome, the efficacy of any modality is likely to be poor and the incidence of clinical recurrences increased. Offering counseling and testing for immunodeficiency virus is included in the routine clinical management of papillomaviral infection prior to treatment in many centers.

Juvenile Laryngeal Papillomatosis

There is usually great maternal concern about genital warts and their association with juvenile laryngeal papillomatosis. There is a particular association with HPV types 6 and 11 (Shah and co-workers, 1986). The frequency of perinatal papillomavirus transmission is unknown, and the route of transmission is unproven. The detection of virus in neonatal peripheral blood mononuclear cells and amnionic fluid raises the possibility that there may be intrauterine infection prior to delivery (Armbruster-Moraes and associates, 1993; Tseng and colleagues, 1992). Furthermore, treatment of visible warts or cesarean delivery have not been proven to decrease the risk of perinatal HPV transmission (Smith and co-workers, 1991).

Given the rarity of juvenile laryngeal papillomatosis—less than 1 per 100,000—and the relative frequency of genital infection—about 3 percent—elective cesarean delivery to prevent laryngeal papillomatosis is not justifiable. Although the risk of perinatal papillomaviral transmission is unknown, Shah and colleagues (1986) have estimated that it may be as high as 1 per 1000 in affected pregnancies. Watts and co-workers (1994) prospectively have followed a cohort of infants whose mothers had papillomavirus infection during pregnancy. Although no cases of certain perinatal transmission have occurred, the upper limit of the risk estimate was 3 percent. Operative delivery should be reserved for obstetric indications or vaginal obstructive viral lesions.

PERIANAL ABSCESS

Anorectal abscesses occasionally complicate pregnancy and must be promptly diagnosed and treated. Most infections begin in the anal glands between the internal and external anal sphincter muscles. Fecal and cutaneous bacteria cause an abscess in the intersphincteric space that spreads into one of several potential spaces filled with areolar tissue or fat. The most common locations of spread are perianal, ischiorectal, intersphincteric, and supralevator, respectively. A pilonidal abscess should be excluded prior to incision and drainage, for they are often multilocular. Rarely, Crohn disease may present as a perineal or perianal abscess or fistula. It is imperative to make the correct diagnosis before drainage, preferably with appropriate surgical consultation.

The perianal abscess is usually superficial and small, but causes significant pain on ambulation or with Valsalva maneuvers. A tender, indurated, erythematous mass is palpable at the anal verge, and there may be fever. The clinician should be alert for signs of septicemia and necrotizing fasciitis, especially with delayed treatment and in immunocompromised women.

Surgical drainage usually is performed under local anesthesia. One technique creates a cruciate incision over the abscess followed by exploration, drainage, and irrigation of the cavity. The "dog ear" edges of the opening may be excised to permit continued drainage during healing. The abscess may be packed with narrow gauze strips or a drain placed for the first 24 hours. Oral or parenteral antimicrobials are unnecessary in most immunocompetent patients, but postoperative Sitz baths or local hydrotherapy may be beneficial. After resolution of the acute infection, the existence of an anal fistula should be excluded.

SUMMARY

Initial treatment of most genital tract infections in pregnancy will consist of medical managment. Development of a bacterial abscess, as may occur with infections of the Bartholin's gland or in the perirectal area, often require surgical incision and drainage. Such patients may require hospitalization for continued local wound treatment as well as for systemic antibiotics. Response to therapy is usually rapid; however, such infections can become fulminant and result in rapid deterioration of maternal condition. Viral condylomata acuminata that obstruct the birth canal or present substantial risk of hemorrhage during parturition may also merit surgical excision using electrocautery or laser.

REFERENCES

Aghajanian A, Bernstein L, Grimes DA. Bartholin's duct abscess and cyst: a case-control study. South Med J 1994;87:26.

Anderson PG, Christensen S, Detlefsen GU, Kern-Hansen P. Treatment of Bartholin's abscess. Marsupialization versus incision, curettage and suture under antibiotic cover. A randomized study with 6 months' follow-up. Acta Obstet Gynecol Scand 1992;71:59.

Armbruster-Moraes E, Ioshimoto LM, Leao E, Zugaib M. Letter to the Editor. Detection of human papillomavirus deoxyribonucleic acid sequences in amniotic fluid during different periods of pregnancy. Am J Obstet Gynecol 1993;169:1074.

Azzan BB. Bartholin's cyst and abscess: a review of treatment of 53 cases. Br J Clin Pract 1978; 32:101.

Berger BJ, Hussain F, Roistacher K. Bacterial infections in HIV-infected patients. Infect Dis Clin North Am 1994;8:449.

Bergman A, Bhatia NN, Broen EM. Cryotherapy for treatment of genital condyloma during pregnancy. J Reprod Med 1984;29:432.

Brook I. Aerobic and anaerobic microbiology of Bartholin's abscess. Surg Gynecol Obstet 1989; 169:32.

Carson GD, Smith LP. *Escherichia coli* endotoxic shock complicating Bartholin's gland abscess. Can Med Assoc J 1980;122:1397.

Centers for Disease Control and Prevention. 1993 Sexually Transmitted Diseases Treatment Guidelines. MMWR 1993;42(No. RR-14).

Cheetham DR. Bartholin's cyst: marsupialization or aspiration? Am J Obstet Gynecol 1985; 152:569.

Cho JY, Ahn MO, Cha KS. Window operation: an alternative treatment method for Bartholin gland cysts and abscesses. Obstet Gyencol 1990; 76:886.

Cruikshank SH, McLauchlan L. A de novo case of vulvar synergistic necrotizing fascitis. Obstet Gynecol 1987;69:516.

Davies JW. Bartholin cyst: a simple method for its restoration to function. Surg Gynecol Obstet 1948;86:329.

Davis GD. Management of Bartholin duct cysts with the carbon dioxide laser. Obstet Gynecol 1985;65:279.

Felix JC, Wright TC. Analysis of lower genital tract lesions clinically suspicious for condylomata using in situ hybridization and the polymerase chain reaction for the detection of human papillomavirus. Arch Pathol Lab Med 1994;118:39.

Ferenczy A. Treating genital condyloma during pregnancy with the carbon dioxide laser. Am J Obstet Gynecol 1984;148:9.

Ferenczy A, Mitao M, Nagai N, et al. Latent papillomavirus and recurring genital warts. N Engl J Med 1985;313:784.

Ferenczy A. HPV-associated lesions in pregnancy and their clinical complications. Clin Obstet Gynecol 1989;32:191.

Frölich EP, Schein M. Necrotizing fascitis arising from Bartholin's abscess. Isr J Med Sci 1989; 25:644.

Gary R, Jones R. Relationship between cervical condylomata, pregnancy and subclinical papillomavirus infection. J Reprod Med 1985;30:393.

Goldberg JE. Simplified treatment for disease of Bartholin's gland. Obstet Gynecol 1970;35:109.

Heath J. Methods of treatment for cysts and abscesses of Bartholin's gland. Commentary. Br J Obstet Gynaecol 1988;95:321.

Jacobson P. Vulvovaginal (Bartholin) cyst: treatment of marsupialization. W J Surg 1950; 58:707.

Jacobson P. Marsupialization of vulvovaginal (Bartholin) cysts: report of 140 patients with 152 cysts. Am J Obstet Gynecol 1960;79:73.

Johnson JJ, Burnett AF, Willet GD, et al. High frequency of latent and clinical human papillomavirus cervical infections in immunocompromised human immunodeficiency virus-infected women. Obstet Gynecol 1992;79:321.

Kirby P, Corey L. Genital human papillomavirus infections. Infect Dis Clin North Am 1987; 1:123.

Koutsky LA, Galloway DA, Holmes KK. Epidemiology of genital human papillomavirus infection. Epidemiol Rev 1988;10:122.

Lashgari M, Keene M. Excision of Bartholin duct cysts using the CO_2 laser. Obstet Gynecol 1986;67:735.

Lee VH, Rankin JS, Alpert S, et al. Microbiological investigations of Bartholin's gland abscesses and cysts. Am J Obstet Gynecol 1977;129:150.

Lopez-Zeno JA, Ross E, O'Grady P. Septic shock complicating drainage of a Bartholin gland abscess. Obstet Gynecol 1990;76:915.

Macho JR, Schecter WP. Surgical care of HIV-infected patients. Infect Dis Clin North Am 1992;6:745.

Matsunaga J, Bergman A, Bhatia NN. Genital condylomata acuminata in pregnancy: effectiveness, safety and pregnancy outcome following cryotherapy. Br J Obstet Gynecol 1987;94:168.

Oliphant MM, Anderson GV. Management of Bartholin-duct cysts and abscesses. Obstet Gynecol 1960;16:476.

Rader JS, Leake JF, Dillon MB, Rosenshein NB. Ultrasonic surgical aspiration in the treatment of vulvar disease. Obstet Gynecol 1991;77:573.

Rando RF, Lindheim S, Hasty L, et al. Increased frequency of detection of human papillomavirus deoxyribonucleic acid in exfoliated cervical cells during pregnancy. Am J Obstet Gynecol 1989;161:50.

Saul HM, Grossman MB. The role of chlamydia trachomatis in Bartholin's gland abscess. Am J Obstet Gynecol 1988;158:76.

Shah K, Haskins K, Polk BF, et al. Rarity of cesarean delivery in cases of juvenile-onset respiratory papillomatosis. Obstet Gynecol 1986; 68:795.

Shah KV, Kashima HK, Buscema J. Reducing mortality from respiratory papillomas. Contemp Obstet Gynecol 1987;29:65.

Shearin RS, Boehlke J, Karanth S. Toxic shock-like syndrome associated with Bartholin's gland abscess: case report. Am J Obstet Gynecol 1989;160:1073.

Spitzer M, Krumholz BA, Seltzer VL. The multicentric nature of disease related to human papillomavirus infection of the female lower genital tract. Obstet Gynecol 1989;73:303.

Smith EM, Johnson SR, Cripe TP, et al. Perinatal vertical transmission of human papillomavirus and subsequent development of respiratory papillomatosis. Ann Otol Rhinol Laryngol 1991; 100:479.

Swenson RM, Michaelson TC, Daly MJ, Spaulding EH. Anaerobic bacterial infections of the female genital tract. Obstet Gynecol 1973;42:538.

Tseng CJ, Lin CY, Wang RL, et al. Possible transplacental transmission of human papillomaviruses. Am J Obstet Gynecol 1992;166:35.

Vermund SH, Kelley KF, Klein RS, et al. High risk of human papillomavirus infection and cervical squamous intraepithelial lesions among women with symptomatic human immunodeficiency virus infection. Am J Obstet Gynecol 1991; 165:392.

Watts DH, Koutsky LA, Holmes KK, et al. Genital expression during and after pregnancy and perinatal transmission of human papillomavirus (Abst). Presented at the Annual Meeting of Infectious Diseases Society for Obstetrics and Gynecology. Monterrey, CA. August 1994.

Word B. New instrument for office treatment of cyst and abscess of Bartholin's gland. JAMA 1964;190:167.

Wright TC, Richart RM, Ferenczy A. Electrosurgery for HPV-related diseases of the lower genital tract. New York: Arthur Vision, 1991.

Zuspan ZP, Quilligan EJ. Surgery and related complications of pregnancy. Douglas-Stromme Operative Obstetrics. 5th ed. Norwalk, CT: Appleton & Lange, 1988:243.

CHAPTER 18

Cesarean Section

Cesarean section is defined as delivery of an infant, alive or dead, through an abdominal uterine incision. Cesarean section is the most common operation performed in the United States; approximately one million cesarean deliveries were performed in this country in 1991, accounting for one-quarter of all live births (National Hospital Discharge Survey, 1991).

Perhaps no other surgical or medical procedure has generated as much controversy as cesarean delivery, and the operation continues to be debated both in the scientific and lay press and media. Such controversy arises from several factors. The performance of cesarean section to many women involves disruption of the natural birth process and invokes a host of psychologic and emotional issues quite apart from the medical goal of a healthy mother and infant. Further, both for the individual and society, cesarean section has enormous cost implications. In 1992, the average total charge for vaginal delivery was $4,720.00 compared to $7,826.00 for cesarean section (Source Book of Health Insurance Data, 1993). These factors have been further complicated by a paucity of obstetric literature clearly defining the fetal benefits of cesarean section, especially in cases of malpresentation and "fetal distress." Ethical and emotional considerations, as well as the issue of informed consent, often hinder the construction of appropriate clinical trials. Rational decision making in these settings is often further complicated by potential legal ramifications. Failure to perform cesarean section is the dominant claim in obstetric malpractice litigation in the United States today, accounting for roughly one-half of all claims from 1988 to 1989 (American College of Obstetricians and Gynecologists, 1988). In 1992, allegations that poor obstetric care resulted in cerebral palsy accounted for 53 percent of all claims against obstetrician-gynecologists, with an average of $549,000 indemnity per paid file (Physicians Insurance Association of America, 1992). The impact of such awards upon a physician and the confusion arising from the apparent differences between legal standard of care and data-based reasonable medical care further complicate the issue (Porreco, 1990; Sandberg, 1984; DeMott and Sandmire, 1990).

HISTORY

The concept of delivery of a living child through an abdominal incision is an ancient one: reference to such births are readily found in the folklore and mythology of both Eastern and Western cultures. Abdominal delivery of an infant following death of the mother was codified in both Roman and early Christian law. Scattered unverified reports of abdominal delivery in living women with the survival of both mother and infant exist even prior to the nineteenth century (Gabert and Bey, 1988; Boley, 1991; Sewell, 1993). However, it was not until the pioneering work of Morton in the use of diethyl ether for operative anesthesia in 1846 and the introduction of carbolic acid antisepsis by Lister some 20 years later that cesarean delivery could begin to be approached in a uniform manner as a potential option for childbirth (Sewell, 1993). Early success in cesarean section was further compromised by the widespread belief that once incised, uterine muscle could not be safely sutured, principally out of fear of infection. Against this background, a series of 22 cesarean deliveries performed in Paris prior to 1876 demonstrated a 100 percent maternal mortality, mostly due to infection or hemorrhage (Sewell, 1993). The first successful cesarean delivery in the British Empire was performed between 1815 and 1821 (Miller, 1992).

The first major surgical advance in the technique of cesarean section was introduced by Porro in 1876 (Miller, 1992). Influenced by the prevailing concept of non-suturing of uterine incisions, Porro introduced a technique in which the uterine fundus was amputated following hysterotomy and the stump marsupialized to the anterior abdominal wall. Although drastic by today's standards, the Porro technique resulted in a dramatic decline in maternal mortality associated with this operative abdominal delivery (Speert, 1958).

Throughout most of the nineteenth century, cesarean section was seen as an operation of last resort. The concept that maternal outcome might be improved by earlier intervention prior to fetal death or maternal infection was initially proposed by Dr. Robert Harris of Philadelphia. In 1887, Harris published a series of nine women "delivered" by being gored by bulls and 12 women delivered by standard cesarean section. The observation of a 56 percent maternal survival in the gored group compared to an 8 percent survival in those surgically delivered led Harris to conclude "a far better showing for the cow-horn than the knife."

The era of modern cesarean began when Max Saenger (1882) introduced the technique of suturing the uterus with silver wire following hysterotomy. The Saenger classical cesarean became the mainstay for the next half century. Nevertheless, the Porro operation remained popular for many years and in one series from the Eastern United States in 1922, 25 percent of cesarean sections were performed as Porro cesarean hysterectomies (Harris, 1922). In 1926 Kerr introduced a downward curving transverse incision on the lower uterine segment. This was modified by Pfaneuf (1931) into the present day, upward-curving low transverse uterine incision. With the subsequent development of antibiotic therapy and modern blood banking techniques, cesarean section has evolved into one of the safest of major operative procedures.

CESAREAN SECTION RATE

In the United States, the rate of cesarean delivery increased dramatically in the decades from 1960 to 1990 (Fig. 18–1). Nationally, 4.5 percent of births in 1965 were performed by cesarean section. The rate then increased progressively from 15 percent in 1980 to 25 per-

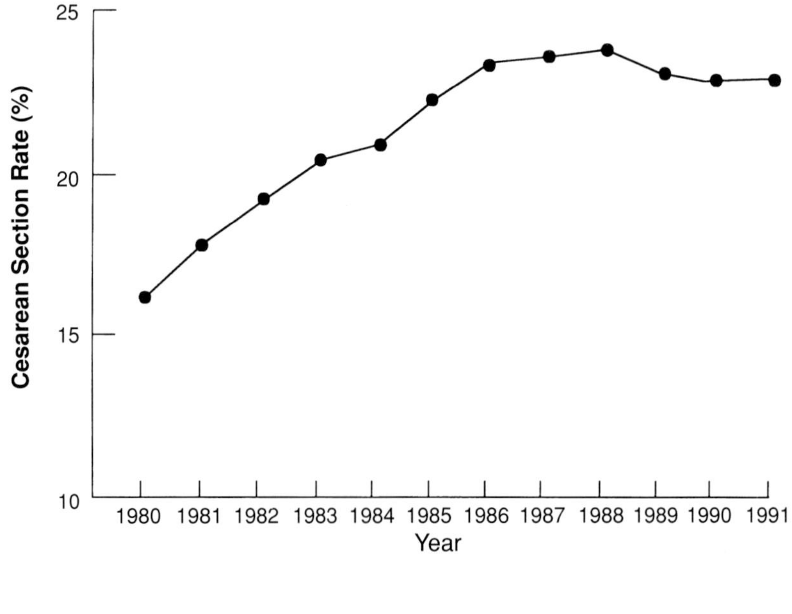

Figure 18–1. The cesarean section rate for the United States, 1980 through 1991. (Adapted from Notzon and colleagues, 1987, and Taffel and associates, 1991).

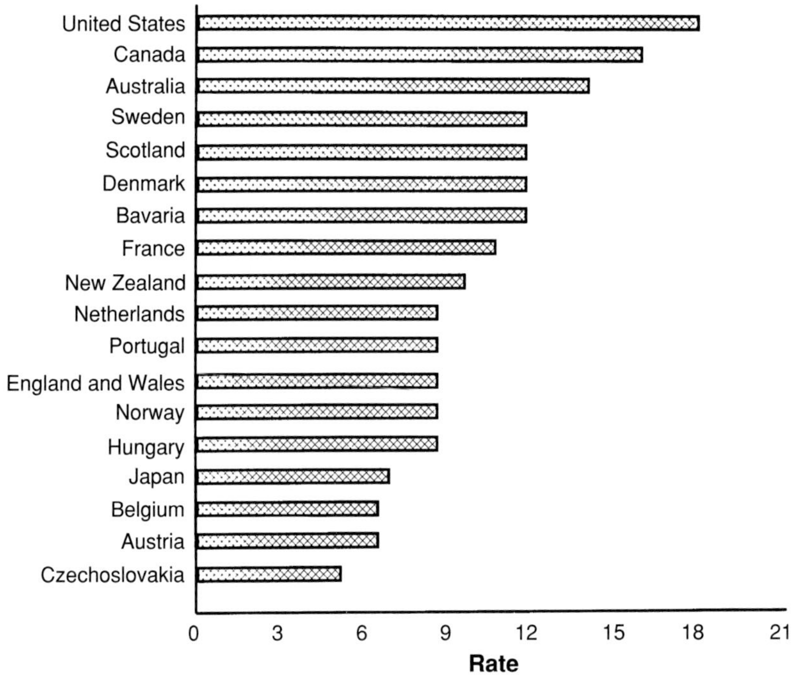

Figure 18–2. Cesarean section rates per 100 hospital deliveries in selected countries, 1981.

cent in 1988 (Taffel and associates, 1987, 1991; cesarean childbirth, 1981). Since 1988 the frequency of cesarean section appears to have plateaued; a 22.7 percent cesarean section rate was seen in 1990 and a 23.5 percent rate in 1991 among slightly over 4 million live births (National Hospital Discharge Survey, 1991). Current data reflects a marked regional disparity with a high number of cesarean births (27.6%) being performed in the South as compared with 19.8 percent for Western states, 21.8 percent for the Midwest, and 22.6 percent for the Northeast. In 1991, 65 percent of cesareans were primary and 35 percent were repeat procedures (National Hospital Discharge Survey, 1991). This increased rate in the United States has been paralleled in many other countries throughout the world, although absolute rates differ greatly (Fig. 18–2) (Thiery, 1989; Anderson, 1989; Notzon, 1987; Bergsjo, 1983; O'Driscoll, 1983; Mor-Yosef, 1990; and their colleagues).

Tables 18–1 and 18–2 detail the cesarean rates by indication from 1980 through 1989 in the United States (Taffell, 1987, 1991; Myers, 1990). Labor dystocia is the most common indication for cesarean delivery, accounting for roughly 16 percent of all births and 31 percent

TABLE 18–1. CESAREAN SECTION RATES[a] FOR SELECTED INDICATIONS IN THE UNITED STATES

	1980		1985		Increase 1980 to 1988	
Indication	*Rate*	*%*	*Rate*	*%*	*Rate*	*%*
Repeat cesarean	4.9	30	9.0	36	4.1	50
Dystocia	4.8	29	7.6	31	2.8	34
Fetal distress	0.8	5	2.3	9	1.5	18
Breech	2.0	12	2.5	10	0.5	6
All other	4.0	24	3.3	14	–0.7	–8
Totals	16.5	100	24.7	100	8.2	100

[a]Cesarean sections per 100 deliveries for stated indication.
Modified from Taffel and associates (1987, 1991) and Myers and Gleicher (1990).

TABLE 18–2. CESAREAN SECTION RATES FOR VARIOUS COMPLICATIONS

	Percentage of All Deliveries		Percent by Cesarean Section	
	1980	*1989*	*1980*	*1989*
Fetopelvic disproportion	4.1	4.2	96	99
Obstructed labor	1.1	4.3	26	66
Abnormal labor or inertia	3.0	7.4	54	43
Breech presentation	3.2	4.0	67	84
Fetal distress	1.7	8.8	67	46
Previous cesarean	5.1	10.4	97	82

Adapted from Taffel and colleagues (1991).

of all cesareans. This indication is followed in order of frequency by repeat cesarean, fetal distress, malpresentation, and miscellaneous causes such as placenta previa. While these rates reflect nationwide trends, individual indications vary considerably from institution to institution in terms of relative contribution to the overall cesarean rate (Sanchez-Ramos, 1990; Hage, 1988; Pridijian, 1991; and their associates). Coincident with the increase in cesarean sections in the United States has been a dramatic decline in the perinatal mortality rate. While superficial consideration may suggest cause and effect, a similar trend in perinatal mortality has been seen outside the United States with little or no change in cesarean rate (Fig. 18–3) (O'Driscoll and Foley, 1983). Such considerations have led many both within and outside the medical community to question whether one-quarter of all infants in the United States would have demonstrated worse outcome had they been born vaginally.

It is not possible to comprehensively catalog all appropriate indications for cesarean delivery. However, 75–80 percent of cesarean sections are performed for one of the following four indications.

Repeat Cesarean

For many years, the scarred uterus was felt to contraindicate labor out of fear of uterine rupture. Indeed, with a classical uterine incision, roughly 12 percent of patients will suffer rupture if given a subsequent trial of labor. One-third of patients with a classic

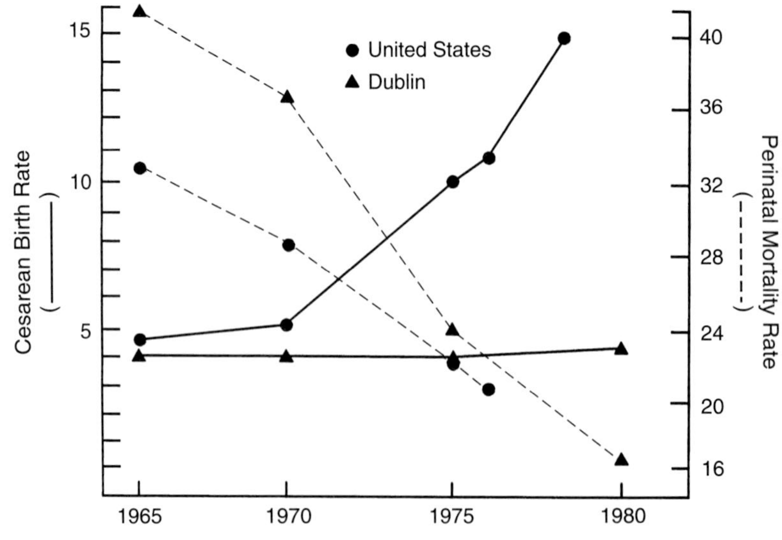

Figure 18–3. Cesarean birth rates per 100 deliveries are represented by solid lines and perinatal mortality rates per 1000 deliveries by broken lines for the United States (circles), according to Bottoms and co-workers (1980), and for the National Maternity Hospital, Dublin (triangles). (Modified from O'Driscoll and Foley, 1983).

cesarean who suffer uterine rupture, do so prior to labor (Haplerin, 1988; Rosen, 1991; and their colleagues). However, in the past 15 years, numerous studies have documented the relative safety for most patients of trial of labor after a low-transverse cesarean section (Flamm, 1990; Farmakides, 1987; Pruett, 1988; Paul, 1985; Farmer, 1991; Phelan, 1987; DeMuylder, 1990; O'Sullivan, 1981; Miller, 1994; and their associates). Efforts to encourage vaginal birth after cesarean (VBAC) appear to be the most productive approach to lowering the cesarean section rate (Porreco, 1990; Sandberg, 1984; Sanchez-Ramos, 1990; Hage, 1988; Pridijian, 1991; DeMuylder, 1990; and their colleagues). In considering VBAC, however, several factors bear special consideration.

Type of Uterine Incision

Patients with transverse scars confined to the lower uterine segment have minimal risk of symptomatic scar separation during a subsequent pregnancy, and that risk does not appear to be affected by the route of delivery (Rosen, 1991; Miller, 1994; and their co-workers). A recent meta-analysis concluded that the risk of scar separation is 1.8 percent with a trial of labor versus 1.9 percent for elective repeat cesarean (Rosen and associates, 1991). One study involving over 8000 deliveries documented a rate of scar separation of 0.5 percent among patients delivering vaginally, compared to 1.8 percent undergoing repeat cesarean (O'Sullivan and co-workers, 1981). Another study involving 17,521 births to women with prior cesarean sections reported that 1.1 percent had an asymptomatic uterine dehiscence and 0.7 percent sustained uterine rupture (Miller and Paul, 1994). Uterine scar rupture occurred in 0.5 percent of women with one prior cesarean section, in 1.3 percent of women with two prior cesarean sections, and in 1.1 percent of women with three or more prior cesarean deliveries. Although anecdotal reports of catastrophic scar separations do exist, the available data do not allow the conclusion that scar separation is more frequent in women undergoing a trial of labor (Rosen, 1991; Jones, 1991; Pitkin, 1991; Scott, 1991; and their colleagues). Thus, until additional data allow accurate identification of women at risk for symptomatic scar separation, it appears reasonable to encourage a trial of labor in most women with a low-transverse scar while focusing efforts upon ways to decrease the primary cesarean rate (American College of Obstetricians and Gynecologists, 1988). Patients with more than one prior cesarean should not be discouraged from trial of labor, although data regarding exact risks and benefits of this approach is not as extensive (American College of Obstetricians and Gynecologists, 1988; Pruett, 1988; Phelan, 1987, 1989; Miller, 1994; and their co-workers).

In the past several years, the VBAC rate has increased steadily to 24.2 percent in 1991 as compared to 8.5 percent in 1986 (National Hospital Discharge Summary, 1991; Shiono and co-workers, 1987). Fifty-eight percent of women offered VBAC accept this option (American College of Obstetricians and Gynecologists, 1990b). Because 600,000 primary cesareans are performed annually, continued encouragement of VBAC will be important in addressing the overall cesarean section rate.

VBAC in women with a vertical scar confined to the lower uterine segment (low-vertical) has been more controversial. Nevertheless, VBAC is a reasonable option provided the scar is limited to the relatively noncontractile lower uterine segment. In a meta-analysis of 170 patients laboring with a low vertical scar, the risk of scar dehiscence was not different from patients laboring with a prior low transverse incision (Rosen and associates, 1991). A uterine incision that has extended into the upper contractile portion of the myometrium is a contraindication to subsequent labor. Such scars have approximately a 12 percent incidence of symptomatic, and often catastrophic, rupture during labor (Haplerin, 1988; Rosen, 1991; and their colleagues). Ideally, these women are delivered by cesarean section upon demonstration of fetal pulmonary maturity prior to the onset of labor. They should be warned of the hazards of unattended labor and of the signs of possible uterine rupture (American College of Obstetricians and Gynecologists, 1990a). If the extent of the scar is unknown or poorly documented, trial of labor is probably not a reasonable approach. In preparing an operative report following any vertical uterine incision, it is important to document the exact extent of the scar in a clear and concise fashion.

Indication for Prior Cesarean

The success rate for VBAC depends greatly upon the indication for the previous cesarean (Table 18–3) (Pruett, 1988; Clark, 1984; Jarrell,

TABLE 18–3. TRIAL OF LABOR RELATED TO INDICATIONS FOR A PREVIOUS CESAREAN SECTION

		Indication for Primary Cesarean Section			
Study	**Overall Success for Trial of Labor No. (%)**	*Dystocia*[a] *No. (%)*	*Breech No. (%)*	*Fetal Distress No. (%)*	*Other No. (%)*
Clark and colleagues, 1984	240/308 (78)	39/61 (64)	81/94 (86)	31/38 (61)	69/52 (75)
Jarrell and associates, 1986	142/216 (66)	42/78 (54)	54/72 (75)		
Mootabar and co-workers, 1984	161/296 (54)	77/163 (47)			75/123 (61)
Paul and collaborators, 1985	614/751 (82)	245/319 (77)	103/135 (91)	56/67(84)	
Vengadasalam, 1986	176/271 (65)	38/82 (46)	33/42 (79)	68/91 (75)	37/56 (52)
Flamm and co-workers, 1990	4291/5733 (75)	1268/1951 (65)	1014/1138 (89)	564/773 (73)	1445/1871 (77)
Totals	5624/7575 (74)	1709/2654 (64)	1305/1481 (88)	719/969 (74)	1626/2142 (76)
Total nonrecurring = 627/810 (79)					

[a]Includes cephalopelvic disproportion and failure to progress.

1986; Vengadasalam, 1986; Duff, 1987; Flamm, 1988; Seitchik, 1982; and their associates). Given the current primary cesarean rate, women laboring following a previous cesarean section for all indications other than labor dystocia appear to have no greater risk of repeat cesarean section than does the background population. Most studies do document a significant increase in the rate of repeat cesarean delivery among women whose previous cesarean was for labor arrest or dystocia (Paul and co-workers, 1985). Still, in one series, 69 percent of women with a prior cesarean for dystocia following unsuccessful stimulation with oxytocin had a subsequent vaginal delivery (Seitchik and Ramakrishna, 1982). The type of dystocia, if known, is clearly a factor in determining the appropriateness of VBAC of labor in such patients. For example, a woman whose operative report describes a cesarean section in the latent phase for "failure to progress" is clearly different from the woman with a clinically borderline pelvis who reached complete dilatation and pushed with the fetus at –1 station for 3 hours. Even in this patient, a subsequent trial of labor may be an appropriate option.

Elective Sterilization

Desire for permanent sterilization in a woman with a prior cesarean section is not an indication for a repeat operation. The morbidity of vaginal birth and postpartum tubal ligation is considerably less than that of repeat cesarean section.

Oxytocin

A critical analysis of available data demonstrates no evidence that the use of oxytocin should be modified in the woman laboring with a prior low-transverse uterine incision (Rosen, 1991; Flamm, 1990; and their associates). In the largest series of uterine ruptures reported to date, Miller and Paul (1994) found that oxytocin was used in 79 (68%) of the 117 cases of uterine rupture. In women with one prior cesarean section oxytocin was used in 52 (74%) of 69 ruptures; with two prior cesarean deliveries it was used in 26 (67%) of the 39 ruptures. Attention to the possibility of rupture is important where labor is induced or augmented with oxytocin.

Epidural Anesthesia

The use of epidural anesthesia has been controversial in the past out of fear that it might mask the pain of uterine rupture. However, less than 10 percent of women with scar separation experience pain and bleeding, and fetal heart rate decelerations are by far the most likely sign of uterine rupture (Flamm and associates, 1988, 1990). Several studies attest to the safety of properly conducted epidural anesthesia; the presence of a low-transverse scar should not affect its use or non-use (Flamm, 1988, 1990; Paul, 1985; Farmer, 1991; and their colleagues).

Examining the Scar

While some obstetricians routinely document the integrity of the old scar by palpation following successful VBAC, such uterine exploration is felt to be unnecessary by many authors with extensive experience in the procedure. It is unknown what effect, if any, the documentation of an asymptomatic scar separation should have on subsequent reproduction or route of delivery. There is general agreement that surgical correction of a scar dehiscence is necessary only if significant bleeding is encountered and that asymptomatic, non-bleeding separations do not require exploratory laparotomy.

Timing of Elective Repeat Cesarean

The American College of Obstetricians and Gynecologists has established guidelines for timing an elective repeat cesarean delivery. According to these suggestions, elective delivery may be considered at or beyond 39 weeks gestation if the following criteria are met:

1. Normal menstrual cycles.
2. No recent use of oral contraceptives.
3. One of the following is present:
   - fetal heart tones auscultated by 10 menstrual weeks
   - positive pregnancy test by 4 menstrual weeks
   - ultrasound confirming menstrual dates prior to 20 weeks' gestation.

In all other instances, fetal pulmonary maturity must be documented by amniotic fluid analysis before elective repeat cesarean is undertaken.

Labor Dystocia

Labor dystocia is the most frequent indication for primary cesarean delivery in the United States. An analysis of labor dystocia as a contributing factor to the cesarean rate is difficult, however, because of the heterogeneity inherent in the condition. Descriptive terms vary from the precise definitions promulgated by Friedman, for example, secondary arrest of dilatation, arrest of descent, to the more ambiguous and commonly used terms of cephalopelvic disproportion and failure to progress (Friedman, 1978). While both the cesarean delivery performed after 8 hours of contractions at 3 cm dilatation and that performed for arrest of descent after 3 hours of pushing with uterine contractions demonstrating 300 Montevideo units are commonly classified as "failure to progress," the strength of the diagnosis and its meaning for subsequent deliveries are no doubt very different. Not surprisingly, efforts to reduce cesarean sections for "failure to progress" has met with less success than has been achieved for repeat cesarean deliveries (Taffel and co-workers, 1987, 1991). Cesarean section for labor dystocia in the latent phase of labor is commonly performed but rarely justified.

Fetal Distress

Electronic fetal heart rate monitoring (EFHRM) and elegant descriptions of various fetal heart rate (FHR) patterns and their association with fetal oxygenation and acid base status occurred in the 1970s (Martin, 1979; Parer, 1980; Murata, 1982; Khazin, 1971; Wood, 1967; Kubli, 1969; and their colleagues). These developments raised hope that recognition of subtle indicators of "uteroplacental insufficiency" and timely cesarean section would eliminate or greatly reduce childhood neurologic abnormalities including cerebral palsy. Recognition of various FHR patterns was seen as the key to diagnosing "fetal distress" (and preventing neurologic damage) despite (1) its relatively poor specificity in the prediction of an abnormal newborn, (2) a lack of scientific foundation for defining "normal" and "abnormal" newborn acid-base status, and (3) widespread disagreement among "experts" in the field regarding FHR interpretation (Cohen, 1982; Bowe, 1970; Lumley, 1971; Tejani, 1976; Sykes, 1982; Ruth, 1988; and their co-workers). Many of the clinical opinions extrapolated from the initial basic science observations lacked one fundamental underpinning: while the correlation existed between certain FHR patterns, fetal acid-base status, and abnormal newborn outcome, no data existed to document that abdominal delivery of an infant exhibiting such patterns would alter long-term outcome. With a paucity of scientific data, and very few appropriately designed studies, an entire industry was developed around EFHRM, and many proponents believed in the technology so strongly that they suggested that randomized clinical trials would be unethical. Beginning with the work of Havercamp in 1976, however, several studies began to cast doubt upon many of the fundamental assumptions of FHR monitoring.

It is now well established that patient management based upon EFHRM neither reduces the risk of cerebral palsy, nor improves any measurable indices of newborn outcome compared to intermittent auscultation of the fetal heart rate (American College of Obstetricians and Gynecologists, 1992; Freeman, 1985; Freeman, 1988; Freeman, 1990; Grant, 1989; MacDonald, 1985; Shy, 1990; Banta, 1979; Leveno, 1986; and their associates). Such data, coupled with the observations that many subtle patterns demonstrated by EFHRM (variability, late decelerations) are not reliably detected by auscultation suggests that while these patterns may in some cases indicate preexisting fetal abnormalities, operative intervention on the basis of such patterns does not improve subsequent neurologic function and long-term outcome (American College of Obstetricians and Gynecologists, 1992; Freeman, 1985; Freeman, 1988; Freeman, 1990; Grant, 1989; MacDonald, 1985; Shy, 1990; Banta, 1979; Leveno, 1986; Miller, 1984; Schifrin, 1992; Nelson, 1986; and their associates). Thus, it is not surprising that despite the ubiquitous utilization of EFHRM in Western industrialized countries in the past two decades, and a significant increase in the cesarean section rate, there has been no change in the rate of cerebral palsy (Hagberg, 1984; Stanley, 1988; Niswander, 1988; Melone, 1991; and their associates). Indeed, Shy and co-workers (1990), in a prospective randomized trial, demonstrated a significant *increase* in cerebral palsy among monitored premature fetuses.

The previously normal fetus, with rare exception, has the capacity to tolerate subtle episodes of contraction-induced hypoxia and manifest heart rate patterns not detectable by intermittent auscultation without incurring neurologic damage. The developmentally abnormal fetus appears to have a greater propensity to exhibit abnormal heart rate findings by electronic monitoring during labor compared to its neurologically intact counterpart. Importantly, no evidence exists to suggest that these patterns indicate ongoing and remedial neurologic damage. In fact, available evidence strongly suggests the opposite. In addition, two studies specifically examining the relationship between the quality of obstetric care in general and the "appropriateness" of fetal heart rate pattern management found no relationship between either of these measurements of care and the risk of subsequent cerebral palsy (Melone, 1991; Niswander, 1984; and their colleagues). In the absence of dramatic fetal heart rate changes reflecting events such as placental abruption or cord accident, both of which would be apparent by simple auscultation, there is no evidence to suggest that cesarean section reduces long-term neurologic morbidity.

The American College of Obstetricians and Gynecologists has recommended that facilities performing obstetric care have the capability of initiating a cesarean delivery within 30 minutes of the decision for operation (Standards for Obstetric-Gynecologic Services, 1989). This recommendation addresses facilities and does not govern clinical decision making. Misinterpretations of this guideline are common. There is no nationally recognized standard of care that codifies an acceptable time interval for performance of cesarean delivery. In most instances, operative delivery is not necessary within this 30-minute time frame. In cases of cesarean for indications such as labor arrest, a timely cesarean often will involve an interval considerably in excess of 30 minutes. On the other hand, when faced with an acute, catastrophic deterioration in fetal condition, cesarean may be indicated as rapidly as possible, and purposeful delays of any time period would be inappropriate.

Breech Presentation

Fetuses presenting as breech are at increased risk of cord prolapse and head entrapment if delivered vaginally compared to those presenting as vertex. Nevertheless, prospective controlled trials suggest that with proper selection, certain fetuses may deliver vaginally in breech presentations with minimal risk (Barlow, 1986; Benson, 1972; Christian, 1990; Collea, 1980; Flanagan, 1987; Gimovsky, 1983, 1989; Jaffa, 1981; Svenningsen, 1985; Woodward, 1969; and their associates). In many of these studies increased death rates or permanent neurologic damage was seen in the group delivered vaginally, yet small numbers precluded statistical significance. One meta-analysis suggests a significant increase in both perinatal mortality (*odds ratio 3.86*) and traumatic morbidity (*odds ratio 3.96*) for planned vaginal delivery versus planned cesarean section (Cheng and Hannah, 1993). When compared to the maternal risks of cesarean section, such small increases in fetal risks may be acceptable. With appropriate informed consent, carefully selected fetuses meeting established criteria may undergo a trial of labor (American College of Obstetricians and Gynecologists, 1986). However, concern for fetal injury, as well as the infrequency with which a breech fetus meets the established criteria for a trial of labor, make it unlikely that significant reductions in the cesarean section rate will come from a more liberal approach to vaginal breech delivery.

Demographic Considerations

Various demographic characteristics of patients and of physicians have been related to the risk of having a cesarean section. Gould and associates (1989) described a primary cesarean section rate of 22.9 percent from high-income patients compared to 13.2 percent for patients in a low socioeconomic group. Gordon and colleagues (1991) identified a relative risk of 2.5 for cesarean section in women age 35 and older, and concluded that maternal age alone may influence a physician's decision for cesarean delivery. Berkowitz and colleagues (1989) concluded that older, more experienced physicians perform significantly fewer cesarean sections for dystocia and have a higher percentage of forceps and vaginal breech deliveries. DeMott and Sandmire (1992) concluded that the frequency of unnecessary cesareans may be safely reduced by using oxytocin more frequently and in higher doses, allowing second stages of labor to continue longer, and performing more forceps deliveries. In a 4-year study of 9480 deliveries, these authors concluded that physicians employing such techniques had a 300 percent reduction in cesarean section for nonprogressive labor with no adverse effect on perinatal outcome.

Unfortunately, the above referenced practice styles and preferences, although medically sound, remain principle sources of obstetric malpractice loss in the United States

(American College of Obstetricians and Gynecologists, 1990b; Physicians Insurance Association of America, 1992). Several studies have documented the direct effect of malpractice fears on increased cesarean section rate (Physicians Insurance Association of America, 1992; Porreco, 1990; Sandberg, 1984; DeMott and Sandmire, 1992). As Sandberg (1984) has aptly observed

> . . . to persist in the attempt to obtain a living and normal neonate by vaginal delivery and, by using impeccable logic, extensive knowledge, broad experience, and perfect judgment, to win, gains one little—a good result was expected . . . to have avoided the challenge and to have opted, without further expenditure of time or thought, for cesarean section, and to have won, is to have performed to the standard expected . . . In short, from the medicolegal vantage point, there is little to gain and a lot to lose from persisting in the attempt to deliver vaginally and from not doing a cesarean section. Conversely, by recommending cesarean section, medicolegal safety is nearly assured.

Stated a decade ago, these medicolegal concerns have not been comprehensively addressed, and until they are many unnecessary cesareans will continue to be performed in the United States.

The Ideal Rate

The concept of an ideal cesarean section rate is meaningless; the operation has become so safe for women that virtually any rate would be justifiable if such increases were reflected consistently in improved newborn outcomes. However, if outcome is not improved, one is hard pressed to justify the economic impact of cesarean delivery to include longer length of stay, use of more medical resources, longer convalescence, and direct cost as reflected in hospital associated cost as well as indirect cost associated with loss of earnings during convalescence. Several studies have documented the feasibility of achieving significant reductions in institutional cesarean section rates without any increase in perinatal morbidity or mortality (Porreco, 1990; DeMott, 1992; Sanchez-Ramos, 1990; Hage, 1988; Pridijian, 1991; DeMuylder, 1990; Shiono, 1987; Dillon, 1992; and their co-workers). These programs, aimed at reducing unnecessary cesareans, have focused upon educational efforts and peer review, encouraging VBAC and restricting cesarean sections for labor dystocia to patients meeting strictly defined criteria. Such efforts, along with increased understanding of the proper use and limitations of EFHRM, may further reduce inappropriate cesarean deliveries.

MATERNAL MORTALITY AND MORBIDITY

Maternal mortality has decreased dramatically in the past 50 years, from 650 per 100,000 live births in 1940 to 14.1 per 100,000 live births in 1988 (Titus, 1940; Rochat, 1988). Historically, the major sources of operative mortality in women undergoing cesarean section were anesthetic accidents (including aspiration), hemorrhage, and infection. With the widespread use of conduction anesthesia, the availability of potent antibiotics, and modern blood banking techniques, deaths from aspiration, infection, and hemorrhage are now less common. Today, thromboembolic events are the major cause of direct maternal death in the United States, accounting for one-quarter of deaths in women whose pregnancies are beyond the mid-trimester (Rochat, 1988).

Maternal death directly associated with cesarean section is rare. Frigoletto and associates (1980) reported a series of 10,000 consecutive cesarean sections with no maternal deaths. Sachs and co-workers (1988) observed only 7 deaths as a direct result of cesarean section in over 121,000 cesarean sections performed between 1976 and 1984. While Lilford and colleagues (1990) documented a sevenfold increase in the relative risk for maternal mortality with cesarean section, most deaths were associated with complicated nonelective cesarean deliveries. Indeed, the relative risk of death for elective cesarean section under epidural anesthesia was actually *lower* than that associated with all vaginal births.

Although maternal death is an infrequent sequel of cesarean section, morbidity is increased dramatically with this procedure compared to vaginal delivery. Principle sources of morbidity are endomyometritis, hemorrhage, urinary tract infection, and nonfatal thromboembolic events. These factors, as well as the increased recovery time associated with cesarean section, results in a twofold increase in total cost for cesarean section compared to vaginal delivery (Source Book of Health Insurance Data, 1993).

While such figures attest to the relative safety of properly conducted cesarean section, it should be remembered that the decision to perform a cesarean section must always be a conscious decision to incur a small but real risk of operative maternal death for either fetal or maternal benefit. Such a decision should only be made with proper scientific backing.

BIRTH TRAUMA

Although cesarean section is often performed in select cases of malpresentation or known excessive fetal size in an effort to avoid birth trauma, it is incorrect to assume that cesarean section provides a guarantee against such injury. Numerous reports attest to the occurrence of Erb palsy, skull fractures, and fractures of long bones in infants delivered by cesarean section (Skajaa, 1987; Kaplan, 1987; Alexander, 1987; Vasa, 1990; and their associates). DeMott and Sandmire (1992) also demonstrated a relative risk of 4.5 for transient tachypnea of the newborn in term infants delivered by cesarean section compared to those delivered vaginally. The very nature of human childbirth makes it a potentially traumatic procedure, and birth injury will continue to occur despite optimal obstetric care.

TECHNIQUE OF CESAREAN SECTION

A cesarean section begins with an abdominal incision, discussed in detail in Chapter 4. Following entry into the peritoneal cavity, the position of the uterus, superior extent of the bladder, and character of the lower uterine segment are assessed.

Choice of Uterine Incision

A low-transverse incision is most commonly performed. A vertical incision may be considered under a few specific circumstances, including:

1. A known back-down transverse lie. Under these circumstances, it may not be possible to successfully grasp the fetal feet and effect delivery through a low-transverse incision without risking trauma to either the uterus or the fetus. Intraoperative intraabdominal version to either breech or vertex presentation is an option that may sometimes allow avoidance of a vertical uterine incision.
2. A premature breech or transverse fetus with a narrow or poorly developed thick lower uterine segment. Under these circumstances, a lower segment incision may not provide ample space to allow atraumatic delivery of the fetal head. A vertical uterine incision can be extended superiorly as needed to facilitate delivery.
3. Select uterine abnormalities. Leiomyomata occasionally involve the lower uterine segment to such an extent that a low-transverse incision is impossible. Structural abnormalities such as uterus didelphis may also be associated with a lower uterine segment insufficient for delivery of the infant through a transverse uterine incision.

Given the clear superiority and strength of low-transverse compared to an upper segment vertical uterine incision, we do not feel that a prior vertical incision is an indication for the same type of incision during subsequent operative delivery.

Technique of Low-transverse Cesarean Section

The visceral peritoneum overlying the uterus is grasped with forceps just above the superior margins of the bladder and incised with Metzenbaum scissors (Fig. 18–4). This peritoneum is then undermined laterally with the scissors and incised to the left and right of the midline (Fig. 18–5). In a primary cesarean the peritoneum is easily undermined and incised; when difficulty is encountered, the incision may be too high and a reevaluation of the anatomic position of the bladder may allow a lower incision to be made. The inferior margin of the incised parietal peritoneum is then grasped with the forceps or a Kelly clamp and undermined with the forefinger. This maneuver results in the development of the potential space between the bladder and the lower uterine segment and creation of a bladder flap (Fig. 18–6). The dissecting forefinger should always be directed with the finger tip exerting

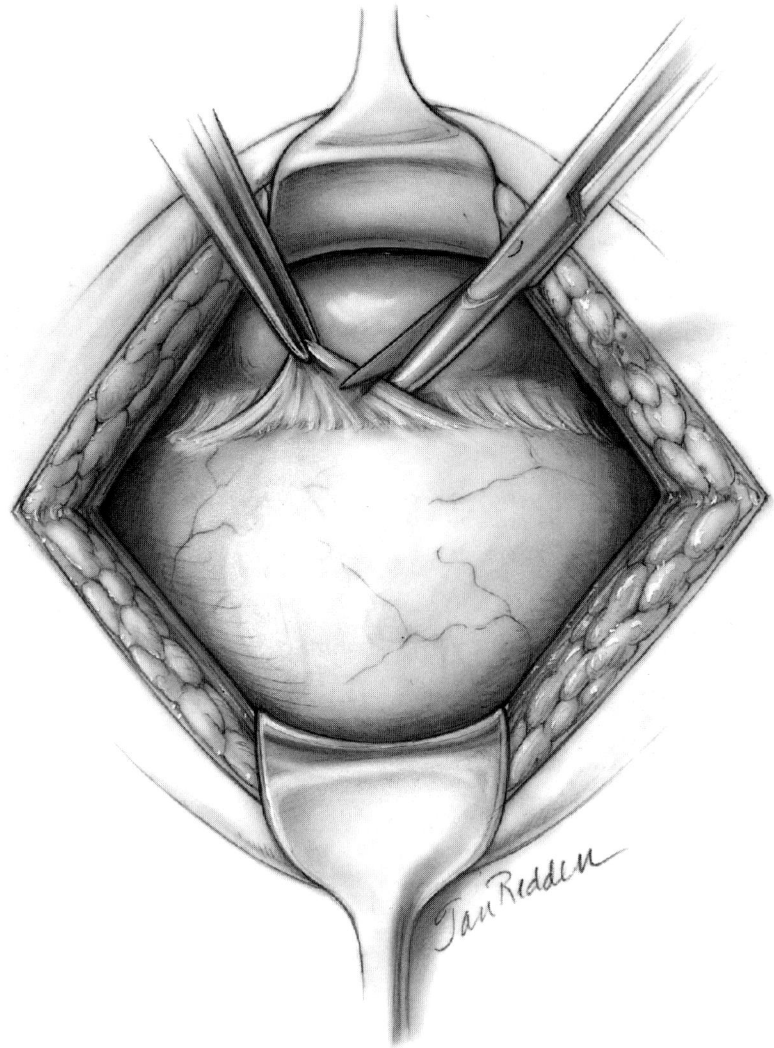

Figure 18–4. The visceral peritoneum is grasped just above the bladder and incised in the midline.

pressure on the lower uterine segment rather than the posterior surface of the bladder (Fig. 18–7A) to minimize the risk of inadvertent blunt cystotomy. Care must also be taken not to dissect too far laterally where vessel injury can lead to profuse bleeding. When a prior procedure has resulted in scarring of the bladder flap, sharp dissection may be necessary (Fig. 18–7B). Extreme caution must be taken under such circumstances to minimize the risk of inadvertent cystotomy.

Following creation of the bladder flap, a bladder blade is placed to keep the bladder out of the operative field and a Richardson retractor is placed superiorly to facilitate adequate exposure (Fig. 18–8). The lower uterine segment is then incised with a scalpel in the midline just below the former area of attachment of the bladder peritoneal reflection. Great care must be taken to avoid cutting too deeply and lacerating the fetus. Often blood obscures the operative field at this stage and continuous suction by the assistant is invaluable in clearing the field and allowing a safe incision. When suction is insufficient, firm pressure with sponge sticks above and/or below the

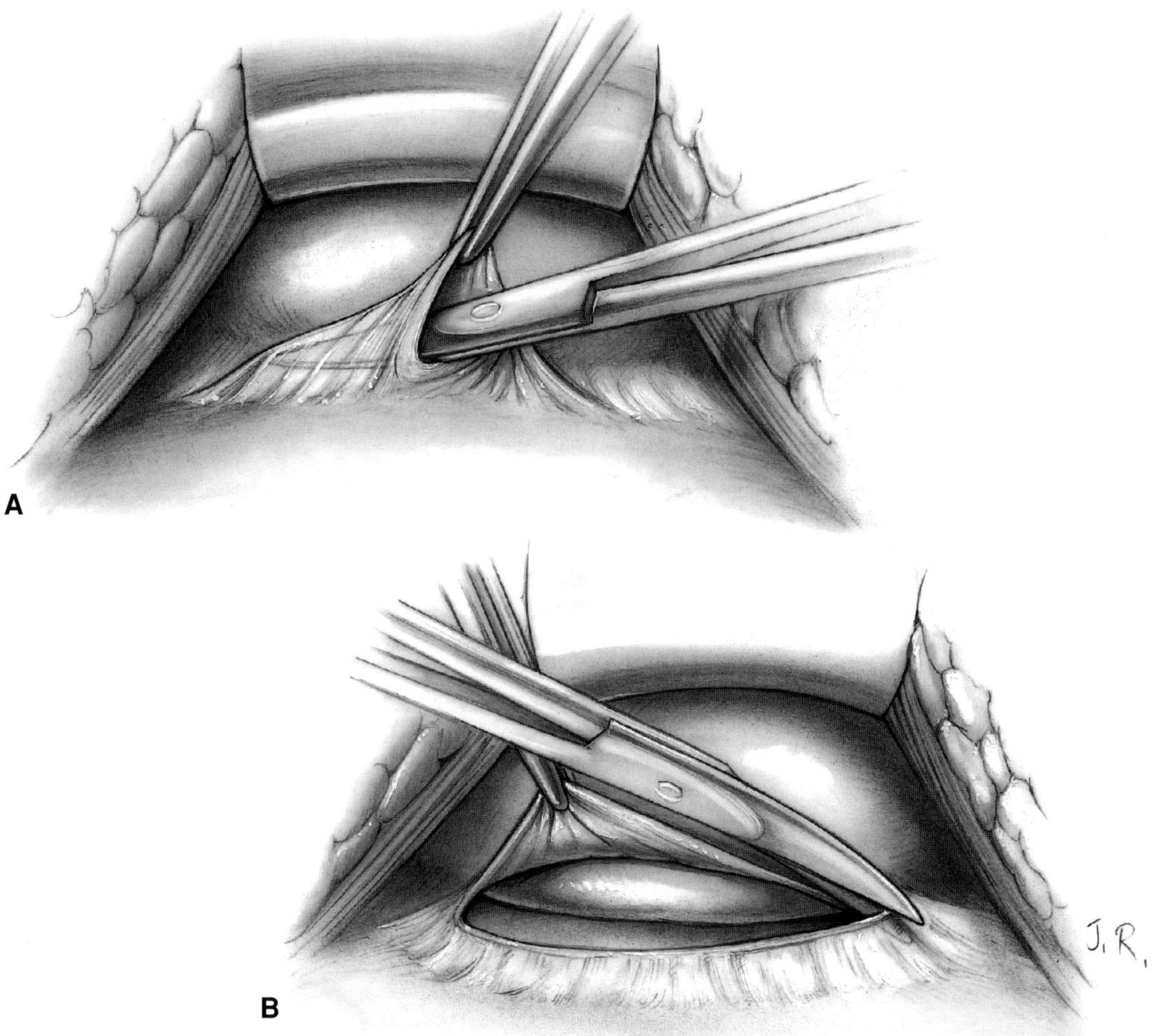

Figure 18–5. **A.** The visceral peritoneum is undermined and **B.** incised laterally with Metzenbaum scissors.

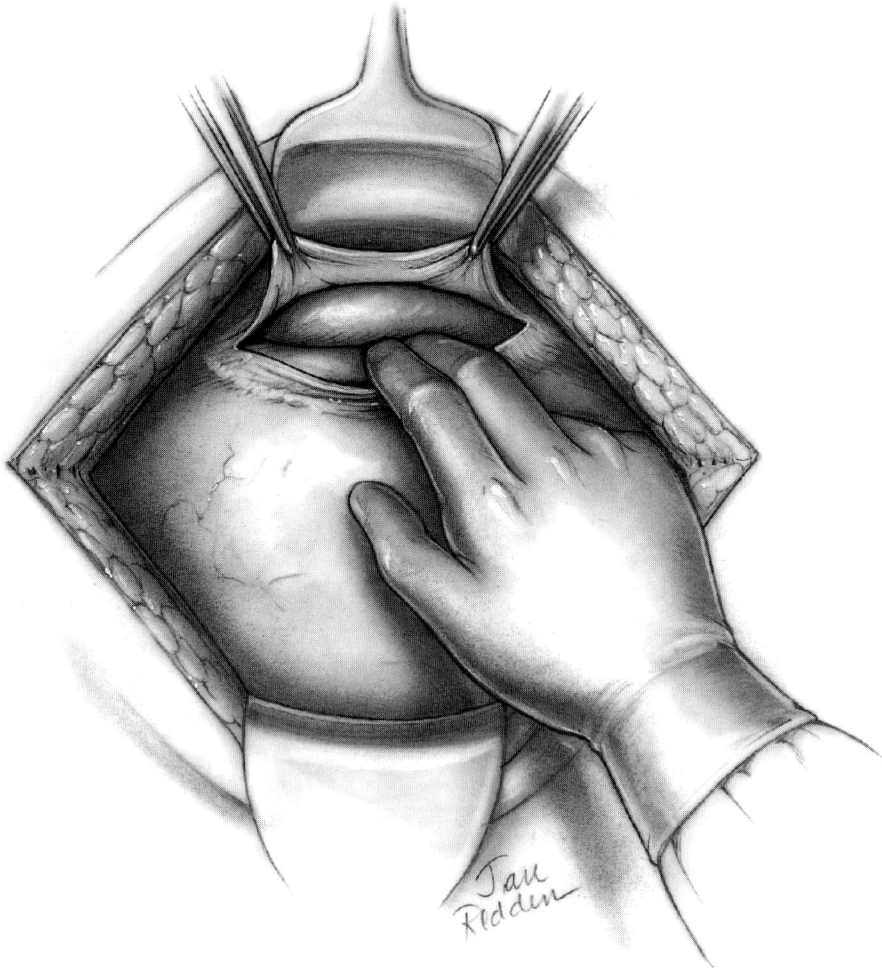

Figure 18–6. The bladder flap is created with the operator's index and forefinger as the potential space between bladder and uterus is developed.

incision margin may slow the bleeding sufficiently to allow visualization. Alternatively, the remaining myometrium may be penetrated bluntly with the finger or the back of the scalpel handle. In incising the myometrium, the amnion and chorion are also usually ruptured.

The surgeon has two choices for extending the uterine incision (Fig. 18–9A, B). One option is to sharply extend the lower segment opening by placing two fingers into the uterine cavity through the midline between the uterine wall and the fetal presenting part. The surgeon then places bandage scissors between the uterine wall and the fingers, and the uterine wall is incised laterally and slightly cephalad. In making this incision, it is essential to be oriented to the usual dextrorotation of the uterus in order to keep the incision centered and avoid inadvertent extension laterally onto the uterine vessels.

A second option is to extend the incision bluntly by tearing the myometrium with the fingers. Using this technique, the surgeon's forefingers are placed in the margins of the

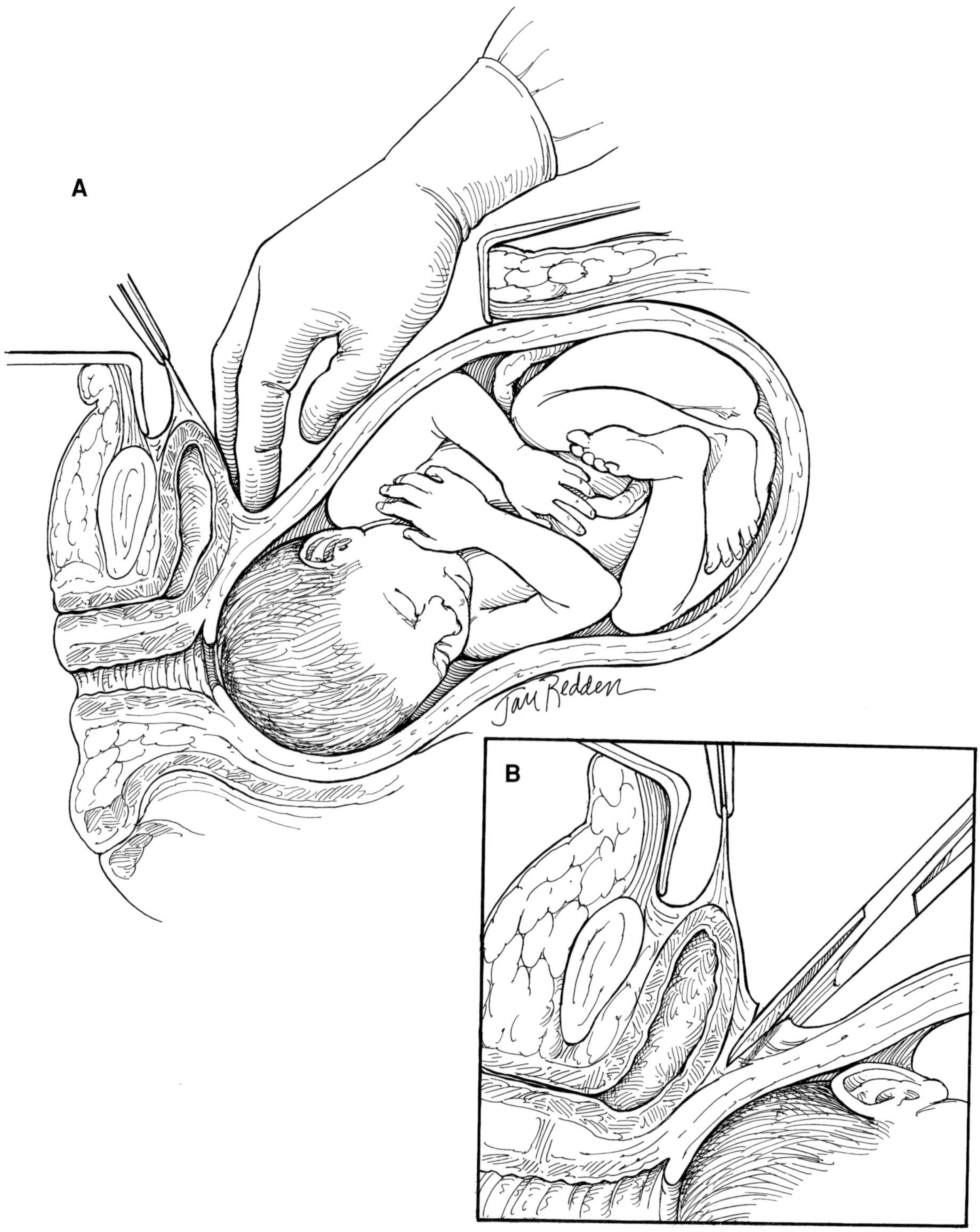

Figure 18–7. A. As the bladder flap is developed, pressure is kept against the uterus, rather than against the bladder. **B.** Adhesions are encountered in developing the bladder flap during a repeat cesarean section. The adhesions are taken down sharply with Metzenbaum scissors.

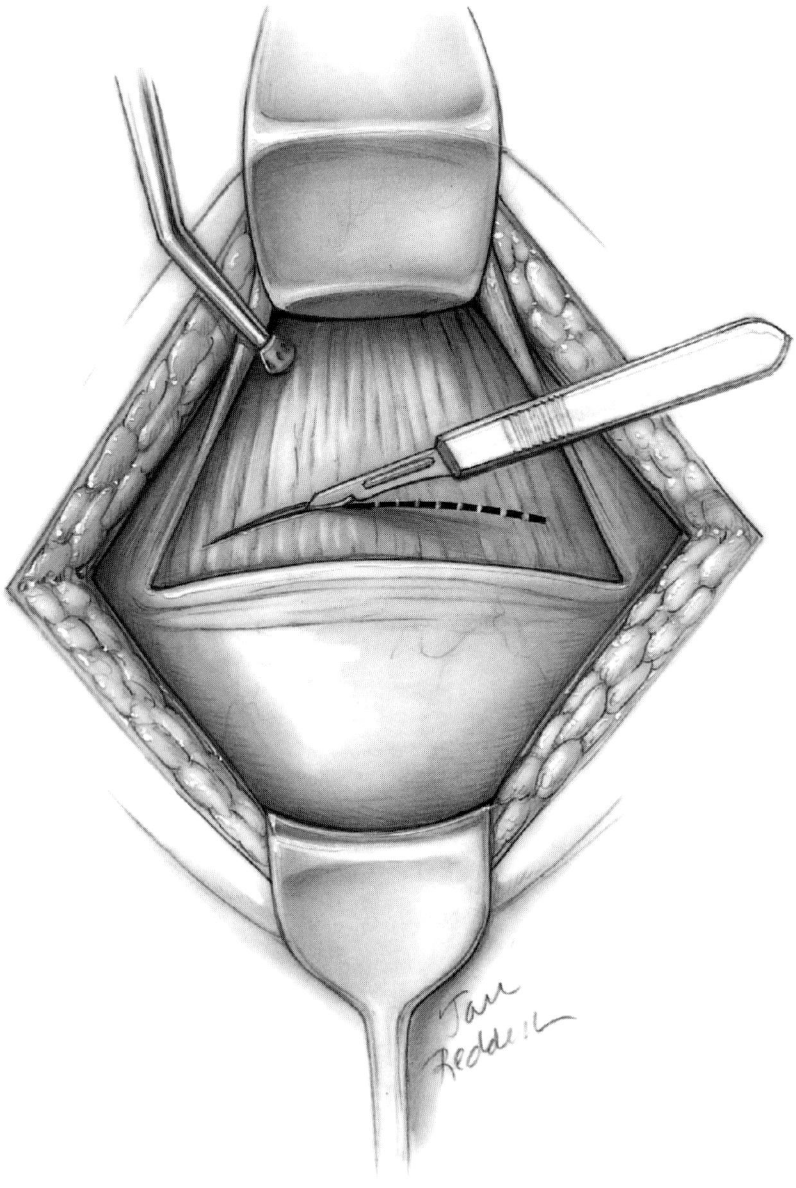

Figure 18–8. A bladder blade is placed to retract the bladder inferiorly while a Richardson retractor retracts the tissues of the abdominal wall cephalad. The lower uterine segment is incised sharply. The operative field is kept free of blood and amniotic fluid by continuous suction.

central lower segment incision and swept laterally and upward. Advantages of this technique include both speed and decreased bleeding from the myometrial edges compared to the sharp technique. Disadvantages include the necessity for a thin lower uterine segment and higher likelihood of extension of the uterine incision into the broad ligament if the fingers are swept too far laterally. At this point, the amnion/chorion may be ruptured with an Allis clamp if they have not already ruptured.

At the time of membrane rupture, the assistant administers continuous suction in

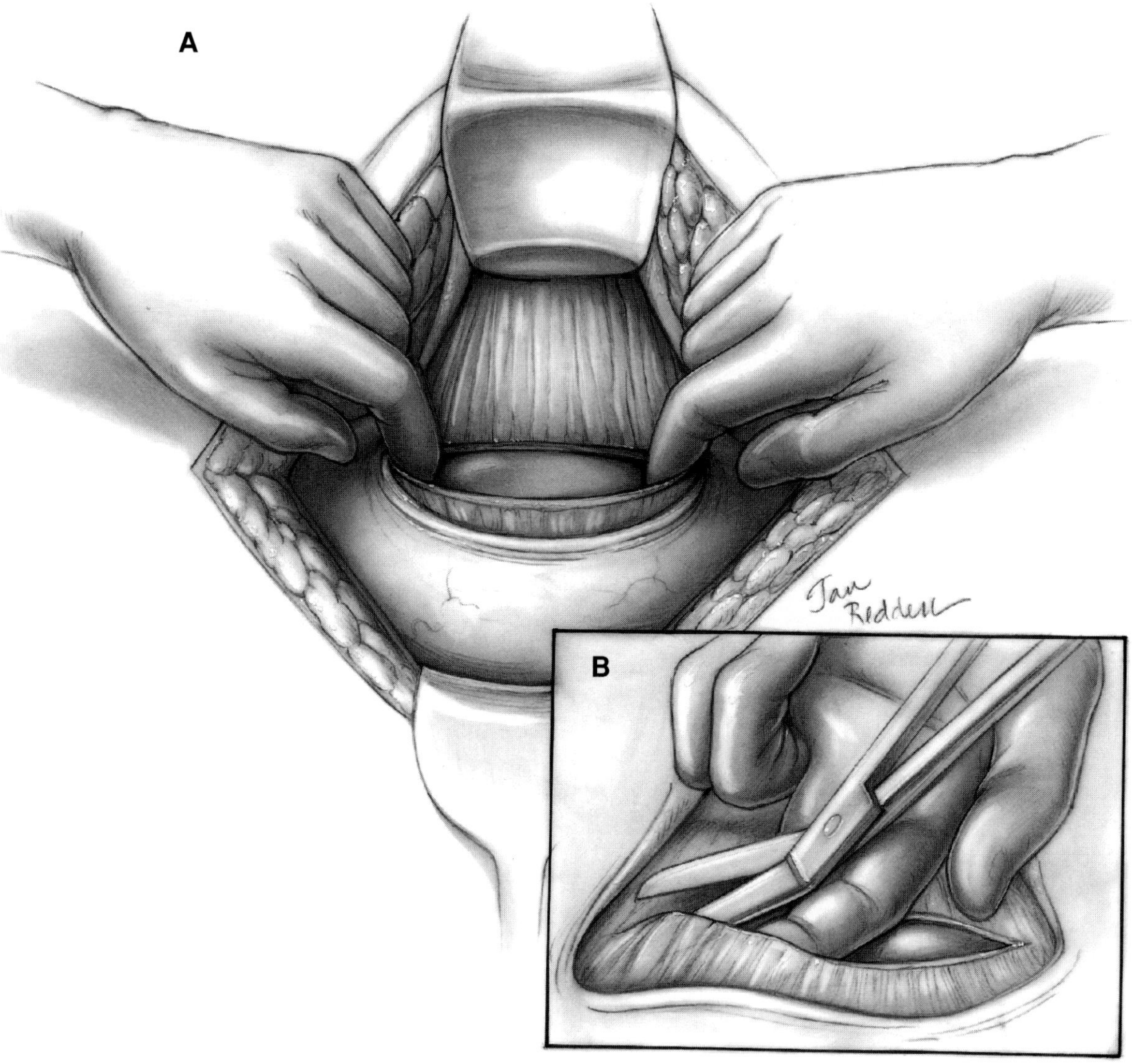

Figure 18–9. A. The incision in a well-developed (thin) lower uterine segment is extended laterally and cephalad with the fingers. **B.** The incision in a thicker lower uterine segment is extended laterally with bandage scissors.

the area of the uterine incision to free the field of blood and amniotic fluid. In vertex presentations, the surgeon then places the dominant hand into the lower uterine segment between the anterior uterine wall and the fetal head, lifting and flexing the head to bring the occiput into the line of incision (Fig. 18–10). If difficulty is encountered at this stage, the surgeon should check to be sure he is lifting the occiput rather than the sinciput or brow toward the incision. If the head is deeply engaged, an assistant may exert pressure vaginally to lift the fetal head toward the incision (Fig. 18–11). At all times, the surgeon should avoid flexing his or her wrists and thereby using the lower margin of the incision as a fulcrum. Failure to heed this instruction may result in broad ligament lacerations. Some surgeons have found the application of a vacuum or forceps valuable in

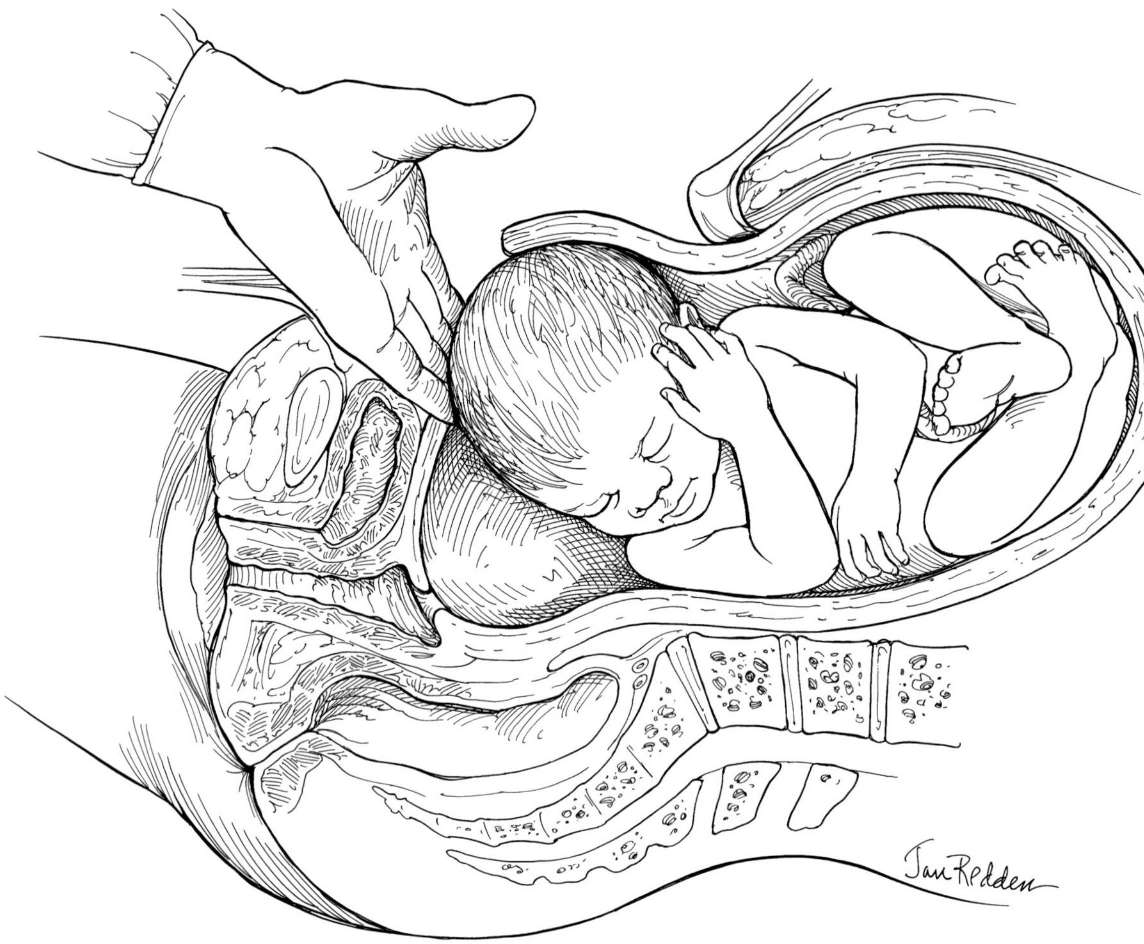

Figure 18–10. The fetal occiput is lifted toward the incision. Care is taken not to use the lower uterine segment as a fulcrum in order to avoid lacerations.

difficult cases of extraction of the fetal head (Fig. 18–12A–C).

As the occiput is brought into the incision, the assistant exerts fundal pressure, thus facilitating expulsion of the head through the incision (Fig. 18–13). At this point, the remaining delivery proceeds similar to a vaginal birth. The oropharynx and nares are cleared with a suction bulb or a DeLee trap connected to wall suction. The surgeon then delivers the anterior shoulder by gentle downward traction on the head followed by delivery of the posterior shoulder. The body is then delivered (Fig. 18–14).

The fetus is laid on the maternal abdomen while the umbilical cord is clamped and cut, and then is given to the health care provider responsible for the newborn. Occlusive type forceps (Pennington, Ovum, etc.) are then placed at the angles of the incision and any other sites of major bleeding to obtain temporary hemostasis while the placenta is removed. A dilute solution of oxytocin, 20–40 units/1000 cc of crystalloid solution, is now administered.

The placenta may now be delivered by shearing it manually from the uterine attachment (Fig. 18–15). An alternative technique is

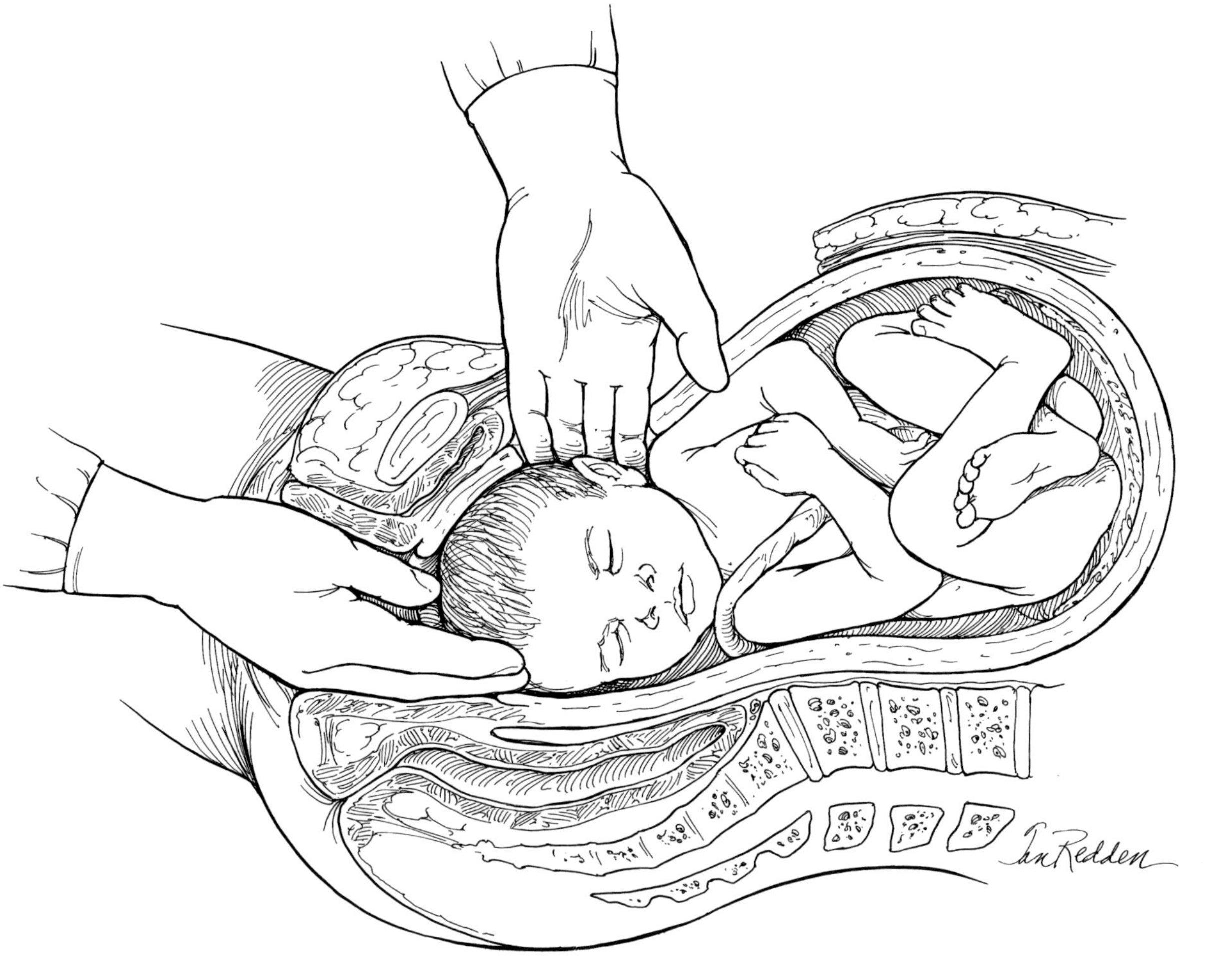

Figure 18–11. The fetal head is deeply engaged. Delivery is facilitated as an assistant places a hand in the vagina and lifts the head toward the surgeon's hand.

to exert gentle traction on the umbilical cord and await spontaneous delivery. While the former technique is probably more common, McCurdy and associates (1992) in a prospective randomized trial demonstrated a mean 300 cc reduction in directly measured blood loss and a sevenfold reduction in postpartum endometritis in the group with spontaneous placental removal. Queenan and Nakamoto (1964) also demonstrated a reduction in the risk of Rh sensitization with spontaneous as opposed to manual placental removal. The interior of the uterus is then wiped manually with a laparotomy sponge to ensure complete removal of the placenta and membranes.

Attention is next directed toward uterine incision closure. The angles of the incision are identified and an absorbable No. 0 or No. 1 suture is begun just beyond one angle and run the length of the incision using a continuous locking suture technique (Fig. 18–16A). Traditionally, a second layer of suture is then placed, imbricating the first (Fig. 18–16B). However, when hemostasis is adequate with a single layer closer, a second layer may not be necessary. Hauth and co-workers (1992) in a prospective randomized study compared single- with traditional double-layer closure and found a significant decrease in operative time with no increase in postoperative complica-

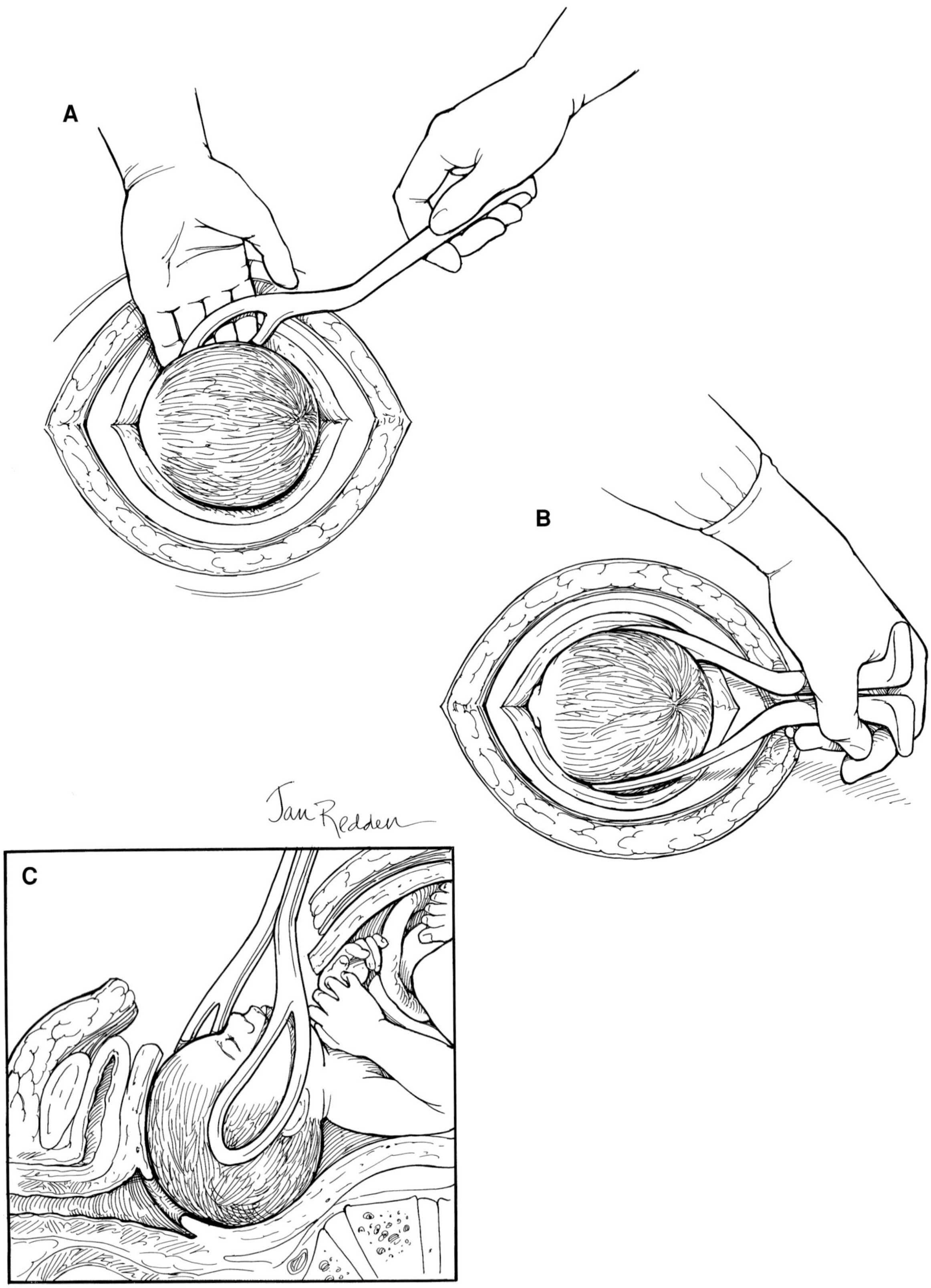

Figure 18–12. Forceps may be applied in a number of ways to assist delivery of the head at the time of cesarean section. **A.** A single blade assists in elevation of the head. **B.** Lauf divergent forceps are placed upon the head as for vaginal forceps delivery, and the occiput then elevated toward the incision. **C.** In occiput posterior presentation, forceps may be placed as shown and the head flexed toward the incision.

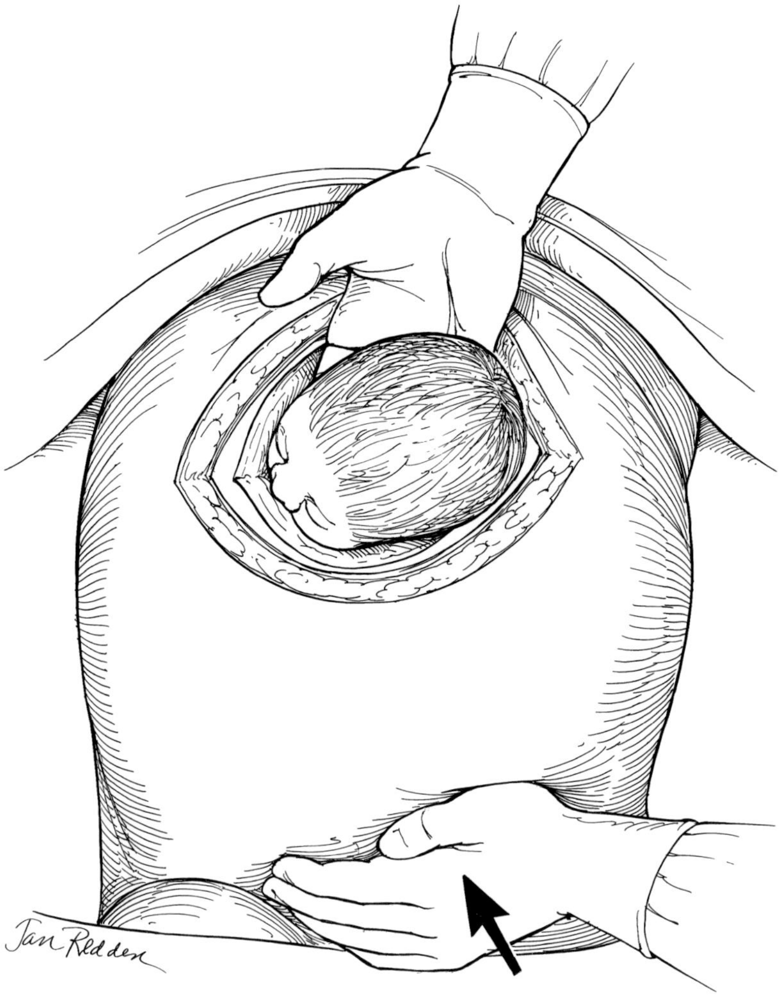

Figure 18–13. Delivery of the fetal head is assisted by fundal pressure. Fundal pressure should not be used before the occiput has entered into the uterine incision.

tions in the group undergoing single-layer closure. Additional interrupted or figure-of-eight absorbable sutures may be placed along the incision line if necessary to complete hemostasis. The uterine closure may be performed either with the uterus within the peritoneal cavity or following removal of the uterus through the abdominal incision. Exteriorization of the uterus provides additional exposure for closure of the uterine incision and facilitates abdominal exploration and tubal ligation. Hershey and Quilligan (1978) demonstrated no difference in postoperative febrile morbidity with the routine exteriorization of the uterus. Such a technique could potentially cause temporary "kinking" of the uterine blood supply, which may result in an increased pulse pressure and hemorrhage after the uterus has been returned to the peritoneal cavity. Thus, if exteriorization is employed, the incision line should be carefully inspected for hemostasis following replacement of the uterus into the abdominal cavity.

Hemostasis of the incision line must be complete. In many instances, minor bleeding points are most effectively addressed by direct

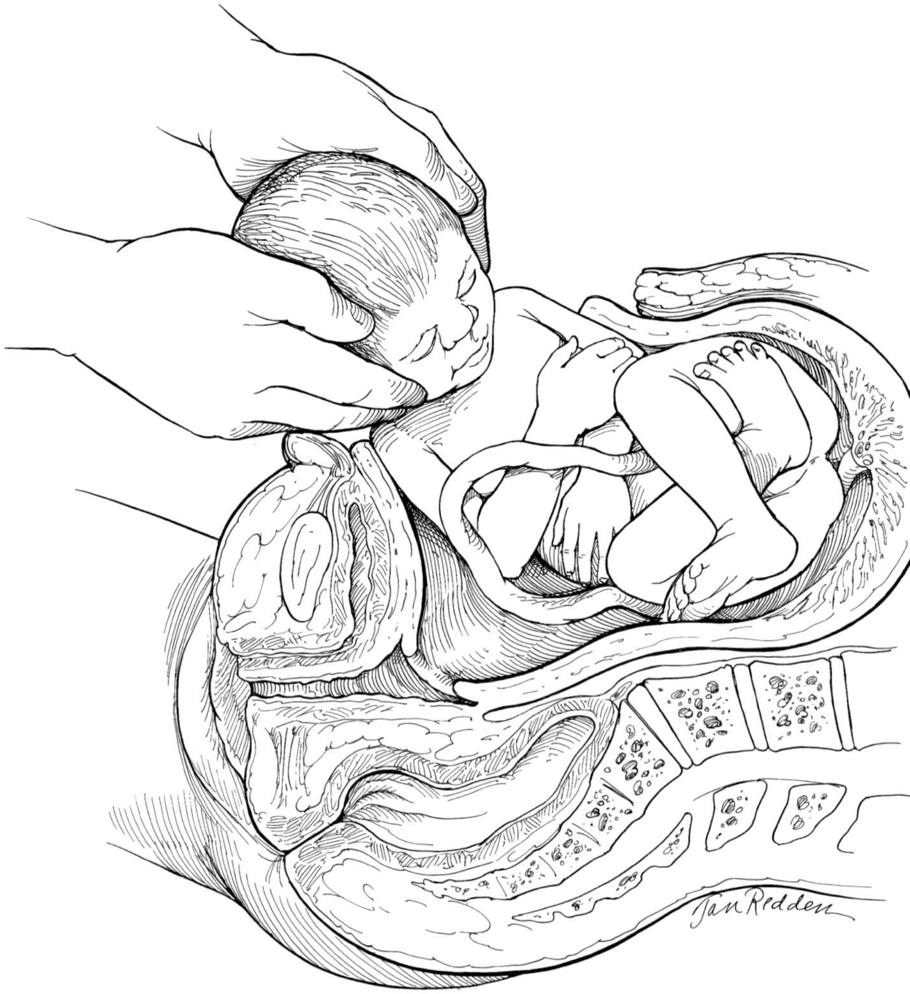

Figure 18–14. The body is delivered after the mouth and nares have been suctioned thoroughly.

compression and hemostasis via platelet aggregation and clot formation rather than by placement of additional sutures, which may create more bleeding points. In this regard, it is well to recall that "The greatest enemy of good is better." After achievement of hemostasis, the adnexa and appendix are examined. Tubal ligation may be performed at this time, if indicated.

The abdominal cavity may be irrigated if desired, especially in cases of chorioamnionitis or when extensive spillage of meconium has occurred. Many surgeons close the bladder flap by approximating visceral peritoneum with a running suture of 3-0 chromic or a similar absorbable material; however, such closure is probably not necessary. Similarly, while the parietal peritoneum may be closed with a fine continuous running absorbable suture, Hull and Varner (1991) demonstrated reduced need for postoperative analgesia and quicker return of bowel function when both the visceral and parietal peritoneum were left open. Similar findings were reported by Pietrantoni and colleagues (1991). When left undisturbed, peritoneal defects demonstrate mesothelial integrity within 48 hours and indistinguishable healing with no scar by 5 days (Buckman, 1976; Elkins, 1987; Ellis, 1962, 1977; McFadden, 1983; Tulandi, 1988;

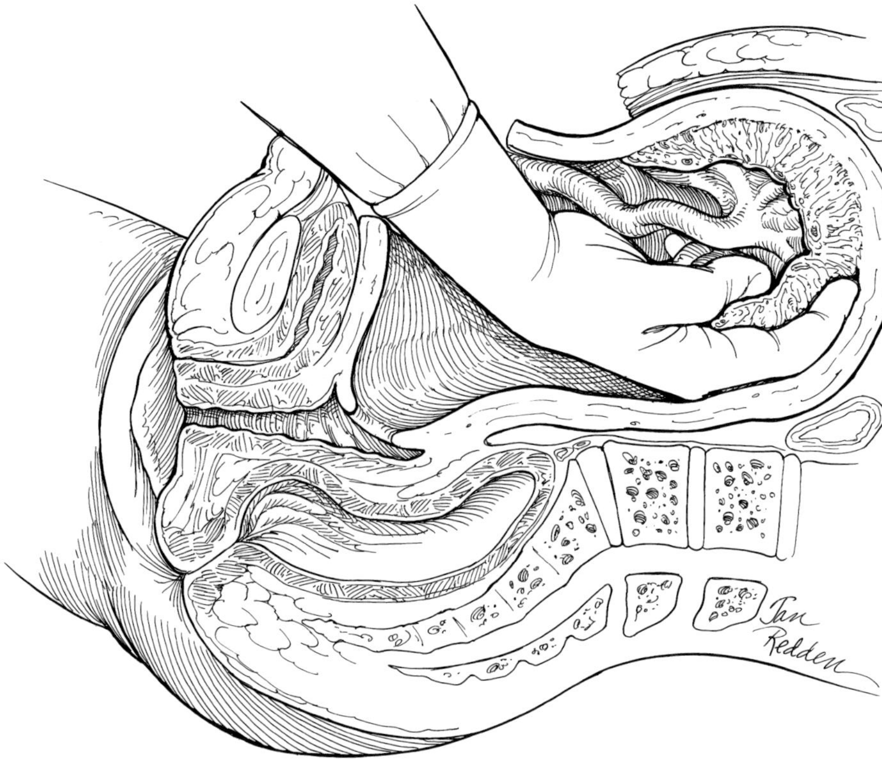

Figure 18–15. The placenta is delivered by shearing it manually from its uterine attachment.

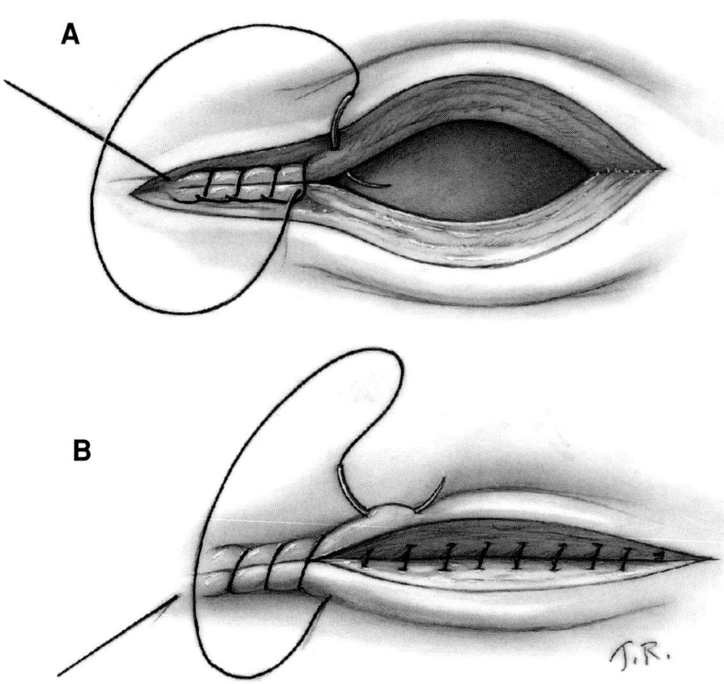

Figure 18–16. A. Initial running-locking closure of the uterine incision. **B.** A second, imbricating layer is closed over the initial suture line.

and their associates). Closure of peritoneal surfaces, even with minimally reactive suture materials, results in increased tissue reaction and may result in increased adhesion formation. Nonclosure of the peritoneum after gynecologic surgery does not increase adhesion formation as judged by findings at the time of second-look laparotomy (Tulandi and co-workers, 1988). While these principles have long been recognized by general surgeons, their discussion has until recently been uncommon in the obstetric literature. Data now supports that the closure of peritoneal surfaces should be abandoned. Abdominal closure next proceeds as outlined in Chapter 4.

Extraperitoneal Cesarean Section

Extraperitoneal cesarean section was originally designed to avoid peritoneal contamination in the pre-antibiotic era, it is uncommonly performed today (Norton, 1946; McCall, 1949; Waters, 1959). A randomized clinical trial comparing extraperitoneal cesarean and standard intraperitoneal cesarean plus prophylactic antibiotics showed no advantage to the extraperitoneal approach (Wallace and associates, 1984).

Low Vertical and Classical Incisions

Following creation of a bladder flap, the lower uterine segment is incised vertically in the midline and the incision carried inferiorly first and then superiorly, either with a scalpel or with bandage scissors, until the incision is deemed adequate for atraumatic delivery of the fetus (Fig. 18–17). It is of utmost importance to document in a clear fashion the extent of the incision and whether or not the contractile upper segment myometrium was entered. Incision closure is carried out as described for low-transverse incisions. Rarely, however, will a single-layer closure be adequate to obtain hemostasis with a vertical incision; often, a three-layer closure is necessary.

Uterine Staples

Absorbable surgical staples have been introduced for use in uterine closure at cesarean section. In experimental animals, the use of such staples was not associated with subsequent impairment of fertility (Bond and colleagues, 1989). A retrospective study of 62 patients undergoing uterine closure with absorbable staples suggested decreased operating time for primary cesarean section and a significant reduction in blood loss, endomyometritis, and hospital stay compared to standard closure techniques (Burkett and associates, 1989). However, the retrospective nature of this study and the possibility that patients experiencing massive hemorrhage or at high risk for infection or other peripartum complications might be excluded from closure with the newer device weakens the study's conclusions. A subsequent prospective randomized controlled trial confirmed the findings of shortened operating time with the use of staples, but found no improvement in any other indices of maternal morbidity (Villeneuve and co-workers, 1990). These authors concluded that their data did not support the routine use of this costly (approximately $200) device.

Prophylactic Antibiotics

Numerous studies attest to the value of prophylactic antibiotic administration for the prevention of endomyometritis and wound infection in high-risk patients undergoing cesarean delivery. In a review of 25 such trials, Duff (1987) concluded that women undergoing cesarean section in labor or following rupture of membranes should receive a single 2-g dose of ampicillin or a first-generation cephalosporin following clamping of the umbilical cord. A second dose may be given 3–4 hours later, although the value of the second dose is not well established (see Chapter 38). The choice of antibiotic should usually be predicated on cost, with the least expensive agent used.

Patients at special risk for infectious morbidity include those with ruptured membranes of at least 6 hours' duration, in whom the risk of endometritis may approach 85 percent in some populations (Cunningham and associates, 1978). Additional risk factors include multiple vaginal examinations, nulliparity, and low gestational age (Chang and Newton, 1992). Administration of prophylactic antibiotics has been shown to decrease the risk of endometritis, pelvic and wound abscess, and pelvic thrombophlebitis (DePalma and coworkers, 1982).

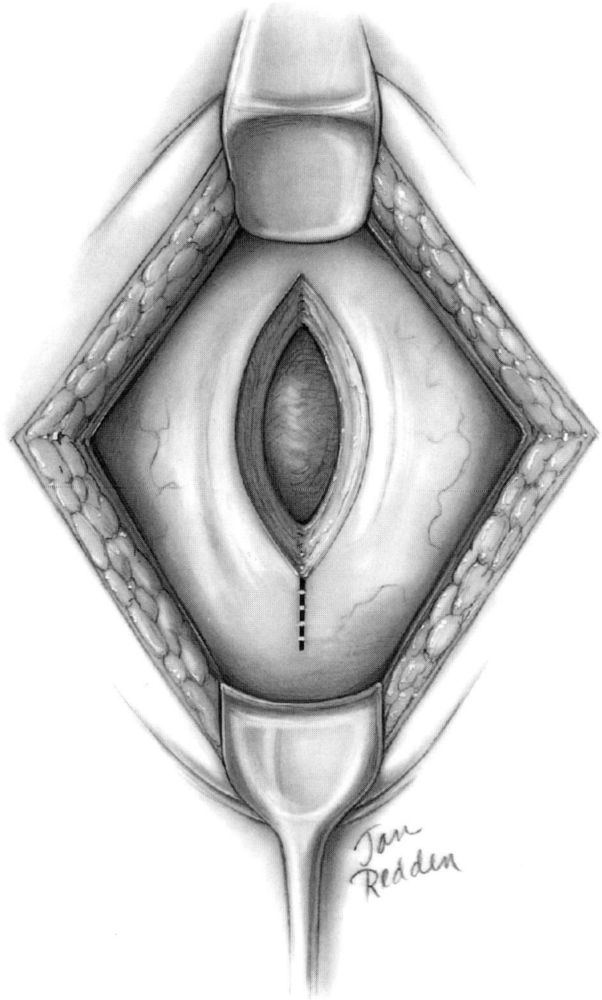

Figure 18–17. A vertical uterine incision.

CESAREAN SECTION — THE SURGICAL ASSISTANT

An interested and competent surgical assistant is essential to the performance of cesarean section. Proper assistance can reduce operating time and blood loss and minimize the risk of complications by providing adequate exposure for incisions and suture placement. The assistant should at all times be attentive and aggressively strive to facilitate the technical aims of the principle surgeon. Table 18–4 details the responsibilities of the surgical assistant at various stages of cesarean section.

SPECIAL PROBLEMS

Delivery of Breech Presenting Fetus

For a fetus presenting as a breech or back-up transverse lie, the first step is to find and grasp a foot and deliver it and the leg through the incision. It is essential to be sure of limb identification, as delivery of an arm at this stage may be difficult to reverse and hinders prompt extraction of the infant. The second foot is grasped as soon as identified. Generally, traction on the first foot brings the contralateral lower limb into the operative field. At this point, the surgeon grasps both feet and proceeds in a manner similar to that

TABLE 18–4. RESPONSIBILITIES OF THE PRIMARY SURGEON AND SURGICAL ASSISTANT

Primary Surgeon	Surgical Assistant(s)
Makes incision down to fascia.	Keeps field clear of blood with laparotomy sponge. Clamps/coagulates significant bleeding vessels with Kelly clamps and electrocautery.
Opens fascia.	Retracts fat laterally with Richardson type retractor to facilitate facial incision.
Develops fascial plane unilaterally.	Develops fascial plane contralaterally.
Divides pyramidalis muscles inferiorly.	Retracts to expose pyramidalis insertion inferiorly with Richardson type retractor.
Incises parietal peritoneum.	Retracts superficial tissues superiorly and inferiorly with Richardson type retractor.
Creates bladder flap.	Retracts superficial tissues superiorly with Richardson retractor. Places bladder blade beneath bladder flap and retracts bladder inferiorly.
Incises uterus and extends uterine incision.	Moves Richardson retractor laterally as needed to facilitate exposure for incision. Operates suction device to keep field clear of blood and amniotic fluid.
Elevates fetal occiput into incision.	On command, exerts fundal pressure to deliver head through incision and facilitate delivery of body.
Delivers placenta, explores uterus.	Places occlusive type forceps on bleeding margins of incision. Continues suction as needed to free abdomen of amniotic fluid and blood.
Closes uterine incision.	"Follows" suture facilitating locking of the stitch. Cuts sutures as necessary.
Closes fascia.	Retracts superficial tissues with Richardson type retractor. Follows and cuts sutures as necessary.
Closes skin.	Assists depending upon closure type.

employed for vaginal breech extraction (see Chapter 10). It must be emphasized that cesarean delivery is no guarantee against birth trauma associated with extraction of the fetus in breech or transverse lie. Gentle and appropriate techniques for delivery of the arms and head as outlined in Chapter 10 remain essential. Undue traction or hyperextension of the head must be avoided. Fetal injury may occur with the use of improper technique or attempted delivery of the head through too small an incision, especially with a premature fetus.

Unstable Lie

The fetus may change positions between the time of preoperative assessment and delivery. This is especially common in premature infants, multiple gestations, and pregnancies complicated by hydramnios. It is important to quickly assess the lie after the uterus has been opened, especially in nonvertex presentations. There should be no hesitation in converting a low-transverse incision into a "J" or hockey stick type incision if there is any question of the ability of the operator to effect atraumatic delivery through the initial incision line. "T"-shaped incisions are the least preferred as healing may be impaired; but if needed they should be employed.

Trapped Head or Body in a Nonvertex Presentation

In addition to extending the surgical incision, a variety of pharmacologic maneuvers are available to effect uterine relaxation and avoid traumatic delivery. These include: terbutaline sulfate, 0.125–0.25 mg intravenously or subcutaneously or halothane in concentrations of 2 percent or greater. Either approach generally results in dramatic uterine relaxation within seconds to minutes of administration and may facilitate atraumatic delivery in difficult cases. The use of these agents, however, has been associated with increased blood loss at the time of cesarean (Gilstrap and colleagues, 1987).

Placenta Directly Beneath the Incision

It is not standard procedure to locate the placenta by ultrasound prior to the operation. Therefore, this complication is generally unexpected and manifests itself by heavy bleeding as an attempt is made to enter the uterus. There is no especially effective solution to this problem except to move quickly. At times the placenta may be retracted laterally; in other instances the incision is carried through the placenta. In these circumstances some of the observed hemorrhage may be fetal. If difficulty is encountered in extracting the fetus, the cord may be clamped prior to delivery of the fetus, beyond which time further placental disruption becomes moot. The pediatrician should be alert to the possibility of fetal blood loss during delivery.

Unexpected Pathology

Exploration of the pelvic organs and appendix is an important part of any cesarean section. Leiomyomata are commonly encountered. Except in cases of pedunculated leiomyomata with extremely thin stalks, they should categorically not be excised at the time of cesarean section. Even large leiomyomata may exhibit a dramatic reduction in size during the postpartum period. The increased vascularity associated with pregnancy further contraindicates myomectomy at this time.

Ovarian pathology encountered at the time of cesarean section is managed as in the nonpregnant patient. Cystic tumors that are persistent into late pregnancy cannot be considered functional (see Chapter 22).

Appendectomy is indicated if inspection suggests acute or chronic inflammation. The wisdom of performing incidental appendectomy at cesarean section has been widely debated (Gilstrap, 1991). Parsons and associates (1986), however, demonstrated no increase in postpartum morbidity with incidental appendectomy performed at the time of cesarean section, and found that 20 percent of appendices so removed were abnormal on pathologic examination.

Perimortem Cesarean

Perimortem cesarean section refers to emergency abdominal delivery in a woman suffering cardiac arrest. Recommendations for perimortem cesarean under these circumstances are based upon the following observations:

1. Cessation of maternal cardiac activity results in complete cessation of uterine perfusion, and eventual total fetal anoxia.
2. Even when cardiopulmonary resuscitation is performed in an ideal manner, cardiac output is, at best, 30 percent of normal (Bircher, 1981; MacKenzie, 1964; Maier, 1986; and their associates).
3. Under conditions of cardiogenic shock (such as during CPR), available maternal blood is shunted from nonvital organs (including the uterus) to maintain perfusion of the maternal myocardium, brain, and adrenal glands.
4. Patient survival following in-hospital cardiac arrest is uncommon (Niemann, 1992). In a review of 42 reports, McGrath (1987) found a mean survival to discharge rate of 13.8 percent. In a more recent series, after careful exclusion of patients with respiratory arrest only, Blackhall and associates (1992) found that only 3.1 percent of patients with in-hospital cardiac arrest survived to be discharged.
5. Maternal resuscitation may be hindered by vena caval compression, which results in diminished blood return to the right atrium. Venous returns may be enhanced by delivery.
6. A review of perimortem cesarean suggests that delivery within 5 minutes from the time of cardiac arrest results in optimal newborn outcome (Weber, 1971; Katz and co-workers, 1986).

It follows from the above principles that emergency perimortem cesarean should be considered *immediately* upon diagnosis of maternal cardiac arrest, assuming the fetus is of sufficient gestational age to warrant delivery. Bedside cesarean should be performed unless spontaneous maternal pulse has been restored before the cesarean can be initiated. Such action is extremely unlikely to be detrimental to the mother, and may avoid fetal damage or death. In applying this principle, several caveats should be observed:

1. Maternal well-being must supersede that of the fetus. Thus, if insufficient manpower is available to both perform cesarean section and simultaneously assure optimal maternal resuscitative effects, delivery would not be appropriate.
2. The grim prognosis for patients with cardiac arrest does not extend to those who may be hypotensive but have not experienced frank arrest or lethal dysrhythmia (ventricular fibrillation, asystole, or electromechanical dissociation). Under such circumstances, additional blood loss associated with a major abdominal operation may harm the mother, and the decision for cesarean must be individualized. Clearly, under such circumstances, the specifics of the situation will determine the proper course of action.
3. Facilities for bedside cesarean section may not be immediately available within 5 minutes. No standard of care exists defining a maximum allowable time to delivery under these circumstances.

SUMMARY

Cesarean section is the most common and controversial operation in obstetrics. Despite efforts to constrain the trend for more and more operative abdominal deliveries, for the foreseeable future it is unlikely that fewer than one million cesarean deliveries will be performed annually in the United States. The concept of VBAC and its implementation is an advance in the practice of obstetrics, as is peer review of all operative abdominal deliveries. The majority of cesarean deliveries can be accomplished via a low transverse uterine incision, the incision with the least maternal morbidity. Because cesarean sections are usually performed for fetal indications as opposed to maternal indications, there should be no hesitancy to employ a low-vertical, or even classical, uterine incision if necessary to prevent fetal trauma or injury. In all instances attention to sound surgical principles with minimal traumatization of tissues and good hemostasis will optimize maternal outcome.

REFERENCES

Alexander J, Gregg JE, Quinn MW. Femoral fractures at caesarean section. Case reports. Br J Obstet Gynaecol 1987; 94:273.

American College of Obstetricians and Gynecologists. Management of breech presentation. Technical bulletin No. 95. Washington, DC: 1986.

American College of Obstetricians and Gynecologists, Committee on Obstetrics. Maternal and Fetal Medicine: Guidelines for vaginal delivery after a previous cesarean birth. No. 64, October 1988.

American College of Obstetricians and Gynecologists, Committee on Obstetrics. Maternal and Fetal Medicine: Assessment of fetal maturity prior to repeat cesarean delivery or elective induction of labor. No 77, January 1990a.

American College of Obstetricians and Gynecologists. Vaginal birth after cesarean section: Report of 1990 survey of ACOG's membership, August 1990b.

American College of Obstetricians and Gynecologists. Fetal and neonatal neurologic injury. Technical bulletin No. 163, January 1992.

Anderson GM, Lomas J. Recent trends in cesarean section rates in Ontario. Can Med Assoc J 1989; 141:1049.

Banta HD, Thacker SB. Assessing the costs and benefits of electronic fetal monitoring. Obstet Gynecol Surv 1979; 34:627.

Barlow K, Larsson G. Results of a five-year prospective study using a feto-pelvic scoring system for term singleton breech delivery after uncomplicated pregnancy. Acta Obstet Gynecol Scand 1986; 65:315–9.

Benson WL, Boyce DC, Vaughn DL. Breech delivery in the primigravida. Obstet Gynecol 1972; 40:417-28.

Bergsjo P, Schmidt E, Pusch D. Differences in the reported frequencies of some statistical interventions in Europe. Br J Obstet Gynecol 1983; 90:628.

Berkowitz GS, Fiarman GS, Mojica MA, et al. Effect of physician characteristics on the cesarean birth rate. Am J Obstet Gynecol 1989; 161:146.

Bircher N, Safar P. Comparison of standard and "new" closed chest CPR and open-chest CPR in dogs. Crit Care Med 1981; 9:384.

Blackhall LJ, Ziogas A, Azen SP. Low survival rate after cardiopulmonary resuscitation in a county hospital. Arch Intern Med 1992; 152:2045.

Boley JP. The history of cesarean section. J Can Med Assoc 1991; 145:319.

Bond SJ, Harrison MR, Slotnick RN, et al. Cesarean delivery and hysterotomy using an absorbable stapling device. Obstet Gynecol 1989; 74:25.

Bottoms SF, Rosen MG, Sokol RJ. The increase in the cesarean birth rate. N Engl J Med 1980; 302:559.

Bowe ET, Beard RW, Finster M, et al. Reliability of fetal blood sampling. Am J Obstet Gynecol 1970; 107:279.

Buckman RF Jr, Buckman PD, Hufnagel HV, Gervin AS. A physiologic basis for the adhesion-free healing of deperitonealized surfaces. J Surg Res 1976; 21:67.

Burkett G, Jensen LP, Lai A, O'Sullivan MJ, Yasin S, Beydoun, McLeod AGW. Evaluation of surgical staples in cesarean section. Am J Obstet Gynecol 1989;161:540.

Cesarean childbirth. NIH publication No. 82-2067. Bethesda, MD: Department of Health and Human Services, 1981.

Chang PL, Newton ER. Predictors of antibiotic prophylactic failure in post-cesarean endometritis. Obstet Gynecol 1992; 80:117.

Cheng M, Hannah M. Breech delivery at term: a critical review of the literature. Obstet Gynecol 1993; 82:605.

Christian SS, Brady K, Read JA, Kopelman JN. Vaginal breech delivery: a 5-year prospective evaluation of a protocol using computed tomographic pelvimetry. Am J Obstet Gynecol 1990;163:848.

Clark SL, Eglinton GS, Beall M, Phelan JP. Effect of indication for previous cesarean section on subsequent delivery outcome in patients undergoing a trial of labor. J Reprod Med 1984; 29:22.

Cohen AB, Klapholz H, Thompson MS. Electronic fetal monitoring and clinical practice. A survey of obstetric opinion. Med Decis Making, 1982; 2:79.

Collea JV, Chein C, Quilligan EJ. The randomized management of term frank breech presentation: a study of 208 cases. Am J Obstet Gynecol 1980; 137:235–4.

Cunningham FG, Hauth JC, Strong JD, Kappus SS. Infectious morbidity following cesarean section: comparison of two treatment regimens. Obstet Gynecol 1978; 52:656.

DeMott RK, Sandmire HF. The Green Bay cesarean section study. I. The physician factor as a determinant of cesarean birth rates. Am J Obstet Gynecol 1990; 162:1593.

DeMott RK, Sandmire HF. The Green Bay cesarean section study. II. The physician factor as a determinant of cesarean birth rates for failed labor. Am J Obstet Gynecol 1992; 166:1799.

DeMuylder X, Thiery M. The cesarean delivery rate can be safely reduced in a developing country. Obstet Gynecol 1990; 75:60.

DePalma RT, Cunningham FG, Leveno KJ, Roark ML. Continuing cesarean delivery: the three-dose perioperative antimicrobial therapy. Obstet Gynecol 1982; 60:53.

Dillon WP, Choate JW, Nusbaum ML, et al. Obstetric care and cesarean birth rates: a program to monitor quality of care. Obstet Gynecol 1992; 80:731.

Duff P. Prophylactic antibiotics for cesarean delivery: a simple cost-effective strategy for prevention of postoperative morbidity. Am J Obstet Gynecol 1987; 157:794.

Elkins TE, Stovall TG, Warren J, et al. A histological evaluation of peritoneal injury and repair: implications for adhesion formation. Obstet Gynecol 1987; 70:225.

Ellis H. The aetiology of post operative abdominal adhesions, an experimental study. Br J Surg 1962; 50:10.

Ellis H, Heddle R. Does the peritoneum need to be closed at laparotomy? Br J Surg 1977; 64:733.

Farmakides G, Duvivier R, Schulman H, et al. Vaginal birth after two or more previous cesarean sections. Am J Obstet Gynecol 1987; 154:565.

Farmer RM, Kirschbaun T, Potter D, et al. Uterine rupture during trial of labor after previous cesarean section. Am J Obstet Gynecol 1991; 165:996.

Flamm BL, Lim OW, Jones C, et al. Vaginal birth after cesarean section: results of multicenter study. Am J Obstet Gynecol 1988; 158:1079.

Flamm BL, Newman LA, Thomas SJ, et al. Vaginal birth after cesarean delivery: results of a 5-year multicenter collaborative study. Obstet Gynecol 1990; 76:750.

Flanagan TA, Mulchahey KM, Korenbrot CC, et al. Management of term breech presentation. Am J Obstet Gynecol 1987; 156:1492.

Freeman J (ed). Prenatal and Perinatal Factors Associated with Brain Disorders. US Department of Health and Human Services, Public Health Service, National Institutes of Health, NIH publication No. 85-1149, 1985.

Freeman JM, Nelson KB. Intrapartum asphyxia and cerebral palsy. Pediatrics 1988; 82:240.

Freeman R. Intrapartum fetal monitoring—a disappointing story. N Engl J Med 1990; 322:624.

Friedman EA. Labor, clinical evaluation and management. New York: Appleton, 1978.

Frigoletto FD Jr, Ryan KJ, Phillipee M. Maternal mortality rate associated with cesarean section: an appraisal. Am J Obstet Gynecol 1980; 136:969.

Gabert HA, Bey M. History and development of cesarean operation. Obstet Gynecol Clin North Am 1988; 15:591.

Gilstrap LC, Hauth JC, Hankins GDV, Patterson AR. Effect of type of anesthesia on blood loss at cesarean section. Obstet Gynecol 1987; 69:328.

Gilstrap LC III. Elective appendectomy during abdominal surgery. JAMA 1991; 265:1736.

Gimovsky ML, Wallace RL, Schifrin BS, Paul RH. Randomized management of the non-frank breech presentation at term: a preliminary report. Am J Obstet Gynecol 1983; 146:34.

Gimovsky ML, Petrie RH. The intrapartum management of the breech presentation. Clin Perinatol 1989; 16:975.

Gordon D, Milberg J, Daling J, Hickok D. Advanced

maternal age as a risk factor for cesarean delivery. Obstet Gynecol 1991; 77:493.

Gould JB, Davey B, Stafford RS. Socioeconomic differences in rates of cesarean section. N Engl J Med 1989; 321:233.

Grant A, O'Brien N, Joy MT, et al. Cerebral palsy among children born during the Dublin randomized trial of intrapartum monitoring. Lancet 1989; 2:1233.

Hagberg B, Hagberg G, Olow I. The changing panorama of cerebral palsy in Sweden. IV. Epidemiological trends 1959–78. Acta Paediatrica Scand 1984; 73:433.

Hage ML, Helms MJ, Hammond WE, Hammond CB. Changing rates of cesarean delivery: the Duke experience, 1978–1986. Obstet Gynecol 1988; 72:98.

Haplerin ME, Moore DC, Hannah WJ. Classical versus low-segment transverse incision for preterm cesarean section: maternal complications and outcome of subsequent pregnancy. Br J Obstet Gynecol 1988; 95:990.

Harris JW. A study of the results obtained in sixty-four cesarean sections terminated by supravaginal hysterectomy. Bull Johns Hopkins Hosp 1922; 33:318.

Harris RP. Cattle horn lacerations of the abdomen and uterus in pregnant women. Am J Obstet Dis Women Child 1887; 20:43.

Hauth JC, Owen J, Davis RO, et al. Transverse uterine incision closure: one versus two layers. Am J Obstet Gynecol 1992; 166:398. Abstract 444.

Havercamp AD, Thompson HE, McFee JG, et al. The evaluation of continuous fetal heart rate monitoring in high-risk pregnancy. Am J Obstet Gynecol 1976; 125:310.

Hershey DW, Quilligan EJ. Extraabdominal uterine exteriorization at cesarean section. Obstet Gynecol 1978; 52:189.

Hull DB, Varner MW. A randomized study of closure of the peritoneum at cesarean delivery. Obstet Gynecol 1991; 77:818.

Jaffa AJ, Peyser MR, Ballas S, Toaff R. Management of term breech presentation in primigravidae. Br J Obstet Gynaecol 1981; 88:721.

Jarrell MA, Ashmead GG, Mann LI. Vaginal delivery after cesarean section—a five year study. Obstet Gynecol 1986; 65:628.

Jones RO, Nagashima AW, Hatnett-Goodman MM, Goodlin RC. Rupture of low transverse cesarean scars during trial of labor. Obstet Gynecol 1991; 77:815.

Kaplan M, Dollberg M, Wajntraub G, Itzchaki M. Fractured long bones in a term infant delivered by cesarean section. Pediatr Radiol 1987; 17:256.

Katz VL, Dotters DJ, Droegemuller W. Perimortem cesarean delivery. Obstet Gynecol 1986; 68:571.

Kerr JMM. The technic of cesarean section with special reference to the lower uterine segment incision. Am J Obstet Gynecol 1926; 12:729.

Khazin AF, Hon EH, Yeh S-Y. Biochemical studies of the fetus. V. Fetal pCO_2 and Apgar scores. Obstet Gynecol 1971; 38:535.

Kubli FW, Hon E, Khazin AF, Takemura H. Observations on heart rate and pH in the human fetus during labor. Am J Obstet Gynecol 1969; 104:1190.

Leveno KJ, Cunningham FG, Nelson S. Prospective comparison of selective and universal electronic fetal monitoring in 34,995 pregnancies. N Engl Med 1986; 315:615.

Lilford RJ, Van Coeverden de Groot HA, Moore PJ, Bingham P. The relative risks of caesarean section (intrapartum and elective) and vaginal delivery: a detailed analysis to exclude the effects of medical disorders and other acute pre-existing physiological disturbances. Br J Obstet Gynaecol 1990; 97:883.

Lumley J, McKinnon L, Wood C. Lack of agreement on normal values for fetal scalp blood. J Obstet Gynaecol Br Commonw 1971; 78:13.

MacDonald D, Grant A, Sheridan-Pereira M, et al. The Dublin randomized control trial of intrapartum fetal heart rate monitoring. Am J Obstet Gynecol 1985; 152:524.

MacKenzie GJ, Taylor SH, MacDonald AH, et al. Hemodynamic effects of external cardiac compression. Lancet 1964; i:1345.

Maier GW, Newton JR Jr, Wolfe JA, et al. The influence of manual chest compression rate as hemodynamic support during cardiac arrest. Circulation 1986; 74(Suppl IV):51.

Martin CB Jr, DeHaan J, Van der Wildt B, et al. Mechanisms of late decelerations in the fetal heart rate. Europ J Obstet Gynecol Reprod Biol 1979; 9/6:361.

McCall ML. Extraperitoneal cesarean section in the profoundly infected patient. Am J Obstet Gynecol 1949; 57:520.

McCurdy CM Jr, Magann EF, McCurdy CJ, Saltzman AK. The effect of placental management at cesarean delivery on operative blood loss. Am J Obstet Gynecol 1992; 167:1363.

McFadden PM, Peacock EE Jr. Preperitoneal abdominal wound repair: Incidence of dehiscence. Am J Surg 1983; 145:213.

McGrath RB. In-house cardiopulmonary resuscitation after a quarter of a century. Ann Emerg Med 1987; 16:1365.

Melone PJ, Ernest JM, O'Shea MD Jr, Klinepeter KL. Appropriateness of intrapartum fetal heart rate management and risk of cerebral palsy. Am J Obstet Gynecol 1991; 165:272.

Miller DA, Paul RH. Vaginal birth after cesarean section: a ten year experience. Obstet Gynecol 1994; 84:255.

Miller FC, Pearse KE, Paul RH. Fetal heart rate pattern recognition by the method of auscultation. Obstet Gynecol 1984; 64:332.

Miller JM. First successful cesarean section in the British empire. Am J Obstet Gynecol 1992; 166:269.

Mootabar H, Dwyer JF, Surur F, Dillon TF. Vaginal delivery following previous cesarean section in 1983. Int J Gynaecol Obstet 1984; 22:155.

Mor-Yosef S, Samueloff A, Modan B, et al. Ranking the risk factors for cesarean: logistic regression analysis of a nationwide study. Obstet Gynecol 1990; 75:944.

Murata Y, Martin CB Jr, Ikenoue T, et al. Fetal heart rate accelerations and late decelerations during the course of intrauterine death in chronically catheterized rhesus monkeys. Am J Obstet Gynecol 1982; 144:218.

Myers SA, Gleicher N. US cesarean section rate: good news or bad? N Engl J Med 1990; 323:200.

National Hospital Discharge Survey. Rates of cesarean delivery—United States, 1991. Morbid Mortal Weekly Rev; 42:285.

Nelson KB, Ellenberg JH. Antecedents of cerebral palsy. N Engl J Med 1986; 315:81.

Niemann JT. Cardiopulmonary resuscitation. N Engl J Med 1992; 327:1075.

Niswander KR. Does substandard care cause cerebral palsy. Contemp Pediatr, Jan 1988:56.

Niswander K, Elbourne D, Redman C, et al. Adverse outcome of pregnancy and the quality of obstetric care. Lancet 1984; 2:827.

Norton JF. A paravesical extraperitoneal cesarean section technique with analysis of 160 pararescale extraperitoneal cesarean sections. Am J Obstet Gynecol 1946; 51:519.

Notzon FC, Placek PJ, Taffel SM. Comparisons of national cesarean section rates. N Engl J Med 1987; 316:386.

O'Driscoll K, Foley M. Correlation of decrease in perinatal mortality and increase in cesarean section rates. Obstet Gynecol 1983; 61:1.

O'Sullivan MJU, Fumia F, Holsinger K, McLeod AGW. Vaginal delivery after cesarean section. Clin Perinatol 1981; 8:131.

Parer JT, Krueger TR, Harris JL. Fetal oxygen consumption and mechanisms of heart rate response during artificially produced late decelerations of fetal heart rate in sheep. Am J Obstet Gynecol 1980; 136:478.

Parsons AK, Sauer MY, Parsons MT, et al. Appendectomy at cesarean section: a prospective study. Obstet Gynecol 1986; 68:479.

Paul RH, Phelan JP, Yeh S-Y. Trial of labor in the patient with a prior cesarean birth. Am J Obstet Gynecol 1985; 151:297.

Pfaneuf LE. The technique of the transverse cervical cesarean section. Surg Gynecol Obstet 1931; 53:202.

Phelan JP, Clark SC, Diaz F, et al. Vaginal birth after cesarean section. Am J Obstet Gynecol 1987; 157:1510.

Phelan JP, Ock Ahn M, Diaz F, et al. Twice a cesarean, always a cesarean? Obstet Gynecol 1989; 73:161.

Physicians Insurance Association of America, data sharing system. Report No. 4, 1992, Pennington, NJ.

Pietrantoni M, Parsons MT, O'Brien WF, et al. Peritoneal closure or non-closure at cesarean. Obstet Gynecol 1991; 77:293.

Pitkin RM. Once a cesarean? Obstet Gynecol 1991; 77:939.

Porreco RP. Meeting the challenge of the rising cesarean birth rate. Obstet Gynecol 1990; 75:133.

Pridijian G, Hibbard JU, Moawad AH. Cesarean: changing the trends. Obstet Gynecol 1991; 77:195.

Pruett KM, Kirshon B, Cotton DB, Poindexter AN III. Is vaginal birth after two or more cesarean sections safe? Obstet Gynecol 1988; 72:163.

Queenan JT, Nakamoto M. Postpartum immunization: the hypothetical hazard of manual removal of the placenta. Obstet Gynecol 1964; 23:392.

Rochat RW, Koonin LM, Atrash HK, et al. Maternal mortality in the United States: Report for the maternal mortality collaborative. Obstet Gynecol 1988; 72:91.

Rosen MG, Dickinson JC, Westhoff CL. Vaginal birth after cesarean: a meta-analysis of morbidity and mortality. Obstet Gynecol 1991; 77:465.

Ruth VJ, Raivo ICU. Perinatal brain damage: predictive value of metchohe analysis and the Apgar score. Br Med J 1988; 297:24.

Sachs BP, Yeh J, Acker D, et al. Cesarean section-related maternal mortality in Massachusetts, 1954–1985. Obstet Gynecol 1988; 71:385.

Saenger M. Der Kaiserschnitt bei Uterusfibromen. Leipzig, 1882.

Sanchez-Ramos L, Kaunitz AM, Peterson HB, et al. Reducing cesarean sections at a teaching hospital. Am J Obstet Gynecol 1990; 163:1081.

Sandberg EC. Trial of labor following previous cesarean section. Am J Obstet Gynecol 1984; 149:41.

Schifrin BS, Amsel J, Burdorf G. The accuracy of auscultating detection of fetal cardiac decelerations: a computer simulation. Am J Obstet Gynecol 1992; 166:566.

Scott JR. Mandatory trial of labor after cesarean delivery: an alternative viewpoint. Obstet Gynecol 1991; 77:811.

Seitchik J, Ramakrishna RV. Cesarean delivery in nulliparous women for failed oxytocin-augmented labor: route of delivery in subsequent pregnancy. Am J Obstet Gynecol 1982; 143:393.

Sewell JE. Cesarean section—a brief history. A brochure to accompany an exhibition on the history of cesarean section at the National Library of Medicine 30 April 1993 to 31 August 1993. American College of Obstetricians and Gynecologists, Washington, DC, 1993.

Shiono PH, Fielden JF, McNellis D, et al. Recent trends in cesarean birth and trial of labor rates in the United States. JAMA 1987; 257:494.

Shy KK, Luthy DA, Bennett FC, et al. Effects of electronic fetal heart rate monitoring, as compared with periodic auscultation, on the neurologic development of premature infants. N Engl J Med 1990; 322:588.

Skajaa K, Hansen ES, Bendix J. Depressed fracture of the skull in a child born by cesarean section. Acta Obstet Gynecol Scand 1987; 66:275.

Source Book of Health Insurance Data, Health Insurance Association of America, Medical Economics, Orodell, NJ, 1993.

Speert H. Eduardo Porro and cesarean hysterectomy. Surg Gynecol Obstet 1958; 106:245.

Standards for Obstetric-Gynecologic Services, 7th ed. Washington, DC: American College of Obstetricians and Gynecologists 1989:37.

Stanley FJ, Watson L. The cerebral palsies in Western Australia; trends, 1968 to 1981. Am J Obstet Gynecol 1988; 158:89.

Svenningsen NW, Westgren M, Ingemarsson I. Modern strategy for the term breech delivery—study with a 4-year follow-up of the infants. J Perinatol Med 1985; 13:117.

Sykes GS, Johnson P, Ashworth F, et al. Do Apgar scores indicate asphyxia? Lancet 1982; 1:494.

Taffel SM, Placek PJ, Liss T. Trends in the United States cesarean section rate for the 1980–1985 rise. Am J Public Health 1987; 77:955.

Taffel SM, Placek PJ, Moien M, Kosary CL. 1989 US cesarean section rate steadies—VBAC rises to nearly one in five. Birth 1991; 18:73.

Tejani M, Mann L, Bhakthavathsalan A, et al. Correlation of fetal heart rate patterns and fetal pH with neonatal outcome. Obstet Gynecol 1976; 48:460.

Thiery M, Derom R, Buekens P. Frequency of cesarean deliveries in Belgium. Biol Neonate 1989; 55:90.

Titus P. The management of obstetric differences. St. Louis: C.V. Mosby. 1940:1.

Tulandi T, Hum HS, Gelfand MM. Closure of laparotomy incisions with or without peritoneal suturing and second-look laparoscopy. Am J Obstet Gynecol 1988; 158:536.

Vasa R, Kim MR. Fracture of the femur at cesarean section: case report and review of literature. Am J Perinatol 1990; 7:46.

Vengadasalam D. Vaginal delivery following cesarean section. Singapore Med J 1986; 37:396.

Villeneuve MG, Khalife S, Marcoux S, Blanchet P. Surgical staples in cesarean section: a randomized controlled trial. Am J Obstet Gynecol 1990; 163:1641.

Wallace RC, Eglinton GS, Yonekura ML, et al. Extraperitoneal cesarean section: a surgical form of infection prophylaxis? Am J Obstet Gynecol 1984; 148:172.

Waters EG. Supravesical extraperitoneal cesarean section: Water's type. Clin Obstet Gynecol 1959; 2:258.

Weber CE. Postmortem cesarean section: review of the literature and case reports. Am J Obstet Gynecol 1971; 110:158.

Wood C, Ferguson R, Leeton J, et al. Fetal heart rate and acid-base status in the assessment of fetal hypoxia. Am J Obstet Gynecol 1967; 98:62.

Woodward RW, Callahan WE. Breech labor and delivery in the primigravida. Obstet Gynecol 1969; 34:260.

CHAPTER 19

Obstetric Hysterectomy

Obstetric hysterectomy refers to surgical removal of the pregnant or recently pregnant uterus. The term includes hysterectomy with the pregnancy in situ as well as operations related to complications of delivery. This chapter focuses on peripartum hysterectomy including cesarean hysterectomy and postpartum hysterectomy. Peripartum hysterectomy is an indispensable tool for management of intractable obstetric hemorrhage unresponsive to other treatment (see Chapter 26). The procedure may be lifesaving and should be within the capabilities of all obstetric consultants. Peripartum hysterectomy can be a formidable operation, particularly when performed for a life-threatening emergency, and skills necessary for its performance are best acquired with an experienced mentor during scheduled nonemergency cases.

HISTORY

Obstetric hysterectomy was developed in the late eighteenth century to make it possible for women to survive cesarean delivery. The history of obstetrics must be contemplated to understand better the place and importance of this operation. Cesarean deliveries were uniformly fatal until the late nineteenth century. Until that time bleeding and infections were untreatable complications. There were no intravenous fluids, antimicrobial drugs, blood transfusions, or respiratory and circulatory support. Anesthetics were limited or nonexistent, and surgical antisepsis was not widely practiced. Obstetricians lacked the knowledge and techniques to perform safe pelvic surgery. For example, before Sanger's 1882 monograph, the uterine incision after cesarean delivery was not closed, which allowed lochia to flow freely into the peritoneal cavity.

Pelvic deformities from nutritional deficiencies or infectious diseases were common until the early twentieth century. Sexually active women with deformed pelves had no reliable contraception, and mothers with very small or distorted pelves labored to exhaustion and died along with their babies. Helpless attendants used fetal destructive operations to attempt to save the mothers, who often had extensive pelvic soft tissue injuries if they survived.

The concepts that enabled the development of obstetric hysterectomy were developed in the late eighteenth century by Joseph Cavallini of Florence. In 1768, he used animal experiments to disprove the prevailing idea that the uterus was an essential organ for life, and he removed the uterus successfully in pregnant and nonpregnant animals (Durfee, 1969). Investigators in Germany and England in the early 1800s concluded that abdominal delivery in animals was less dangerous if they removed the uterus after delivery (Young, 1944). These experiments prepared the way for safe cesarean delivery as well as for obstetric hysterectomy.

The earliest documented human peripartum hysterectomy was performed in 1868 by

Horatio Robinson Storer of Boston (Bixby, 1869). Storer was America's first specialist in diseases of women, and he was confronted by a woman whose labor was obstructed by a large uterine tumor. The baby was already dead, but the tumor prevented any fetal destructive procedures. Storer performed cesarean delivery and because of life-threatening hemorrhage, he removed the uterus with its "fibrocystic tumor the size of a baby's head." Ligatures around the cervix and the tumor pedicle controlled bleeding. The cervical stump was seared with a hot iron and returned to the pelvis, after which the abdominal wound was closed with silver wire. The patient recovered from the chloroform anesthetic but died 3 days later.

Eduardo Porro (1876) published the first case report to describe a patient who survived hysterectomy after cesarean delivery. For this reason, some clinicians still refer to cesarean hysterectomy as the "Porro operation." Before this case, Porro had previously performed an emergency cesarean delivery in a woman with obstructed labor from a rachitic pelvis. She had died, as had almost every woman after abdominal delivery. Determined to improve the safety of cesarean delivery, Porro repeatedly rehearsed cesarean hysterectomy in the animal laboratory.

Isaac Taylor of New York performed the first Porro operation in the United States in 1880 (Durfee, 1969). The woman died of a pulmonary embolism 3 weeks after an otherwise successful operation. In 1878, E. Richardson reported the first maternal survival after a Porro operation in the United States. In 1880, Robert P. Harris reviewed the world literature on cesarean hysterectomy. He collected 50 cases from seven countries. The maternal mortality rate was 58 percent and the fetal survival rate was 86 percent. In 1884, Clement Godson of England reviewed a total of 134 cases. At that time, two-thirds of the most common indications for surgery still was a contracted pelvis due to rickets. He reported a maternal mortality rate of 45 percent with death usually due to peritonitis (27%), shock (12%), and septicemia (6%).

European surgeons modified the Porro procedure in an attempt to reduce operative risks and improve outcomes. Tait (1890) of England published changes that were widely adopted. The Tait-Porro operation enjoyed increasing popularity, and indications for the procedure expanded beyond absolute emergencies as surgical techniques improved. Two events in 1900 illustrate a division of opinion about obstetric hysterectomy that continues to the present. Reed (1900) was of the opinion that cesarean hysterectomy was properly performed only with life-threatening circumstances. In the same year, Duncan and Targett (1900) of England reported the first elective sterilization by cesarean hysterectomy. While conservative surgeons clung to the "emergency only" philosophy, aggressive surgeons extended indications to gynecologic disorders and sterilization (Lash and Cummings, 1935). In 1937, Wilson reported that almost 10 percent of women in Rochester undergoing cesarean delivery also had a hysterectomy for myoma or sterilization.

Experiences with cesarean hysterectomy at Charity Hospital at New Orleans began in 1938. The first 30 years' experiences were reported by Barclay (1970) and Mickal and associates (1969) to support the use of planned obstetric hysterectomy. Since then, the ongoing Charity Hospital experiences have been reported periodically (Bey and co-workers, 1992; Gonsoulin and associates, 1991; Plauché and colleagues, 1981, 1983). Morbidity and mortality figures for obstetric hysterectomy steadily improved during these years. Subsequently, Davis (1951) of Chicago championed elective cesarean hysterectomy. He reported a 20 percent incidence of hysterectomy in a series of 736 cesarean deliveries. John Weed (1959) later reported that 20 percent of 400 women who had previous cesarean deliveries later required hysterectomy for gynecologic disorders. The mean time between delivery and hysterectomy was 6.3 years. Those who favored elective cesarean hysterectomy often cited these data.

Those who reserved peripartum hysterectomy for life-threatening emergencies also found persuasive support. Brenner and colleagues (1970) concluded that complications outweighed benefits if hysterectomy was performed for sterilization. These and others held that tubal ligation after either cesarean or vaginal delivery was safer. The literature of the 1970s and 1980s reflected continuing controversy about the appropriate use of obstetric hysterectomy. Cesarean hysterectomy versus cesarean tubal ligation for sterilization was commonly debated, though no controlled comparative data existed. Certainly, reports from university services contained many catastrophic emergency cases (Chestnut and associates, 1984; Clark and colleagues, 1984; Plauché and co-workers, 1983). While conservative obstetricians called attention to the excessive blood loss, transfusions, and other complications in these reports, a number of reports of planned cesarean hysterectomy supported the opposite view with few complications (Dyer and colleagues, 1953; Schneider and Tyrone, 1968; Ward and Smith, 1965).

Bey and colleagues (1993) performed a prospective comparative study of 82 elective cesarean hysterectomies and 102 matched cesarean tubal ligations. They found significantly greater blood loss and operating time in the hysterectomy patients but significantly greater febrile morbidity in the tubal ligation patients. Blood transfusion, mean hospital stay, and perioperative complications were not significantly different between these two groups.

Currently, enthusiasm for nonemergency peripartum hysterectomy varies by region across the United States. Some obstetric services regularly perform the operation when obstetric indications for cesarean delivery coexist with gynecologic indications for hysterectomy. Other obstetric services reserve peripartum hysterectomy for major obstetric emergencies. These variations reflect legitimate differences of professional opinion and training experience.

CLASSIFICATION

Table 19–1 offers a classification for obstetric hysterectomy. Careful classification considers the timing, indication, extent, and circumstances associated with each case. Peripartum hysterectomies include those following cesarean delivery (cesarean hysterectomy) and those following vaginal delivery (postpartum hysterectomy). Either operation may be subtotal, total, or radical, with or without removal of one or both adnexa. Each operation may be further characterized by the indication for which it was performed. Each may be identified as an emergency, an indicated nonemergency, or an elective case. Only when all these factors are considered can valid conclusions be drawn about comparative risks and outcomes.

TABLE 19–1. CLASSIFICATION OF OBSTETRIC HYSTERECTOMY

Antepartum hysterectomy—fetus in situ
- Subtotal—with or without adnexectomy
- Total—with or without adnexectomy
- Radical—with or without node dissection and/or adnexectomy

Peripartum hysterectomy
- Cesarean hysterectomy—after cesarean delivery
  - Subtotal—with or without adnexectomy
  - Total—with or without adnexectomy
  - Radical—with or without node dissection and adnexectomy
- Postpartum hysterectomy—after vaginal delivery
  - Subtotal—with or without adnexectomy
  - Total—with or without adnexectomy

Each classification may be further subdivided by indication and into emergency, indicated nonemergency, and elective categories.

INDICATIONS FOR OBSTETRIC HYSTERECTOMY

Emergency Indications

Table 19–2 gives many of the published indications for obstetric hysterectomy. Emergency indications are less common than in the past, as there are now alternative treatments that are less invasive for many problems that formerly required surgery. For example, obstructed labors are currently managed by cesarean delivery long before uterine rupture or severe infections develop as they did in earlier years.

Contemporaneously, hysterectomies are performed as final efforts to stop intractable hemorrhage. In 1964, Bowman and colleagues reported that 55 percent of cesarean hysterectomies at Charity Hospital were done for postpartum hemorrhage and two-thirds of these were for uterine atony. While modern medical management controls most cases of uterine atony, some unresponsive cases still require hysterectomy as a lifesaving measure. Recently, uterine atony was the indication for 20 percent of emergency peripartum hysterectomies reported by Stanco and colleagues (1993) from Los Angeles County Hospital and Zelop and associates (1993) from Harvard.

Ruptured uterus is the second most common indication for emergency hysterectomy for hemorrhage. In the Los Angeles report

TABLE 19–2. INDICATIONS FOR OBSTETRIC HYSTERECTOMY

Obstetrical Emergencies
- Hemorrhage
  - Ruptured uterus
    - Spontaneous
      - Previous uterine scar
      - Previous intact uterus
    - Traumatic
    - Extratubal ectopic pregnancy rupture
      - Cornual pregnancy
      - Intramural pregnancy
      - Cervical pregnancy
      - Diverticular pregnancy
  - Expanding pelvic hematoma
  - Placental disorders
    - Placenta accreta, increta, and percreta
    - Placenta previa complications
    - Abruptio placentae complications
  - Postpartum hemorrhage
    - Intractable uterine atony
    - Inverted uterus
- Sepsis
  - Chorioamnionitis with sepsis
  - Myometrial abscesses

Indicated Nonemergencies
- Coexisting gynecologic disorders
  - Leiomyomas
  - Cervical intraepithelial neoplasia
  - Early invasive cervical malignancy
  - Ovarian malignancies

Elective Cases
- Multiple or defective previous cesarean scars
- Gynecologic disorders
  - Previous endometriosis, pelvic inflammatory disease, irregular and heavy menses, pelvic adhesions
- Request for sterilization by hysterectomy

cited above, all uterine ruptures that required emergency hysterectomy were in women with previous cesarean section scars. Similarly, 60 percent of emergency hysterectomies in the Harvard series were done in women who previously had cesarean deliveries. A previous cesarean section increases the likelihood of placenta previa, placenta accreta, scar dehiscence, and overt uterine rupture, and each of these diagnoses increases the risk for emergency hysterectomy (Leung and colleagues, 1993; Zelop and co-workers, 1993).

There has been great interest in the risk of uterine rupture during trials of vaginal birth after cesarean section. Uterine rupture required hysterectomy in 1 of 555 trials of labor cited in the recent review by Stanco and colleagues (1993) while Leung and co-workers (1993) reported scar rupture requiring laparotomy in 70 of 8513 cases (1 in 122). In earlier years, uterine scar dehiscence discovered at repeat cesarean section was a common indication for hysterectomy. For example, almost half of the Charity Hospital cases in the first three decades were performed for a defective scar. Contemporary management is now quite different, as experience has accrued that scars that appear thin and minor dehiscences do not mandate uterine removal.

Major scar dehiscences and overt ruptures can be managed either by repair or by hysterectomy. Catastrophic uterine ruptures, particularly of the unscarred uterus, most often require hysterectomy; however, there is a recent trend for repair in selected cases (Plauché, 1991). The decision of uterine repair versus removal depends on the extent of uterine damage, condition of the woman, and her wish for more pregnancies. The available operating environment and the surgeon's experience and training also play important roles in the decision.

Placental disorders are the third most frequent cause of emergency obstetric hysterectomy for bleeding. Most of these are from placenta accreta with or without an associated previa. Placenta accreta has increased in frequency as an emergent indication for hysterectomy, and 65 percent of emergency procedures in the Harvard series were performed for this reason (Zelop and co-workers, 1993).

Severe uterine infections that formerly required cesarean hysterectomy usually respond to modern antimicrobial therapy. Sepsis from chorioamnionitis is rare because of aggressive management of prematurely ruptured membranes. Tinga (1986) reported several women with neglected infections that developed myometrial abscesses or intractable uterine atony that required hysterectomy and pelvic drainage.

Nonemergency Indications

Peripartal hysterectomy is more controversial when performed for reasons other than obstetric emergencies. These indicated but nonemergent procedures are performed when women requiring cesarean delivery also have a gynecologic disorder that is usually managed by hysterectomy. These have been variously termed nonemergency, planned, or anticipated cesarean hysterectomies (Plauché, 1991; Zelop and colleagues, 1993). The rationale is to perform both cesarean delivery and hysterectomy for gynecologic disease during the same hospital stay with a single procedure and anesthetic.

Currently, uterine leiomyomas and cervical intraepithelial neoplasia are common indications (Plauché, 1991). McNulty (1984) reviewed a 10-year experience with 80 planned cesarean hysterectomies performed in several California private hospitals. The most prevalent diagnoses in this series were uterine leiomyomas (25%) and defective scars after previous cesarean operations (28%). Another 25 percent had other benign gynecologic conditions, 5 percent had a pelvic malignancy, and the remainder of cases were elective. These are similar to the 5-year British experience reported by Sturdee and Rushton (1986). Conversely, Yancey and associates (1993) reported that abnormal gynecologic bleeding (34%) or chronic pelvic pain (32%) constituted the most common indicators.

Park and Duff (1980) reported a series of planned cesarean hysterectomies from Walter Reed Army Medical Center, most of which were radical operations in women referred for cervical cancer. Hoffman and colleagues (1993) described 37 cesarean hysterectomies for early cervical neoplasia complicating pregnancy. Other malignancies occasionally require cesarean hysterectomy, for example, operations to control metastatic breast cancer or ovarian cancer diagnosed during pregnancy or at delivery.

Elective

Completely elective obstetric hysterectomies are the most controversial. McNulty (1984) reported that many of the women in his California series elected hysterectomy after multiple vaginal (15%) or cesarean (15%) deliveries. Multiple previous cesarean deliveries was the diagnosis in a fourth of cases in the early years of the Charity Hospital series (Mickal and colleagues, 1969; Plauché, 1986). Importantly, these groups did not encourage primary abdominal delivery to create opportunities for surgical sterilization by hysterectomy.

OPERATIVE TECHNIQUE

General Considerations

There are a number of anatomic and physiologic changes in pregnant women that increase the likelihood of intraoperative problems. The uterus, of course, is markedly enlarged and pelvic blood vessels are large and tortuous. Collateral circulation enlarges vessels that are normally of little concern during gynecologic surgery. Pelvic tissues are edematous and more friable than in nonpregnant women. Rapid control of all vascular supply to the uterus is essential. Dilated vessels and multiple collaterals require careful dissection. Extra clamps are necessary to avoid retrograde blood loss from severed blood vessels. The distal two-thirds of clamps hold tissues and vessels with maximum security. Clamps on vascular pedicles should be manipulated as little as possible. All pedicles should be inspected several times for hemostasis before completing the case.

Obstetric surgeons should develop several methods to quickly control severe uterine bleeding. In some emergency cases, when it may seem impossible to stop blood loss, manual aortic compression controls bleeding long enough to clear the operating field and identify specific bleeding points. Bilateral internal iliac artery ligation reduces arterial bleeding from the uterine, vesical, and pudendal vessels. Pressure packs reduce venous bleeding. An umbrella pack that exits through the vagina to some form of traction can compress veins causing troublesome bleeding deep in the pelvis after hysterectomy. Remember that bleeding within the abdomen may come from damage to other abdominal organs, particularly the spleen and liver.

The bulky uterus is difficult to manipulate during obstetric surgery. It cannot be safely manipulated by means of clamps on friable adnexal structures. A tumor tenaculum placed on the uterine fundus is an efficient traction device. A finger in the apex of a vertical cesarean incision also provides effective traction and manipulation.

The bladder wall becomes edematous and friable during labor and is easily injured by blunt dissection. The bladder can also be injured by rotating movements of bladder retractors held under tension. Assistants should release traction before repositioning bladder retractors. A laparotomy sponge placed between the retractor blade and the bladder helps avoid injury.

There are often dense adhesions between the bladder and the lower uterine segment in women with previous cesarean section scars. Metzenbaum scissors with the curve turned downward away from the bladder can be used to accomplish meticulous sharp dissection. When blunt dissection is required, rolled umbilical tape in the tip of a Kelly clamp is used with small, focused movements. Avoid gross rolling or pushing motions with large sponges.

Bladder injuries are sometimes difficult to detect. One method is to search for small or hidden perforations of the posterior bladder wall by filling the bladder with sterile colored or opaque solutions. One such “contrast solution” is milk from presterilized nursery bottles drawn into a bulb syringe. The circulating nurse attaches the syringe to the urethral catheter and fills the bladder with 200–300 mL of milk. The milk is easily seen flowing from small defects in the bladder wall. Milk can be used repeatedly during a case because it does not stain tissues.

In elective cases, colored bladder solutions can be prepared before surgery. Sterile milk or an ampule of indigo carmine or methylene blue is placed into a 1-L bag of normal saline. The intravenous tubing can be connected to the transurethral catheter with an adapter. Lifting the bag fills the bladder and lowering the bag drains the bladder into a closed system.

Bladder defects are repaired promptly using a two-layer closure with absorbable suture (see Chapter 28). Undetected, unrepaired bladder injuries may result in fistulas.

The ureter in pregnancy is dilated and sluggish. The ureter and bladder may be damaged or displaced by trauma, hematomas, or pelvic tumors. The surgeon should be aware of the proximity of the ureter at all phases of the operation. Dissect the course of the ureter if there is any question of its safety. If necessary, open the dome of the bladder and insert retrograde ureteral catheters to ensure ureteral integrity. Repair and support any identified ureteral injury by standard methods along with expert intraoperative consultation.

The vaginal wall in pregnancy is friable and edematous, particularly if the woman has been in labor. Firm traction on clamps attached to the vagina will tear the tissues. When the cut edges of the vaginal cuff are under tension during surgery, the vaginal epithelium tends to separate from the vascular subepithelial layer. Avoid postoperative bleeding by incorporating all vaginal layers in the cuff closure.

Sutures may cut through friable pedicles unless tightened carefully. Pedicles shrink in size as edema subsides after delivery. Single circumferential sutures may allow vessels to escape control. Transfixing sutures improve hemostatic control when edema subsides. Hematomas can result if transfixing sutures are used alone without circumferential proximal ties.

Traction or twisting of clamps on vascular pedicles may strip pedicles away from adjacent tissues. This opens blood vessels that are difficult to clamp and suture without injury to nearby structures, particularly the ureter and bladder. Clamps should be supported, not manipulated, during suturing.

Meticulous hemostatic and aseptic technique reduces infectious complications. Careful hemostasis at the vaginal cuff prevents postoperative bleeding and cuff hematomas. Infected cuff hematomas may suppurate to form cuff abscesses. Prophylactic antimicrobials are recommended for women who have been in labor (see Chapter 38). Treatment is given for obvious infections. Avoid bacteria-laden lochia spills during surgery, especially when opening the vagina. In grossly infected cases, the skin and subcutaneous tissues may be left open under surgical dressings. Delayed closure after antimicrobial treatment reduces the risk of wound suppuration and dehiscence.

Consider surgical drains at sites that may collect blood or tissue fluids after surgery. Complete surgical hemostasis, when it can be attained, is preferable to surgical drainage. Place drains near, but not directly upon, the sites of bladder or large bowel injury and repair.

The Original Porro Hysterectomy

Porro's original technique is described for its historical interest and for contrast with current methods. Porro carefully followed nineteenth century surgical techniques. The amphitheater was heated to a precise 18 degrees centigrade. The surgeons washed their hands with dilute carbolic acid. Chloroform anesthesia was induced and a 12-cm vertical midline infraumbilical incision was made. A vertical uterine incision allowed delivery of a 3300 g female by version and extraction. Attempts at manual and suture control of bleeding after removal of the placenta were unsuccessful. He wrote: "It was providential that we had made all the preparations necessary for hysterectomy; otherwise the patient would surely have died." An assistant elevated the uterus out of the abdominal wound. Porro slipped the wire noose of a Cintrat constrictor over the uterus and over both fallopian tubes and ovaries. He tightened the loop about the lower uterus for hemostasis. He sliced the uterus and adnexa away. He drained the cul de sac through the vagina and placed additional drains in the abdominal wound. The cervical stump was treated with perchloride of iron. Both cervical stump and Cintrat constrictor were exteriorized onto the abdominal wall. The abdominal wound was closed around these with silver wire mass sutures. The operation lasted 26 minutes.

The exteriorized constriction device was left on the cervical stump under dressings for 4 days. The wound sutures were removed on the seventh postoperative day. The ischemic cervical pedicle detached 7 days later. The woman left the hospital on the fortieth postoperative day.

Contemporary Tourniquet Method

Some surgeons still use a tourniquet around the lower uterine segment for hemostasis, as did Porro and his successors. The following method for peripartum hysterectomy is attributed to Leon Gaillard of Louisiana State University School of Medicine: Cesarean delivery is performed as usual. The assistant elevates the uterus out of the abdominal cavity. The operator transilluminates the broad ligaments to identify avascular spaces. Kelly clamps are placed through these windows on each side below the level of the uterine incision. A tourniquet is passed through the two openings in the broad ligament to encircle the uterus below the hysterotomy incision. The tourniquet can be a rubber catheter, heavy Penrose drain, or plastic intravenous tubing. The tourniquet is drawn very tight and secured by an Ochsner (Kocher) clamp at the back of the uterus. Hysterectomy then proceeds using the chosen technique.

The tourniquet helps to control postcesarean blood loss from the uterine vessels. It does not control collateral circulation from the ovarian vessels. The delayed ligation technique described next offers another method to rapidly control both uterine and collateral blood supply.

Delayed Ligation Technique

Dyer and colleagues (1953) described the delayed ligation technique as performed on the Tulane Obstetric Service of Charity Hospital of New Orleans. Other surgeons have modified the method over a period of years to address operative problems. This technique quickly controls all vascular supply to the uterus. The operating principles are simple. Each vascular pedicle supplying the uterus is clamped and severed between clamps. The clamped pedicles drop from the operative field as the operator proceeds quickly from one pedicle to the next, delaying suture ligation until all six vascular bundles are controlled. This technique gains complete hemostasis very quickly. The delayed ligation technique is well suited to nonemergency and elective cases and can be used for many emergency cases.

Preoperative Preparation

Preoperative evaluation includes careful assessment of the woman and her fetus. Complicating conditions or illnesses, hemodynamic stability, and coagulation status are particularly important. The blood bank is asked to prepare the appropriate blood replacement products. Blood transfusion usually begins before surgery in unstable patients; however, surgical hemostasis must not be delayed if bleeding continues.

An experienced surgical team is assembled consisting of a nurse circulator, surgical technician, anesthesiologist, assistant surgeon, and principal surgeon. Hemodynamic support and anesthetic technique are discussed. The situation is discussed with the woman and her family and informed consent is obtained. Prophylactic antibiotics are ordered before or during surgery for women who have been in labor or who are otherwise at risk for infection. An indwelling Foley catheter with a large balloon is placed to empty the bladder and monitor urine output. This also helps to identify the bladder neck during later dissection.

When time permits, details of the operation are reviewed with the team to assure maximum efficiency. Instruments and sutures can be chosen before the operation begins. A single suture such as 0 chromic or 00 polyglycolic suture on a general closure needle usually suffices for most phases of the operation. A single type of suture expedites the work of both surgical technician and circulating nurse.

Surgery can be performed through either vertical or transverse abdominal wall incisions. Adequate visualization of the operative site is essential (see Chapter 4). The fastest method is the vertical incision below the umbilicus. This incision offers good exposure to explore the entire abdomen and is easily extended. The pregnant uterus restricts general examination of the abdomen early in the case. Complete abdominal exploration should be done at some time during the procedure.

Operative Technique

Cesarean delivery is performed as usual except that the incision in the vesicouterine fold is extended to meet each round ligament 2–3 cm from the uterine wall (Fig. 19–1). A vertical uterine incision is preferable, particularly if the lower uterine segment is narrow. After delivery of the infant and placenta, the edges of the vertical incision are approximated with three or four towel clips. This gains rapid hemostasis and reduces lochia spill (Fig. 19–2). Approximation of the uterine edges with a mass running suture is equally effective but takes longer.

The round ligaments are divided between straight Ochsner (Kocher) clamps placed 2 and 3 cm from the uterus (Fig. 19–3). This

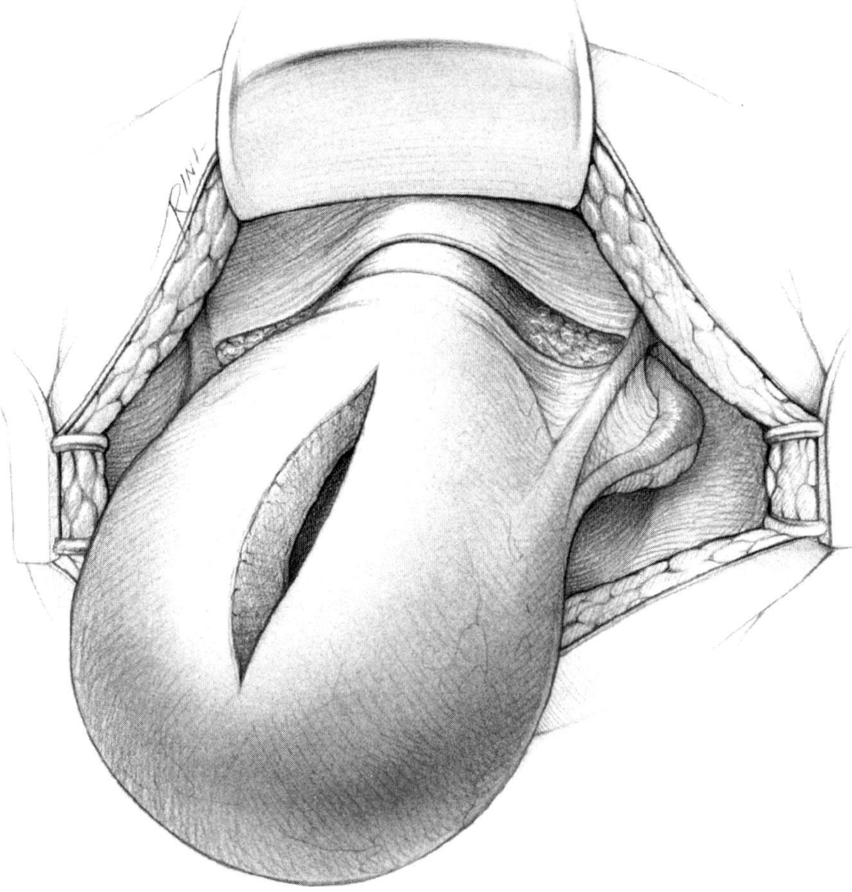

Figure 19–1. Prior to cesarean hysterectomy, the peritoneal incision made for the cesarean operation is extended to the round ligaments.

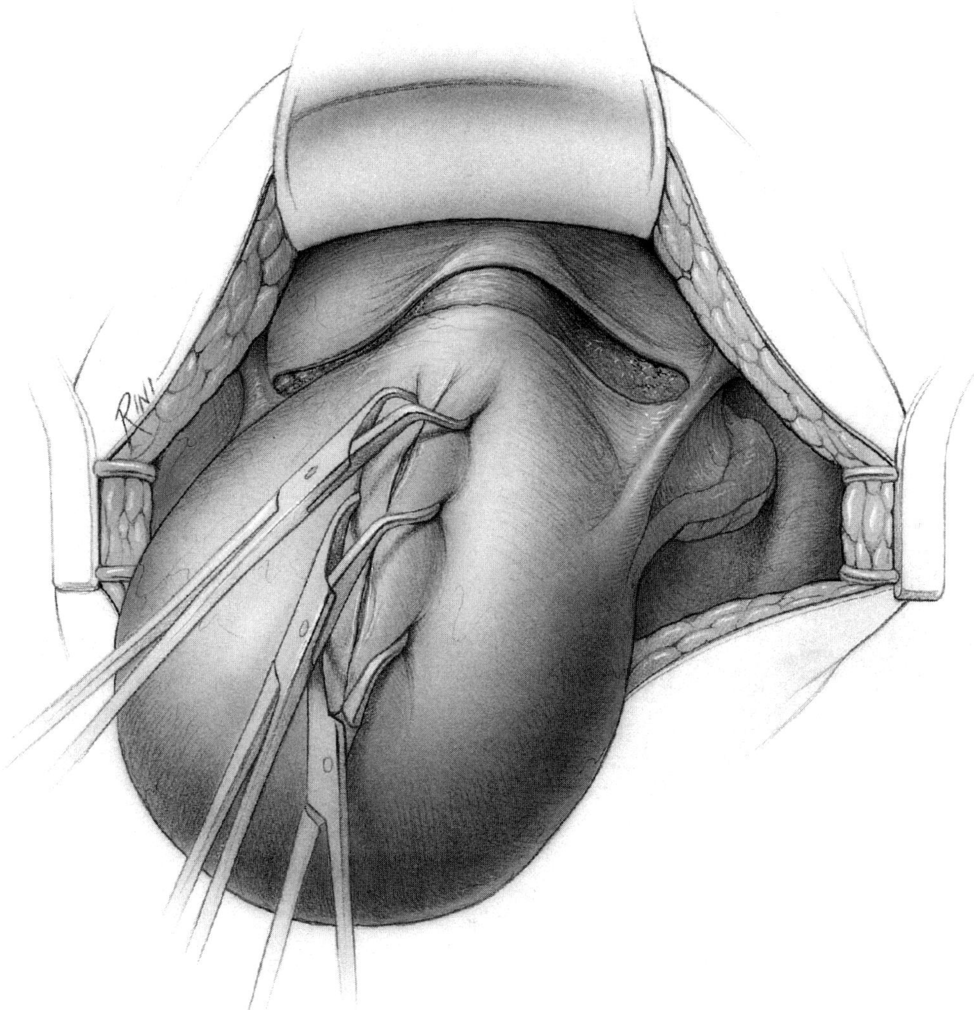

Figure 19–2. Towel clamps are used to quickly close the edges of the cesarean incision and to control bleeding. Alternatively, a single-layer running-locking suture can be placed to quickly close the uterine incision and gain hemostasis.

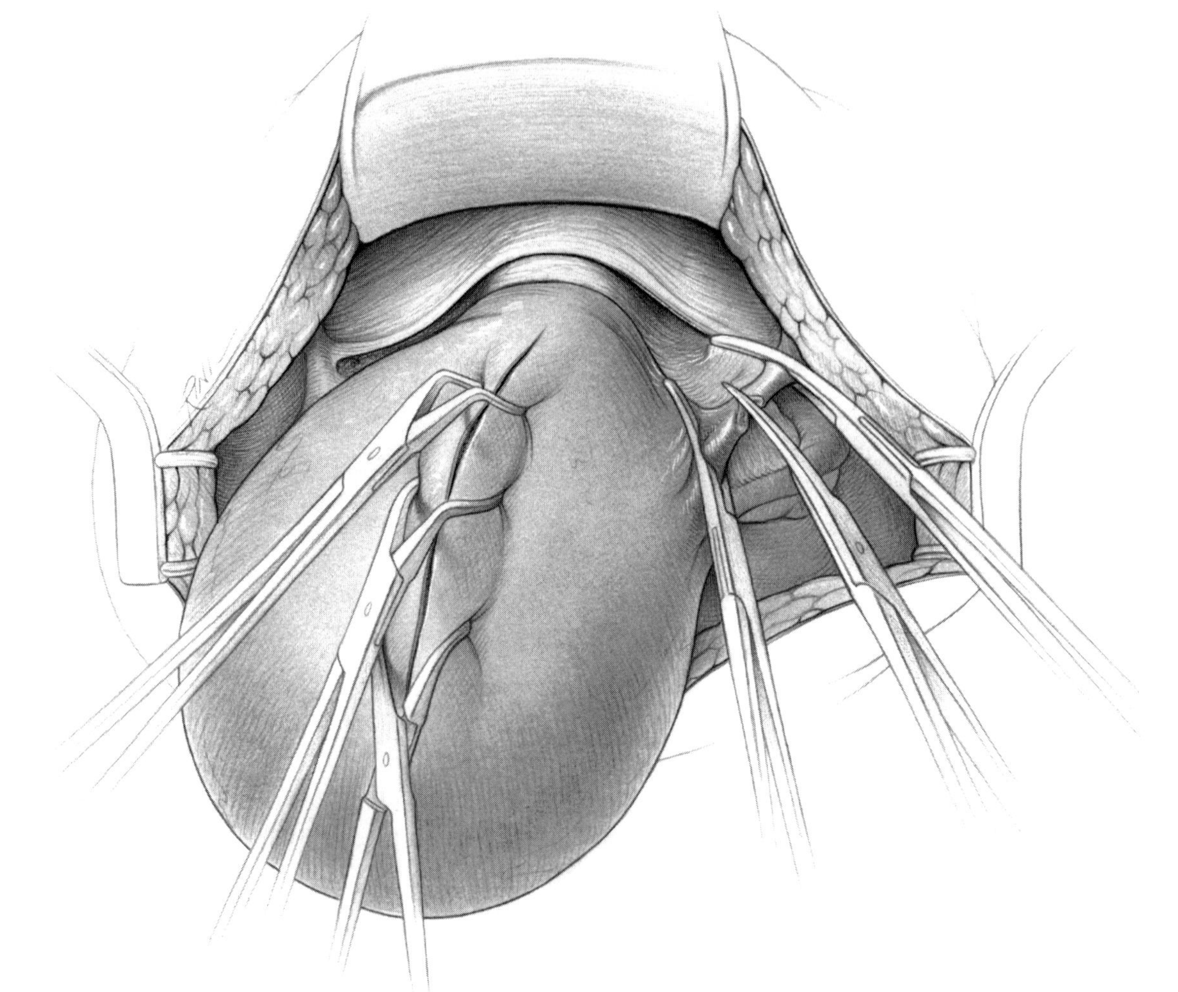

Figure 19–3. The right round ligament is doubly clamped with Oschner (Kocher) clamps. It is divided between clamps with scissors and the pedicle is then dropped, to be sutured later. In elective and non-emergent cases, the lateral pedicle can be secured with an absorbable suture. Attention is directed to placing the suture initially beneath the round ligament, following which it is passed directly through the round ligament, ensuring that Sampsons's artery is ligated.

includes Sampson's artery that courses parallel to the round ligament. The distal round ligament pedicle and clamp are left in the lateral pelvic cavity to be sutured later.

An avascular window in the right broad ligament is identified and a curved Kelly clamp is pushed through the chosen site and then opened to enlarge the aperture (Fig. 19–4). The proximal Ochsner clamp on the right round ligament is repositioned to encompass all adnexal structures near the uterus (Fig. 19–5). Two additional Ochsner clamps are placed across the utero-ovarian ligament and fallopian tube 1 cm lateral to the first clamp. The tips of all of these adnexal clamps lie within the opening in the broad ligament to assure control of all blood vessels. The adnexal pedicle is cut between

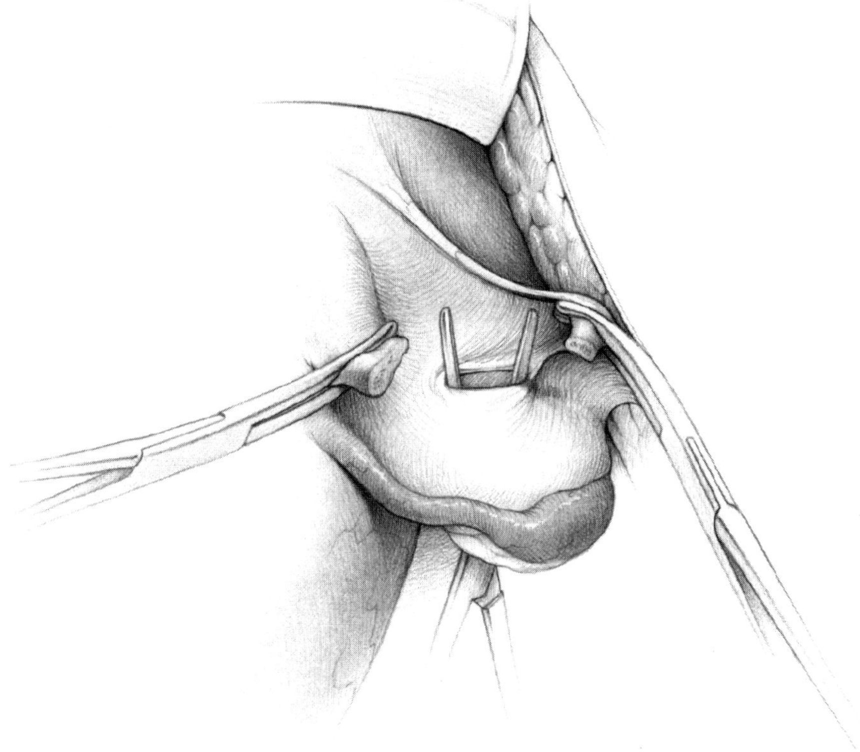

Figure 19–4. A Kelly clamp is thrust through an avascular portion of the right broad ligament. The opening is enlarged by opening the clamp.

the proximal and two distal clamps. The distal pedicle and clamps are placed aside to be sutured later.

The right uterine vessels are exposed as the assistant retracts the uterus upward. The posterior leaf of the broad ligament is incised medially from the previous opening to the posterior wall of the uterus. Loose connective tissue is dissected around from the uterine vessels (Fig. 19–6). A Heaney clamp is placed on the isolated uterine artery and vein at a level below the cesarean incision near the junction of the cervix and uterus. The clamp is placed higher on the uterine wall if there is distortion of anatomic relationships by broad ligament hematoma or tumor. The right uterine vascular pedicle is not severed at this time, and attention is directed to the left side of the dissection.

The left round ligament and adnexal pedicles are clamped and cut as on the right side. The left uterine vessels are skeletonized and doubly clamped. All major blood vessels supplying the uterus are now controlled.

The next step in delayed ligation technique is to replace all clamps with suture ligatures, beginning with the last clamps placed. A Heaney or Ochsner clamp is placed on the left uterine vessels above the dissection to control collateral back bleeding before the vessels are divided. The upper portion of the uterine vascular pedicle is incised and shaped with a small scalpel blade leaving a small amount of tissue distal to the clamp to prevent the escape of tissues from the clamp (Fig. 19–7A). Dissection extends beyond the tip of the first clamp but not past the second.

A suture needle is passed beneath the tip of the distal (back) clamp. This clamp is then removed as the first throw of a surgeon's knot

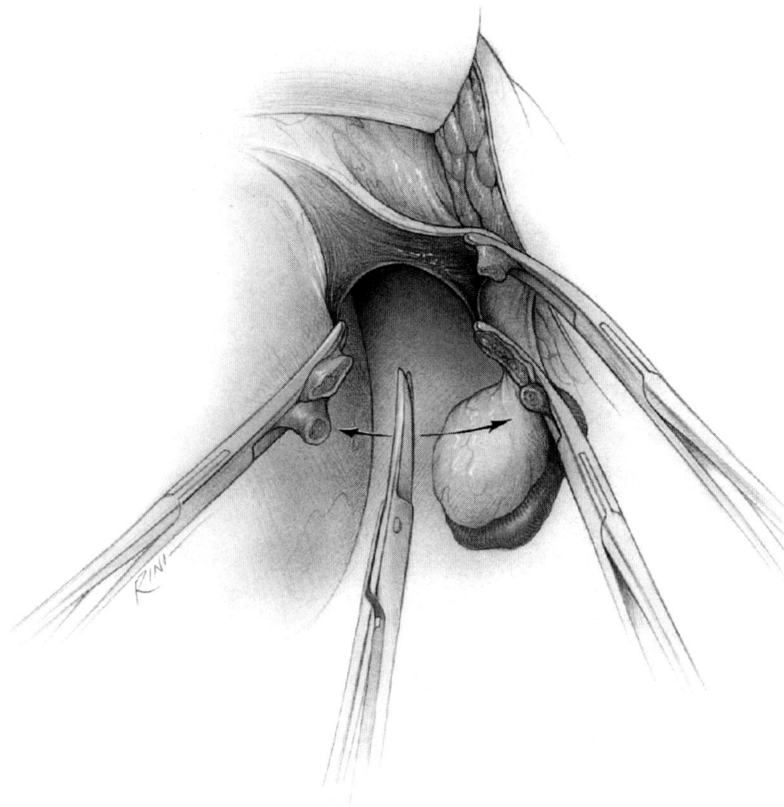

Figure 19–5. The right fallopian tube and utero-ovarian ligament are doubly clamped with Oschner (Kocher) clamps. The medial round ligament clamp is replaced to encompass all adnexal structures. The adnexal pedicle is then divided between the medial clamp and the two lateral clamps (dotted line). The pedicle is dropped, to be sutured later.

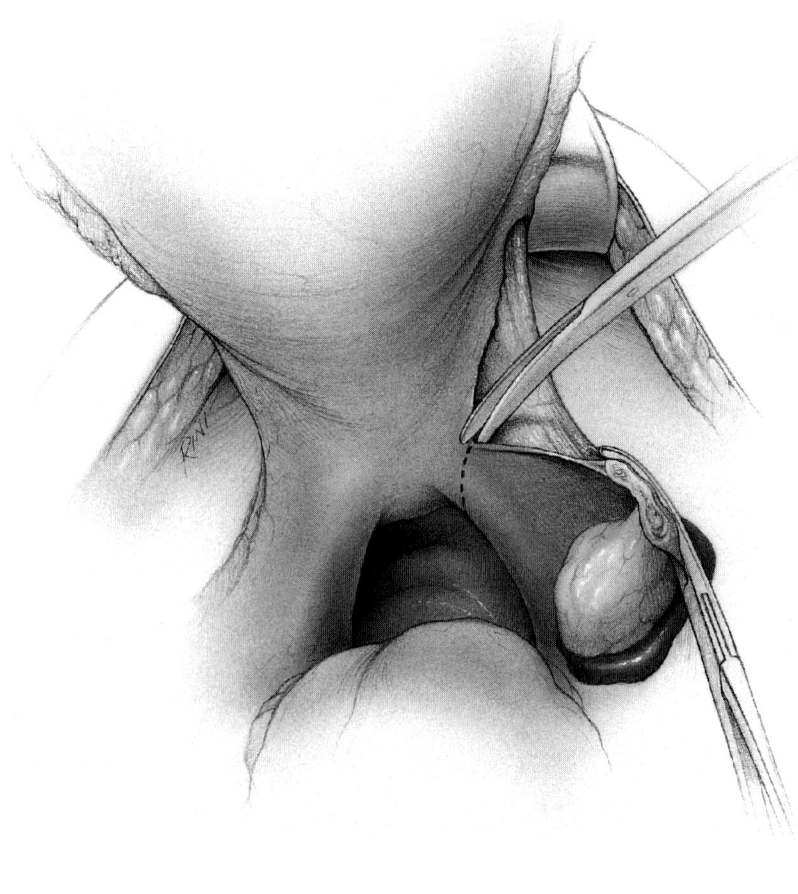

Figure 19–6. The posterior peritoneal leaf of the right broad ligament is incised (dotted line) to expose the right uterine vascular pedicle.

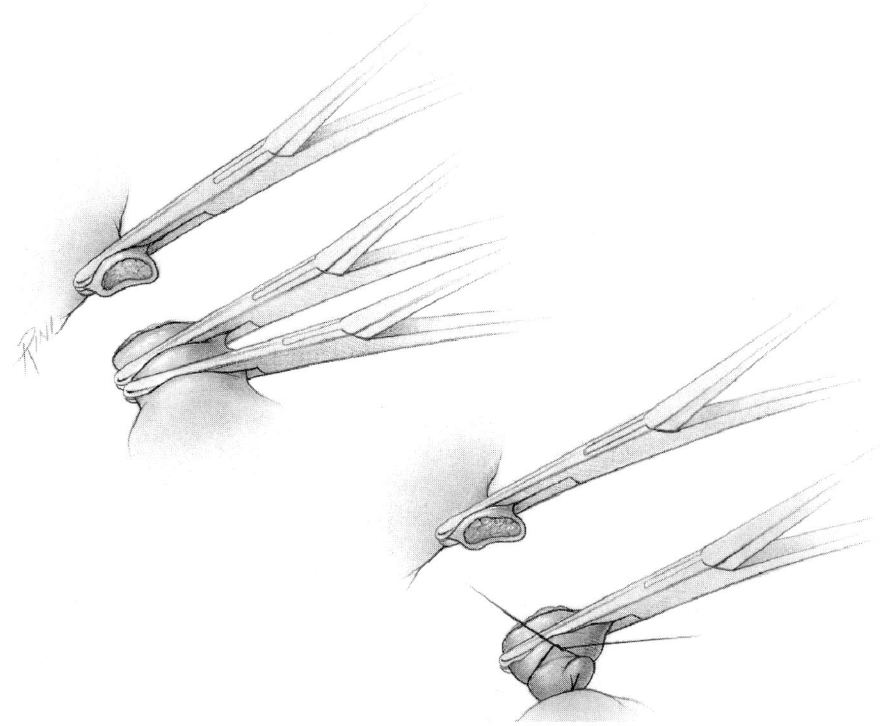

Figure 19–7. The uterine vascular pedicle has been secured with two Heaney clamps. An additional clamp has been placed above the dissection to control retrograde bleeding. The pedicle has been severed. **A.** The proximal clamp is replaced with a simple suture. **B.** The remaining clamp is replaced with a Heaney transfixing suture.

is slowly tightened. A second suture—a Heaney stitch—passes beneath the tip of the remaining clamp, around the back of the clamp, and through the center of the pedicle (Fig. 19–7B). This suture is tied behind the second clamp as the assistant removes the clamp.

The clamp on the left round ligament is replaced with a single transfixing suture (Fig. 19–8). The left adnexal pedicle receives two sutures (Fig. 19–9). The distal (back) clamp is replaced with a ligature around the entire pedicle. The suture is carefully tightened at the indentation where the clamp expressed edema from the pedicle. A second suture is passed through the center of the pedicle between this ligature and the remaining clamp. This suture is passed around both sides of the clamp and tied as the assistant removes the clamp.

Returning to the right side of the dissection, the circumferential ligature and transfixing suture is placed on the right adnexal pedicle. The right round ligament receives a single transfixing suture. A second Heaney clamp is placed above the previous clamp on the right uterine vascular bundle and a third higher clamp to control back bleeding. The right uterine vascular pedicle is developed and sutured as described for the left. All vessels to the uterus are now securely tied.

For supracervical hysterectomy, the fundus of the uterus is amputated next. Total hysterectomy is usually performed in stable patients, but removing the fundus improves exposure. When the fundus is amputated, Ochsner (Kocher) clamps are placed to control bleeding and provide traction and manipulation of the remaining cervix.

The operating team has focused intensely on operative details to this point. It is time for a brief respite while the surgeon explores the bowel and other abdominal organs. The surgeon packs the bowel out of the pelvic cavity with tagged laparotomy sponges. Care is

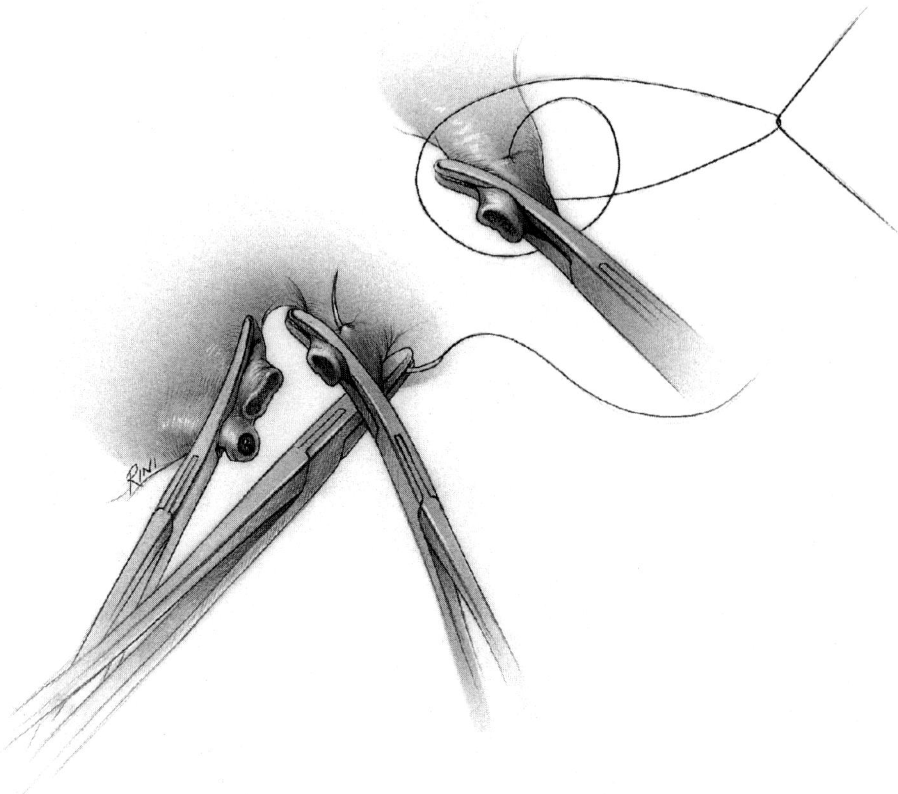

Figure 19–8. Each round ligament is secured with a single transfixing suture. Shown is the suture being passed directly through the round ligament initially, following which it is passed beneath the round ligament and then tied. The medial segment can be left clamped or secured with a large surgical clip.

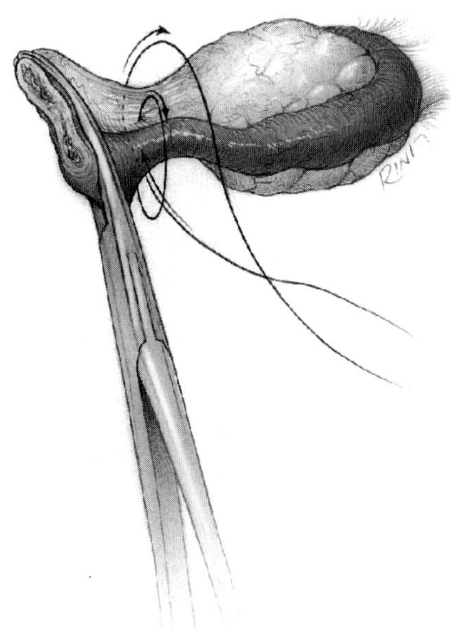

Figure 19–9. Each adnexal pedicle is secured by replacing the distal clamp with a circumferential suture and the proximal clamp with a transfixing suture. Shown is the transfixing suture.

taken not to disturb ligated vascular pedicles during packing. The surgeon positions a self-retaining abdominal wall retractor—either an O'Conner-O'Sullivan retractor for thin patients or a large Balfour retractor for obese women.

Cervical resection requires further mobilization of the bladder. The vesico-uterine serosal flap is elevated and the posterior bladder wall is detached from the upper cervix (Fig. 19–10). A plane of thin connective tissue normally permits easy finger dissection. If dense adhesions are present, usually from prior uterine surgery, these are dissected cautiously with fine scissors and small pushing movements to avoid bladder injury. Dissection is kept near the midline because lateral dissection often causes troublesome venous bleeding.

The cervix is then resected from its attachments to the cardinal ligaments, uterosacral ligaments, and the vagina. The cardinal ligaments are successively clamped where they

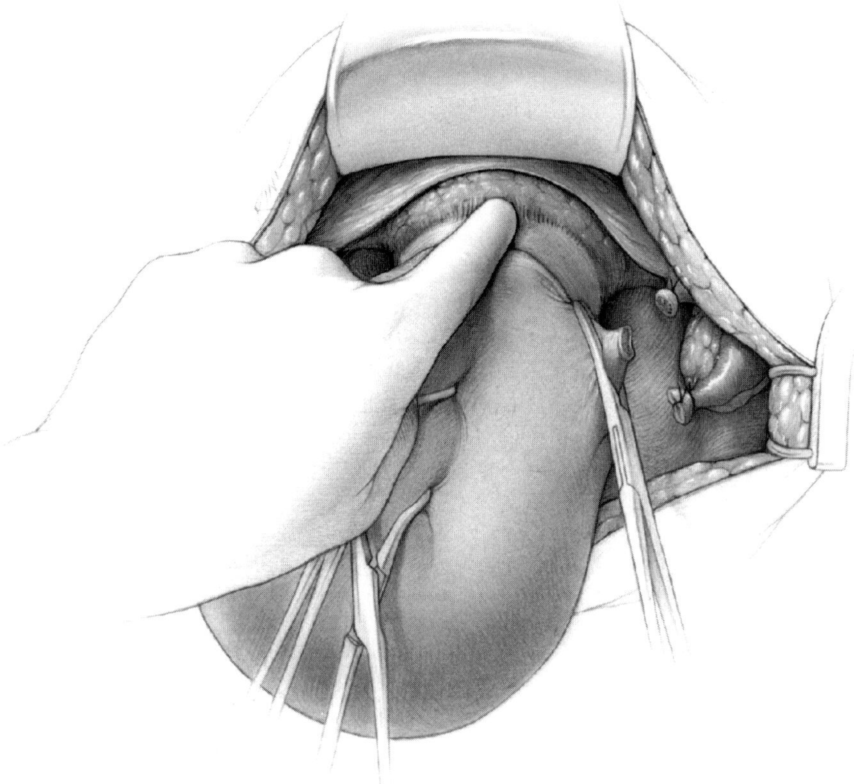

Figure 19–10. Dissection of the cervix begins by separating the bladder from the lower uterus and upper cervix. Loose areolar tissues are easily dissected with the gloved finger. Dense adhesions require sharp scissor dissection.

meet the cervix (Fig. 19–11). Each straight Oschner (Kocher) instrument application encloses 1–1.5 cm of cardinal ligament. The jaws of the instrument slide off the body of the cervix as they close to assure the most medial placement of the clamp. A scalpel blade incises the pedicle to the tip of the clamp. A suture is then passed exactly beneath the tip of the clamp and the tie tightened slowly down the back of the clamp as it is removed.

Alternating sides maintains a symmetrical dissection. Each cardinal ligament pedicle is clamped medial to the previous one. The ureter progressively falls further from the dissection with each step. Two or three pedicles are usually necessary to complete the resection of the cardinal ligaments on each side.

The uterosacral ligaments insert on the posterior aspect of the lower cervix. These ligaments may be either stretched and attenuated or thick and edematous. The uterosacral ligaments are clamped, cut, and sutured separately if they are large or under tension. Otherwise, they are incorporated into the cardinal ligament pedicles.

Bilateral cardinal ligament dissection continues to the lowest extent of the cervix. The upper vagina is palpated between the thumb and forefinger to identify the location of the cervix. The cervix may be difficult to feel if it was recently effaced and dilated. In that case, a doubly gloved hand palpates the lowest extent of the cervix from within the cervical canal. The outer glove is discarded to reduce contamination of the operative site.

Using a suction and clean laparotomy sponge in the cul-de-sac, assistants prepare for potential contamination before the vagina is opened. The posterior vaginal wall is opened transversely just below the cervix with large curved Mayo scissors (Fig. 19–12). Under direct vision, one blade of the scissors is

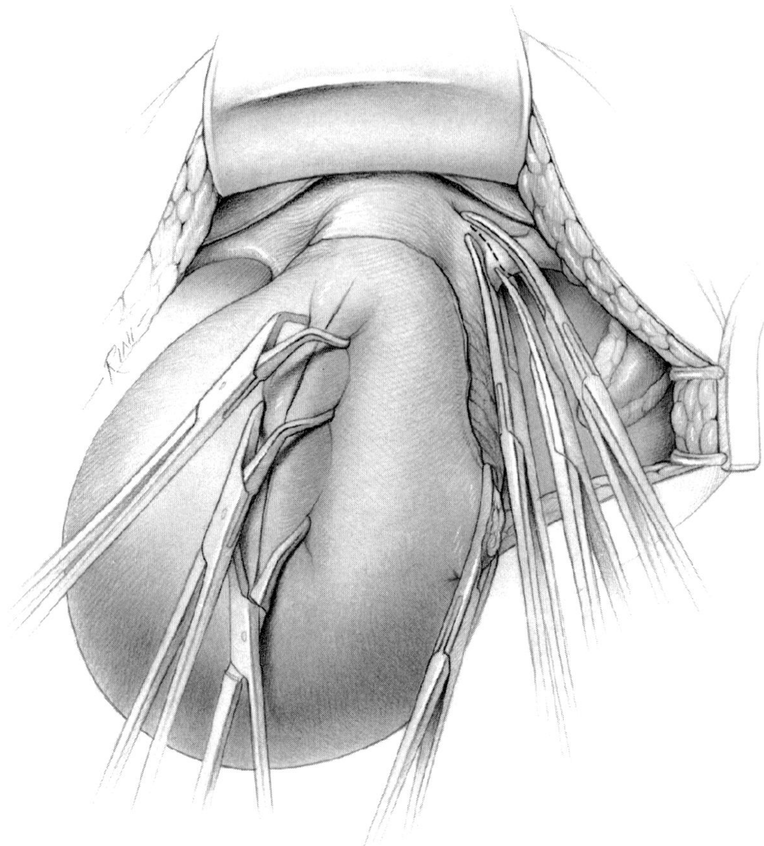

Figure 19–11. The upper cardinal ligament is clamped as close to the cervix as possible. A second clamp above the dissection controls retrograde bleeding. The cardinal ligament is severed with scissors (dotted line). It will next be secured with a single circumferential suture. Cardinal ligament dissection is completed by developing several such pedicles on each side of the dissection.

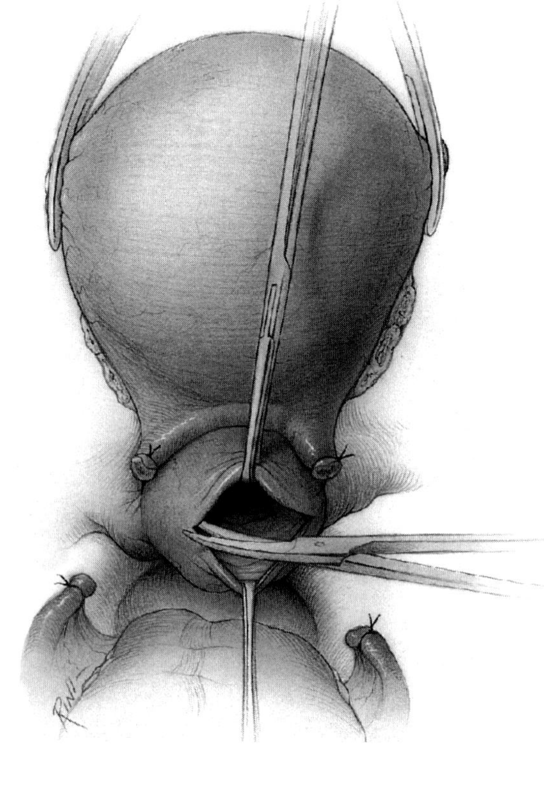

Figure 19–12. The posterior upper vagina is incised with scissors. The uterus and cervix will be dissected from its last attachments by circumferential dissection of the upper vagina.

placed within the vaginal cavity and the circumference of the cervix is resected at its junction with the vagina. Direct visualization assures removal of the entire cervix, preservation of the full length of the vagina, and safety of the bladder. The surgeon can easily resect an extra length of upper vagina when clinically necessary.

Assistants grasp the vaginal edges with Allis clamps at 6, 3, 12, and 9 o'clock as the vaginal incision progresses. Gentle upward tension on these clamps reduces the spill of contaminated material from the upper vagina. Care is taken not to tear delicate vaginal tissues.

The vaginal cuff may be closed or left open. Many favor closing the vaginal cuff when there is good hemostasis, no infection, and no injury to bowel or bladder. The open technique is chosen when excess drainage is anticipated to collect in the pelvis or if overt infection is present.

Suspension of the vaginal cuff is important in all cases. Support sutures at each lateral vaginal angle successively incorporate the anterior vaginal wall, cardinal ligament pedicles, round ligament pedicle, uterosacral ligament, and posterior vaginal wall (Fig. 19–13). When tied, these sutures bring together ligaments that supply strong support to the upper vagina.

In closed cuff technique, the vaginal cuff suture begins at the apex opposite the operator. After the support suture is tied, the needle arm of the suture is used to approximate the anterior and posterior vaginal walls, progressing toward the operator (Fig. 19–13). Each pass of the needle incorporates the full thickness of both anterior and posterior vaginal walls. Closure is completed with a tie to the support suture at the vaginal apex on the near side.

For the open vaginal cuff technique, the anterior and posterior vaginal edges are

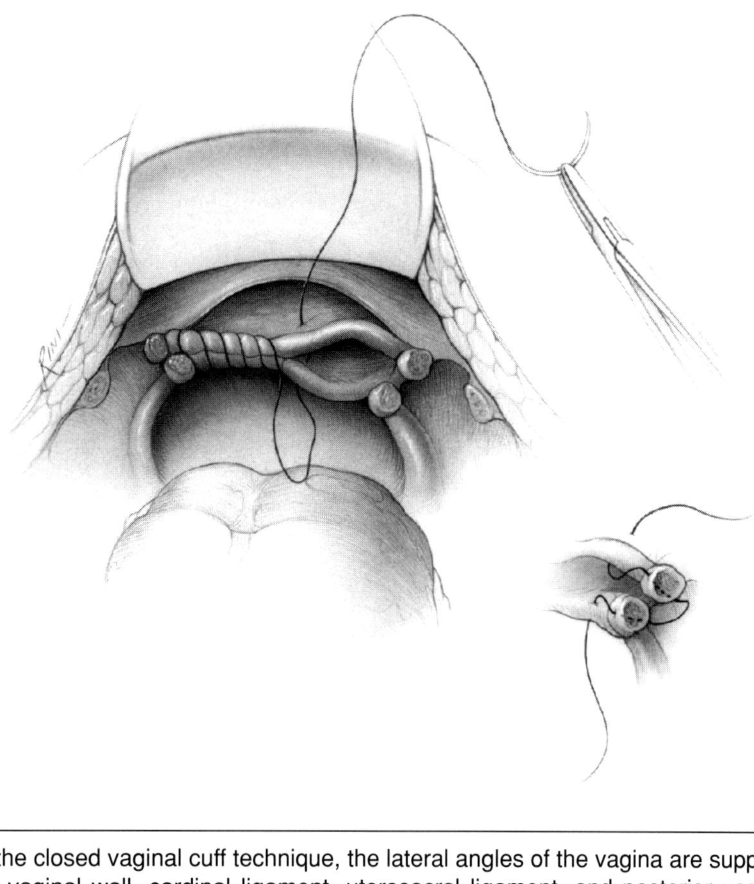

Figure 19–13. For the closed vaginal cuff technique, the lateral angles of the vagina are supported by sutures that include the anterior vaginal wall, cardinal ligament, uterosacral ligament, and posterior vaginal wall. The upper vagina is closed with a running suture approximating the anterior and posterior vaginal walls.

oversewn individually with continuous hemostatic stitches (Fig. 19–14). All layers of the vagina are included in each pass of the suture and support sutures are placed at each vaginal angle. At the conclusion of suturing, a small opening remains at the center of the vagina.

Surgical drainage is established in cases of incomplete hemostasis, extensive pelvic infection, peritonitis, or repair of injuries to the urinary tract or large bowel. Suction sump drainage that exits through a separate stab wound in the anterior abdominal wall is preferable for most pelvic drainage. Drains that exit through the vagina provide only gravity drainage and permit entrance of bacteria from the vagina.

At the conclusion of the cuff closure, if bladder integrity is in question, then the bladder is filled with sterile milk or dye solution as described above. Any defects in the bladder wall are repaired with a two-layer closure using absorbable suture.

The operative site is irrigated and each pedicle is inspected for hemostasis. The pelvic peritoneum is closed, leaving all pedicles outside the peritoneal cavity (Fig. 19–15). Many contemporary surgeons choose not to reperitonealize the pelvis. All sponges and instruments are removed, and after the sponge, needle, and instrument count is reported as correct, the abdominal wall is closed (see Chapter 4).

Concurrent Ligation Technique

The concurrent ligation technique is the familiar technique used for most gynecologic hysterectomies. Each vascular and tissue pedicle is ligated as it is developed. The sequence of pedicle development is similar to the delayed ligation method previously described. The concurrent ligation technique is most useful in complicated cases when hematomas or tumors obscure or distort anatomic relationships. The technique is applicable to many emergency peripartum hysterectomy cases where dissec-

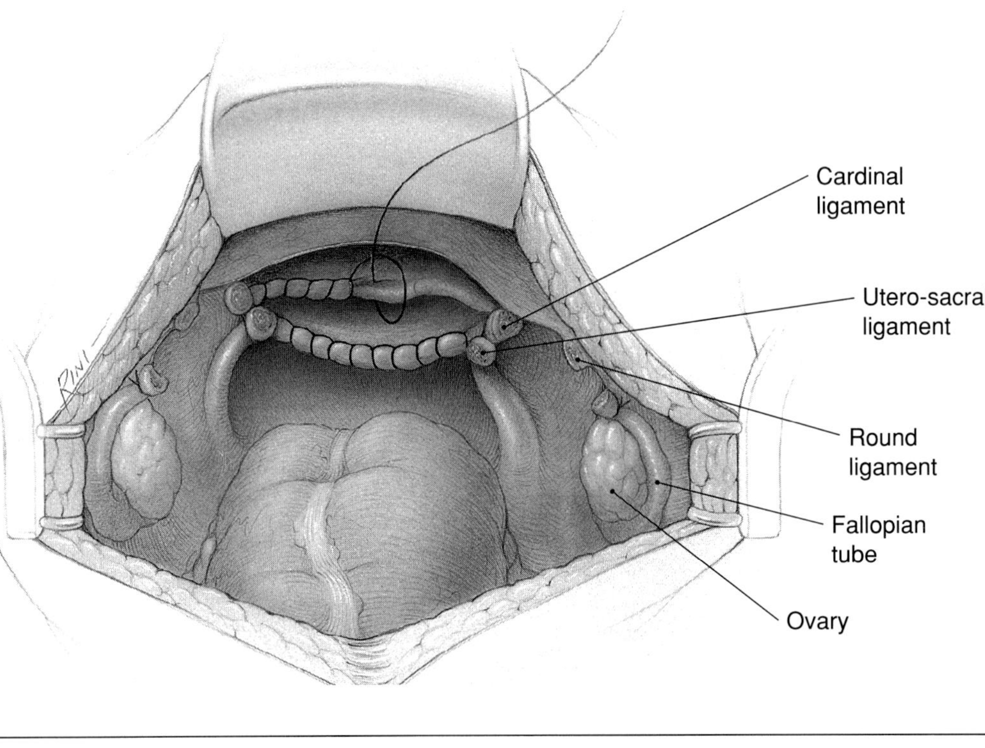

Figure 19–14. For the open vaginal cuff technique, support sutures are placed at each vaginal angle. The anterior vaginal cuff and posterior vaginal cuff are oversewn with separate running locked sutures. The upper vagina remains open.

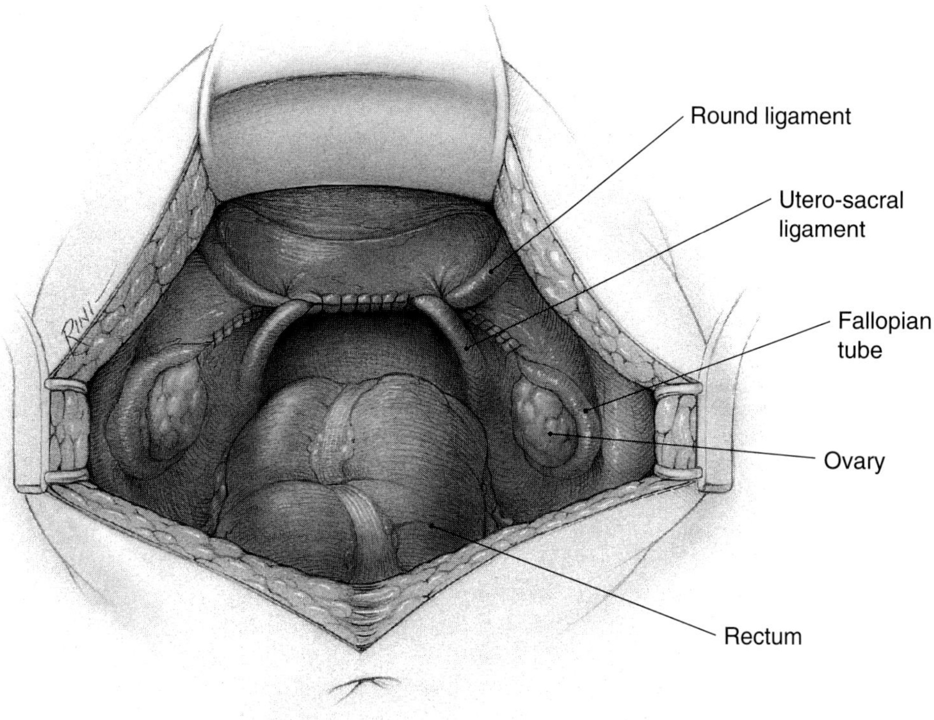

Figure 19–15. The peritoneum is closed with a running suture that leaves all pedicles outside the peritoneal cavity.

tion lends itself to sequential clamping, cutting, and ligating. Concurrent ligation has the disadvantage in elective cases of taking longer than the delayed ligation technique to control all the blood supply to the uterus.

COMPLICATIONS

Complications of obstetric hysterectomy must be assessed by separating direct surgical complications from complications attributable to preexisting disease or injury. As shown in Table 19–3, there is significant morbidity and mortality associated with these major operations. In emergency cases, the risks of obstetric catastrophe often outweigh the risks of the procedure. Direct procedural risk can be more clearly defined in elective cases. A comparison of maternal morbidity in women who underwent cesarean section with either hysterectomy or tubal ligation is shown in Table 19–4.

TABLE 19–3. MORBIDITY AND MORTALITY WITH OBSTETRIC HYSTERECTOMY

	Private Series[a]	Training Center *(Louisiana State University)*	
		1954–1985[b]	*1990–1992*[c]
	(n = 543)	*(n = 1335)*	*(n = 82)*
Blood transfusion (%)	32	63	23
Operative complications (%)	11	19	4
Febrile morbidity (%)	13	41	50
Total morbidity (%)	21	53	n.s.
Deaths	0	7	1

[a]*From Plauché (1981), Schneider (1968), Ward (1965) and their colleagues.*
[b]*From Plauché (1986) and Plauché and associates (1983).*
[c]*From Bey and co-workers (1992).*

TABLE 19–4. MATERNAL MORBIDITY COMPARISONS OF CESAREAN SECTION AND BILATERAL TUBAL LIGATION VERSUS CESAREAN HYSTERECTOMY

	Tubal Ligation (*n*=103)	Hysterectomy (*n*=82)	Significance
Hematocrit (volumes %)			
Preoperative	35.4 ± 3.9	35.2 ± 3.6	ns
Postoperative	31.4 ± 3.9	30.4 ± 4.8	ns
Estimated blood loss (mL)	718 ± 364	1201 ± 474	.001
Hematocrit change (volumes %)	4.5 ± 3.4	6.0 ± 4.4	.01
Operating time (min)	73.5 ± 26.4	114 ± 37	.001
Hospital stay (days)	5.0 ± 1.5	5.1 ± 2.4	ns
Blood transfusion (%)	21	23	ns
Febrile morbidity (%)	68	50	.01
Complications (%)			
Intraoperative	0.97	3.7	ns
Postoperative	4.9	12.2	ns

Data adapted from Bey and colleagues (1992).

Mortality Risk

Wingo and colleagues (1985) examined the mortality risk for all hysterectomies in the United States from data collected by the Commission on Professional and Hospital Activities during 1979–80. They identified 477 deaths among 317,389 women undergoing abdominal hysterectomy for a mortality rate of 12 per 10,000 procedures. The mortality risk for 5435 women who had hysterectomies for pregnancy complications was 29.2 per 10,000. These investigators did not correct for disease-related mortality, nor did they separate the various types of obstetric hysterectomies. They also did not separately report the outcomes with elective cesarean hysterectomy. A review of several large series of obstetric hysterectomies estimates that about 40 percent of maternal deaths can be ascribed to operative rather than pregnancy complications (Clark, 1984; Davis, 1951; Park, 1980; Weed, 1959, and their colleagues).

Emergency obstetric hysterectomies historically have the most complications and highest mortality rate (Plauché, 1991). Two recent studies illustrate current mortality risks. Stanco and associates (1993) reported one maternal death among 123 emergency cases from the University of Southern California. Zelop and co-workers (1993) reported no maternal deaths in 117 emergency cases from Harvard.

The Louisiana State University obstetric hysterectomy series contains approximately equal numbers of elective and emergency cases. Mortality rates show significant changes over the years of case collection (Plauché, 1992a). In the first 30 years of the series, 7 of 1335 women died after obstetric hysterectomy (52.4 per 10,000 cases). There has been only one death in the last 15 years during which time 435 cases were reported (23 per 10,000 cases). Three of these eight women who died were moribund on admission due to prior hemorrhage or sepsis. One woman died of advanced pelvic malignancy and one from postoperative sepsis. The most disturbing cases were three in which fatal retroperitoneal bleeding was not recognized early in the postoperative course. The maternal mortality rate in the Louisiana State University series, corrected for obstetrical complications, is 13.5 per 10,000 cases.

Maternal death is a rare event in series of elective cesarean hysterectomy cases. For example, there were no maternal deaths recorded in 543 cesarean hysterectomies reported by three private practice groups in New Orleans (McNulty, 1984; Schneider and Tyrone, 1968; Ward and Smith, 1965). Park and Duff (1980) surveyed 11 series of planned cesarean hysterectomy cases without a maternal death. They concluded that correction for underlying obstetric catastrophe yields a mortality rate for cesarean hysterectomy comparable to that of cesarean section or abdominal hysterectomy alone.

Morbidity Risks

The clinical risks for obstetrical hysterectomies are influenced by the patient population, environmental conditions, associated diseases, and the experience of the operating team. In Table 19–3, reports from private practitioners performing mostly elective cases are compared with reports from supervised training environments where half of cases were emergencies. The private groups recorded 20 percent shorter operating times, 50 percent fewer patients transfused, 42 percent fewer intraoperative complications, and a third of the febrile and total morbidity rates reported by training hospitals.

Operative Complications

The two most frequent operative complications of obstetric hysterectomy are hemorrhage and urinary tract injury (Table 19–5). Both problems may be present before surgery or may occur during the procedure.

Control of blood loss during obstetric hysterectomy depends on meticulous hemostatic surgical technique and careful management of all vascular pedicles. A common cause of blood loss related to surgical technique is loss of control of a uterine or adnexal vascular pedicle. Uterine vessels usually escape control during manipulation of clamps or tying of sutures. The resulting bleeding either collects in the operating field or forms an expanding broad ligament hematoma. Another common source of intraoperative blood loss is "back bleeding" from severed pedicles. Back bleeding from collateral circulation is controlled by clamping distal vessels before incising pedicles.

Adnexal bleeding during or after surgery may be encountered for several reasons. An ovarian vessel may be torn during manipulation of the adnexal pedicle. A suture may pierce a vessel that is not controlled by a proximal tie or clamp. An ovarian vessel under tension may retract out of a ligature around a shrinking pedicle. Any of these may result in an expanding adnexal or retroperitoneal hematoma. Unilateral salpingo-oophorectomy is often necessary to control the expansion of the hematoma.

Zelop and colleagues (1993) reported a 17 percent incidence of adnexectomy for bleeding among 117 women undergoing emergency peripartum hysterectomy. Adnexal hematomas required unilateral adnexectomy in 6 percent of cases reported from Charity Hospital by Plauché and colleagues (1983). Securing the

TABLE 19–5. OPERATIVE PARAMETERS AND COMPLICATIONS WITH 189 ELECTIVE CESAREAN HYSTERECTOMIES (LOUISIANA STATE UNIVERSITY 1984–1991)

	Number	Percent
Estimated surgical blood loss	1016 ± 396 mL	
Operating time	109 ± 27 min	
Cases requiring blood replacement		18
Hospital stay	4.6 ± 1.8 days	
Intraoperative complications		2.1
Inadvertent cystotomy	3	(1.6)
Retroperitoneal hematoma	1	(0.5)
Postoperative complications		31
Cuff cellulitis	29	(15)
Urinary tract infection	13	(6.9)
Wound infection	9	(4.8)
Wound dehiscence	2	(0.9)
Cuff bleeding	2	(0.9)
Pneumonitis	2	(0.9)
Ileus	1	(0.4)

Compiled from LSU units at University Medical Center, Lafayette, LA; Earl K. Long Hospital, Baton Rouge, LA; and Charity Hospital, New Orleans, LA.

adnexal pedicle first with an encircling suture followed by a distal transfixing suture has reduced the incidence of postoperative adnexal bleeding requiring reoperation at Charity Hospital to less than 1 percent.

Urinary tract structures are subject to injury during several procedural steps. Unrecognized injuries before or during surgery can become serious postoperative problems. Surgical injuries usually do not cause lasting disability if they are recognized and repaired. Operative bladder injury most often occurs while dissecting the bladder from a scarred lower uterine segment. The bladder may also be injured by inclusion in a vaginal cuff clamp or suture. Cross clamping the upper vagina increases the risk of trauma to the tented lateral bladder wall. The traumatized bladder wall may undergo necrosis with development of a urinary fistula. Vaginal cuff cellulitis or abscess also increase this risk. Plauché and associates (1983) reported a 3 percent incidence of bladder injury among 108 private patients with a prior cesarean section undergoing elective cesarean hysterectomy. In the emergency cases reported by Stanco and coworkers (1993), 3.2 percent had urinary tract injuries and there was a 10 percent incidence of either intentional cystotomy or passage of a ureteral stent. Zelop and colleagues (1993) reported a 7.7 percent incidence of operative cystotomy and 2.5 percent occurrence of ureteral injury requiring stenting among 117 emergency peripartum hysterectomies.

Plauché (1992a) reported a 0.44 percent incidence of ureteral injury in a review of over 5,000 published cases. There is particular risk to the ureter when hematomas or tumors distort the pelvic anatomy. The surgeon should attempt to identify preoperative displacement or injury to the ureter. Intraoperative ureteral injury may occur during dissection of adnexal structures, uterine vessels, or cardinal ligaments. The safety of the ureter is partially ensured by visualization, palpation, and dissection of its course. Dissection within the cardinal and broad ligaments in pregnant women requires care and experience. The risk of injury to the lower ureter may be reduced by placing clamps exactly against the wall of the cervix, always medial to previous pedicles. High ureteral injury is prevented by visualizing the course of the ureter before clamping adnexal pedicles.

Postoperative Complications

Bleeding and infection are the more common serious postoperative complications (Table 19–5). In Table 19–6 are listed the most frequent postoperative complications in a review of more than 5000 obstetric hysterectomies. Vaginal bleeding immediately postoperatively usually is from inadequate control of blood vessels in the cuff. A uterine vessel that has escaped its ligature can also cause vaginal bleeding but more often develops a broad ligament hematoma. Late postoperative vaginal bleeding may be from trauma to the vaginal cuff or drainage of a cuff hematoma.

Bleeding within the abdomen after obstetric hysterectomy is usually from uterine or adnexal vessels that have escaped suture control. Bleeding may be within the peritoneal cavity or in the retroperitoneal space. Patients with intraperitoneal bleeding show signs of peritoneal irritation. Bleeding from uterine vessels usually collects as a hematoma in the broad ligament. Enlarging broad ligament hematomas may dissect into the large presacral space or the retroperitoneal spaces along the lateral pelvic walls. Adnexal vessels may bleed into the peritoneal cavity or may form a hematoma in the infundibulopelvic ligament and retroperitoneal flank spaces. Bleeding into large retroperitoneal spaces is difficult to detect even when blood loss is extensive.

TABLE 19–6. POSTOPERATIVE COMPLICATIONS OF OBSTETRIC HYSTERECTOMY REPORTED IN 5185 CASES FROM 1951 TO 1984

Complications	Percent
Febrile morbidity	35
Vaginal cuff abscess or hematoma	12.1
Urinary tract infections	9.3
Wound abscess or dehiscence	5.0
Pulmonary complications	4.1
Postoperative bleeding requiring surgery	3.3
Vaginal pack or suture	(1.7)
Laparotomy	(1.6)
Urinary fistulas	0.57
Vesicovaginal	(0.46)
Ureterovaginal	(0.09)
Other	(0.02)
Thromboembolism	0.52
Intestinal obstruction	0.33

From Plauché (1992b).

Stable small hematomas in asymptomatic patients usually require no treatment. Reoperation may be necessary if hematomas are large or growing in size and are not accessible to vaginal drainage. Patients who are hemodynamically unstable should be carefully evaluated for intra-abdominal bleeding. Sonography, computed tomography, or magnetic resonance imaging may be helpful in evaluation. Transfusions are given as indicated and laparotomy is planned if imaging reveals a large or expanding hematoma. Reexploration is considered if vital signs become unstable or serial hematocrit values fall after transfusion. Surgical treatment of pelvic hematomas includes evacuation, securing any visible bleeding vessels, and placing adequate surgical drains (Plauché, 1992a).

Laparotomy for internal bleeding after obstetric hysterectomy was required in 1.6 percent of the Louisiana State University series (Plauché, 1986). Park and Duff (1980) reoperated for internal bleeding in 1 percent of cases, Stanco and colleagues (1993) in 4 percent of cases, and Zelop and associates (1993) in 2.6 percent of cases.

Infections are among the most common complications after obstetric hysterectomy. Febrile morbidity was reported in 10–50 percent of reviewed studies (Plauché, 1992b; Stanco and associates, 1993; Yancey and colleagues, 1993). The reviews describe febrile morbidity rates exceeding 33 percent for emergency procedures (Zelop and co-workers, 1993). Conversely, cases performed before labor have only a 10 percent febrile morbidity. The most common infections are those of the urinary tract as well as wound infections of the vaginal cuff or abdominal incision.

The incidence of postoperative urinary tract infections is proportional to the duration that indwelling catheters remain in place. These are documented in 10–20 percent of most series (Park and Duff, 1980; Plauché, 1986). Policies encouraging prophylactic antimicrobials and early removal of catheters have reduced urinary tract infections on the Louisiana State University Service to 6 percent (Bey and colleagues, 1992).

After hysterectomy, many bacteria colonize the region above the vaginal cuff. Cuff hematomas often become infected. The Louisiana State University series reported a 13 percent incidence of vaginal cuff hematoma or infection (Plauché, 1986). Park and Duff (1980) reported a 9 percent incidence of pelvic or cuff cellulitis and a 5 percent incidence of abscess either of the vaginal cuff or in the pelvis.

Clinical findings of a cuff abscess or infected hematoma include fever and a tender mass above the cuff. It is usually possible to drain midline abscesses or hematomas through the vaginal cuff. Symptoms and signs rapidly resolve after adequate drainage. Brisk bleeding from injury to major vessels may occur if an attempt is made to drain a lateral pelvic hematoma or abscess that does not point near the midline of the vaginal cuff.

Abdominal incisional infection or dehiscence occurs in 3–9 percent of obstetrical hysterectomies (Plauché, 1986; Stanco and associates, 1993; Yancey and colleagues, 1993). Wound complications may be reduced by careful hemostasis, avoidance of bacterial contamination of the operative site, and prophylactic antibiotics.

SUMMARY

While infrequently performed, the obstetrical hysterectomy should be a part of every obstetrician's armamentarium. When performed, they are often under adverse conditions such as catastrophic uterine rupture or refractory uterine atony and life-threatening maternal hemorrhage. Under such emergency circumstances, it is thus not surprising that the rate of injury to the bladder or ureters and of requirement for blood transfusion is increased over that of routine cesarean section or scheduled interval hysterectomy. Intraoperatively, any concerns of bladder or ureter injury should be thoroughly investigated and resolved prior to closing the abdominal cavity. In cases of severe hemorrhage or disseminated intravascular coagulopathy, use of the supracervical hysterectomy should be considered in lieu of a total hysterectomy as it will decrease operative time as well as the extent of surgical dissection and potential bleeding areas.

REFERENCES

Barclay DL. Cesarean hysterectomy: Thirty years experience. Obstet Gynecol 1970; 35:120.

Bey M, Pastorek JGII, Lu P. Comparison of morbidity in cesarean section hysterectomy versus cesarean section tubal ligation. Presented at annual meeting of District VII, American College of Obstetricians and Gynecologists, St. Louis, Sept 1993.

Bixby GH. Extirpation of the puerperal uterus by abdominal section. J Gynaec Soc Boston 1869; 1:223.

Bowman EA, Barclay DL, White LC. Cesarean hysterectomy: an analysis of 1,000 consecutive operations. Bull Tulane Med Faculty 1964; 23:75.

Brenner P, Sall S, Sonnenblick B. Evaluation of cesarean section hysterectomy as a sterilization procedure. Am J Obstet Gynecol 1970; 108:335.

Chestnut DH, Eden RD, Gall SA, Parker RT. Peripartum hysterectomy: a review of cesarean and postpartum hysterectomy. Obstet Gynecol 1984; 65:792.

Clark SL, Yeh SY, Phelan JP, Bruce S, Paul RH. Emergency cesarean hysterectomy for obstetric hemorrhage. Obstet Gynecol 1984; 64:376.

Davis ME. Complete cesarean hysterectomy—logical advance in modern obstetric surgery. Am J Obstet Gynecol 1951; 62:838.

Duncan W, Targett JH. Porro-caesarean hysterectomy with retro-peritoneal treatment of the stump in a case of fibroids obstructing labour; with remarks upon the relative advantages of the modern Porro operation over the Sanger caesarean in most other cases requiring abdominal section. Trans Obstet Soc Lond 1900; 42:244.

Durfee RB. Evolution of cesarean hysterectomy. Clin Obstet Gynecol 1969; 12:575.

Dyer I, Nix GF, Weed JC. Total hysterectomy at cesarean section and the immediate puerperal period. Am J Obstet Gynecol 1953; 65:517.

Godson C. Porro's operation. Br Med J 1884; 1:142.

Gonsoulin W, Kennedy R, Guidry K. Elective versus emergency cesarean hysterectomy cases in a residency program setting: a review of 129 cases from 1984 to 1988. Am J Obstet Gynecol 1991; 165:91.

Harris RP. Results of the first fifty cases of caesarean ovaro-hysterectomy: 1869–1880. Am J Med Sci 1880; 80:129.

Hoffman MS, Roberts WS, Fiorica JV, et al. Elective cesarean hysterectomy for treatment of cervical neoplasia: an update. J Reprod Med 1993; 38:186.

Lash AF, Cummings WC. Report on the outcome of caesarean hysterectomy. Am J Obstet Gynecol 1935; 30:199.

Leung AS, Farmer RM, Leung EK, et al. Risk factors associated with uterine rupture during trial of labor after cesarean delivery: a case control study. Am J Obstet Gynecol 1993; 168:1358.

McNulty JV. Elective cesarean hysterectomy—revisited. Am J Obstet Gynecol 1984; 149:29.

Mickal A, Begneaud WP, Hawes TP. Pitfalls and complications of cesarean section hysterectomy. Clin Obstet Gynecol 1969; 12:660.

Park RC, Duff WP. Role of cesarean hysterectomy in modern obstetric practice. Clin Obstet Gynecol 1980; 23:601.

Plauché WC, Gruich FG, Bourgeois MO. Hysterectomy at the time of cesarean section: analysis of 108 cases. Obstet Gynecol 1981; 58:459.

Plauché WC, Wycheck JG, Ianessa MJ, et al. Cesarean hysterectomy on the LSU Service of Charity Hospital, 1975–1981. South Med J 1983; 76:1261.

Plauché WC. Cesarean hysterectomy. In: J Schiarra (ed), Gynecology and Obstetrics, Vol. 2, Ch. 84 1986:1.

Plauché WC. Surgical problems involving the pregnant uterus: uterine inversion, uterine rupture and leiomyomas. In: WC Plauché, JC Morrison, MJ O'Sullivan, Surgical Obstetrics. Philadelphia: WB Saunders. 1991:231.

Plauché WC. Obstetric genital trauma. In: WC Plauché, J Morrison, MJ O'Sullivan, Surgical Obstetrics. Philadelphia: WB Saunders. 1992a: 383.

Plauché WC. Peripartal hysterectomy. In: WC Plauché, J Morrison, MJ O'Sullivan, Surgical Obstetrics. Philadelphia: WB Saunders 1992b: 447.

Porro E. Dell'amputazione utero-ovarica come complemento ditaglio cesareo. Ann Univ Med e Chir 1876; 237:289.

Reed CAL. Caesarean hysterectomy indications. Am J Obstet 1900; 42:71.

Richardson E. Caesarean section with removal of uterus and ovaries after the Porro-Muller method. Am J Med Sci 1878; 81:36.

Sanger M. Der Kaiserschnitt bei Uterusfibromen nebst Verleichenden Methodik der Sectio Caesarea und der Porro Operation. Leipzig, Germany: Englemann, 1882.

Schneider GT, Tyrone CH. Cesarean total hysterectomy: experience with 160 cases. South Med J 1968; 59:927.

Stanco LM, Schrimmer DB, Paul RH, Mishell DR Jr. Emergency peripartum hysterectomy and associated risk factors. Am J Obstet Gynecol 1993; 168:879.

Sturdee DW, Rushton DI. Caesarean and post-partum hysterectomy 1968–1983. Br J Obstet Gynecol 1986; 93:270.

Tait L. Address on the surgical aspect of impacted labour. Br Med J 1890; 1:657.

Tinga D. Hysterectomy after cesarean section. The treatment of last resort for serious infections. East Afr Med J 1986; 63:362.

Ward SV, Smith H. Cesarean total hysterectomy: combined section and sterilization. Obstet Gynecol 1965; 26:858.

Weed JC. The fate of the postcesarean uterus. Obstet Gynecol 1959; 14:780.

Wingo PA, Huezo CM, Rubin GL, et al. The mortality risk associated with hysterectomy. Am J Obstet Gynecol 1985; 152:803.

Yancey MK, Harlass FE, Benson W, Brady K: The perioperative morbidity of scheduled cesarean hysterectomy. Obstet Gynecol 1993; 81: 206.

Young JH. Caesarean section. The history and development of the operation from earliest times. London: H.K. Lewis & Co. Ltd., 1944: 93–105.

Zelop CM, Harlow BL, Frigoletto FD Jr, et al. Emergency peripartum hysterectomy. Am J Obstet Gynecol 1993; 168:1443.

CHAPTER 20

Postoperative Complications

Because cesarean section is the most commonly performed obstetric surgical procedure, most postoperative complications in obstetrics are encountered after this operation. Pelvic infection is most commonly encountered, but other less common conditions that cause excessive morbidity and mortality include aspiration pneumonia, deep venous thrombosis, and pulmonary embolism.

DIFFERENTIAL DIAGNOSIS OF FEVER

Most persistent fevers after childbirth are caused by genital tract infection. This especially is likely if the preceding labor was attended by extensive vaginal or uterine manipulation, prolonged membrane rupture, or intrauterine electronic monitoring. Regardless, every postpartum woman whose temperature rises to 38°C should be evaluated for extrapelvic causes of fever as well as for puerperal infection. Filker and Monif (1979) reported that only 21 percent of febrile women (first 24 hours) delivered vaginally were found to have infection in contrast to 72 percent of those delivered by cesarean section. Some extragenital causes of puerperal fever include **respiratory complications, pyelonephritis, intense breast engorgement, bacterial mastitis, thrombophlebitis,** and in cases of laparotomy, **incisional wound abscess.**

Respiratory complications most often are seen within the first 24 hours following delivery, and almost invariably are in women delivered by cesarean section or given general anesthesia for vaginal delivery. Complications include atelectasis, aspiration pneumonia, or occasionally, bacterial pneumonia. Atelectasis is best prevented with the use of routine coughing and deep breathing on a fixed schedule, usually every 4 hours for at least 24 hours following the administration of general anesthesia. Hypoventilation causes alveolar collapse. Airway obstruction from thick secretions and diminished cough reflex increase this possibility. Fever associated with atelectasis is thought to be due to infection with normal flora that proliferate distal to the obstructing lesion. Roberts and colleagues (1988) have shown that fever and x-ray findings of atelectasis correlate in only half of cases. Because of severe sequelae, the possibility of aspiration must be suspected in the woman with severe or persistent pulmonary findings. These women most often will develop a high spiking fever, varying degrees of respiratory wheezing, and in most instances, obvious signs of hypoxemia.

Pyelonephritis may be difficult to diagnose postpartum. In the typical case, bacteriuria, pyuria, costovertebral angle tenderness, and spiking temperature clearly indicate renal infection; however, the clinical picture varies. For example, in the puerperal woman the first sign of renal infection may be a temperature elevation, but costovertebral angle tenderness may not develop until later. The clinical diagnosis is confirmed by demonstrating bacteriuria microscopically and by urine culture.

Empirical therapy is begun without waiting for culture results.

Breast engorgement commonly causes a brief temperature elevation. About 15 percent of all postpartum women develop fever from breast engorgement, rarely exceeding 39°C in the first few postpartum days. The fever characteristically lasts no longer than 24 hours. In contrast, the elevated temperature of bacterial mastitis develops later and usually is sustained. It is associated with other signs and symptoms of breast infection that become overt within 24 hours.

Superficial or deep venous thrombophlebitis of the legs may cause temperature elevations in the puerperal woman. The diagnosis is made by the observation of a painful, swollen leg, usually accompanied by calf tenderness, or occasionally femoral triangle area tenderness. Treatment is given with intravenous heparin therapy.

ASPIRATION PNEUMONITIS

Aspiration of acidic gastric contents during anesthesia for delivery can cause severe chemical pneumonitis, primarily as the consequence of the necrotizing effects of hydrochloric acid. Thus, it is another cause of adult respiratory distress syndrome. The aspiration of gastric contents is not limited to anesthesia for delivery. For example, treatment of eclampsia with large doses of morphine, barbiturates, or diazepam has been followed by the aspiration of gastric contents and a poor maternal outcome. In one study done to evaluate diazepam given for eclampsia, Crowther (1990) reported that 3 of 27 women developed pneumonic infiltrates presumably from aspiration while heavily sedated! Pneumonitis from inhalation of gastric contents has been the most common cause of anesthetic death in obstetrics. In its survey of over 2700 maternal deaths between 1979 and 1986, the Centers for Disease Control identified inhalation of gastric contents to be associated with at least a fourth of all anesthetic deaths (Atrash and colleagues, 1990). The aspirated material from the stomach may contain undigested food and thereby cause airway obstruction and tissue damage that, unless promptly relieved, may prove rapidly fatal. Although gastric juice is likely to contain less particulate matter during fasting, it is extremely acidic and capable of inducing a lethal chemical pneumonitis.

Prophylaxis

Important to effective prophylaxis are (1) fasting for at least 6 and preferably 12 hours before anesthesia, (2) use of agents to reduce gastric acidity during the induction and maintenance of general anesthesia, (3) skillful tracheal intubation accompanied by pressure on the cricoid cartilage to occlude the esophagus, and (4) at completion of the operation, extubation with the mother awake and lying on her side with head lowered, and (5) utilization of regional anesthetic techniques when appropriate.

Fasting

Steps should be taken to lessen the likelihood of danger from aspiration of both particulate matter and acidic gastric secretions. These measures should be included also for women for whom conduction analgesia is planned. For elective obstetric procedures, fasting for 12 hours usually rids the stomach of undigested food but not necessarily of acidic liquid. Sutherland and colleagues (1986) studied women undergoing early pregnancy termination or minor gynecologic surgery and showed that despite overnight fasting, the mean stomach juice volume was 20 mL with a pH of 1.6. In women at term undergoing elective cesarean section, Lewis and Crawford (1987) showed that women given a light meal of only tea and toast had twice the volume of gastric contents as fasted controls at 4 hours, and particulate matter was identified in 20 percent. Gastric emptying in labor is even more retarded, and women in early labor should be advised to fast before coming to the hospital, and certainly thereafter. Despite these precautions, it should be assumed that any woman in labor has both gastric particulate matter and acidic contents.

Antacids

The practice of administering antacids shortly before induction of anesthesia probably has done more to decrease mortality from obstetric anesthesia than any other single practice. It is essential that the antacid disperse promptly throughout all of the gastric contents to neutralize the hydrogen ion effectively. It is equally important that the antacid, if aspirated, not incite comparably serious pulmonary problems.

Gibbs and Banner (1984) reported that 30 mL of 0.3 *M* sodium citrate with citric acid (Bicitra), given about 45 minutes before surgery, neutralized gastric contents (mean volume 70 mL) in nearly 90 percent of women undergoing cesarean section. Thus, a popular method is to routinely administer 30 mL of Bicitra within a few minutes of the anticipated time of anesthesia induction, either general or by major regional block. If more than 1 hour passes between the first dose and anesthesia induction, then a second dose is given.

Magnesium hydroxide, or milk of magnesia, also effectively neutralizes gastric acid (Wheatley and colleagues, 1979), and its favorable effects last long enough for cesarean section to be completed. However, Gibbs and associates (1979) demonstrated in dogs that pulmonary instillation of a suspension of milk of magnesia and aluminum hydroxide can induce pneumonitis; thus, most prefer Bicitra as described.

Cimetidine, given sometime before general anesthesia for delivery, also has been recommended (Hodgkinson and colleagues, 1983). At least 30–60 minutes are required after parenteral administration to decrease gastric acidity to relatively safe levels. Therefore, in emergency situations, either an antacid or antacid plus cimetidine should be used (Moir, 1983). Thorburn and Moir (1987) studied 100 women undergoing emergency cesarean section who were given cimetidine, 200 mg intravenously, along with 30 mL of sodium citrate orally. The time interval from cimetidine administration to induction of general anesthesia was 5–208 minutes. None of the women had a gastric pH of less than 2.7 and all but one had a pH of 3.0 or higher.

Ranitidine, a histamine H_2-antagonist, can be given the night before surgery and will result in decreased gastric action through the next morning. This agent might prove useful when given along with a second dose on the morning of surgery for scheduled elective cesarean sections (Burchman, 1992). Yau and associates (1992), in a study of 49 women undergoing cesarean section who received ranitidine and sodium citrate, reported that only one (2%) had an intragastric pH of less than 2.5 and a volume greater than 25 mL.

Intubation

Various positions have been tried to minimize aspiration before and during tracheal intubation and cuff inflation, but the disadvantages from positions other than supine outweigh any advantage. Cricoid pressure from the time of induction of anesthesia until intubation should be performed by a trained associate. In special instances, intubation may be performed with the mother awake. In these cases, local anesthesia usually is applied. Appropriately applied topical spray generally will not significantly depress the laryngeal reflex.

Extubation

At the completion of the surgical procedure, the tracheal tube may be safely removed only if the woman is conscious to a degree to follow commands and is capable of maintaining oxygen saturation with spontaneous respiration.

Pathophysiology

Aspiration pneumonitis associated with obstetric anesthesia was described by Mendelson in 1946. Teabeaut (1952) demonstrated experimentally that if the pH of aspirated fluid was below 2.5, severe chemical pneumonitis developed. Additional characteristics of gastric acid that intensify pulmonary damage include large volume and particulate matter. In one study the pH of gastric juice of nearly half of women tested intrapartum without treatment was below 2.5 (Taylor and Pryse-Davies, 1966). The right mainstem bronchus usually offers the simplest pathway for aspirated material to reach the lung parenchyma, and therefore the right lower lobe most often is involved. In severe cases, there is bilateral widespread involvement.

The woman who aspirates may develop evidence for respiratory distress immediately or as long as several hours after aspiration, depending in part upon the material aspirated, the severity of the process, and the acuity of the attendants. Aspiration of a large amount of solid material causes obvious signs of airway obstruction. Smaller particles without acidic liquid may lead to patchy atelectasis and later to bronchopneumonia.

When highly acidic liquid is inspired, decreased oxygen saturation along with tachypnea, bronchospasm, rhonchi, rales, atelectasis, cyanosis, tachycardia, and hypotension are likely to develop. At the sites of injury, protein-rich fluid containing numerous erythrocytes exudes from capillaries into the lung interstitium and alveoli to cause decreased pulmonary compliance, shunting of blood, and severe hypoxemia. Radiographic changes may not appear immediately and they may be quite variable, although the right lobe most often is affected. Therefore, a chest x-ray alone should not be used to exclude aspiration.

Treatment

In recent years, the methods recommended for treatment of aspiration have changed appreciably, indicating that previous therapy was not very successful. Suspicion of aspiration of gastric contents demands very close monitoring for evidence of any pulmonary damage.

Suction and Bronchoscopy

Immediately following suspected aspirations, as much as possible of the inhaled fluid should be immediately wiped out of the mouth and removed from the pharynx and trachea by suction. Saline lavage may further disseminate the acid throughout the lung and is not recommended. If large particulate matter is inspired, prompt bronchoscopy may be indicated to relieve airway obstruction. Otherwise, bronchoscopy not only is unnecessary but may contribute to morbidity and mortality.

Corticosteroids

There is no clinical or experimental evidence that appreciable benefits accrue from the use of corticosteroids in aspiration pneumonitis (Bynum and Pierce, 1976). Nonetheless, the clinical impression of some has been that the immediate intravenous administration of 500 mg of methylprednisolone sodium succinate (Solu-Medrol), with repeated doses of 250 mg every 8 hours for 24 hours, is beneficial. It has not been the practice of the authors to use steroids.

Oxygen and Ventilation

Oxygen delivered through a tracheal tube in increased concentration by intermittent positive pressure may be required to raise and maintain the arterial Po_2 at 60 mm Hg or higher and the arterial oxygen saturation (Sao_2) at 90 percent or higher. Frequent suctioning is necessary to remove secretions, including edema fluid. In severe cases, adult respiratory distress syndrome develops. Mechanical ventilation that produces positive end-expiratory pressure may prove lifesaving by preventing the complete collapse of the now surfactant-poor lung on expiration.

Antimicrobials

Although the likelihood of bacterial contamination and infection from aspiration is appreciable, the use of antimicrobials prophylactically is controversial (Bynum and Pierce, 1976). Bartlett and associates (1974) identified anaerobic bacteria in 50 of 54 cases of pneumonia caused by aspiration. They concluded that anaerobes play a key role in most cases of infection after aspiration, and they suggested the use of clindamycin or chloramphenicol for those anaerobes not sensitive to penicillin. Most do not give antimicrobials unless there is clinical evidence of infection.

INFECTIONS FOLLOWING CESAREAN DELIVERY

Delivery by cesarean section places the woman at extraordinary risk for developing uterine infection. The incidence of metritis following surgical delivery varies with socioeconomic factors, and over the years this has been altered substantially by the common use of perioperative antimicrobials. For example, Cunningham and associates (1978) found an overall incidence of about 50 percent in women at a county hospital delivered by cesarean section who were not given prophylactic antimicrobials. Duration of labor and membrane rupture, multiple cervical examinations, and internal fetal monitoring are important determinants of infection morbidity. Women with all of these factors delivered for cephalopelvic disproportion, who were not given perioperative prophylaxis, had an incidence of serious pelvic infection that was nearly 90 percent (DePalma and colleagues, 1982; Gilstrap and Cunningham, 1979). Serious infections are much less common with the use of perioperative antimicrobials, and this is discussed in detail in Chapter 38.

Bacteriology

Organisms that contaminate and invade surgical incisions and lacerations typically are those that normally colonize the cervix, vagina, and perineum. Most of these bacteria are of relatively low virulence, and seldom do they initiate infection in healthy tissues. Although more virulent bacteria may be introduced from exogenous sources, in modern obstetrics an epidemic of serious puerperal sepsis rarely develops, as virulent bacteria usually are not carried from person to person during labor, delivery, or early in the puerperium. However, at least one epidemic from group A β-hemolytic streptococcus has been well documented in the past 25 years (Jewett and associates, 1968). Moreover, there have been several recent reports of this organism in association with postpartum genital tract infections and a toxic shock-like syndrome (Cone and associates, 1987; Dotters and Katz, 1991; Nathan and co-workers, 1993; Whitted and colleagues, 1990).

Common Pathogens

In the great majority of instances, bacteria responsible for pelvic infection are those that normally reside in the bowel and also commonly colonize the perineum, vagina, and cervix. Bacteria commonly responsible for female genital tract infections are shown in Table 20–1. Usually, multiple species of bacteria are isolated, and although typically considered to be of relatively low virulence, these bacteria may become pathogenic as a result of hematomas and devitalized tissue. Under the circumstances, their pathogenicity now is enhanced sufficiently to cause uterine infection with extensive pelvic cellulitis, abscesses, peritonitis, and suppurative thrombophlebitis.

TABLE 20–1. BACTERIA COMMONLY RESPONSIBLE FOR FEMALE GENITAL INFECTIONS

Aerobes
Group A, B, and D streptococci
Enterococcus
Gram-negative rods—*E. coli, Klebsiella,* and *Proteus* species
Staphylococcus aureus
Anaerobes
Peptococcus species
Peptostreptococcus species
Bacteroides bivius, B. fragilis, B. disiens
Clostridium species
Fusobacterium species
Other
Mycoplasma hominis
Chlamydia trachomatis

From American College of Obstetricians and Gynecologists, (1988).

Although the cervix and lower genital tract routinely harbor such bacteria, the uterine cavity usually is sterile before rupture of the amnionic sac. As the consequence of labor and delivery and associated manipulations, the amnionic fluid and perhaps the uterus commonly become contaminated with anaerobic and aerobic bacteria. For example, Gilstrap and Cunningham (1979), from cultures of amnionic fluid obtained at cesarean section performed in women in labor with membranes ruptured more than 6 hours, identified the following bacteria: anaerobic and aerobic organisms in 63 percent, anaerobes alone in 30 percent, and aerobes alone in 7 percent. Predominant anaerobic organisms were gram-positive cocci (*Peptostreptococcus* and *Peptococcus*), 45 percent; *Bacteroides,* 9 percent; and *Clostridium,* 3 percent. Gram-positive aerobic cocci also were common (*Enterococcus,* 14 percent; group B *Streptococcus*, 8 percent). *Escherichia coli* comprised 9 percent of isolates. An average of 2.5 organisms was identified from each specimen.

These observations serve to emphasize the polymicrobial nature of genital tract infections associated with delivery, and especially cesarean section. Gibbs (1987) reemphasized the importance of these organisms, and reported an increasing prevalence of *Bacteroides bivius* as a cause of female pelvic infection. Walmer and colleagues (1988) more recently provided evidence for the role of *Enterococcus* in the pathogenesis of these infections.

Bacterial Cultures

Precise identification of bacteria specifically responsible for any puerperal infection may be quite difficult. Even results of cultures of uterine specimens obtained by using double-lumen catheters are unclear. Using these techniques, Gibbs and associates (1975), like Hite and co-workers (1947) three decades before, cultured one or more pathogens from the uterine cavity in 70 percent or more of clinically healthy puerperal women. For these reasons, routine pretreatment genital tract cultures in women with puerperal infection are of little clinical utility.

Appropriately performed anaerobic and aerobic blood cultures obtained before antimicrobials are given may be useful to identify some of these pathogens. Blood cultures were positive in 13 percent of women treated at

Parkland Hospital for postoperative pelvic infections (Cunningham and colleagues, 1978) and 24 percent of those from Los Angeles County Hospital (diZerega and co-workers, 1979).

Pathogenesis

The pathogenesis of uterine infection following cesarean section is that of an infected surgical incision. Bacteria that colonized the cervix and vagina gain access to amnionic fluid during labor, and postpartum they invade devitalized uterine tissue. Invariably, with uterine infections that follow cesarean sections, there is myometritis with parametrial cellulitis. Hence, the term *metritis* is more descriptive than endometritis.

Clinical Course

The clinical picture of metritis varies with the extent of the disease, and whenever fever persists postpartum, uterine infection should be suspected. The degree of temperature elevation probably is proportional to the extent of infection, and when confined to the endometrium (decidua) and superficial myometrium, the cases are mild and there is minimal fever. With more severe infection, the temperature often exceeds 38.3°C. Chills may accompany fever and suggest bacteremia, which may be documented in nearly 20 percent of women with uterine infection following cesarean delivery. The pulse rate typically follows the temperature curve.

The woman usually complains of abdominal pain, and afterpains may be bothersome. There is tenderness on one or both sides of the abdomen and parametrial tenderness is elicited upon bimanual examination. Even in the early stages, an offensive odor may develop, long regarded as an important sign of uterine infection. However, in many women, foul-smelling lochia is found without other evidence for infection. Conversely, some infections, and notably those due to group A β-hemolytic streptococci, frequently are associated with scanty, odorless lochia. Leukocytosis may range from 15,000 to 30,000 cells per μL, but in view of the physiologic leukocytosis of the early puerperium, these findings are difficult to interpret.

Treatment of Metritis

Post-cesarean section metritis is treated with a parenterally administered broad-spectrum antimicrobial(s). Improvement will follow in 48–72 hours in nearly 90 percent of women treated with one of the regimens discussed below. Persistence of fever after this interval mandates a careful search for causes of refractory pelvic infection, although nonpelvic sources occasionally are found. Complications of metritis that cause persistent fever despite appropriate therapy include parametrial phlegmons, surgical incisional and pelvic abscesses, and septic pelvic thrombophlebitis.

Following a successful response to the initial intravenous antimicrobial regimen, it had become common practice in the past to send the woman home with oral antibiotics to complete a prearranged course of therapy. Data to support this practice is lacking, and the usual contemporary practice is to discharge the woman without further therapy after she has been afebrile for at least 24 hours. Indeed, Dinsmoor and colleagues (1991) found no differences in infection-related complications when oral antibiotic therapy was combined with placebo for women discharged following successful intravenous therapy.

Principles of Antimicrobial Treatment

Although few, if any, antimicrobial regimens are effective against all of these putative pathogens of pelvic infection, treatment is directed against at least most of the polymicrobial and mixed flora that are listed in Table 20–1 and that typically cause puerperal infections. Fortunately, selection of an agent(s) effective against the most common pathogens usually proves suitable. Because, as described above, material for culture frequently is impractical to obtain, antimicrobial therapy is empirical.

β-Lactam antimicrobials have spectra that include activity against many anaerobic pathogens and have been used successfully for decades to treat these infections. Many of the popular and effective multiagent regimens include a drug from this group, although some are effective when used alone. Examples include some cephalosporins (cefoxitin, cefoperazone, cefotetan, cefotaxime, and others) and extended-spectrum penicillins (piperacillin, ticarcillin, and mezlocillin). β-Lactam antimicrobials are inherently safe, and except for allergic reactions, they are free of major toxicity. Another advantage is the cost-effectiveness of administering only one drug. The **β-lactamase inhibitors,** clavulinic acid and sulbactam, have been combined with ampicillin, amoxicillin, and ticarcillin to extend their spectra, and these also have been proven effective.

In 1979, diZerega and colleagues compared the effectiveness of clindamycin plus gentamicin with penicillin G plus gentamicin given for treatment of pelvic infections following cesarean section. Women given the **clindamycin–gentamicin** regimen had a favorable response 95 percent of the time, and this regimen now is considered by most to be the standard by which others are measured. Unfortunately, clindamycin, like most other regimens effective against anaerobic flora, may induce **pseudomembranous colitis** by overgrowth of resistant enterotoxin-producing *Clostridium difficile.* If severe, such colitis may be life-threatening and treatment with vancomycin or metronidazole is given along with supportive measures. Walmer and colleagues (1988) later provided evidence that enterococcal infections may be associated with clinical failure of the clindamycin–gentamicin regimen. While 93 percent of women from whom enterococci were not isolated responded to this regimen, only 82 percent with enterococcal infections responded. The incidence of wound infection was much higher in women with enterococcal infections compared with those without (16 vs 3%). Diligent monitoring of the impact of enterococcal isolates for these infections is needed.

Although some recommend that serum gentamicin levels periodically be monitored, it is not necessary to measure peak and trough serum concentrations in most women. Because the potential for nephrotoxicity and ototoxicity is worrisome with gentamicin in the event of diminished glomerular filtration, such women can be given a combination of clindamycin and a second-generation cephalosporin. Others have recommended a combination of clindamycin and aztreonam, a monobactam compound with activity against gram-negative aerobic pathogens similar to the aminoglycosides (American College of Obstetricians and Gynecologists, 1988).

Metronidazole has superior in vitro activity against most anaerobes and is recommended by some to be given intravenously in combination with either gentamicin or tobramycin, especially if an abscess is suspected. **Chloramphenicol** remains a potent antimicrobial in vitro against most anaerobes that cause pelvic infections. Given intravenously along with one of the ß-lactam antimicrobials, it provides excellent coverage for severe pelvic sepsis. It can be given safely with impaired renal function, but unfortunately deaths due to irreversible bone marrow suppression follow in about 1 in 20,000 courses of therapy. As with any of these regimens, its benefits must be weighed against these adverse effects.

Imipenem is a carbapenem that has broad-spectrum coverage against the majority of organisms associated with metritis. It is used in combination with cilastatin, which inhibits the renal metabolism of imipenem. Although this antibiotic most certainly will be effective in the vast majority of cases of metritis following cesarean section, it seems reasonable to reserve it for more serious infections such as pelvic abscesses and for primary antibiotic failures.

COMPLICATIONS OF UTERINE INFECTIONS

In about 90 percent of women, metritis responds within 48–72 hours to treatment with one of the regimens discussed above. In the others, any of a number of complications may arise.

Wound Infections

The incidence of abdominal incisional infections following cesarean section has been reported to range from 3 to 15 percent with an average of 7 percent (Faro, 1990). When prophylactic antibiotics are given, the incidence is 2 percent or less. According to Soper and coworkers (1992), wound infection is the most common cause of antimicrobial failure in women given therapy for metritis. Risk factors for abdominal wound infections include obesity, diabetes, corticosteroid therapy, immunosuppression, anemia, and poor hemostasis with hematoma formation.

Abdominal incisional abscesses that develop in women delivered by cesarean section usually cause fever beginning on the fourth postoperative day or so. In most cases, these are preceded by uterine infection, and there is persistent fever despite adequate antimicrobial therapy. Erythema and drainage also may be present. Organisms causing these infections usually are the same as those isolated from amnionic fluid at the time of cesarean section, but hospital-acquired pathogens must be suspected (Emmons and colleagues, 1988; Gilstrap and Cunningham, 1979).

When cellulitis first manifests, treatment with antimicrobials may be effective in suppressing infection. As indicated above, most women with incisional wound infections following cesarean section have already been given prophylactic antimicrobials intraoperatively or were treated for metritis. An obvious hematoma or abscess requires drainage on discovery. In those women in whom an abscess is not initially apparent, observation and antimicrobial therapy is appropriate. With continuing infection the incision will become tender and more swollen and the woman will have persistent fever. In some cases, the wound opens spontaneously.

Treatment of an abscess includes surgical drainage of all purulent material. Frequently, there are loculations of pus. In most cases, the entire length of the wound must be explored with disruption of all layers to the fascia. Careful inspection for fascial integrity is

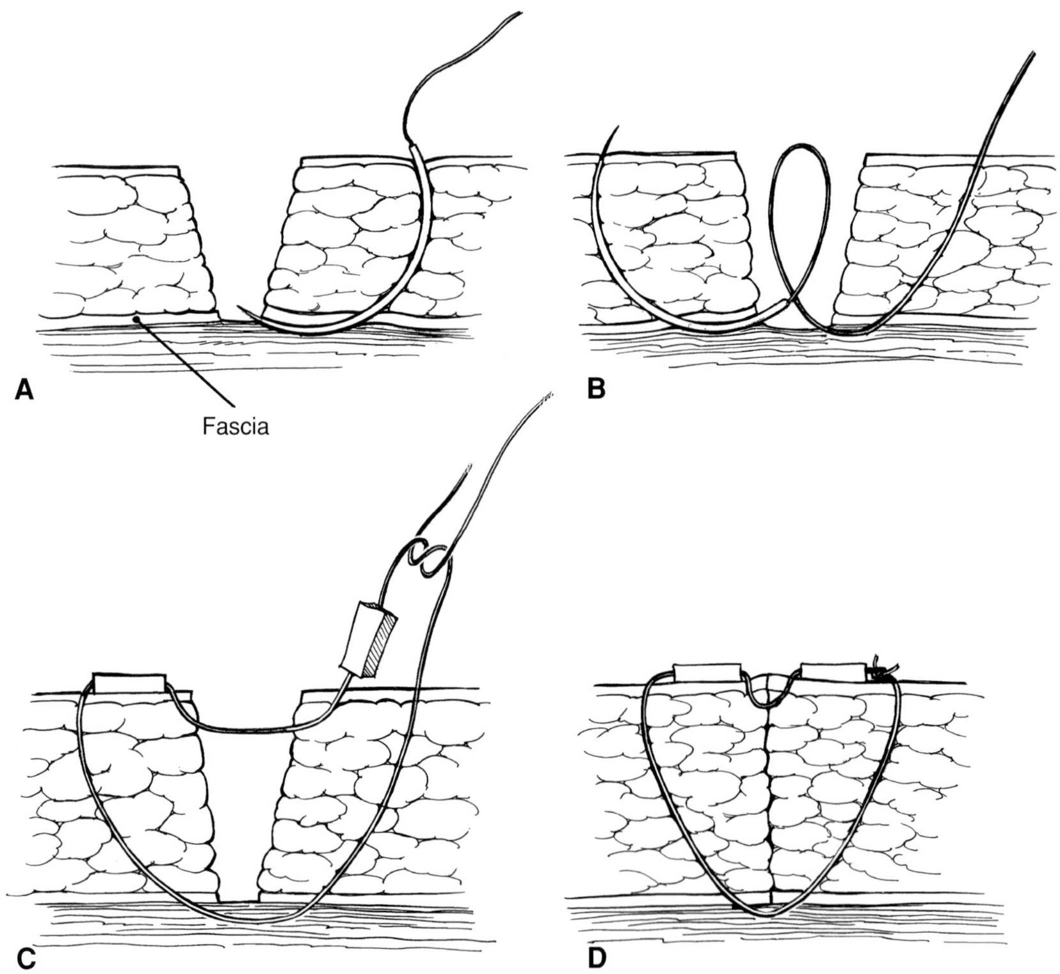

Figure 20–1. Technique of en bloc wound reclosure. **A.** The needle is passed from a point on the skin 3–4 cm from the wound edge through the superior part of the fascia at the wound base. **B.** The needle is withdrawn from the wound base, reintroduced into the fascia at the point from which it emerged with the first pass, and brought out through the skin at a point 3–4 cm from the opposite wound edge. **C.** Rubber suture guards are loaded onto the suture, the suture is brought across the incision incorporating the dermis and epidermis of the wound margins, and a second suture guard is loaded. **D.** The suture is tied, closing the wound. (Modified from Walters and colleagues, 1990, with permission.)

paramount when the wound is first drained. If the fascial layer is intact, then debridement and local wound care is appropriate. In some cases, inspection and debridement are initially carried out in the operating room because extensive debridement and exploration requires major anesthesia.

After vigorous debridement of all necrotic tissue and drainage of purulent material, the wound cavity is packed with moistened sterile gauze. Some prefer to soak the gauze in povidone-iodine solution. This dressing should be changed at least daily, and preferably twice daily, with appropriate debridement at the time of dressing change. Whirlpool hydrotherapy may also be useful in achieving effective debridement and hastening the time to reclosure. Hydrotherapy is carried out in a Hubbard tank with chlorinated water (5 ppm) once or twice weekly.

Healing by secondary intention takes several weeks to months depending on the size and depth of the wound. An aesthetically preferable method of management is to allow healthy pink granulation tissue to form—usually about 4–6 days—after which the wound edges are apposed with Steri-strips or nonabsorbable suture. Walters and associates (1990) reported that the mean time to healing in six women randomized to second intention was 72 days. They recommended en bloc reclosure of disrupted incisions. The method, shown in Figure 20–1, was not employed for a minimum of 4 days after daily debridement and dressing changes three times a day. The size of the wound cavity is inconsequential, and if it is large because of excessive debridement of subcutaneous tissue, the wound edges can be apposed with steri-strips and the woman instructed to return in 1 week. If the strips come off, then she and her family are instructed to continue cleaning the wound as they were taught in the hospital. When she returns, Steri-strips are replaced or suture material is used to appose the skin edges.

Wound Dehiscence

Wound disruption or dehiscence or "burst abdomen" refers to separation of an abdominal wound involving the fascial layer. Its incidence following obstetric surgery is rare. Indeed, Gallup and colleagues (1990) used a mass running closure in 285 women with midline incisions who were at high risk for wound disruption and encountered only one such complication. These closures are discussed in detail in Chapter 4.

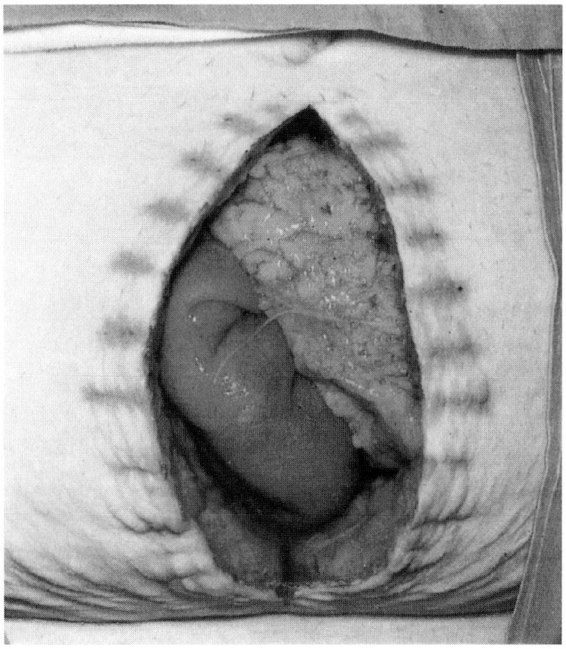

Figure 20–2. Wound dehiscence 7 days after cesarean section. After the skin sutures were removed, the wound fell apart. Bowel and omentum are apparent. (From Beischer and MacKay, 1981, with permission.)

Most disruptions do not manifest until about the fifth postoperative day. The usual presenting sign is a serosanguinous discharge. Infection may coexist. In some women, dehiscence becomes apparent when the skin sutures or clips are removed and evisceration follows (Fig. 20–2).

The incision is closed in the operating room usually using general anesthesia. If there is normal distention, conduction analgesia may be sufficient. As shown in Figure 20–3, surgical debridement is carried out first, followed by secondary fascial closure. Most surgeons prefer myofascial approximation as described in Chapter 4 and shown in Figure 20–3.

Necrotizing Fasciitis

A rare but frequently fatal complication of cesarean section wound infections is deep soft tissue infection involving muscle and fascia. Such infections may extend from any infection adjacent to myofascial edges, and this includes

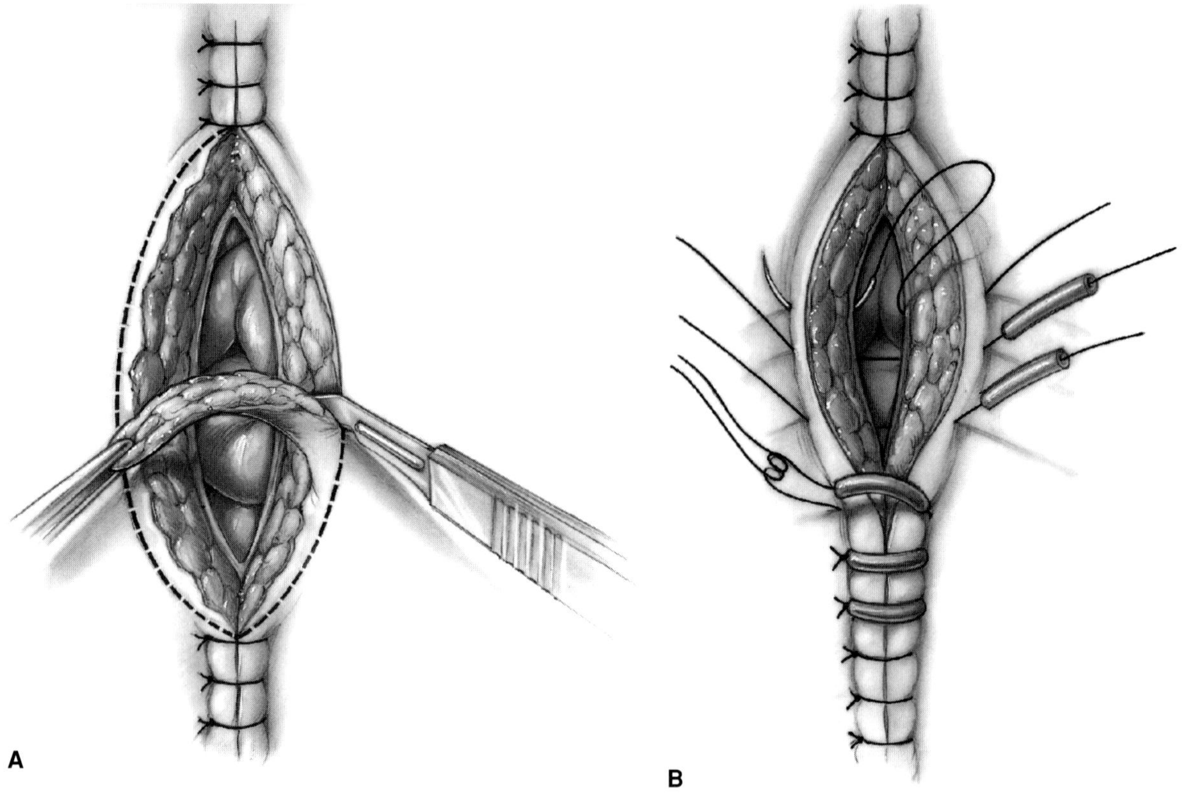

Figure 20–3. A. Sharp debridement of abdominal wound dehiscence. **B.** Through-and-through closure of wound shown in **A.**

surgical incisions or other wounds. They are seen also with vulvar infections in diabetic and immunocompromised women, but they develop rarely in otherwise healthy women. In obstetrics, these severe infections are more commonly encountered in episiotomy and other perineal wounds (see Chapter 7).

Early skin changes usually include erythema, tenderness, and edema. Frequently, these are accompanying systemic symptoms of fever, malaise, and generalized toxicity. Initially the skin may be intact, but as gangrene progresses, the skin becomes discolored and vesicles and crepitance appear accompanied by cutaneous anesthesia and skin necrosis.

Bacteria that cause these serious perineal infections appear to be similar to those that cause other pelvic infections, but anaerobes predominate. Gram-positive anaerobic cocci or *Clostridium perfringens* usually are isolated along with aerobic cocci, *B. fragilis* group or *E. coli* (Thompson and associates, 1993). *S. pyogenes* and group B streptococci may cause necrosis (McHenry and associates, 1984; Sutton and colleagues, 1985).

Necrotizing fasciitis of the surgical incision may involve any of the several superficial or deep perineal fascial layers, and thus it may extend over the abdominal wall. From their review, Thompson and colleagues (1993) reported that these severe infections also may follow episiotomy, mini-laparotomy, diagnostic laparoscopy, and suprapubic catheter placement. Clinical symptoms vary, and frequently it is difficult to differentiate superficial infections from deep fascial ones. A high index of suspicion, with surgical exploration if the diagnosis is uncertain, may be lifesaving. Stamenkovic and Lew (1984) recommend biopsy of the fascial edges with frozen section microscopic examination when the diagnosis is uncertain. Certainly, if myofascitis progresses, the woman becomes very ill from septicemia, there is profound hemoconcentration from capillary leakage with circulatory failure, and death soon follows.

Aggressive surgical treatment is carried out emergently and includes wide debridement of all infected tissue (Nolan and colleagues, 1994). This is performed in the operating room using general anesthesia. These infections are usually associated with tremendous endothelial cell damage from bacterial toxins. Thus there is hemoconcentration and capillary leakage. Debridement may include extensive abdominal wall debridement with unroofing and excision of abdominal fascia as shown in Figure 20–3. It is important to incise all infection with debridement carried peripherally until there is no loss of resistance to blunt probing and until the tissue bleeds easily. Split-thickness skin grafts are used later to repair the defects. Mortality is virtually universal without surgical treatment, and it approaches 50 percent even if aggressive excision is performed.

Peritonitis

Uterine infection may extend by way of the lymphatics to reach the abdominal cavity to cause peritonitis. This complication rarely is seen today with prompt therapy, but may be encountered with infections following cesarean section when there is uterine incisional necrosis and dehiscence. Also rare, late in the course of pelvic cellulitis, a parametrial or adnexal abscess may rupture and produce catastrophic generalized peritonitis. This is a grave complication, and typically, fibrinopurulent exudate binds loops of bowel to one another, and locules of pus may form between the loops. The cul-de-sac and subdiaphragmatic space may then be sites for abscess formation.

Clinically, puerperal peritonitis resembles surgical peritonitis except that abdominal rigidity usually is less prominent. Pain may be severe. Marked bowel distention is a consequence of paralytic ileus. It is important to identify the cause of the generalized peritonitis. If the infection began in the uterus and extended into the peritoneum, the treatment usually is medical. Conversely, peritonitis as the consequence of a bowel lesion or its appendages usually is best treated surgically. Antimicrobial therapy should include those agents most likely effective against *Peptostreptococcus, Peptococcus, Bacteroides, Clostridia,* and aerobic coliforms. Septicemic shock may supervene.

Intravenous fluid and electrolyte replacement are important because with generalized peritonitis large amounts of fluid are sequestered in the lumen and the wall of the gastrointestinal tract and, at times, in the peritoneal cavity. Vomiting, diarrhea, and fever also contribute appreciably to fluid and electrolyte loss. The volumes of fluid and the amounts of electrolytes necessary to replace what is sequestered in the abdomen, aspirated from the gut, and lost through diaphoresis usually are quite large but must not be so massive as to produce circulatory overload. Because paralytic ileus usually is a prominent feature, the gastrointestinal tract should be decompressed by continuous nasogastric suction. Oral feeding is withheld throughout the course of treatment until bowel function returns and flatus is expelled.

Purulent exudate between loops of bowel, or between bowel and other organs, may cause intestinal kinking, following which symptoms of mechanical bowel obstruction will supervene. Surgical decompression may be necessary. Surgery is not indicated early in the course of the disease, although abscesses may form at various sites and need to be drained, and mechanical intestinal obstruction may need to be relieved.

Adnexal Infections

Most often with puerperal infections the fallopian tubes are involved only with perisalpingitis without subsequent tubal occlusion and sterility. An **ovarian abscess** rarely develops as a complication of puerperal infection, presumably from bacterial invasion through a rent in the ovarian capsule (Wetchler and Dunn, 1985). The abscess usually is unilateral and women typically present 1–2 weeks after delivery. In many cases, rupture causes peritonitis, which prompts surgical exploration. Unless peritonitis is apparent, initially intravenous antimicrobial agents are given, but surgical drainage usually becomes necessary.

Parametrial Phlegmon

In some women in whom metritis develops following cesarean delivery, parametrial cellulitis is intensive and forms an area of induration, termed a **phlegmon,** within the leaves of the broad ligament (Fig. 20–4). These infections are the most common cause of persistent fever despite prompt and adequate treatment of pelvic infections that complicate cesarean section (DePalma and colleagues, 1982). Such areas of cellulitis more often are unilateral, and while frequently they may remain limited to the base of the broad ligament, if the inflammatory reaction is more intense, celluli-

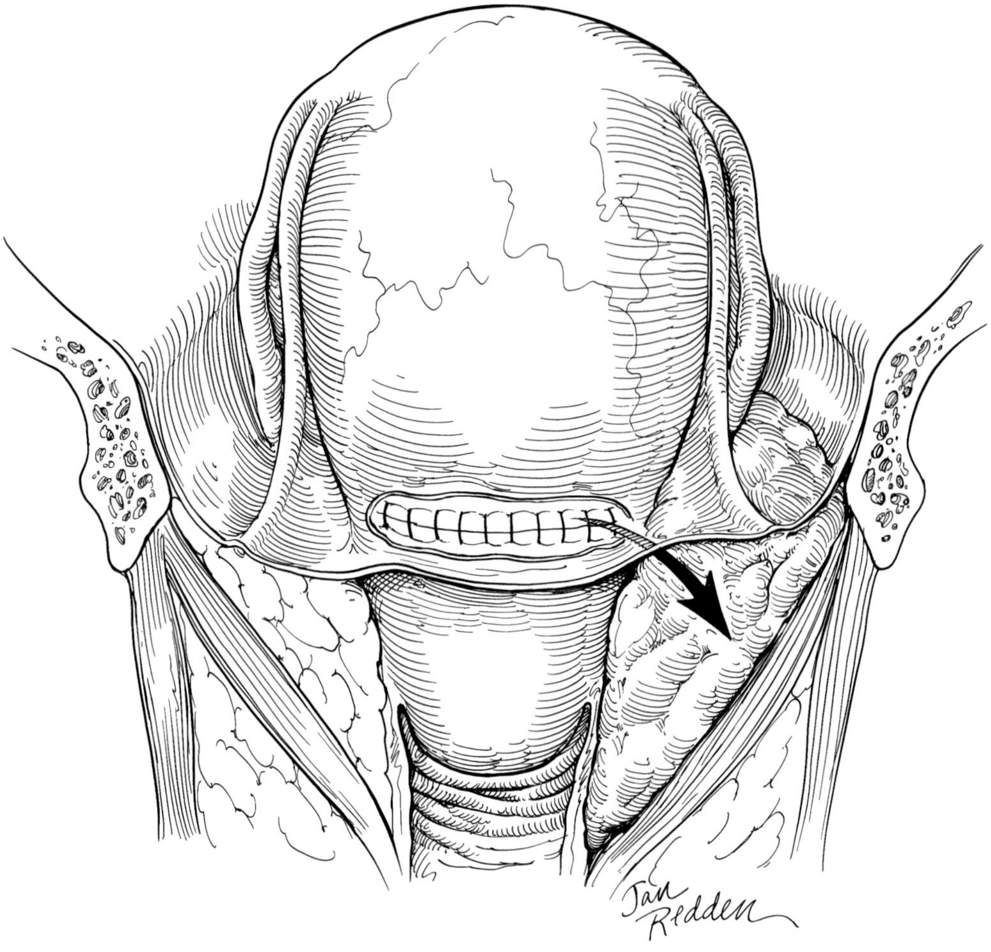

Figure 20–4. Parametrial phlegmon. Cellulitis in the left parametrium begins adjacent to the cesarean section incision and extends to the pelvic sidewall. On pelvic examination, the phlegmon is palpable as a firm, three-dimensional mass.

tis extends along natural lines of cleavage. The most common form of extension is directly laterally, along the base of the broad ligament, with a tendency to extend to the lateral pelvic wall. The uterus is pushed toward the opposite side and is fixed. Occasionally, high intraligamentous exudates spread from the region of the uterine cornua to the iliac fossa. Posterior extension may involve the rectovaginal septum with the development of a firm mass posterior to the cervix. Rarely, involvement of the connective tissue anterior to the cervix results in cellulitis of the space of Retzius with extension upward and beneath the anterior abdominal wall.

Fortunately rare, intensive cellulitis of the uterine incision may cause necrosis and separation with extrusion of purulent material into the peritoneal cavity. Clinical findings then are as described above for peritonitis. Frequently, the first symptoms of peritonitis are those of **adynamic ileus,** which usually is absent or mild following uncomplicated cesarean section. Puerperal metritis with pelvic cellulitis typically is a retroperitoneal infection, and evidence for peritonitis should alert the physician to the possibility of uterine incisional necrosis with dehiscence, or less commonly a bowel injury or other lesion.

In the majority of women who develop a parametrial phlegmon, clinical response follows continued treatment with one of the intravenous antimicrobial regimens previously discussed. As long as the initial regimen has been appropriately chosen, and if there is no evidence of clinical deterioration, especially

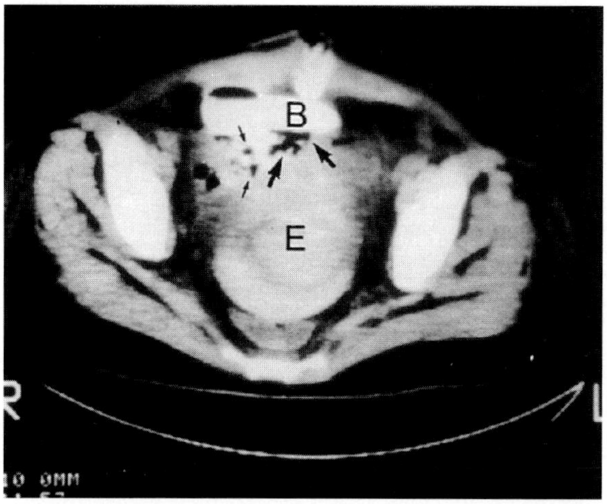

Figure 20–5. Pelvic computed tomography showing uterine necrosis with gas (arrows) in the infected cesarean section incision. B, bladder; E, endometrial cavity. (From Cunningham and colleagues, 1993, with permission.)

peritonitis, then the same regimen may be continued, or an alternate regimen chosen. Women with a phlegmon usually remain febrile for 5–7 days, and in some cases, even longer. Absorption of the induration follows, but it may take several weeks to dissipate completely.

Evaluation of pelvic infections using sonography has been less than satisfactory because ultrasound generally is poor for soft tissue imaging. Frequently, these areas of cellulitis have ultrasonic characteristics suggesting an abscess, but as discussed above, surgical drainage of a phlegmon is inadvisable. Brown and colleagues (1991) described the use of computed tomography in 74 women to assess refractory pelvic infections, and there was at least one abnormal radiologic finding in three-fourths of these women. Lev-Toaff and colleagues (1991) reported similar findings in 31 women using ultrasound along with computed tomography or magnetic resonance imaging. Only two of these women had negative findings. Sometimes, as shown in Figure 20–5, evidence for uterine incisional dehiscence is detected. It is important that these x-ray findings be interpreted along with the clinical course, because apparent uterine separations seen radiographically may resolve spontaneously. In that case, these are presumed to represent either infection without dehiscence or normal healing. Twickler and colleagues (1991) reported that myometrial incisional defects can be visualized radiographically in women after cesarean section who have no other evidence for infection, dehiscence, or other complications.

Surgery is reserved for women in whom uterine incisional necrosis is suspected or who fail to respond to medical therapy. Hysterectomy and surgical debridement usually are difficult, and often there is appreciable blood loss. Frequently, the cervix and lower uterine segment are involved with an intensive inflammatory process that extends to the pelvic sidewall to encompass one or both ureters, and supracervical hysterectomy should be considered. The adnexa are seldom involved, and depending on their appearance, one or both ovaries may be conserved.

Pelvic Abscess

Rarely, despite prompt and appropriate antimicrobial treatment for metritis, a parametrial phlegmon will suppurate, forming a fluctuant broad ligament mass that may point above the Poupart ligament. In these circumstances the woman may not have worsening of symptoms, but fever persists. Should the abscess rupture into the peritoneal cavity, life-threatening peritonitis may develop as previously described. More likely, these abscesses will dissect anteriorly and may be amenable to needle drainage directed by computed tomography (Fig. 20–6). Occasionally they dissect posteriorly through the retroperitoneal space to the rectovaginal septum, where surgical drainage is easily effected by colpotomy incision (Fig. 20–7).

THROMBOEMBOLIC DISEASE

According to the Consensus Conference sponsored by the National Institutes of Health (1986), venous thromboembolism in normal pregnancy and the puerperium is five times as likely as in nonpregnant women of similar age. Certainly, venous thrombosis and pulmonary embolism remain a major cause of maternal death in the United States (Grimes, 1994). Kaunitz and colleagues (1985) found that thrombotic pulmonary embolism caused 13 percent of 2,067 nonabortion-related direct maternal deaths in the United States from

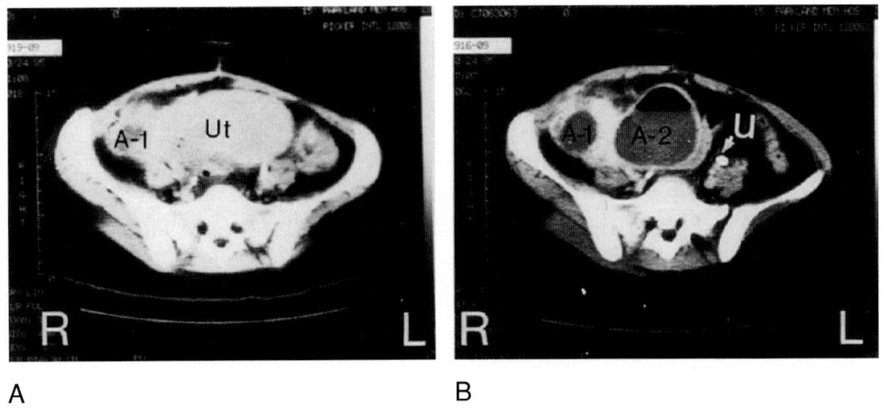

Figure 20–6. Pelvic computed tomography showing two large pelvic abscesses. **A.** One abscess cavity (A-1) is within the right broad ligament adjacent to the puerperal uterus (Ut). **B.** The large abscess in the center (A-2) is bounded caudad by the uterine fundus and the smaller cavity (A-1) on the patient's right. The left ureter (U) is shown by the arrow. (From Cunningham and colleagues, 1993, with permission.)

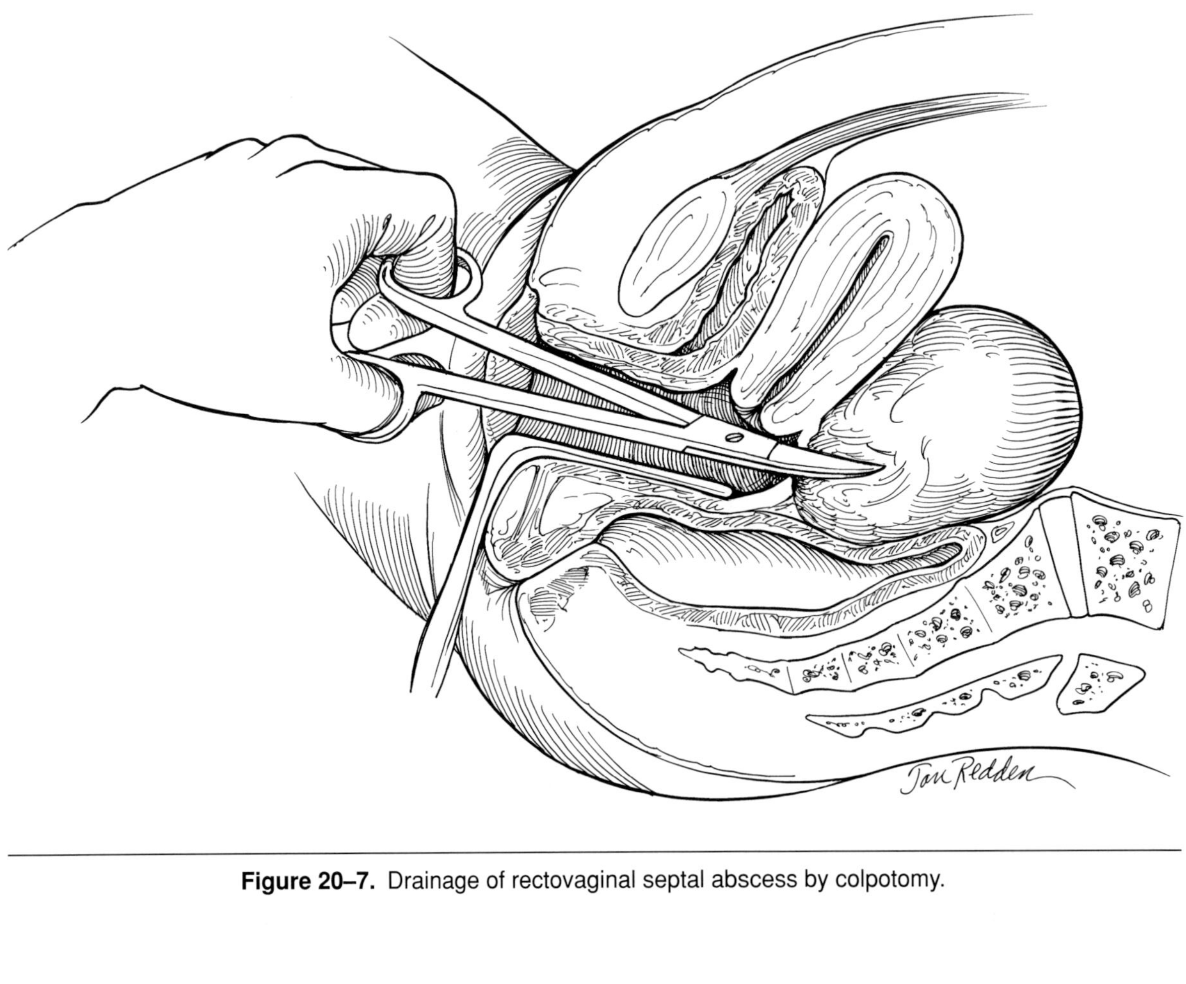

Figure 20–7. Drainage of rectovaginal septal abscess by colpotomy.

1974 through 1978. Sachs and associates (1987) reported that pulmonary embolism is now the second most common cause of maternal mortality in Massachusetts.

In the past, thromboembolic diseases were considered unique to the puerperium; however, this is no longer true. In recent years, there has been a decrease in the frequency of deep venous thrombosis and thromboembolism during the puerperium, but perhaps an increase antepartum. For example, Henderson and co-workers (1972) described 20 cases that developed antepartum among 29,770 pregnancies, but during the same period, only 16 were identified postpartum. Observations from Parkland Hospital indicate even more of a propensity for antepartum disease (Cunningham and associates, 1993). During the 2½-year period ending June 1991, 17 of 20 cases of deep venous thrombosis or pulmonary embolism were identified antepartum.

Undoubtedly, the frequency of venous thromboembolic disease during the puerperium decreased remarkably when early ambulation became practiced widely. Stasis is probably the strongest single predisposing event to deep vein thrombosis and, therefore, should be kept to a minimum. Venous thrombosis with a significant potential for generating pulmonary emboli may originate in the deep veins of the thigh or pelvis. A thrombosis confined to the deep veins of the calf, or that involves only the superficial veins of the leg or thigh, is very unlikely to generate a pulmonary embolus.

More recently, attention has been directed to a number of isolated deficiencies of proteins involved either in coagulation inhibition or in the fibrinolytic system. In some women these deficiencies can lead to hypercoagulability and recurrent venous thromboembolism. For example, according to Hellgren and associates (1989), up to 70 percent of women with hereditary deficiency of antithrombin-III may experience thromboembolic complications during pregnancy. Trauscht-Van Horn and associates (1992) reported that a third of 15 protein-C deficient women developed thromboembolism during pregnancy. Heijboer and colleagues (1990) studied the prevalence of isolated coagulation protein deficiencies in 277 consecutive nonpregnant outpatients with venographically proven acute deep vein thrombosis. Overall, 8.3 percent of these patients had deficiencies of **antithrombin-III, protein C, protein S,** or **plasminogen,** compared with 2.2 percent of age- and sex-matched controls without thrombosis. They concluded that such screening was not cost-effective in these nonpregnant patients, but similar studies during pregnancy are lacking.

Superficial Venous Thrombosis

Antepartum or postpartum thrombosis limited strictly to the superficial veins of the saphenous system is treated with analgesia, elastic support, and rest. If it does not soon subside, or if deep venous involvement is suspected, appropriate diagnostic measures are taken, and heparin is given if deep vein involvement is confirmed. Superficial thrombophlebitis is typically seen in association with superficial varicosities or as a sequela to intravenous catheterization.

Deep Venous Thrombosis

The incidence of deep venous thrombosis, both antepartum and postpartum, has decreased. For example, in the study from Parkland Hospital cited above, in the 2½-year period ending June 1991, of the nearly 35,000 women delivered there were 17 cases of deep venous thrombosis, for an incidence of about 1 in 2000. This low incidence of proven thrombosis likely is due in part to improved techniques to confirm as well as exclude thrombosis suspected clinically.

The signs and symptoms of deep venous thrombosis involving the lower extremity vary greatly, depending in large measure upon the degree of occlusion and the intensity of the inflammatory response. Ginsberg and colleagues (1992) reported an amazing tendency for left-leg involvement in pregnant women. Indeed, of 60 consecutive antepartum women, 58 had isolated left-leg thrombosis and it was bilateral in the other two. Classical puerperal thrombophlebitis involving the lower extremity, sometimes called **phlegmasia alba dolens** or **milk leg,** is abrupt in onset, with severe pain and edema of the leg and thigh. The thrombus typically involves much of the deep venous system from the foot to the iliofemoral region. Occasionally, reflex arterial spasm causes a pale, cool extremity with diminished pulsations. More likely, there may be appreciable volume of clot yet little reaction in the form of pain, heat, or swelling. Importantly, calf pain, either spontaneous or in response to squeezing, or to stretching the Achilles tendon (Homans' sign), may be caused by a strained muscle or a contusion. The latter may be common during the early puerperium as the consequence of inappropriate contact between the calf and the delivery table leg holders.

Diagnosis

Venography or **phlebography** remains the standard for confirmation of the clinical diagnosis of deep venous thrombosis. In most studies, it has been shown that by using this technique at least half of clinically suspected cases do not have a thrombosis, thereby obviating the need for anticoagulation and its hazards. Venography is not without complications, and indeed the method itself may induce thrombosis (Fig. 20–8). Because of this, there has been renewed interest in noninvasive methods to confirm the clinical diagnosis.

In nonpregnant patients, **impedance plethysmography** apparently has promise, both as a screening method and for diagnosis. In a study from Amsterdam (Huisman and colleagues, 1986), 471 consecutive patients in whom deep venous thrombosis was clinically suspected were screened with serial impedance plethysmography, and if positive, they underwent venography. All patients in whom plethysmography was normal did well without treatment. Hull and colleagues (1985) presented similarly optimistic data, but emphasized that serial plethysmography was imperative when deep venous thrombosis was suspected clinically, the initial examination was negative, and venography was not to be done. They also reported that calf-vein thrombosis likely would be missed using plethysmography alone.

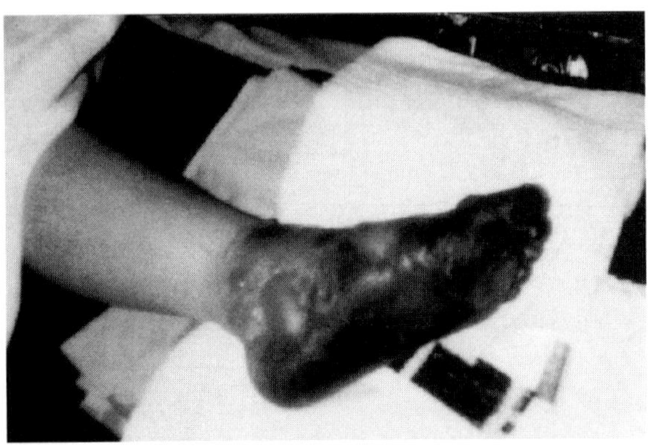

Figure 20–8. Aseptic gangrene of the foot that followed extravasation of contrast material injected intravenously under pressure preparatory to performing ascending venography. Partial foot amputation later was necessary. The patient did not have a venous thrombosis. (From Cunningham and colleagues, 1993, with permission; photograph courtesy of Dr. Tom Lowe.)

Hull and associates (1990b) later reported their experiences with serial plethysmography in 152 pregnant women referred for clinically suspected deep vein thrombosis. Plethysmography was abnormal in only 13 women (9%); 12 of these 13 subsequently underwent venography, and proximal-vein thrombosis was confirmed in 11. Importantly, none of the 139 with negative findings had venous thromboembolism on long-term follow-up. From these findings, it seems reasonable to use impedance plethysmography for screening in pregnant women in whom thrombosis is suspected, but if the examination is abnormal, then a confirmatory study is recommended.

Real-time B-mode ultrasonography, during which venous compressibility is assessed, is yet another noninvasive method to detect proximal deep vein thrombosis. Lensing and colleagues (1989) evaluated 220 consecutive nonpregnant patients with clinically suspected deep venous thrombosis. They compared contrast venography with real-time ultrasonography and evaluated the **common femoral** and **popliteal veins** for full compressibility (no thrombosis) and noncompressibility (thrombosis). Both of these vessels were fully compressible in 142 of 143 patients with normal venograms (specificity, 99%). All 66 patients with proximal-vein thrombosis had noncompressible femoral or popliteal veins, or both (sensitivity, 100%). Lensing and co-workers further reported that intraluminal echogenicity and venous distention during the Valsalva maneuver were relatively inaccurate. Although they found ultrasonography to be highly accurate and simple, they cautioned against its widespread clinical use as the sole diagnostic test for clinically suspected thrombosis until the safety of withholding anticoagulation in patients with negative tests was evaluated.

With the addition of duplex and color Doppler ultrasound technology, similar sensitivities can be found with shorter examination times (Scott and colleagues, 1990). Real-time sonography, coupled with duplex and color Doppler ultrasound, has tremendous potential to diagnose deep venous thrombosis of the lower extremities, but its role in the evaluation of pelvic vein thrombosis is less clear. **In pregnant women, thrombosis frequently originates in the iliac veins.** Using real-time and Doppler ultrasound along with impedance plethysmography, complete but not partial iliac vein occlusion can be detected (Hull and colleagues, 1990b). In a prospective evaluation of color-flow imaging in conjunction with compression ultrasonography, Polak and Wilkinson (1991) reported an incidence of symptomatic deep venous thrombosis of 7 per 10,000 deliveries, which was similar to the incidence in a retrospective cohort group (11 of 26,196 deliveries) in which the diagnosis was confirmed by venography.

Magnetic resonance imaging also has been utilized more recently for diagnosis of symptomatic deep venous thrombosis. This technique allows for excellent delineation of anatomic detail above the inguinal ligament, and phase images can be used to diagnose the presence or absence of pelvic vein flow. An additional advantage is the ability to image in coronal and sagittal planes. Erdman and coworkers (1990) reported that magnetic resonance imaging was 100 percent sensitive and 90 percent specific for detection of venographically proven deep venous thrombosis in nonpregnant patients. Furthermore, in 44 percent of patients without deep venous thrombosis, they were able to demonstrate nonthrombotic conditions to explain the clinical findings that originally had suggested venous thrombosis. Examples include cellulitis, edema, hematomas, or superficial phlebitis.

Computed-tomographic scanning also may be used to assess these findings. It is more widely available but it requires contrast agents and ionizing radiation.

Pulmonary Embolism

In many cases, but certainly not all, clinical evidence for deep venous thrombosis of the legs precedes pulmonary embolization. In others, especially those that arise from deep pelvic veins, the woman usually is asymptomatic until symptoms of embolization develop (Fig. 20–9). The mortality rate of treated acute pulmonary embolism is about 3 percent, and most of these are fatal within the first week (Carson and associates, 1992). The incidence of pulmonary embolism associated with pregnancy has varied widely and has been reported to be from 1 in 2700 deliveries (Stamm, 1960) to less than 1 in 7000 deliveries (Mengert, 1945). Recent experiences from Parkland Hospital are more consonant with Mengert's earlier observations and indicate that pulmonary embolism is quite uncommon (Cunningham and associates, 1993). In a 2½-year period, during which time nearly 35,000 women gave birth, there were only four cases of pulmonary embolism; two were antepartum and two were postpartum, one immediately after delivery and one 4 weeks later. Unfortunately, the latter woman succumbed to a massive saddle embolism.

Diagnosis

Chest discomfort, shortness of breath, air hunger, tachypnea, or obvious apprehension are signs and symptoms that should alert the physician to a strong likelihood of pulmonary embolism. The most common abnormality in one study was a respiratory rate of greater than 16 per minute (Bell and Simon, 1977). Its frequency was so striking that a lower respiratory rate was felt to exclude the diagnosis. Examination of the chest may yield findings such as an accentuated pulmonic closure sound, rales, or friction rub. Right axis deviation may or may not be evident in the electrocardiogram. Even with massive pulmonary embolism, signs, symptoms, and laboratory data to support the diagnosis of pulmonary embolism may be deceivingly unspecific. In one study pulmonary angiography was used to identify 90 patients with a massive embolism (Wenger and colleagues, 1972). Although at least two lobar arteries were obstructed, the classic triad of hemoptysis, pleuritic chest pain, and dyspnea was noted in only 20 percent.

Controversy still exists regarding the safest, least invasive technique that can accurately diagnose pulmonary embolism. Some investigators believe that **ventilation–perfusion scintigraphy** is adequate. These scans use a small dose of a radioactive agent, usually technetium (Tc^{99m}) macroaggregated albumin administered intravenously. A lung scan may not provide a definite diagnosis because many other conditions—for example, pneumonia or local bronchospasm—can cause perfusion defects. Ventilation scans with inhaled $xenon^{133}$ or $technetium^{99m}$ were added to per-

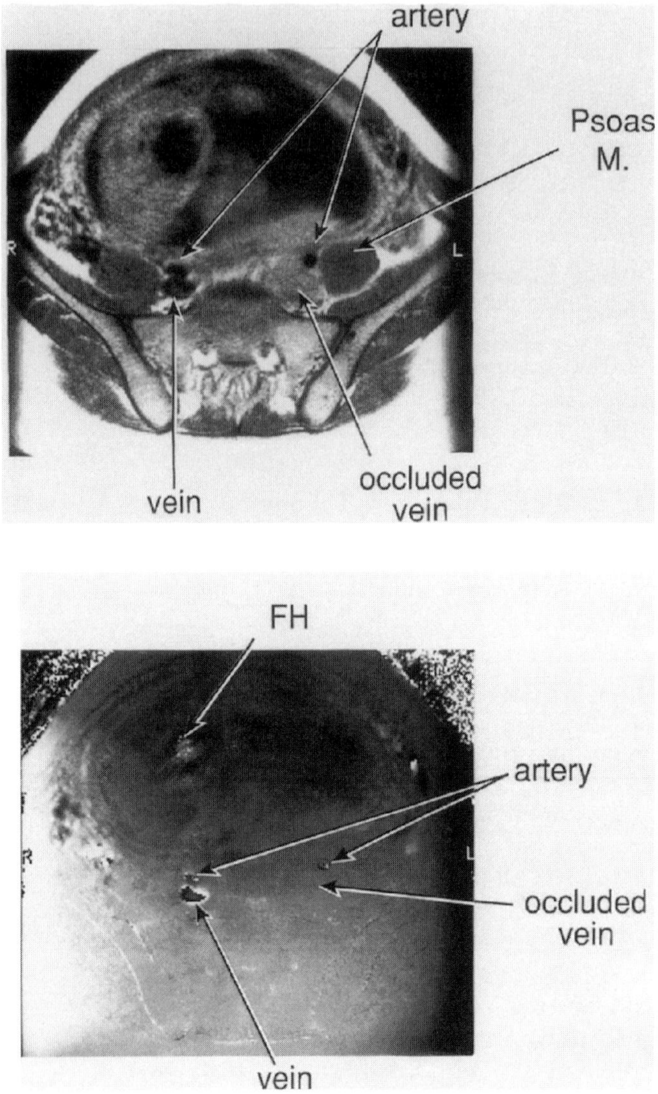

Figure 20–9. Magnetic resonance images through the pelvis of a 26-week pregnant woman who presented with symptoms of pulmonary embolism but without clinically apparent deep venous thrombosis of the lower extremities. Top, T_1-weighted image showing occlusion of left common iliac vein. Bottom, phase image that demonstrates flow and therefore shows right common iliac artery and vein patency, arterial patency on the left, but lack of signal from the occluded left common iliac vein. Because flow is detected by this method, fetal heart motion (FH) is also visualized. (From Cunningham and associates, 1993, with permission; photographs courtesy of Dr. Diane Twickler.)

fusion scans in the hope that ventilation would be abnormal, but perfusion normal, in areas of pneumonia or hypoventilation. Reporting data from the Hamilton District Thromboembolism Programme, Hull and associates (1990b) concluded that ventilation scanning increased the probability of an accurate diagnosis of pulmonary embolus in patients with **large perfusion defects** and **ventilation mismatches,** but that normal ventilation–perfusion was *not* helpful in ruling out pulmonary embolism. They reported that pulmonary angiography was necessary in most patients with perfusion abnormalities because the diagnosis of pulmonary embolism could not be made or excluded with sufficient accuracy in such patients.

Because of these uncertainties, the National Heart, Lung and Blood Institute commissioned the Prospective Investigation of Pulmonary Embolism Diagnosis (PIOPED, 1990). This study was designed to determine the sensitivities and specificities of ventilation–perfusion scans to diagnose pulmonary embolism. This prospective investigation included 933 patients of whom 931 underwent scintigraphy and 755 pulmonary angiography; 33 percent of the 755 patients studied angiographically had pulmonary embolism. While almost all patients with an embolism had abnormal scans of high, intermediate, or low probability, so did most without embolism (sensitivity, 98%; specificity, 10%). Of 116 patients with high-probability scans, 88 percent had an embolism seen on angiography, but only a minority of patients with a pulmonary embolism had a high-probability scan (sensitivity, 41%; specificity, 97%). Of 322 with intermediate-probability scans, 33 percent had an embolism on angiography, and for those with a low-probability scan, the figure was 12 percent. **Importantly, 4 percent of patients with a near normal to normal scan had pulmonary embolism detected by angiography.**

The PIOPED investigators concluded that a high-probability scan usually indicates pulmonary embolism, but that only a small number of patients with emboli have a high-probability scan. A low-probability scan combined with a strong clinical impression that embolism is unlikely makes the possibility of pulmonary embolism remote. Similarly, near-normal or normal scans make the diagnosis very unlikely. Finally, an intermediate-probability scan is of no help in establishing the diagnosis. Thus, the scan combined with clinical assessment permits a noninvasive diagnosis or exclusion of pulmonary embolism for only a minority of patients. Bone (1990) suggested that diagnostic accuracy could be improved by combining the results of ventilation–perfusion scans with noninvasive studies of the deep leg veins. He emphasized that when there is significant doubt, pulmonary angiography should be done. **Because half of pulmonary emboli during pregnancy arise from the pelvic veins, this approach using leg vein studies clearly has limitations.** As discussed previously, magnetic resonance imaging shows great promise for visualizing thromboses arising in pelvic veins (Erdman and colleagues, 1990).

If there is suspicion of pulmonary embolism, most pursue vigorously verification of the clinical diagnosis (Fig. 20–10). Initial evaluation includes a chest radiograph, and if this is not suggestive of another diagnosis, then a ventilation–perfusion lung scan is performed. If the scan is completely normal, this is taken as evidence against embolism, and the workup is considered complete. Conversely, a high-probability scan such as that shown in Figure 20–11, in concert with a chest radiograph showing no corresponding abnormalities, for example, a pneumonic infiltrate, is considered diagnostic of embolization, and therapy is begun. For cases in which the diagnosis is still in doubt after these measures, pulmonary angiography is performed.

Management of Postpartum Thromboembolism

Deep Venous Thrombosis

Treatment of deep venous thrombosis consists of anticoagulation, bed rest, and analgesia.

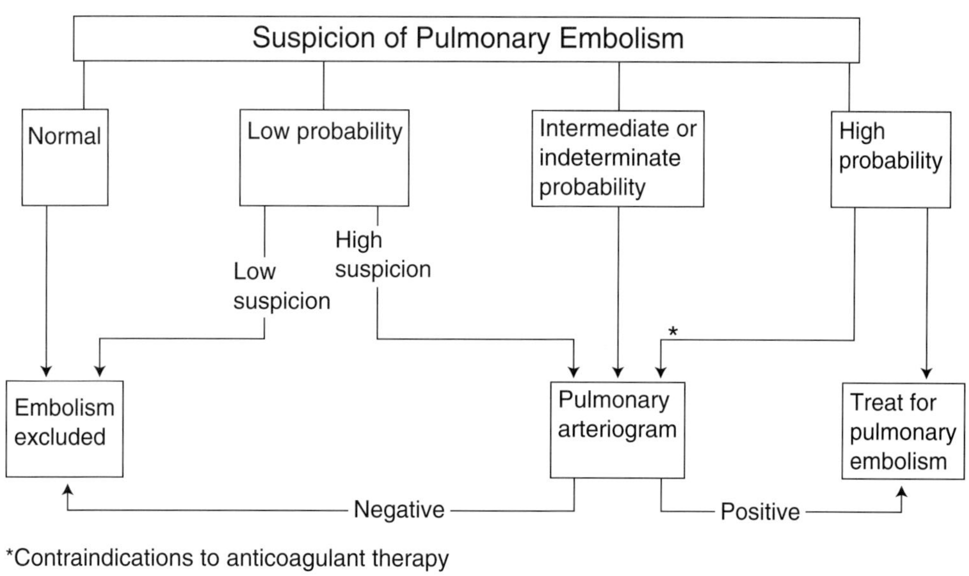

Figure 20–10. Evaluation of possible pulmonary embolism. (Modified from Senior, 1988, with permission.)

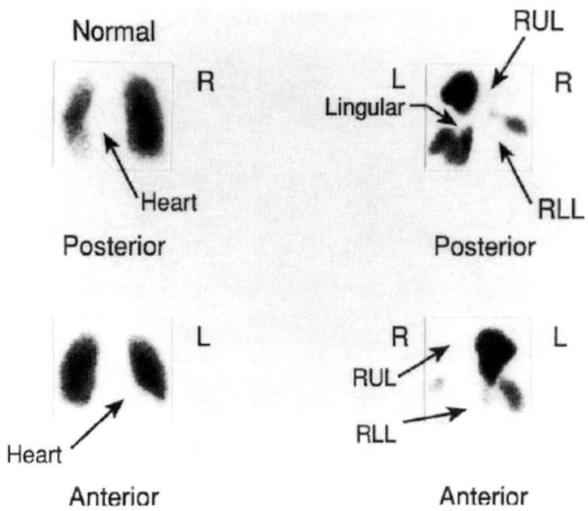

Figure 20–11. Abnormal ventilation–perfusion scintigraphy showing pulmonary emboli compared with a normal scan. Left, anterior-posterior view of normal ventilation scan showing homogeneous distribution of $xenon^{133}$. Right, anterior-posterior view of perfusion scan showing large nonperfused areas (arrows). There is virtually no perfusion of the right upper and lower lobes, and very little perfusion of the right middle lobe. The absence of lingular lobe perfusion is evident on the left side. (From Cunningham and colleagues, 1993, with permission; photographs courtesy of Dr. Diane Twickler.)

Most often, the pain soon is relieved by these measures. After the signs and symptoms have completely abated, graded ambulation should be started with the legs fitted with elastic stockings, and anticoagulation continued. Recovery to this stage usually takes about 7–10 days.

Anticoagulation is achieved initially with intravenous heparin such that the activated partial thromboplastin time is prolonged to 1.5–2.5 times the laboratory control value (Hirsh, 1991a). Hull and co-workers (1986) reported the results of a randomized clinical trial in which they compared continuous intravenous heparin with intermittent subcutaneous heparin for proximal vein thrombosis in 115 nonpregnant patients. Although each group received a total of approximately 30,000 units of heparin per day, most of those given the drug subcutaneously had an initial anticoagulant response below the target range, and importantly, nearly 20 percent had recurrent thromboembolism compared with only 5 percent of those given heparin intravenously. All patients in this study were given warfarin beginning on the sixth or seventh day of heparin therapy, and heparin was continued for a total of 10 days. More recently, the Ontario group (Hull and associates, 1990a) demonstrated that if intravenous heparin and oral warfarin are initiated simultaneously, then heparin can be discontinued safely after only 5 days. Warfarin is contraindicated in antepartum patients.

Low-Molecular-Weight Heparin

Clinical experience with low-molecular-weight heparin has accrued over the past decade (Fejgin and Lourwood, 1994). This is a family of derivatives of commercial heparin that average about 4000–5000 daltons compared with about 12,000–16,000 daltons for conventional heparin. One such preparation, *logipram*, was shown safe and effective for treatment of proximal-vein thrombosis in nonpregnant patients (Hull and co-workers, 1992). Various other preparations, all of which are pharmacologically unique, have been shown effective in preventing and treating deep-vein thrombosis, but with fewer bleeding complications. Other advantages are daily administration and that certain of these subcutaneously administered drugs do not have to be monitored (Hull and Pineo, 1992). Their use in pregnant women has been limited. Gillis and associates (1992) described six pregnant women given *enoxaparim.*

Pulmonary Embolism

Treatment for pulmonary embolism is similar to that for deep venous thrombosis, but with less well-documented results. In general, heparin is given in a similar fashion for deep venous thrombosis or pulmonary embolism, whether antepartum or postpartum. Considerable controversy exists as to which regimen is best, and several are widely used, effective, and considered acceptable (Mohr and colleagues, 1988; Weiner, 1985). Heparin commonly is administered by continuous intravenous infusion, and most recommend starting with a dose of 1000 U/hour after an initial bolus dose of 5000–10,000 U. Intermittent intravenous injections of 5000 U every 4 hours or 7500 U every 6 hours are preferred by others. Finally, heparin may be given subcutaneously in doses of 10,000 U every 8 hours or 20,000 U every 12 hours. The common theme of these regimens is that the total daily heparin dose is between 25,000 and 40,000 U. Although low-dose heparin has been used to treat deep-vein thrombosis and to prevent thromboembolism, its use with documented pulmonary embolism is limited (Hull and Pineo, 1992).

The most serious complication with any of these regimens is hemorrhage, which is more likely if there has been recent surgery or lacerations, such as with delivery. Troublesome bleeding also is more likely if the heparin dosage is excessive. Conversely, thrombus extension or embolization is more likely if heparin dosage is inadequate. Unfortunately, many management schemes using laboratory testing to identify whether heparin dosage is sufficient to inhibit further thrombosis, yet not cause serious hemorrhage, have been discouraging (Moser, 1991).

Whole blood clotting times have long been used and more recently measurement of the plasma partial thromboplastin time has been popularized. The two tests often correlate poorly. An important test that will aid in detecting hemorrhage is the frequent measurement of the hematocrit. Clinical improvement without hemorrhage is the desired goal. It is important to remember that heparin is being administered whenever blood is to be drawn or medications are ordered to be given parenterally. Serious hemorrhage may occur, especially when arterial blood is drawn for blood gas analyses.

Therapy with heparin as described may be discontinued in the postpartum woman after 10 days to 2 weeks if the disease process has clearly abated and there is no evidence of underlying chronic venous abnormalities that would predispose to venous thrombosis and no evidence of underlying cardiopulmonary dysfunction. If a switch to warfarin therapy is planned, heparin is discontinued after the prothrombin time is considered therapeutically prolonged (Gallus and colleagues, 1986).

Long-Term Therapy

During the past several years, considerable controversy has arisen concerning the most effective agent and its duration of use for long-term therapy to prevent recurrent thromboembolism (Hirsh, 1991a,b). In nonpregnant patients, Hull and co-workers (1982a) reported that heparin was as effective as oral warfarin when heparin was administered subcutaneously every 12 hours with the dose adjusted to prolong the activated partial thromboplastin time to 1.5 times the control value when measured 6 hours after injection. Furthermore, heparin therapy was associated with a lower risk of bleeding. Subsequently, Hull and colleagues (1982b) reported that by decreasing the dosage of warfarin, bleeding complications could be reduced to the level achieved with heparin and yet the effectiveness of the two agents remained comparable.

Warfarin is the drug of choice for long-term treatment or prophylaxis in the postpartum period when consideration is given to the cost of heparin, the problem of administration, and the possibility of heparin-induced thrombocytopenia or osteoporosis (Hirsh, 1991a). The exact incidence of these latter two with heparin use is unclear. Thrombocytopenia probably occurs in less than 6 percent of patients given porcine heparin, while osteoporosis appears to be associated with heparin doses of greater than 20,000 U/day for periods longer than 6 months (Hirsch, 1991a).

Vena Caval Filters

In the very infrequent circumstances where heparin therapy fails to prevent recurrent pulmonary embolism from the pelvis or legs, or when embolism develops from these sites despite heparin given for their treatment, then vena caval interruption is indicated. In the past, vena caval ligation or plication was preferred; however, this procedure, which requires extensive surgical dissection in an area that is highly vascular during pregnancy and the puerperium, has been replaced largely by use of a **vena caval filter.** Greenfield and Michna (1988) recommend suprarenal placement during pregnancy and Hux and colleagues (1986) described the use of the Greenfield filter in five pregnant women and another who was 3 days postpartum. Their indications for filter placement, which is inserted through either the jugular or femoral vein, were bleeding, thrombocytopenia, or recurrent embolization in women who were anticoagulated with heparin.

Good experiences have been reported with the use of a **bird's nest filter,** such as that shown in Figure 20–12. In a multi-institutional trial, Roehm and colleagues (1988) described its use in 568 nonpregnant patients at risk for pulmonary embolism. The prevalence of clinically suspected recurrent embolism was 2.7 percent and that of inferior vena caval occlusion was 2.9 percent.

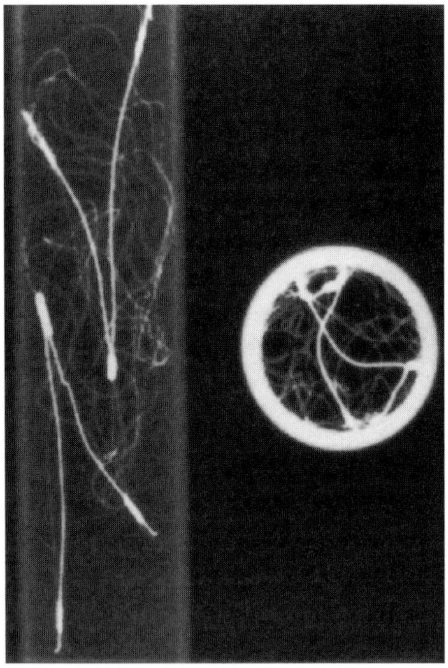

Figure 20–12. Lateral and axial radiographs of modified bird's-nest filter, which has been placed into a 2.5-cm-diameter plastic tube. (From Roehm and colleagues, 1988, with permission.)

SUMMARY

Women undergoing cesarean delivery may develop a number of postoperative complications that occur in any patient undergoing major surgery. Fortunately, serious complications are uncommon. When they occur, prompt recognition and treatment combined with the usual good health of these young women result in a salutary outcome. Persistent fever postoperatively may be due to aspiration pneumonitis, urinary infections, or peritonitis, but in most cases is due to pelvic infection. Serious complications of these infections may ensue. These include incisional wound infections—sometimes with dehiscence—as well as pelvic and intraabdominal abscesses. Another important and potentially life-threatening complication is deep venous thrombosis, which may lead to pulmonary embolization.

REFERENCES

American College of Obstetricians and Gynecologists. Antimicrobial therapy for obstetric patients. Tech Bull No. 117, June 1988.

Atrash HK, Koonin LM, Lawson HW, et al. Maternal mortality in the United States, 1979–1986. Obstet Gynecol 1990; 76:1055.

Barss VA, Schwartz PA, Green MF, et al. Use of the subcutaneous heparin pump during pregnancy. J Reprod Med 1985; 30:899.

Bartlett JG, Gorbach SL, Finegold SM. The bacteriology of aspiration pneumonia. Am J Med 1974; 56:202.

Beischer NA, MacKay EV. Color Atlas of Gynecology. Sydney: W.B. Saunders, 1981:167.

Bell WR, Simon TL, DeMets DL. The clinical features of submassive and massive pulmonary emboli. Am J Med 1977; 62:355.

Bergqvist A, Bergqvist D, Hallbook T. Deep vein thrombosis during pregnancy. A prospective study. Acta Obstet Gynecol Scand 1983; 62:443.

Bone RC. Ventilation/perfusion scan in pulmonary embolism. "The emperor is incompletely attired." JAMA 1990; 263:2794.

Brown CEL, Dunn DH, Harrell R, et al. Computed tomography for evaluation of puerperal infections. Surg Gynecol Obstet 1991; 172:285.

Burchman CA. Maternal aspiration. In: Ostheimer GW, ed. Manual of Obstetric Anesthesia. 2nd ed. New York: Churchill Livingstone, 1992:161.

Bynum LJ, Pierce AK. Pulmonary aspiration of gastric contents. Am Rev Respir Dis 1976; 114:1129.

Carson JL, Kelley MA, Duff A, et al. The clinical course on pulmonary embolism. N Engl J Med 1992; 326:1240.

Cone LA, Woodard DR, Schlievert PM, Tomory GS. Clinical and bacteriologic observations of a toxic shock-like syndrome due to *Streptococcus pyogenes*. N Engl J Med 1987; 317:146.

Crowther C. Magnesium sulphate versus diazepam in the management of eclampsia: a randomized controlled trial. Br J Obstet Gynaecol 1990; 97:110.

Cunningham FG, Hauth JC, Strong JD, Kappus SS. Infectious morbidity following cesarean: comparison of two treatment regimens. Obstet Gynecol 1978; 52:656.

Cunningham FG, MacDonald PC, Gant NF, et al. Williams Obstetrics, 19th ed. Norwalk, CT: Appleton & Lange, 1993.

DePalma RT, Cunningham FG, Leveno KJ, Roark ML. Continuing investigation of women at high risk for infection following cesarean delivery. Obstet Gynecol 1982; 60:53.

Dinsmoor MJ, Newton ER, Gibbs RS. A randomized, double-blind placebo-controlled trial of oral antibiotic therapy following intravenous antibiotic therapy for postpartum endometritis. Obstet Gynecol 1991; 77:60.

diZerega G, Yonekura L, Roy S, et al. A comparison of clindamycin-gentamicin and penicillin-gentamicin in the treatment of post-cesarean section endomyometritis. Am J Obstet Gynecol 1979; 134:238.

Dotters DJ, Katz VL. Streptococcal toxic shock

associated with septic abortion. Obstet Gynecol 1991; 78:549.

Emmons SL, Krohn M, Jackson M, Eschenbach DA. Development of wound infections among women undergoing cesarean section. Obstet Gynecol 1988; 72:559.

Erdman WA, Jayson HT, Redman HC, et al. Deep venous thrombosis of extremities: role of MR imaging in the diagnosis. Radiology 1990; 174:425.

Faro S. Soft tissue infections. In: Gilstrap LC, Faro S, eds. Infections in Pregnancy. New York: Wiley-Liss, 1990:75.

Fejgin MD, Lourwood DL. Low molecular weight heparins and their use in obstetrics and gynecology. Obstet Gynecol Surv 1994; 49:424.

Filker R, Monif GRG. The significance of temperature during the first 24 hours postpartum. Obstet Gynecol 1979; 53:359.

Gallup DG, Nolan TE, Smith RP. Primary mass closure of midline incisions with a continuous polyglyconate monofilament absorbable suture. Obstet Gynecol 1990; 76:872.

Gallus A, Jackaman J, Tillett J, et al. Safety and efficacy of warfarin started early after submassive venous thrombosis or pulmonary embolism. Lancet 1986; 2:1293.

Gibbs RS, O'Dell TN, MacGregor RR, et al. Puerperal endometritis: a prospective microbiologic study. Am J Obstet Gynecol 1975; 121:919.

Gibbs CP, Schwartz DJ, Wynne JW, et al. Antacid pulmonary aspiration in the dog. Anesthesiology 1979; 51:380.

Gibbs CP, Banner TC. Effectiveness of Bicitra I Pr as a preoperative antacid. Anesthesiology 1984; 61:97.

Gibbs RS. Microbiology of the female genital tract. Am J Obstet Gynecol 1987; 156:491.

Gillis S, Shushan A, Eldor A. Use of low molecular weight heparin for prophylaxis and treatment of thromboembolism in pregnancy. Int J Gynecol Obstet 1992; 39:297.

Gilstrap LC III, Cunningham FG. The bacterial pathogenesis of infection following cesarean section. Obstet Gynecol 1979; 53:545.

Ginsberg JS, Brill-Edwards P, Burrows RF, et al. Venous thrombosis during pregnancy: Leg and trimester of presentation. Thromb Haemost 1992; 67:519.

Greenfield LJ, Michna BA. Twelve-year clinical experience with the Greenfield vena caval filter. Surgery 1988; 104:706.

Grimes DA. The morbidity and mortality of pregnancy: Still risky business. Am J Obstet Gynecol 1994; 170:1489.

Heijboer H, Brandjes DPM, Buller HR, et al. Deficiencies of coagulation-inhibiting and fibrinolytic proteins in outpatients with deep-vein thrombosis. N Engl J Med 1990; 323:1512.

Hellgren M, Trenhgborn L, Abildgaard U. Pregnancy in women with congenital antithrombin III deficiency: Experience of treatment with heparin and antithrombin. Gynecol Obstet Invest 1989; 14:127.

Henderson SR, Lund CJ, Creasman WT. Antepartum pulmonary embolism. Am J Obstet Gynecol 1972; 112:476.

Hirsh J. Heparin. N Engl J Med 1991a; 324:1565.

Hirsh J. Oral anticoagulant drugs. N Engl J Med 1991b; 324:1865.

Hite KE, Hesseltine HC, Goldstein L. A study of the bacterial flora of the normal and pathologic vagina and uterus. Am J Obstet Gynecol 1947; 53:233.

Hodgkinson R, Bhatt M, Kim SS, et al. Neonatal neurobehavioral tests following cesarean section under general and spinal anesthesia. Am J Obstet Gynecol 1978; 132:670.

Hodgkinson R, Glassenberg R, Joyce TH, et al. Comparison of cimetidine (Tagamet) with antacid for safety and effectiveness in reducing gastric acidity before elective cesarean section. Anesthesiology 1983; 59:86.

Huisman MV, Büller HR, Ten Cate JW, Vreeken J. Serial impedance plethysmography for suspected deep venous thrombosis in outpatients: The Amsterdam general practitioner study. N Engl J Med 1986; 314:823.

Hull R, Delmore T, Carter C, et al. Adjusted subcutaneous heparin versus warfarin sodium in the long-term treatment of venous thrombosis. N Engl J Med 1982a; 306:189.

Hull R, Hirsh J, Jay R, et al. Different intensities of oral anticoagulant therapy in the treatment of proximal-vein thrombosis. N Engl J Med 1982b; 307:1676.

Hull R, Hirsh J, Carter CJ, et al. Diagnostic efficacy of impedance plethysmography for clinically suspected deep-vein thrombosis: A randomized trial. Ann Intern Med 1985; 102:21.

Hull RD, Rascob GE, Hirsh J, et al. Continuous intravenous heparin compared with intermittant subcutaneous heparin in the initial treatment of proximal-vein thrombosis. N Engl J Med 1986; 315:1109.

Hull RD, Raskob GE, Carter CJ. Serial impedance plethysmography in pregnant patients with clinically suspected deep-vein thrombosis. Clinical validity of negative findings. Ann Intern Med 1990a; 112:664.

Hull RD, Raskob GE, Rosenbloom D, et al. Heparin for 5 days as compared with 10 days in the initial treatment of proximal venous thrombosis. N Engl J Med 1990b; 322:1260.

Hull RD, Raskob GE, Pineo GF, et al. Subcutaneous low-molecular-weight heparin compared with continuous intravenous heparin in the treatment of proximal-vein thrombosis. N Engl J Med 1992; 326:975.

Hull RD, Pineo GF. Treatment of venous thromboembolism with low molecular weight heparins. Hematology/Concology Clin North Am 1992; 6:1095.

Hux CH, Wapner RJ, Chayen B, et al. Use of the Greenfield filter for thromboembolic disease in pregnancy. Am J Obstet Gynecol 1986; 155:734.

Jewett JF, Reid DE, Safon LE, Easterday CL. Childbed fever: A continuing entity. JAMA 1968; 206:344.

Kaunitz AM, Hughes JM, Grimes DA, et al. Causes of maternal mortality in the United States. Obstet Gynecol 1985; 65:605.

Lensing AWA, Prandoni P, Brandjes D, et al. Detection of deep-vein thrombosis by real-time B-mode ultrasonography. N Engl J Med 1989; 320:342.

Lev-Toaff AS, Baka JJ, Toaff ME, et al. Diagnostic imaging in puerperal febrile morbidity. Obstet Gynecol 1991; 78:50.

Lewis M, Crawford JS. Can one risk fasting the obstetric patient for less than 4 hours? Br J Anaesth 1987; 59:312.

McHenry CR, Brandt CP, Protrowski JJ, et al. Idiopathic necrotizing fasciitis: Recognition, incidence, and outcome of therapy. Am Surg 1994; 60:490.

Mendelson CL. The aspiration of stomach contents into the lungs during obstetric anesthesia. Am J Obstet Gynecol 1946; 52:191.

Mengert WF. Venous ligation in obstetrics. Am J Obstet Gynecol 1945; 50:467.

Mohr DN, Rhu JH, Litin SC, Rosenow EC III. Recent advances in the management of venous thromboembolism. Mayo Clin Proc 1988; 63:281.

Moir DD. Cimetidine, antacids, and pulmonary aspiration. J Anesthesiol 1983; 59:81.

Moser KM. Pulmonary thromboembolism. In: Wilson JD, Braunwald E, Isselbacher JK, et al, eds. Harrison's Principles of Internal Medicine. 12th ed. New York: McGraw-Hill, 1991:1090, Chap 213.

National Institutes of Health Consensus Development Conference. Prevention of venous thrombosis and pulmonary embolism. JAMA 1986; 256:744.

Nolan TE, King LA, Smith RP, Gallup DC. Necrotizing surgical infection and necrotizing fasciitis in obstetrics and gynecology. So Med J 1994; 86:1363.

PIOPED Investigators. Value of the ventilation/perfusion scan in acute pulmonary embolism: results of the Prospective Investigation of Pulmonary Embolism Diagnosis (PIOPED). JAMA 1990; 263:2753.

Polak JF, Wilkinson DL. Ultrasonographic diagnosis of symptomatic deep venous thrombosis in pregnancy. Am J Obstet Gynecol 1991; 165:625.

Roberts J, Barnes W, Pennock M, Browne G. Diagnostic accuracy of fever as a measure of postoperative pulmonary complications. Heart Lung 1988; 17:166.

Roehm JOF, Johnsrude IS, Barth MH, Gianturco C. The bird's nest inferior vena cava filter. Progress report. Radiology 1988; 168:745.

Sachs BP, Brown DA, Driscoll SG, et al. Maternal mortality in Massachusetts: trends and prevention. N Engl J Med 1987; 316:667.

Scott LM, Zawin ML, Taylor KJW. Doppler US. Part II: Clinical applications. Radiology 1990; 174:310.

Senior RM. Pulmonary disease. In: Wyngaarden JB, Smith LH Jr, eds. Cecil Textbook of Medicine. Philadelphia: Saunders, 1988:445.

Shy KK, Eschenbach DA. Fatal perineal cellulitis from an episiotomy site. Obstet Gynecol 1979; 52:293.

Soper DE, Brockwell WJ, Dalton HP. The importance of wound infection in antibiotic failures in the therapy of postpartum endometritis. Surg Gynecol Obstet 1992; 174:265.

Stamenkovic I, Lew PD. Early recognition of potentially fatal necrotizing fascitis: the use of frozen-section biopsy. N Engl J Med 1984; 310:1689.

Stamm H. Obstetrical and gynecological mortality due to embolism in Central Europe and Scandinavia. Geburtshilfe Frauenheilkd 1960; 20:675.

Sutherland AD, Stock JG, Davies JM. Effects of preoperative fasting on morbidity and gastric contents in patients undergoing day-stay surgery. Br J Anaesth 1986; 58:876.

Sutton GP, Smirz LR, Clark DH, Bennett JE. Group B streptococcal necrotizing fasciitis arising from an episiotomy. Obstet Gynecol 1985; 66:733.

Taylor G, Pryse-Davies J. The prophylactic use of antacids in the prevention of the acid pulmonary aspiration syndrome. Lancet 1966; 1:288.

Teabeaut JR II. Aspiration of gastric contents: an experimental study. Am J Pathol 1952; 28:51.

Thompson CD, Brekken AL, Kutteh WH. Necrotizing fasciitis: A review of management guidelines in a large obstetrics and gynecology teaching hospital. Infec Dis Obstet Gynecol 1993; 1:16.

Thorburn J, Moir DD. Antacid therapy for emergency cesarean sections. Anesthesia 1987; 42:352.

Trauscht-Van Horn JJ, Capeless EL, Easterling TR, Bovill EG. Pregnancy loss and thrombosis with protein C deficiency. Am J Obstet Gynecol 1992; 167:968.

Twickler DM, Setiawan AT, Harrell RS, Brown CEL. CT appearance of the pelvis after cesarean section. Am J Radiol 1991; 156:523.

Walmer D, Walmer KR, Gibbs RS. Enterococci in post-cesarean endometritis. Obstet Gynecol 1988; 71:159.

Walters MD, Dombroski RA, Davidson SA, et al. Reclosure of disrupted abdominal incisions. Obstet Gynecol 1990; 76:597.

Weiner CP. Diagnosis and management of thromboembolic disease during pregnancy. Clin Obstet Gynecol 1985; 28:107.

Wenger NK, Stein PD, Willis PW III. Massive acute

pulmonary embolism: the deceivingly nonspecific manifestations. JAMA 1972; 220:843.
Wetchler SJ, Dunn LJ. Ovarian abscess. Report of a case and a review of the literature. Obstet Gynecol Surv 1985; 40:476.
Wheatley RG, Kallus FT, Reynolds RC, Giesecke AH. Milk of magnesia is an effective pre-induction antacid in obstetrical anesthesia. Anesthesiology 1979; 50:514.
Wheeless CR. Atlas of Pelvic Surgery. 2nd ed. Philadelphia: Lea & Febiger, 1988; 375.
Whitted RW, Yeomans ER, Hankins GDV. Group A β-hemolytic streptococcus as a cause of toxic shock. A case report. J Reprod Med 1990; 35:558.
Yau G, Kan AF, Gin T, Oh TE. A comparison of omeprazole and ranitidine for prophylaxis against aspiration pneumonitis in emergency cesarean section. Anesthesia 1992; 47:2.

CHAPTER 21

Evaluation of the Surgical Abdomen

Abdominal surgical illnesses complicating pregnancy require the interaction of the obstetrician, surgeon, anesthesiologist, and frequently the internist, as well as other subspecialists and superspecialists. Because pregnancy does not make a woman immune to any disease, the obstetrician must have a working knowledge of common surgical diseases that may befall women during childbearing years. Likewise, nonobstetricians should be familiar with the effects that medical and surgical diseases have on the pregnant woman, or vice versa. Importantly, normal pregnancy-induced physiologic changes must be interpreted vis-à-vis their effects on underlying nonobstetric disorders. Changes induced by pregnancy in many laboratory tests should also be considered.

The purpose of this chapter is to review generalizations concerning the interaction of pregnancy with some of the more common surgical abdominal diseases and to suggest a rational approach to their management along with the care of the woman and her pregnancy. A commonly recurring theme will be that a woman should never be penalized **because** she is pregnant. Put another way: If a proposed medical or surgical regimen is different simply because the woman is pregnant, then can this be justified? This approach still allows individualization of care for most surgical disorders that complicate pregnancy and should always be remembered, especially when dealing with the myriad consultants who often are asked to see these women.

EFFECT OF SURGERY AND ANESTHESIA ON PREGNANCY OUTCOME

If complications of the surgical disorders per se are taken into account, there is very little evidence to suggest that an otherwise technically uncomplicated surgical and anesthetic procedure will increase adverse pregnancy outcome. For example, complications from perforative appendicitis with gross peritonitis are associated with increased maternal and perinatal morbidity and mortality even if surgical procedures and anesthetic management are flawless. Contrariwise, if these procedures themselves have complications, then these can adversely affect pregnancy outcome. For example, if the woman who undergoes uncomplicated surgery for appendicitis suffers vomiting with aspiration of acidic gastric contents, then resulting respiratory failure may cause fetal death, preterm labor, or both, as well as significant maternal morbidity and even mortality.

Mazze and Källén (1989) studied the effects of 5405 nonobstetric surgical procedures performed in 720,000 pregnant Swedish

TABLE 21–1. TYPES OF NONOBSTETRIC OPERATIONS IN 5405 SWEDISH WOMEN

Type of Operation	Percent of Procedures by Trimester			Total	Percent
	First (*n* = 2252)	*Second* (*n* = 1881)	*Third* (*n* = 1272)	(*n* = 5405)	
Central nervous system	7	6	6	323	6
Head and neck	8	6	10	419	8
Heart and lung	0.7	0.8	0.6	40	0.7
Abdominal	20	30	23	1331	25
Gynecologic and urologic	11	23	24	1008	19
Laparoscopy	34	1.2	6	868	16
Orthopedic	9	9	14	558	10
Endoscopy	4	11	9	406	8
Skin	4	3	4	202	4
Others	4	4	6	250	5

Adapted from Mazze and Källén (1989).

women from 1973 to 1981. Surgery was performed most commonly in the first trimester—41 percent compared with 35 percent in the middle trimester and 24 percent in the third. Shown in Table 21–1 are the most common operations listed by trimester. Abdominal surgery comprised a fourth of all operations and another 19 percent were accounted for by gynecologic and urologic procedures. Laparoscopic procedures were done in 16 percent of these women with almost 90 percent being done in the first trimester. While laparoscopy was the most commonly performed first-trimester operation, appendectomy was the most common procedure in the second trimester.

The types of anesthesia administered to these 5405 women are given in Table 21–2. Over half of these procedures were done using general anesthesia, and in 98 percent of these, nitrous oxide supplemented by another inhalation agent or intravenous medication was used.

To determine the effects of these diseases and their surgical and anesthetic managements in pregnancy outcome, these 5405 pregnancies in the Swedish report were compared with the total database of 720,000 pregnancies for the 9-year period. As shown in Table 21–3, there was a significantly increased incidence of low-birthweight and preterm infants as well as neonatal deaths by 7 days in these women who had undergone surgery. Importantly, the stillbirth and congenital malformation rates were not increased significantly. Mazze and Källén concluded that nonobstetrical surgery

TABLE 21–2. TYPES OF ANESTHESIA FOR SURGERY IN 5405 PREGNANT WOMEN

Types of Anesthesia	Percent by Trimester			Total	Percent
	First (2252)	*Second* (1881)	*Third* (1272)		
General	65	51	41	2929	54
Spinal or epidural	3	5	6	255	5
Infiltration	4	6	6	278	5
Nerve block	1	2	3	114	2
Topical	1	2	3	55	1
Unknown	25	34	41	1732	32

Adapted from Mazze and Källén (1989).

TABLE 21–3. BIRTH OUTCOMES IN 5405 PREGNANT WOMEN UNDERGOING NONOBSTETRIC SURGERY

Birth Outcome	Trimester (Observed/Expected)			Total	Significance
	First	*Second*	*Third*		
Stillborn	1.1	1.7	1.5	1.4	N.S.
Death by 7 days	1.4	3.2	1.9	2.1	$p<.05$
Congenital malformation	1.0	0.9	1.5	1.1	N.S.
Birthweight < 1500 g	1.7	3.2	1.5	2.2	$p<.05$
Birthweight < 2500 g	1.4	1.8	2.2	2.0	$p<.05$

Adapted from Mazze and Källén (1989).

during pregnancy is not without hazard. They attributed excessive perinatal morbidity to the disease itself rather than to adverse effects of surgery and anesthesia.

PHYSIOLOGIC CHANGES OF THE GASTROINTESTINAL TRACT DURING PREGNANCY

During normal pregnancy the gastrointestinal tract and its appendages undergo anatomic and functional changes that can alter appreciably the criteria for diagnosis and treatment of several diseases to which they are susceptible. For example, nausea and vomiting are frequent symptoms early in normal pregnancy, but if these symptoms are erroneously attributed to normal physiologic changes, then gastrointestinal disease can be overlooked. Conversely, persistent nausea and vomiting in late pregnancy always should prompt a search for underlying pathology. In another example, heartburn is reported in half of women at some time during pregnancy, especially in late gestation. **During advanced pregnancy, symptoms of gastrointestinal disease become difficult to assess and physical findings are greatly obtunded by the large uterus and its contents.**

The small bowel has diminished motility during pregnancy. Parry and associates (1970) showed that small intestinal transit time was about 60 hours in women 12–20 weeks pregnant compared with 52 hours in nonpregnant controls. They showed that the colon undergoes muscular relaxation as well, and this was accompanied by increased absorption of water and sodium. Both of these predispose to constipation. According to Anderson and Whichelow (1985), almost 40 percent of women complain of constipation at some time during pregnancy, and 20 percent do so in the third trimester. While symptoms usually are only mildly bothersome, pregnant women occasionally are encountered who developed megacolon from impacted stool. Although these latter women almost invariably have abused stimulatory laxatives, Sheld (1987) described a woman with recurrent megacolon during pregnancy related to **Hirschsprung disease.** Preventative measures include a high-fiber diet along with prescription of bulk-forming laxatives when there is mild constipation.

Most obstetricians, but not most internists or surgeons, are aware that upper abdominal pain—epigastric or right upper quadrant—can be an ominous sign of severe preeclampsia. An ultrasonic examination negative for gallstones or a normal serum amylase value do not serve to exclude serious disease, but rather may support the diagnosis of severe preeclampsia or eclampsia.

While many gastrointestinal disorders are best managed by medical treatment, laparotomy and surgical treatment may be lifesaving for certain conditions, a common example being acute appendicitis. Nearly 1 of every 500–1000 pregnant women will undergo laparotomy. Cited previously were the Swedish data reported by Mazze and Källén (1989). Abdominal surgery was performed in 1,331 of 720,000 pregnancies—about 1 in every 500 pregnancies. Allen and colleagues (1989) reported that they performed abdominal sur-gery in 90 women during nearly 41,500 pregnancies cared for at their institution over a 17-year period. At Parkland Hospital during 1989 through 1991, 62 abdominal operations unrelated to pregnancy were carried out in nearly 45,000 pregnant women (Cunningham and associates, 1993). While about half of these were for adnexal masses, most of the remainder were for gastrointestinal lesions.

DIAGNOSTIC TECHNIQUES

Confirmative diagnosis of most gastrointestinal lesions cannot be made by physical examination alone. Gastrointestinal radiography usually is avoided during pregnancy. The advent of fiberoptic endoscopic instruments for examination of the upper gastrointestinal tract as well as the colon has revolutionized the diagnosis and management of many of these conditions. Endoscopy particularly is well-suited for use in the pregnant woman. **Upper gastrointestinal endoscopy** permits evaluation of the esophagus, stomach, and duodenum. With specialized instruments, the proximal jejunum can be studied, and the ampulla of Vater can be cannulated to perform retrograde cholangiopancreatography. **Colonoscopy** is used to view the entire colon and the distal ileum and is invaluable in diagnosis and management of inflammatory bowel disease. Diagnostic and therapeutic uses of gastrointestinal endoscopy were reviewed by Morrissey and Reichelderfer (1991).

A variety of sophisticated noninvasive imaging modalities occupy a preeminent role in medicine and serve as invaluable aids to diagnosis and treatment. Advances in technology have allowed improved image quality and resolution, and consequently, indications and potential applications for these procedures constantly are increasing. Obviously, caution is observed when obtaining imaging studies during pregnancy to protect the developing embryo-fetus from potential harmful effects. In all cases, imaging during pregnancy should provide the best diagnostic test with the least harmful effect on the developing conceptus. Radiation hazards of some techniques are considered potentially too harmful, and they are thus proscribed for use in the pregnant woman.

Techniques used to evaluate gastrointestinal diseases include **ultrasonography,** which has a crucial role in evaluation of some of these diseases, especially those involving the gallbladder. Although frequently useful, **computed tomography** must be limited in its application because of radiation exposure. **Magnetic resonance imaging** has proved invaluable for evaluating the abdomen and retroperitoneal space during pregnancy. The principal drawback of this technique is its great expense and limited availability.

The limitations of these techniques must be realized, along with the knowledge that their use during pregnancy for evaluation of many gastrointestinal disorders has not been validated. However, while none of these procedures should be considered routine during pregnancy, they likewise should not be withheld if indicated.

Ionizing Radiation

When discussing ionizing radiation, the most important image is the x-ray image. X-rays are very short wavelengths on the electromagnetic spectrum that behave as bundles of energy called **photons** (Curry and colleagues, 1990). Ionization refers to the ability of x-rays to excite atoms by detaching electrons as the x-rays pass through a substance. There are several methods to measure the effects of x-ray. Standard terms used are the **exposure** in air, measured in Roentgens, the **dose** to tissue in rads, and the **relative effective dose** to tissue measured in rems. For diagnostic x-rays, the dose that is expressed in **rad** and the relative effective dose that is expressed in **rem** are the same, and these units can be used interchangeably. For the sake of consistency, all doses subsequently discussed are expressed in traditional units of rad or rem instead of their modern units, **Gray (Gy)** or **Sievert (Sv).**

Dosimetry

Dosimetry refers to the assignment of dose from the ionizing radiation of a particular study. The dose is calculated based on many factors, including the type of study, type of equipment, distance of organ in question from the source of radiation, thickness of body part penetrated, and individual methods of the radiologist performing the study (Wagner and associates, 1985). Because of the tremendous variability of these factors, assignment of an average dose is imprecise (Taylor and co-workers, 1979).

Fetal Risk of Ionizing Radiation

The harmful effects of ionizing radiation can be direct or indirect with three principal biologic effects: (1) cell killing, which affects embryogenesis, (2) carcinogenesis secondary to mutation activation of an oncogene, and (3) genetic effects secondary to mutation in a germ cell (Brent, 1989; Committee on Biological Effects, 1990; Hall, 1991). The harmful fetal effects of ionizing radiation have been studied extensively in the case of cell damage with resultant dysfunction of embryogenesis, both in the animal model and in human studies of Japanese atomic bomb survivors (Committee on Biological Effects, 1990; Gaulden and Murry, 1980).

At 8–15 weeks' gestation, the embryo is most susceptible to radiation-induced mental retardation. This risk is probably a nonthreshold linear function of dose with the following incidence of severe mental retardation: 4 percent at 10 rad, 20 percent at 50 rad, 40 percent at 100 rad, and 60 percent at 150 rad (Committee on Biological Effects, 1990; Hall, 1991).

The American College of Radiology holds the official view that no single diagnostic procedure results in a radiation dose that threatens the well-being of the developing embryo or fetus (Hall, 1991). Cumulative doses from multiple procedures, however, may enter that harmful range, especially at 8–15 weeks' gestation. At 16–25 weeks, the risk is less, and there is no proven risk in humans at 0–8 weeks or at greater than 25 weeks (Committee on Biological Effects, 1990).

Plain X-ray Films

To put the fetal risk into perspective, it is important to consider the dosimetry of x-ray procedures, realizing that the average is a crude estimate. The dose for some commonly used standard plain film x-rays is shown in Table 21–4.

Fluoroscopy and Angiography

Assignment of dosimetry for fluoroscopic and angiographic procedures is much more difficult because of variations in the number of x-ray films obtained, fluoroscopy time, and the percentage of fluoroscopy time the fetus is in the radiation field. Some of these values are given in Table 21–5, and their range is quite variable.

Computed Axial Tomography

This has become an important imaging modality for evaluation of most organ systems. Simply put, computed tomography involves multiple exposures of very thin x-ray beams in a 360° circle with computerized interpretations of these exposures. The result is an axial (and occasionally sagittal) image of a portion of the body, referred to as a **slice.** Multiple slices of the targeted body part are obtained along the length of the entire organ or of the area in question. For example, routine cranial tomography is performed with 10–15 slices, each 10 mm thick, to show the entire brain in an axial projection. Many variables in a given tomographic study will affect the calculations of radiation doses, especially the slice thickness and number of slices obtained. If a study is performed with and without contrast, twice as many images are obtained over the target area; therefore, the dose to that area is doubled.

Newer generation tomographic equipment is more sensitive and flexible than older systems. When compared with less directed x-ray

TABLE 21–4. DOSE OF THE UTERUS FOR COMMON RADIOLOGIC PROCEDURES

Study	View	Films/Study	Dose/Study (mrad)
Skull	AP, PA, Lat	4.1	< .05
Chest	AP, PA, Lat	1.5	0.02–0.07
Mammogram	CC, Lat	4.0	7–20
Lumbar spine	AP, Lat	2.9	51–126
Abdomen	AP, PA, Lat	1.7	122–245
Pyelogram	AP, PA, Lat	5.5	686–1398
Hip	AP, Lat	2.0	103–213

AP, anterior-posterior; PA, posterior-anterior; Lat, lateral; CC, cranial-caudad.
From Twickler and colleagues (1992).

TABLE 21–5. REPRESENTATIVE DOSES TO UTERUS/EMBRYO FROM COMMON FLUOROSCOPIC PROCEDURES

Procedure	Total Dose to Uterus (mrad)	Fluoroscopic Exposure Time (sec)	Cinegraphic Exposure Time (sec)
Cerebral angiography	< 10	—	—
Cardiac angiography	65	223 (SD = 118)	49 (SD = 9)
Single vessel PTCA	60	1023 (SD = 952)	32 (SD = 7)
Double vessel PTCA	90	1186 (SD = 593)	49 (SD = 13)
Upper gastrointestinal series	56	136	—
Barium swallow	6	192	—
Barium meal	8	228	—
Barium enema	1945–3986	289–311	—
Small bowel series with upper gastrointestinal series	2,132 (SD = 2700)	684 (SD = 282)	— —

PTCA, percutaneous transluminal coronary angioplasty; SD, standard deviation.
From Twickler and colleagues (1992).

equipment, however, there is less exposure from scatter, and therefore areas not directly scanned have less risk of radiation exposure. All of this information has been compiled in Table 21–6 to provide dosimetry calculations for various tomographic studies. The low dose from cranial tomography is because of the distance of the fetus from the maternal head. As the target scanned is closer to the fetus—for example, the chest—there is more exposure. When the fetus is within the area scanned—for example, the pelvis—exposure is greatest.

Ultrasound

Ultrasound employs sound wave transmission at certain frequencies to image the body. There is a potential for tissue damage at very high intensities from heat and cavitation (Dakins, 1991; Merritt, 1989; Wells, 1986). For clinical purposes, in the low-intensity range of real-time imaging, no fetal risks have been demonstrated in 25 years of its use (American Institute of Ultrasound in Medicine, 1988). There is no contraindication to ultrasound imaging of maternal organs during pregnancy.

TABLE 21–6. ESTIMATED MAXIMUM FETAL DOSES FROM COMPUTED TOMOGRAPHIC SCANS

	Fetal Dose (Rad) at Gestational Age (Weeks)				
Study	*0–14*	*15–24*	*25–29*	*30–34*	*35–42*
Head (10 slices × 10 mm thick)	<0.05	<0.05	<0.05	<0.05	<0.05
Chest (10 slices × 10 mm thick)	<0.10	<0.10	<0.10	<0.10	<0.10
Abdomen (10 slices × 10 mm (5 mm gaps)	2.6	2.2–2.4	2.3	2.0–2.1	1.7
Lumbar spine (5 slices × 10 mm thick)	3.5	2.8–3.2	3.0	2.6–2.7	2.3
Pelvimetry (1 slice × 10 mm thick, including lateral scout)	—	—	—	—	0.25

From Twickler and co-workers (1992).

Magnetic Resonance Imaging

Magnetic resonance imaging has emerged as a major imaging modality in recent years because of its resolution, its ability to characterize tissue, and its reproduction of information in three planes (axial, sagittal, and coronal). Rather than ionizing radiation, magnetic resonance employs powerful magnets to temporarily alter the energy state of hydrogen protons in molecules, especially water. Through a series of acquisitions, information about the location and characteristics of these hydrogen protons can be obtained as they return to their normal state (Curry and associates, 1990).

Several investigations have been directed to the safety of magnetic resonance imaging. To date, there are no reported harmful effects of its use in pregnancy, including mutagenic effects (Geard and colleagues, 1984; McRobbie and Foster, 1985; Schwartz and Crooks, 1982; Thomas and Morris, 1981). No deleterious effects have been reported in diagnostic systems that use less than 2 tesla (a measure of magnetic field strength). Nonetheless, the National Radiological Protection Board advises against imaging in the first trimester unless termination of pregnancy is probable (Garden and co-workers, 1991).

In a number of studies magnetic resonance imaging has been employed in the management of maternal complications of pregnancy (Angtuaco, 1992; McCarthy, 1985; Weinreb, 1985, 1986; and their co-workers). It is useful particularly to evaluate suspected maternal intra-abdominal and retroperitoneal pathology. As discussed in Chapter 20, it is useful to evaluate suspected venous thrombosis. Because this technology does not use ionizing radiation, it is preferred over computed tomography to evaluate pelvic masses in the pregnant woman. Magnetic resonance imaging may allow for better visualization because of its multiplanar potential as well as better tissue characterization using T_1- and T_2-weighted images in most organ systems.

PARENTERAL NUTRITION

For some of the gastrointestinal disorders that will be discussed, parenteral feeding or **hyperalimentation** may be considered. Its purpose is to provide nutrition when the gastrointestinal tract must be kept quiescent. Peripheral venous access may be adequate for short-term supplemental nutrition, which derives calories from isotonic fat solutions. Jugular or subclavian venous catheterization is necessary for **total parenteral nutrition** because its hyperosmolarity requires rapid dilution in a high-flow system. These solutions provide up to 24–40 kcal/kg, principally as hypertonic glucose solution; they frequently cause thrombophlebitis if infused by peripheral vein. Madan and colleagues (1992) reported that these hyperosmolar solutions may be infused through a peripheral vein with a low risk of thrombophlebitis if an ultrafine-bore silicone catheter is used. Greenspoon and associates (1993) described peripheral placement of a silicone catheter advanced into the superior vena cava. In three women, parenteral nutrition was carried out for 28–137 days without complications or the need to replace the catheter.

A number of complications are associated with parenteral nutrition (Howard, 1991). Major mechanical complications from gaining intravenous access include pneumothorax, hemothorax from injury to subclavian vessels, brachial plexus injury, and catheter malpositions. Greenspoon and colleagues (1989) described a maternal death from cardiac tamponade 7 days after successful placement of a subclavian venous catheter for hyperalimentation in a woman with hyperemesis gravidarum. Metabolic complications may be avoided by slowly increasing the dietary prescription to avoid fluid overload, osmotic diuresis, and massive electrolyte shifts due to insulin secretion. Late metabolic complications include gallstones and hepatic cholestasis. Catheter-induced sepsis is an important source of morbidity, and infection must be treated vigorously. Greenspoon and associates (1994) reviewed the effects of lipid-containing parenteral nutrition and found no association with preterm labor or preeclampsia. Kirby and colleagues (1988) reviewed the use of total parenteral nutrition for a variety of indications in 55 pregnant women (Table 21–7). Gastrointestinal disorders were the most common indication, and the duration of parenteral feeding ranged from conception to delivery with a mean of 4.8 weeks. Their observations were similar to those reported earlier in reviews by Catanzarite and associates (1986) and Lee and colleagues (1986). Complications were identified in about one-third of these women, and one that is particularly worri-

TABLE 21–7. SOME REPORTED CONDITIONS IN WHICH TOTAL PARENTERAL NUTRITION HAS BEEN USED DURING PREGNANCY

Anorexia nervosa
Appendiceal rupture
Bowel obstruction
Burns
Cholecystitis
Crohn disease
Cystic fibrosis
Diabetic complications
Esophageal injury
Esophagocolonogastrostomy
Hyperemesis gravidarum
Jejunoileal bypass
Leukemia
Partial hepatectomy
Pancreatic cancer
Pancreatitis
Paroxysomal nocturnal hemoglobinuria
Persistent abdominal pain
Short bowel syndrome
Ulcerative colitis

Modified from Kirby and colleagues (1988) with permission.

some is the reversible **Wernicke–Korsakoff psychosis,** which may complicate up to 10 percent of cases. Lee and colleagues (1986) emphasize that parenteral nutrition for the woman with diabetic gastroenteropathy is particularly hazardous, and they reported one antepartum maternal death and four other women with deteriorating renal function. Sepsis also is common. Nutritional support currently costs up to $500 per day. Catanzarite and colleagues (1986) rightly caution that, because of these various potential problems, informed consent with patient participation in decision making is vital.

UPPER GASTROINTESTINAL LESIONS

Peptic Ulcer

There are conflicting data regarding gastric physiology during pregnancy. According to Hytten (1991), there is consensus that gastric secretion and motility are reduced, but there is considerably increased mucus secretion. From these observations, it is not surprising that active peptic ulcer disease is uncommon during pregnancy. In the past 20 years at Parkland Hospital, Cunningham and associates (1993) have cared for nearly 200,000 pregnant women and have encountered only two women with presumed symptomatic peptic ulcer. Obviously, complications such as perforation or hemorrhage are even more rare. Published experiences indicate that women with a symptomatic peptic ulcer most often note considerable improvement during pregnancy. Clarke (1953) studied 313 pregnancies in 118 women with proven ulcer disease and reported a clear remission in almost 90 percent. These benefits were short-lived, and within 3 months of delivery symptoms had recurred in over half. By the end of 2 years, almost every woman had suffered a recurrence.

Upper Gastrointestinal Bleeding

Occasionally, especially during early pregnancy, nausea and vomiting may be accompanied by worrisome upper gastrointestinal bleeding. The obvious concern is that there is a bleeding peptic ulceration; however, most of these women have minute linear mucosal tears near the gastroesophageal junction, or so-called **Mallory–Weiss** tears. These women usually respond promptly to conservative measures that include iced-saline irrigations, topical antacids, and intravenously administered cimetidine. In some instances, blood transfusions are needed. **Endoscopy, if indicated, should not be withheld because of pregnancy.** It may be important to distinguish this from the more dangerous **Boerhaave syndrome,** which is esophageal rupture caused by greatly increased esophageal pressure from retching.

Esophageal Varices

Esophageal varices may complicate portal venous hypertension that results from cirrhosis or from extrahepatic portal vein obstruction. Postnecrotic hepatitis and chronic alcoholism account for almost all cases of portal hypertension due to liver disease in young women. About an equal number of cases of esophageal varices, at least in pregnant women, are caused by **extrahepatic portal hypertension.** About half of these are idiopathic, but a number arise as a complication of umbilical vein catheterization in the neonate. With increasing salvage of very small preterm infants who survive to childbearing age, this entity is expected to be encountered more commonly during pregnancy.

Whatever its underlying cause, portal vein pressure rises from its normal of 10–15 mm Hg to exceed 30 mm Hg. This leads to formation of collateral circulation, which carries blood to the systemic circulation. Drainage is via the gastric, intercostal, and other veins ultimately to the esophageal system, where varices develop. Bleeding from varices usually is near the gastroesophageal junction. Bleeding can be torrential, and blood and clotting factors are given as needed. In some cases, bleeding can be stopped with a triple-lumen tube, but this is not always successful. Emergency shunting procedures may be necessary, but these are associated with high mortality. Recently, endoscopically guided **sclerotherapy** has been used for control of acute hemorrhage, and some have found it preferable in preventing subsequent bleeding episodes.

Varices in Pregnancy

Bleeding from esophageal varices causes much of the maternal mortality associated with cirrhosis. Britton (1982) reviewed outcomes in 160 pregnancies complicated by cirrhosis or varices or both (Table 21–8). Bleeding was common when pregnancy was complicated by varices, regardless of whether there was cirrhosis. Conversely, mortality depended heavily on varices associated with cirrhosis. While maternal mortality from bleeding in women with cirrhosis was 18 percent, in those without cirrhosis it was only 2 percent. As expected, perinatal mortality was common.

TABLE 21–8. OUTCOMES IN 160 PREGNANCIES COMPLICATED BY CIRRHOSIS OR ESOPHAGEAL VARICES OR BOTH

Outcome	Patients With Cirrhosis	Varices Without Cirrhosis
Patients	53	38
Varices	33/53	38/38
Pregnancies	83	77
Bleeding during pregnancy at risk	13/21 (62%)	25/54 (46%)
Operation during pregnancy	5	2
Pregnancy outcome		
Losses		
Abortions	14	10
Stillborn	4	5
Neonatal death	3	2
Vaginal delivery	59	43
Cesarean section	11	11
Maternal mortality	7	2

Modified from Britton (1982) with permission.

Sclerotherapy

In recent years, endoscopically directed injection of a sclerosing solution has been used to control variceal bleeding. Such sclerotherapy is at least 90 percent effective in controlling hemorrhage in nonpregnant patients. When used repeatedly, it decreases the number of subsequent bleeding episodes. This has now been successfully used during pregnancy (Kochhar and colleagues, 1990; Pauzner and associates, 1991). Preliminary results from Parkland Hospital with sclerotherapy also have been successful for esophageal variceal bleeding but less so for gastric varices (Cunningham and colleagues, 1993).

INTESTINAL LESIONS

Ostomy and Pregnancy

Women with a colostomy or an ileostomy may develop complications during pregnancy. Gopal and colleagues (1985) described 82 pregnancies in 66 women following ostomy, usually done for inflammatory bowel disease. Although stomal dysfunction was common, it responded to conservative management in all cases. Bowel obstruction developed in six women and in three surgery was necessary. Ileostomy prolapse was surgically corrected in three women during pregnancy or at cesarean section, and in a fourth postpartum. The cesarean section rate was 37 percent, and one third of these were done because of prior abdominoperineal resection.

Recently, colectomy with mucosal proctectomy and ileal pouch–anal anastomosis has become the procedure of choice for surgical treatment of ulcerative colitis and familial colonic polyposis. According to Santos and Thompson (1993), pouchitis and small bowel obstruction are common long-term complications. Successful pregnancies have been described in women with an ileoanal pouch following colectomy for ulcerative colitis (Metcalf and colleagues, 1986; Nelson and associates, 1989). The experiences of these investigators lead them to believe that vaginal delivery is acceptable in these women, and they recommend a mediolateral episiotomy. Kohler and co-workers (1991) have described deterioration of anal function and increased bowel movements during pregnancy, but reported resolution a few months postpartum.

Intestinal Obstruction

The incidence of bowel obstruction during pregnancy probably is not different from that for the general population. According to Davis and Bohon (1983), the incidence of intestinal obstruction during pregnancy was between 1 in 2500–3500 deliveries. In most experiences from large obstetric services, however, the incidence is much lower. From their review, Perdue and associates (1992) cite an incidence that varied from 1 in 66,500 to 1 in 1500 deliveries. As shown in Table 21–9, most cases—probably 60–70 percent—are due to adhesions from previous pelvic surgery, including cesarean section, after which omental adhesions to the uterine incision may cause obstruction. Volvulus is another common cause.

Ludmir and associates (1989) reported a case of spontaneous small bowel obstruction in a woman with triplets. Kohn and colleagues (1944) reported a remarkable case in which the same woman was operated upon for volvulus four times, three of the operations having been performed in the course of two pregnancies. In one-third of the cases reported by Harer and Harer (1958), delivery by cesarean section was necessary to obtain proper exposure. Volvulus, especially of the cecum, has been observed early in the puerperium after cesarean section (Pratt and colleagues, 1981).

TABLE 21–9. CAUSES OF INTESTINAL OBSTRUCTION DURING PREGNANCY AND THE PUERPERIUM IN 66 WOMEN

Cause	Number (%)
Adhesions	39 (60)
First trimester (1)	
Second trimester (13)	
Third trimester (18)	
Postpartum (7)	
Volvulus	15 (25)
Midgut (3)	
Cecal (3)	
Sigmoid (7)	
Ileus	5 (8)
Intussusception	3 (5)
Hernia, carcinoma, appendicitis	4 (6)

Adapted from Perdue and colleagues (1992).

Intestinal obstruction is a grave complication of pregnancy and results most frequently from pressure of the growing uterus on intestinal adhesions. According to Davis and Bohon (1983), there are three times when obstruction is more likely: around midpregnancy, when the uterus becomes an abdominal organ; at term, when the fetal head descends; and immediately postpartum, when there is an acute change in the uterine size. From their review, Perdue and colleagues (1992) found that 80 percent of women had nausea and vomiting. Importantly, abdominal pain, either continuous or colicky, was found in 98 percent of these women. Abdominal tenderness was encountered in 70 percent. While characteristic high-pitched intestinal rushes may be heard, they reported abnormal bowel sounds in only 55 percent.

Limited x-ray examinations, including plain abdominal films, and those following administration of soluble contrast medium, either orally or by enema, should be performed if obstruction is suspected. Perdue and associates (1992) reported that 38 of 42 pregnant women in whom x-rays were performed had radiographic evidence of obstruction.

The mortality rate with intestinal obstruction can be very high, principally because of errors in diagnosis, delayed diagnosis, reluctance to operate during pregnancy, and inadequate preparation for surgery. With unrelenting obstruction there is bowel distension with subsequent perforation (Fig. 21–1). Of the 66 pregnancies in their review, Perdue and associates (1992) found a 6 percent maternal mortality rate and 26 percent fetal mortality rate. Two of the four mothers who died had adhesive obstruction late in pregnancy and one each had sigmoid or cecal volvulus.

Pseudo-obstruction of the colon, or **Ogilvie syndrome,** is caused by adynamic colonic ileus; about 10 percent of all reported cases follow delivery. The syndrome is characterized by massive abdominal distention with cecal dilation found on x-ray studies (Fig. 21–2). Although unusual, the large bowel may rupture, and decompression is recommended when the bowel becomes distended to 10–12 cm. Laparotomy or cecostomy may be indicated, but colonoscopy for decompression has

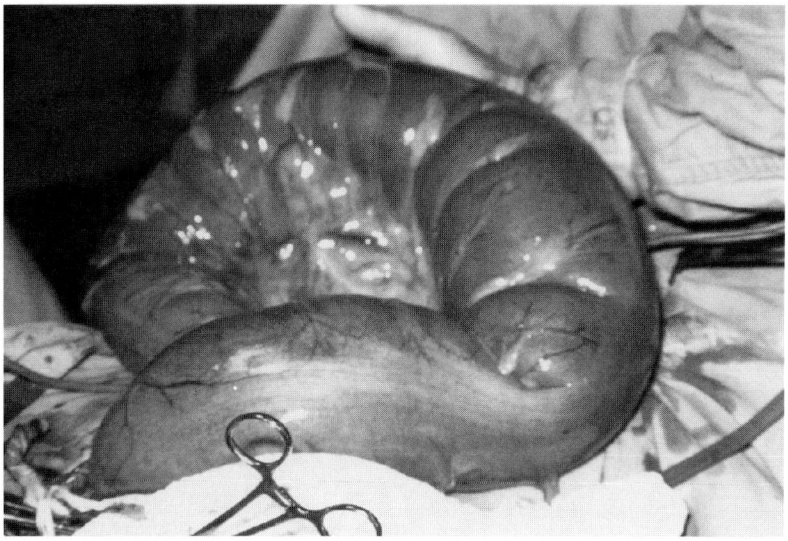

Figure 21–1. Laparotomy for bowel obstruction in a woman 28 weeks pregnant. Sigmoid volvulus was successfully reduced before perforation developed. (Photograph courtesy of Dr. Lowell Davis.)

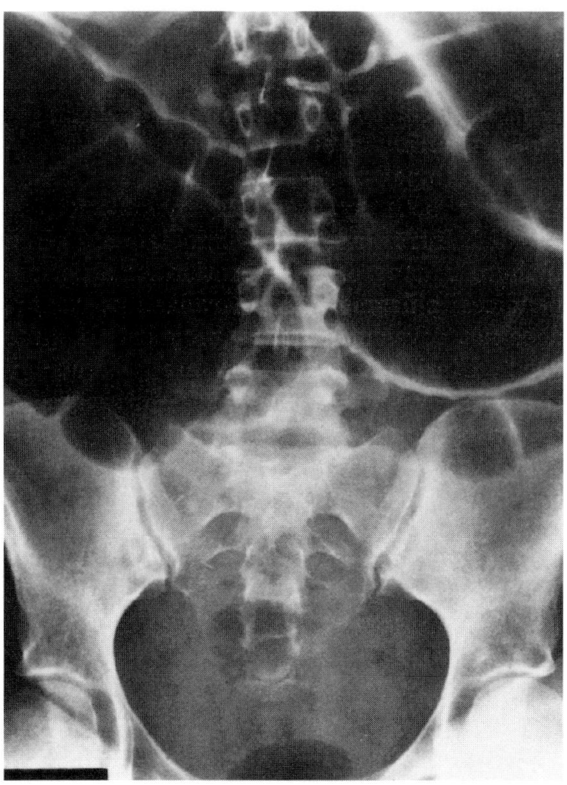

Figure 21–2. Flat abdominal x-ray showing massively dilated colon with thin haustra and nonedematous septae, suggesting pseudoobstruction. (From Davis and Bohon, 1983, with permission.)

been described in a woman 2 days following cesarean section (Moore and associates, 1986).

Appendicitis

Pregnancy does not predispose to appendicitis, but reflects the general prevalence of the condition. Mazze and Källén (1991) described findings from 720,000 Swedish registry deliveries and reported that 778—about 1 in 1000 pregnancies—of these women underwent appendectomy during pregnancy. Appendicitis was confirmed in 65 percent or 1 in 1440 pregnancies.

Pregnancy often makes diagnosis of appendicitis more difficult for the following reasons: (1) Anorexia, nausea, and vomiting that accompany normal pregnancy are fairly common symptoms of appendicitis. (2) As the uterus enlarges, the appendix commonly moves upward and outward toward the flank, so that pain and tenderness may not be prominent in the right lower quadrant (Fig. 21–3). (3) Some degree of leukocytosis is the rule during normal pregnancy. (4) During pregnancy especially, other diseases, such as pyelonephritis, renal colic, placental abruption, and degeneration of a uterine myoma, may be readily confused with appendicitis. (5) Pregnant women, especially those late in gestation, frequently do not have symptoms considered "typical" for nonpregnant patients with appendicitis.

As the appendix is pushed progressively higher by the growing uterus, containment of

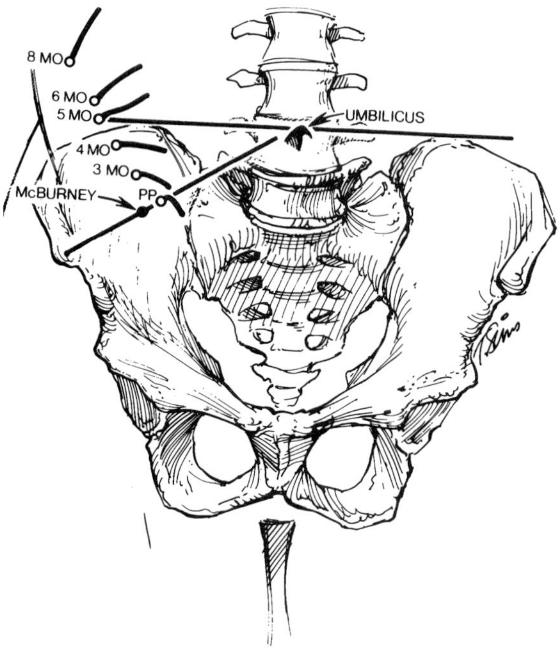

Figure 21–3. Changes in position of the appendix as pregnancy advances (MO, month; PP, postpartum). (From Cunningham and colleagues, 1993, with permission.)

infection by the omentum becomes increasingly unlikely and appendiceal rupture causes generalized peritonitis. These complications are more common if treatment is delayed and gangrene supervenes. Acute appendicitis in the last trimester, therefore, may carry a poor prognosis, and it is worth emphasizing that in some series **maternal mortality approaches 5 percent** (DeVore, 1980). Increased mortality is due to surgical delay (Cunningham and McCubbin, 1975; Sharp, 1994).

Appendicitis increases the likelihood of abortion or preterm labor, especially if there is peritonitis. Pregnancies further advanced are at greater risk. For example, Mazze and Källén (1991) found that spontaneous labor ensued with greater frequency if surgery for appendicitis was performed after 23 weeks' gestation. Fetal loss is increased in most series, and overall it is about 15 percent. In the Swedish study, fetal loss was 22 percent if surgery was performed after 23 weeks' gestation (Mazze and Källén, 1991).

Diagnosis and Management

Persistent abdominal pain and tenderness are the most reproducible findings. If appendicitis is suspected, then treatment, regardless of the stage of gestation, is immediate surgical exploration by either laparoscopy or laparotomy (Chap. 29). The diagnosis is principally clinical, and few laboratory tests are helpful. Graded compression using ultrasound imaging has been demonstrated to be effective in diagnosis of appendicitis in nonpregnant patients (Puylaert and colleagues, 1987). In our experience, because of cecal displacement and uterine interposition, compression ultrasonography is less accurate for diagnosis of appendicitis during pregnancy. **Even though diagnostic errors sometimes lead to the removal of a normal appendix, it is better to operate unnecessarily than to postpone intervention until generalized peritonitis has developed.** In most reports, the diagnosis is verified in about half of women who undergo surgical exploration. In the Swedish study of 778 women surgically explored for suspected appendicitis, the diagnosis was confirmed in 64 percent (Mazze and Källén, 1991). In the first trimester, 77 percent of diagnoses were correct; however, in the latter two trimesters, only 57 percent of diagnoses were confirmed at surgery. Cesarean section is seldom indicated at the time of appendectomy, and aside from local tenderness, a recent abdominal incision presents no problem during labor and vaginal delivery.

It is important during surgery and recovery that both hypoxia and hypotension be avoided. Intravenous antimicrobials are given if there is gangrene, perforation, or a periappendiceal phlegmon. If generalized peritonitis does not develop, then the prognosis is quite good. Uterine contractions are common if there is peritonitis. While some recommend tocolytic agents for these women, there is evidence that pulmonary permeability edema is increased when they are given to women with sepsis (de Veciana and colleagues, 1994).

In some women, undiagnosed appendicitis will stimulate preterm labor. While the large uterus helps to contain infection locally, after delivery when the uterus rapidly empties, the walled-off infection is disrupted with spillage of free pus into the peritoneal cavity. In these cases, an acute surgical abdomen is encountered within a few hours postpartum.

Simply because it is coincidental, appendicitis during the early puerperium is rare. In some cases, especially with early appendicitis, diagnosis is particularly difficult because of the normally robust leukocytosis as well as the frequency of other puerperal disorders with similar signs and symptoms. Anorexia with any evidence of peritoneal irritation such as distention and adynamic ileus should suggest appendicitis. Puerperal pelvic infections typically do not cause peritonitis (see Chap. 20).

DISEASES OF THE GALLBLADDER AND PANCREAS

Gallbladder Physiology During Pregnancy

Gallbladder kinetics during pregnancy using real-time sonography have been investigated by Braverman and associates (1980). After the first trimester, both gallbladder volume during fasting and residual volume after contracting in response to a test meal were twice as great as in nonpregnant subjects. Incomplete emptying may result in retention of cholesterol crystals, a prerequisite for cholesterol gallstones. **Biliary sludge,** probably a forerunner to gallstones, immediately was seen ultrasonically in a fourth of nearly 300 postpartum women. A year later, only 4 percent had persistent sludge. These findings are supportive of the view that pregnancy increases the risk of gallstones. Presumably, the very high progesterone levels that characterize the second and third trimester are responsible for diminished gallbladder motility. Singletary and colleagues (1986) documented that gallbladder tissue has both nuclear and cytosolic receptors for estrogens and progesterone. Progesterone has been shown to impair the gallbladder response to exogenously administered cholecystokinin in experimental animals. Other factors include an increased bile acid pool size, decreased enterohepatic circulation, and increased cholic acid/chenodeoxycholic acid ratio (Scott, 1992).

Cholelithiasis

In the United States, 20 percent of women over age 40 have gallstones. Over 80 percent of stones contain cholesterol, and its oversecretion into bile is thought to be a major factor in their pathogenesis. Biliary sludge, which may increase during pregnancy, is an important precursor to gallstone formation. The cumulative risk of a patient with silent gallstones to require surgery for symptoms or complications is about 1–2 percent per year; it is 10 percent at 5 years, 15 percent at 10 years, and 18 percent at 15 years (Greenberger and Isselbacher, 1991). For these reasons, many believe that prophylactic cholecystectomy is not warranted for asymptomatic stones.

A number of nonsurgical approaches have been used for gallstone disease. These include oral bile acid therapy with chenodeoxycholic acid, extracorporeal shock wave lithotripsy, and contact dissolution with methyl tert-butyl ether placed directly into the gallbladder. There is no experience with any of these methods during pregnancy, and they currently are not recommended.

Asymptomatic Gallstones During Pregnancy

Because of their prevalence in the general population, it is perhaps expected that gallstones would be relatively common findings in asymptomatic pregnant women. Indeed, an incidence of ultrasonically visualized asymptomatic stones of 2.5–5 percent during pregnancy or the puerperium has been reported in over 800 women (Chesson, 1985; Maringhini, 1987; Stauffer, 1982; and their colleagues). Although ideal treatment for silent stones is debated, pregnancy is not the appropriate time for surgical removal if they remain asymptomatic.

Acute Cholecystitis

Acute cholecystitis usually develops when there is obstruction of the cystic duct. Bacterial infection plays a role in 50–85 percent of these acute inflammatory conditions. In over half of patients with acute cholecystitis, a history of previous right upper quadrant pain from cholelithiasis is elicited. With acute disease, pain is accompanied by anorexia, nausea and vomiting, low-grade fever, and mild leukocytosis. Ultrasonography can be used to visualize stones as small as 2 mm, and false-positive and false-negative rates for diagnosing gallstones are about 2–4 percent (Greenberger and Isselbacher, 1991). Ultrasonic examination confirms gallstones in about 90 percent of patients (Fig. 21–4).

About 75 percent of nonpregnant patients with acute cholecystitis respond to medical therapy consisting of nasogastric suction, intravenous fluids and antimicrobials, and analgesics (Greenberger and Isselbacher, 1991). The remaining 25 percent require cholecystec-

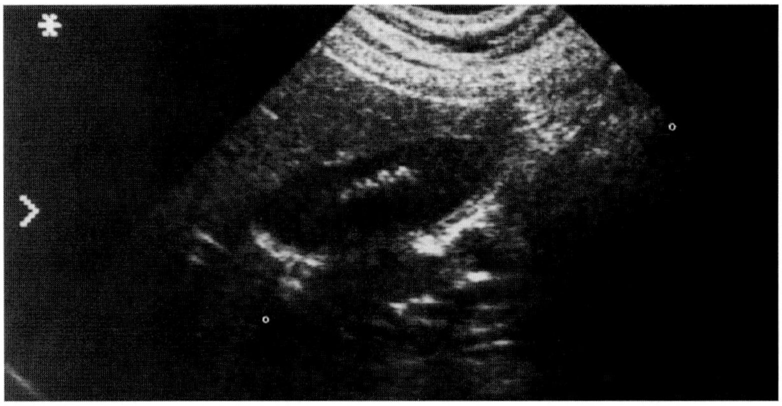

Figure 21–4. Multiple floating gallstones visualized in a woman 26 weeks pregnant. (From Cunningham and colleagues, 1993, with permission; photograph courtesy of Dr. Diane Twickler.)

tomy for persistent pain or gangrene, empyema, or perforation of the gallbladder.

Management

In general, acute cholecystitis during pregnancy or the puerperium is managed in a manner similar as for nonpregnant women. Landers and colleagues (1987) reported their experiences with 30 women with acute cholecystitis complicating pregnancy. The incidence was about 1 in 1000 deliveries. Gallstones were successfully visualized in 96 percent of women undergoing ultrasonic scanning. Although 21 of these women presented for care before the third trimester, these investigators elected medical therapy in 25. Such therapy was successful in 21, and the other four women required cholecystectomy for persistent or worsening pain. In 5 of 30 women, cholecystectomy was performed primarily.

Dixon and colleagues (1987) preferred more aggressive surgical management and performed cholecystectomy in 18 of 44 women with acute cholecystitis or cholelithiasis with biliary colic. The women treated surgically did well, and in contrast, 15 of the 26 patients managed medically had recurrent disease during pregnancy. Multiple hospitalizations were common in the latter group and two women required prolonged total parenteral nutrition during late pregnancy. Similarly, Hiatt and associates (1986) performed cholecystectomy and cholangiography during pregnancy in 9 of 26 women with acute cholecystitis. These women all did well.

Stones obstructing the common bile duct can be removed using **endoscopic retrograde cholangiopancreatography (ERCP)** along with sphincterotomy. This procedure has been used in pregnant women, but experiences are limited (Baillie and colleagues, 1990). **Laparoscopic cholecystectomy** is evolving in this country as the primary operation for gallbladder disease, but there currently is little experience with the technique during pregnancy. While Gadacz and Talamini (1991) list pregnancy as an absolute contraindication, uncomplicated laparoscopic cholecystectomy was described by Pucci and Seed (1991) in a woman 31 weeks pregnant. Subsequently, Elerding (1993) and Morrell and colleagues (1992) described the technique in 10 pregnant women. Three women were in the first trimester, six in the second, and one was 28 weeks pregnant (See Chap. 29).

It seems reasonable to consider cholecystectomy for acute cholecystitis diagnosed early in pregnancy. If cholecystectomy is to be performed during pregnancy, many consider the second trimester to be the optimal time because the risk of abortion is lower and that of preterm labor and delivery is reduced; moreover, the uterus is not yet large enough to impinge on the operative field. **Regardless, when surgery is thought to be indicated in the pregnant women, procrastination should be avoided.** Delay can only place the woman and her fetus in greater jeopardy. At times, gallbladder drainage may be the procedure of choice. Recent surgery does not complicate labor except for incisional discomfort.

Acute Pancreatitis

In nonpregnant patients, acute pancreatitis most likely is associated with chronic alcohol ingestion, but during pregnancy, cholelithiasis is a more common predisposing condition. Why inflammation is triggered is unclear, but there is activation of pancreatic enzymes followed by autodigestion characterized by cellular membrane disruption and proteolysis, edema, hemorrhage, and necrosis. There are a number of associated causes. In addition to alcohol abuse and cholelithiasis, pancreatitis is encountered more commonly in the postoperative patient, and it is associated with trauma, certain metabolic conditions including acute fatty liver of pregnancy, familial hypertriglyceridemia, some viral infections, or drug use.

Clinically, acute pancreatitis is characterized by mild to incapacitating epigastric pain, nausea and vomiting, and abdominal distention. Patients usually are in distress and have low-grade fever and tachycardia; hypotension is common. Findings include abdominal tenderness, and up to 10 percent of patients have associated pulmonary findings. Serum amylase levels three times upper normal values are confirmatory, but there is no correlation with their degree of elevation and severity of disease. In fact, usually by 48–72 hours, serum amylase levels return to normal despite evidence for continuing pancreatitis. Other conditions may cause hyperamylasemia, and measurement of serum lipase activity increases the diagnostic yield. There usually is leukocytosis, and 25 percent of patients have hypocalcemia. Serum bilirubin and aspartate aminotransferase levels usually are elevated somewhat.

A number of prognostic factors may be used to predict severity of the disease. These include respiratory failure, shock, need for massive colloid replacement, hypocalcemia of less than 8 mg/dL, or dark hemorrhagic fluid on paracentesis. If three of the first four features are documented, survival is only 30 percent.

Complications

In some cases, a pancreatic **phlegmon** develops and imaging studies may be necessary to distinguish this from a pseudocyst or abscess. Sonography will usually confirm a **pseudocyst,** but differentiation between an abscess and phlegmon is more difficult, even if computed tomography is used. A **pancreatic abscess** (Fig. 21–5), must be drained or mortality is high. Pseudocysts develop in perhaps 15 percent of all patients following acute inflammation, and although at least half subside spontaneously, persistent pseudocysts should be drained because they may rupture subsequently with disastrous results.

Pancreatitis During Pregnancy

Pregnancy does not appear to predispose to pancreatitis, and its incidence reflects that of otherwise healthy young women. The incidence of pancreatitis was reported by Ramin and colleagues (1995) and Swisher and associates (1994) to be about 1 in 1500–2000 pregnancies. As discussed previously, these women seldom have associated alcoholism; however, **cholelithiasis** commonly coexists (Block and Kelly, 1989). Associated biliary disease was found in 65 percent of 35 pregnant women with pancreatitis reported by Ramin and coworkers (1995). Certainly, the predisposition of pregnancy toward gallstone formation may link pregnancy indirectly with pancreatitis.

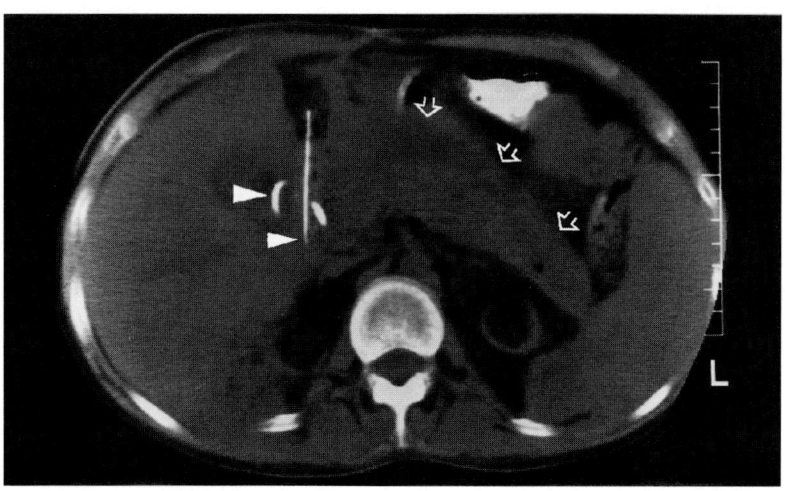

Figure 21–5. Computed tomograph showing pancreatic abscess (arrows) containing air. The nasogastric and enteric feeding tubes are seen in the duodenum (arrowheads). (Photograph courtesy of Dr. Diane Twickler.)

In a small number of pregnant women with pancreatitis, there is an associated **familial hyperlipidemic syndrome,** usually hypertriglyceridemia (Nies and Dreiss, 1990). Sanderson and colleagues (1991) described a woman in whom aggressive dietary therapy and intermittent intravenous glucose feedings ostensibly prevented recurrent pancreatitis in her fourth term pregnancy. Watts and associates (1992) described two pregnant women with hypertriglyceridemia due to familial lipoprotein lipase deficiency.

Diagnosis

Pancreatitis is diagnosed during pregnancy using the same criteria as in nonpregnant patients. Ramin and colleagues (1995) reported that 34 of 35 pregnant women with pancreatitis complained of nausea, vomiting, and abdominal pain. Forty percent of these 35 women had midepigastric pain with back radiation. Despite earlier reports, Strickland and colleagues (1984) found no significant change in serum amylase levels in 413 normal women studied at various stages of gestation and again 6 weeks postpartum. Ordorica and associates (1991) confirmed these findings and showed also that serum lipase levels were not changed during normal pregnancy. Thus, serial determinations of serum amylase and lipase activity remain the best methods to confirm the clinical diagnosis of pancreatitis. Block and Kelly (1989) reported that in all 21 pregnant or recently pregnant women with pancreatitis, serum amylase exceeded 1500 IU/L. In Ramin's study the mean serum amylase level was 1367 U/L (range, 111–4560) and the mean serum lipase level was 7974 U/L (range, 295–41,825) (Ramin and colleagues, 1995). They also confirmed that serum amylase values do not correlate with the severity of disease.

Management

The principles of therapy are the same as for nonpregnant patients. Management is medical and includes analgesics for pain, intravenous hydration, and measures to decrease pancreatic secretion by proscribing oral intake. Nasogastric suction has not been shown to improve the outcome in mild to moderate disease. Antimicrobials are not indicated unless there is evidence of established infection. In most patients, acute pancreatitis is self-limited, and in 90 percent inflammation subsides within 3–7 days after treatment. For patients with unrelenting disease, intensive supportive therapy is given, and laparotomy with debridement and drainage may be lifesaving (Fernandez-del-Castillo and colleagues, 1993).

In pregnant women, mild inflammation usually subsides in response to conservative therapy. In the Parkland Hospital series, all 35 women responded to conservative treatment and were hospitalized for a mean of 8.5 days (Ramin and colleagues, 1995). In women with severe disease, fetal loss is high because of associated hypovolemia, hypoxia, and acidosis. Because more than half of cases are associated with gallstone disease, consideration is given to cholecystectomy after inflammation subsides. Block and Kelly (1989) described their experience with 11 women with antepartum gallstone pancreatitis. One woman re-quired cholecystectomy shortly after admission for persistent pancreatitis. Women in whom pancreatitis was encountered before the third trimester underwent cholecystectomy after acute inflammation subsided. In four of five women in the third trimester, surgery was postponed until after delivery. Swisher and colleagues (1994) have described similar results.

SUMMARY

Intraabdominal surgical disorders are difficult to evaluate in the pregnant woman, especially after midpregnancy. In many cases, persistent abdominal pain without accompanying symptoms may herald a life-threatening disorder such as a perforated viscus. When interpreting physical findings and laboratory values in the woman suspected to have abdominal pathology, the physician must consider the normal physiological changes of pregnancy. In cases with an uncertain diagnosis, it may be safer to perform exploratory laparotomy lest an early inflamed appendix suppurates and ruptures with catastrophic sequela. Above all, if her treatment is modified, it must be remembered that a woman should not be penalized because she is pregnant.

REFERENCES

Allen JR, Helling TS, Langenfeld M. Intraabdominal surgery during pregnancy. Am J Surg 1989; 158:567.

American Institute of Ultrasound in Medicine: AIUM bioeffects considerations for the safety of diagnostic ultrasound. J Ultrasound Med 1988; 7:S1.

Anderson AS, Whichelow MJ. Constipation during pregnancy: dietary fibre intake and the effect of fibre supplementation. Hum Nutr: Appl Nutr 1985; 39A:202.

Angtuaco TL, Shah HR, Mattison DR, Quirk JG. MR imaging in high-risk obstetric patients: a valuable complement to US. Radiographics 1992; 12:91.

Baillie J, Cairns SR, Putnam WS, Cotton PB. Endoscopic management of choledocholithiasis during pregnancy. Surg Gynecol Obstet 1990; 171:1.

Block P, Kelley TR. Management of gallstone pancreatitis during pregnancy and the postpartum period. Surg Gynecol Obstet 1989; 168:426.

Boyce RA. Enteral nutrition in hyperemesis gravidarum: a new development. J Am Diet Assoc 1992; 92:733.

Braverman DZ, Johnson ML, Kern F Jr. Effects of pregnancy and contraceptive steroids on gallbladder function. N Engl J Med 1980; 302:362.

Brent RL. The effect of embryonic and fetal exposure to x-ray, microwaves, and ultrasound: counseling the pregnant and nonpregnancy patient about these risks. Semin Oncol 1989; 16:347.

Briggs GG, Freeman RK, Yaffee SJ. Drugs in Pregnancy and Lactation, 2nd ed. Baltimore, Williams & Wilkins, 1986.

Britton RC. Pregnancy and esophageal varices. Am J Surg 1982; 143:421.

Castillo CF, Rattner DW, Warshaw AL. Acute pancreatitis. Lancet 1993; 342:475.

Castro LDP. Reflux esophagitis as the cause of heartburn in pregnancy. Am J Obstet Gynecol 1967; 98:1.

Catanzarite VA, Arguright K, Mann BA, Brittain VL. Malnutrition during pregnancy: consider parenteral feeding. Contemp Ob/Gyn 1986; 27:110.

Cheng Y-S. Pregnancy in liver cirrhosis and/or portal hypertension. Am J Obstet Gynecol 1977; 128:812.

Chesson RR, Gallup DG, Gibbs RL, et al. Ultrasonographic diagnosis of asymptomatic cholelithiasis in pregnancy. J Repro Med 1985; 30:921.

Clark DH. Peptic ulcer in women. Br Med J 1953; 2:1254.

Cohen S. The sluggish gallbladder of pregnancy. N Engl J Med 1980; 302:397.

Cohen S, Harris LD. Does hiatus hernia affect competence of the gastroesophageal sphincter? N Engl J Med 1971; 284A:1053.

Committee on Biological Effects of Ionizing Radiation, National Research Council. Other somatic and fetal effects. In: Beir V; Effects of Exposure to Low Levels of Ionizing Radiation. Washington, DC: National Academy Press, 1990.

Cunningham FG, McCubbin JH. Appendicitis complicating pregnancy. Obstet Gynecol 1975; 45:415.

Cunningham FG, MacDonald PC, Gant NF, et al, eds. Williams Obstetrics, 19th ed. East Norwalk, CT: Appleton & Lange, 1993.

Curry TS III, Dowdey JE, Murry RC Jr: Christensen's Physics of Diagnostic Radiology, 4th ed. Philadelphia: Lea & Febiger, 1990:1, 470.

Dakins DR: US output deliberations hinge on thermal effects. Diagn Imaging, May 1991.

Davis MR, Bohon CJ. Intestinal obstruction in pregnancy. Clin Obstet Gynecol 1983; 26:832.

de Veciana M, Towers CV, Major CA, et al. Pulmonary injury associated with appendicitis during pregnancy: who is at risk? Am J Obstet Gynecol 1994; 171:1008.

DeVore GR. Acute abdominal pain in the pregnant patient due to pancreatitis, acute appendicitis, cholecystitis, or peptic ulcer disease. Clin Perinatol 1980; 7:349.

Dixon NF, Faddis DM, Silberman H. Aggressive management of cholecystitis during pregnancy. Am J Surg 1987; 154:294.

Elerding SC. Laparoscopic cholecystectomy in pregnancy. Am J Surg 1993; 165:625.

Fernández-del-Castillo C, Rattner DW, Warshaw AL. Acute pancreatitis. Lancet 1993; 342:475.

Gadacz TR, Talamini MA. Traditional versus laparoscopic cholecystectomy. Am J Surg 1991; 161:336.

Garden AS, Griffiths RD, Weindling AM, Martin PA. Fast-scan magnetic resonance imaging in fetal visualization. Obstet Gynecol 1991; 164:1190.

Gaulden ME, Murry RC. Medical radiation and possible adverse effects on the human embryo. In: Meyn RE, Withers HR (eds), Radiation Biology in Cancer Research. New York: Raven Press, 1980:277.

Geard CR, Osmak RS, Hall EJ, et al. Magnetic resonance imaging and ionizing radiation: a comparative evaluation in-vitro of oncogenic and genotoxic potential. Radiology 1984; 152:199.

Gopal KA, Amshel AL, Shonberg IL, et al. Ostomy and pregnancy. Dis Colon Rectum 1985; 28:912.

Greenberger NJ, Isselbacher KJ. Diseases of the gallbladder and bile ducts. In: Wilson JD, Braunwald E, Isselbacher KJ, et al, eds. Harrison's Principles of Internal Medicine, 12th ed. New York: McGraw-Hill, 1991: (chap 258) 1358.

Greenspoon JS, Masaki DI, Kurz CR. Cardiac tamponade in pregnancy during central hyperalimentation. Obstet Gynecol 1989; 73:465.

Greenspoon JS, Safarik RH, Hayashi JT, Rosen DJD. Parenteral nutrition during pregnancy. J Reprod Med 1994; 39:87.

Greenspoon JS, Rosen DJD, Ault M. Use of the peripherally inserted central catheter for parenteral nutrition during pregnancy. Obstet Gynecol 1993; 81:831.

Hall EJ. Scientific view of low-level radiation risks. Radiographics 1991; 11:509.

Harer WB Jr, Harer WB Sr. Volvulus complicating pregnancy and the puerperium: a report of three cases and review of the literature (37 references cited). Obstet Gynecol 1958; 12:399.

Hiatt JR, Hiatt JCG, Williams RA, Klein SR. Biliary disease in pregnancy: strategy for surgical management. Am J Surg 1986; 151:263.

Howard LJ. Parenteral and enteral nutrition therapy. In: Wilson JD, Braunwald E, Isselbacher KJ, et al, eds. Harrison's Principles of Internal Medicine, 12th ed. New York: McGraw-Hill, 1991; chap 75:427.

Hytten FE. The alimentary system. In: Hytten F, Chamberlain G, eds. Clinical Physiology in Obstetrics. London: Blackwell Scientific, 1991; chap 5:137.

Kirby DF, Fiorenza V, Craig RM. Intravenous nutritional support during pregnancy. J Parent Enterent Nutr 1988; 12:72.

Kochhar R, Goenka MK, Mehta SK. Endoscopic sclerotherapy during pregnancy. Am J Gastroenterol 1990; 85:1132.

Kohler LW, Pemberton JH, Zinsmeister AR, et al. Quality of life after proctocolectomy: a comparison of Brooke ileostomy. Gastroenterology 1991; 101:679.

Kohn SG, Briele HA, Douglass LH. Volvulus complicating pregnancy. Am J Obstet Gynecol 1944; 48:398.

Landers D, Carmona R, Crombleholme W, Lim R. Acute cholecystitis in pregnancy. Obstet Gynecol 1987; 69:131.

Lee RV, Rodgers BD, Young C, et al. Total parenteral nutrition during pregnancy. Obstet Gynecol 1986; 68:563.

Levine MG, Esser D. Total parenteral nutrition for the treatment of severe hyperemesis gravidarum: maternal nutritional effects and fetal outcome. Obstet Gynecol 1988; 72:102.

Ludmir J, Samuels P, Armson BA, Torosian MH. Spontaneous small bowel obstruction associated with a spontaneous triplet gestation: a case report. J Reprod Med 1989; 34:985.

Madan M, Alexander DJ, McMahon MJ. Influence of catheter type on occurrence of thrombophlebitis during peripheral intravenous nutrition. Lancet 1992; 339:101.

Maringhini A, Marcenò MP, Lanzarone F, et al. Sludge and stones in gallbladder after pregnancy: prevalence and risk factors. J Hepatol 1987; 5:218.

Mayberry JF, Atkinson M. Achalasia and pregnancy. Br J Obstet Gynaecol 1987; 94:855.

Mazze RI, Källén B. Reproductive outcome after anesthesia and operation during pregnancy: a registry study of 5405 cases. Obstet Gynecol 1989; 161:1178.

Mazze RI, Källén B. Appendectomy during pregnancy: a Swedish registry study of 778 cases. Obstet Gynecol 1991; 77:835.

McCarthy SM, Stark DD, Filly RA, et al. Obstetrical magnetic resonance imaging: Maternal anatomy. Radiology 1985; 154:421.

McRobbie D, Foster MA. Pulsed magnetic field exposure during pregnancy and implications for NMR foetal imaging: a study with mice. Magn Reson Imaging 1985; 3:231.

Merritt CRB. Ultrasound safety: what are the issues? Radiology 1989; 173:304.

Metcalf AM, Dozois RR, Kelly KA. Sexual function in women after proctocolectomy. Ann Surg 1986; 204:624.

Moore JG, Gladstone NS, Lucas GW, et al. Successful management of post-cesarean-section acute pseudoobstruction of the colon (Ogilvie's syndrome) with colonoscopic decompression. A case report. J Reprod Med 1986; 31:1001.

Morrell DG, Mullins JR, Harrison PB. Laparoscopic cholecystectomy during pregnancy in symptomatic patients. Surgery 1992; 112:856.

Morrissey JF, Reichelderfer M. Gastrointestinal endoscopy. N Engl J Med 1991; 325:1142.

Nelson H, Dozois RR, Kelly KA, et al. The effect of pregnancy and delivery on the ileal pouch–anal anastomosis functions. Dis Colon Rectum 1989; 32:384.

Nies BM, Dreiss RJ. Hyperlipidemic pancreatitis in pregnancy: a case report and review of the literature. Am J Perinatol 1990; 7:166.

Ordorica SA, Frieden FJ, Marks F, et al. Pancreatic enzyme activity in pregnancy. J Reprod Med 1991; 36:359.

Östman JIC. Update of pancreatic transplantation. Ann Med 1991; 23:101.

Parry E, Shields R, Turnbull AC. Transit time in the small intestine in pregnancy. J Obstet Gynaecol Br Commonw 1970; 77:900.

Pauzner D, Wolman I, Niv D, et al. Endoscopic sclerotherapy in extrahepatic portal hypertension in pregnancy. Am J Obstet Gynecol 1991; 164:152.

Perdue PW, Johnson HW Jr, Stafford PW. Intestinal obstruction complicating pregnancy. Am J Surg 1992; 164:384.

Pratt AT, Donaldson RC, Evertson LR, Yon JL Jr. Cecal volvulus in pregnancy. Obstet Gynecol 1981; (Suppl) 57:37.

Pucci RO, Seed RW. Case report of laparoscopic cholecystectomy in the third trimester of pregnancy. Am J Obstet Gynecol 1991; 165:401.

Puylaert JBCM, Rutgers PH, Lalisang RI, et al. A prospective study of ultrasound in the diagnosis of appendicitis. N Engl J Med 1987; 317:666.

Ramin K, Richey S, Ramin S, Cunningham FG. Acute pancreatitis in pregnancy. Am J Obstet Gynecol 1995 (in press).

Rigler LG, Eneboe JB. Incidence of hiatus hernia in pregnant women and its significance. J Thorac Surg 1935; 4:262.
Sanderson SL, Iverius P-H, Wilson DE. Successful hyperlipemic pregnancy. JAMA 1991; 265:1858.
Santos MC, Thompson JS. Late complications of the ileal pouch–anal anastomosis. Am J Gastroenterol 1993; 88:3.
Satin AJ, Twickler D, Gilstrap LC. Esophageal achalasia in late pregnancy. Obstet Gynecol 1992; 79:812.
Schreyer P, Caspi E, El-Hindi JM, Eschar J. Cirrhosis—Pregnancy and delivery: a review. Obstet Gynecol Surv 1982; 37:304.
Schwartz JL, Crooks LE. NMR imaging produces no observable mutations or cytotoxicity in mammalian cells. Am J Radiol 1982; 139:5.
Scott LD. Gallstone disease and pancreatitis in pregnancy. Gastroenterol Clin No Am, 1992; 21:803.
Sharp HT. Gastrointestinal surgical condition during pregnancy. Clin Obstet Gynecol 1994; 37:306.
Sheld HH. Megacolon complicating pregnancy. J Reprod Med 1987; 32:239.
Singletary BK, Van Thiel DH, Eagon PK. Estrogen and progesterone receptors in human gallbladder. Hepatology 1986; 6:574.
Stauffer RA, Adams A, Wygal J, Lavery JP. Gallbladder disease in pregnancy. Am J Obstet Gynecol 1982; 144:661.
Steven MM. Progress report: pregnancy and liver disease. Gut 1981; 22:592.
Steven MM, Buckley JD, Mackay IR. Pregnancy in chronic active hepatitis. Q J Med 1979; 48:519.
Strickland DM, Hauth JC, Widish J, et al. Amylase and isoamylase activities in serum of pregnant women. Obstet Gynecol 1984; 63:389.
Swisher SG, Hunt KK, Schmit PJ, et al. Management of pancreatitis complicating pregnancy. Ann Surg 1994; 160:759.
Taylor KW, Patt NL, Johns HE. Variations in x-ray exposures to patients. J Can Assoc Radiol 1979; 30:6.
Thomas A, Morris PG. The effects of NMR exposure on living organisms, a microbial assay. Br J Radiol 1982; 55:615.
Twickler DM, Clarke G, Cunningham FG. Diagnostic Imaging in Pregnancy. Supplement No 18 to Cunningham FG, et al. William's Obstetrics, 18th ed, 1992.
Wagner LK, Lester RG, Saldana LR. Exposure of the Pregnant Patient to Diagnostic Radiation. Philadelphia: JB Lippincott, 1985:40, 61.
Watson WJ, Gaines TE. Third-trimester colectomy for severe ulcerative colitis. J Reprod Med 1987; 32:869.
Watts GF, Morton K, Jackson P, Lewis B. Management of patients with severe hypertriglyceridaemia during pregnancy: report of two cases with familial lipoprotein lipase deficiency. Br J Obstet Gynaecol 1992; 99:163.
Weinreb JC, Brown CE, Lowe TW, et al. Pelvic masses in pregnant patients: MR and US imaging. Radiology 1986; 159:717.
Weinreb JC, Lowe TW, Santos-Ramos R, et al. Magnetic resonance imaging in obstetric diagnosis. Radiology 1985; 154:157.
Wells PNT. The prudent use of diagnostic ultrasound. Br J Radiol 1986; 59:1143.

CHAPTER 22

Adnexal Masses

Pelvic masses during pregnancy have historically posed diagnostic and therapeutic dilemmas for the physician. The first published case of successful surgical removal of an ovarian cyst in a pregnant woman was by Burd in 1846; the patient survived the operation, but aborted a few days later (McKerron, 1906). J. Marion Sims was the first to report the surgical removal of an ovarian tumor from a patient 3 months pregnant who survived and eventually delivered a living child (McKerron, 1906). Among 720 pregnant women with surgically treated adnexal masses reported by McKerron (1906), the maternal mortality rate was 21 percent and the fetal mortality rate was 50 percent.

In later series where patients with adnexal masses during pregnancy were treated expectantly, a 26 percent maternal mortality rate occurred secondary to hemorrhage, torsion, or suppuration with peritonitis (Patton, 1906). In 1920 Spencer reported that in pregnant patients managed expectantly, 11 percent of adnexal masses underwent torsion, 2.3 percent underwent rupture with significant intra-abdominal hemorrhaging, 14.5 percent underwent suppuration, and 5.5 percent caused significant dystocia leading to cesarean delivery. Caverly (1931) subsequently reported a 30 percent spontaneous abortion rate with expectant management of adnexal masses.

As a result of the above observations, "expectant management until the second trimester" became the standard therapy for adnexal masses occurring during pregnancy beginning in the early 1900s. Any mass that persisted into the second trimester was removed surgically. This regimen gained popular acceptance not only because of the high maternal complication rate if the mass was not removed, but also because of the significant (3–7%) risk of ovarian malignancy in any adnexal mass occurring with pregnancy.

Numerous series of pregnant patients with adnexal masses have been reported since 1900 and include those of Caverly (1931), Wilson (1937), Hamilton and Higgins (1949), Grimes (1954), Booth (1963), Beischer (1971), Ballard (1984), Struyk and Treffers (1984), Hess (1988), and their associates. Since McKerron's monograph was published in 1906, the risk of maternal and fetal mortality has diminished dramatically. Following the introduction of antibiotics and modern blood banking techniques, reports have indicated a low risk of maternal complications and no maternal deaths with elective removal of a persistent adnexal mass. Despite these improvements, adnexal masses during pregnancy still pose clinical and therapeutic dilemmas for clinicians.

INCIDENCE

The reported incidence of adnexal masses occurring with pregnancy has varied considerably. Prior to the use of ultrasound evaluation, the incidence was estimated to be between 1 in 81 and 1 in 2500 pregnancies (Grimes,

1954; Hass, 1949; Gustafson, 1954; and their colleagues). The highest incidence of adnexal masses was reported by Grimes and co-workers (1954) at 1 in 81, or 1.2 percent of pregnancies, in their series of 49 masses reported from private practice. Diagnosis was dependent primarily on clinical evaluation. Since the introduction of ultrasound, the incidence has still varied considerably from 1 of 42 to 1 of 640 pregnancies (Thornton and Wells, 1987; Hogston and Lilford, 1986; Lavery and associates, 1986; Nelson and co-workers, 1986; Jubb, 1963). Thornton and Wells (1987) reported one cyst in every 346 deliveries, 62 percent of which required removal for various reasons. Hogston and Lilford (1986) identified 1 cyst in every 42 pregnancies. They noted that only 45 percent of 137 cysts had been identified by pelvic examination alone; the remainder were found at the time of ultrasound exams. Eighty-eight percent of all clinically identified masses were greater than 6 cm; however, 13 percent of such masses were not detected by clinical exam. Clearly, ultrasound has increased the identification of adnexal masses in pregnancy, but should be used in conjunction with a thorough physical examination. The combination of physical and sonographic examination will detect most of the 0.5–2.2 percent of pregnancies complicated by an adnexal mass.

The percentage of adnexal masses that are malignant has also varied in the literature. A review of the English literature by Jubb revealed only 24 cases of primary ovarian carcinoma in pregnancy (Jubb, 1963). At the time, ovarian carcinoma in pregnancy was thought to be rare. Roberts' (1983) review of adnexal masses in pregnancy revealed a 2.2–8 percent malignancy rate, which has been supported by other authors (Struyk, 1984; Haas, 1949; Gustafson, 1954; Thornton, 1987; Hogston, 1986; Roberts, 1983; Hess, 1988; Creasman, 1971; and their associates). The highest rate (8.6 percent) was noted in Thornton's series (Thornton, 1987). Therefore it is prudent to consider malignancy whenever evaluating adnexal masses in pregnancy due to its frequent occurrence and serious consequences.

INITIAL RECOGNITION

The recognition of an adnexal mass in pregnancy depends upon a careful history, a thorough physical examination, and clinical suspicion. In Dgani and associates' review (1989), patients with malignant adnexal masses occurring with pregnancy presented with symptoms of pelvic pain, abdominal distention, or pelvic pressure. In contrast, most benign adnexal masses occurring with pregnancy are asymptomatic. Pelvic examination in the first trimester affords the clinician the best opportunity to assess the adnexa and identify a mass. After the first trimester the increased uterine size and changing location of the adnexa interfere with identification of adnexal abnormalities by either physical or ultrasonographic examination. An attempt should be made to view and evaluate the adnexa as a routine part of obstetric ultrasound examinations, especially those performed in the first trimester, when visualization is best achieved (American College of Obstetricians and Gynecologists, 1993).

Whenever an adnexal mass is identified, pelvic examination should include assessment of uterine and adnexal size and the presence of uterine, adnexal, or cul de sac irregularity. Additionally, the mobility of the mass should be determined. A rectal examination should also be performed to evaluate the posterior cul-de-sac for masses, tenderness, or fixation of the uterus or adnexa. All patients with a pelvic mass should have a stool guaiac test performed.

Often pelvic masses are identified during pregnancy as an incidental finding during an ultrasound examination performed for other indications. Ultrasound evaluation of the adnexal mass should include size, location, origin, and specific characteristics including echogenicity, presence or absence of septa, septal characteristics, and the presence or absence of excrescences. As Meire and coworkers' (1978) study revealed, these characteristics aid in distinguishing between benign and malignant disease (Table 22–1). The ultrasound examination also should include an evaluation to exclude hydatidiform or partial molar pregnancy, conditions that may be the source of large theca lutein cysts in response to high serum HCG concentrations.

EVALUATION

Further evaluation of adnexal masses in gravidas includes basic laboratory, ultrasono-

TABLE 22–1. ULTRASOUND CHARACTERISTICS OF OVARIAN MASSES

Benign	Malignant
Less than 5 cm	Greater than 5 cm
Unilocular	Multilocular with thin septa and nodules
Anechoic	Hyperechoic
Multilocular with thin septa and no nodules	Multilocular with thick septa with or without nodules
Mobile	Fixed

graphic, and/or radiographic evaluation. In general, a complete blood count, urinalysis, complete chemistry panel, and ultrasound examination should be obtained on all patients with adnexal masses. Tumor markers may be considered if malignancy is suspected. Magnetic resonance imaging or other radiographic studies should be considered in those adnexal masses that remain confusing after an initial evaluation.

Tumor Markers

The most common tumor marker used when evaluating an adnexal mass in a nonpregnant patient is the serum CA125. In nonpregnant patients who have a level greater than 65 U/mL, ovarian malignancy was predicted with a sensitivity of 91 percent (Malkasian and colleagues, 1988; Patsner, 1989, 1991). Thirty-five units per milliliter is considered the maximum normal value for CA125. CA125 also is elevated in other disease states including endometriosis, peritonitis, salpingitis, tuberculosis as well as with certain other metastatic nongynecologic and gynecologic cancers (Patsner, 1989). Unfortunately, during pregnancy CA125 is not as sensitive a marker as it is in the non-pregnant patient. Increased levels of CA125 have been found in both the first and second trimesters of pregnancy (Seki, 1986; Touitou, 1989; and their associates). Touitou and co-workers' study noted that if immunoradiometric assay (IRMA) was used instead of the standard enzyme immunoassay (EIA), the false-positive rates for pregnancy were different (Touitou and co-workers, 1989). Specifically, concentrations that exceeded the usual cutoff level of 35 U/mL were observed during pregnancy by IRMA in only 2.8 percent of gravidas, whereas 12.5 percent, 3.1 percent, and 8.3 percent of normal pregnant women had elevated concentrations in the first, second, and third trimesters, respectively, when EIA was used (Touitou and colleagues, 1989). If CA125 is to be used, it is important to identify the type of assay being performed.

Sialyl SSEA-1 antigen is currently undergoing evaluation as an ovarian tumor marker. Of note is that when combined with CA125 in pregnant patients, this antigen has rare false-positive values (Iwanari and associates, 1990). In Kobayashi and Kawashima's study, the combination of Sialyl SSEA-1 and CA125 did not increase the ovarian cancer detection rate, but when both were increased in the serum of pregnant women, the presence of a malignant ovarian tumor was highly likely (Kobayashi and Kawashima, 1990).

A quantitative beta human chorionic gonadotropin (β HCG) level may also be used as a tumor marker for a molar pregnancy or to exclude ectopic pregnancy as an etiology of adnexal mass. If the β HCG level is greater than 1000 U/L (International Reference Preparation, IRP) and transvaginal ultrasound (5-9 MHz probe) reveals no gestational sac, ectopic pregnancy should be considered. Serial HCGs should double approximately every 48 hours in a normal singleton gestation between 4 and 9 weeks' gestation (Hay, 1988). In Cacciatore's study (1990a) a serum HCG level of 1000 U/L combined with transvaginal sonographic identification of an adnexal mass was diagnostic of an ectopic pregnancy with a sensitivity of 97 percent and a specificity of 99 percent.

Another common test, maternal serum alpha-fetoprotein, can also be used as a tumor marker in pregnancy or as an indicator of an extrauterine pregnancy as the etiology of adnexal masses. Maternal serum alpha-fetoprotein is elevated in neural tube or other fetal defects, multiple gestations, germ cell tumors, gastrointestinal tumors, and extrauterine pregnancies (Gonsoulin, 1990; Barett, 1990; and their colleagues). Alpha-fetoprotein levels may be greater than 1000 ng/mL with maternal germ cell or gastrointestinal tumors (Gonsoulin and associates, 1990).

Ultrasound

Sonographic evaluation of the female pelvis is often extremely useful when an adnexal mass is identified (Lavery, 1986; Meire, 1978; Fleischer, 1990; Guy, 1988; Coleman, 1992; and their associates). In the first trimester of pregnancy, transvaginal sonography provides better resolution and closer proximity to the pelvic organs than does transabdominal sonography (Coleman, 1993; Lande, 1988; Lewitt, 1990; Burry, 1993; and their co-workers). With transvaginal ultrasound, significantly more direct signs of an ectopic pregnancy are seen than are seen with abdominal techniques (Weigel, 1993). Positive predictive values for ectopic pregnancy are 93.5 percent for an extrauterine double ring, 90.7 percent for inhomogeneous adnexal masses with simultaneous echogenic fluid in the cul-de-sac and, 79.3 percent for isolated inhomogeneous adnexal masses. The predictive values for indirect sonographic hints of suspected extrauterine pregnancy are 78.4 percent for an empty uterine cavity and 87.3 percent for echogenic cul-de-sac fluid.

After the uterus has left the true pelvis, transabdominal ultrasonography is preferentially (Lande and colleagues, 1988) performed. An ultrasonographic evaluation should include size, location, and characteristics of the mass. Characteristics include the echogenicity, loculation, density or thickness of septa, presence or absence of solid nodules, evidence of invasion of the capsule or fixation of the mass. When all of these criteria are considered, ultrasound can permit a correct differentiation of malignant from nonmalignant ovarian cysts in up to 91 percent of cases (Meire, 1978) (Table 22–2). Most cysts that are anechoic and less than 5 cm will not be malignant (Meire and co-workers, 1978). However, when all anechoic lesions in pregnancies are evaluated, 5 percent have the potential to be malignant (Moyle and associates, 1983).

Despite the importance of ultrasound, its limits also must be appreciated. Comparing laparoscopy to ultrasound, Mikkelsen and Felding (1990) noted that ultrasound had an 82.1 percent positive predictive ability, but only a 46.9 percent negative predictive ability. However, as previously noted, when correlated with human chorionic gonadotropin levels of 1,000 IRP units/L or greater, transvaginal

TABLE 22–2. DIFFERENTIAL DIAGNOSIS OF PELVIC MASSES OCCURRING DURING PREGNANCY

Uterine	Adnexal	Other
Leiomyoma	Primary ovarian neoplasm	Urologic origin
Leiomyosarcoma	Benign	Distended bladder
Uterine wall hematoma	Malignant	Pelvic or accessory kidney
Placenta increta/percretta	Metastatic ovarian neoplasm	Neoplasm
Congenital anomalies	Infection/abscess	Benign
Uterine incarceration	Ectopic pregnancy	Malignant
	Tubal	Urachal cyst
	Ovarian	Gastrointestinal origin
	Primary fallopian tube neoplasm	Infection/abscess
	Tubal leiomyomata	Appendicitis
	Endometriosis/endometrioma	Diverticulitis
		Inflammatory bowel disease
		Neoplasm
		Benign
		Malignant
		Stool in colon
		Lymphatic system
		Benign inflammatory node
		Lymphoma/leukemia
		Accessory or ectopic spleen
		Neurofibromatosis/neural neoplasm
		Striated muscle sarcoma
		Hematoma
		Abdominal pregnancy
		Articles intentionally placed in the vagina

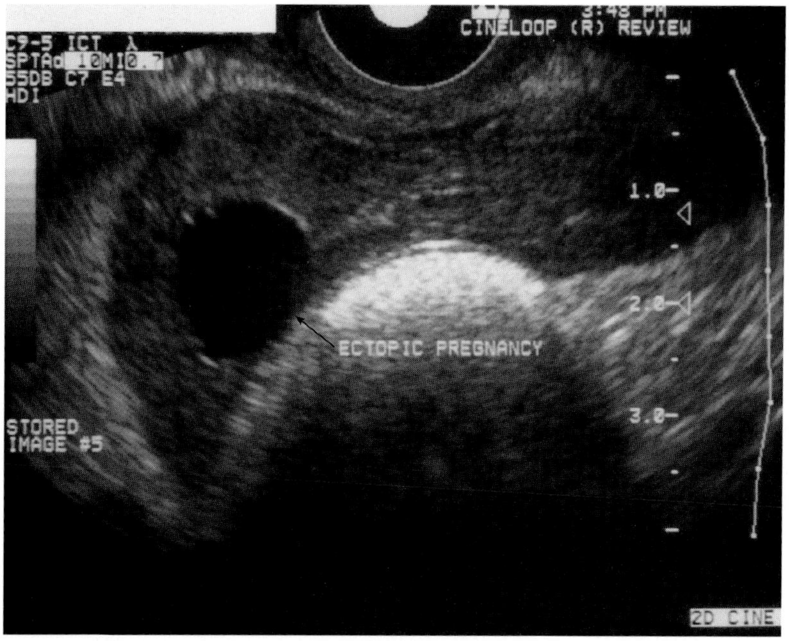

Figure 22–1. Ultrasonographic image of an ectopic pregnancy. (Courtesy Advanced Technology Laboratories (ATL), Bothwell, Washington.)

ultrasonography is particularly sensitive and specific for evaluating the pelvis for potential ectopic pregnancy (Cacciatore, 1990a,b; Coleman, 1992; Athey, 1991; Stabile, 1988; and their associates). (Figs. 22–1 and 22–2).

Color and pulse Doppler flow studies in combination with two-dimensional ultrasound might be used in the future to evaluate pelvic masses (Schiller and Grant, 1992). Taylor and associates (1989) compared conventional sonography with duplex Doppler evaluation for the diagnosis of ectopic pregnancies. The positive predictive values were 47 percent for imaging alone and 85 percent for Doppler. Negative predictive values were 60 percent and 81 percent, respectively. An initial study by Kurjak and associates (1990) shows some correlation between pelvic mass blood flow and evidence of malignancy. Neovascularization was detected in 6 of 10 cases of uterine fibroma and in 2 cases of ovarian cancer. In 6 cases of benign ovarian pathol-

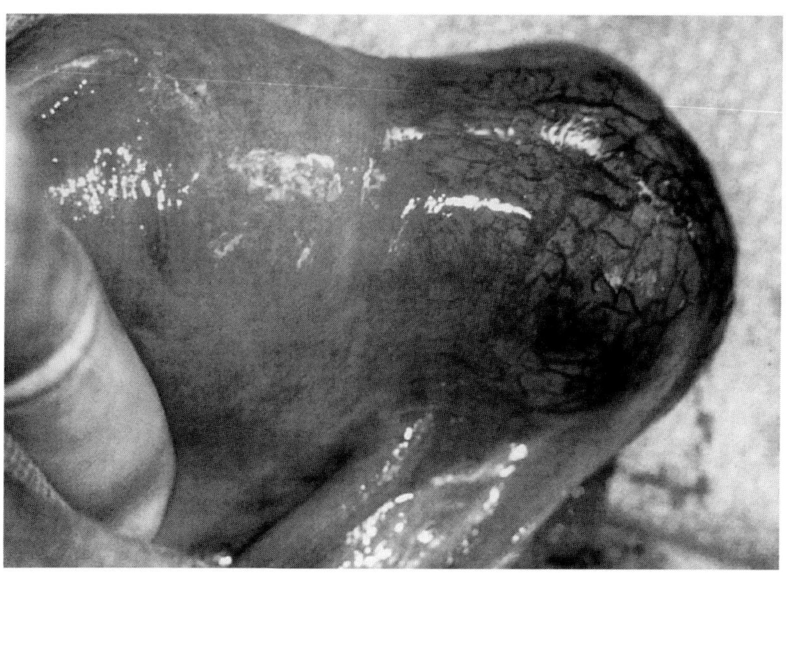

Figure 22–2. Cornual ectopic pregnancy initially identified via ultrasonographic evaluation.

ogy, no abnormal blood supply could be seen. Lower impedance and higher blood velocity due to neovascularization was directly correlated with the cases of malignancy (Kurjak and co-workers, 1990).

Magnetic Resonance Imaging (MRI)

MRI should be considered a useful diagnostic adjunct to ultrasonographic evaluation for an adnexal mass complicating pregnancy. Although there are few reported cases of adnexal masses undergoing MRI in pregnancy, those that have been studied reveal MRI to be a valuable complement to ultrasonography (Kier, 1990; Lubbers, 1988; and their colleagues). MRI is particularly good at identifying the origin of the pelvic mass, its contents (particularly absence of hemorrhage), and degenerative or malignant changes (Fig. 22–3) (Kier, 1990; Lubbers, 1988; Dooms, 1986; Al-Awanhi, 1991; Nyberg, 1987; and their associates). MRI is also useful in diagnosing or distinguishing uterine leiomyomata from more serious pathology and thus preventing unnecessary surgical exploration. One small series reported five pregnant women with adnexal masses suspected to be leiomyomas who underwent MRI. Four patients had evidence of leiomyoma and one had a benign cystic teratoma. All avoided laparotomy because of the almost certain radiologic findings of a benign process (Curtis and co-workers, 1993). MRI appears safe for use in pregnancy (Kier, 1990; Lubbers, 1988; Dooms, 1986; Al-Awanhi, 1991; Nyberg, 1987; Geard, 1984; Wolff, 1980; and their associates; National Radiological Protection Board, 1983). However, despite the lack of evidence of hazards to the embryo or fetus, the British National Radiological Protection Board (1983) suggested that "It might be prudent to exclude women from MRI scanning during the first trimester." Additionally, the National Institutes of Health Consensus Development Conference on MRI recommended that "MRI scanning in pregnancy should be used during the first trimester only when there is a clear medical indication that it offers definitive advantages over other tests" (Kier and co-workers, 1990).

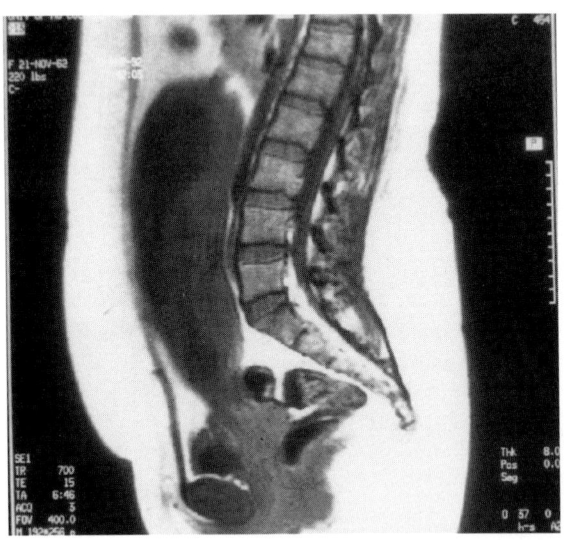

Figure 22–3. MRI scan of the pregnant uterus demonstrating an elongated uterus high in the abdomen. This patient was initially diagnosed as an abdominal pregnancy via ultrasonographic evaluation.

Computed Tomography (CT)

CT is less desirable than MRI when attempting to further define and characterize an ultrasonographically identified cyst. CT uses ionizing radiation and provides minimal discriminatory information because most pelvic masses have a nonspecific appearance (Kier and associates, 1990). CT scanning of adnexal masses occurring with pregnancy should be reserved for those patients for whom additional diagnostic information is required, but who are not candidates for MRI.

Other radiographic procedures such as intravenous pyelography (IVP), barium enema (BE), and abdominal series, for example, may be required if colonic or urologic malignancy is suspected (Peters and associates, 1990; Kvale and Heuch, 1991). However, in pregnancy radiographic studies should be used with caution and as infrequently as possible. Brent (1986) recommends that exposure be limited to 5 rads or less.

DIFFERENTIAL DIAGNOSIS

Pelvic masses may arise from the uterus itself or be extrauterine in origin (Table 22–2). Extrauterine masses may arise from bowel, bladder, fallopian tubes, ovaries, or other abdominal organs. They can be grouped into four separate categories based on ultrasonographic evaluation: simple unilocular cysts, simple multilocular cysts, complex masses, and solid masses (Table 22–3). This sono-

TABLE 22–3. SONOGRAPHIC CATEGORIES OF PELVIC MASSES

Simple Unilocular Cysts	Simple Multilocular Cysts	Complex Masses	Solid Masses
Corpus luteum	Hydrosalpinx	Abscess: appendiceal, ovarian, tubo-ovarian, bowel	Fibroma, thecoma, Brenner's tumor
Distended bladder	Malignancy	Bowel with fecal material	Granulosa cell tumor
Endometrioma	Molar pregnancy	Degenerating myoma	Leiomyomata
Hydrosalpinx	Mucinous cystadenoma	Ectopic pregnancy	Malignant tumors
Paraovarian cyst	Multicystic ovary	Endometrioma	
Serous cystadenoma	Small bowel with fluid	Granulosa cell tumor	
	Theca leutein cyst	Hemorrhage and/or necrosis with cystic or solid tumors	
		Hydrosalpinx	
		Malignant tumor	
		Pelvic kidney	
		Teratoma (dermoid cyst)	

graphic classification can narrow the differential diagnosis of the pelvic mass; however, many of the disease processes may fit into more than one sonographic category. For instance, a hydrosalpinx may appear as a unilocular cyst but more often will have the appearance of a complex mass. Similarly, a granulosa cell tumor may appear as a solid or as a complex mass. Ovarian masses are the most commonly identified extrauterine mass (Table 22–4). The specific ovarian lesion most often identified is a mature or benign cystic teratoma (Fig. 22–4). In multiple series with 509 combined ovarian masses surgically removed in pregnancy, 32 percent were teratomas. The next most common mass was either a mucinous or serous cystadenoma (Fig. 22–5). The third most common adnexal mass was a corpus luteum cyst.

The clinician must always be aware of the risk of malignancy, particularly in masses greater than 5 cm. Of ovarian masses discovered during pregnancy, 2–8 percent will be malignant (Grimes, 1954; Ballard, 1984; Struyk, 1984; Hess, 1988; Gustafson, 1954; White, 1973; McGowan, 1983; Ashkenazy, 1988; Munnell, 1963; and their colleagues). Combining studies results in a malignancy

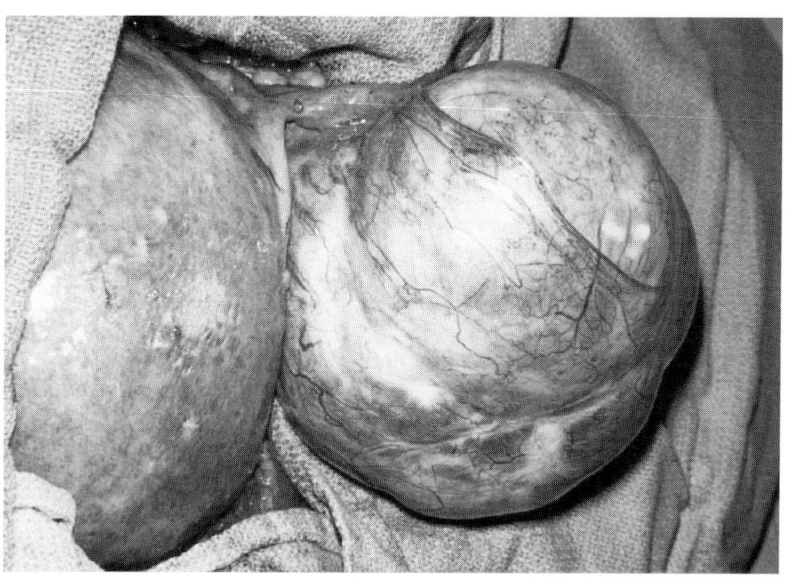

Figure 22–4. Teratoma in early pregnancy that underwent acute torsion.

TABLE 22–4. PELVIC MASSES REMOVED IN PREGNANCY (N = 509)

	Ashkenazy (1988)	Ballard (1984)	Grimes (1954)	Gustafson (1954)	Haas (1949)	Hess (1988)	Hogston (1986)	Struyk (1984)	Thornton (1987)	White (1973)	Total of 509	%
Teratoma (dermoid cyst)	9	49	11	18	4	14	4	25	20	8	162	31.8
Cystadenomas (serous and mucinous)	10	21	5	14	5	14	4	25	22	12	132	25.9
Corpus luteum	4	4	12	4	1	7	4	4	6	7	53	10.4
Functional cyst	4	8	14	0	2	6	4	1	6	2	47	9.3
Paraovarian cyst	2	8	2	2	0	3	2	9	6	1	35	6.9
Other	0	4	3	0	2	2	0	1	12	2	26	5.1
Endometrioma	3	7	1	2	2	2	1	1	2	2	23	4.5
Malignancy	2	2	0	2	1	2	1	3	7	3	23	4.5
Fibroma	4	1	1	1	0	0	0	0	0	1	8	1.6

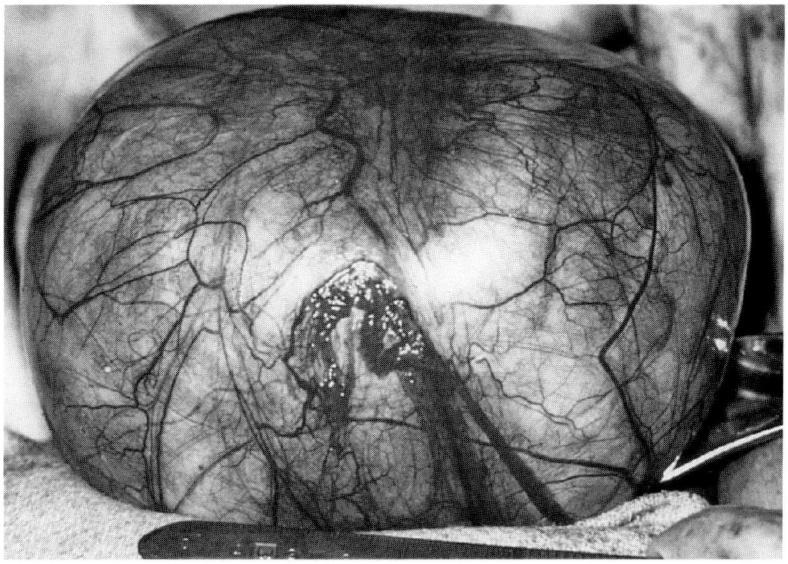

Figure 22–5. Serous cystadenoma electively removed at 15 weeks' gestation.

rate of 4.5 percent (Table 22–4). The incidence of ovarian malignancy in pregnancy has been reported to be between 1 in 1,800 (Munnell, 1963; the most often quoted source) and 1 in 25,000 pregnancies (Dgani, 1989; Ashkenazy, 1988; Munnell, 1963; Tawa, 1964; Chung, 1973; Wilson, 1937; Dougherty, 1950; Ballard, 1984; and their associates).

Leiomyomas

Leiomyomas are the most common pelvic mass associated with pregnancy (Figs. 22–6 through 22–8). They occur in 0.3–2.6 percent of pregnancies and usually have no clinical significance (Bezjian, 1984). The usual sonographic appearance of a leiomyoma is a relatively hypoechoic mass lying within the uterine wall with a distinct capsule. Leiomyomas may develop cystic areas as a result of red degeneration, demonstrate echogenic rims corresponding to areas of calcification, or demonstrate heterogeneity (Fleischer, 1990; Lev-Toaff, 1987; and their co-workers) (Figs. 22–9 and 22–10). They also may be pedunculated and separate from the uterus. In a 1987 study, Lev-Toaff and associates evaluated the behavior of leiomyomas in pregnancy. Contrary to the popularly held belief that fibroids enlarge during

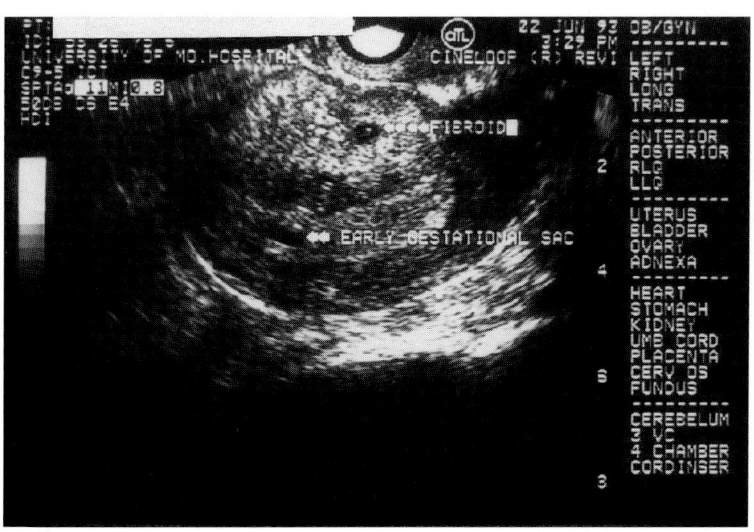

Figure 22–6. Sonographic image of a fibroid uterus with an early gestational sac. Note that the fibroid has a well-delineated capsule.

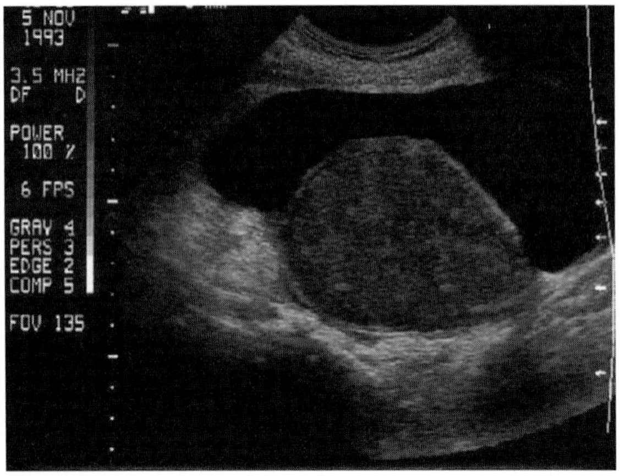

Figure 22–7. Sonographic image of a pedunculated leiomyoma in early pregnancy.

pregnancy and regress in the puerperium, Lev-Toaff and co-workers noted that in the second trimester, smaller fibroids increased in size, but larger fibroids decreased. During the third trimester all fibroids, regardless of their initial size, decreased in size (Lev-Toaff, 1987; Ahavoni, 1988; and their associates). Ahavoni and co-workers (1988) noted no increase in size in 78 percent of fibroids detected during pregnancy. Those fibroids that enlarged increased no more than 21 percent. At 6 weeks postpartum, size was the same as that documented during pregnancy.

Leiomyomas may cause severe abdominal pain during pregnancy. This may result from acute torsion of a pedunculated fibroid or so-called red degeneration of the fibroid. Leiomyomas also may increase the risk of first trimester abortion, malpresentation of the fetus, preterm labor, abruptio placenta, and retained placenta (Cunningham and colleagues, 1993). Myomectomy is generally considered inadvisable during pregnancy unless the fibroid is pedunculated. If greater dissection is required for myomectomy, the bleeding may be profuse and the uterus may need to be sacrificed to control hemorrhage (Bezjian, 1984).

Uterine Abnormalities

Bicornuate or other uterine anomalies, blind uterine horn pregnancy, incarceration of the gravid uterus (Hess and associates, 1989), and persistent retroversion are other uterine causes of pelvic masses in pregnancy. These usually can be diagnosed by history, physical examination, and sonographic evaluation (Jackson and associates, 1988; Flienger, 1986), but at times may require MRI to establish the diagnosis.

Simple Unilocular Cysts

Simple unilocular cysts have anechoic internal echoes: clear, sharp, smooth borders, and round configurations sonographically (Lavery, 1986; Fleischer, 1990; Bezjian, 1984; and their colleagues). These cysts may range in size

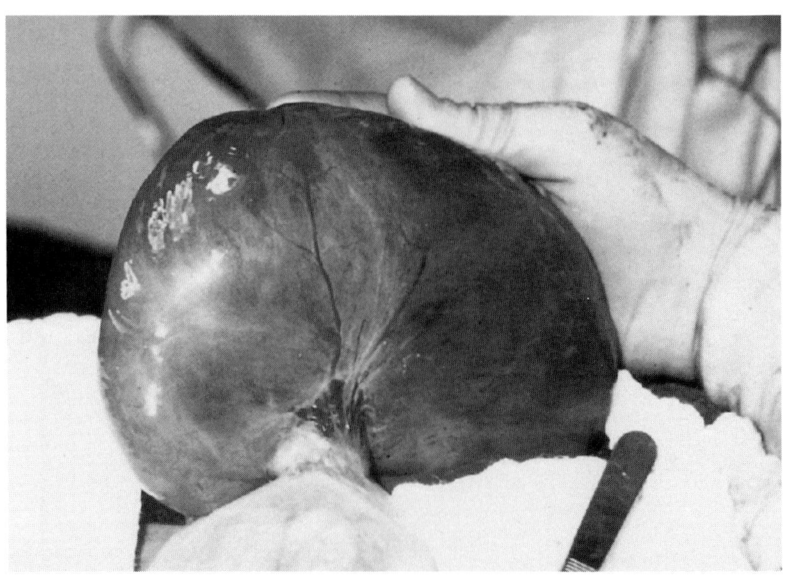

Figure 22–8. Pedunculated fibroid from Fig. 22–7, which underwent acute torsion in pregnancy.

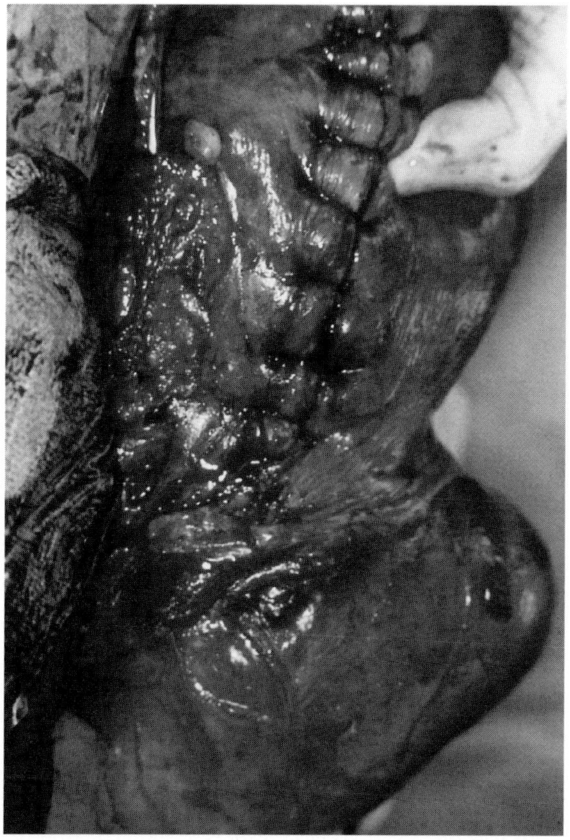

Figure 22–9. Vaginal delivery was obstructed by a large leiomyoma of the left lower uterine segment, requiring delivery by cesarean section.

from 3 to 25 cm (Lavery, 1986; Nelson, 1986; Fleischer, 1990; and their co-workers). The most common cause of a simple unilocular cyst in early pregnancy is the corpus luteum cyst. The corpus luteum generally ranges in size from 2 to 6 cm. While corpus luteum cysts are common in early pregnancy, they usually resolve by 16 weeks of pregnancy (Thornton, 1987; Lavery, 1986; Fleischer, 1990; and their colleagues). In Thornton and Wells' study (1987), 38 percent of unilocular adnexal masses in pregnancy resolved by 16 weeks of gestation. Rarely do these cysts have internal echoes and septae secondary to internal hemorrhage or separation of the luteinized lining from the wall of the cyst. While the purpose of the corpus luteum is to support the pregnancy during the first trimester, the corpus luteum is not necessary to support the pregnancy after the seventh week of gestation (Csapo and co-workers, 1973). Most—but not all—corpus luteum cysts resolve in the second trimester.

Other etiologies for simple unilocular cysts are serous cystadenomas, paraovarian cysts, borderline malignancies, hydrosalpinges, distended bladder, and endometriomas. Cystadenomas can range in size from 4 to 35 cm when presenting as a simple cyst (Thornton, 1987; Lavery, 1986; Fleischer, 1990; Bezjian, 1984; and their associates). Paraovarian cysts may present at any size and can occasionally be identified as separate from the ovaries. Hydrosalpinges are generally tubular in con-

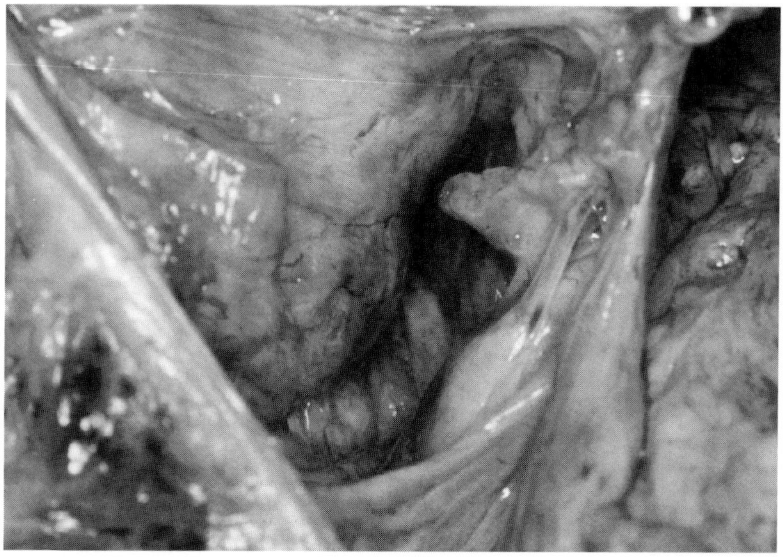

Figure 22–10. On cut section the heterogeneity of the leiomyomata is obvious and demonstrates why the mass had a complex appearance on sonographic evaluation. The tumor was benign.

figuration; a history of pelvic inflammatory disease, endometriosis, or prior surgery may suggest this diagnosis. Of most concern when a unilocular cyst is detected is a borderline or malignant tumor. In Thornton and Wells' study (1987), there were three borderline malignancies: diameters 8, 12, and 18 cm with an echo-free simple cystic pattern. According to Meire and associates (1978) ultrasound can delineate benign from malignant ovarian neoplasms in only 90 percent of patients. A clinician cannot assume that a cyst is benign solely because of a simple echo-free pattern, particularly if the mass's diameter is greater than 5 cm and has persisted into the second trimester.

Simple Multilocular Cysts

Simple multilocular cysts present with anechoic centers, but septations are noted. The differential diagnosis includes mucinous cystadenoma, theca lutein cyst, multicystic ovary, malignancy, hydrosalpinx, small bowel with fluid, and gestational trophoblastic disease (molar pregnancy).

Cystadenomas, the second most common cause of a pelvic mass in pregnancy, range in size from 8 to 35 cm (Ballard, 1984; Gustafson and associates, 1954; Tawa, 1964). As in all large cysts identified in pregnancy, cystadenomas have an increased risk for torsion. Additionally, when they rupture, the patient can develop pseudomyxoma peritonei. Thus great care must be taken to remove cystadenomas intact (Bezjian, 1984).

Theca lutein cysts are commonly associated with multiple gestation, trophoblastic disease, and ovulation induction. Theca lutein cysts average 7 cm in diameter (Gains, 1965; Montz and associates, 1988). Prior to ovulation induction therapy, most theca lutein cysts were associated with gestational trophoblastic disease (Montz and co-workers, 1988). Their most common complications include torsion and hemoperitoneum (Montz and colleagues, 1988). Ascites is rare in theca lutein cysts secondary to hydatidiform mole, choriocarcinoma, or multiple gestation, but frequently associated with ovarian hyperstimulation syndrome (OHS), which occurs in 1.8–23 percent of cycles when ovulation induction has been performed (Rizk and Aboulghar, 1991). The severe form of OHS, ovarian enlargement greater than 5 cm, may include pulmonary edema and massive ascites, and occurs less than 1.8 percent of the time (Rizk and Aboulghar, 1991). With ovulation induction, the diagnosis should be obvious based on patient history, prior ultrasound evaluation, presence of bilateral ovarian cysts, and ascites. Moderate and severe cases are treated conservatively with correction of fluid and electrolyte imbalances, avoidance of pelvic examination, and prevention of thromboembolism (Rizk and Aboulghar, 1991). Surgical therapy should be limited to cases of torsion, rupture, or ectopic pregnancy (Rizk and Aboulghar, 1991). The natural progression for these cysts due to all etiologies is spontaneous resolution in late pregnancy or the postpartum period (Montz, 1988; Rizk, 1991; Wajda, 1989; King, 1991; and their associates).

Complex Masses

Complex ultrasonographic masses include the most common ovarian mass present after the first trimester, mature cystic teratomas. Teratomas, in older literature referred to as dermoid cysts, typically have diameters greater than 5 cm (Table 22–4). They most often present with a pattern of echogenic foci with acoustic shadowing situated within a predominantly cystic mass (Lavery and co-workers, 1986). The typical acoustic shadowing can be due to fat or bone. Occasionally, the variable echogenic nature of a teratoma can cause it to be confused with loops of bowel. In order to differentiate between adnexal mass or bowel, a good physical examination is a must. Serial ultrasound examination is also useful.

Granulosa cell tumors, while uncommon, usually present as complex ultrasonographic masses. These tumors present as solid and cystic neoplasms in which the cyst may contain hemorrhagic fluid. The stage of the tumor is the most important prognostic factor. When confined to the ovary, granulosa cell tumors have an excellent prognosis. If disease is confined to the ovary, removal of only the affected ovary is possible (Czernobilsky, 1987).

Ectopic pregnancies and tubo-ovarian complexes must be considered when a complex mass is identified even if an intrauterine pregnancy has already been noted. Although simultaneous intrauterine and ectopic pregnancies are rare, the clinician should keep the possibility in mind, particularly in a patient who has undergone ovulation induction. Bello and colleagues (1986) have reported the incidence of combined ectopic and intrauterine pregnancies as 1 in 3899 to 15,000.

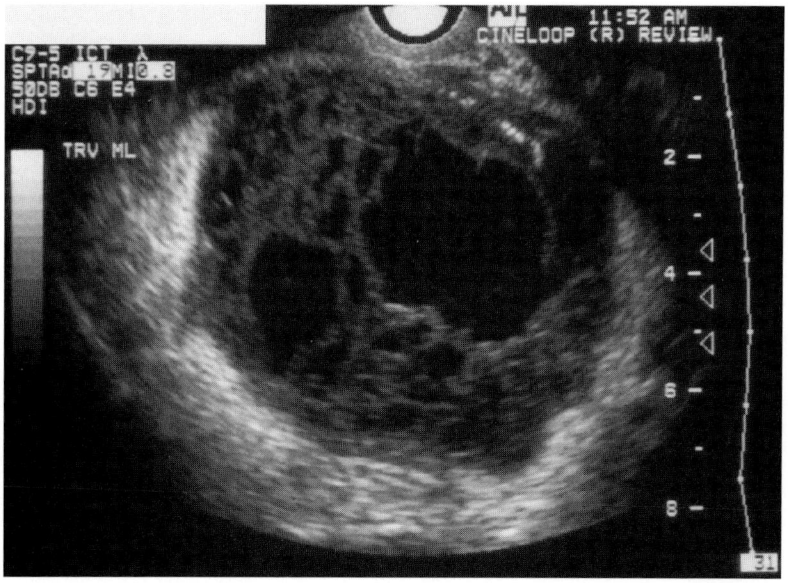

Figure 22–11. Sonographic image of a tubo-ovarian abscess.

Acute pelvic inflammatory disease and tubo-ovarian complexes or abscess (Fig. 22–11) are complex masses rarely considered in pregnancy. When they occur, the gravida usually will present with localized abdominal tenderness, fever, and an elevated white blood cell count. Pelvic inflammatory disease occurs most commonly in the first trimester before the uterine cavity becomes totally occluded at 12 weeks' gestation. Other mechanisms that can cause abscess formation include recrudescence of preexisting PID, instrumentation, hematogenous or lymphatic spread into the area, or spread from a contiguous structure such as appendicitis or diverticulitis (Blanchard and associates, 1987). Ovarian abscesses may result from hematogenous spread from distant foci, contiguous spread from adjacent organs such as the uterus, fallopian tube, appendix or intestine, or lymphatic spread from adjacent structures such as appendix, bowel, or cervical lymphatics (Halpin, 1988). Additionally, diverticular disease is a common cause of adnexal abscesses in the older gravida.

Solid Masses

Solid masses have a more limited differential diagnosis, which includes benign fibroma, thecoma, Brenner's tumor, or other malignancy. Fibromas composed of spindle cells represent 4 percent of all ovarian tumors and also may be associated with Meigs syndrome (Czernobilsky, 1987). Thecomas are approximately one-third as common as granulosa cell tumors in the general population and therefore rare in pregnancy. Only 10 percent of all thecomas appear in patients under age 30 (Young and Scully, 1987). Brenner tumors, which constitute only 1.7 percent of all ovarian neoplasms, vary in size from microscopic to 2–8 cm in diameter. These tumors are rarely metaplastic, proliferating, or malignant (Young and Scully, 1987).

Because 2–8 percent of all adnexal masses in pregnancy are carcinomas, malignant neoplasia must be suspected in all cases involving solid or complex masses. Although most ovarian cancers are epithelial in origin, more germ cell tumors are identified in pregnant patients due to their youth (Creasman, 1971; Novak, 1975; Dgani, 1989; Chung, 1973; and their associates). Sarcoma is a rare solid tumor occurring in pregnancy (Fig. 22–12). In a case report Kyoto and colleagues (1989) noted that while the sarcoma actively invades the endometrial cavity, it does not invade the amnion and chorion, and the membranes appear to protect the fetus.

COMPLICATIONS OF ADNEXAL MASSES MANAGED WITHOUT SURGICAL EXPLORATION

Torsion has been noted by various authors to occur at a rate of 7 to 28 percent of all pelvic masses diagnosed in pregnancy (Ballard, 1984; Struyk and Treffers, 1984; Hess and co-

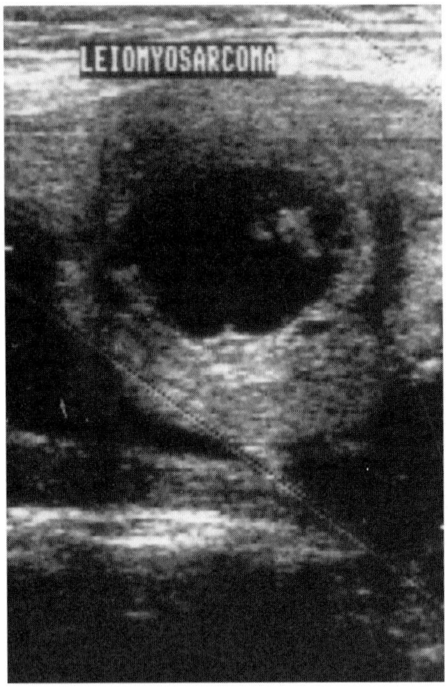

Figure 22–12. Sonographic image of a leiomyosarcoma identified in early pregnancy. Note that the amnion is not invaded by the tumor.

workers, 1988; Roberts, 1983; McGowan, 1983; Wilson, 1937). The lowest rate of torsion, 0.8 percent, was found by Hogston and Lilford (1986) in a study using ultrasound to diagnose all cysts in pregnancy. Because most studies are biased toward symptomatic patients, this low rate is not surprising. If symptoms prompt the evaluation that discovers the adnexal mass, it is accordingly not surprising that the rate of torsion is higher than that in asymptomatic patients with a mass.

Impedance to labor has been extensively discussed. Munnell (1963) stated that dystocia was the primary reason cysts were removed in pregnancy. In some series, the incidence of labor dystocia has been as high as 75 percent; in others, almost nonexistent (Struyk and Treffers, 1984; Munnell, 1963). Dystocia is rarely caused by small masses.

Roberts (1983) noted that ovarian mass rupture had been responsible for a majority of the maternal deaths related to adnexal masses. The worst prognosis occurs from rupture of a teratoma with subsequent reactive peritonitis. Great care should be taken to remove teratomas intact. The rate of rupture from symptomatic cysts varies from 6 to 12 percent (Dooms, 1986; Nyberg, 1987; and their associates).

Infarction can present as an acute abdomen. One review indicates that infarction may occur in 13 percent of adnexal masses in pregnancy (Dougherty and Lund, 1950). In a more recent review, infarction alone occurred in 2 percent of adnexal masses; however, if torsion were included, the percentage would be much higher (Hess and colleagues, 1988).

Infection or abscess of adnexal cysts is reported by Struyk and Treffers (1984) to occur in 4 percent of adnexal masses in pregnancy. Most infections occur in the postpartum period.

TREATMENT

Treatment is aimed at achieving the best maternal and fetal outcome. Since the introduction of ultrasound, increasing numbers of adnexal masses are being identified in the first trimester. In an asymptomatic patient, management should proceed along a logical progression such as that in Figure 22–13. This algorithm attempts to balance the risk of maternal and fetal complications from torsion, hemorrhage, infarction, abscess formation, and malignancy against the surgical complications associated with exploratory laparotomy.

The fear of fetal wastage remains a major consideration regarding timing for surgical removal of adnexal masses presenting in pregnancy. When reviewing fetal wastage in association with general surgical procedures during pregnancy, tremendous variation exists. Many investigators noted increased fetal loss when an acute intra-abdominal process occurred (Mazze and Källén, 1991; Allen and associates, 1989; Saunders and Mailton, 1973). Additionally, Hess and associates (1988) found that when surgery for an adnexal mass was delayed until the onset of symptoms, the pregnancy prognosis was worse than when surgery had been performed electively, without regard to the trimester. Fetal loss reported by Gustafson and co-workers (1954) was 30 percent with adnexal surgery; however, most of these losses occurred in patients with preoperative threatened abortions. Novak and colleagues (1975) reported a 33 percent fetal loss, and Levine and Diamond (1961) a 45 percent fetal loss; however, neither detailed the cir-

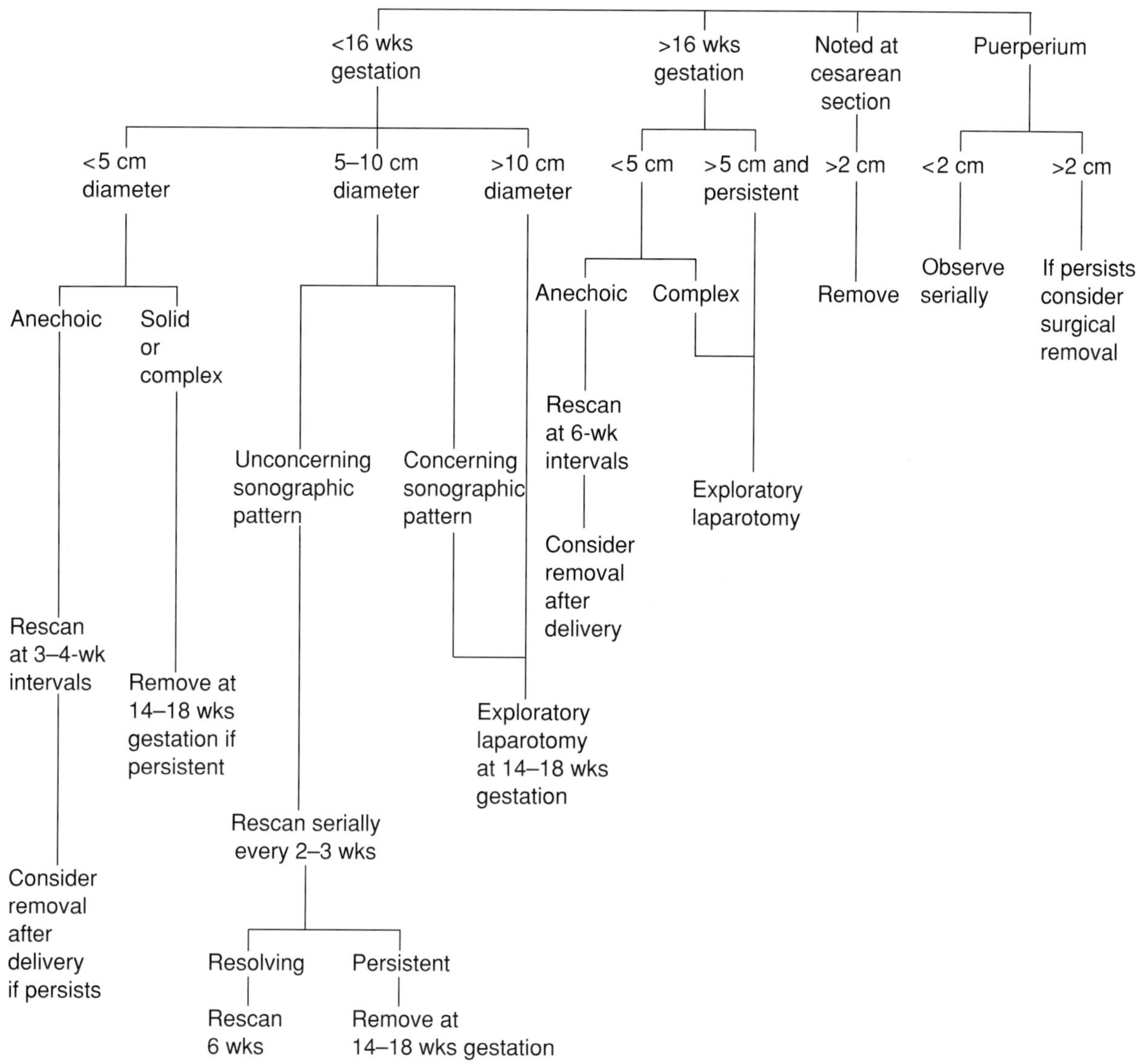

Figure 22–13. Treatment algorithm for asymptomatic masses occurring with pregnancy (unrelated to ovulation induction).

cumstances surrounding the abortions. Among 12 patients who underwent adnexal surgery in the first trimester, Saunders and Mailton (1973) reported a fetal wastage of 44 percent. Many other studies report normal to low fetal wastage. Rabinerson and associates (1992) found no fetal loss after adnexectomy in pregnancies less than 8 weeks. Ashkenazy and associates (1988) reported no increase in fetal loss over the background population risk. White (1973) noted a fetal loss rate of 18 percent that corrected to 12 percent when ectopic and molar pregnancies were eliminated. Another study noted a fetal loss rate of 13 percent that when corrected for molar pregnancies, ectopics, and hysterectomy performed for malignancy was only 2.5 percent (Grimes and co-workers, 1954). Thus, while there is no consensus on the fetal loss rate directly attributable to first trimester adnexal surgery, the rate probably is not greater than the 15 percent background risk of spontaneous abortion.

When ovarian surgery is necessary in the first trimester, some authors advocate progesterone supplementation to replace progesterone production loss by the corpus luteum.

Other believe that there is no place for progesterone therapy. Csapo and colleagues (1973) concluded that the corpus luteum is nonessential after the seventh week of gestation. In contrast, Ashkenazy and co-workers (1988) found improved pregnancy outcome when 500 mg of hydroxy progesterone caproate was given intramuscularly every week until the twenty-fifth week of pregnancy. In Ashkenazy and associates' review there was no risk of teratogenesis to the fetus. At this time there are no clear guidelines concerning progesterone therapy. Because its use is associated with little or no risk, we generally provide progesterone supplementation if the operation is performed prior to 12 weeks' gestation.

When the pregnant patient presents with an adnexal mass and an acute abdomen, the decision to operate should not be delayed. Hemorrhage and abscess should be treated in the usual fashion. Torsion can present a special surgical case with 7–28 percent of ovarian masses so presenting. Unfortunately, and often due to unimpressive signs and symptoms, the diagnosis may be delayed (Bider and co-workers, 1991). In 30 percent of the cases of adnexal torsion, the preoperative diagnosis is incorrect (Bider and associates, 1991; Shalev and Peley, 1993). Unless torsions are treated expeditiously, peritonitis and death can result. General opinion has been that because the unwinding of a necrotic adnexa may increase the risk of thromboembolism and infection, the adnexa should be removed en-block. However, recent studies that include pregnant patients indicate that adnexal torsion can be safely managed by a simple unwinding of the adnexa even when it appears to be hemorrhagic and ischemic, but not when necrotic (Shalev, 1990, 1993; Bider, 1991; and their co-workers). These investigators reported minimal postoperative complications, no evidence of infection, and no evidence of thromboembolic disease.

The timing of surgical intervention for asymptomatic cysts is controversial. Since up to 60 percent of all first trimester masses may be functional cysts (Struyk and Treffers, 1984), most authors recommend observation in the first trimester because a large number of cysts will resolve (Thornton, 1987; Rodin, 1989; Nelson, 1986; Gains, 1965; Roberts, 1983; Struyk, 1984; Lavery, 1986; Hess, 1988; and their co-workers). In the first trimester, if a cyst is less than 5 cm in size, anechoic, or a simple cyst without septations, it is usually functional. Cysts between 5 and 10 cm with anechoic centers and no septa generally can be safely observed in the first trimester (Thornton and Wells, 1987; Rodin and associates, 1989). Such management schemas are not perfect, and an occasional borderline malignancy will be missed (Thornton and Wells, 1987). Cysts that contain internal echos and are greater than 5 cm should be removed due to a risk of malignancy and low likelihood of spontaneous resolution (Ashkenazy and associates, 1988; Thornton and Wells, 1987). Cysts greater than 10 cm or with internal septations or varying echogenicity rarely resolve. Unless the cyst is a theca lutein cyst due to ovulation induction, most authors recommend removal. No surgery should be delayed in the first trimester if there is suspicion of peritonitis, torsion, infarction, or infection. Struyk and Treffers (1984) have recommended removing all possibly malignant adnexal cysts between 16 and 20 weeks of gestation. Others recommend removal of all cysts greater than 6 cm that persist into the second trimester (Roberts, 1983; Hess and co-workers, 1988; Thornton and Wells, 1987). Ashkenazy and colleagues (1988) are some of the few authors who recommend removal of all ovarian masses identified during pregnancy regardless of the trimester.

Some adnexal masses will not be identified until the time of cesarean section performed for other obstetric indications. At the time of cesarean section, Koonings and associates (1988) advised the removal of all masses including those smaller than 5 cm. In his study, only 2 of 41 masses smaller than 5 cm were simple functional cysts while 3 of 41 that were greater than 5 cm were functional cysts. The rest of the tumors were benign, but fell into categories such as teratoma, cystadenomas, fibromas, endometriomas, and hydatid cysts of Morgagni.

Occasionally, the mass will be identified in the puerperium. As soon as the mass is identified, it should be evaluated. In the postpartum period, the mass will not be a functional cyst in the majority of cases (McGowan, 1989). There is no reason to delay treatment unless the patient is unstable or, a poor surgical candidate, or the patient and clinician want to wait for a laparoscopic approach when the uterus has involuted. Standard therapy includes laparotomy with cystectomy. Attempts to salvage the ovary should be made if malignancy is not suspected. If malignancy is suspected or even seems a remote possibility, cytologic washings of the peritoneum should be obtained. (See Chap. 27.)

Aspiration and cytologic evaluation of cyst content has been supported by some authors as a way to treat ovarian or adnexal masses in pregnancy, particularly those that are anechoic, unilocular, and less than or equal to 5 cm (Rodin, 1989; Khaw, 1990; Hassan, 1990; Worthen, 1990; and their associates). Khaw and Walker (1990) and Rodin and co-workers (1989) caution against aspiration of cysts with diameters greater than 5 cm because malignancies can be missed even with anechoic smooth wall cysts. Rodin and associates (1989) found that although benign lesions were diagnosed accurately 94 percent of the time, 6 percent of the time a malignant lesion was misdiagnosed by the combination of ultrasound and cytologic evaluation. Other investigators do not recommend aspiration owing to the risk of malignancy (Harwitz, 1988; Hess, 1988; Buckley, 1989; and their co-workers). As Buckley (1989) noted, even when a cyst is benign, it is impossible for the pathologist to cytologically distinguish between serous cystadenoma, peritubular cysts, paraovarian cysts, hyposalpinx, and functional cysts. All of these contain a similar cell population, and cytologic examination alone fails to identify malignant cysts in 6 percent of the cases (Buckley, 1989). Therefore, at this time we do not recommend aspiration of ovarian cysts. As ultrasonography and cytopathology become more refined, aspiration of ovarian cysts may become adequate for diagnosis and therapy in the future.

Other issues connected with laparotomy for removal of ovarian cysts include the possibility of preterm labor and/or maternal infection. At this time, opinions are mixed concerning routine peri- and postoperative tocolysis, and there have been no controlled studies that adequately assess the issue. No firm recommendation can be made based on the literature. If tocolysis is elected, a continuous infusion of magnesium sulfate is suitable. Caution is advised in the use of indomethacin because it might lead to bleeding problems due to interference with platelet function.

Ashkenazy and colleagues (1988) evaluated maternal infection and noted that two-thirds of women undergoing adnexal surgery in pregnancy had low-grade temperatures lasting for more than 48 hours. Of these cases, 42 percent had infertility problems later in life. He accordingly recommends that preoperative antibiotics be given. Since preoperative and perioperative antibiotics carry a low potential for complications, this recommendation appears reasonable.

SUMMARY

In pregnancy therapy for an adnexal cyst that may be malignant can prove difficult in the best of circumstances. If an adnexal mass proves to be malignant and the pregnancy is less than 24–26 weeks' gestation, most authors agree that the patient should be treated as if she were not pregnant (McGowan, 1989; Thornton and Wells, 1987; Hess and associates, 1988; Roberts, 1983; Struyk and Treffers, 1984). However, unless the malignancy is obvious, frozen tissue diagnosis should not be used to make intraoperative decisions. If a tumor of low malignant potential or a dysgerminoma is identified, unilateral oophorectomy may be sufficient until hysterectomy can be performed at a later date (Thornton and Wells, 1987; McGowan, 1983). In these cases, if the patient wishes to have additional children, it may be appropriate to do a unilateral oophorectomy and allow vaginal delivery with the plan to remove the remaining ovary and the uterus after childbearing has been completed (McGowan, 1983). If the pregnancy is greater than 24–26 weeks and malignancy is suspected, some authors recommend that the mass be observed until after 34–37 weeks' gestation (McGowan, 1989; Struyk and Treffers, 1984). The infant should then be delivered via cesarean hysterectomy in a tertiary care center followed by surgical extirpation of the adnexae, tumor debulking, and appropriate postsurgical therapy. Transfer to a tertiary care center affords the mother and fetus the best access to comprehensive care from specialists in maternal–fetal medicine, neonatal intensive care, and gynecologic oncology.

Whenever malignancy is suspected, an oophorectomy should be performed in a manner appropriate for a malignant carcinoma. Peritoneal washing should be performed in the cul-de-sac, at the level of the diaphragm, and at the lateral gutters for cytologic evaluation. A thorough manual exploration of the abdomen should also be performed. Proceeding to further staging such as omentectomy, node sampling, and so on is not recommended unless cancer is proven (Hess and co-workers, 1988; Thornton and Wells, 1987; Roberts, 1983; Dgani and associates, 1989; McGowan, 1983). All gravidas should be advised of the approximate 5 percent risk of malignancy when an adnexal mass persists into the second trimester of pregnancy. Prior to proceeding with exploratory laparotomy, the patient's desires for method of therapy (i.e., pregnancy sacrifice with hysterectomy and tumor debulking versus debulking and awaiting cesarean hysterectomy with final therapy at 34–37 weeks' gestation, etc.) should be extensively discussed.

Although adnexal masses in pregnancy pose therapeutic and diagnostic dilemmas, consensus exists in many areas of their management. The clinician cannot afford to ignore an adnexal mass or pelvic mass identified in pregnancy. Expectant management, tried in the past, is associated with serious sequelae for mother and fetus. Surgical intervention may be necessary in many cases, as outlined in the body of this chapter. Clinician and patient should in no case ignore the small but real potential for malignancy, even in these young women.

REFERENCES

Ahavoni A, Reiter A, Golan D, et al. Patterns of growth of uterine leiomyomas during pregnancy. A prospective longitudinal study. Br J Obstet Gynaecol 1988;95:510.

Al-Ahwani S, Assem M, Belal A, et al. Magnetic resonance imaging of abnormal uterine masses. J Belge Radiol 1991;74:19.

Allen JR, Helling TS, Langenfeld M. Intraabdominal surgery during pregnancy. Am J Surg 1989; 158:567.

American College of Obstetricians and Gynecologists. Ultrasonography in pregnancy. Technical Bulletin No. 187. Washington, DC: December 1993.

Ashkenazy M, Kessler I, Czernobilsky B, et al. Ovarian tumors in pregnancy. Int J Gynecol Obstet 1988;27:79.

Athey PA, Lamki N, Matyas MA, et al. Comparison of transvaginal and transabdominal ultrasonography in ectopic pregnancy. Can Assoc Radiol J 1991;42:349.

Ballard CA. Ovarian tumors associated with pregnancy termination patients. Am J Obstet Gynecol 1984;149:384.

Barett RJ, Harper MA, Marshall RB. Tuboovarian pregnancy associated with elevated maternal serum α-fetoprotein. J Reprod Med 1990;35:277.

Beischer NA, Buttery BW, Fortune DW, et al. Growth and malignancy of ovarian tumors in pregnancy. Aust NZ J Obstet Gynaecol 1971; 11:208.

Bello G, Schonholz D, Mosipur J, et al. Combined pregnancy: the Mount Sinai experience. Obstet Gynecol Surv 1986;41:603.

Bezjian AA: Pelvic masses in pregnancy. Clin Obstet Gynecol 1984;27:402.

Bider D, Mashiach S, Dulitzky M, et al. Clinical, surgical and pathological findings of adnexal torsion in pregnant and nonpregnant women. Surg Gynecol Obstet 1991;173:363.

Blanchard AC, Pastorek JG, Weeks T. Pelvic inflammatory disease during pregnancy. South Med J 1987;80:1363.

Booth RT. Ovarian tumors in pregnancy. Obstet Gynecol 1963;21:189.

Brent RL. The effects of embryonic and fetal exposure to x-ray, microwaves, and ultrasound. Clin Perinatol 1986;13:615.

Buckley CH. Is needle aspiration of ovarian cysts adequate for diagnosis? Br J Obstet Gynaecol 1989;96:1021.

Burry KA. Transvaginal ultrasonographic findings in surgically verified ectopic pregnancy. Am J Obstet Gynecol 1993;168:1796.

Cacciatore B. Can the status of tubal pregnancy be predicted with transvaginal sonography? Radiology 1990a;177:481.

Cacciatore B, Stenman OH, Ilostalo P. Diagnosis of ectopic pregnancy by vaginal ultrasonography in combination with a discriminatory serum hCG level of 1000 iu/l (IRP). Br J Obstet Gynaecol 1990b;97:904.

Caverly CE. Ovarian cysts complication pregnancy. Am J Obstet Gynecol 1931;21:566.

Chung A, Birnbaum SJ. Ovarian cancer associated with pregnancy. Obstet Gynecol 1973;41:211.

Coleman BG. Transvaginal sonography of adnexal masses. Radiol Clin North Am 1992;30:677.

Creasman WT, Rutledge F, Smith J. Carcinoma of the ovary associated with pregnancy. Obstet Gynecol 1971;38:111.

Csapo AL, Pulkkinen MO, and Wiest WG. Effects of lutectomy and progesterone replacement in early pregnant patients. Am J Obstet Gynecol 1973;115:759.

Cunningham FG, MacDonald PC, Gant NF, et al. Williams Obstetrics, 19th ed. Norwalk, CT: Appleton & Lange, 1993.

Curtis M, Hopkins MP, Zarlingo T, et al. Magnetic resonance imaging to avoid laparotomy in pregnancy. Obstet Gynecol 1993;82:833.

Czernobilsky B. Blaustein's Pathology of the Female Genital Tract, 3rd ed. New York: Springer-Verlag, 1987.

Dgani R, Shoham Z, Alar E, et al. Ovarian carcinoma during pregnancy. Gynecol Oncol 1989; 33:326.

Dooms GC, Hricak H, Txcholakoff D. Adnexal structures: MR imaging. Radiology 1986;158:639.

Dougherty CM, Lund CJ. Solid ovarian tumors complicating pregnancy: A clinical-pathology study. Am J Obstet Gynecol 1950:261.

Fleischer AC, Shah DM, Entman SS. Sonographic evaluation of maternal disorders during pregnancy. Radiol Clin North Am 1990;28:51.

Fliegner JRH. Uncommon problems of double uterus. Med J Aust 1986;145:510.

Gains JA. Medical, Surgical and Gynecologic Complications of Pregnancy, 2nd ed. Baltimore: Williams & Wilkins, 1965.

Geard CR, Osmak RS, Hall EJ, et al. Magnetic resonance and ionizing radiation: a comparative evaluation in vitro of oncogenic and genotoxic potential. Radiology 1984;152:199.

Gonsoulin W, Mason B, Carpenter RJ. Colon cancer in pregnancy with elevated maternal serum α-fetoprotein level at presentation. Am J Obstet Gynecol 1990;163:1172.

Grimes WH, Bartholomew RA, Calvin ED, et al. Ovarian cysts complicating pregnancy. Am J Obstet Gynecol 1954;68:594.

Gustafson GW, Gardiner SH, Stout FE. Ovarian tumors complicating pregnancy. Am J Obstet Gynecol 1954;67:1210.

Guy RL, King E, Ayers AB. The role of transvaginal ultrasound in the assessment of the female pelvis. Clin Radiol 1988;39:669.

Haas RL. Pregnancy and adnexal cysts. Am J Obstet Gynecol 1949;58:283.

Halpin TF. Ovarian abscess in pregnancy. Infect Surg 1988; September:523.

Hamilton HG, Higgins RS. Ovarian tumors in pregnancy. Surg Gynecol Obstet 1949;80:525.

Harwitz A, Yagel S, Zion I, et al. The management of persistent clear pelvic cysts diagnosed by ultrasonography. Obstet Gynecol 1988;72:320.

Hassan MA, Jenkins DM. Needle aspiration of simple ovarian cysts in pregnancy. Br J Obstet Gynaecol 1990;97:89.

Hay DL. Placental histology and the production of human choriogonadotropin and its subunits in pregnancy. Br J Obstet Gynaecol 1988;95:1268.

Hess LW, Peaceman A, O'Brien WF, et al. Adnexal masses occurring with intrauterine pregnancy. Am J Obstet Gynecol 1988;158:1029.

Hess LW, Nolan TE, Martin JN Jr, et al. Incarceration of the retroverted gravid uterus: report of four patients managed with uterine reduction. South Med J 1989; 82:310.

Hogston P, Lilford RJ. Ultrasound study of ovarian cysts in pregnancy: prevalence and significance. Br J Obstet Gynaecol 1986;93:625.

Iwanari O, Miyako J, Dare Y, et al. Clinical evaluations of the tumor marker siayl SSEA-1 antigen for clinical gynecological disease. Gynecol Obstet Invest 1990;29:214.

Jackson D, Elliott JP, Pearson M. Asymptomatic uterine retroversion at 36 weeks' gestation. Obstet Gynecol 1988;77:466.

Jubb ED. Primary ovarian carcinoma in pregnancy. Am J Obstet Gynecol 1963;85:345.

Khaw KT, Walker WJ. Ultrasound guided fine needle aspiration of ovarian cysts: diagnosis and treatment in pregnant and non-pregnant women. Clin Radiol 1990;41:105.

Kier R, McCarthy SM, Scoutt LM, et al. Pelvic masses in pregnancy and MR imaging. Radiology 1990;176:709.

King PA, Lopes A, Tang MHY, et al. Theca-lutein ovarian cysts associated with placental chorioangioma. Case report. Br J Obstet Gynaecol 1991;98:322.

Kobayashi H, Kawashina Y. Clinical usefulness of serum sialyl SSEA-1 antigen levels in patients with epithelial ovarian cancer. Gynecol Obstet Invest 1990;30:52.

Koonings PP, Lawrence P, Wallace R. Incidental adnexal neoplasms at cesarean section. Obstet Gynecol 1988;72:767.

Kurjak A, Jurkovic D. Alfirevic Z, et al. Transvaginal color Doppler imaging. J Clin Ultrasound 1990;18:227.

Kvale G, Heuch I. Is the incidence of colorectal cancer related to reproduction? Int J Cancer 1991;47:390.

Kyoto Y, Inatomi K, Abe T. Sarcoma associated with pregnancy. Am J Obstet Gynecol 1989;161:94.

Lande IM, Hill MC, Cosco FE, et al. Adnexal and cul-de-sac abnormalities: transvaginal sonography. Radiology 1988;166:325.

Lavery J, Koontz WL, Layman L, et al. Sonographic evaluation of the adnexa during early pregnancy. Surg Gynecol Obstet 1986;163:319.

Lev-Toaff AS, Coleman BG, Arger PH, et al. Leiomyomas in pregnancy: sonographic study. Radiology 1987;164:375.

Levine W, Diamond B. Surgical procedures during pregnancy. Am J Obstet Gynecol 1961;81:1046.

Lewitt N, Thaler L, Rotten S. The uterus: a new look with transvaginal sonography. J Clin Ultrasound 1990;18:331.

Lubbers PR, Izuno C, Goff WB, et al. Magnetic resonance imaging of pelvic masses complicating pregnancy. J Am Osteopath Assoc 1988;88:1010.

Malkasian GD, Knapp RC, Lavin PT, et al. Preoperative evaluation of serum CA125 levels in premenopausal and postmenopausal patients with pelvic masses. Am J Obstet Gynecol 1988; 159:341.

Mazze RI, Källén B. Appendectomy during pregnancy: a Swedish Registry Study of 778 cases. Obstet Gynecol 1991;97:835.

McGowan L. Surgical diseases of the ovary in pregnancy. Clin Obstet Gynecol 1983;26:843.

McGowan L. Adnexal masses. Female Patient 1989;14:50.

McKerron RG. Pregnancy, Labor, and Childbirth with Ovarian Tumors. New York: Redman, 1906.

Meire HB, Furrant P, Guha T. Distinction of benign from malignant ovarian cysts by ultrasound. B J Obstet Gynaecol 1978;85:893.

Mikkelsen AL, Felding C. Laparoscopy and ultrasound examination in women with acute pelvic pain. Gynecol Obstet Invest 1990;30:162.

Montz FJ, Schlaerth JB, Morrow CP. The natural history of theca lutein cysts. Obstet Gynecol 1988;72:247.

Moyle JW, Rochester D, Sider L, et al. Sonography of ovarian tumors: predictability of tumor type. Am J Roentgenol 1983;141:985.

Munnell EW. Primary ovarian cancer associated with pregnancy. Clin Obstet Gynecol 1963;6:983.

National Radiological Protection Board Ad Hoc Advisory Group on Nuclear Magnetic Resonance Clinical Imaging. Revised guidance on acceptable limits of exposure during nuclear magnetic resonance clinical imaging. Br J Radiol 1983;56:974.

Nelson MJ, Cavalieri R, Graham D, Sander R. Cysts in pregnancy discovered by sonography. J Clin Ultrasound 1986;14:509.

Novak ER, Lambrou CD, Woodruff JD. Ovarian tumors in pregnancy. Obstet Gynecol 1975; 46:401.

Nyberg DA, Porter BA, Olds MO, et al. MR imaging of hemorrhagic adnexal masses. J Comput Assist Tomogr 1987;11:664.

Patsner B. Promise and pitfalls of CA-125 in gynecology. Am J Gynecol Health 1989;3:13.

Patsner B. How serum CA-125 serves as tumor marker. Contemporary Ob/Gyn 1991:37.

Patton CL. Adnexal tumors in pregnancy. Surg Gynecol Obstet 1906;3:413.

Peters RK, Pike MC, Chang WWL, Mack TM. Reproductive factors and colon cancers. Br J Cancer 1990;61:741.

Rabinerson D, Toharm, Pomerantz M, et al. Persistence of a normal pregnancy after an early lutectomy. J Reprod Med 1992;37:749.

Rizk B, Aboulghar M. Modern management of ovarian hyperstimulation syndrome. Hum Reprod 1991;6:1082.

Roberts JA. Management of gynecologic tumors during pregnancy. Clin Perinatol 1983;10:369.

Rodin A, Coltart TM, Chapman MG. Needle aspiration of simple ovarian cysts in pregnancy. Br J Obstet Gynaecol 1989;96:994.

Saunders P, Mailton PJD. Laparotomy during pregnancy: an assessment of diagnostic accuracy and fetal wastage. Br Med J 1973;3:165.

Schiller VL, Grant EG. Doppler ultrasonography of the pelvis. Radiol Clin North Am 1992;30:735.

Seki K, Kikuchi Y, Uesato T, Kuto K. Increased serum CA 125 levels during the first trimester of pregnancy. Acta Obstet Gynecol Scand 1986; 65:583.

Shalev E, Peley D. Laparoscopic treatment of adnexal torsion. Surg Gynecol Obstet 1993; 176:448.

Shalev E, Rahav D, Romano S. Laparoscopic relief of adnexal torsion in early pregnancy. Br J Obstet Gynaecol 1990;97:834.

Spencer CP. Pregnancy and ovarian cysts. Br Med J 1920;1:179.

Stabile I, Campbell S, Grudinskas JG. Can ultrasound reliably diagnose ectopic pregnancy? Br J Obstet Gynaecol 1988;95:1247.

Struyk APHB, Treffers PE. Ovarian tumors in pregnancy. Acta Obstet Gynecol Scand 1984;63:421.

Taylor KJ, Ramos IM, Feyock AL, et al. Ectopic pregnancy: duplex Doppler evaluation. Radiology 1989;173:93.

Tawa K. Ovarian tumors in pregnancy. Am J Obstet Gynecol 1964;90:511.

Thornton JG, Wells M. Ovarian cysts in pregnancy: does ultrasound make traditional management inappropriate? Obstet Gynecol 1987;69:717.

Touitou Y, Bogdan A, Darbois Y. CA 125 (ovarian cancer associated antigen) in cancer and pregnancy. Anticancer Res 1989;9:1805.

Wajda KJ, Lucas JG, Marsh WL. Hyperreactio luteinalis: benign disorder masquerading as an ovarian malignancy. Arch Pathol Lab Med 1989;113:921.

Weigel M, Friese K, Schmitt W, et al. Welchen Vorhersagewert hat die sonographische Diagnostik bei Verdacht auf Extrauteringraviditat in der klinischen Routine? Zentral Gynakol 1993; 115:228.

White KC. Ovarian tumors in pregnancy: a private hospital ten year survey. Am J Obstet Gynecol 1973;116:544.

Wilson KM. Pregnancy complicated by ovarian and paraovarian tumors. Am J Obstet Gynecol 1937;34:977.

Wilson KM. Pregnancy complicated by ovarian and paraovarian tumors. Am J Obstet Gynecol 1937;34:977.

Wolff S, Crooks LE, Brown P, et al. Tests for DNA and chromosomal damage induced by nuclear magnetic resonance imaging. Radiology 1980; 136:707.

Worthen MJ, Genning J, Miller J. Percutaneous aspiration of the persistent cystic mass of pregnancy. J Clin Ultrasound 1990;18:117.

Young RH, Scully RE. Blansteins Pathology of the Female Genital Tract, 3rd ed. New York: Springer-Verlag, 1987.

CHAPTER 23

Abdominal Pregnancy

An abdominal pregnancy is an ectopic pregnancy in the truest sense because it is a pregnancy lying totally outside of the reproductive tract (Fig. 23–1). There are few obstetrical complications that portend the need for massive blood transfusions more than this form of ectopic pregnancy. Costa and colleagues (1991) provided an excellent review on this topic. According to them, Arab writer Albucasis in 963 AD was probably the first to describe an abdominal pregnancy. He described the discharging of fetal parts through the abdominal wall. The first record of a "true primary peritoneal pregnancy" was by Gallabin (1903). Since then, the literature is replete with articles on this subject. Fortunately, this complication is rare.

INCIDENCE AND ETIOLOGY

The incidence of abdominal pregnancy has been reported to range from 1 in 3300 to 1 in 25,000 births (Beacham and associates, 1962; Cunningham and colleagues, 1993). Atrash and associates (1987), using data from the Centers for Disease Control's Abortion and Ectopic Pregnancy Mortality Surveillance Systems and the National Hospital Discharge Survey from 1970 to 1983, reported 5221 abdominal pregnancies and 47,869,951 deliveries for a ratio of 10.9 per 100,000 births. The rate appears to have increased with the availability of assisted reproductive techniques such as in vitro fertilization and gamete intrafallopian transfer (Ferland and associates, 1991; Vignali and colleagues, 1990). Moreover, the frequency of all ectopic pregnancies in the United States has increased over the past three decades (Costa and coworkers, 1991). Atrash and colleagues (1987) have estimated that there are approximately 9.2 abdominal pregnancies for every 1000 ectopic pregnancies.

Abdominal pregnancy has also been reported to be associated with endometriosis, tuberculosis, as well as use of intrauterine devices (Børlum and Blom, 1988; Goldman and colleagues, 1988; Vignali and associates, 1990). Durukan and associates (1990) reported a case of abdominal pregnancy 10 years after treatment for pelvic tuberculosis.

In most cases, an abdominal pregnancy arises as a secondary implantation from a ruptured tubal pregnancy (Fig. 23–2). Very rarely, primary implantation may occur on the peritoneal surface (Fig. 23–3). For example, Goldman (1988) and Thomas (1991) and their colleagues reported a total of six cases of documented primary abdominal pregnancy.

An abdominal pregnancy may implant anywhere in the abdominal or pelvic cavity. Implantation is probably more common in adjacent pelvic surfaces such as the posterior aspect of the broad ligament and uterus (Figs. 23–1 and 23–4). As shown in Figures 23–5 and 23–6, the site of implantation may involve extrapelvic organs such as the small and large intestine, liver, and spleen (Martin, 1988; Salinas, 1985; and their associates).

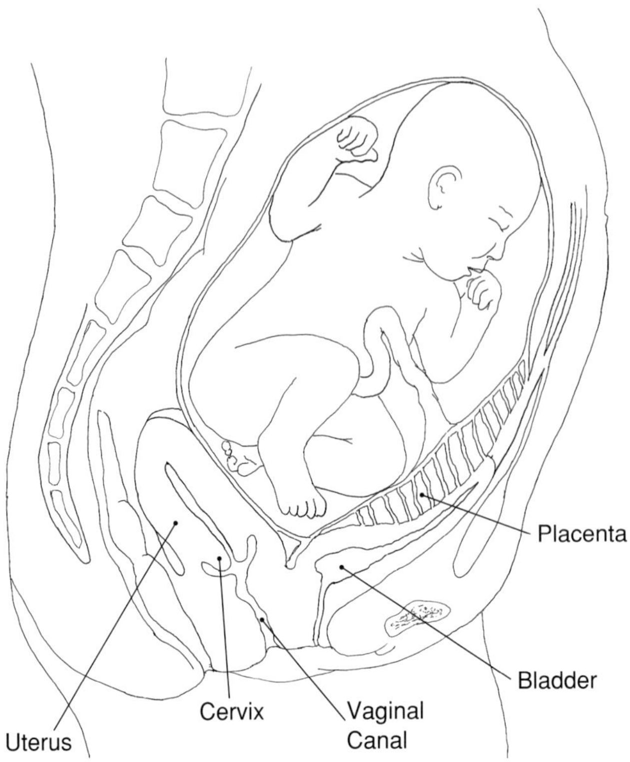

Figure 23–1. Abdominal pregnancy at term. Placenta is implanted on bladder and anterior abdominal wall. The enlarged, flattened uterus is located posteriorly in the cul-de-sac. Cervix and vagina are also dislodged posteriorly by the pregnancy.

DIAGNOSIS

The early diagnosis of abdominal pregnancy is difficult at best, and there must be a high index of suspicion if the diagnosis is to be made preoperatively. Because abdominal pregnancy is a life-threatening condition in most cases, it is of paramount importance to entertain the diagnosis when considering the differential for abdominal pain during pregnancy. Most often abdominal pregnancy is an incidental finding at the time of sonography or at laparotomy for other suspected conditions. Women with abdominal pregnancies who present in the first trimester may manifest signs and symptoms similar to those of a ruptured tubal pregnancy. These include amenorrhea, abdominal pain, abnormal bleeding, and a positive pregnancy test (Alto, 1990).

Diagnosis after the first trimester presents a much greater challenge and may be in error in many cases (Costa and colleagues, 1991). For example, in one report by Rahman and associates (1982) involving 10 women, a diagnostic error rate of 60 percent was reported. Delke and colleagues (1982) reported their experience with 10 cases of abdominal pregnancy. Nine of these had a history consistent with a ruptured tubal pregnancy or abortion in early pregnancy. Abdominal pregnancy was suspected in five of these women and the correct diagnosis was made between 16 and 24 weeks gestation. However, in the remaining five women, there was a considerable delay in diagnosis.

Symptoms

Like the symptoms of an early tubal pregnancy, women with abdominal pregnancy often experience abdominal pain, nausea and vomiting, general malaise, amenorrhea, and abnormal early pregnancy bleeding (Table 23–1). Abdominal pain was present in all women with an abdominal pregnancy reported

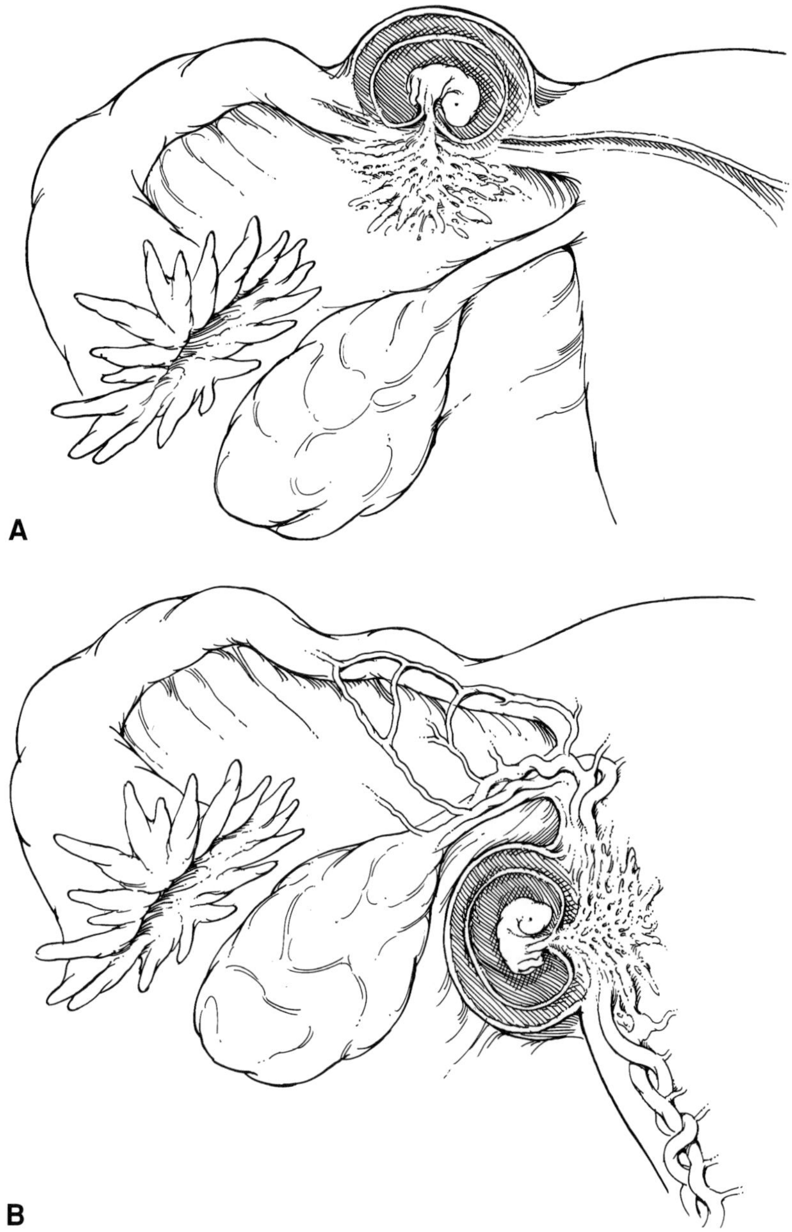

Figure 23–2. Secondary abdominal pregnancy. **A.** There is partial abortion from a tubal, cornual, or uterine pregnancy. **B.** Placental growth continues outside original confines.

by both Rahman (1982) and Delke (1982) and their colleagues. Moreover, abdominal pain was a complaint in almost 80 percent of women reviewed by Costa and associates (1991). Other clinical symptoms include flatulence, constipation, and diarrhea. Unfortunately, many of the symptoms associated with abdominal pregnancy are also commonly present in women with an intrauterine pregnancy. Interestingly, fetal movement, which is most often considered a reassuring sign in pregnancy, may be associated with significant pain in 40 to 50 percent of women with an abdominal pregnancy (Rahman and associates, 1982; Costa and colleagues, 1991). Some women may simply complain that "the pregnancy does not feel right" (Cunningham and coworkers, 1993).

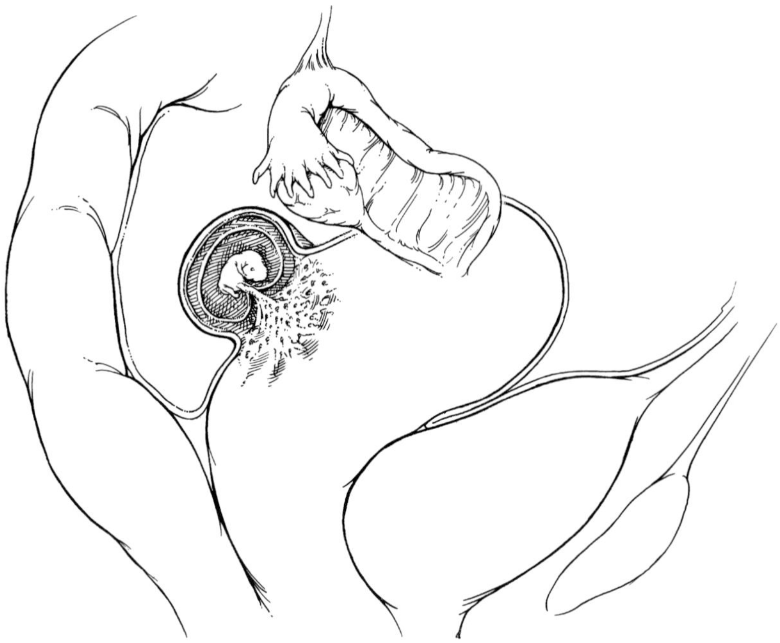

Figure 23–3. Primary abdominal pregnancy, characterized by peritoneal implantation of the blastocyst.

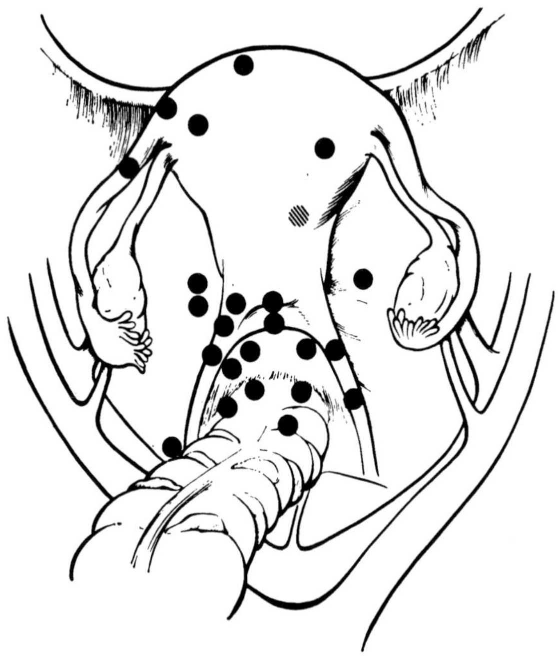

Figure 23–4. Sites of reported primary pelvic peritoneal pregnancies. (From Friedrich and Rankin, 1968, with permission.)

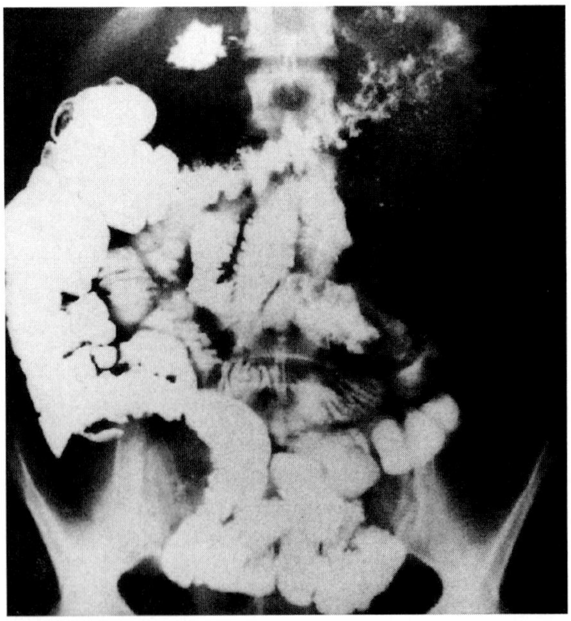

Figure 23–5. Barium small-bowel follow-through showing extrinsic compression of terminal ileum and cecum from the abdominal pregnancy. (From Salinas and colleagues, 1985, with permission.)

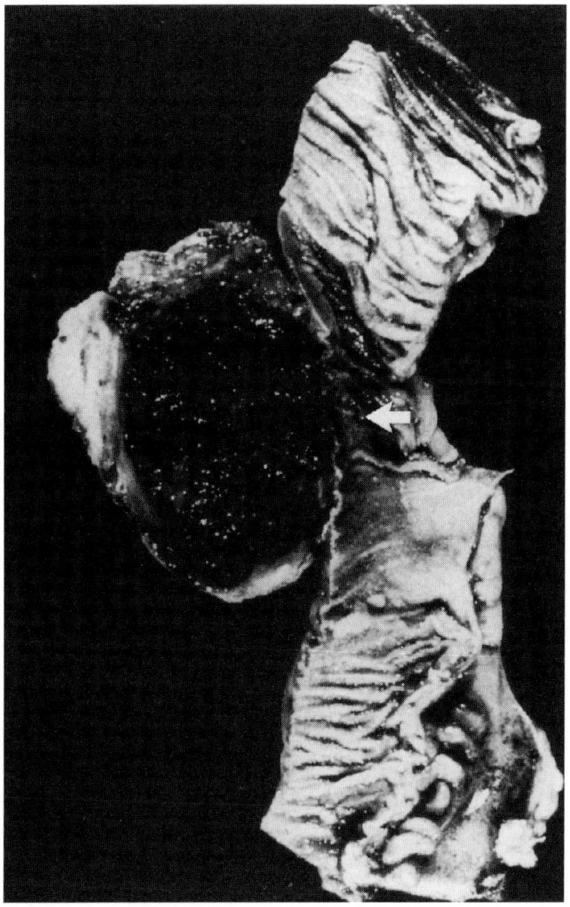

Figure 23–6. Resection of ileum and mass containing organized blood clots. Both were cut sagittally. Arrow shows opening to lumen. (From Salinas and colleagues, 1985, with permission.)

Physical Findings

There are few, if any, conclusive or pathognomic findings or signs on physical examination in women with abdominal pregnancies. In the series reported by Rahman and colleagues (1982) abdominal tenderness (100 percent), abnormal fetal position (70 percent), and cervical displacement (40 percent), were the most frequent clinical findings.

Although the ease of palpation of fetal parts and position is often listed as a useful finding for the diagnosis of abdominal pregnancy, in actual clinical practice it is not very reliable. Palpation of fetal parts is relatively easy in many women with normal pregnancies. One sign that might cause an increased suspicion is failure of abdominal massage over the pregnancy to stimulate contractions as

TABLE 23–1. SYMPTOMS OF ABDOMINAL PREGNANCY

	Percent with Symptoms		
Symptoms	*Rahman et al (1982)*	*Delke et al (1982)*	*Costa et al (1991)*
Amenorrhea	—	100	—
Abdominal pain	100	100	79
Nausea and vomiting	70	40	20
General malaise	40	—	20
Painful fetal movements	40	—	48
Abnormal uterine bleeding	—	70	31

TABLE 23–2. ULTRASONIC FEATURES IN 20 WOMEN WITH AN ABDOMINAL PREGNANCY

	Number (Percent)
Uterus and fetus separate	18 (90)
Ectopic placenta	15 (75)
Oligohydramnios	9 (45)
Fetal parts in close proximity to maternal abdominal wall	5 (25)
Abnormal fetal lie	5 (25)
Poor placental visualization	5 (25)
Maternal bowel gas blocking visualization	5 (25)
Failure to visualize myometrium between fetus and maternal bladder	5 (25)
Failure to visualize myometrium between placenta and maternal bladder	3 (15)
Placenta previa appearance	2 (10)
Maternal peritoneal fluid	2 (10)

Source: Adapted from Stanley and colleagues (1986), with permission.

occurs with most normal pregnancies (Cunningham and associates, 1993).

Laboratory and Ultrasound Findings

There are few, if any, laboratory tests that are diagnostic of abdominal pregnancy; indeed, most of the routine tests are normal. Delke and colleagues (1982) reported that 4 of 10 women had anemia defined as a hemoglobin level less than 11 g/dL. Abdominal pregnancy has been reported to be associated with a marked elevation of maternal serum alphafetoprotein (Hage and associates, 1988; Tromans and colleagues, 1984).

The most useful examination for the diagnosis of abdominal pregnancy is ultrasonography, which has largely replaced other radiologic tests used in the past. Importantly, ultrasonic diagnosis of abdominal pregnancies may be missed in up to half of cases (Costa and colleagues, 1991). Stanley and co-workers (1986) have summarized the ultrasonic features in 20 abdominal pregnancies (Table 23–2). The three most common findings were a fetus separate from the uterus (90 percent), an ectopic placenta (75 percent), and oligohydramnios (45 percent). Examples of ultrasound findings are shown in Figures 23–7 and 23–8. It is again emphasized that the most significant finding is identification of the gestational sac or fetus outside of the uterine cavity.

Magnetic resonance imaging may be used for the diagnosis of abdominal pregnancy (Figs. 23–9 and 23–10). Although computerized tomography may be superior to magnetic resonance imaging for this diagnosis (Costa and associates, 1991), it is generally not used because of the risk of fetal radiation exposure.

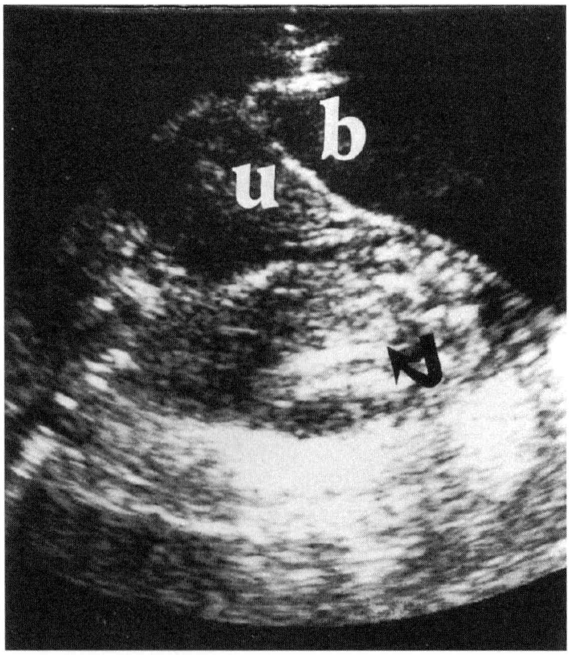

Figure 23–7. Ultrasound examination shows the posterior location of the ectopic fetus (arrow) beneath the bladder (b) and uterus (u). (From Martin and colleagues, 1990, with permission.)

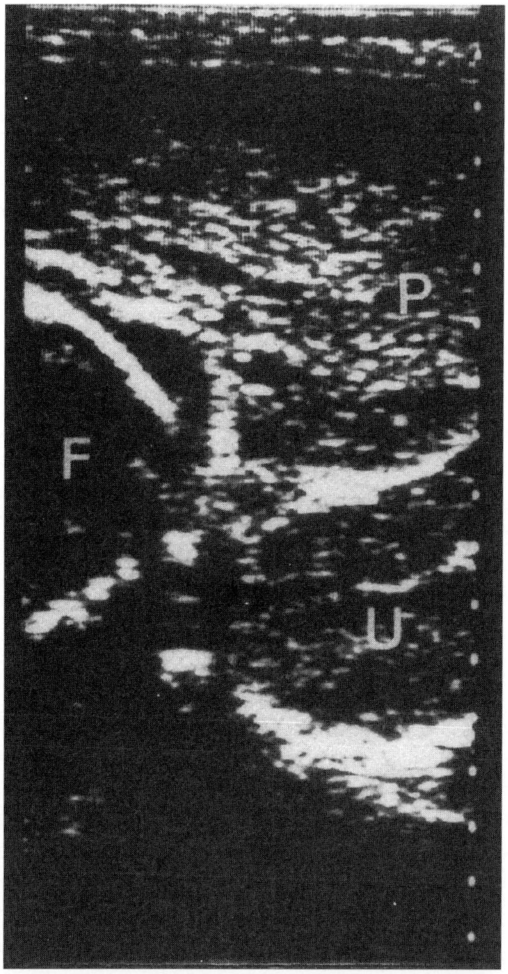

Figure 23–8. On longitudinal ultrasound the uterus (U) is separate from the placenta (P) and the fetal head (F). (From Ombelet and associates, 1988, with permission.)

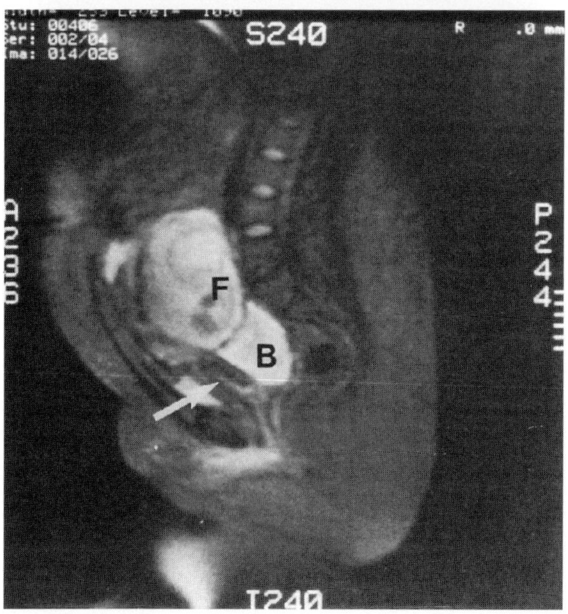

Figure 23–9. Sagittal magnetic resonance imaging spin echo image (T_2 weighted) at 18 weeks' gestation. The fetus (F) is in breech presentation. Blood (B) is present in the cul-de-sac. The arrow points to the uterus, anterior to the gestational sac. (From Hage and co-workers, 1988, with permission.)

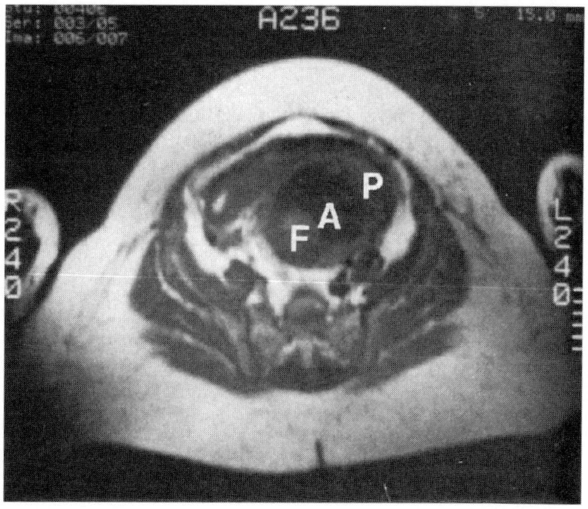

Figure 23–10. Transverse magnetic resonance imaging spin echo image (T_1 weighted) at 18 weeks' gestation. The gestational sac is composed of the placenta (P), fetus (F), and amnionic fluid (A). (From Hage and co-workers, 1988, with permission.)

Oxytocin stimulation has been suggested by some as an aid in the diagnosis of abdominal pregnancy (Cabbad, 1985; Cross, 1951; Golan, 1985; Hertz, 1977; Martin, 1988; and their colleagues). Although the lack of response to oxytocin indeed would seem to be the case in most women with an abdominal pregnancy, there have been reports in which uterine contractions were detected (Costa and colleagues, 1991; Golan and associates, 1985). Moreover, Orr and associates (1979) reported a negative oxytocin challenge test in a woman with an abdominal pregnancy.

Management

Clinical management of abdominal pregnancy is summarized in Table 23–3. Some have suggested that surgical management of abdominal pregnancy be delayed in selected cases until fetal viability has been achieved (Cartwright, 1986; Golz, 1984; Hage, 1988; and their associates). However, such procrastination may be dangerous and life-threatening in many of these women because massive hemorrhage may develop from spontaneous placental separation. For these reasons, most recommend immediate surgical intervention once the diagnosis of abdominal pregnancy is suspected or confirmed (Cunningham, 1993; Hallatt, 1985; Pelosi, 1988; Strafford, 1977; and their colleagues). It seems reasonable to perform immediate surgical intervention even if the fetus is nonviable or has died. Importantly, massive hemorrhage may be encountered even when the diagnosis is made preoperatively and timely surgical intervention is carried out. Hemorrhage follows placental separation and is secondary to the inability of the "placental bed" blood vessels to undergo constriction as they normally do with an intrauterine pregnancy.

TABLE 23–3. SUGGESTED MANAGEMENT PROTOCOL FOR ABDOMINAL PREGNANCY

- Preoperative preparation if possible
  - Two large-bore intravenous infusion systems
  - 4–6 units of blood available
  - Availability of clotting factors
  - Skilled surgeon
- Surgical intervention once diagnosis is made
- Generous midline abdominal incision
- Incision of amnionic sac, if intact, and careful removal of fetus
- Clamp cord and leave placenta in place if possible
- Removal of placenta if separated with hemorrhage
  - Attempt ligation of vessels
  - Cautery
  - Selective angiographic embolization of bleeding vessels

For all of the foregoing reasons, it is of paramount importance to be prepared for hemorrhage when the diagnosis of abdominal pregnancy is made or suspected preoperatively. Two large-bore (14- or 16-gauge) intravenous needles capable of rapid infusion should be inserted. At least 4–6 units of blood should be readily available, along with various blood components for clotting factors to include fresh frozen plasma, cryoprecipitate, and platelets. An experienced surgeon should be readily available as well.

The abdomen is entered through a generous midline incision. An intact amnionic sac can often be identified (Fig. 23–11A). If possible, the amnionic sac should be carefully incised and the fetus carefully removed without disturbing the placenta (Fig. 23–11B,C). Following delivery of the fetus, the question arises as to the most appropriate management of the placenta. In a review of 101 cases of abdominal pregnancy, Hreshchyshyn and associates (1961) reported that the placenta was removed, either partially or completely, in about 70 percent of cases. However, great care must be employed if the placenta is to be removed. Prior to making any attempts at removal, it is important to be able to ligate the major blood supply to the placenta. If the placenta is attached to the back of the uterus and broad ligament, it may be possible to remove the placenta and perform a hysterectomy for control of bleeding if the woman does not desire future fertility.

In the majority of cases, it is best to leave the placenta in place and make no attempt to remove it. Even partial removal may result in life-threatening, uncontrollable hemorrhage. Following delivery of the fetus, the cord should be cut and ligated as close to the placenta as possible and the placenta left undisturbed. Although methotrexate has been given by some in the past, it may lead to placental necrosis and abscess formation and it is currently not recommended (Cunningham and associates, 1993; Rahman and colleagues, 1982). Other complications of leaving the placenta in situ includes ileus, peritonitis, intestinal obstruction, prolonged hospitalization, and

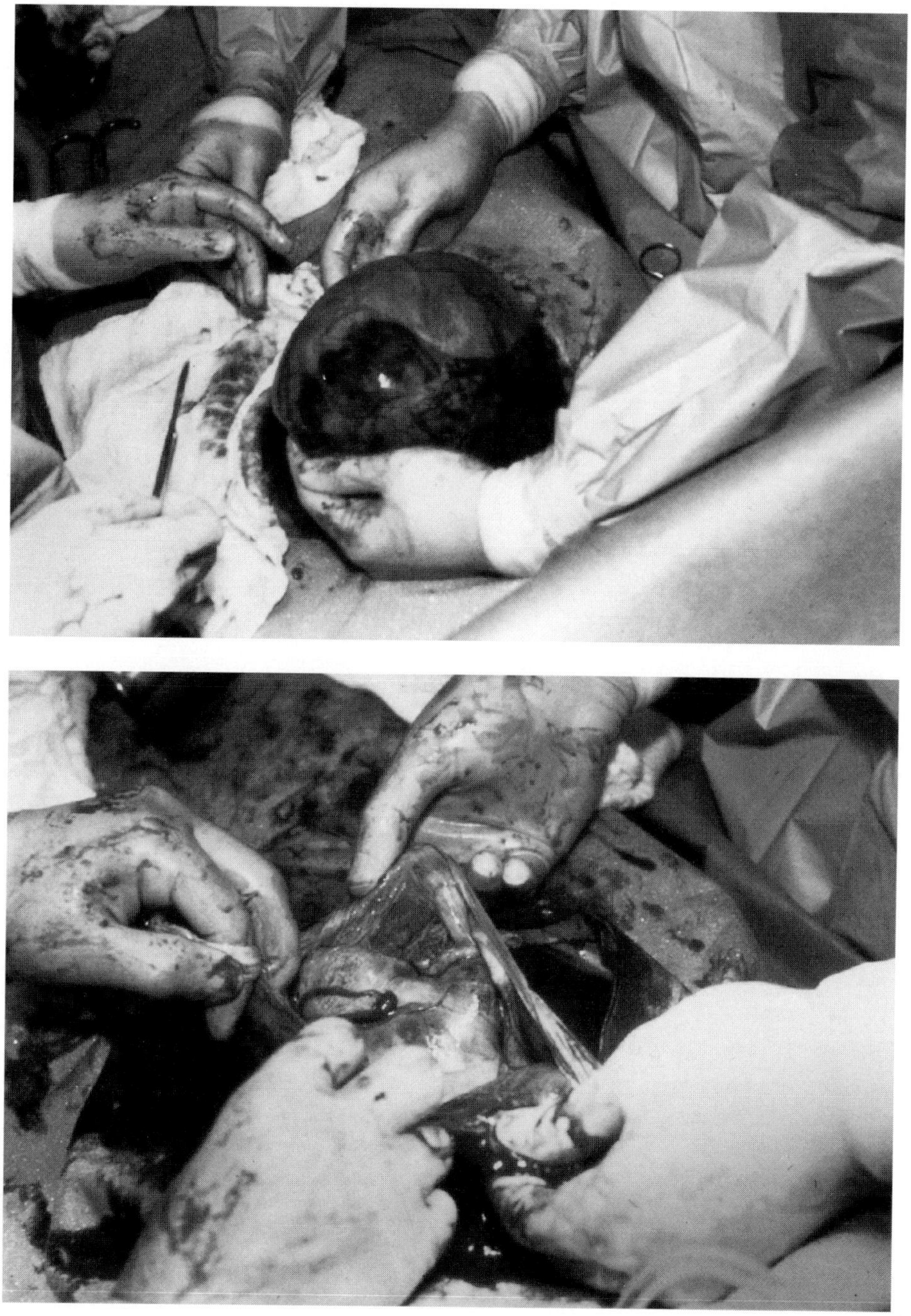

A

B

Figure 23–11 A. Intact amnionic sac in a woman with a viable abdominal pregnancy. **B.** Amnionic sac has been opened. (Courtesy of Dr. George Wendel.) (continued)

subsequent laparotomies (Delke and colleagues, 1982). Although abscesses, adhesions, and other complications may develop if the placenta is left in place—with or without methotrexate therapy—these complications can usually be managed with antibiotics and surgery later when life-threatening hemorrhage is a lesser risk. In most cases, placental absorption is a slow process and takes several months to years for completion. An example of this is shown in Figure 23–12, in which Belfar and colleagues (1986) serially monitored the involuting placental mass after fetal delivery, the process taking more than 5 years!

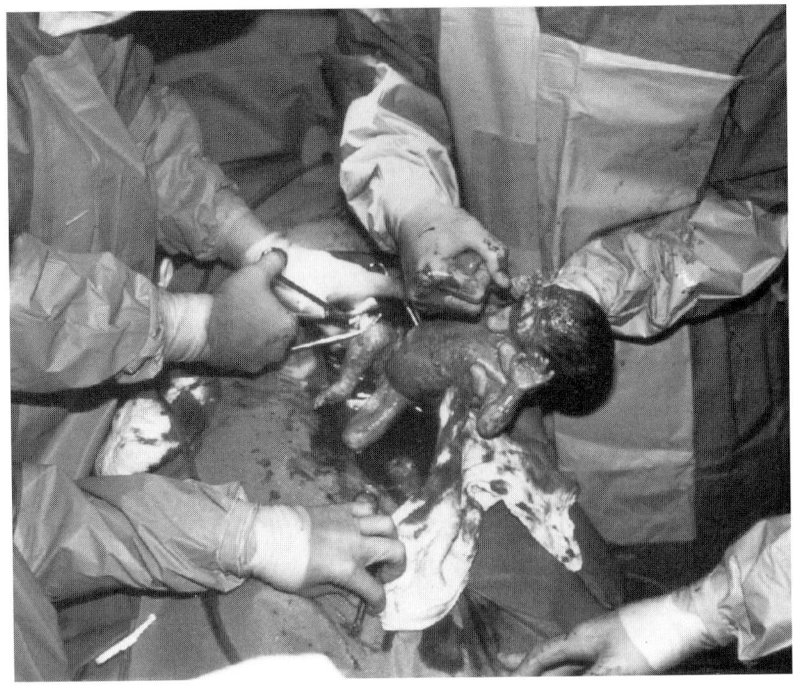

C

Figure 23–11. (continued) **C**. Viable 2155-g fetus is delivered. (Courtesy of Dr. George Wendel.)

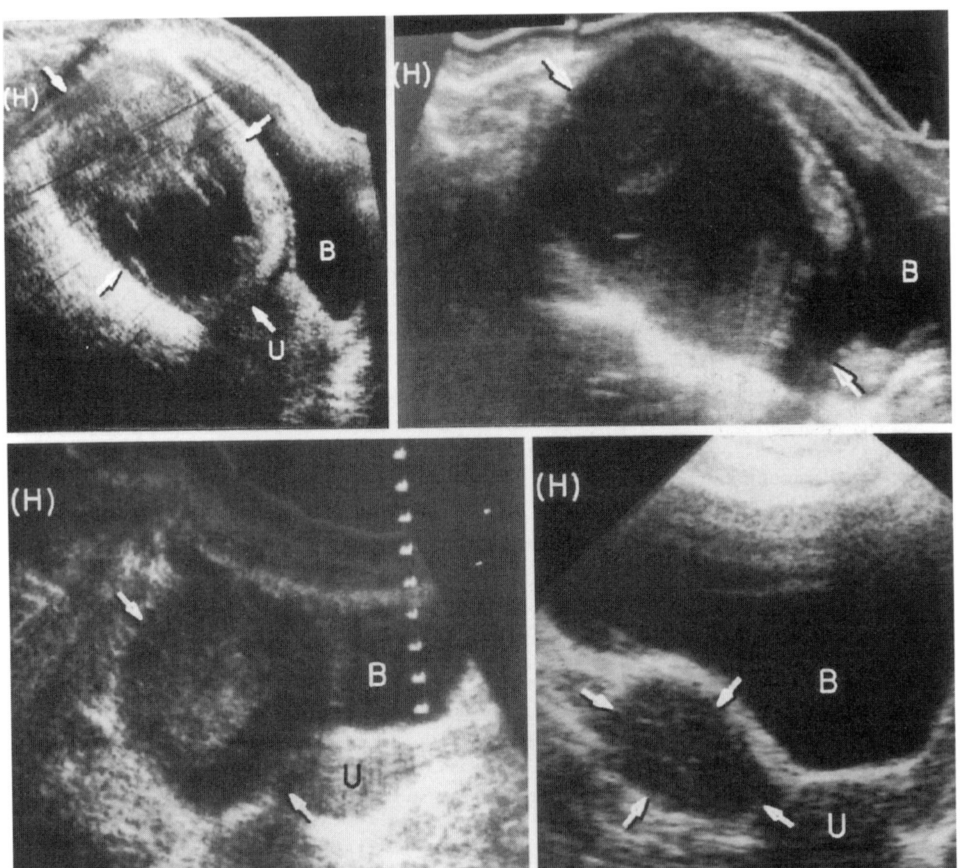

Figure 23–12. Placental mass **A** (top left) one month, **B** (top right) 2 months, **C** (bottom left) 1 year, 6 months, and **D** (bottom right) 5 years, 7 months after fetal delivery. **A, C,** and **D** are midline scans that demonstrate the placental mass to assume a hyperechoic texture as it involuted. **B** is a scan somewhat to the right of the midline, demonstrating the abrupt and brief increase in volume at 2 months postoperatively accompanied by a generalized decrease in the echogeneity of the placental tissue mass. B, bladder; U, uterus; arrows, placental tissue mass; (H), toward patient's head. (From Belfar and colleagues, 1986, with permission.)

In some women with life-threatening hemorrhage following placental separation, selective embolization of the placental bed bleeding sites using pelvic angiography may prove life-saving (Martin and associates, 1990). Emboli of shredded Gelform are usually used to occlude the bleeding vessels. These techniques are described in detail in Chapter 26.

Outcome

In their review, Hreshchyshyn and colleagues (1961) cited the report by Harris in 1887, who described a maternal mortality rate of 90 percent. Fortunately, mortality from abdominal pregnancy has decreased significantly—from 5.3 percent in the period of 1932 to 1961 to 0.5 percent from 1979 to 1982 (Atrash and colleagues, 1987). As expected, hemorrhage is the most common cause of mortality. Although mortality has decreased, maternal morbidity remains high, usually from infection and adhesions (Costa and associates, 1991).

The outcome for the fetus is poor in most cases of abdominal pregnancy. Perinatal mortality was reported earlier to be as high as 95 percent (Beachham and colleagues, 1962). More recently, a perinatal survival of 5–25 percent has been reported (Martin and McCaul, 1990). Congenital malformations have been reported in 20–40 percent of newborns of abdominal pregnancies (Beacham, 1962; Hallatt, 1985; Rahman, 1982; and their colleagues). Many of these "malformations" are actually deformations, that is, compression anomalies, caused by oligohydramnios and the constrictive milieu.

SUMMARY

Abdominal pregnancy will be encountered in approximately 1 of every 10,000 pregnancies. Diagnosis is difficult as symptoms often mimic those of tubal ectopic pregnancy. Once the diagnosis is made, the fetus should be delivered abdominally and if possible, the placenta should be left undisturbed. Hemorrhage is the greatest risk to the mother's life, and the health care team must be prepared to address it in a timely fashion.

REFERENCES

Alto WA. Abdominal pregnancy. Am Fam Physician 1990; 41:209.

Atrash HK, Friede A, Hogue CJR. Abdominal pregnancy in the United States: frequency and maternal mortality. Obstet Gynecol 1987; 69:333.

Beacham WD, Hernquist WC, Beacham DW, Webster HD. Abdominal pregnancy at Charity Hospital in New Orleans. Am J Obstet Gynecol 1962; 84:1257.

Belfar HL, Kurtz AB, Wapner RJ. Long-term follow-up after removal of an abdominal pregnancy: ultrasound evaluation of the involuting placenta. J Ultrasound Med 1986; 5:521.

Børlum K-G, Blom R. Primary hepatic pregnancy. Int J Gynecol Obstet 1988; 27:427.

Cabbad MF, Minkoff H, Faustin D. Fetal heart rate decelerations after oxytocin infusion in an abdominal pregnancy. Obstet Gynecol 1985; 66(S):2S.

Cartwright PS, Brown JE, Davis RJ, et al. Advanced abdominal pregnancy associated with fetal pulmonary hypoplasia: report of a case. Am J Obstet Gynecol 1986; 155:396.

Costa SD, Presley J, Bastert G. Advanced abdominal pregnancy. Obstet Gynecol Surv 1991; 46:515.

Cross JB, Lester WM, McCain J. The diagnosis and management of abdominal pregnancy with a review of 19 cases. Am J Obstet Gynecol 1951; 62:303.

Cunningham FG, MacDonald PC, Gant NF, et al. Williams Obstetrics, 19th ed. Norwalk, CT: Appleton & Lange, 1993:710.

Delke I, Veridiano NP, Tancer ML. Abdominal pregnancy: Review of current management and addition of 10 cases. Obstet Gynecol 1982; 60:200.

Durukan T, Urman B, Yarali H, et al. An abdominal pregnancy 10 years after treatment for pelvic tuberculosis. Am J Obstet Gynecol 1990; 163:594.

Ferland RJ, Chadwick DA, O'Brien JA, Granai CO III. An ectopic pregnancy in the upper retroperitoneum following in vitro fertilization and embryo transfer. Obstet Gynecol 1991; 78:544.

Friedrich ED Jr, Rankin CA Jr. Primary pelvic peritoneal pregnancy. Obstet Gynecol 1968; 31:649.

Gallabin AL. Primary abdominal pregnancy (Trans London Obstet Soc, 1896, 5:38) Br Med J 1903; 1:664.

Golan A, Sandbank O, Andronikou A, Rubin A. Advanced extrauterine pregnancy. Acta Obstet Gynecol Scand 1985; 64:21.

Goldman GA, Dicker D, Ovadia J. Primary abdominal pregnancy: Can artificial abortion, endometriosis and IUD be etiological factors? Eur J Obstet Gynecol Reprod Biol 1988; 27:139.

Golz N, Kramer D, Robrecht D, Mast H. (Abdominal pregnancy. Case report and review of the literature). Die abdominale Gravidität. Fallbericht und Literaturubersicht. Geburtsh Frauenheilkd 1984; 44:816.

Hage ML, Wall LL, Killam A. Expectant management of abdominal pregnancy. A report of two cases. J Reprod Med 1988; 33:407.

Hallatt JG, Grove JA. Abdominal pregnancy: A study of twenty-one consecutive cases. Am J Obstet Gynecol 1985; 152:444.

Hertz RH, Timor-Tritsch I, Sokol RJ, Zador I. Diagnostic studies and fetal assessment in advanced extrauterine pregnancy. Obstet Gynecol 1977; 50(S):62S.

Hreshchyshyn MM, Bogen B, Loughran CH. What is the actual present-day management of the placenta in late abdominal pregnancy? Analysis of 101 cases. Am J Obstet Gynecol 1961; 81:302.

Martin JN Jr, McCaul JF IV. Emergent management of abdominal pregnancy. Clin Obstet Gynecol 1990; 33:438.

Martin JN Jr, Ridgway LE III, Connors JJ, et al. Angiographic arterial embolization and computed tomography-directed drainage for the management of hemorrhage and infection with abdominal pregnancy. Obstet Gynecol 1990; 76:941.

Martin JN, Sessums JK, Martin RW, et al. Abdominal pregnancy: Current concepts of management. Obstet Gynecol 1988; 71:549.

Ombelet W, Vandermerwe JV, Van Assche FA. Advanced extrauterine pregnancy: Description of 38 cases with literature survey. Obstet Gynecol Surv 1988; 43:386.

Orr JW, Huddleston JF, Knox GE, et al. False negative oxytocin challenge test associated with abdominal pregnancy. Am J Obstet Gynecol 1979; 133:108.

Pelosi MA, Apuzzio J. Surgical management of abdominal pregnancy. Contemp Obstet Gynecol 1988; 31:144.

Rahman MS, Al-Suleiman SA, Rahman J, Al-Sibai MH. Advanced abdominal pregnancy—observations in 10 cases. Obstet Gynecol 1982; 59:366.

Salinas A, Guelrud M, Toledano A, Dreiling DA. Abdominal pregnancy causing massive lower gastrointestinal bleeding: Case report. Mt Sinai J Med 1985; 52:371.

Stanley JH, Horger EO III, Fagan CJ, et al. Sonographic findings in abdominal pregnancy. Am J Roentgenol 1986; 147:1043.

Strafford JC, Ragan WD. Abdominal pregnancy. Review of current management. Obstet Gynecol 1977; 50:548.

Thomas JS Jr, Willie JO, Clark JFJ. Primary peritoneal pregnancy: A case report. J Natl Med Assoc 1991; 83:635.

Tromans PM, Coulson R, Lobb MO, Abdulla U. Abdominal pregnancy associated with extremely elevated serum α-fetoprotein: Case report. Br J Obstet Gynaecol 1984; 91:296.

Vignali M, Busacca M, Brigante C, et al. Abdominal pregnancy as a result of gamete intrafallopian transfer (GIFT) and subsequent treatment with methotrexate: Case report. Int J Fertil 1990; 35:280.

CHAPTER 24

Ectopic Pregnancy

Ectopic pregnancy is an important public health concern worldwide. Complications from ectopic gestations are major causes of maternal morbidity and mortality during early pregnancy. A clear understanding of the factors that contribute to the development of ectopic pregnancy, the current methods of establishing its early diagnosis, and appropriate management strategies are essential. Appropriate diagnosis and management will have a major impact with respect to morbidity and mortality as well as enhancement and conservation of reproductive potential.

EPIDEMIOLOGY AND INCIDENCE

The incidence and case-fatality rate of ectopic pregnancy in the United States has been monitored since 1970 by the Centers for Disease Control (CDC) through the National Center for Health Statistics (NCHS), which collects data from the National Hospital Discharge Survey (NHDS). As shown in Figure 24–1, the rate of ectopic pregnancy per 1000 reported pregnancies has increased fourfold from 4.5 to 16.8 between 1970 and 1987. When reported per 1000 live births, this represents a fivefold increase from 4.8 to 23.1. Both of these methods of reporting ectopic pregnancy rates have the inherent risk of overestimating the actual rate because spontaneous losses, illegal pregnancy terminations, and stillbirths are excluded from the denominator. The traditional method of reporting ectopic pregnancy rates uses a constant denominator—all women aged 15 to 44—and therefore more accurately estimates the rate, taking into consideration patterns of contraceptive use, sexual activity, and fluctuations in the spontaneous and induced abortion rate within the general population that are not biased by individual risks (Doyle and colleagues, 1991). When expressed in this manner, the rate of ectopic pregnancy from 1970 to 1987 has increased slightly more than threefold from 4.2 to 15.3 per 10,000 women aged 15–44 (Table 24–1). More recent data from 1989 show that approximately 88,400 women were hospitalized for ectopic pregnancy (Centers for Disease Control, 1992). The rate of ectopic pregnancy per 10,000 women aged 15–44 was 15.5. In that same report, the case-fatality rate from 1970 to 1989 declined by over 90 percent, from 35.5 to 3.8 deaths per 10,000 ectopic pregnancies.

Within specific populations of women, those over 35 years had the highest rate of ectopic pregnancy at 20.5 per 1000 reported pregnancies. More striking are the race-specific rates of ectopic pregnancies per 1000 pregnancies. From 1970 to 1987, nonwhite women had a rate of 14.2 ectopic pregnancies per 1000 reported pregnancies compared with 9.7 in white women. As shown in Table 24–2, the case-fatality rate of 17.5 in nonwhite women during this time period was 3.3 times that for white women. According to the 1989 figures from the Centers for Disease Control (1992), the rate of ectopic pregnancy was 32 percent higher in nonwhite women, with a case fatality rate five times that of white women.

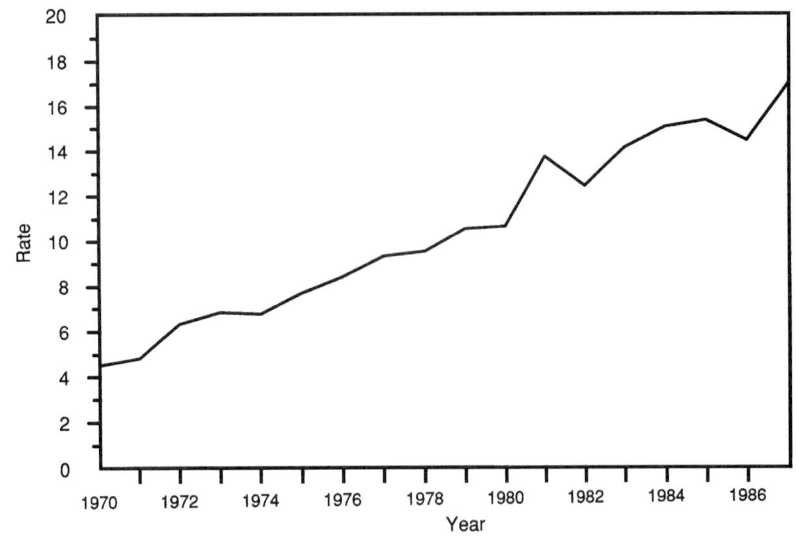

Figure 24–1. Ectopic pregnancy rates by year (per 1000 total pregnancies) in the United States, 1970–1987. (From Centers for Disease Control, 1990.)

ETIOLOGY

Factors that have been implicated in the pathogenesis of ectopic pregnancy include (1) an increased prevalence of pelvic inflammatory disease, (2) tubal sterilization, (3) tubal surgery such as salpingostomy, tubal anastomosis, and tuboplasty, (4) assisted reproductive technologies, (5) use of the intrauterine device, (6) diethylstilbestrol (DES) exposure, (7) use of low-dose progestational agents, (8) chromosomal aberrations in the conceptus, and (9) improvements in diagnostic techniques.

TABLE 24–1. NUMBER AND RATE OF ECTOPIC PREGNANCIES BY YEAR IN THE UNITED STATES FROM 1970 TO 1987

Year	Number[a]	Rate[b]
1970	17,800	4.5
1971	19,300	4.8
1972	24,500	6.3
1973	25,600	6.8
1974	26,400	6.7
1975	30,500	7.6
1976	34,600	8.3
1977	40,700	9.2
1978	42,400	9.4
1979	49,900	10.4
1980	52,200	10.5
1981	68,000	13.6
1982	61,800	12.3
1983	69,600	14.0
1984	75,400	14.9
1985	78,400	15.2
1986	73,700	14.3
1987	88,000	16.8
Total	877,400[c]	10.7

[a]Rounded to nearest hundred.
[b]Rate per 1000 pregnancies (live births, legally induced abortions, and ectopic pregnancies).
[c]Because of rounding, the total differs from the sum of the numbers.
From Centers for Disease Control (1990).

Sexually Transmitted Diseases

The most common cause of tubal damage by deciliation, tubal adhesions, and fimbrial infection is pelvic inflammatory disease. Causative organisms are *Chlamydia trachomatis, Neisseria gonorrhoeae,* and mixed aerobic–anaerobic infections (McCormack, 1994). Westrom and associates (1981) reported that the incidence of tubal obstruction after one, two, or three episodes of salpingitis rose from 13 to 35 to 75 percent respectively. Equally important was the risk of extrauterine pregnancy, which was sixfold greater in women with laparoscopically proven salpingitis as compared with controls. Chow and associates (1990) demonstrated that evidence for past chlamydial infection is associated with more than a twofold risk of ectopic pregnancy. Chlamydia—unlike gonorrhea and polymicrobial infections—is a clinically mild disease, and there is often an associated delay in diagnosis. It has been suggested, but not proven, that early treatment of pelvic infections may limit the course of the disease, the extent of tubal damage, and fertility impairment. In

TABLE 24–2. NUMBER OF DEATHS DUE TO ECTOPIC PREGNANCY AND CASE-FATALITY RATES BY RACE AND YEAR IN THE UNITED STATES FROM 1970 TO 1987

	Number			Rate[a]		
Year	*White*	*Black and Other*	*Total*	*White*	*Black and Other*	*Total*
1970	28	35	63	21.7	72.1	35.5
1971	21	40	61	15.1	74.9	31.7
1972	28	20	48	16.2	27.7	19.6
1973	25	21	46	15.1	23.4	18.0
1974	20	31	51	10.1	47.0	19.4
1975	19	31	50	8.8	34.9	16.4
1976	11	28	39	4.4	28.7	11.3
1977	15	29	44	5.2	24.5	10.8
1978	13	24	37	4.4	18.7	8.7
1979	20	25	45	5.7	17.2	9.0
1980	22	24	46	6.0	15.4	8.8
1981	15	19	34	3.1	9.7	5.0
1982	19	24	43	3.8	19.3	7.0
1983	17	20	37	3.3	11.2	5.3
1984	14	15	39	2.7	10.8	5.2
1985	11	22	33	2.1	8.4	4.2
1986	17	19	36	3.3	7.6	4.9
1987	17	13	30	2.6	4.8	3.4
Total	332	440	782	5.3	17.5	8.9

[a]Deaths from ectopic pregnancy per 10,000 ectopic pregnancies.
Source: Nederloff and colleagues (1990).

particular, early treatment of chlamydial infections may prevent these sequelae altogether (Hillis and associates, 1993).

Tubal Sterilization

Tubal sterilization failures are estimated at a rate of 2–4 per 1000. From 5 to 20 percent of women with an ectopic pregnancy will have had a tubal sterilization procedure (Holt and colleagues, 1991; Tatum and Schmidt, 1977; Wolf and Thompson, 1980). The overall risk of ectopic pregnancy in women who have undergone tubal sterilization is lower than that in a comparable group of women who use no contraception (DeStefano and co-workers, 1982). Nonetheless, 10–75 percent of pregnancies in women who have had previous tubal ligations will be ectopic (Kjer and Knudsen, 1989; McCausland, 1980). Laparoscopic and other interval tubal sterilization procedures have a higher rate of ectopic pregnancy, attributed in part to incomplete tubal occlusion with recanalization or fistula formation.

Tubal Surgery

Previous tubal surgery, whether reconstructive or to evacuate an ectopic pregnancy, places a woman at increased risk for ectopic pregnancy. In a summary of the literature with respect to pregnancy rates after microsurgical procedures, Soules (1986) found that ectopic pregnancy rates varied between 2 and 7 percent, while uterine pregnancy rates exceeded 50 percent. The extent of tubal disease and reconstructive surgery obviously influences these data. Others have reported ectopic pregnancy rates from 12 to 20 percent (Lavy and colleagues, 1987; Tomazevic and Rubic-Pucey, 1992). A woman who undergoes a linear salpingostomy for an ectopic pregnancy has a 15 percent incidence of a recurrent ectopic pregnancy. Conservative treatment in women with an occluded or absent contralateral fallopian tube has an incidence of a recurrent ectopic pregnancy of 20 percent (Thornton and associates, 1991).

Intrauterine Contraceptive Device

The studies of the association between users of contraceptive devices and ectopic pregnancy have yielded conflicting results. While some investigators have reported that women who are device users have an increased risk of ectopic pregnancy, this is seen only with prolonged use (Ory, 1981; Sivin, 1991; Vessey and colleagues, 1979). Others have demonstrated that device users compared with non-contraceptive users do not have an increased ectopic pregnancy ratio. However, its use is associated with an increased risk when compared with users of other contraceptive methods (Franks and co-workers, 1990; Rossing and colleagues, 1993).

Assisted Reproductive Technologies

Controlled ovarian hyperstimulation has been associated with an increased risk of ectopic pregnancy (Fernandez and associates, 1991). Assisted reproductive technologies similarly have increased rates. The Society for Assisted Reproductive Technology (1993), through the National IVF Registry, reported that in 1991 the ectopic pregnancy rate per clinical pregnancy was 5.5 percent for in vitro fertilization, 2.9 percent for gamete intrafallopian transfer, and 4.5 percent for zygote intrafallopian transfer. The ectopic pregnancy rate per transfer ranged from 1 to 1.4 percent. The mechanism of ectopic pregnancy in women undergoing superovulation may be a result of excessive estrogen interfering with tubal transport. Additionally, in these procedures, embryos may reflux into damaged fallopian tubes, or direct intratubal placement of transfer catheters may result in tubal damage.

Other Causes

Pathologic conditions of the fallopian tube such as salpingitis isthmica nodosa and diethylstilbestrol (DES) exposure may be causative for ectopic pregnancy (DeCherney and colleagues, 1981a; Honore, 1978).

PATHOLOGY AND ANATOMY

Over 95 percent of ectopic pregnancies implant in the fallopian tube, 2.5 percent are in the cornua of the uterus, and 2.5 percent are in other locations, which include the ovary, cervix, and abdomen (Fig. 24–2). Most tubal pregnancies are located in the ampulla. Budowick and associates (1980) demonstrated that an ampullary conceptus rapidly erodes through the tubal mucosa into the surrounding adventitia with subsequent extraluminal

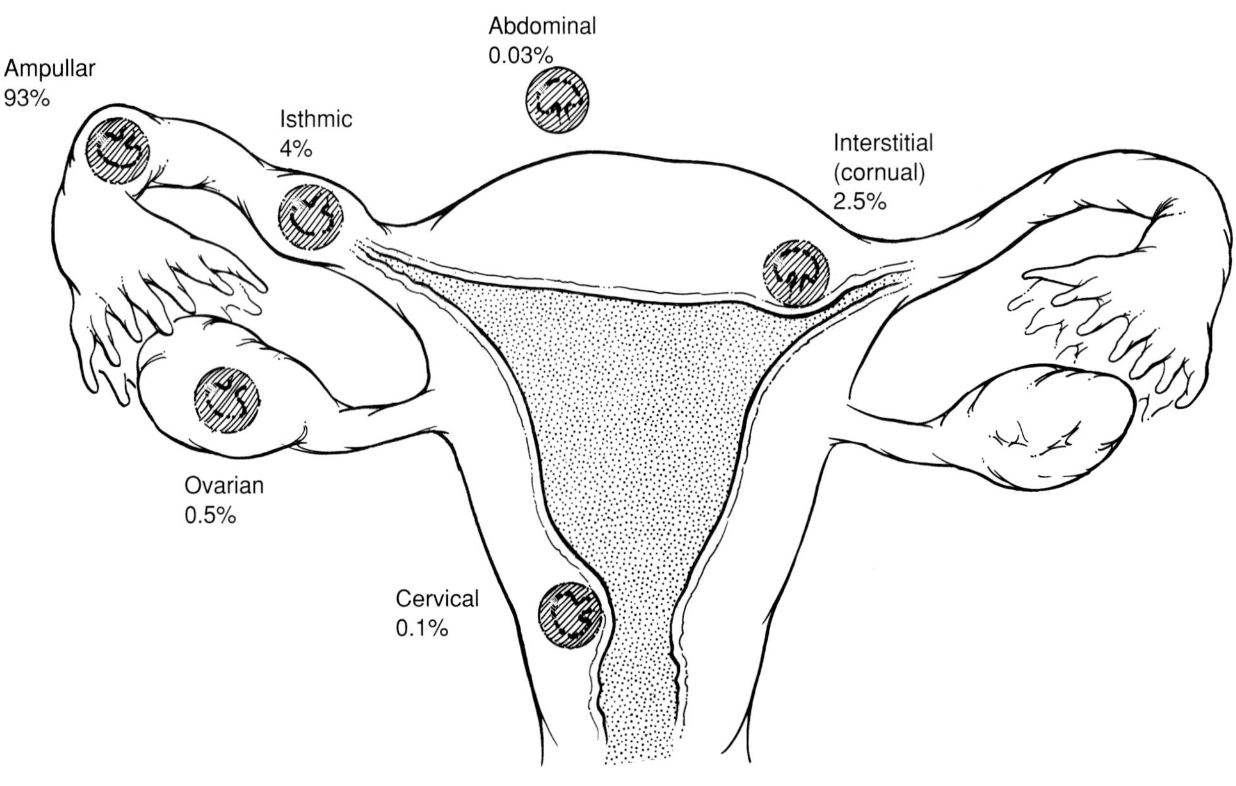

Figure 24–2. Site and incidence of ectopic pregnancy. (Modified from Maheux, 1986, with permission.)

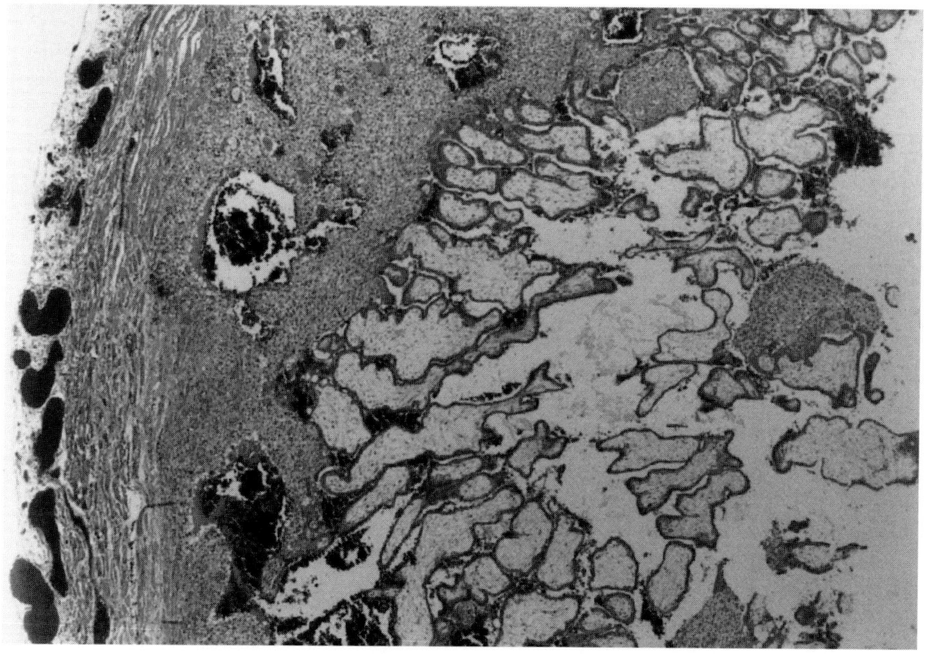

Figure 24–3. Low-power photomicrograph of a tubal ectopic gestation. The villi and trophoblast are growing in a directional pattern toward the submucosa and muscularis, implicating this area as the site of implantation. The lack of the decidual layer is characteristic of ectopic gestations. (Photo courtesy of Christopher M. Zahn, MD.)

growth. Conversely, Senterman and associates (1988) demonstrated that ampullary gestations were intraluminal in 56 percent of cases, extraluminal in 7 percent, and both extra- and intraluminal in 37 percent (Fig. 24–3). Isthmic gestations were equally distributed between the extra- and intraluminal locations. Extraluminal growth results in mucosal damage at the implantation site with otherwise minimal destruction of the mucosa and muscularis. Intraluminal growth results in more mucosal destruction. Mixed growth results in the greatest tissue destruction and is most commonly seen with isthmic pregnancies.

Interstitial or **cornual pregnancy** such as that shown in Figure 24–4, constitutes about 2–4 percent of ectopic implantations (Dorfman and colleagues, 1984). The interstitial portion of the fallopian tube is approximately 1 cm in length and is surrounded by myometrium. Greater distensibility of the cornua results in more extensive trophoblastic invasion, increased vascularity, and delayed diagnosis, which is associated with increased maternal morbidity and mortality.

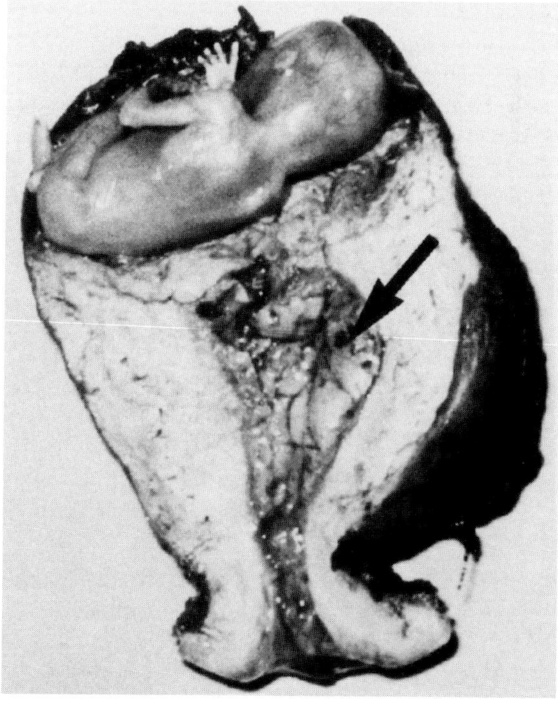

Figure 24–4. Interstitial pregnancy. Abundant decidua (arrow) fills the uterine cavity.

Ovarian pregnancy accounts for approximately 2.5 percent of ectopic gestations and has an estimated incidence of 1 in 7000 deliveries (Grimes and co-workers, 1983). Criteria for diagnosis of an ovarian pregnancy were defined by Spiegleberg in 1878 and require that (1) the fallopian tube, including the fimbriae ovarica, on the affected side be intact, (2) the fetal sac occupy the position of the ovary, (3) the ovary be connected to the uterus by the ovarian ligament, and (4) definite ovarian tissue be found in the sac wall.

A case of **cervical pregnancy** is shown in Figure 24–5. In order to diagnose cervical pregnancy, Rubin in 1911 established the criteria that (1) cervical glands be present opposite the placental attachment site, (2) the attachment of the placenta to the cervix be located below the entrance of the uterine vessels, (3) fetal parts must not be present in the uterine corpus, and (4) the placental attachment to the cervix must be intimate. While this is a pathologic diagnosis, Paalman (1959) established clinical criteria that require (1) a closed internal os, (2) products of conception completely confined within and firmly attached to the endocervix, (3) uterine bleeding in the absence of cramping, and (4) a soft enlarged cervix equal to or larger than the uterine fundus. Cervical pregnancy has been estimated to have an incidence ranging from 1 in 1000 in Japan to 1 in 18,000 in some American studies (Parente and co-workers, 1983; Shinagawa and Nagayama, 1969).

Abdominal pregnancy usually results from tubal abortion and secondary nidation. Studdiford in 1942 defined that primary abdominal pregnancy gestations (1) must exist in the presence of normal fallopian tubes and ovaries and (2) in the absence of uteroplacental fistulas and (3) must be diagnosed early enough to eliminate the possibility of secondary nidation. These are discussed in detail in Chapter 23.

Heterotopic pregnancy—the coexistence of both an intrauterine and extrauterine gestation—is a rare obstetric phenomenon, with a reported worldwide incidence of 1 in 30,000. In their review, Reece and associates (1983) reported an incidence of 1 in 8000 at the Sloan Hospital for Women. They postulated that this high incidence was related to an increased incidence of salpingitis; however, tubal surgery, ovulation induction, and multiple embryo transfer with in vitro fertilization procedures also are factors in heterotopic pregnancies (Svare and co-workers, 1993). In either case, a high index of suspicion is necessary to identify and manage these women.

CLINICAL FINDINGS

Women with an ectopic pregnancy will either present with acute symptoms that demand immediate diagnosis and management, or because of certain risk factors, will be diagnosed after prospective determination of serial serum chorionic gonadotropin levels prior to

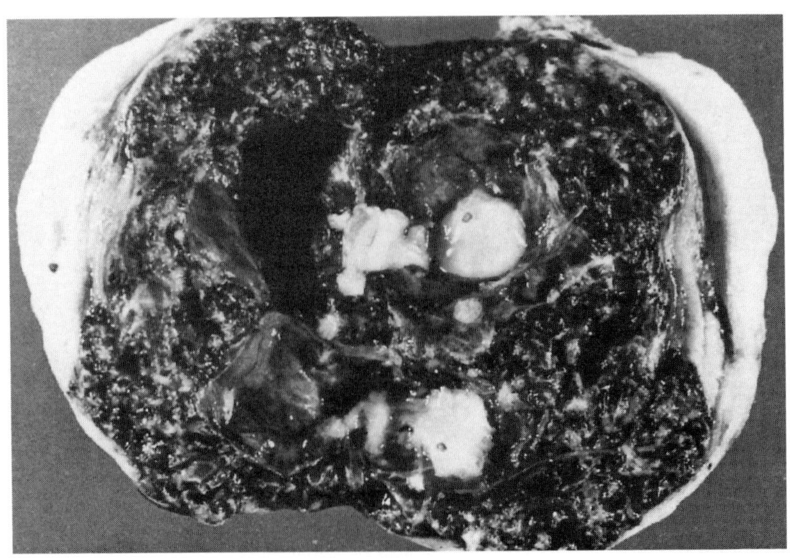

Figure 24–5. Cervical pregnancy.

the onset of symptoms. Early diagnosis relies on the clinical ability to first suspect the diagnosis and then proceed with the appropriate diagnostic tests.

Signs and Symptoms

The location of the ectopic pregnancy influences clinical symptoms. Typically, abdominal pain and bleeding after missed menses are common symptoms in tubal gestations (Kallenberger and colleagues, 1978). Pain results from distension of the tubal serosa, whereas abnormal bleeding represents decidual shedding as a result of abnormal chorionic gonadotropin production and insufficient luteal support. Rarely a woman presents with syncopal episodes. Less than 5 percent of women with an ectopic pregnancy present with hypovolemic shock from acute blood loss. A more typical presentation is the woman with a normal pulse, but who has abdominal tenderness with guarding and rebound tenderness that results from peritoneal irritation by blood. On pelvic examination, the uterus may be normal to slightly enlarged and an adnexal mass may be palpable in half of cases. Histologic evaluation of tissue that is passed vaginally may disclose the **Arias-Stella phenomenon** (Fig. 24–6), often with an associated decidual cast.

Diagnosis

For the woman who presents with an acute abdomen in the emergency room, a rapid qualitative serum chorionic gonadotropin level determination and transvaginal ultrasonography may be useful. In the absence of ultrasonic documentation of either an intrauterine or extrauterine gestation, the diagnosis is not definitive. In some cases, culdocentesis is valuable to diagnose ectopic pregnancy. A positive culdocentesis productive of nonclotting blood, in association with a positive pregnancy test, corresponds with ectopic pregnancy in 99 percent of cases and is sufficient evidence for surgical treatment (Romero and colleagues, 1985a). Alternative diagnoses to consider with a positive culdocentesis include ruptured ovarian cyst, ruptured endometrioma, and bleeding from other causes. The hematocrit determination of cul-de-sac fluid is usually greater than 15 volumes percent with an ectopic preg-

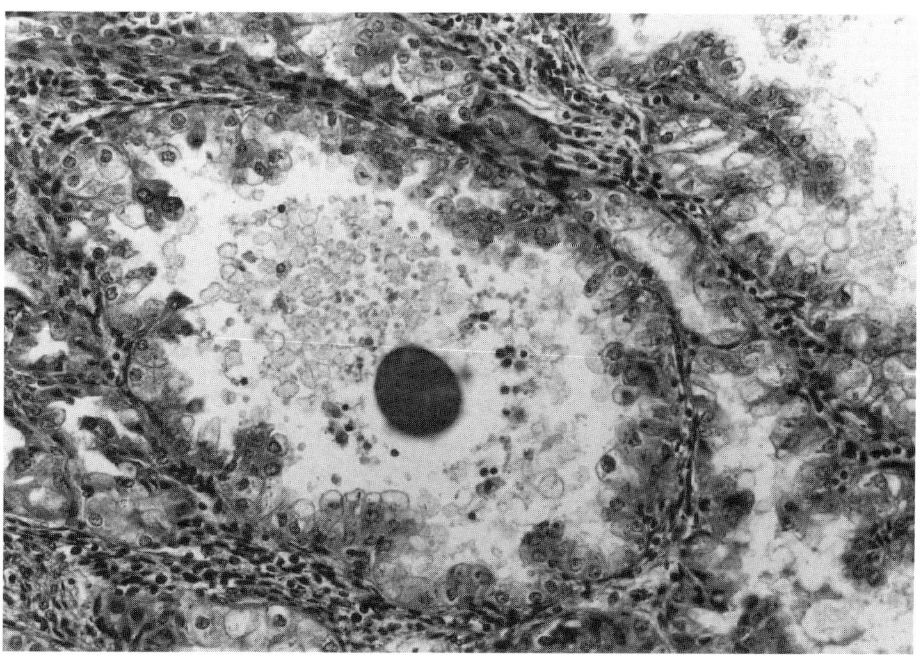

Figure 24–6. Arias-Stella phenomenon. The endometrial glands are hypersecretory, depicted by dilated, tortuous glands with minimal intervening decidualized stroma. In contrast to normal secretory endometrial glands, the nuclei are atypical; characterized by an increased nuclear-cytoplasmic ratio and hyperchromasia. (Photo courtesy of Christopher M. Zahn, MD.)

nancy, while a hematocrit of less than 15 suggests cyst fluid. In many cases, the ectopic pregnancy will be ruptured, or more commonly there is bleeding from the distal end of the tube. A negative culdocentesis is the finding of serous fluid, whereas no fluid or blood is considered a non-diagnostic result. Both require further evaluation to rule out ectopic pregnancy.

In the woman who is clinically stable or has presented early, the use of quantitative serum chorionic gonadotropin levels, transvaginal ultrasound, and diagnostic laparoscopy may all play a role in confirming the diagnosis. The ability to accurately and quickly determine serum levels of the β-subunit of chorionic gonadotropin has revolutionized the clinical management of ectopic pregnancy. It is important to be aware of the standard that is used to determine the serum levels. In 1974, the World Health Organization introduced a new standard that used a highly purified gonadotropin preparation to establish the International Reference Preparation (IRP). This standard replaced the second International Standard (IS), which used a heterogeneous gonadotropin preparation. Serum levels determined by the IRP are approximately twice the value of those calculated by the second International Standard (Bangham and Storring, 1982). With the use of either the radioimmunoassay (RIA) or the radioreceptor assay (RRA) for the β-subunit, issues such as cross-reactivity with luteinizing hormone have been eliminated. Because the sensitivity of the assay is 5 mIU/mL, a negative serum determination virtually rules out ectopic pregnancy (Romero and co-workers, 1986).

With a normal pregnancy, serum chorionic gonadotropin levels can be expected to increase by at least 66 percent in 2 days (Table 24–3), although there are some reports that these levels have a doubling time of 1.5 to 1.87 days (Kadar and associates, 1993). In a woman who is hemodynamically stable, but at risk for an ectopic pregnancy, the value of serial chorionic gonadotropin levels cannot be overemphasized. Abnormal pregnancies such as a blighted ovum, missed abortion, and ectopic pregnancy will be associated with serum levels that either rise inappropriately or decline, and these pregnancies require further evaluation.

Determination of the threshold serum level of chorionic gonadotropin above which an intrauterine gestation should be seen has greatly facilitated the ability to diagnose ectopic pregnancy. Kadar and colleagues (1980) established a threshold level of 6,500 mIU/mL (IRP). When the serum level exceeded that value, the absence of an intrauterine gestational sac was associated with an ectopic pregnancy in 86 percent of cases. Furthermore, this criteria had a sensitivity of 100 percent, a specificity of 96 percent, and a negative predictive value of 100 percent. Absence of a gestational sac using abdominal ultrasonography in a woman whose level is below 6000 mIU/mL is a nondiagnostic finding that requires further evaluation (Romero and associates, 1985b).

TABLE 24–3. LOWER LIMIT FOR THE PERCENTAGE INCREASE OF SERUM CHORIONIC GONADOTROPIN LEVELS DURING EARLY INTRAUTERINE PREGNANCY

Sampling Interval (Days)	Percentage Increase in Serum β-hCG from Initial Value
1	29
2	66
3	114
4	175
5	255

Modified from Kadar and colleagues (1981).

Using transvaginal ultrasound, an intrauterine gestational sac may be visible when the serum chorionic gonadotropin value exceeds 1000–1500 mIU/mL (IRP). However, the discriminatory zone should be established at individual institutions (Bateman and associates, 1990; Cacciatore and co-workers, 1990; Keith and colleagues, 1993). The clinical correlation between serum chorionic gonadotropin levels and transvaginal ultrasonography allows for the confident diagnosis of ectopic pregnancy about 1 week earlier than previously possible by using transabdominal sonography (Aleem and co-workers, 1990).

Serum progesterone levels serve as an adjunct to chorionic gonadotropin determinations and may be useful to confirm an abnormal pregnancy. In two retrospective studies, a single serum progesterone level less than 15 ng/mL was associated with an ectopic pregnancy, while a level greater than 20 ng/mL was associated with normal pregnancy (Matthew and colleagues, 1986; Yeko and associates, 1987). Stovall and co-workers (1989, 1992) demonstrated that a serum progesterone level less than 5 ng/mL resulted in a sensitivity for spontaneous abortion of 75 percent and ectopic pregnancy of 40 percent. The specificity, however, was 100 percent, and this prompted these investigators to recommend curettage for earlier diagnosis of an abnormal pregnancy in an effort to obviate unnecessary laparoscopy. In this scheme, laparoscopy was reserved for women with a negative curettage. Such management allows possible consideration for medical treatment in asymptomatic women.

Transvaginal Ultrasonography and Color Doppler

The development of transvaginal ultrasound has greatly facilitated the diagnosis of ectopic gestation. In comparison with transabdominal ultrasound in which frequencies of 3 MHz are employed, higher frequencies of 5–7 MHz may be used. This improves resolution because the vaginal probe is in closer proximity to the pelvic organs. Transvaginal sonography facilitates identification of the uterus and both ovaries; thus imaging of an ectopic gestational sac distinct from the ovary is enhanced (Fleischer, 1990; Nyberg, 1987; Shapiro, 1988; Timor-Tritsch, 1989; and their many colleagues). With the use of transvaginal ultrasound, an intrauterine gestational sac can first be visualized by 5 weeks' gestation or with a serum chorionic gonadotropin level between 1000 and 1500 mIU/mL (Aleem and associates, 1990). This is approached with caution, however, as the intrauterine gestational sac may be confused with the pseudogestational sac often seen with ectopic pregnancies. Although it is impossible to definitively identify an intrauterine gestation until a fetal pole is present, the double decidual sac has been shown to be present in 98 percent of cases (Nyberg and co-workers, 1983). Definitive diagnosis of an ectopic gestation requires the identification of fetal heart activity. Presumptive identification of an ectopic gestation may be made when there is no evidence of an intrauterine gestation combined with appropriate serum chorionic gonadotropin levels above the discriminatory zone, or if there is evidence of either an adnexal gestational sac or a non-specific adnexal mass distinct from the ovary (Fig. 24–7). Timor-Tritsch and associates (1989) have concluded that the "tubal ring," representing the unruptured, thickened tubal wall, is important in making the diagnosis. Ultrasonic findings that are highly suggestive of an ectopic gestation are listed in Table 24–4.

Recently, improvements in the diagnosis of ectopic pregnancy have concentrated on duplex Doppler techniques. Color flow Doppler imaging of vascular patterns in the adnexae are displayed simultaneously with conventional B-mode images. This allows identification of both normal and pathologic structures. Trophoblastic flow typically gives a high-veloc-

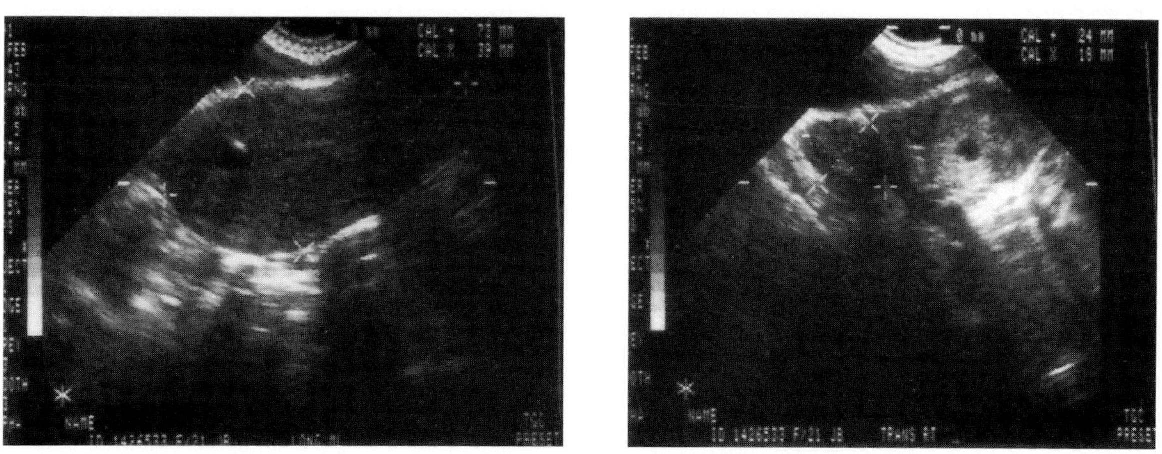

Figure 24–7. Vaginal sonogram of an ectopic pregnancy demonstrating an empty uterus and an ectopic gestational sac separate from the ovary.

TABLE 24–4. ULTRASONIC FINDINGS IN 47 WOMEN WITH ECTOPIC PREGNANCY

Ultrasonic Findings	No. of Cases (%)
Uterine	
Thickened endometrium	20 (43)
Pseudogestational sac	7 (15)
Adnexal	
Tubal ring	23 (49)
With living embryo	10 (21)
With embryo and yolk sac	4 (8)
With dead embryo	2 (4)
With yolk sac	3 (6)
Without embryo and yolk sac	7 (15)
Corpus luteum	16 (34)
Nonspecific adnexal mass	13 (28)
Dilated tube	9 (19)
Peritoneal cavity	
Simple fluid	22 (47)
Particulate fluid	13 (28)

Modified from Fleischer and colleagues (1990).

ity, low-impedance signal. This was initially described by Taylor and colleagues (1989) with respect to intrauterine pregnancies; however, it is also applicable to tubal pregnancies. Thus, a low-impedance pattern, separate from the ovary, is sufficient to suggest placental flow and an ectopic pregnancy. Pellerito and colleagues (1992), using transvaginal ultrasound with endovaginal color flow imaging, increased the sensitivity of detection of an ectopic pregnancy from 55 to 95 percent. Others have reported similar results (Jurkovic and associates, 1992; Kurjak and co-workers, 1991). Color Doppler can potentially be used to identify the viability and perhaps the invasiveness of the trophoblast. The clinical utility of endovaginal color Doppler in assisting clinical diagnostic and therapeutic decisions is yet to be determined.

Laparoscopy

Laparoscopy provides a direct visual diagnosis of ectopic pregnancy. Clearly, in instances where the diagnosis is highly suspected, and other diagnostic modalities are equivocal, laparoscopy allows a definitive diagnosis and simultaneous removal of the ectopic pregnancy surgically. Importantly, in very early pregnancy with extremely low serum chorionic gonadotropin levels, the tube may be only minimally distorted, and the ectopic pregnancy may not be visible. These early pregnancies are unlikely to be symptomatic; thus caution should be exercised to prevent premature surgical evaluation. Finally, in women with significant pelvic adhesive disease that prohibits visualization of the pelvis laparoscopically, laparotomy is appropriate.

SURGICAL MANAGEMENT

The management of tubal ectopic pregnancies has evolved over the years with a definite trend toward a more conservative approach in appropriate circumstances. This trend in part developed because of earlier diagnosis of ectopic pregnancies and the data demonstrating a subsequent intrauterine pregnancy rate that approximates 60 percent (Thornton and colleagues, 1991). Certain prerequisites must be satisfied before an ectopic pregnancy is managed conservatively. These include an assessment to ensure hemodynamic stability, as well as a careful examination of the ectopic gestation in the tube, as outlined in Table 24–5.

Hemodynamic stability is essential for conservative management. Women at risk for ectopic pregnancy who have been closely observed during the first trimester and are diagnosed prior to becoming symptomatic are often candidates for such management. The woman who presents with acute symptoms may also be considered for conservative management if she is hemodynamically stable and blood loss is estimated to be less than 500 mL. Conversely, the woman who presents in shock, regardless of her desire for future fertility, should be managed as an emergency and gen-

TABLE 24–5. INDICATIONS FOR CONSERVATIVE SURGICAL MANAGEMENT OF TUBAL ECTOPIC PREGNANCY

Hemodynamic stability
Unruptured fallopian tube
Ruptured fallopian tube with minimal tubal destruction
Location in the ampulla of the fallopian tube
Size ≤5 cm
Easily accessible
Patient desires future pregnancy

erally is not a candidate for conservative surgery.

DeCherney and colleagues (1980) have demonstrated that ruptured ectopic pregnancies may be managed conservatively if the tube is not severely damaged. In these cases, debridement is done and the site of rupture extended to remove any remaining trophoblast. The site of implantation may influence the choice of surgical procedure. Ectopic gestations located in the ampullary and infundibular portion of the tube are amenable to linear salpingostomy. With regard to size, ectopic pregnancies between 3 and 6 cm have been managed conservatively (DeCherney and colleagues, 1981b; Vermesh and associates, 1989). When the ectopic pregnancy is too large, however, complications such as hemorrhage have been reported (Cartwright and coworkers, 1986). The current recommendation is to establish an upper limit of 4–5 cm when contemplating conservative management. Finally, the fallopian tube should be accessible, especially when considering a laparoscopic approach. The presence of extensive adhesions and the potential for extensive adhesiolysis to incite bleeding in the setting of an ectopic gestation may be relative contraindications for laparoscopic management. A proposed algorithm for the laparoscopic management of ectopic pregnancy is presented in Figure 24–8.

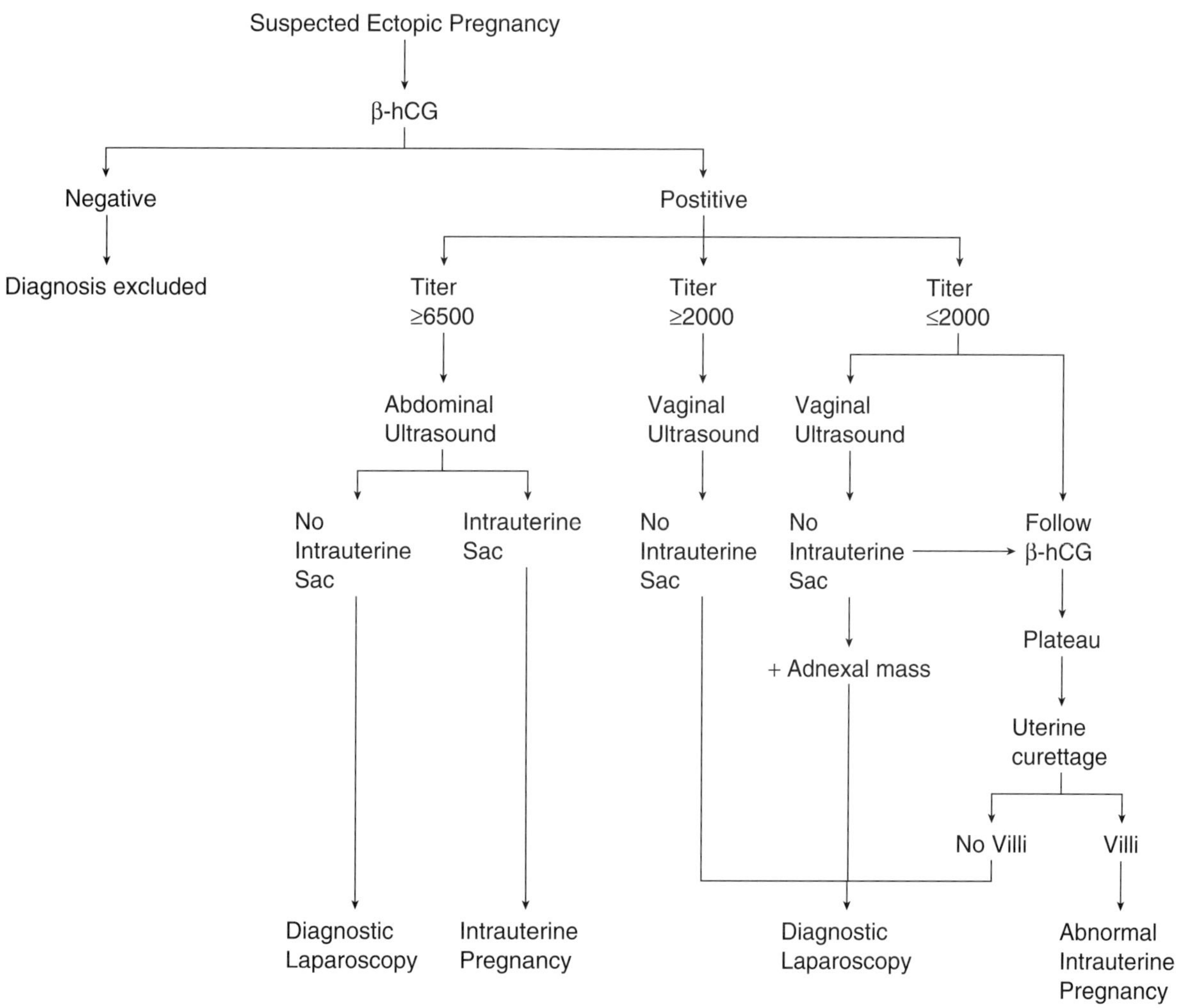

Figure 24–8. Algorithm illustrating the surgical management of ectopic pregnancy.

Linear Salpingostomy

The technique of linear salpingotomy for the treatment of an early recognized ectopic pregnancy was first described by Stromme in 1953. Linear salpingostomy is a similar procedure in which the tubal defect is left to heal by secondary intent; this procedure may be performed either at laparoscopy or at laparotomy. A laparoscopic approach depicted in Figure 24–9 is now described: Either the double- or triple-puncture technique may be used. The double-puncture technique allows introduction of an operative laparoscope through a primary subumbilical incision. A secondary suprapubic puncture is then made for introduction of the accessory trocar through which atraumatic grasping forceps are introduced to stabilize the pregnancy. Instruments may then be placed through the operating channel of the operative laparoscope. If laser is used, a third puncture often is necessary to place a smoke evacuator and to retract the bowel. When a nonoperative laparoscope is used, a triple-puncture technique is necessary for the introduction of operative instruments through the third port.

The hemoperitoneum is aspirated and the pelvis irrigated to detect the site of active bleeding. After careful inspection with special attention to the status of the contralateral fallopian tube, atraumatic grasping forceps are introduced through the suprapubic trocar sleeve and the tube containing the ectopic gestation is grasped distally to stabilize it. Vasopressin may be injected along the antimesenteric border of the ectopic gestation to assist with hemostasis (Fig. 24–9A) (DeCherney and Diamond, 1987; Semm and Mettler, 1988). Alternatively, when laparotomy is performed, bleeding may be controlled by compression of the mesosalpingeal vessels (DeCherney and associates, 1980). Before relieving the compression, hemostasis may be achieved with needlepoint cautery. Schinfield and Reedy (1988) described the technique of ligating the mesosalpingeal vessels whereby a single ligature of 3-0 chromic catgut was placed. Paulson and Sauer (1990) prefer to ligate the infratubal vessel—the tubal branch of the ovarian artery that runs along the mesenteric border for the entire length of the tube and finally anastomoses with the ovarian branch of the uterine artery. The principle behind these techniques is to decrease the pulse pressure to allow a clot to form at the ectopic site. Potential benefits of the technique are less tissue damage as a result of minimal cauterization or suturing. Adequate collateral blood supply prevents total devascularization of the salpingostomy site such that healing is not compromised.

A 2-cm incision is made on the antimesenteric border overlying the ectopic gestation at the point of maximal bulge (Fig. 24–9B). This incision may be made with needlepoint electrocautery, scissors, or using a carbon dioxide, Argon, or KTP-532 laser. Products of conception often spontaneously extrude through the incision; however, in many cases the trophoblast will need to be gently removed by teasing it from its bed with grasping forceps (Fig. 24–9C). Undoubtedly, there will be evidence of residual tissue in the ectopic bed, however, tissue that is not easily removed should not be aggressively debrided because significant bleeding may ensue. The bed of the ectopic gestation is then irrigated and additional hemostasis achieved with cautery (Fig. 24–9D).

Products of conception may then be removed easily by placing them in the Endobag (Ethicon Corp.), which is introduced through a 10-mm accessory trocar sleeve. Alternatively, products may be removed utilizing the 10-mm Semm spoon forceps (Karl Storz, Endoscopy-America, Inc.). These forceps enable the operator to grasp the trophoblast and remove it intact. Alternately, the specimen may be divided with scissors to facilitate removal of smaller pieces through the trocar sleeve.

Segmental Resection

As discussed before, isthmic ectopic gestations grow intraluminally or have a mixed pattern of growth. As a result of increased destruction of tubal architecture, linear salpingostomy is not the procedure of choice. Tubal fistula formation and obstruction are complications of isthmic linear salpingostomies (DeCherney and colleagues, 1984; DeCherney and Boyers, 1985). Thus, the procedure of choice for an isthmic ectopic pregnancy is segmental resection, with tubal anastomosis performed later when there is less tissue hyperemia, edema, and potential for infection. This procedure may be performed at laparotomy or at laparoscopy and involves ligation or cauterization of the tube immediately proximal and distal to

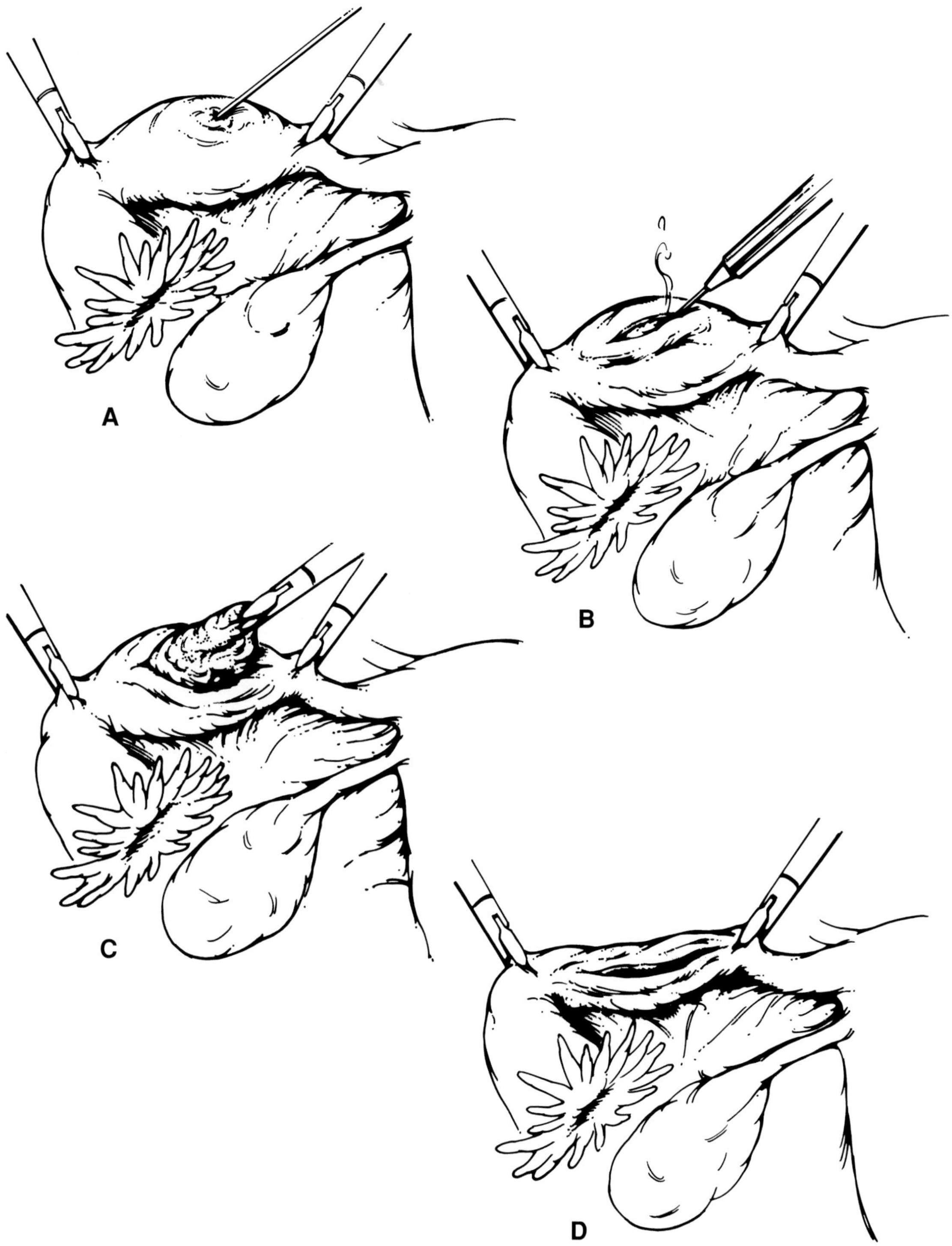

Figure 24–9. Technique of linear salpingostomy. **A.** Injection of vasopressin along the antimesenteric border of the ectopic mass. **B.** Incision is made over the ectopic bed. **C.** Products of conception are grasped with forceps and gently removed from the ectopic bed. **D.** Appearance of tube at completion of the linear salpingostomy.

the ectopic gestation and removing the involved segment of fallopian tube.

Salpingectomy

Salpingectomy is a radical surgical procedure and may be performed at the time of laparoscopy or at laparotomy (Dubuisson and associates, 1987). Considerations to proceed with this procedure include the size and location of the ectopic pregnancy, the desire for future childbearing, the status of the contralateral fallopian tube, and the reproductive history. Salpingo-oophorectomy was once the surgical procedure of choice; however, attempts are now made to preserve as much ovarian tissue as possible for subsequent in vitro fertilization and embryo transfer. The technique of salpingectomy involves placing suture ligatures along the mesosalpinx and cross-clamping the fallopian tube at the cornua at laparotomy. Alternatively, at laparoscopy, the mesosalpinx is cauterized and the tube may either be cauterized or an Endoloop (Ethicon Corp.) ligature placed before excision.

Reproductive Outcome After Tubal Surgery

Salpingectomy

Dubuisson and colleagues (1990) followed 125 women who had laparoscopic salpingectomy and who desired fertility. Of those women with a normal contralateral fallopian tube, almost half had a subsequent liveborn, while 20 percent had an ectopic pregnancy in the contralateral tube. When the contralateral tube was abnormal, however, a fourth each had a liveborn or an ectopic pregnancy. Others have reported birth rates that range from 15 to 60 percent with repeat ectopic pregnancy rates of 5–15 percent (DeCherney, 1979; Mitchell, 1989; Silva, 1993; Tuomivaara, 1988; and their colleagues). Wide variations in these rates may reflect presence or absence of disease in the contralateral tube and history of infertility.

Linear Salpingostomy

There have been a number of studies that have examined the reproductive outcome of women who have undergone conservative tubal surgery. Data exist with respect to surgery performed at the time of laparotomy as well as for that performed at laparoscopy, and comparisons have been made with radical surgical procedures. Table 24–6 is a compilation of many of these studies with regard to pregnancy rates after laparoscopic salpingostomy. The intrauterine pregnancy rate averaged 56 percent with a range of 25–77 percent. The ectopic pregnancy rate averaged 16 percent and ranged from none to 33 percent. Impor-

TABLE 24–6. REPRODUCTIVE OUTCOME FOLLOWING LAPAROSCOPIC LINEAR SALPINGOSTOMY

Study	Year	Number	Number Attempting Conception	Pregnancies (%)	
				Intrauterine	*Ectopic*
Bruhat et al	1980	43	18	14 (77)	1 (5)
DeCherney et al	1981b	18	16	8 (50)	0
Pouly et al	1986	321	118	76 (64)	26 (22)
Cartwright et al	1986	27	8	3 (38)	2 (25)
DeCherney and Diamond	1987	79	69	36 (52)	7 (10)
Silva	1988	8	6	4 (66)	2 (33)
Vermesh	1989	30	18	9 (50)	1 (5)
Mitchell	1989	13	12	3 (25)	4 (33)
Keckstein et al	1990	22	16	7 (44)	3 (19)
Lundorff et al	1992	48	42	22 (52)	3 (7)
Silva et al	1993	80	60	36 (60)	11 (18)
Ory et al	1993	80	33	17 (52)	8 (24)
Totals and means		689	416	235 (56)	68 (16)

tantly, the incidence of subsequent infertility in this group of women approximated 20–25 percent. Randomization to either salpingostomy by laparoscopy or laparotomy results in comparable rates of intrauterine pregnancies and ectopic pregnancies (Bruhat and associates, 1980; Lundorff and colleagues, 1992). The trend for a higher recurrence of ectopic pregnancy after laparotomy that was noted in both studies may be reflective of a lower rate of adhesion formation and reformation that has been demonstrated with laparoscopic procedures (Lundorff and co-workers, 1991).

Pregnancy rates after linear salpingostomy in a woman with only one remaining fallopian tube also have been reported. A review of 233 such women is presented in Table 24–7. While 55 percent of women desiring conception were able to conceive an intrauterine pregnancy, 20 percent experienced a recurrent ectopic pregnancy and 25 percent were infertile.

The final question relates to reproductive outcome following two ectopic pregnancies. Clausen and colleagues (1992) demonstrated that in those women with at least one patent fallopian tube, 32 percent experienced at least one more ectopic pregnancy, 26 percent experienced an intrauterine pregnancy, and 52 percent were subsequently infertile. This high rate of a third ectopic pregnancy is similar to the findings of others and should be discussed when presenting management options to these women (DeCherney and associates, 1985; Tulandi, 1988; Uotila and co-workers, 1989).

TABLE 24–7. REPRODUCTIVE OUTCOME FOLLOWING LINEAR SALPINGOSTOMY IN WOMEN WITH ABSENT OR OCCLUDED CONTRALATERAL FALLOPIAN TUBES

Study	Year	Number	Number Desiring Conception	Pregnancies (%)	
				Intrauterine	*Ectopic*
Stromme	1953	5	5	2 (40)	2 (40)
Tompkins[a]	1956	1	1	1 (100)	0
Vehaskari	1967	9	8	6 (75)	1 (13)
Barclay	1961	8	8	1(13)	1 (13)
Ploman and Wicksell	1969	7	7	3 (43)	2 (28)
Jarvinen et al	1972	10	10	6 (60)	3 (30)
Stangel et al	1976	2	2	2 (100)	0
Bukovsky et al	1979	1	1	1 (100)	0
DeCherney and Kase	1979	6	6	4 (66)	0
Giana et al	1979	51	2	1 (50)	0
Henri-Suchet et al	1979	14	14	8 (57)	2 (15)
Wilson	1979	1	1	1 (100)	0
Bruhat et al	1980	5	5	3 (60)	0
Stangel and Gomel	1980	5	4	1 (25)	1 (50)
DeCherney et al	1982	15	15	8 (53)	3 (20)
Langer et al	1982	8	8	5 (63)	2 (25)
Valle and Lifchez	1983	13	11	11 (100)	0
DeCherney et al	1985	1	1	0	0
Oelsner et al	1986	18	17	7 (41)	6 (35)
Pouly et al	1986	24	24	11 (46)	7 (29)
Smith et al	1987	1	1	1 (100)	0
Tulandi[b]	1988	24	16	8 (50)	3 (19)
Total		233	167	91 (55)	34 (20)

[a]Bilateral linear salpingostomies.
[b]Single fallopian tube; two previous ectopic gestations.
Thornton and colleagues (1991).

POSTOPERATIVE MANAGEMENT CONCERNS

Persistent Ectopic Pregnancy

Conservative management of ectopic pregnancy allows for the removal of the majority of viable trophoblastic tissue. The remaining trophoblast generally will undergo degeneration; however, it is capable of proliferation, resulting in persistently elevated levels of serum gonadotropin, recurrence of a symptomatic pelvic mass, and in some circumstances, delayed hemorrhage (DiMarchi and associates, 1987). As conservative surgical management of ectopic gestation has evolved, persistent ectopic pregnancy has become an increasingly important complication (Seifer and colleagues, 1991). It is imperative that women who have had a linear salpingostomy undergo weekly serum chorionic gonadotropin assessment until negative. An increase or plateau warrants further assessment and possible treatment. Surgical management considerations include a second salpingostomy, segmental resection, or salpingectomy; however, medical management with methotrexate is an attractive and effective option (Higgins and Schwartz, 1986; Kenisberg and colleagues, 1987).

Management of D-Negative Women

The American College of Obstetricians and Gynecologists (1990) recommends that women undergoing treatment for an ectopic pregnancy be considered as at risk for D-sensitization and receive 50 µg of anti-D immunoglobulin if they are Rh-negative.

Medical Management with Methotrexate

Medical management of ectopic pregnancy was initially reported by Tanaka and associates (1982), who described treatment of an unruptured interstitial pregnancy with a 15-day course of methotrexate. Since that time, a number of investigators have reported success with methotrexate given for both primary and secondary treatment of ectopic gestation (Ichinoe, 1987; Ory, 1986; Rodi, 1986; Sauer, 1987; and their colleagues). The single-dose regimen described by Stovall and associates (1991) has evolved as the currently accepted medical regimen for women who satisfy the criteria listed in Table 24–8. Contraindications to medical management include women who are symptomatic and those who have ectopic pregnancies that exceed 4 cm in size. Although medical management of ectopic pregnancies with fetal cardiac activity is considered a relative contraindication, successful treatment has been reported (Stovall and Ling, 1993).

TABLE 24–8. INDICATIONS FOR MEDICAL MANAGEMENT OF ECTOPIC PREGNANCY WITH METHOTREXATE

Abnormal serum chorionic gonadotropin levels (β-hCG)
Asymptomatic patient
No intrauterine pregnancy demonstrated:
Transvaginal ultrasound (β-hCG ≥ 1000–1500 mIU/mL)
Abdominal ultrasound (β-hCG ≥ 6500 mIU/mL)
Absence of adnexal mass or visible adnexal mass ≤4 cm
No chorionic villi on curettage
Reliable, conscientious patient

The current recommendation for medical management of ectopic pregnancy was developed by Stovall and associates (1991) and involves treatment with single-dose methotrexate, 1.0 mg/kg given intramuscularly on an outpatient basis. Before treatment, laboratory evaluation includes serum chorionic gonadotropin, liver enzymes, serum creatinine levels, hemogram with platelet count, and blood type and Rh status. Characteristically, the serum chorionic gonadotropin level will increase within the first 4 days of treatment; however, there is usually a decline of 15 percent or greater by post-treatment day 7. When the decline is less than 15 percent, a second course of methotrexate is given. Serum chorionic gonadotropin levels may take up to 70 days to revert to negative and the rate of decline is apparently slower with higher initial values.

Patients are informed that medical treatment fails in about 5 percent of cases. They are counseled that they may experience lower abdominal pain that may represent tubal rupture. Thus, abdominal pain, weakness, dizziness, or syncope are reported immediately and evaluated. These women are counselled to avoid intercourse, alcohol, and vitamins that contain folic acid until the serum chorionic gonadotropin level is negative. Reassurance may also be given that the chemotherapeutic side effects seen with methotrexate, that is, gastritis, nausea and vomiting, stomatitis, elevated liver enzymes, thrombocytopenia, and leukopenia are virtually eliminated with the single-dose regimen.

In their most recent prospective study of 121 women treated, Stovall and Ling (1993) reported a 94 percent success rate. Of 62 women treated with methotrexate, 51 (82 percent) had a post-treatment hysterosalpingogram that demonstrated tubal patency on the involved side. Of the 49 women who attempted pregnancy, 39 (80 percent) conceived; 87 percent were intrauterine and 13 percent were ectopic pregnancies.

SUMMARY

Ectopic pregnancy has been an increasingly important public health problem worldwide. Fortunately, the use of high resolution ultrasonography and B-HCG subunit assays have reduced the case fatality rate by more than 90 percent over the last 20 years. The great majority of ectopic pregnancies are now identified before rupture, and well before the accumulation of a massive hemoperitoneum and cardiovascular instability. Accordingly, they are candidates for laparoscopic management. Laparoscopy offers the advantage of minimal intraoperative manipulation, less adhesion formation, more rapid recovery, reduced hospital stays, and monetary savings. The disadvantage of laparoscopic management is the increased rate of persistent ectopic pregnancy relative to that seen with laparotomy. Equally effective as laparoscopy is the use of methotrexate for medical management of ectopic pregnancies that are diagnosed prior to the onset of symptoms and that are less than or equal to 4 cm in size.

REFERENCES

Aleem FA, DeFazio M, Gintautas J. Endovaginal sonography for the early diagnosis of intrauterine and ectopic pregnancies. Hum Reprod 1990; 5:755.

American College of Obstetricians and Gynecologists. Prevention of D isoimmunization. ACOG Technical Bulletin No.147, 1990.

Bangham DR, Storring PL. Standardization of human chorionic gonadotropin, hCG subunits and pregnancy tests. Lancet 1982; 1:8628.

Barclay SDeC. Conservative surgery in tubal ectopic gestation. Aust NZ J Surg 1961; 31:51.

Bateman BG, Nunley NC, Colp LA, et al. Vaginal sonography findings and hCG dynamics of early intrauterine and tubal pregnancies. Obstet Gynecol 1990; 75:421.

Bruhat MA, Manhes H, Mage G, Pouly JL. Treatment of ectopic pregnancy by means of laparoscopy. Fertil Steril 1980; 33:411.

Budowick M, Johnson TRB, Genadry R, et al. The histopathology of the developing tubal ectopic pregnancy. Fertil Steril 1980; 34:169.

Bukovsky I, Langer R, Herman A, Caspi E. Conservative surgery for tubal pregnancy. Obstet Gynecol 1979; 33:709.

Cacciatore B, Stenman U, Ylostalo P. Diagnosis of ectopic pregnancy by vaginal ultrasonography in combination with a discriminatory serum hCG level of 1000 IU/L(IRP). Br J Obstet Gynecol 1990; 97:904.

Cartwright PS, Herbert CM, Maxson WS. Operative laparoscopy for the management of tubal pregnancy. J Reprod Med 1986; 31:589.

Centers for Disease Control. Current trends: ectopic pregnancy—United States 1987. Morbid Mortal Weekly Rev 1990; 39:401.

Centers for Disease Control. Current trends: ectopic pregnancy—United States 1988–1989. Morbid Mortal Weekly Rev 1992; 41:591.

Chow JM, Yonekura L, Richwald GA, et al. The association between chlamydia trachomatis and ectopic pregnancy. JAMA 1990; 263:3164.

Clausen I, Frost L, Borlum K-G. Reproductive outcome following two ectopic gestations: results after conservative surgery. Int J Fertil 1992; 37:204.

DeCherney AH, Boyers SP. Isthmic ectopic pregnancy: segmental resection as the treatment of choice. Fertil Steril 1985; 44:307.

DeCherney AH, Cholst I, Naftolin F. Structure and function of the fallopian tubes following exposure to diethylstilbestrol (DES) during gestation. Fertil Steril 1981a; 36:741.

DeCherney AH, Diamond MP. Laparoscopic salpingostomy for ectopic pregnancy. Obstet Gynecol 1987; 70:948.

DeCherney AH, Kase N. The conservative surgical management of unruptured ectopic pregnancy. Obstet Gynecol 1979; 54:451.

DeCherney AH, Maheux R. Modern management of tubal pregnancy. In: Leventhal JM et al, eds. Current Problems in Obstetrics and Gynecology. Chicago: Chicago Year Book Medical Publishers, 1983.

DeCherney AH, Maheux R, Naftolin F. Salpingostomy for ectopic pregnancy in the sole patent oviduct: reproductive outcome. Fertil Steril 1982; 37:619.

DeCherney AH, Naftolin F, Graebe R. Isthmic ectopic pregnancy segmental resection as the treatment of choice. Fertil Steril 1984; 41:45S.

DeCherney AH, Polan ML, Kort H, Kase N. Microsurgical technique in the management of tubal ectopic pregnancy. Fertil Steril 1980; 34:324.

DeCherney AH, Romero R, Naftolin F. Surgical management of unruptured ectopic pregnancy. Fertil Steril 1981b; 35:21.

DeCherney AH, Silidker JS, Mezer HC, Tarlatzis BC. Reproductive outcome following two ectopic pregnancies. Fertil Steril 1985; 43:82.

DeStefano F, Peterson HB, Layde PM, Rubin GL. Risk of ectopic pregnancy following tubal sterilization. Obstet Gynecol 1982; 60:326.

DiMarchi JM, Kosasa TS, Kobara TV, Hale RW. Persistent ectopic pregnancy. Obstet Gynecol 1987; 70:555.

Dorfman SF, Grimes DA, Cates W, et al. Ectopic pregnancy mortality, United States, 1979 to 1980: clinical aspects. Obstet Gynecol 1984; 64:386.

Doyle MB, DeCherney AH, Diamond MP. Epidemiology and etiology of ectopic pregnancy. Obstet Gynecol Clin North Am 1991; 18:1.

Dubuisson JB, Aubriot FX, Cardone V. Laparoscopic salpingectomy for tubal pregnancy. Fertil Steril 1987; 47:225.

Dubuisson JB, Aubriot FX, Foulot H, et al. Reproductive outcome after laparoscopic salpingectomy for tubal pregnancy. Fertil Steril 1990; 53:1004.

Fernandez H, Coste J, Job-Spira N. Controlled ovarian hyperstimulation as a risk factor for ectopic pregnancy. Obstet Gynecol 1991; 78:656.

Fleischer AC, Pennell RG, McKee MS, et al. Ectopic pregnancy: features at transvaginal sonography. Radiology 1990; 174:375.

Franks AL, Beral V, Cates W, Hogue CSR. Contraception and ectopic pregnancy risk. Am J Obstet Gynecol 1990; 163:1120.

Giana M, Dolfin GC, Siliguini PN. Trahamento chirurgico conservative in 51 caza de gravidenza tubarica. Minerva Ginecol 1979; 30:99.

Grimes HG, Nosal RA, Gallagher JC. Ovarian pregnancy: a series of 34 cases. Obstet Gynecol 1983; 61:174.

Henri-Suchet J, Tesquier L, Loffredo V. Chirurgie conservatrice de la grossesse extrauterine. In: Oviducte et Sterilie. Paris; Masson, 1979:393.

Higgins KA, Schwartz MB. Treatment of persistent trophoblastic tissue after salpingostomy with methotrexate. Fertil Steril 1986; 45:427.

Hillis SD, Joesoef R, Marchbanks PA, et al. Delayed care of pelvic inflammatory disease as a risk factor for impaired fertility. Am J Obstet Gynecol 1993; 188:1503.

Holt VL, Chu J, Daling JR, et al. Tubal sterilization and subsequent ectopic pregnancy. A case control-study. JAMA 1991; 226:242.

Honore LH. Salpingitis isthmica nodosa in female infertility and ectopic tubal pregnancy. Fertil Steril 1978; 29:164.

Ichinoe K, Wake N, Shinkai N, et al. Nonsurgical therapy to preserve oviduct function in patients with tubal pregnancies. Am J Obstet Gynecol 1978; 156:484.

Jarvinen PA, Nummi S, Peitila K. Conservative operative treatment of tubal pregnancy with postoperative daily hydrotubations. Acta Obstet Gynecol Scand 1972; 51:169.

Jurkovic D, Bourne TH, Jauniaux E, et al. Transvaginal color Doppler study of blood flow in ectopic pregnancies. Fertil Steril 1992; 57:68.

Kadar N, Bohrer M, Kemman E, Sheldon R. A prospective, randomized study of the chorionic gonadotropin-time relationship in early gestation: clinical implications. Fertil Steril 1993; 60:409.

Kadar N, DeVore G, Romero R. The discriminatory hCG zone. Its use in sonographic evaluation for ectopic pregnancy. Obstet Gynecol 1980; 50:156.

Kadar N, et al. A method of screening for ectopic pregnancy and its indications. Obstet Gynecol 1981; 58:162.

Kallenberger DA, Ronk DA, Jimerson GK. Ectopic pregnancy: a 15-year review of 160 cases. South Med J 1978; 71:758.

Keckstein J, Hepp S, Schneider V, et al. The contact Nd:YAG laser: a new technique for conservation of the fallopian tube in unruptured ectopic pregnancy. Br J Obstet Gynaecol 1990; 97:352.

Keith SC, London SN, Weitzman GA, et al. Serial transvaginal ultrasound scans and β-human chorionic gonadotropin levels in early singleton and multiple pregnancies. Fertil Steril 1993; 59:1007.

Kenisberg D, Porte J, Hull M, Spitz IM. Medical treatment of residual ectopic pregnancy: RU 486 and methotrexate. Fertil Steril 1987; 47:702.

Kjer JJ, Knudsen LB. Ectopic pregnancy subsequent to laparoscopic sterilization. Am J Obstet Gynecol 1989; 160:1202.

Kurjak A, Zalud I, Schulman H. Ectopic pregnancy. Transvaginal color Doppler of trophoblastic flow in questionable adnexa. J Ultrasound Med 1991; 10:685.

Langer R, Bukovsky I, Herman A, et al. Conservative surgery for tubal pregnancy. Fertil Steril 1982; 38:427.

Lavy G, Diamond MP, DeCherney AH. Ectopic pregnancy. Its relationship to tubal reconstructive surgery. Fertil Steril 1987; 47:543.

Lundorff P, Hahlin M, Kallfelt B, et al. Adhesion formation after laparoscopic surgery in tubal pregnancy, a randomized trial versus laparotomy. Fertil Steril 1991; 59:911.

Lundorff P, Thorburn J, Lindblom B. Fertility outcome after conservative surgical treatment of ectopic pregnancy evaluated in a randomized trial. Fertil Steril 1992; 57:998.

Maheux R. Ectopic pregnancy. In: DeCherney AH, Polan ML, eds. Reproductive Surgery, Chicago: Chicago Year Book Medical Publishers, 1986.

Matthew CP, Coulson PB, Weld RA. Serum progesterone levels as an aid in the diagnosis of ectopic pregnancy. Obstet Gynecol 1986; 68:390.

McCausland A. High rate of ectopic pregnancy following laparoscopic tubal coagulation failures. Am J Obstet Gynecol 1980; 136:97.

McCormack WM. Pelvic inflammatory disease. N Engl J Med 1994; 330:115.

Mitchell DE, McSwain HF, Peterson HB. Fertility after ectopic pregnancy. Am J Obstet Gynecol 1989; 161:576.

Nederloff KP, Lawson HW, Saftlas AF, et al. Ectopic pregnancy surveillance—United States 1970–1987. Morbid Mortal Weekly Rev 1990; 39:9.

Nyberg DA, Laing FC, Filly RA, et al. Ultrasonographic differentiation of the gestational sac of early intrauterine pregnancy from the progestational sac of ectopic pregnancy. Radiology 1983; 146:755-759.

Nyberg DA, Mack LA, Brooke JR, Laing FC. Endovaginal sonographic evaluation of ectopic pregnancy. A prospective study. AJR 1987; 149:1181.

Oelsner G, Rabinovitch O, Morad J, et al. Reproductive outcome after microsurgical treatment of tubal pregnancy in women with a single fallopian tube. J Repro Med 1986; 31:483.

Ory SJ, Nnadi E, Herrmann R, et al. Fertility after ectopic pregnancy. Fertil Steril 1993; 60:231.

Ory SJ, Villanueva AL, Sand PK, Tamura RK. Conservative treatment of ectopic pregnancy with methotrexate. Am J Obstet Gynecol 1986; 154:1299.

Ory HW. Women's health study: ectopic pregnancy and intrauterine contraceptive devices: new perspectives. Obstet Gynecol 1981; 57:137.

Paalman RJ, McElin TW. Cervical pregnancy. Am J Obstet Gynecol 1959; 77:1261.

Parente JT, Ou CS, Levy J, Legatt E. Cervical pregnancy analysis: a review and report of five cases. Obstet Gynecol 1983; 62:79.

Paulson RJ, Sauer MV. Conservative surgical treatment of ectopic pregnancy: avoiding partial salpingectomy. J Reprod Med 1990; 35:22.

Pellerito JS, Taylor KJW, Quedens-Case C, et al. Ectopic pregnancy: evaluation with endovaginal color flow imaging. Radiology 1992; 183:407.

Pouly JL, Manhes H, Mage G, et al. Conservative laparoscopic treatment of 321 ectopic pregnancies. Fertil Steril 1986; 46:1093.

Reece EA, Petrie RH, Sirmans MF, et al. Combined intrauterine and extrauterine gestations: a review. Am J Obstet Gynecol 1983; 146:323.

Rodi IA, Sauer MV, Gorrill MJ, et al. The medical treatment of unruptured ectopic pregnancy with methotrexate and citrovorum rescue: preliminary experience. Fertil Steril 1986; 46:811.

Romero R, Copel JA, Kadar N, et al. Value of culdocentesis in the diagnosis of ectopic pregnancy. Obstet Gynecol 1985a; 65:519.

Romero R, Kadar N, Copel JA, et al. The value of serial human chorionic gonadotropin testing as a diagnostic tool in ectopic pregnancy. Am J Obstet Gynecol 1986; 155:392.

Romero R, Kadar N, Jeanty P, et al. The value of the discriminatory hCG in the diagnosis of ectopic pregnancy. Obstet Gynecol 1985b; 66:357.

Rossing MA, Daling JR, Voigt LF, et al. Current use of an intrauterine device and risk of tubal pregnancy. Epidemiology 1993; 4:252.

Rubin IC. Cervical pregnancy. Surg Gynecol Obstet 1911; 13:625.

Sauer MV, Gorrill MJ, Rodi IA, et al. Nonsurgical management of unruptured ectopic pregnancy: an extended clinical trial. Fertil Steril 1987; 48:752.

Schinfield JS, Reedy G. Mesosalpingeal vessel ligation for conservative treatment of ectopic pregnancy. Am J Obstet Gynecol 1988; 159:939.

Seifer DB, Diamond MP, DeCherney AH. Persistent ectopic pregnancy. Obstet Gynecol Clin North Am 1991:153.

Semm K, Mettler L. Local infiltration of ornithine 8-vasopressin (POR) as a vasoconstrictive agent in surgical pelviscopy. Endoscopy 1988; 20:298.

Senterman M, Rawle J, Tulandi T. Histopathologic study of ampullary and isthemic ectopic pregnancy. Am J Obstet Gynecol 1988; 159:939.

Shapiro B, Cullen M, Taylor K, DeCherney AH. Transvaginal ultrasonography for the diagnosis of ectopic pregnancy. Fertil Steril 1988; 50:425.

Shinagawa S, Nagayama M. Cervical pregnancy as a possible sequela of induced abortion: a report of 19 cases. Am J Obstet Gynecol 1969; 105:292.

Silva PD. A laparoscopic approach can be applied to most cases of ectopic pregnancy. Obstet Gynecol 1988; 72:944.

Silva PD, Schaper AM, Rooney B. Reproductive outcome after 143 laparoscopic procedures for ectopic pregnancy. Obstet Gynecol 1993; 81:710.

Sivin I. Dose and age dependent ectopic pregnancy risks with intrauterine conception. Obstet Gynecol 1991; 78:291.

Smith HO, Toledo AA, Thompson JD. Conservative surgical management of isthmic ectopic pregnancies. Am J Obstet Gynecol 1987; 157:604.

Society for Assisted Reproductive Technology. The American Fertility Society. Assisted reproductive technology in the United States and Canada: 1991 results from the Society for Assisted Reproductive Technology generated from The American Fertility Society Registry. Fertil Steril 1993; 59:956.

Soules MR. Infertility surgery. In: DeCherney AH, ed. Reproductive Failure. New York: Churchill Livingstone, 1986:177.

Spiegleberg O. Zur causitik der ovarialshuvangerschaft. Arch Gynaekol 1878; 13:73.

Stangel JJ, Gomel V. Techniques in conservative surgery for tubal gestation. Clin Obstet Gynecol 1980; 23:1221.

Stangel JJ, Reyniak V, Stone ML. Conservative surgical management of tubal pregnancy. Obstet Gynecol 1976; 48:241.

Stovall TG, Ling FW. Single-dose methotrexate: an expanded clinical trial. Am J Obstet Gynecol 1993; 168:1759.

Stovall TG, Ling FW, Carson SA, Buster JE. Methotrexate treatment of unruptured ectopic pregnancy: a report of 1000 cases. Obstet Gynecol 1991; 77:749.

Stovall TG, Ling FW, Carson SA, Buster JE. Serum progesterone of uterine curettage with differential diagnosis of ectopic pregnancy. Fertil Steril 1992; 57:456.

Stovall TG, Ling FW, Cope BJ, Buster JE. Preventing ruptured ectopic pregnancy utilizing a single serum progesterone. Am J Obstet Gynecol 1989; 160:1425.

Stromme WB. Salpingotomy for tubal pregnancy. Obstet Gynecol 1953; 1:472.

Studdiford WE. Primary peritoneal pregnancy. Am J Obstet Gynecol 1942; 44:487.

Sultana CJ, Easley K, Collins RL. Outcome of laparoscopic versus traditional surgery for ectopic pregnancies. Fertil Steril 1992; 57:285.

Svare J, Norup P, Thomsen SG, et al. Heterotopic pregnancies after in vitro fertilization and embryo transfer—a Danish survey. Hum Reprod 1993; 8:116.

Tanaka T, Hayashi H, Kutsuzawa T, et al. Treatment of interstitial ectopic pregnancy with methotrexate: a report of a successful case. Fertil Steril 1982; 37:851.

Tatum HJ, Schmidt FH. Contraceptive and sterilization practices and extrauterine pregnancy: a realistic perspective. Fertil Steril 1977; 28:407.

Taylor KW, Ramos IM, Feyock AL, et al. Ectopic pregnancy—duplex Doppler evaluation. Radiology 1989; 173:93.

Thornton KL, Diamond MP, DeCherney AH. Linear salpingostomy for ectopic pregnancy. Obstet Gynecol Clin North Am 1991; 18:95.

Timor-Tritsch IE, Yeh MN, Peisner DB, et al. The use of transvaginal ultrasonography in the diagnosis of ectopic pregnancy. Obstet Gynecol 1989; 161:157.

Tomazevic T, Rubic-Pucey M. Ectopic pregnancy following the treatment of tubal infertility. J Reprod Med 1992; 39:611.

Tompkins P. Preservation of fertility by conservative surgery for ectopic pregnancy: principles and report of case. Fertil Steril 1956; 7:448.

Tulandi T. Reproductive performance of women after two tubal ectopic pregnancies. Fertil Steril 1988; 50:164.

Tuomivaara L, Kauppila A. Radical or conservative surgery for ectopic pregnancy? A follow-up study of fertility of 323 patients. Fertil Steril 1988; 50:580.

Uotila J, Heinonen PK, Punnonen R. Reproductive outcome after multiple ectopic pregnancies. Int J Fertil 1989; 34:102.

Valle JA, Lifchez AS. Reproductive outcome following conservative surgery for tubal pregnancy in women with a single fallopian tube. Fertil Steril 1983; 39:316.

Vehaskari A. Interstitial pregnancy following homolateral salpingectomy with cornual resection. Ann Chirg Gynaecol Fem 1967; 56:99.

Vermesh M. Conservative management of ectopic gestation. Fertil Steril 1989; 51:559.

Vermesh M, Presser SC. Reproductive outcome after linear salpingostomy for ectopic gestation: a prospective 3-year follow-up. Fertil Steril 1992; 57:682.

Vermesh M, Silva PD, Rosen GF, et al. Management of unruptured ectopic gestation by linear salpingostomy: a prospective, randomized clinical trial of laparoscopy versus laparotomy. Obstet Gynecol 1989; 73:400.

Vessey MP, Yeates D, Flavel R. Risk of ectopic pregnancy and duration of use of an intrauterine device. Lancet 1979; 2:501.

Westrom L, Bengtsson LPM, Mardh PA. Incidence, trends and risks of ectopic pregnancy in a population of women. Br Med J 1981; 282:15.

Wilson PC. Successful birth after previous tubal ectopic pregnancies. Med J Aust 1979; 2:660.

Wolf GC, Thompson NJ. Female sterilization and subsequent ectopic pregnancy. Obstet Gynecol 1980; 55:17.

Yeko TR, Gorrill MJ, Hughes LH, et al. Timely diagnosis of early ectopic pregnancy using a single blood progesterone measurement. Fertil Steril 1987; 48:1048.

CHAPTER 25

Female Sterilization

The worldwide popularity of surgical sterilization has increased dramatically in the last few decades. In the United States alone, more than 1 million people undergo a sterilization operation each year. The most recent US National Survey of Family Growth estimates that by 1988, 39 percent of all women aged 15–44 who were using some form of contraception had either been sterilized or reported that their partner had been sterilized. Among married women aged 15–44, 49 percent reported that they or their partner had been sterilized; this percentage was more than double that reported in a comparable survey of married women conducted in 1973 (Mosher, 1990).

TRENDS IN USE OF TUBAL STERILIZATION

Tubal sterilization was uncommon in the United States prior to 1970. The number of tubal sterilizations in US hospitals increased dramatically, however, from approximately 200,000 in 1970 to approximately 700,000 in 1977 (DeStefano and associates, 1982a). The numbers of tubal sterilizations performed in hospitals began to decrease after 1977, with a corresponding increase in the number of tubal sterilizations performed in out-of-hospital facilities. By 1987, approximately one-third of all tubal sterilizations in the United States were performed on an outpatient basis (Schwartz and associates, 1989).

The rapid increase in popularity of outpatient tubal sterilization occurred concurrently with the increasing popularity of laparoscopy for tubal sterilization. The prevalence of tubal sterilization by laparoscopy increased from less than 1 percent in 1970 to approximately 33 percent by 1975 (Peterson and co-workers, 1981). This trend was accompanied by a decrease in hospital stay for tubal sterilization from 6.5 nights in 1970 to 4.0 nights in 1975–1978 (Layde and co-workers, 1981). Of the estimated 215,000 tubal sterilizations that required no overnight stay in 1987, 79 percent were performed by laparoscopy (Schwartz and associates, 1989).

TIMING OF STERILIZATION

Tubal sterilization can be performed concurrent with pregnancy termination (cesarean section, vaginal delivery, or induced abortion) or on an interval basis. The timing of sterilization may influence the surgical approach and method of tubal occlusion. For example, most procedures performed post-vaginal delivery are minilaparotomy procedures with subumbilical incisions and partial salpingectomies. Interval procedures can be performed either by laparoscopy or minilaparotomy, although the former is more common. The timing of sterilization may also influence the choice of anesthesia. For example, sterilizations performed with cesarean sections will require no separate anesthesia; some postpartum procedures are performed immediately following vaginal delivery using the same anesthesia, and others are performed during the same hospitalization using separate anesthesia. Interval sterilizations are usually performed under either general or local anesthesia.

ANESTHESIA

Postpartum

Sterilization in the postpartum period can be performed using regional anesthesia, general anesthesia, or local anesthesia. When sterilization is performed immediately postpartum and epidural anesthesia has been used, a sterilization procedure can usually be performed with the same epidural anesthetic. Spinal anesthesia is often used for postpartum sterilization. When general anesthesia is used, care should be taken to avoid aspiration. Postpartum women are at increased risk for aspiration due to delayed gastric emptying.

Interval Sterilization

Although sterilization is usually performed under general anesthesia, local anesthesia is a safe and appropriate alternative (Peterson 1987, Bordahl 1993; and their many colleagues). Local anesthesia can be accomplished using lidocaine (0.5%) or bupivacaine (0.5%) with a 20-gauge spinal needle and injecting the anesthetic in a layer-by-layer fashion for periumbilical analgesia. Aspiration before injection will avoid intravascular instillation. After entry into the peritoneal cavity, lidocaine (1%) or bupivacaine (0.5%) can be dripped onto each fallopian tube before tubal occlusion. Alternatively, local anesthetic can be injected into the mesosalpinx to reduce the pain of tubal manipulation (Thompson and associates, 1987). Spielman and colleagues (1983) have shown that use of up to 240 mg of lidocaine or 100 mg of bupivacaine will provide sufficient analgesia for tubal sterilization at safe blood levels well below demonstrated toxicity.

SURGICAL APPROACH

Surgical approach to tubal sterilization is influenced by whether the procedure is being performed on a postpartum or on an interval basis. Sterilizations after vaginal delivery are performed through a minilaparotomy incision at the level of the uterine fundus, usually subumbilically. Interval sterilizations are performed by laparoscopy or minilaparotomy. Culdotomy is now rarely performed in the United States, primarily because it is associated with greater infectious morbidity than procedures performed using either laparoscopy or minilaparotomy.

The choice of surgical approach influences the choice of methods of tubal occlusion. For example, most procedures performed via minilaparotomy use some type of partial salpingectomy technique as the method of tubal occlusion. Most laparoscopic sterilizations use either coagulation, application of silicone rubber bands, or application of clips as the method of tubal occlusion.

Modified Pomeroy

The method of tubal occlusion used by Pomeroy was described in 1930 by his colleagues, 4 years after his death (Bishop and Nelms, 1930). The Pomeroy technique as originally described included grasping the fallopian tube in its midportion and then ligating the loop of tube thus created with a double strand of No. 1 chromic catgut suture. As with all methods of tubal occlusion, it is critical that the fallopian tube be conclusively identified. This can be accomplished by visualizing the fimbriated portion of the tube and identifying the round ligament as a separate structure. The original description of the Pomeroy technique noted the importance of using absorbable sutures so that the tubal ends would separate quickly after surgery. This rationale is the main reason that the most popular modification of the Pomeroy technique involves the use of No. 1 plain catgut suture instead of chromic catgut suture. In performing the procedure, care should be taken to make the loop of fallopian tube sufficient in size to assure that complete transection of the tubal lumen will occur. After the loop of fallopian tube is ligated, the mesosalpinx of the ligated loop should be perforated using scissors (Fig. 25–1). Each ligated portion of the tube is then individually transected (Fig. 25–2). It is important not to resect the fallopian tube so close to the suture that the remaining portion of the fallopian tube slips out of the ligature and causes delayed bleeding. After the procedure, complete transection of the fallopian tube can be assured by passing a chromic suture through the lumen of the resected specimen.

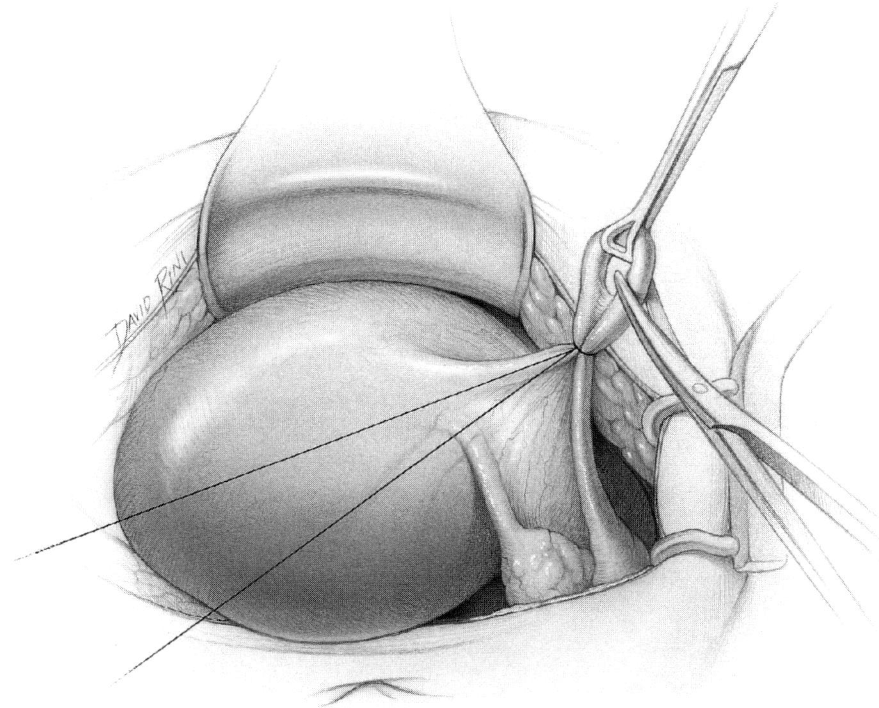

Figure 25–1. Pomeroy Tubal Ligation. Midportion of tube is grasped and elevated with a Babcock clamp. The base of the loop of tube is tied with plain catgut suture and a window in the mesosalpinx is created with the tips of the scissors.

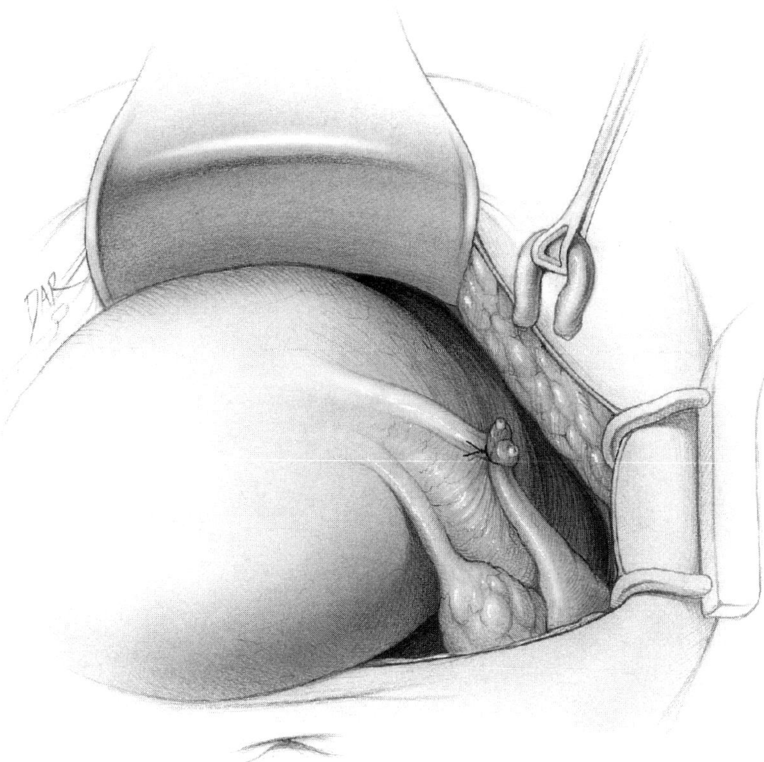

Figure 25–2. Pomeroy Tubal Ligation (continued). Each limb of the tubal loop is individually cut, and the tubal segment is removed. After hemostasis is assured, the long tails of the suture ligature are cut. If operating through a minilaparotomy incision, the tubal stumps will then retract back into the abdominal cavity.

The Parkland Method

In the Parkland Method of partial salpingectomy (Cunningham and associates, 1993), the tube is first conclusively identified and then grasped in its midportion. A hemostat is used to bluntly create a window in the avascular portion of the mesosalpinx just beneath the tube. The window is stretched to approximately 2.5 cm in length by opening the hemostat (Fig. 25–3). Ligatures of No. 0 chromic catgut are then passed through the window, and ligation of a proximal and distal portion of the fallopian tube is performed. The intervening segment of tube (approximately 2 cm) is then resected. In contrast with the modified Pomeroy technique, in which the resected portion of tubes are ligated together and then separated after the suture weakens, immediate separation of the tubal ends is accomplished with this method (Fig. 25–4).

The Irving Procedure

Irving first reported his sterilization technique in 1924 and later, in 1950, reported a modification of his original procedure (Irving, 1950). In the modified procedure, a window is created in the mesosalpinx and the fallopian tube is doubly ligated with No. 1 chromic catgut. The fallopian tube is then divided approximately 4 cm from the uterotubal junction; the two free ends of the ligation stitch on the proximal tubal segment are held long. The proximal portion of the fallopian tube is dissected free from the mesosalpinx and then buried into an incision into the myometrium of the posterior uterine wall, near the uterotubal junction. This is accomplished by first creating a tunnel approximately 2 cm in length with a mosquito clamp (Fig. 25–5). The two free ends of the ligation stitch on the proximal tubal segment are then separately threaded onto a curved needle, brought deep into the myometrial tunnel, and brought out through the uterine serosa (Fig. 25–6). Traction is then placed on the sutures to draw the proximal tubal stump into the myometrial tunnel; tying the free sutures fixes the tube in that location (Fig. 25–7). The opening of the myometrial incision is plicated closed using fine absorbable sutures, taking care not to strangulate or damage the fallopian tube. No treatment of the distal tubal stump is neces-

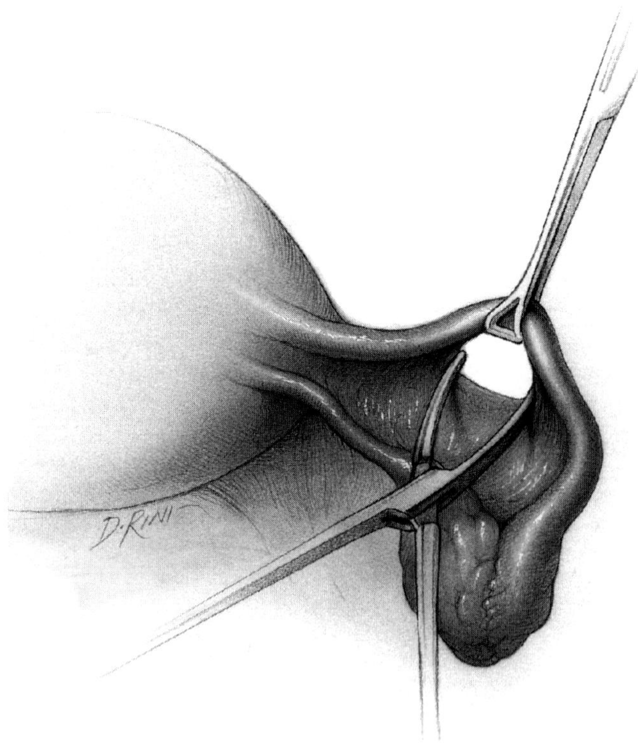

Figure 25–3. Parkland Method. An opening in the mesosalpinx is made and then stretched using a hemostat.

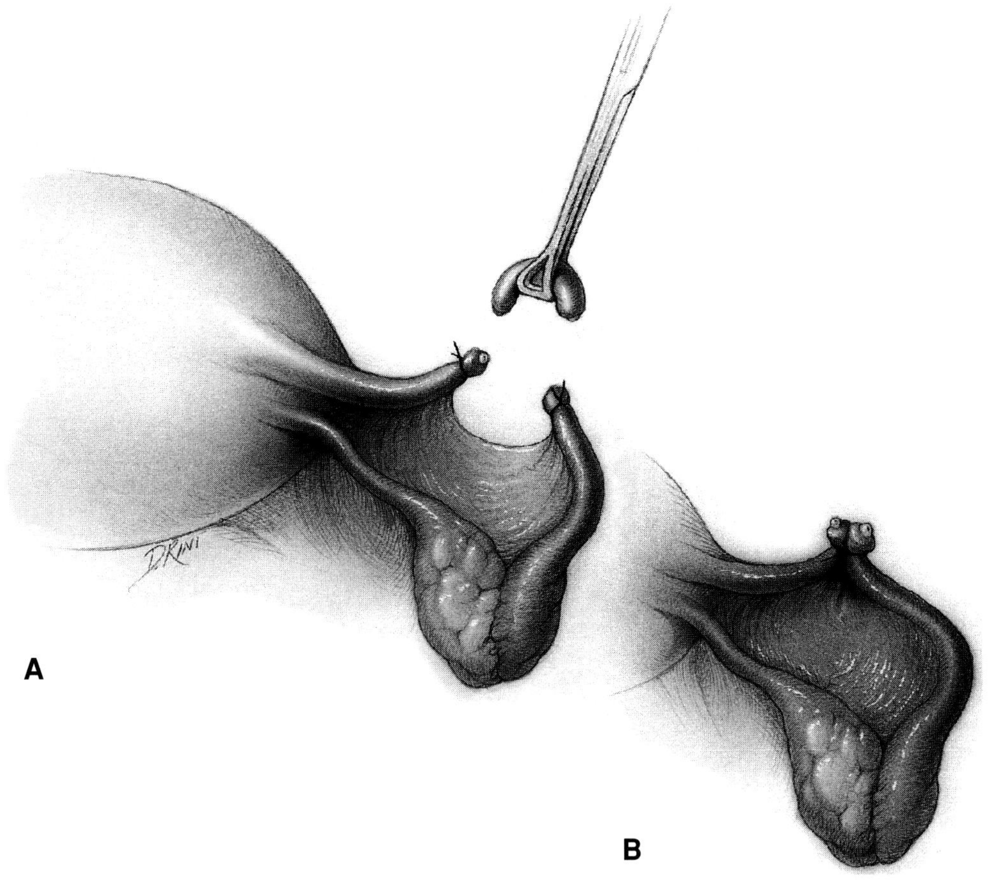

Figure 25–4. Parkland Method (continued). **A.** Proximal and distal chromic ties are applied, and the intervening tubal segment is removed. End result of Parkland method, with the immediate separation of the tubal stumps is shown. **B.** Contrasted with the end result of the Pomeroy method, shown here, where the cut tubal ends are held in proximity.

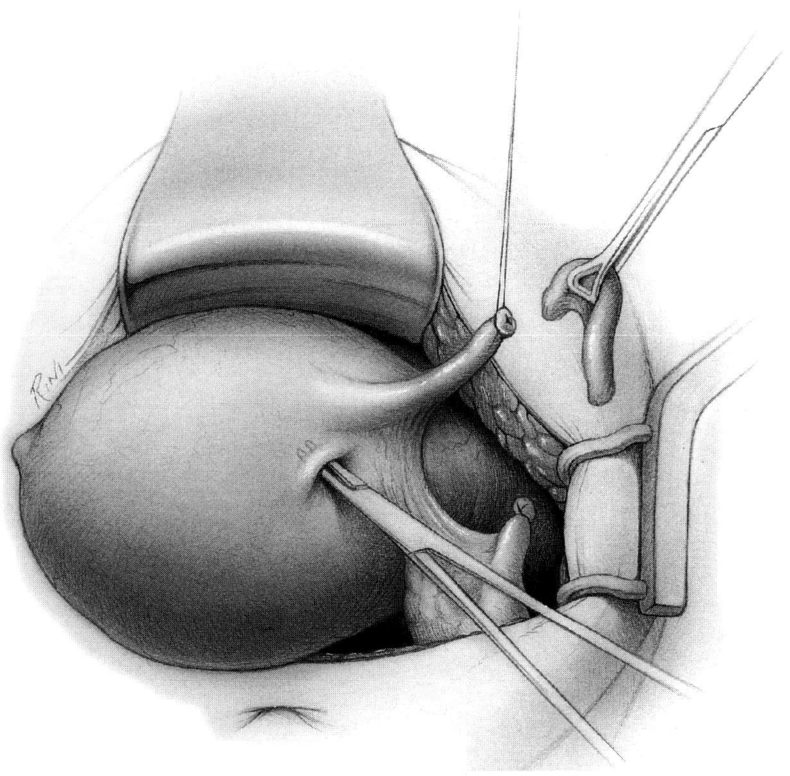

Figure 25–5. Irving Method. Tube is tied and cut at a location giving sufficient length for the proximal tubal segment to be turned back and buried into uterus. Mosquito clamp bluntly prepares tunnel in myometrium for tube burial.

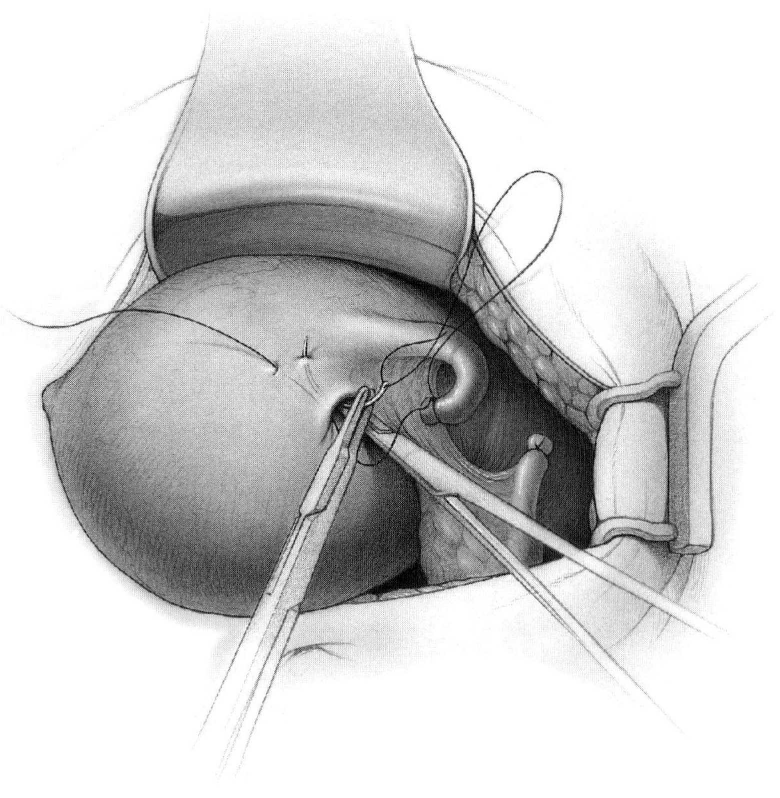

Figure 25–6. Irving Method (continued). Suture tails from the proximal tube ligature are held long, individually loaded onto a needle, and each brought deep into the myometrial tunnel and out through the uterine serosa.

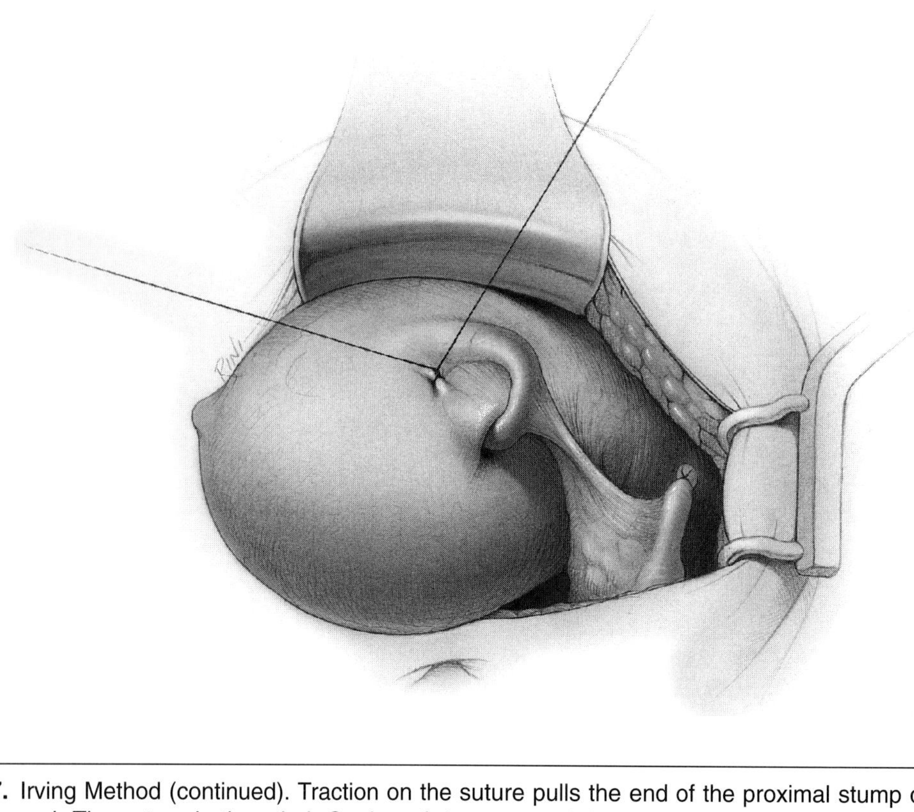

Figure 25–7. Irving Method (continued). Traction on the suture pulls the end of the proximal stump deep into the myometrial tunnel. The suture is then tied. Gaping of the myometrial tunnel around the tube, if present, can be approximated with fine absorbable suture, taking care to not damage or constrict the tube.

sary, but some choose to bury that segment in the mesosalpinx.

The Uchida Procedure

Uchida first described his procedure in 1961 and later modified it in 1975. In the Uchida procedure, the fallopian tube is grasped approximately 6–7 cm from the uterotubal junction. A 1:1000 epinephrine in saline solution is injected subserosally and the serosa is then incised. The muscular portion of the fallopian tube is grasped with a clamp and divided. The serosa over the proximal tubal segment is bluntly dissected toward the uterus, exposing approximately 5 cm of the proximal tubal segment (Fig. 25–8). The tube is then ligated with chromic suture near the uterotubal junction, and approximately 5 cm of the tube is resected. The shortened proximal tubal stump is allowed to retract into the mesosalpinx. The serosa around the opening in the mesosalpinx is sutured in a purse string with a fine absorbable stitch; when the suture is tied, the mesosalpinx is gathered around the distal tubal segment. This both ligates the distal tubal segment and fixes it in a position open to the abdominal cavity (Fig. 25–9). Although Uchida added fimbriectomy to the procedure in 1975, some surgeons choose to omit this step and to excise only 1 cm of fallopian tube (rather than the recommended 5 cm) in order to increase the likelihood that any future attempt at tubal reanastomosis will be successful.

Unipolar Coagulation

Initially, all laparoscopic sterilizations were performed with unipolar coagulating instruments. However, with reports of electrical complications, particularly thermal bowel injury, the popularity of the unipolar coagulation approach dropped dramatically when alternative methods of tubal occlusion (bipolar coagulation and mechanical devices) became available in the mid-1970s.

As much as 5 cm of tube can be destroyed with a single burn using the unipolar coagulating system. Thus, the isthmic-ampullary portion of fallopian tube should be grasped with the unipolar coagulating forceps at least 5 cm from the uterus. The tube should be

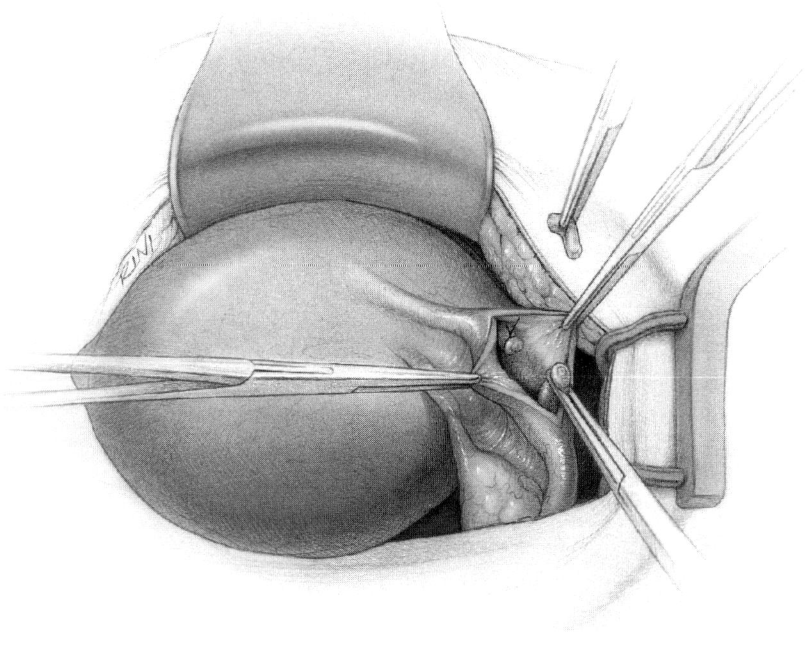

Figure 25–8. Uchida Method. After subserosal injection with dilute epinephrine (not shown), the serosa over the antimesenteric side of the tube is incised longitudinally, and the muscular tube is identified. A hemostat is held on the distal tubal segment, and the proximal segment is ligated. The intervening segment of tube is cut and removed. The proximal stump, with ligature, is then allowed to retract back into the mesosalpinx.

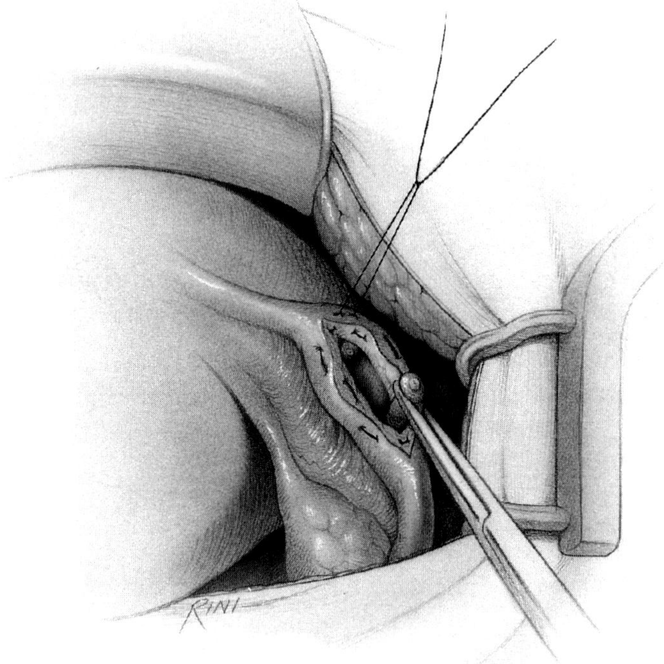

Figure 25–9. Uchida Method (continued). The purse string suture applied along the edge of the opened tubal serosa is tied, and the hemostat on the distal tube is removed. This closes the proximal tube in a retroperitoneal position, and simultaneously fixes and ligates the cut end of the distal tube in an extraperitoneal location.

identified with certainty. The jaws of the grasping forceps should completely encircle the fallopian tube and include a portion of the mesosalpinx as well. The fallopian tube should be carefully elevated from adjacent structures ensuring that bowel, bladder, vessels, and other structures are well away from the grasping forceps before current is applied. Current should be applied for approximately 5 seconds. The current should then be turned off before the grasping forceps is drawn back into the laparoscope. If a second burn is necessary, it should be applied to the proximal tubal stump and not to the distal tubal stump. In such a case, current should be applied for 3–4 seconds. The most proximal centimeter of the tube should not be coagulated, as thermal injury to this area theoretically increases the risk of tuboperitoneal fistula formation.

Some injuries to abdominal structures with use of unipolar coagulating instruments have occurred because the coagulating forceps came into direct contact with those structures. These injuries can also occur with bipolar coagulating systems. However, other injuries have occurred because of electrical properties unique to the unipolar electrocoagulation system. The two most noteworthy are injuries related to attachment of the ground plate and injuries related to use of nonconducting trocar sheaths.

In unipolar coagulating systems, both jaws of the grasping forceps are an active electrode, and the return electrode is the ground plate underneath the patient's buttocks. The patient is, therefore, an integral part of the electrical circuit. If the ground plate has only a small surface area, the electrical current will have sufficient density as it exits the body to have a thermal effect. Modern ground plates are sufficiently large to avoid this effect, but incomplete attachment of the ground plate could create a small surface area. Some but not all unipolar generators have built-in circuitry that will sense whether the ground plate is fully or only partly attached. To reduce the risk of electrical injury, care should be taken to assure that the ground plate is properly attached.

Use of a nonconductive trocar sheath with unipolar coagulation can result in thermal injury attributable to capacitive coupling (Soderstrom, 1978). Metal trocar sheaths, which conduct current, allow for dissipation of current over the broad surface area between the metal sheath and the abdominal wall. Plastic or fiberglass sheaths will not permit such safe low density grounding. Consequently, the capacitively charged laparoscope will be able to discharge current by contact with intraabdominal structures such as bowel. For this reason, metal trocar sheaths should be used with unipolar coagulating systems.

Should thermal injury of the bowel occur, it is important to recognize that the injury will extend well beyond the visibly damaged area. Small burns of the serosa of the bowel may not require repair; hospitalization for 5–7 days for observation to rule out peritonitis is required. If peritonitis is suspected, laparotomy is required. If burns to the bowel occur that are large or extend beyond the serosa, the damaged bowel should be resected instead of being oversewn. Oversewing the damaged area may result in delayed perforation and peritonitis. Segmental resection of the bowel with margins of 5 cm on either side of the burn lesion is recommended (Wheeless, 1992).

Bipolar Coagulation

The use of bipolar coagulation for tubal sterilization was reported by Rioux and Cloutier in 1974. With bipolar coagulation, one jaw of the grasping forceps is the active electrode and the other jaw is the return electrode. Although any structure coming into contact with both jaws of the forceps (including bowel) could be coagulated, the electrical properties of the bipolar system provide a safety advantage over the unipolar system. Bipolar coagulation results in a more discrete and limited injury to the fallopian tube than occurs with unipolar coagulation. Therefore, to maximize the effectiveness of bipolar coagulation, care needs to be taken to assure complete coagulation of at least 3 cm of the isthmic portion of the fallopian tube. To accomplish this, the isthmic portion of the fallopian tube should be grasped and elevated away from adjacent structures. The fallopian tube should be identified with certainty. The grasping forceps should completely encircle the fallopian tube and cover a portion of the mesosalpinx. The portion of the tube thus grasped should then be coagulated completely, followed by coagulation of at least two additional contiguous areas proximal to the first coagulated area (Kleppinger, 1983) (Fig. 25–10). Theoretically, as with unipolar coagulation, the most proximal 3 cm of the fallopian tube should not be coagulated, to reduce the risk of tuboperitoneal fistula formation.

It is important to recognize that complete coagulation of the isthmus cannot be assured merely by observing a "blanching" and "swelling" of the fallopian tube when bipolar coagulation is used. Desiccation of the outer one-third of the fallopian tube can occur without desiccation of the inner one-third of the tube with bipolar coagulation (Soderstrom and associates, 1989). Because inspection alone is insufficient to assure complete coagulation, an optical meter to measure current flow is useful. Some bipolar systems include an optical meter; it can be added to other systems. Presumably, when the tube is desiccated, there are no longer sufficient electrolytes in the tissue to carry current and flow stops. Although use of an optical meter does not guarantee complete coagulation, its proper use will

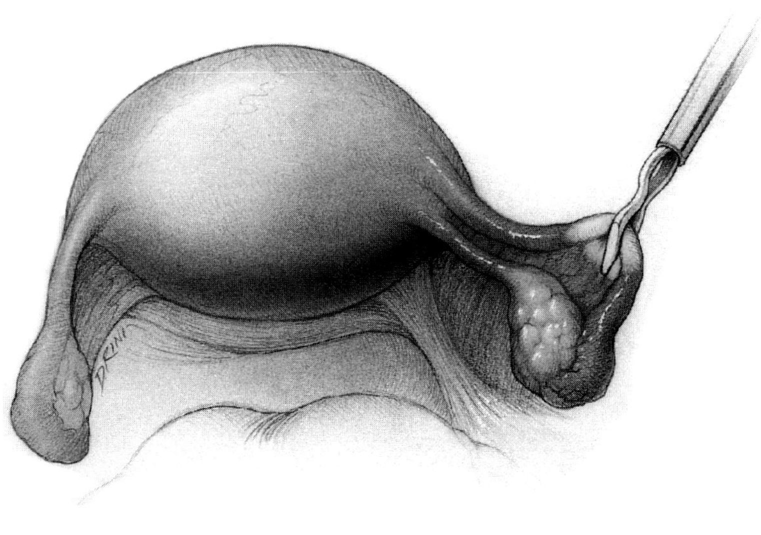

Figure 25–10. Bipolar Method. Bipolar paddles completely grasp the tube and a portion of the underlying mesosalpinx. Proximal 3 cm of the tube should theoretically be avoided.

assure that current is applied to the tube for longer than it would have been if a visual end point (such as blanching and swelling) alone were used; a longer application of current will, in turn, enhance the likelihood of complete coagulation (Soderstrom and co-workers, 1989).

Soderstrom and colleagues (1989) have demonstrated, in experiments with human fallopian tubes, that complete desiccation of the fallopian tube with bipolar systems is more likely when a cutting waveform is used than with coagulation or blend waveforms. They also demonstrated that complete coagulation of the tube with the bipolar system was achieved with the power set at 25 watts in a cutting waveform. It appears, therefore, that adequate coagulation of the fallopian tube with a bipolar system requires sufficient energy (eg, 25 watts in the cutting mode) delivered to the tube over a sufficient period of time (as estimated using a current meter rather than using a visual end point).

Silicone Rubber Bands

Yoon and associates (1974) reported on the use of silicone rubber bands for tubal sterilization. Silicone rubber bands are applied with an endoscopic applicator, which can be inserted either through the operating channel of a laparoscope or through a separate second puncture port. The band is first stretched over the distal end of the applicator; this should be done immediately prior to use. After the grasping tongs have been introduced into the abdominal cavity, they should be extended from within the applicator. The extended tongs should be used to grasp the isthmic portion of the fallopian tube, approximately 3 cm from the uterus. The tube should be conclusively identified; it should ideally be free of adhesions and normal in caliber to reduce the likelihood of surgical complications and to maximize effectiveness. The tube needs to be sufficiently mobile to allow it to be drawn into the applicator (Fig. 25–11). This is accomplished by retracting the tongs back into the applicator, which will close the tongs around the tube and pull the loop of tube into the barrel of the applicator. To reduce the risks of mesosalpingeal hemorrhage and tubal laceration, the tube should be grasped by the extended tongs and slowly elevated into the applicator, while simultaneously advancing the applicator toward the tube. The constricted loop created by the applied band should be sufficiently large that it contains two complete tubal lumens; such a loop will contain approximately 1.5–2 cm of fallopian tube (Fig. 25–12). Damage to the tube appears to be limited to that portion that is enclosed within the band; the adjacent tube appears to be normal within 2 mm from the band (Levinson and co-workers, 1978).

Spring Clip

The use of a spring clip for tubal sterilization was reported by Hulka and colleagues (1973). Application of a spring clip, like application of the silicone rubber band, requires use of an

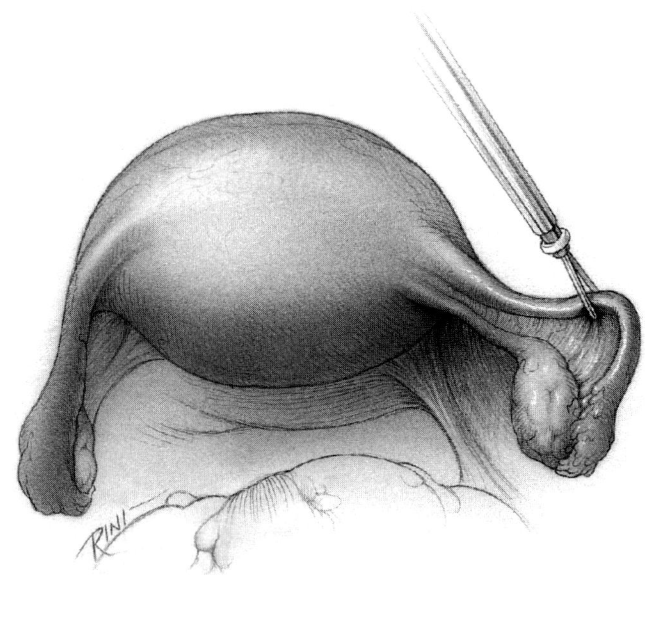

Figure 25–11. Silicone Band. One of the extended tongs is used to gently grasp and lift a mobile and undistorted isthmic portion of tube. Band shown loaded onto end of applicator.

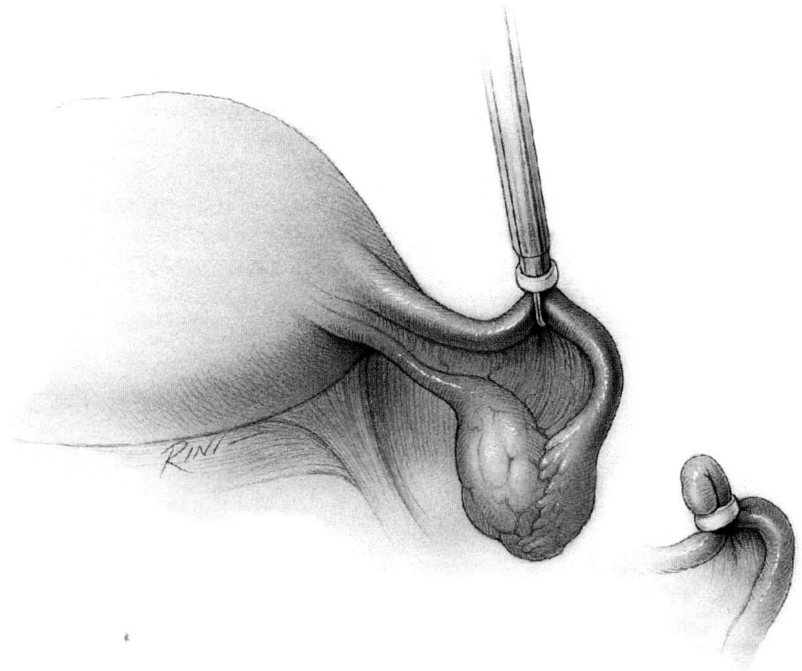

Figure 25–12. Silicone Band (continued). As tongs are gently retracted into barrel of applicator, the entire applicator is advanced toward tube to avoid undue stretching or tearing of the tube. Applicator mechanism then advances band onto base of tubal loop.

endoscopic applicator that can be inserted through the operating channel of the laparoscope or through a second puncture port (Hulka, 1985). Because the clip must be applied exactly perpendicular to the long axis of the fallopian tube, it is helpful to place the tube on stretch using a uterine manipulator and a grasping forceps inserted through the laparoscope. The clip can then be applied through the second puncture cannula. To be effective, the clip must be applied to the proximal isthmus of the fallopian tube, approximately 2 cm

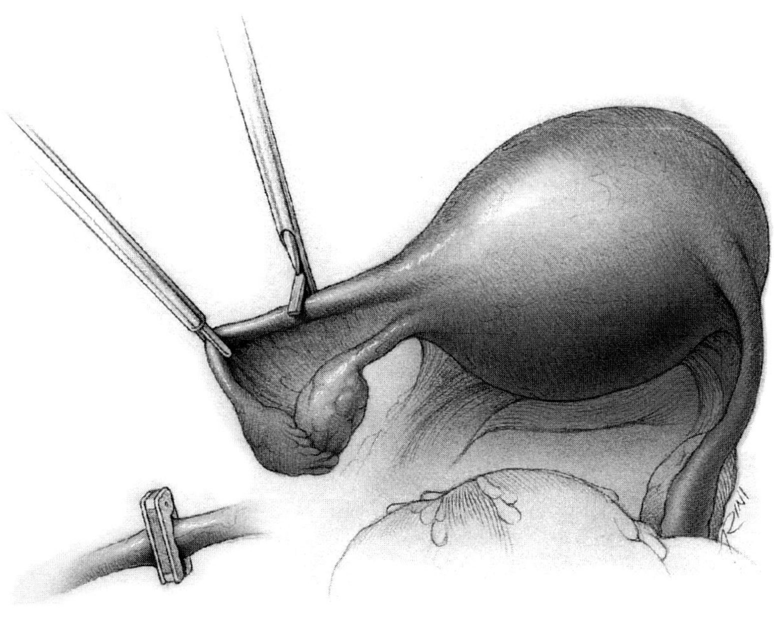

Figure 25–13. Spring Clip. With uterus deviated toward right, the left tube is put on stretch. The applicator applies clip at right angle to an undistorted portion of isthmic tube, approximately 2 cm from the uterus. Tube is seated firmly in the depths of the clip before clip is applied.

from the uterus (Fig. 25–13). As noted, the clip must also be placed precisely at right angles to the tube. In application of the clip, unlike electrocoagulation and application of silicone rubber bands, the tube is not elevated. Correct placement can be assured before the clip is applied by opening and closing the clip until the proper position is achieved. Once the clip is on the proximal isthmus at a 90 degree angle to the tube, it should be fully advanced on the tube until the tube is pressing firmly against the hinge of the clip. When this position is achieved, the tips of the jaws of the clip should extend beyond the tube and into the mesosalpinx. The clip should then be closed and the spring advanced over the clip by the applicator. The clip and tube are then carefully inspected to ensure correct application.

The spring clip, like the silicone rubber band, is most likely to be effective when used to occlude a normal tube. The presence of adhesions will make it difficult to place the tube on sufficient stretch to achieve a proper application; the presence of a thickened or dilated tube will make it more difficult to ensure that the tube is completely occluded by the clip.

COMPLICATIONS

Mortality

Although sterilization-attributable deaths can and do occur, the risk of death from tubal sterilization is remarkably low. The case-fatality rate for tubal sterilization-attributable deaths in the United States is 1–2 deaths per 100,000 procedures (Ecescobedo and associates, 1989). Complications of general anesthesia are the leading cause of death from tubal sterilization in the United States (Peterson and colleagues, 1983). The other major causes of death include sepsis and hemorrhage. Among deaths attributable to these causes in 1977–1981, most deaths attributable to sepsis followed apparent thermal bowel injury during unipolar electrocoagulation; most deaths attributable to hemorrhage followed major vessel lacerations associated with abdominal entry for laparoscopic sterilization (Peterson and associates, 1983).

Morbidity

Major morbidity attributable to tubal sterilization is uncommon, but not rare. The risks and types of morbidity attributable to tubal sterilization appear to vary by surgical approach, method of tubal occlusion, and patient characteristics.

In a multicenter, multinational, randomized trial of minilaparotomy versus laparoscopy for interval sterilization conducted by the World Health Organization, major complications occurred in 1.5 percent of women undergoing minilaparotomy with modified Pomeroy tubal occlusion, and 0.9 percent of women undergoing laparoscopy with electrocoagulation (technique not specified) (World Health Organization, 1982). Complications defined as minor occurred in 11.6 percent of the former group and 6.0 percent of the latter. The most frequently occurring major complication was pelvic infection requiring rehospitalization; this complication occurred with approximately equal frequency between study groups (0.6 percent in the minilaparotomy group and 0.7 percent in the laparoscopy group). The next most frequent complication was injury to abdominal or pelvic organs. Bladder laceration was more common among women undergoing minilaparotomy (2 of 791 women); the single case of organ injury (1 of 819 women) during laparoscopy was an electrocoagulation injury to the small bowel requiring resection of the injured segment.

In a US multicenter collaborative study, major complications occurred among 1.7 percent of women undergoing interval laparoscopic sterilization and among 3.5 percent of women undergoing interval minilaparotomy procedures (incision length ≤ 4 cm) (DeStefano and co-workers, 1983a). The study participants were not randomized, however, and women undergoing interval laparotomy procedures were likely to have been at intrinsically greater surgical risk than women undergoing interval laparoscopy procedures. In that series, risk factors for complications among women undergoing laparoscopic sterilization included a history of pelvic inflammatory disease, previous abdominal or pelvic surgery, obesity, diabetes mellitus, and lung disease. Risk factors for women undergoing interval laparotomy were virtually identical. In addition, however, incision length was identified as an important determinant of the complication rate; women with an incision 7 cm or longer had three times the complication rate of women with shorter incisions (Layde and associates, 1983). In some of these women, incisions that were initially ≤ 4 cm may have been extended to manage complications. However, it is likely that incision length is an independent risk factor for complications, with longer incisions associated with increased morbidity.

Effectiveness

Tubal sterilization is, without doubt, a highly effective method of contraception. Nevertheless, sterilization failures can and do occur. Precise failure rates for each method of tubal occlusion, however, remain unclear. Available data regarding sterilization failures are largely based on the experiences of single clinicians or institutions and evaluate only one or two methods of tubal occlusion. Most also are limited by a small number of study participants and follow-up limited to 1–2 years after the sterilization procedure. No reported studies have systematically evaluated a large number of women sterilized by a variety of methods in which a high percentage of the study participants have been followed for a sufficient period to characterize sterilization effectiveness. One large US multicenter collaborative study, which will provide 10-year follow-up of study participants, suggests that many current estimates of sterilization failure may be substantial underestimates. Preliminary, unpublished data from that prospective study suggests that a substantial percentage of sterilization failures may occur more than 1–2 years after the procedure. Further, one small study from Thailand that included 418 women followed for 6–10 years post-sterilization, found that only one of four pregnancies identified occurred within 2 years after the sterilization procedure (Koetsawang and coworkers, 1990). Two failures occurred at 6 and 7 years, respectively, after the procedure. Thus, cumulative failure rates over time may be substantially greater than suggested by estimates based on 1–2-year follow-up.

Although some uncertainty remains about sterilization failures, it is clear that a substantial percentage of pregnancies after sterilization are pregnancies conceived prior to tubal sterilization (luteal phase pregnancies). Luteal phase pregnancies are estimated to occur in approximately 1–7 per 1000 sterilization procedures (Chi, 1981; Loffer, 1980; Lichter, 1986; and their colleagues). Although luteal phase pregnancies are not true sterilization failures, they nevertheless are often quite disturbing. Strategies for avoiding luteal phase pregnancies have been evaluated. Although routine dilation and curettage will reduce the risk somewhat, performing routine dilation and curettage at the time of sterilization is less effective and more costly than timing the sterilization procedure to occur during the follicular phase of the menstrual cycle and use of highly sensitive hormonal pregnancy tests (Lichter, 1986; Grubb, 1985; Grimes, 1982; and associates).

When true sterilization failures occur, there is an increased likelihood of ectopic gestation (McCausland, 1980; Chi, 1980; Bhiwandiwala, 1982; and their colleagues). In particular, laparoscopic procedures performed by electrocoagulation appear to carry a substantial increased risk, with several reports suggesting that over one-half of pregnancies after unipolar or bipolar coagulation may be ectopic gestations (McCausland, 1980; Kjer and Knudson, 1989). Thus, in any situation where a woman or her clinician suspects that pregnancy after sterilization might have occurred, a sensitive hormonal pregnancy test should be performed and the index of suspicion for an ectopic gestation should be high, particularly if the sterilization was performed by electrocoagulation.

The absolute risk of ectopic pregnancy for a woman after sterilization is a reflection of both the relative likelihood of ectopic pregnancy when pregnancy occurs after sterilization, and the overall likelihood of sterilization failure. Thus, if sterilization failures were extremely rare, an increased relative risk of ectopic pregnancy might have little practical consequence for the individual. However, sterilization failures occur often enough that some women may be at an overall increased risk of ectopic pregnancy relative to the risk they had with the contraceptive method they were using prior to sterilization. One study, based on reported incidence rates of ectopic pregnancy after tubal sterilization, estimated that women undergoing tubal sterilization were at greater cumulative lifetime risk of ectopic pregnancy than women using oral contraceptives or barrier contraceptives. Conversely, sterilized women were estimated to be at lower lifetime risk of ectopic pregnancy than women using an IUD or using no contraceptives (DeStefano and co-workers, 1982b). A subsequent case-control study in Seattle, however, separately evaluated the risk of ectopic pregnancy after interval tubal sterilization and after postpartum sterilization. In that study, both postpartum sterilization and interval sterilization were associated with a lower ectopic pregnancy risk than use of no contraception. However, interval sterilization had an ectopic pregnancy risk equal to IUD use, while postpartum sterilization had a lower ectopic pregnancy risk than IUD use. Further, while postpartum sterilization was comparable to other methods of temporary contraception in risk of ectopic pregnancy, interval sterilization was associated with a much higher risk of ectopic pregnancy than use of oral contraceptives or barrier methods (Holt and colleagues, 1991).

Sterilization failures may be related to characteristics of patients and surgeons as well as to characteristics of the method of tubal occlusion, per se. For example, although data are limited, it is apparent that the presence of dense pelvic adhesions may make it more difficult to properly occlude the fallopian tubes, particularly with application of silicone rubber bands or spring clips. It is also apparent that the success of any method of tubal occlusion requires proper technique. Soderstrom and associates (1989) have determined that many bipolar coagulation failures occur because of incomplete desiccation of the endosalpinx. Stovall and colleagues (1991) identified a high failure rate associated with use of silastic bands and spring clips in a residency training program. Subsequently, the same authors evaluated surgical specimens from 20 women who experienced a sterilization failure and who later underwent bilateral salpingectomy. Improper application of the occlusive device was demonstrated on gross and microscopic evaluation in all 20 cases. There were no broken or apparently defective devices identified (Stovall and co-workers, 1990).

Menstrual Function

Since 1951, when Williams and associates identified menstrual abnormalities among women after tubal sterilization, there has been debate over whether a "post-tubal syndrome" exists. Although the post-tubal syndrome has been variously defined, it usually refers to some combination of menstrual symptoms including menorrhagia, metrorrhagia, abnormalities in cycle length or cycle regularity, and dysmenorrhea. In particular, it has been suggested that those methods of tubal occlusion that cause more tissue destruction, and therefore more disruption of the utero-ovarian blood supply, may be more likely to cause menstrual abnormalities.

Most early studies of the relationship between sterilization and menstrual function failed to account for factors other than sterilization per se that would influence menstrual function, for example, cessation of oral contraceptive use at the time of sterilization. In the more recent prospective studies that account for possible confounding factors, most studies find little or no difference in menstrual function between women before and after sterilization and between sterilized women and nonsterilized controls. Most such studies have assessed menstrual function at 1–2 years after sterilization (Foulkes, 1985; Bhiwandiwala, 1983; DeStefano, 1983b; Rulin, 1985, 1989; and their many associates). In contrast, one well-controlled prospective study found that sterilized women were more likely to experience adverse menstrual changes than nonsterilized controls (Shain and associates, 1989).

Although nearly all recent studies suggest that tubal sterilization does not increase the risk of menstrual abnormalities within 1–2 years after sterilization, several reports that included follow-up beyond 2 years have been somewhat less consistent. DeStefano and colleagues (1985) analyzed data from the Walnut Creek Contraceptive Drug Study and found that sterilized women were no more likely than nonsterilized controls to experience menstrual abnormalities at less than 2 years after sterilization. However, sterilized women were more likely than nonsterilized controls to have adverse menstrual changes 2 or more years after sterilization. In contrast, Rulin and associates (1993) found no differences in menstrual abnormalities between sterilized women and nonsterilized controls at 3–4.5 years after sterilization. Further, in the same study, an increase in dysmenorrhea seen at 1 year after sterilization (Rulin and associates, 1989) was not present at later follow-up (Rulin and co-workers, 1993). A large US multicenter collaborative study evaluated women before and after sterilization and found no difference in menstrual function at 2-year follow-up (DeStefano and co-workers, 1983b). By contrast, some increases in menstrual pain, menstrual bleeding, and menstrual spotting were observed at 5 years after sterilization. However, the latter findings could have been attributable to aging of the cohort and other study limitations (Wilcox and colleagues,

1992). Further, the same study did not support the hypothesis that menstrual changes after sterilization are related to the amount of tissue destruction at the time of sterilization. Specifically, six different menstrual parameters were evaluated for each of six different sterilization techniques. No single technique (including unipolar coagulation—the method causing the most tissue destruction) was more likely than another to be consistently associated with adverse changes (Wilcox and associates, 1992).

Two studies have evaluated the relationship between tubal sterilization and subsequent hospitalization for menstrual disorders. Vessey and co-workers (1983) reported on findings from a large cohort of British women followed for up to 6 years after sterilization. Sterilized women were slightly, but not statistically significantly, more likely than nonsterilized women to be referred to the hospital for management of menstrual problems. Shy and co-workers (1992) found, in a population-based cohort study in Seattle, that sterilized women were 1.6 times more likely (95% confidence interval 1.3–2.1) than women whose husbands underwent vasectomy to be subsequently hospitalized for menstrual disorders. However, like the large US multicenter collaborative study (Wilcox and associates, 1992), the study of Shy and colleagues (1992) failed to support the hypothesis that menstrual abnormalities are related to the amount of tissue destroyed at sterilization. In fact, the risk of menstrual abnormalities after unipolar coagulation in the study was lower than that for all other sterilization methods (Shy and associates, 1992).

Laboratory studies of sterilized women reported to date provide little useful information with respect to the biologic plausibility of a post-tubal syndrome. All such studies have compared serum hormone levels in sterilized women with those of other women and with normal laboratory controls. None have suitably compared hormone levels for the same woman pre- and post-sterilization. At least one study is in progress that will compare women pre- and post-sterilization, and that study should provide useful information.

Hysterectomy After Tubal Sterilization

It appears that at least some sterilized women are more likely than nonsterilized women to undergo subsequent hysterectomy. Although it is likely that this observed increase in hysterectomy for some women is multifactorial, several studies suggest that the threshold for choosing hysterectomy as a treatment option may change after a woman undergoes sterilization. Rulin and associates (1993), for example, found that women undergoing sterilization were approximately twice as likely (4.55% vs 2.17%) as nonsterilized women to undergo hysterectomy at 3–4.5 years after sterilization. However, sterilized women were no more likely to experience menstrual abnormalities than nonsterilized women, suggesting that any increased risk of hysterectomy was unrelated biologically to the sterilization operation.

Three other studies have found that women who are younger at the time of sterilization have a higher risk of later hysterectomy than age-matched nonsterilized controls (Stergachis, 1990; Goldhaber, 1993; Cohen, 1987; and their colleagues). Conversely, all three studies found that women sterilized at older ages had a risk of hysterectomy similar to that for nonsterilized controls. For example, one of these studies found that women sterilized at age 20–29 years were 3.4 times (95% confidence interval 2.4–4.7) more likely to undergo hysterectomy than nonsterilized women (Stergachis and associates, 1990). A second study found that women aged 25–29 at sterilization were 1.6 times (95% confidence interval 1.2–2.3) as likely as nonsterilized women to undergo hysterectomy (Cohen 1987). Both studies, however, found no increase in risk of hysterectomy among women sterilized at age 30 or older.

In the third study, Goldhaber and co-workers (1993) also found the greatest increase in risk of hysterectomy among women sterilized at age 20–24 (relative risk 2.45; 95% confidence interval 1.79–3.36) with the risk declining at older ages such that women sterilized at age 40–49 had no increased risk (relative risk 0.96; 95% confidence interval 0.72–1.28). However, when Goldhaber and colleagues restricted their analysis to women followed for more than 4 years after sterilization, sterilized women had a greater risk of hysterectomy than nonsterilized women in all age categories. They suggested that the elevated risk after 7 years may represent a biologic effect of tubal sterilization that takes years to manifest. However, they found no increase in risk of hysterectomy among those women undergoing sterilization by methods causing more extensive tissue destruction. Thus, any latent biologic effect would have to be one attributable to any type of sterilization procedure.

Regret

Although tubal sterilization is intended to be permanent, some women will ultimately regret having had the procedure. If these women could be identified prior to sterilization, counseling might reduce the likelihood of later regret. Studies of the prevalence and determinants of regret after sterilization are difficult to interpret. Regret in these studies has been varyingly defined and that may, at least partially, be responsible for a wide variety in the prevalence of post-sterilization regret identified across studies. For example, in a review by Philliber and Philliber (1985), the rates of regret after sterilization in this series of studies range from 0 to 18 percent. Studies in the United States have identified rates of regret as low as 0.9 percent (Shain and associates, 1986) and 2.0 percent (Allyn and co-workers, 1986). However, in the 1982 National Survey of Family Growth, 11 percent of sterilized women reported that they would have their sterilizations reversed if it were safe to do so (Henshaw and Singh, 1986). In a large US multicenter collaborative study, 6.2 percent of sterilized women indicated that they had sought information on sterilization reversal (Wilcox and associates, 1991).

Studies have evaluated regret for varying periods of time following sterilization. In general, it appears that the likelihood of a woman's expressing regret after sterilization increases over time. For example, in a large US multicenter collaborative study, the rate of regret at 5-year follow-up (3.1%) was 70 percent greater than the rate of regret at 1-year follow-up (Wilcox and associates, 1991).

Although studies of regret after sterilization are difficult to interpret, they nevertheless suggest several considerations that may be useful in counseling prior to sterilization. In a large US multicenter collaborative study, young age at the time of sterilization was the strongest predictor of regret, regardless of parity or marital status (Wilcox and co-workers, 1991). After adjusting for other risk factors, women who were sterilized at age 20–24 were approximately twice as likely (odds ratio 1.9; 95% confidence interval 1.4–2.5) as women sterilized at age 30–34 to experience regret in a 5-year follow-up study. Young age at sterilization has also been identified as a risk factor for regret in other reports (Henshaw and Singh, 1986; Boring and co-workers, 1988; Marcil-Gratton, 1988; Leader and associates, 1983; Divers, 1984).

Another potentially important finding from the US multicenter collaborative study was the relationship between regret and the timing of sterilization relative to pregnancy. Compared with women having interval sterilization procedures, women undergoing sterilization postvaginal delivery were 40 percent more likely to experience regret (odds ratio 1.4; 95% confidence interval 1.0–2.0) and women undergoing sterilization with cesarean section were approximately twice as likely (odds ratio 2.1; 95% confidence interval 1.5–2.9) to experience regret (Wilcox and co-workers, 1991). Because few other studies have addressed this issue, these findings should be interpreted cautiously.

In sum, regret after sterilization is not rare. Regret will often be the result of life changes that are difficult to predict prior to sterilization, for example, divorce and remarriage. The fact that young age at sterilization is a strong and consistent predictor of later regret is likely a reflection of such life changes.

SUMMARY

Permanent sterilization has been used increasingly worldwide as a means of contraception. The operation is easily performed at the time of cesarean section or alternatively in the early postpartum period. Surgical sterilization also can be performed as an interval procedure by either minilaparotomy or more often by laparoscopy. Although surgical sterilization is a highly effective method of contraception, failure rates for each specific method of tubal occlusion remain unclear; they are probably substantially greater than those suggested by one- to two-year follow-up studies. When pregnancy follows a permanent sterilization procedure, the likelihood of an ectopic pregnancy is substantially increased.

REFERENCES

Allyn DP, Leton DA, Westcott NA, Hale RW. Presterilization counseling and women's regret at having been sterilized. J Reprod Med 1986; 31:1027.

Bhiwandiwala PP, Mumford SD, Feldblum PJ. A comparison of different laparoscopic sterilization occlusion techniques in 24,439 procedures. Am J Obstet Gynecol 1982;144:319.

Bhiwandiwala PP, Mumford SD, Feldblum PJ. Menstrual pattern changes following laparoscopic sterilization with different occlusion techniques: a review of 10,004 cases. Am J Obstet Gynecol 1983;145:684.

Bishop E, Nelms WF. A simple method of tubal sterilization. NY State J Med 1930;30:214.

Bordahl PE, Raeder JC, Nordentoft J, et al. Laparoscopic sterilization under local or general anesthesia? A randomized study. Obstet Gynecol 1993;81:137.

Boring CC, Rochat RW, Becerra J. Sterilization regret among Puerto Rican women. Fertil Steril 1988;49:973.

Chi I-C, Laufe LE, Gardner SD, Tolbert MA. An epidemiologic study of risk factors associated with pregnancy following female sterilization. Am J Obstet Gynecol 1980;136:768.

Chi I-C, Feldblum PJ. Luteal phase pregnancies in female sterilization patients. Contraception 1981;23:579.

Cohen MM. Long-term risk of hysterectomy after tubal sterilization. Am J Epidemiol 1987; 125:410.

Cunningham FG, MacDonald PC, Leveno KJ, et al, eds. Williams Obstetrics, 19th ed. Norwalk, CT: Appleton & Lange, 1993:1353.

DeStefano F, Greenspan JR, Ory HW, Peterson HB. Demographic trends in tubal sterilization: United States, 1970–1978. Am J Public Health 1982a;72:480.

DeStefano F, Peterson HB, Layde PM, Rubin GL. Risk of ectopic pregnancy following tubal sterilization. Obstet Gynecol 1982b;60:326.

DeStefano F, Greenspan JR, Dicker RC, et al. Complications of interval laparoscopic tubal sterilization. Obstet Gynecol 1983a;61:153.

DeStefano F, Huezo CM, Peterson HB, et al. Menstrual changes after tubal sterilization. Obstet Gynecol 1983b;62:673.

DeStefano F, Perlman JA, Peterson HB, Diamond EL. Long-term risks of menstrual disturbances after tubal sterilization. Am J Obstet Gynecol 1985;152:835.

Divers WA. Characteristics of women requesting reversal of sterilization. Fertil Steril 1984;41:233.

Downey, CA. American Association of Gynecologic Laparoscopists, 1983:117.

Ecescobedo LG, Peterson HB, Grubb GS, Franks AL. Case-fatality rates for tubal sterilization in US hospitals, 1979–1980. Am J Obstet Gynecol 1989;160:147.

Foulkes J, Chamberlain G. Effects of sterilization on menstruation. South Med J 1985;78:544.

Goldhaber MK, Armstrong MA, Golditch IM, et al. Long-term risk of hysterectomy among 80,007 sterilized and comparison women at Kaiser Permanente, 1971–1987. Am J Epidemiol 1993; 138:508.

Grimes DA, Peterson HB. Routine performance of dilation and curettage at the time of laparoscopy. J Reprod Med 1982;27:213.

Grubb GS, Peterson HB. Luteal phase pregnancy and tubal sterilization. Obstet Gynecol 1985; 66:784.

Henshaw SK, Singh S. Sterilization regret among US couples. Fam Plann Perspect 1986;18:238.

Holt VL, Chu J, Daling JR, et al. Tubal sterilization and subsequent ectopic pregnancy: a case-control study. JAMA 1991;226:242.

Hulka JF, Fishburne JI, Mercer JP, Omran KF. Laparoscopic sterilization with a spring clip: A report of the first fifty cases. Am J Obstet Gynecol 1973;116:715.

Hulka JF. Textbook of Laparoscopy. Orlando: Grune & Stratton, 1985:84.

Irving FC. Tubal sterilization. Am J Obstet Gynecol 1950;60:1101.

Kjer JJ, Knudson LB. Ectopic pregnancy subsequent to laparoscopic sterilization. Am J Obstet Gynecol 1989;160:1202.

Kleppinger RK. The advantages and safety of bipolar laparoscopic sterilization. In: Phillips JM, ed. Endoscopic Female Sterilization: A Comparison of Methods.

Koetsawang S, Gates DS, Suwanichati S, et al. Long-term follow-up of laparoscopic sterilizations by electrocoagulation, the Hulka clip, and the tubal ring. Contraception 1990;41:9.

Layde PM, Ory HW, Peterson HB, et al. The declining length of hospitalization for tubal sterilizations. JAMA 1981;245:714.

Layde PM, Peterson HB, Dicker RC, et al. Risk factors for complications of interval tubal sterilization by laparotomy. Obstet Gynecol 1983;62:180.

Leader A, Gallan N, George R, Taylor P. A comparison of definable traits in women requesting reversal of sterilization and women satisfied with sterilization. Am J Obstet Gynecol 1983; 145:198.

Levinson CJ, Daily HJ, Skinner SJ. Pathologic changes in the fallopian tube after silastic ring occlusion. In: Phillips JM, ed. Endoscopy in Gynecology. Downey, CA: American Association of Gynecologic Laparoscopists, 1978:180.

Lichter ED, Laff SP, Friedman EA. Value of routine dilation and curettage at the time of interval sterilization. Obstet Gynecol 1986:66:763.

Loffer FD, Pent D. Pregnancy after laparoscopic sterilization. Obstet Gynecol 1980;55:643.

Marcil-Gratton N. Sterilization regret among women in metropolitan Montreal. Fam Plann Perspect 1988;520:222.

McCausland A. High rate of ectopic pregnancy following laparoscopic tubal coagulation failures. Am J Obstet Gynecol 1980;136:97.

Mosher WD. Contraceptive practice in the United States, 1982–1988. Fam Plann Perspect 1990; 22:198.

Peterson HB, Greenspan JR, DeStefano F, et al. The impact of laparoscopy on tubal sterilization in United States hospitals, 1970 and 1975–1978. Am J Obstet Gynecol 1981;140:811.

Peterson HB, DeStefano F, Rubin GL, et al. Deaths attributable to tubal sterilization in the United States, 1977–1981. Am J Obstet Gynecol 1983; 146:131.

Peterson HB, Hulka JF, Spielman FJ, et al. Local versus general anesthesia for laparoscopic sterilization: a randomized study. Obstet Gynecol 1987;70:903.

Philliber SG, Philliber WW. Social and psychological perspectives on voluntary sterilization: a review. Stud Fam Plann 1985;16:1.

Rioux JE, Cloutier D. A new bipolar instrument for tubal sterilization. Am J Obstet Gynecol 1974; 119:737.

Rulin MC, Turner JH, Dunworth R, Thompson DS. Post-tubal sterilization syndrome—a misnomer. Am J Obstet Gynecol 1985;151:13.

Rulin MC, Davidson AR, Philliber SG, et al. Changes in menstrual symptoms among sterilized and comparison women: a prospective study. Obstet Gynecol 1989;74:149.

Rulin MC, Davidson AR, Philliber SG, et al. Long-term effect of tubal sterilization on menstrual indices and pelvic pain. Obstet Gynecol 1993; 82:118.

Schwartz D, Wingo PA, Antarsh L, Smith JC. Female sterilization in the United States, 1987. Fam Plann Perspect 1989;21:209.

Shain RN, Miller WB, Holden AEC. Married women's dissatisfaction with tubal sterilization and vasectomy at first-year follow-up: Effects of perceived spousal dominance. Fertil Steril 1986;45:808.

Shain RN, Miller WB, Mitchell GW, et al. Menstrual pattern change one year after sterilization: results of a controlled, prospective study. Fertil Steril 1989;52:192.

Shy KK, Stergachis A, Grothaus LC, et al. Tubal sterilization and risk of subsequent hospital admission for menstrual disorders. Am J Obstet Gynecol 1992;166:1698.

Soderstrom R. Electrical safety in laparoscopy. In: Phillips JM, ed. Endoscopy in Gynecology. Downey, CA: American Association of Gynecologic Laparoscopists, 1978:306.

Soderstrom RM, Levy BS, Engel T. Reducing bipolar sterilization failures. Obstet Gynecol 1989; 74:60.

Spielman FJ, Hulka JF, Ostheimer, et al. Pharmacokinetics and pharmacodynamics of local analgesia for laparoscopic tubal ligations. Am J Obstet Gynecol 1983;146:821.

Stergachis A, Shy KK, Grothaus LC, et al. Tubal sterilization and the long-term risk of hysterectomy. JAMA 1990;264:2893.

Stovall TG, Ling FW, O'Kelly KR, Coleman SA. Gross and histologic examination of tubal ligation failures in a residency training program. Obstet Gynecol 1990;76:461.

Stovall TG, Ling FW, Henry GM, Ryan GM Jr. Method failures of laparoscopic tubal sterilization in a residency training program: A comparison of the tubal ring and spring-loaded clip. J Reprod Med 1991;36:283.

Thompson RE, Wetchler BV, Alexander CD. Infiltration of the mesosalpinx for pain relief after laparoscopic tubal sterilization with Yoon rings. J Reprod Med 1987;32:537.

Uchida H. Uchida tubal sterilization. Am J Obstet Gynecol 1975;121:153.

Vessey M, Huggins G, Lawless M, et al. Tubal sterilization: Findings in a large prospective study. Br J Obstet Gynaecol 1983;90:203.

Wheeless CR Jr. Tubal sterilization. In: Thompson JD, Rock JA, eds. Te Linde's Operative Gynecology, 7th ed. Philadelphia: JB Lippincott, 1992:343.

Wilcox LS, Chu SY, Eaker ED, et al. Risk factors for regret after tubal sterilization: 5 years of follow-up in a prospective study. Fertil Steril 1991; 55:927.

Wilcox LS, Martinez-Schnell B, Peterson HB, et al. Menstrual function after tubal sterilization. Am J Epidemiol 1992;135:1368.

Williams ED, Jones HE, Merril RE. The subsequent course of patients sterilized by tubal ligation. Am J Obstet Gynecol 1951;61:423.

World Health Organization Task Force on Female Sterilization, Special Programme of Research, Development and Research Training in Human Reproduction. Minilaparotomy or laparoscopy for sterilization: A multicenter, multinational randomized study. Am J Obstet Gynecol 1982; 143:645.

Yoon IB, Wheeless CR, King TM. A preliminary report on a new laparoscopic sterilization approach: the silicone rubber band technique. Am J Obstet Gynecol 1974;120:132.

CHAPTER 26

Management of Postpartum Hemorrhage

Despite widespread recognition of the consequences of obstetric hemorrhage and the availability of modern blood-banking techniques, postpartum bleeding remains a major source of maternal morbidity and mortality, both in the United States and in developing countries. Recent surveys suggest that postpartum hemorrhage accounts for about 10 percent of maternal deaths in the United States (Rochat and colleagues, 1988). If ectopic pregnancy is included, hemorrhage is the leading cause of maternal mortality in this country. In developing countries, obstetric hemorrhage is an even more important cause of maternal death (Harrison, 1989; Rosenfield, 1989).

There is no universally accepted definition of postpartum hemorrhage. Traditionally, blood loss exceeding 500 mL following vaginal delivery has been defined as postpartum hemorrhage. In practice, clinical estimate of blood loss is oftentimes inaccurate and usually significantly less than this value. However, several studies using quantitative techniques of blood loss assessment suggest a *mean* blood loss following uncomplicated vaginal delivery of about 500 mL. This compares with a 1000 mL blood loss for cesarean section, 1,400 mL for elective cesarean hysterectomy, and 3000–3500 mL for emergency cesarean hysterectomy (Table 26–1). In view of such data, it is clearly inappropriate to perpetuate the traditional definition. Unfortunately, in the absence of reliable clinical means to quantify postpartum hemorrhage, a better substitute for the older definition is lacking. In a review of 19 studies of postpartum blood loss, Gahres and associates (1962) found the mean loss following vaginal delivery to range from 50 mL with an average of 450 mL for all series. The American College of Obstetricians and Gynecologists (1989) has suggested that postpartum hemorrhage be defined as a fall in hematocrit peripartum of at least 10 percent or hemorrhage requiring blood transfusion. While such definitions may have research applications, in clinical practice the qualitative recognition and prompt response to excessive blood is of greater importance.

Significant postpartum hemorrhage as defined above is estimated to complicate 2–4 percent of vaginal deliveries and 6 percent of cesarean births (Combs and colleagues, 1991a,b; Mee, 1990). In women delivering vaginally, risk factors for postpartum hemorrhage include prolonged third-stage labor, preeclampsia, episiotomy, previous postpartum hemorrhage, twins, arrest of descent, soft tissue lacerations, oxytocin augmented labor, instrumental vaginal deliveries, nulliparity, Asian or Hispanic ethnicity, and obesity (Combs and associates, 1991a). Risks factors for hemorrhage following cesarean delivery include classical uterine incision, amnionitis, preeclampsia, abnormal labor, general anes-

TABLE 26–1. ESTIMATED MEAN BLOOD LOSS FOR OBSTETRIC PROCEDURES

Procedure	Blood Loss
Vaginal delivery	450
Cesarean section	1000
Elective cesarean hysterectomy	1400
Emergency cesarean hysterectomy	3200

From Clark, 1984; Chestnut, 1985; Gahres, 1962; Gilbert, 1987; Newton, 1961; Pritchard, 1962; and all of their colleagues.

thesia, pre- and postterm delivery, and Hispanic ethnicity (Combs and co-workers, 1991b; Gilstrap and associates, 1987).

An intrinsic lack of constrictor reactivity in the uterine arteries of women with various types of postpartum hemorrhage has also been described (Nelson and Suresh, 1992). It is difficult to separate this deficiency from secondary local effects of hypoxia/ischemia in bleeding hypotensive patients.

HYPOVOLEMIC SHOCK

In general, the hypervolemia with accompanying expanded red cell mass of pregnancy allows the parturient to accommodate normal to even excessive blood loss of vaginal delivery without incurring a postpartum hematocrit decline. In one study, the mean postpartum hematocrit decline was 2.6 ± 4.3 percent and one-third of women had no decline, or an actual increase (Combs and associates, 1991a). Women undergoing cesarean section experience a mean drop in hematocrit of 4.0 ± 4.2 percent after equilibration, but about 20 percent had no decline (Combs and colleagues, 1991b). Even with moderate additional blood loss, venous compensatory mechanisms are invoked that allow the woman to tolerate such hemorrhage without hemodynamic compromise. With continued hemorrhage, however, these mechanisms may be overwhelmed with resultant hypotension, decreased tissue perfusion, cellular hypoxia, and death.

Hypovolemic shock evolves through several stages. Early in the course of massive hemorrhage, there are decreases in mean arterial pressure, cardiac output, central venous pressure, pulmonary capillary wedge pressure, and stroke volume. Increases in arterial venous oxygen content difference reflect a relative increase in tissue oxygen extraction, although overall oxygen consumption falls (Bland and colleagues, 1985; Shoemaker, 1973; Shoemaker and associates, 1979a, b).

Blood flow to capillary beds in various organs is controlled by arterioles, which are resistance vessels that in turn are controlled by the central nervous system. At least 70 percent of total blood volume is contained in venules, which are passive resistance vessels controlled by humoral factors. Catecholamine release during hemorrhage causes a generalized increase in venular tone, resulting in an autotransfusion from this capacitance reservoir. These changes are accompanied by compensatory increases in heart rate, systemic and pulmonary vascular resistance, and myocardial contractility. In addition, there is redistribution of cardiac output and blood volume by selective central nervous system mediated arteriolar constriction. This results in diminished perfusion to the kidneys, splanchnic beds, skin, and uterus with relative maintenance of blood flow to the heart, brain, and adrenal glands (Shoemaker and colleagues 1967; Slater and associates, 1973).

As blood volume deficit exceeds 25 percent, such compensatory mechanisms usually are inadequate to maintain cardiac output and blood pressure. At this point, additional small losses of blood result in rapid clinical deterioration. Despite an initial increase in **total** oxygen extraction by maternal tissue, maldistribution of blood flow results in **local** tissue hypoxia and metabolic acidosis, producing a vicious cycle of vasoconstriction, organ ischemia, and cellular death, leading to loss of capillary membrane integrity and additional loss of intravascular volume (Slater and co-workers, 1973). Increased platelet aggregation is also found in hypovolemic shock, resulting in the release of a number of vasoactive mediators, which cause small vessel occlusion and further impairment of microcirculatory perfusion.

MANAGEMENT

Proper management of postpartum bleeding requires a differential diagnosis and a thorough search for the specific cause of the hemorrhage. Individual diagnoses in the differential diagnosis require specific approaches to management, both in terms of technique and in the rapidity with which such techniques are applied. Proper management of intermittent uterine atony, for example, may at times involve a prolonged period of uterine massage, observation, and continued attempts at pharmacologic reversal. On the other hand, postpartum hemorrhage from placenta accreta will generally require prompt hysterectomy. Errors can be made when the clinician manages "postpartum hemorrhage" without attempts to determine specific etiology.

Fortunately, the causes of severe postpartum hemorrhage are few and, in virtually all cases, will involve one of four factors: uterine atony, retained placenta (including placenta accreta and other abnormal attachment), upper or lower genital tract lacerations, and coagulopathy. For the woman experiencing hemorrhage at the time of cesarean, the cause is often immediately apparent. Table 26–2 presents a management scheme for the evaluation of hemorrhage following vaginal delivery.

Atony

Uterine atony is the most frequent cause of serious postpartum hemorrhage. Risks factors for uterine atony include advanced maternal age and parity, the use of oxytocin for labor augmentation, magnesium sulfate infusion, chorioamnionitis, arrest disorders of labor, and uterine overdistention, as in macrosomia or multiple gestation. In the series described by Clark and colleagues (1984), 80 percent of women undergoing hysterectomy for intractable atony had one or more of these risk factors. Recognition of such factors may allow the clinician to anticipate this problem. Bleeding from atony may be rapid and leave little time for indecision, and there must be a well-established management protocol such as that shown in Table 26–3 designed to reverse atony.

TABLE 26–2. EVALUATION OF POSTPARTUM HEMORRHAGE

1. Palpate the uterus to rule out atony.
2. Inspect the lower genital tract for lacerations.
3. Perform manual and/or instrument curettage to remove retained placenta.
4. Consider causes of coagulopathy.
5. Perform exploratory laparotomy.

TABLE 26–3. MANAGEMENT OF UTERINE ATONY

1. Fundal compression
2. Oxytocin 40 units/liter—rapid infusion
3. 15-methyl PGF_2 α 0.25–1.5 mg intramuscular or intramyometrial[a]
4. Uterine artery ligation
5. Internal iliac artery ligation[b]
6. Hysterectomy

[a]Alternatives include PGE_2 α, 20 mg suppository (rectally), methylergonovine 0.2 mg intramuscularly, and other approaches described in text.
[b]Prerequisites: hemodynamic stability, desirous of future childbearing, operator experience.

If atony is encountered following removal of the placenta, firm compression is exerted on the uterus. This may be performed transabdominally; however, in many cases, bimanual compression will be more effective (Fig. 26–1). Even if atony does not promptly resolve, such compression can often provide temporary effective control of hemorrhage while additional pharmacologic manipulation is attempted, blood products are obtained, and assistance is summoned. Simultaneous with such compression, a dilute solution of 40 units of oxytocin in 1000 mL of crystalloid is infused rapidly. Because rapid crystalloid infusion is the first step in management of such women, the intravenous line can be opened fully. The direct intravenous bolus injection of oxytocin may cause a paradoxical hypotensive response, which could be detrimental to an already hypovolemic patient and is, therefore, contraindicated (Secher and colleagues, 1978).

If these initial attempts to reverse uterine atony are unsuccessful, additional pharmacologic maneuvers are indicated. A number of studies have demonstrated the effectiveness of various prostaglandin preparations in reversing uterine atony. In the United States, the most commonly used is 15-methyl-PGF_2 α, 0.25–1.5 mg. It may be administered as an intramuscular injection, or given directly into the myometrium, transabdominally, or transvaginally. Each method has proponents; a critical review of the available data, however, does not suggest a clear general superiority of any route of injection (Bittino and Garite, 1986; Bruce and co-workers, 1982; Hayashi and associates, 1984; Toppozada and colleagues, 1981).

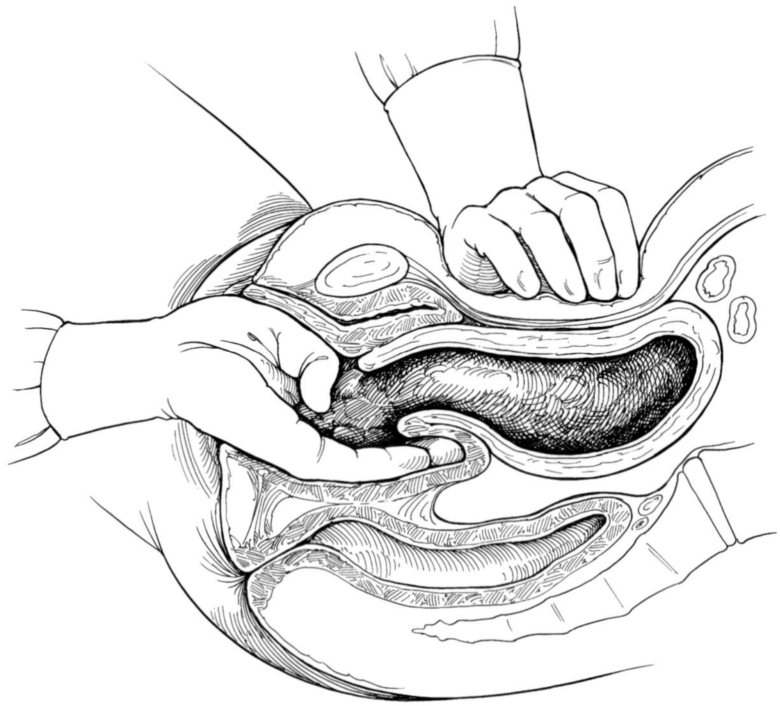

Figure 26–1. Bimanual compression. The vaginal hand should also lift the uterus out of the pelvis and towards the abdominal hand.

If there is hypotension and peripheral muscle perfusion is diminished, direct intrauterine injection may be preferable.

The use of intravaginal or intrarectal 20 mg PGE_2 suppositories has also been described as has the direct intrauterine instillation of a solution of PGE_2 following occlusion of the cervix with a balloon catheter (Hertz and colleagues, 1980; Oleen and Mariano, 1990; Peyser and Kupferminc, 1990). Additional prostaglandin analogues such as PGE_1 have also been used successfully but are not generally available in the United States. The use of uterine packing for atony following failure of pharmacologic therapy is controversial and is discussed in more detail in Chapter 16.

In the past, ergot derivatives, principally methylergonovine in doses of 0.2 mg, were commonly given intramuscularly and repeated as necessary. This drug must be used with caution in a previously hypertensive woman. Intravenous methylergonovine should only be used in cases of life-threatening hemorrhage and is contraindicated if there is underlying hypertension. Although the use of methylergonovine remains acceptable, prostaglandin derivatives have relegated such preparations to less frequent use.

At times, atony may be intermittent and require repeated physical or pharmacologic intervention over a period of several hours. Under such circumstances, the utmost care must be taken both to assess the amount of blood loss and to assure adequate fluid and blood replacement and hemodynamic stability.

If, following the above maneuvers, the patient with atony continues to bleed significantly, exploratory laparotomy is indicated.

Lacerations

Genital tract lacerations are another frequent cause of postpartum hemorrhage. Lower tract injuries with bleeding from the vagina, cervix, or ischiorectal fossa are most commonly encountered following vaginal delivery with an unscarred uterus. Uterine rupture with vaginal and/or intraperitoneal bleeding or a retroperitoneal hematoma is uncommon following vaginal delivery in the absence of a prior uterine scar, but occasionally is encountered in multiparous women.

Following vaginal delivery, careful inspection of the vagina and cervix is mandatory if there is bleeding. Lacerations of the vagina and perineum are addressed as outlined in Chapter 14. Cervical lacerations are common and, in general, are not repaired unless they are bleeding.

Lacerations encountered at the time of cesarean section most commonly result from lateral or inferior extensions of a lower segment transverse incision. Because of the proximity of the uterine vessels to the margins of the standard low transverse incision, such lacerations commonly bleed profusely. In the series by Clark and associates (1984), blood loss associated with hysterectomy for uterine lacerations exceeded that from any other type of hemorrhage. Occasionally, such lacerated vessels may temporarily constrict and retract away from the site of primary laceration. Relaxation following abdominal closure may result in delayed intra- or retroperitoneal bleeding, despite meticulous surgical technique.

The surgical approach to lateral or lateral/inferior lacerations involves awareness of the relative location of uterine vessels, bladder, and ureters (Fig. 26–2). In many cases, the apex of the laceration falls well short of the broad ligament or bladder and repair is straightforward. Hemostasis is achieved with a running locked absorbable suture beginning just beyond the apex of the laceration. When profuse bleeding from the edges of the laceration obscures precise identification of the apex, a running locked absorbable suture placed in one side of the laceration beginning proximally and extending toward the apex may decrease bleeding and facilitate identification of the extent of laceration as the apex is approached (Fig. 26–3).

Two situations may be encountered that call for modification of the standard technique of laceration repair; uterine vessel laceration and extension of the incision into the broad ligament. In the first case, when inspection of the lateral laceration reveals profuse bleeding from the lateral margins, involvement of the uterine veins or artery must be suspected. Occasionally, the transected vessel itself is identified. More commonly, bleeding is profuse and palpation of the myometrium–broad ligament junction confirms extension into the area of the uterine vessels. Hemostatic figure-of-eight sutures may be placed in the area, keeping in mind the proximity of the ureter. Often, however, a single wide suture ligature encompassing the uterine vessels at a point just inferior to the level of the incision may be simpler and result in complete hemostasis. The latter approach is generally preferred to multiple "blind" sutures at the margin of the incision which may give rise to additional bleeding

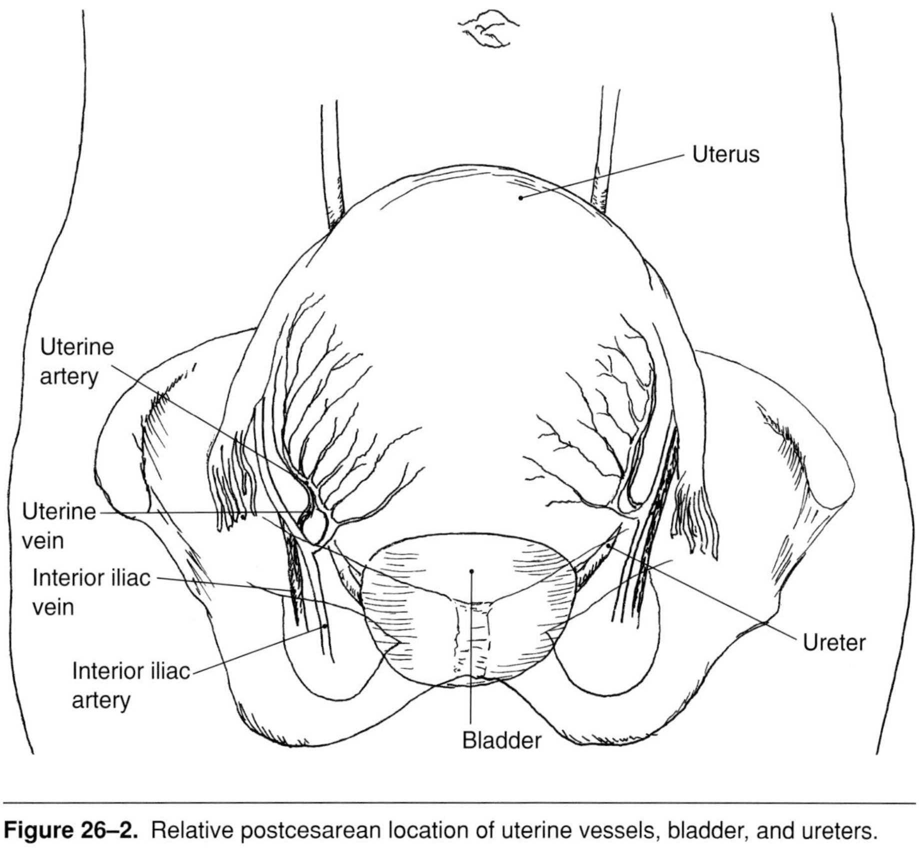

Figure 26–2. Relative postcesarean location of uterine vessels, bladder, and ureters.

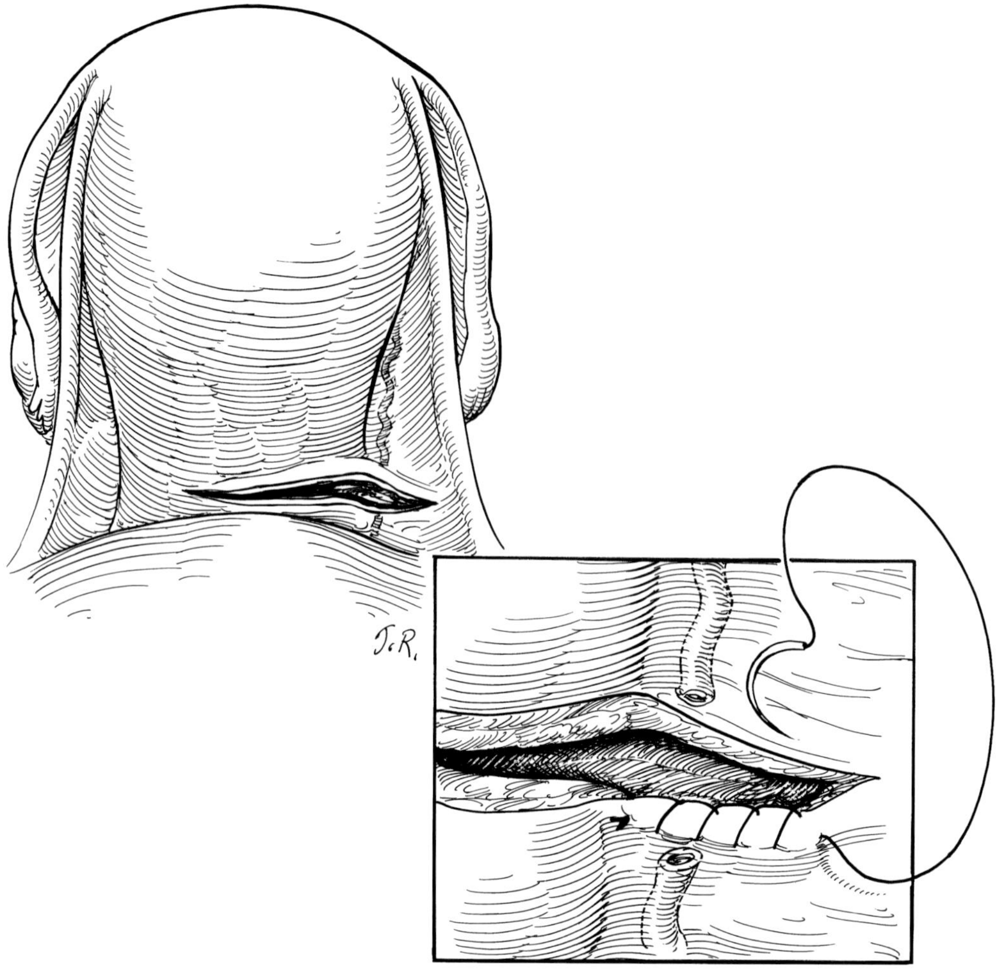

Figure 26–3. Identification of apex of lateral uterine laceration when bleeding obscures direct visualization. A running, locked absorbable suture is placed in one margin and run toward the apex, reducing blood loss and facilitating identification of the laceration apex.

points and endanger the integrity of the ureter (Fig. 26–4).

In the second case, the laceration extends into the broad ligament and the relative position of the laceration apex and ureter will not be clear. This situation is uncommon with direct lateral extensions but is frequently encountered with lateral-inferior extensions. Under such circumstances, it is essential to open the broad ligament and positively identify the course of the ureter prior to suture placement.

Identifying the Ureter

One effective approach is to incise the peritoneum of the broad ligament between the round ligament and fallopian tube. The incision is then extended with Metzenbaum scissors. With experience, the ureter can be readily approached by careful blunt dissection of the areolar tissue in the retroperitoneal space. When difficulty is encountered, the following technique is effective: First, a finger is gently placed into the retroperitoneal space laterally and a pulsating artery identified by palpation. This is usually the external iliac artery. Using a tonsil tip suction device or a small "peanut" sponge stick, the areolar tissue surrounding the external iliac artery is partially cleared and the artery is followed *proximally* to the bifurcation of the common iliac artery. Recalling the course of the ureter on the right or left side (Fig. 26–5), it is now easily identified as it crosses the major arteries. Observation of peristalsis, either spontaneous or induced by gentle pressure with an

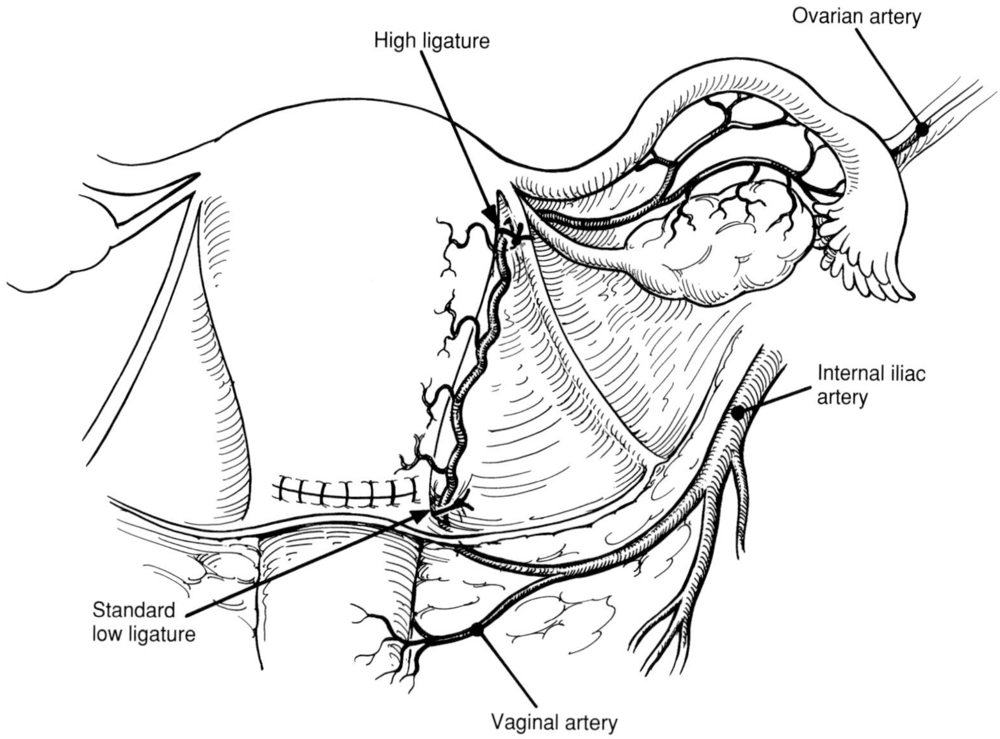

Figure 26–4. Uterine artery ligation performed at approximate level of the utero-ovarian ligament/uterine junction superiorly and just below the uterine incision inferiorly.

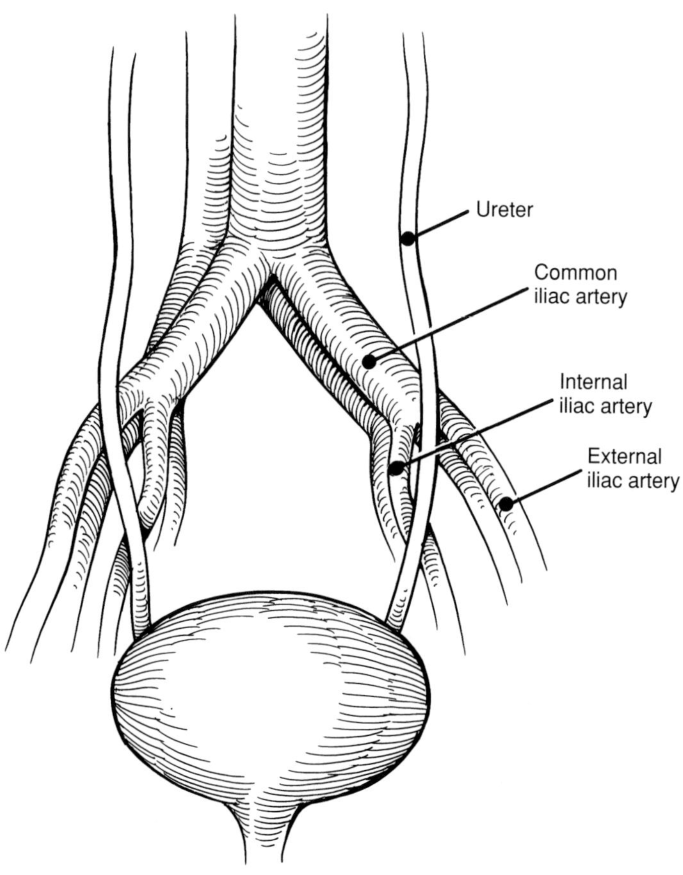

Figure 26–5. Course of ureter at bifurcation of common iliac arteries.

instrument, confirms the identity of the ureter. Following identification, the course of the ureter may be traced distally to the area of laceration and appropriate hemostatic sutures can be placed following direct ureteral visualization in this area. This procedure is generally bloodless; however, occasionally small bleeding vessels may be encountered prior to closure of the retroperitoneal space. Use of a lap sponge and pressure or small hemostatic clips is invaluable in obtaining hemostasis under these circumstances and is often preferable to suture placement or extensive cautery. After hemostasis has been achieved, the peritoneum and broad ligament is closed with a running suture of fine absorbable material.

If the integrity of the ureter is in doubt after hemostasis has been achieved, several approaches are possible. The broad ligament may be opened and the course of the ureter directly identified as above. If the issue remains in doubt, the bladder may be opened longitudinally from an extraperitoneal approach (Fig. 26–6), and the trigone identified. Indigo carmine dye, 5–10 mL injected intravenously, should appear within minutes from both ureteral orifices. If ureteral integrity remains in question, an 8 French catheter may be threaded in a retrograde manner into the ureter under direct observation using a right-angle clamp. If injury is identified, intraoperative urologic consultation will allow the outcome to be optimized. It must be emphasized that there may be ureteral injury despite meticulous surgical technique, often as a result of an unexpected anatomic variation or distortion in the course of the ureter.

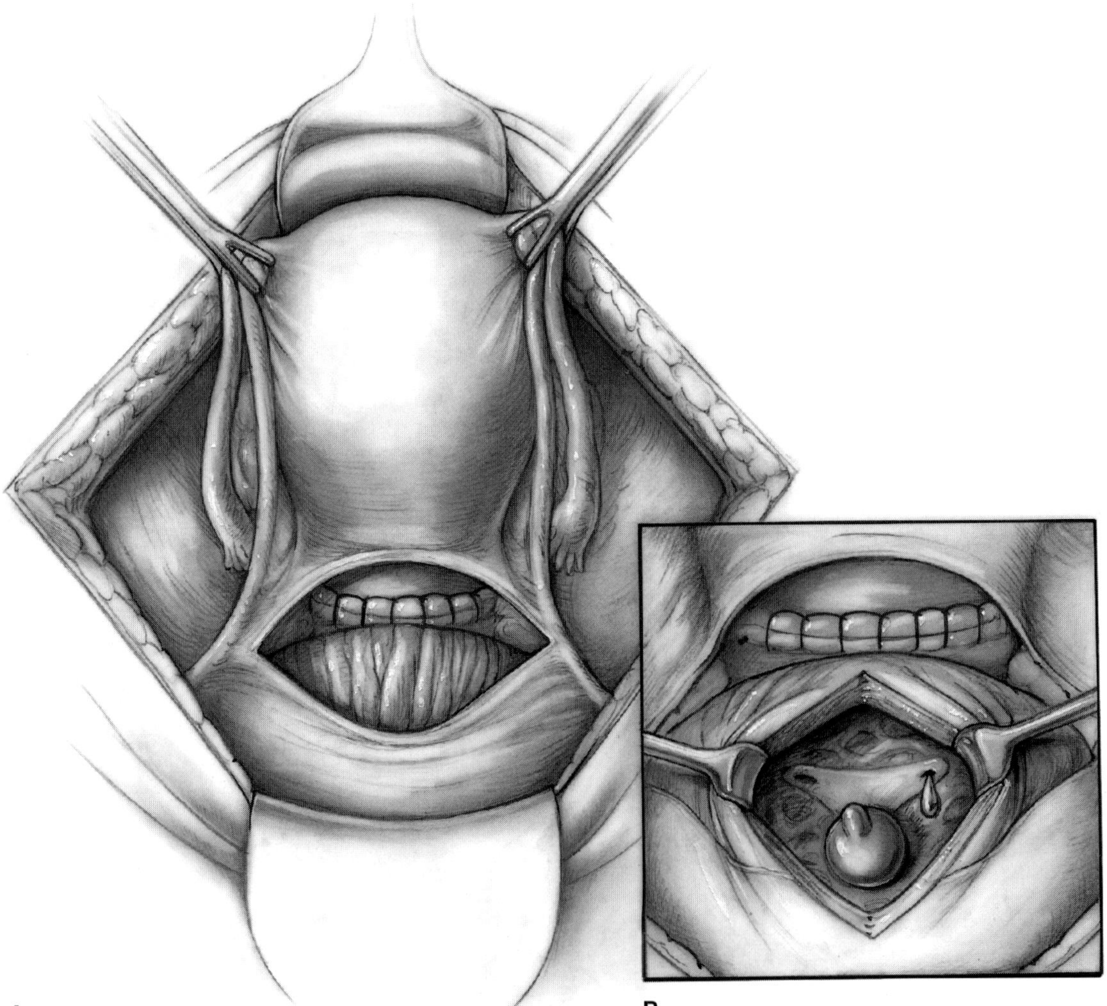

A B

Figure 26–6. A. The bladder is opened extraperitoneally. **B.** The trigone is identified.

Retained Placenta

Following delivery of the infant, delivery of the placenta may be expected. If spontaneous delivery is delayed, manual extraction may be indicated. No data exist to document an ideal duration of the third stage of labor prior to a manual removal; however, in a recent review Combs and Laros (1991) found no increase in hemorrhage until the third stage exceeded 30 minutes.

Following its delivery, the placenta is carefully inspected for integrity of the cotyledons. If there is a suggestion of retained fragments, then manual exploration of the uterine cavity is undertaken. This may be facilitated by wrapping a 4 × 4-inch gauze around one or two fingers. If retained fragments cannot be removed in this manner, curettage using appropriate anesthesia is undertaken with a blunt postpartum curette. When, despite such maneuvers, pieces of placenta remain adherent and are associated with hemorrhage, placenta accreta is diagnosed clinically and exploratory laparotomy is indicated.

Placenta accreta is the second most common indication for emergency hysterectomy for obstetric hemorrhage (Clark and colleagues, 1984). As shown in Figure 26–7, the incidence appears to be increasing. This phenomenon is principally owing to two factors. First, low-transverse cesarean section appears to increase the risk of subsequent placenta previa, although the mechanism of this is not known. Second, there is the well-documented association of placenta accreta with placenta previa and previous cesarean delivery, both of which have increased. In recent reviews of the subject, up to a fourth of women undergoing cesarean for placenta previa in the presence of one or more scars subsequently underwent cesarean hysterectomy for placenta accreta (Clark and associates, 1985a; Weckstein and co-workers, 1987). This risk appears to increase directly with the number of previous uterine incisions. Other risk factors are age and parity.

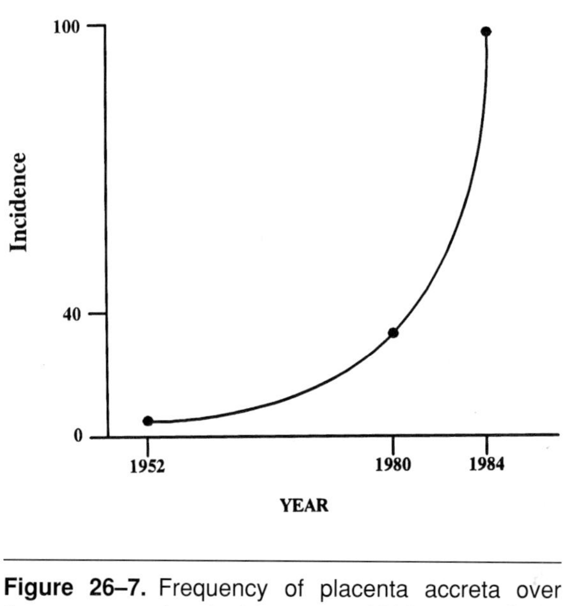

Figure 26–7. Frequency of placenta accreta over time, expressed as incidence per 1000 cases of placenta previa.

Several case reports have suggested that placenta accreta may occasionally be identified prenatally by the use of high-resolution real-time sonography and magnetic resonance imaging (Cox and associates, 1988; Rosemond and Kepple, 1992; Thorp and colleagues, 1991). Unfortunately, false positive and negative rates are high. Further, the prospective utility of such an approach has never been demonstrated nor has clinical benefit been observed compared with the recognition of clinical risk factors alone.

Some authors have reported a relatively high mortality for women with placenta accreta treated by procedures other than hysterectomy. This conclusion, however, has not been borne out by more recent data. In one review, 45 percent of women with clinical placenta accreta were treated with measures other than hysterectomy with no maternal mortality (Clark and co-workers, 1985a). When the accreta is focal, simple excision of the site of trophoblast invasion, oversewing the area with absorbable figure-of-eight sutures, or sharp curettage under direct visualization after hysterotomy may be effective. Nevertheless, except in cases of focal accreta in the hemodynamically stable young woman for whom future childbearing is a major concern, hysterectomy appears to remain the procedure of choice and should be initiated as soon as the diagnosis of placenta accreta is made.

When the placenta invades through the myometrium and uterine wall, placenta percreta is said to exist. At times, the invasion may involve the wall of the bladder. Surgical approaches to this situation are complex and may necessitate urologic consultation (Mechan and colleagues, 1989). There are case reports that describe oversewing and conservative management of placenta percreta diagnosed in early pregnancy at time of exploratory laparotomy performed for other indications (Cox and associates, 1988). Cho and co-workers (1991) also reported a series of women with placenta accreta managed conservatively by placing a series of deep interrupted through and through sutures in a circular pattern surrounding the bleeding implantation site following placental removal.

Dilutional Coagulopathy

Although fresh whole blood is theoretically ideal for the management of serious hemmorhage, in practice it is rarely available. Thus, crystalloid solution and packed red blood cells are the mainstays of volume replacement in patients with obstetric hemorrhage. When blood loss is massive, however, such replacement may result in a depletion of platelets and soluble clotting factors leading to a "dilutional" coagulopathy, impairing hemostasis and further contributing to blood loss. The most frequent coagulation defect found in patients who have experienced blood loss and multiple transfusions is thrombocytopenia (Wilson and associates, 1971). As shown in Table 26–4, because stored whole blood is deficient in factors V, VIII, XI, and platelets, and all soluble clotting factors are absent from packed red blood cells, severe hemorrhage without factor replacement may also lead to a decrease in fibrinogen and prolongation of the prothrombin and partial thromboplastin times. In some cases, frank disseminated intravascular coagulopathy may accompany shock and confuse the distinction between dilutional and consumptive coagulopathy. Fortunately, in most situations encountered in obstetrics, treatment of both is the same.

Although various algorithms have been proposed to guide the replacement of platelets and clotting factors according to the volume of blood loss, patient variability is great. Such component replacement is rarely necessary with the acute replacement of 8–10 units of packed red blood cells or less. However, when blood loss exceeds this amount, consideration should be given to laboratory evaluation of platelet count and fibrinogen levels with replacement predicated on the laboratory values or clinical evidence of bleeding from a coagulopathy.

In the bleeding patient, the platelet count should be kept above 50,000/mL with the infusion of platelet concentrates. A fibrinogen level of less than 100 mg/dL or sufficiently prolonged prothrombin or partial thromboplastin times in a bleeding patient is an indication for fresh frozen plasma administration in doses of 10–15 mL/kg. Following platelet or factor replacement, levels should be followed closely until the patient is stable.

SURGICAL TECHNIQUES

Uterine Artery Ligation

Surgical ligation of the uterine artery is an important part of the obstetrician's arma-

TABLE 26–4. BLOOD PRODUCTS

Product	Volume	Content	Shelf Life
Whole blood	450 mL	All blood components	35 days No granulocytes or platelets after 24 hours. Decreased but functionally adequate levels of factors V and VIII for 1–2 weeks.
Packed red blood cells	250 mL	Red cells	35 days
Fresh frozen plasma	200–250 mL	All stable and labile clotting factors	1 year
Cryoprecipitate	50 mL	Factors V, VIII:c, VIII:von Willebrand, XIII, fibronectin fibrinogen	1 year
Platelets	50 mL (per pack)	Platelets	5 days

mentarium. The ability to properly perform this procedure may reduce blood loss associated with uterine rupture or lacerations and may, under certain circumstances, permit uterine conservation. In a review of over 200 women undergoing bilateral uterine artery ligation for post-cesarean section hemorrhage, O'Leary (1986) found this procedure potentially helpful in 95 percent of cases. Because this was not a controlled series, the actual efficacy of uterine artery ligation in avoiding hysterectomy is not known. Uterine atony was the major indication for vessel ligation. The incidence of significant complications was approximately 1 percent and appeared to be associated with operator inexperience. No urologic injury was observed. Given the low rate of complications, uterine artery ligation is a logical option for some cases of hemorrhage following failure of more conservative therapy.

Technique

Uterine artery ligation is performed using a large tapered needle and No. 0 or No. 1 absorbable suture (Fig. 26–4). The uterus and tubes are elevated, exposing and flattening the broad ligament. The ligature is placed around the ascending uterine artery and accompanying veins at a level just below the site of the standard low-transverse uterine incision. The needle is initially introduced into the myometrium from anterior to posterior approximately 2 cm medial to the lateral margin of the uterus. The needle is removed from the posterior myometrium and redirected from posterior to anterior through an avascular space in the broad ligament. The suture is then securely tied. Depending on the surgeon's position at the operating table, uterine artery ligation may be more easily performed by first going anteriorly through an avascular space in the broad ligament and then posteriorly through the myometrium.

Occasionally, there are anastomoses between branches of the ovarian and uterine arteries in the area of the utero-ovarian ligament. In order to prevent collateral backflow to the ligated uterine artery from these anastomoses, a second ligature is sometimes useful. This ligature is placed at the utero-ovarian ligament/uterine junction. In placing this second ligature, care must be taken to avoid compromising the interstitial portion of the fallopian tube.

Internal Iliac (Hypogastric) Artery Ligation

In the United States, internal iliac artery ligation was first described in the late nineteenth century by Kelly, who used it to control bleeding associated with carcinoma of the cervix. Subsequently, the procedure has been most commonly used in the control of postpartum hemorrhage (Clark and colleagues, 1985b; Evans and McShane, 1985). The anatomy of the internal iliac artery with its anterior and posterior division is detailed in Figure 26–8. Branches of the anterior division provide the major blood supply to organs of the female pelvis. Reports of term pregnancy after bilateral ligation of internal iliac, uterine, and ovarian arteries attest to the abundant collateral blood supply of the female reproductive tract (Mengert and colleagues, 1969).

Unilateral internal iliac artery ligation reduces distal ipsilateral blood flow by only half. A more important clinical effect is an 85 percent diminution of pulse pressure distal to the ligation, thus changing the hemodynamics of the distal arterial tree to one more resembling those of a venous system and amenable to hemostasis via simple clot formation (Burchell, 1968).

There are several uncontrolled reports that have examined the potential efficacy of bilateral internal iliac artery ligation to control obstetric hemorrhage and avoid hysterectomy (Clark and colleagues, 1985b; Evans and McShane, 1985). Reported success rates have ranged from 25 to 60 percent. Data from recent series indicate that ligation is successful in avoiding hysterectomy in approximately half of the cases associated with uterine atony and placenta accreta. Ligation may be far less successful when a uterine or broad ligament laceration is encountered, although occasional efficacy may be seen in these women as well. In some cases, identification and ligation of the lacerated vessels is facilitated by first performing internal iliac artery ligation.

In a series of 19 women undergoing bilateral internal iliac artery ligation for control of otherwise intractable obstetric hemorrhage, there was an increased incidence of ureteral injury and cardiac arrest from blood loss in women undergoing unsuccessful ligation followed by hysterectomy compared with those undergoing primary hysterectomy without prior vessel ligation. However, ureteral in-

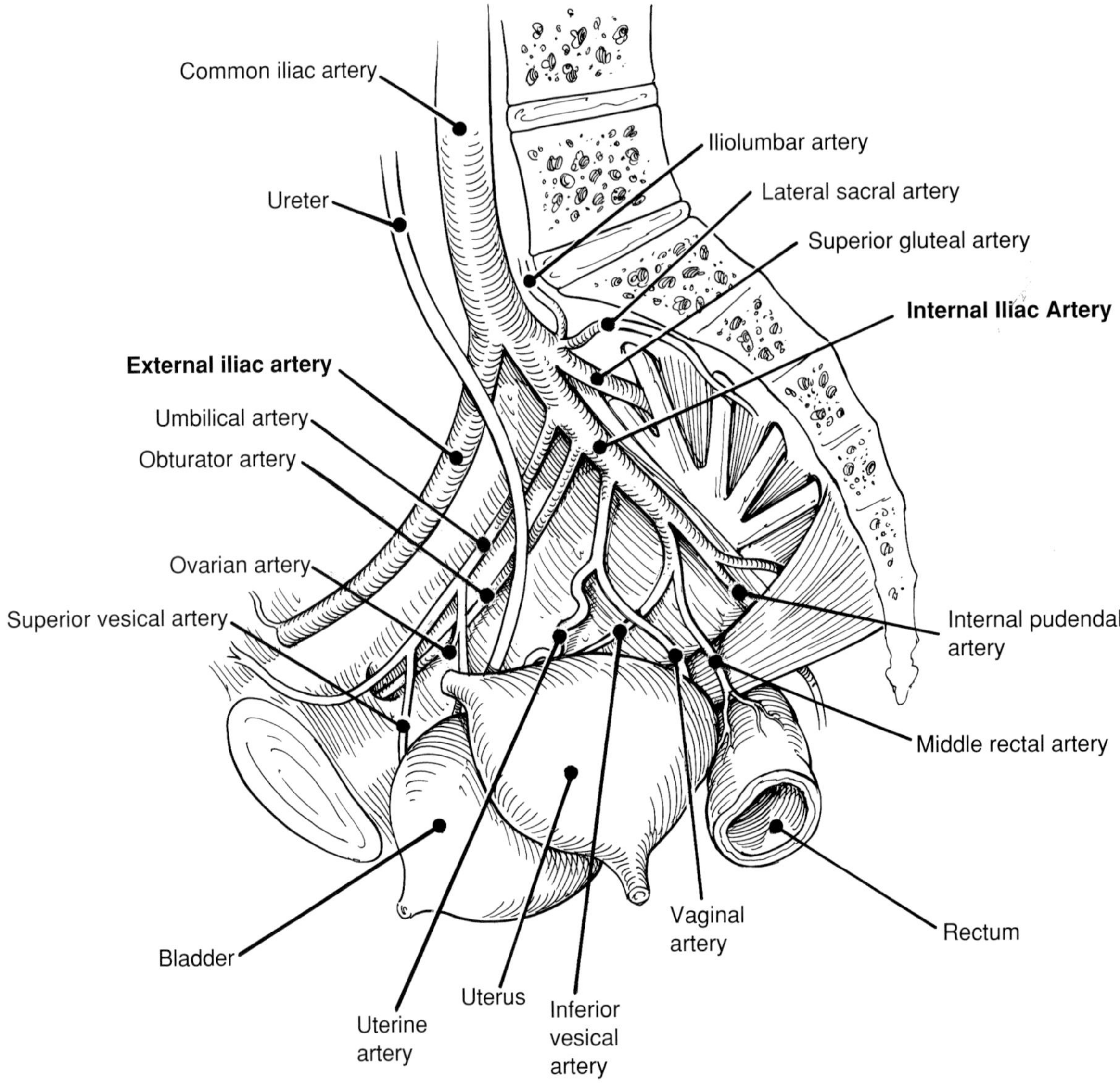

Figure 26–8. The internal iliac (hypogastric) artery.

juries appear to have been surgically related to the hysterectomy rather than to artery ligation. The authors concluded that the prolonged operative time and extensive blood loss after unsuccessful artery ligation may have led to less meticulous surgical technique during the subsequent hysterectomy, resulting in ureteral injury (Clark and colleagues, 1985b). Thus, complications associated with unsuccessful internal iliac artery ligation may be related to delay in hysterectomy rather than with the surgical procedure itself.

Although extensive collateral circulation generally prevents ischemic complications, central pelvic ischemia, breakdown of the perineal skin and episiotomy site, and post-ischemic lower motor neuron damage with weakness of the lower extremities have been reported as sequelae of internal iliac artery occlusion (Braf and Knootz, 1979; Greenwood and associates, 1987). Although such complications are rare, the possibility of atypical collateral circulation must be kept in mind when evaluating the appropriateness of this procedure.

Technique

The retroperitoneal space is entered as shown in Figure 26-9A,B. This may be done either anteriorly between the round and infundibulopelvic ligaments or posteriorly, entering the broad ligament medial to the infundibulopelvic ligament and lateral to the external

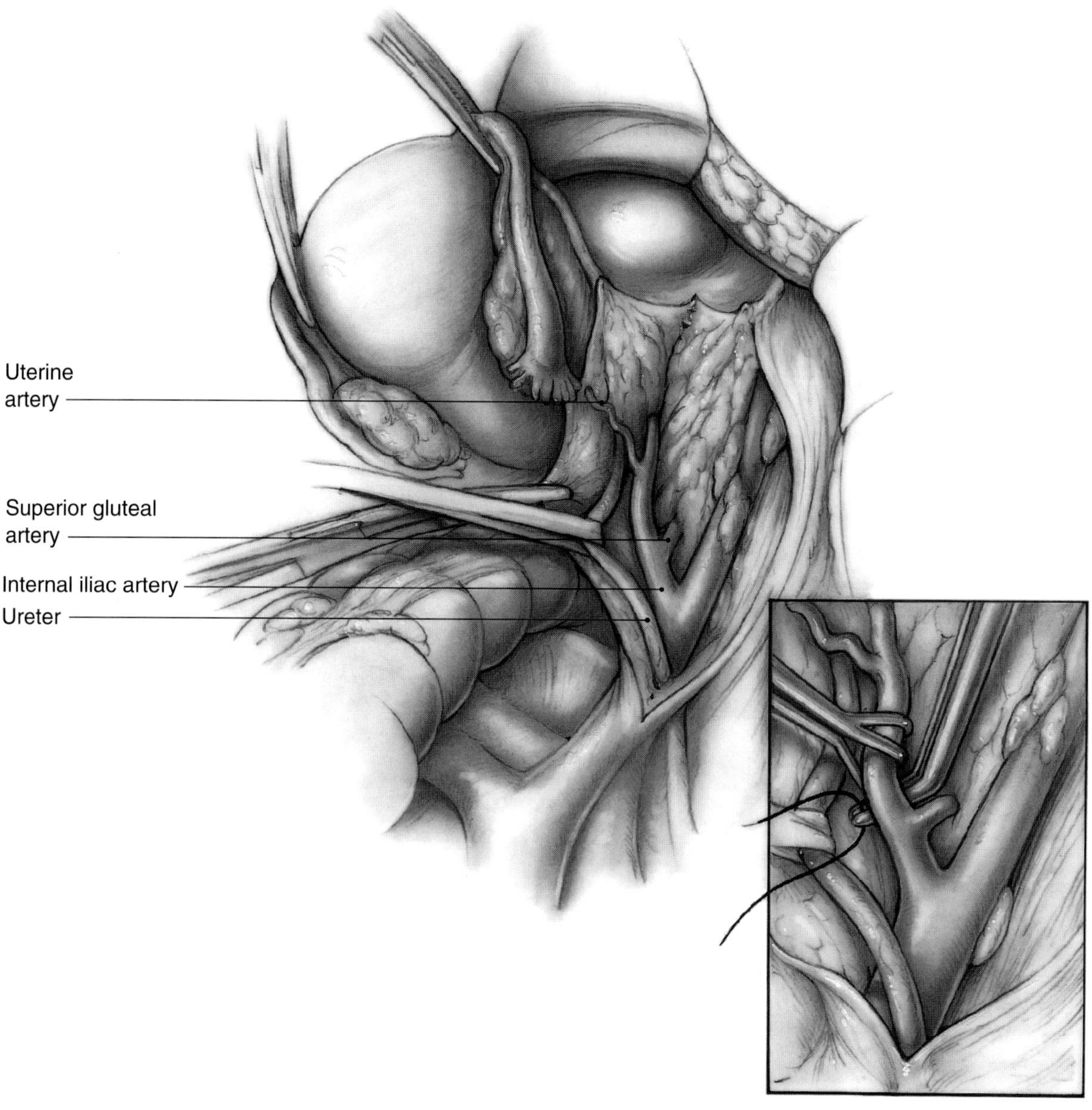

Figure 26–9. A. The retroperitoneal space has been opened, the ureter retracted medially, and the hypogastric artery exposed. **B.** The hypogastric artery is elevated with a large Babcock clamp and the suture is passed beneath the artery.

iliac artery. Next, the ureter is identified and retracted medially. The external iliac artery is located and its course traced proximally to the bifurcation of the common iliac artery. At the bifurcation, the internal iliac artery is found and traced distally. A tonsil tip sucker or "peanut" sponge stick is helpful in this blunt dissection. The areolar tissue surrounding the artery is carefully dissected to free it from the adventicia for a distance of 2–3 cm from the bifurcation. This will result in suture placement distal to the posterior division of the artery. Placement at this point allows the surgeon to avoid distal reversal of blood flow through iliolumbar–lumbar and lateral sacral–middle sacral anastomoses. Ischemic complications related to tissues supplied by branches of the posterior division of the artery may also be minimized in this way. A right-angle clamp is passed beneath the artery. The artery is then double-ligated with nonabsorbable suture, No. 0 or No. 1. The artery is not divided. The retroperitoneal space is then closed with a fine absorbable suture.

Four common errors in surgical technique must be avoided when performing internal iliac artery ligation. The first is misidentification and ligation of the external iliac artery. This is a serious complication, which, if unrecognized and uncorrected, will lead to ischemia and possible loss of the leg. Careful dissection and identification of anatomic landmarks including both external and internal iliac arteries and palpation of femoral pulses following internal iliac artery ligation are essential.

A second potential complication involves laceration of the internal or external iliac veins. These thin-walled structures lie immediately adjacent to the arteries and may be easily lacerated if retroperitoneal dissection has been too vigorous or during passage of the right-angle clamp beneath the internal iliac artery. Such lacerations are often difficult to repair and may result in massive hemorrhage. Passage of the right-angle clamp from lateral to medial and medial to lateral have both been advocated as superior techniques in avoiding laceration of the veins. No data exists to support either position. Perhaps more important is keeping the tip of the clamp against the artery when passed beneath it, and elevation of the artery with a large Babcock clamp, as shown in Figure 26–9B.

A third serious complication is ureteral injury. This may be avoided by properly identifying the ureter and retracting it immediately upon entering the retroperitoneal space.

Finally, a retroperitoneal hematoma may result if hemostasis in the retroperitoneal space has been inadequate or there is a coagulopathy. Meticulous surgical technique is essential to avoid this complication. Small hemostatic clips, manual pressure with a lap sponge, or topical application of thrombin or microfibrillar collagen are extremely helpful in controlling small bleeding vessels within the retroperitoneal space and are often superior to suture ligatures or extensive cautery.

The recent development of radiologic techniques for arterial embolization and the dramatic effectiveness of synthetic prostaglandin preparations in cases of uterine atony have combined to make internal iliac artery ligation an infrequently employed technique. Further, with the trend in the United State toward limitation of family size, "heroic" measures directed at uterine conservation are less commonly indicated. Few individuals currently completing training programs in the United States are sufficiently facile in this operation to complete it safely under emergency conditions. Thus, while ligation may be effective in select cases, its performance is never mandated by standard of care and is, in fact, infrequently justified. The risk/benefit ratio of this procedure in cases of obstetric hemorrhage is probably acceptable only if three criteria are met: the woman must be hemodynamically stable, future childbearing must be an overwhelming concern for the patient, and an experienced operator must be available.

Transvaginal Pressure Pack

In cases of placenta percreta or abdominal pregnancy, bleeding may be diffuse and difficult to control with either suture placement or electrocautery. Following postpartum hysterectomy, similar diffuse bleeding may be encountered, especially when the course is further complicated by dilutional coagulopathy. Under these circumstances, a vaginal pressure pack may provide lifesaving hemostasis. The use of a pelvic pressure pack was originally described by Logothetopulos in 1926. Several reports since that time have described its successful use for obstetric pelvic hemorrhage (Parenta and associates, 1962; Robie and colleagues, 1990). One technique of pressure pack construction was recently described by Hallek and co-workers (1991): A sterile plastic x-ray cassette bag or plastic instrument tray cover is filled with 8 rolls of 4–5-inch gauze tied end-to-end. Alternately, several cloth laparotomy sponges may be tied together. The gauze- or cloth-filled bag is then placed in the pelvis with the opening of the bag and protruding end of the packing material extending through the vaginal cuff or a separate cul-de-sac incision, thus creating a mushroom-shaped pack (Fig. 26–10). The protruding "stalk" is then tied with intravenous tubing attached directly to a 1-liter bag of solution which is hung over the foot of the bed. The pack is removed 24–48 hours later, after the woman is clinically stable.

Angiographic Embolization

Angiographic embolization techniques may in select cases provide an alternative to exploratory laparotomy or hypogastric artery ligation for the control of postpartum hemorrhage. This technique has been described in the control of postpartum vaginal wall hematomas, abdominal pregnancy, retroperi-

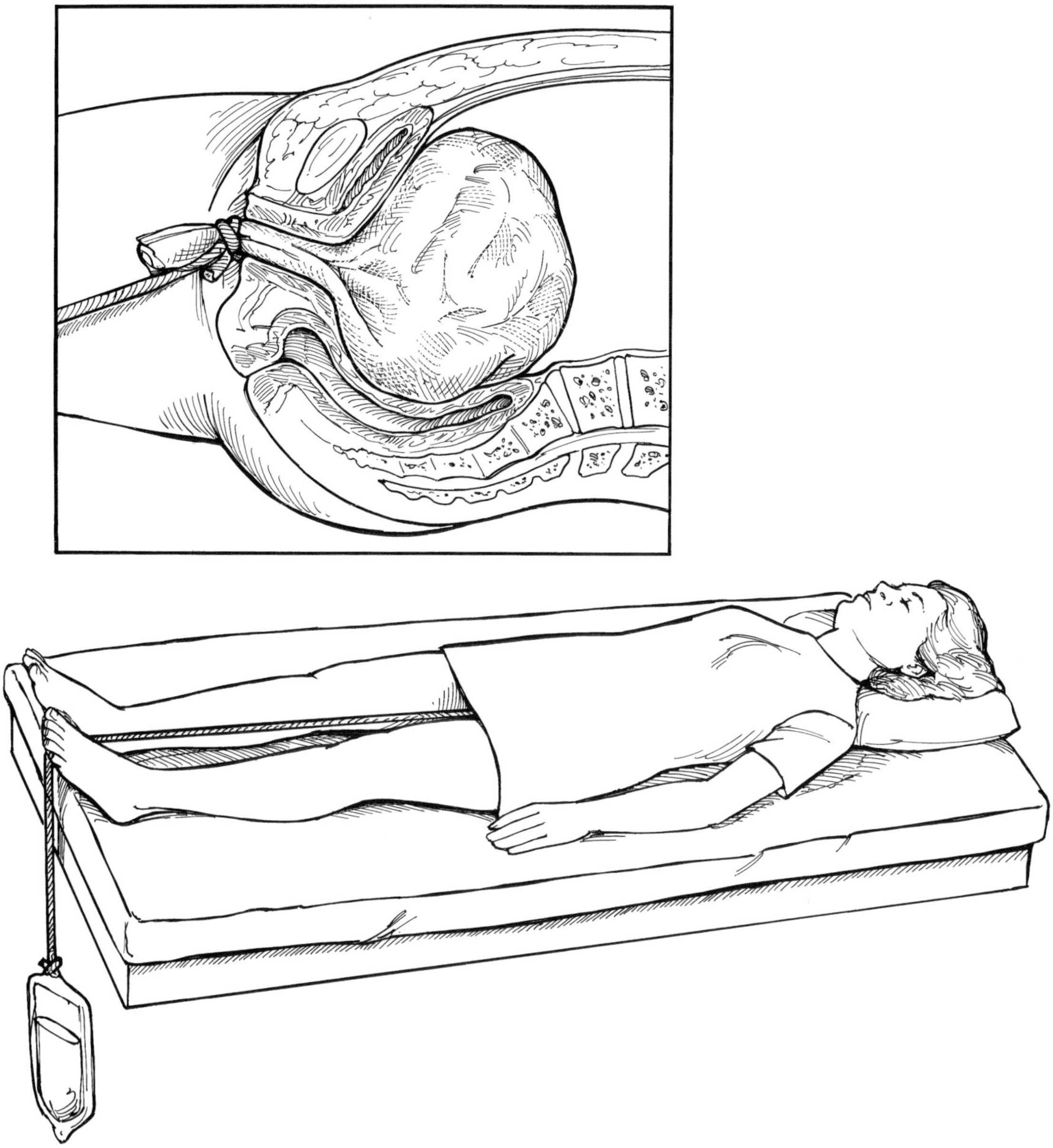

Figure 26–10. Transvaginal pressure pack.

toneal hematomas, and miscellaneous types of postpartum and postcesarean hysterectomy hemorrhage (Chin, 1989; Gilbert, 1992; Greenwood, 1987; Jander, 1980; Kivokoski, 1988; Smith, 1985; Yamashita, 1991; and their many colleagues). It is also used in the control of hemorrhage associated with gynecologic malignancies (Greenwood and associates, 1987).

Using a percutaneous approach under local anesthesia, an aortogram is performed to identify the anatomy of the pelvic vessels as well as specific bleeding sites. The internal iliac artery is then entered under fluoroscopy and a specific bleeding site identified by the appearance of a "blush" or pooling of contrast media in an extravascular site (Fig. 26–11). The bleeding vessel is then selectively catheterized and occluded. Hemostasis may be documented by fluoroscopy. Multiple vessels including bleeding collaterals may be occluded in this manner. Alternately, the anterior division of the hypogastric artery itself may be embolized.

A variety of agents are available for angiographic embolization. The choice is dependent upon the size of the vessel to be occluded and whether short-term or permanent occlusion is

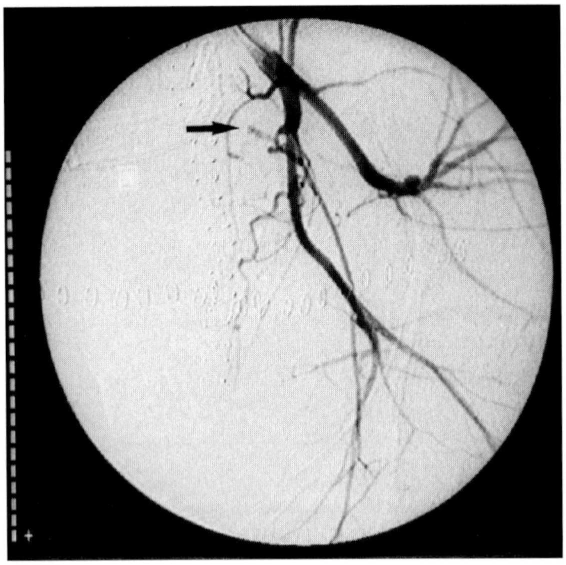

A

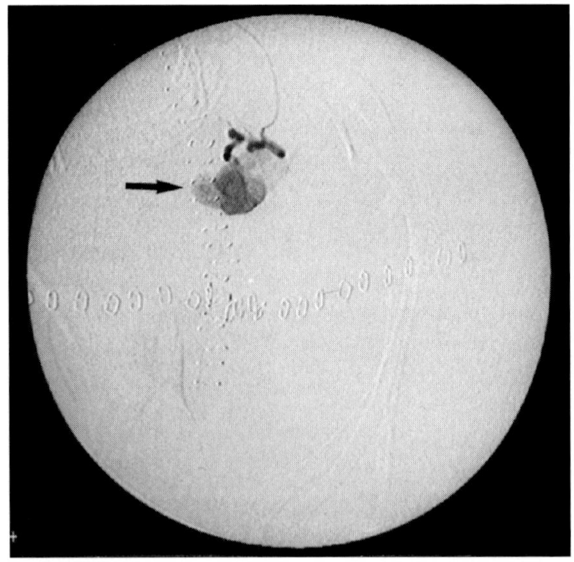

B

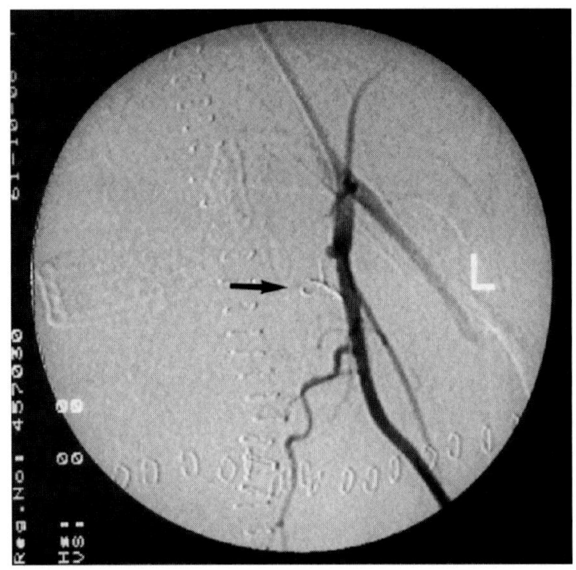

C

Figure 26–11. A. Arteriogram of internal iliac artery, anterior and posterior divisions. Note faint dye blush in region of middle hemmorhoidal branch (arrow). **B.** More selective catheterization of middle hemmorhoidal branch demonstrating extravasation of dye (arrow). **C.** Post embolization film demonstrating coil placement (arrow) and absence of distal flow.

desired. Gianturco wire coils, consisting of a metal coil with numerous attached Dacron fibers to promote thrombus function are available in various sizes and provide permanent occlusion of large vessels. More commonly, small particles of gelfoam are used to promote short-term (10–30 day) occlusion of small bleeding arterial branches. Although surgical internal iliac artery ligation acts principally via a general reduction in pulse pressure, angiographic embolization allows direct occlusion of one or more specific bleeding vessels. This technique also avoids the need for general or conduction anesthesia and the morbidity inherent in surgical exploration.

The primary disadvantage of angiographic technique involves the usual need to transfer a bleeding patient to the radiology suite. Thus, such techniques are not useful in settings of rapid life-threatening hemorrhage, where a direct surgical approach is mandated. Other complications occasionally reported include transient fever and, depending upon the vessel embolized, ischemia of distal tissues (Braf and Knootz, 1979; Greenwood and colleagues, 1987).

SUMMARY

Despite the availability of modern blood banking techniques and the recent introduction of potent agents to combat uterine atony, postpartum hemorrhage remains a significant cause of maternal morbidity and morality throughout the world. The differential diagnosis for postpartum hemorrhage is limited, and the procedures for handling most cases are well-established. However, because postpartum hemorrhage can occur rapidly, and its management often involves difficult decisions regarding preservation of fertility, managing these patients requires caution, judgment, and attention to detail. A critical analysis of the cause of the bleeding, prompt attention to blood and component replacement when necessary, and an aggressive approach to hemostasis will, in most cases, allow an optimal outcome.

REFERENCES

The American College of Obstetricians and Gynecologists. Quality assurance in obstetrics and gynecology. Washington, DC: American College of Obstetricians and Gynecologists, 1989.

Bland RD, Shoemaker WC, Abraham E, Cobo JC. Hemodynamic and oxygen transport patterns in surviving and nonsurviving postoperative patients. Crit Care Med 1985; 13:85.

Braf ZF, Knootz WW Jr. Gangrene of bladder. Complication of hypogastric artery embolization. Urology 1979; 9:670.

Bruce SL, Paul RH, Van Dorsten JP. Control of postpartum uterine atony by intramyometrial prostaglandin. Obstet Gynecol 1982; 59:47S.

Burchell RC. Physiology of internal iliac artery ligation. J Obstet Gynaecol Br Commonw 1968; 75:642.

Buttino L Jr, Garite TJ. The use of 15-methyl F_2 alpha prostaglandin (Prostin 15M) for the control of postpartum hemorrhage. Am J Perinatol 1986; 3:241.

Chestnut DH, Eden RD, Gall SA, Parker RT. Peripartum hysterectomy: a review of cesarean and postpartum hysterectomy. Obstet Gynecol 1985; 65:365.

Chin HG, Scott DR, Resnik R, et al. Angiographic embolization of intractable puerperal hematomas. Am J Obstet Gynecol 1989; 160:434.

Cho JY, Kim SJ, Cha KY, et al. Interrupted circular suture: bleeding control during cesarean delivery in placenta previa accreta. Obstet Gynecol 1991; 78:876.

Clark SL, Koonings P, Phelan JP. Placenta accreta and previous cesarean section. Obstet Gynecol 1985a; 66:89.

Clark SL, Phelan JP, Yeh S-Y, Paul RH. Hypogastric artery ligation for obstetric hemorrhage. Obstet Gynecol 1985b; 66:353.

Clark SL, Yeh S-Y, Phelan JP, et al. Emergency hysterectomy for the control of obstetric hemorrhage. Obstet Gynecol 1984; 64:376.

Combs CA, Laros RK Jr. Prolonged third stage of labor: morbidity and risk factors. Obstet Gynecol 1991; 77:863.

Combs CA, Murphy EL, Laros RK Jr. Factors associated with postpartum hemorrhage with vaginal birth. Obstet Gynecol 1991a; 77:69.

Combs CA, Murphy EL, Laros RK Jr. Factors associated with hemorrhage in cesarean deliveries. Obstet Gynecol 1991b; 77:77.

Cox SM, Carpenter RJ, Cotton DB. Placenta percreta: ultrasound diagnosis and conservative surgical management. Obstet Gynecol 1988; 71:454.

Evans S, McShane P. The efficacy of internal iliac artery ligation in obstetric hemorrhage. Surg Gynecol Obstet 1985; 160:250.

Gahres EE, Albert SN, Dodek SM. Intrapartum blood loss measured with Cr^{51}-tagged erythrocytes. Obstet Gynecol 1962; 19:455.

Gilbert WM, Moore TR, Resnik R, et al. Angiographic embolization in the management of hemorrhage complications of pregnancy. Am J Obstet Gynecol 1992; 166:493.

Gilbert L, Porter W, Brown VA. Postpartum hemorrhage: a continuing problem. Br J Obstet Gynaecol 1987; 94:67.

Gilstrap LC, Hauth JC, Hankins GDV, Patterson AR. Effect of type of anesthesia on blood loss at cesarean section. Obstet Gynecol 1987; 69:328.

Greenwood LH, Glickman MG, Schwartz PE, et al. Obstetric and nonmalignant gynecologic bleeding: treatment with angiographic embolization. Radiology 1987; 164:155.

Hallek M, Dildy GA, Hurley TJ, Moise KJ. Transvaginal pressure pack for life-threatening pelvic hemorrhage secondary to placenta accreta. Obstet Gynecol 1991; 78:938.

Harrison KA. Maternal mortality in developing countries. Br J Obstet Gynaecol 1989; 96:1.

Hayashi RH, Castillo MS, Noah ML. Management of severe postpartum hemorrhage with a prostaglandin F_2 alpha analogue. Obstet Gynecol 1984; 63:806.

Hertz RH, Sokol RJ, Dierker LJ. Treatment of postpartum uterine atony with prostaglandin E_2 vaginal suppositories. Obstet Gynecol 1980; 56:129.

Hurley TJ, Moise KJ Jr. Transvaginal pressure pack for life-threatening pelvic hemorrhage secondary to placenta accreta. Obstet Gynecol 1991; 78:938.

Jander HP, Russinovich NAE. Transcatheter gelfoam embolization in abdomina, retroperitoneal, and pelvic hemorrhage. Radiology 1980; 136:337.

Kivokoski AI, Martin C, Weyman P, et al. Angiographic arterial embolization to control hemorrhage in abdominal pregnancy: a case report. Obstet Gynecol 1988; 71:456.

Logothetopulos K. Eine absolut sichere blutstillungsmethode bei vaginalen und abdominalen gynakologischen operationen. Zentralbl Gynaekol 1926; 50:3202.

Mee HK. Blood transfusion in contemporary obstetric practice. Obstet Gynecol 1990; 75:940.

Meehan FP, Casey C, Costello JN, Connolly CE. Placenta previa percreta with bladder involvement. Review. Obstet Gynecol Surv 1989; 44:835.

Mengert WF, Burchell RC, Blumstein RW, Daskal JL. Pregnancy after bilateral ligation of the internal iliac and ovarian arteries. Obstet Gynecol 1969; 34:669.

Nelson SH, Suresh MS. Lack of reactivity of uterine arteries from patients with obstetric hemorrhage. Am J Obstet Gynecol 1992; 166:1436.

Newton M, Mosey LM, Egli GE, et al. Blood loss during and immediately after delivery. Obstet Gynecol 1961; 17:9.

Oleen MA, Mariano JP. Controlling refractory atonic postpartum hemorrhage with Hemabate sterile solution. Am J Obstet Gynecol 1990; 162:205.

O'Leary JA. Stop of hemorrhage with uterine artery ligation. Contemp Ob/Gyn, 1986; 28:13.

Parenta JT, Dlugi H, Weingold AB. Pelvic hemostasis: a new technic and pack. Obstet Gynecol 1962; 19:218.

Peyser MR, Kupferminc MJ. Management of severe postpartum hemorrhage by intrauterine irrigation with prostaglandin E_2. Am J Obstet Gynecol 1990; 162:694.

Prendiville W, Elbourne D, Chalmers I. The effects of routine oxytocic administration in the management of the third stage of labour: an overview of the evidence from controlled trials. Br J Obstet Gynaecol 1988a; 95:3.

Prendiville WJ, Harding JE, Elbourne DR, Stirrat GM. The Bristol Third Stage Trial: active versus physiological management of third stage of labour. Br Med J 1988b; 297:1295.

Pritchard JA, Baldwin RM, Dickey JC, Wiggins KM. Blood volume changes in pregnancy and the puerperium. II. Red blood cell loss and changes in apparent blood volume during and following vaginal delivery, cesarean section, and cesarean section plus total hysterectomy. Am J Obstet Gynecol 1962; 84:1271.

Robie GF, Morgan MA, Payne GG, Wasemiller-Smith L. Logothetopulos pack for the management of uncontrollable postpartum hemorrhage. Am J Perinatol 1990; 7:327.

Rochat RW, Koonin LM, Atrash HK, Jewett JF. Maternal mortality in the United States: report for the maternal mortality collaborative. Obstet Gynecol 1988; 72:91.

Rosenfield A. Maternal mortality in developing countries. An ongoing but neglected "epidemic." JAMA 1989; 262:376.

Rosemond RL, Kepple DM. Transvaginal color Doppler sonography in the prenatal diagnosis of placenta accreta. Case reports. Obstet Gynecol 1992; 80:508.

Secher NJ, Arnso P, Wallin L. Haemodynamic effects of oxytocin (Syntocinon) and methylergometrine (Methergin) on the systemic and pulmonary circulations of pregnant anaesthetized women. Acta Obstet Gynecol Scand 1978; 57:97.

Shoemaker WC. Pathophysiologic basis of therapy for shock and trauma syndromes. Semin Drug Treat 1973a, 3:211.

Shoemaker WC, Bryan-Brown CW. Resuscitation and immediate care of the critically ill and injured patient. Semin Drug Treat 1973b; 3:249.

Shoemaker WC, Czer LSC. Evaluation of the biologic importance of various hemodynamic and oxygen transport variables. Crit Care Med 1979; 7:424.

Shoemaker WC, Boyd DR, Kim SI, et al. Sequential oxygen transport and acid-base changes after trauma to the unanesthetized patient. Surg Gynecol Obstet 1971; 132:1023.

Shoemaker WC, Printon KJ, Amato JJ, et al. Hemodynamic patterns after acute anesthetized and unanesthetized trauma. Arch Surg 1967; 95:492.

Slater GI, Vladeck BC, Bassin R, et al. Sequential changes in distribution of cardiac output in hemorrhagic shock. Surgery 1973; 73:714.

Smith DC, Wyatt JF. Embolization of the hypogastric arteries in the control of massive vaginal hemorrhage. Obstet Gynecol 1985; 2:204.

Thorp JM Jr, Councell RB, Sandridge DA, Wiest HH. Antepartum diagnosis of placenta previa percreta by magnetic resonance imaging. Case reports. Obstet Gynecol 1991; 80:506.

Toppozada M, El-Bossaty M, El-Rahman HA, El-Din AHS. Control of intractable atonic postpartum hemorrhage by 15-methyl prostaglandin F_2 alpha. Obstet Gynecol 1981; 58:327.

Weckstein LN, Masserman JS, Garite TJ. Placenta accreta: a problem of increasing clinical significance. Obstet Gynecol 1987; 69:480.

Wilson RF, Mammem E, Walt AJ. Eight years of experience with massive blood transfusions. J Trauma 1971; 11:275.

Yamashita Y, Takahashi M, Ito M, Okamura H. Transcatheter arterial embolization in the management of postpartum hemorrhage due to genital tract injury. Obstet Gynecol 1991; 77:160.

CHAPTER 27

Cancer

The diagnosis of cancer complicates approximately one out of every one thousand pregnancies in the United States, and cancer remains the second leading cause of death in women during their reproductive years (Allen and Nisker, 1986; Donegan, 1983; Jacob and Stringer, 1990). The cancers most commonly diagnosed in pregnancy are listed in Table 27–1. The most frequent cancers during pregnancy are the same as occur in nonpregnant women of the same age. This stands to reason, as there is no data suggesting that pregnancy is either a risk factor for nor does it protect against any type of malignancy. In recent years, women have tended to delay pregnancy until the third or fourth decade of life. As this trend continues we may see a change in both the incidence and pattern of cancer diagnosed in pregnancy.

The diagnosis of cancer in a pregnant women creates great emotional turmoil. Regardless of the type of malignancy, therapeutic decision making must consider what is best for the mother and safest for the fetus (Allen and Nisker, 1986; Donegan, 1983; Jacob and Stringer, 1990; Jolles, 1989; Sachs and associates, 1990; Moore and Martin, 1992; Clark, 1991a,b). While a concurrent pregnancy rarely alters the prognosis or treatment of most malignancies, the pregnancy may influence the timing of treatment. Most therapeutic options are associated with risks to the fetus, and frequently it is impossible to develop a treatment strategy that does not compromise optimal treatment of either the cancer or the pregnancy. These complex issues mandate a team approach involving the oncologist, obstetrician, social services, clergy, psychologist, and others individualized to best support the patient and her family. The woman's final decision regarding therapy will integrate the medical data presented to her with her own ethical and religious beliefs. With improvements in overall patient survival using highly aggressive and toxic treatment regimens, these ethical and emotional issues have become increasingly more complex.

Development of treatment strategies for cancer during pregnancy is compromised by lack of clinical data. Due to the relative infrequency of cancer in pregnancy, the database consists of small retrospective reports, anecdotal descriptions, and editorial reviews. Assuming no change in the incidence of cancer in pregnancy, it is unlikely that prospective data regarding the effects of pregnancy on cancer or the effects of any specific cancer and its treatment on fetal outcome will be available. Our goal within these confines is to summarize available clinical data and provide rational treatment options for those malignancies most frequently encountered in pregnant women.

DIAGNOSTIC AND THERAPEUTIC MODALITIES

Physical Examination

The normal anatomic and physiologic changes of pregnancy can compromise the ability to detect pathologic abnormalities and must be

TABLE 27–1 CANCERS MOST FREQUENTLY COMPLICATING PREGNANCY

Site	Cases/1000 Pregnancies
Cervix	0.8
Breast	0.3
Melanoma	0.2
Ovary	0.05
Thyroid	< 0.05
Colorectal	0.02
Leukemia	0.01
Lymphoma	0.01

Modified from Jacob and Stringer (1990).

taken into account when interpreting symptoms and physical findings (Allen and Nisker, 1986; Donegan, 1983; Jacob and Stringer, 1990; Jolles, 1989; Moore and Martin, 1992; Clark, 1991a,b). Many signs and symptoms that would alert the physician to the possibility of malignancy in the nonpregnant patient are frequent events in normal pregnancy and as such do not merit thorough evaluation. For instance, all pregnant women will experience abdominal distention and bloating sensation at some point in pregnancy. Distinguishing normal from abnormal complaints and discomfort of pregnancy still can lead to dangerous delays in the diagnosis of malignancy (Allen and Nisker, 1986; Donegan, 1983; Jacob and Stringer, 1990; Jolles, 1989; Moore and Martin, 1992; Clark, 1991a,b). Other specific examples of these problems will be illustrated as they pertain to the various malignancies discussed.

Diagnostic Radiology

Optimal fetal exposure to radiation is no exposure, yet prudent management of the pregnant patient may necessitate the use of radiographs for prompt diagnosis as well as staging and treatment planning once the diagnosis of cancer has been made. Some of the anatomic and physiologic changes associated with pregnancy may compromise the value of certain radiologic exams such as mammograms (Allen and Nisker, 1986; Donegan, 1983; Jacob and Stringer, 1990; Jolles, 1989; Moore and Martin, 1992; Clark, 1991a,b). Newer methods of imaging such as ultrasonography and magnetic resonance have been proposed as suitable alternatives to x-ray examinations (Kier and associates, 1990).

Radiation-induced damage to the fetus is related to two factors: gestational age at the time of exposure and the radiation dose the fetus receives (Sutcliffe, 1985; Kalter and Warkany, 1983; Timothy, 1986; Brent, 1981; Kinlen and Achejun, 1968; Mole, 1979; Dekaben, 1968; Brill and Forgotson, 1964). The spectrum of radiation effects include fetal death, congenital malformations, developmental and growth retardation, and future malignancy. Radiation exposure at the time of or within 2 weeks of implantation is believed to have an all-or-none effect that may result in embryonic death and abortion (Timothy, 1986). Exposure during the remainder of the first trimester places the fetus at risk for congenital abnormalities as this is the major period of organogenesis. Radiation exposure during the second and third trimesters has been associated with developmental and growth retardation. The dose of radiation required to induce damage is also related to gestational age. The minimal lethal dose of radiation increases from 0.1 Gy at day 1 of life to greater than 1.0 Gy after the first trimester (Brent, 1981). Doses above 0.1 Gy after the second week of life can result in sublethal complications such as malformations or developmental retardation (Brent, 1981). The risk of these complications increases significantly with increasing radiation dose. The potential for the development of childhood malignancies is present in all three trimesters and can occur with doses as low as .01 Gy (Schlono and colleagues, 1980; Harvey and co-workers, 1985; Sweet and Kinzie, 1976). The embryo is at greatest risk for radiation-induced mental retardation at 8–15 weeks' gestation with estimates as low as 4 percent for .1 Gy (10 rad) to as high as 60 percent for 1.5 Gy (150 rad) (Committee on Biological Effects, 1990; Hall, 1991). At the same levels of exposure there is a smaller risk at 16–25 weeks. There appears to be no significant increased risk of mental retardation at gestational ages less than 8 weeks or greater than 25 weeks, even with radiation exposure exceeding 0.5 Gy (50 rads) (Committee on Biological Effects, 1990).

The dose of radiation to the fetus from various diagnostic tests is listed in Table 27–2. In general, the levels of ionizing radiation to the fetus from these exams remains significantly below the doses required for potential damage. With multiple exams and exposures there is an additive effect. As pointed out by

TABLE 27–2 RADIATION DOSES ASSOCIATED WITH DIAGNOSTIC TESTS FREQUENTLY USED IN ONCOLOGY

Test	Estimated Final Exposure
Chest x-ray	< 0.5 mGy
Intravenous pyelogram	< 15.0 mGy
Barium enema	< 40.0 mGy
Upper GI series	< 10.0 mGy
Upper GI series with small bowel series	< 25.0 mGy
K U B	< 5.0 mGy
Mammography	< 0.5 mGy
Computerized tomography	
Head	< 0.5 mGy
Chest	< 10.0 mGy
Abdomen	< 30.0 mGy
Extremity film	< 0.5 mGy

Modified from Kereiakes and Rosenstein (1980).

the American College of Radiology, no single diagnostic test results in a radiation dose significant enough to warrant therapeutic abortion (Hall, 1991).

Tumor Markers

Most of the clinically useful tumor markers are of little value in pregnancy as they are normally elevated in pregnancy (ie, CEA, HCG, AFP). However, elevations above the normal levels of pregnancy may warrant special attention. Evaluations of extremely high alpha-fetoprotein levels during pregnancy have yielded the diagnoses of colon cancer, hepatocellular carcinoma, and germ cell tumors of the ovary (Goldberg and colleagues, 1991; Johnson, 1992; Farahmand and associates, 1991; van der Zee and co-workers, 1991; Gonsoulin and colleagues, 1990; Frederiksen and associates, 1991).

Radiotherapy

Radiation therapy offers the potential for cure in several malignancies. Although the doses of radiation used in cancer therapy are well above the lethal dose for a fetus, use of lead shields and carefully planned dosimetry allow therapeutic doses above the diaphragm and to the extremities without compromising the fetus (Timothy, 1986). Tumors located within the abdomen or pelvis require treatment doses that will result in fetal death.

Chemotherapy

Advances in chemotherapy have increased longevity and survival in women with cancers previously considered incurable. Chemotherapy is a potentially curative treatment in several malignancies that can effect pregnant women, including ovarian cancer, breast cancer, lymphomas, and leukemias.

Chemotherapeutic agents exert their lethal effects on the most rapidly dividing cells in the body. Since fetal cells are rapidly dividing, chemotherapy poses risks to the fetus to include direct fetal toxicity and/or death, congenital malformations, developmental and growth retardation, and the risk of future malignancy (Kalter and Warkany, 1983; Sweet and Kinzie, 1976; Beeley, 1986; Blatt and colleagues, 1980; Doll and co-workers, 1989; Zemlickis and associates, 1992b; Kim and colleagues, 1992). As with radiotherapy, fetal risks are dependent on the gestational age at which treatment is administered. The major period of risk for anomalies is the first 8 weeks of gestation, corresponding to the major period of organogenesis. Doll and associates (1989) compiled an exhaustive review of the literature and reported a 17 percent incidence of fetal malformation with single agent chemotherapy and a 25 percent incidence with multi-agent chemotherapy when the treatment was administered in the first trimester. With the exceptions of the hematopoietic system, the central nervous system, and the fetal eyes, all other major organ systems have developed by the end of the first trimester and are not at risk for teratogenic anomalies when chemotherapy is administered in the second or third trimester. Correspondingly, Doll and associates (1989) were unable to identify any reports of teratogenicity when single agent or multi-agent chemotherapy was administered in the second or third trimesters. Other factors that affect the risk of chemotherapy include the agents used, frequency and dose of therapy, individual susceptibility, and the number of agents used. Folic acid antagonists are the agents most frequently associated with fetal malformations, while the alkylating agents seem to have less potential for teratogenicity (Doll and associates, 1989). Nonteratogenetic effects (ie, fetal effects) such as growth retardation, premature labor, fetal organ toxicity, and an increased stillbirth rate have been associated with antineoplastic agents administered in the second and third trimesters of pregnancy (Sweet and Kinzie, 1976; Blatt and associates, 1980; Doll and co-workers, 1989; Zemlickis and colleagues, 1992b). Data regarding the specific risks of a particular antineoplastic agent is unavailable due to the infrequency of their use in pregnancy. Conclusions regarding the use of these agents in pregnancy must be drawn from theoretical concerns, animal data, and anecdotal reports.

The actual effects of pregnancy on the pharmacokinetics of anticancer drugs remains unknown; however, there are multiple physiologic changes associated with pregnancy that may have a significant effect. These physiologic changes include delayed gastric emptying which may affect the absorption of oral agents. Increased plasma volume, decreased serum albumin, and a decreased oncotic pressure could affect drug distribution, while an increased glomerular filtration rate and increased hepatic metabolism could potentially increase drug clearance. Additionally, the amniotic fluid may serve as a chemotherapeutic sink. In light of these practical and theoretical concerns, adequate dosing of chemotherapeutic agents is unknown.

Surgery

Cancers of the cervix, breast, thyroid, and colon and malignant melanoma have been diagnosed in pregnant women and are all potentially curable with early surgical intervention. With the exception of cervical cancer, pregnancy rarely alters the surgical management of these patients.

The potential risks to the fetus with surgical intervention include: (1) uteroplacental insufficiency from hypotension, hypoxia, or positioning the patient such that the enlarged uterus compresses the vena cava; (2) preterm labor secondary to peritoneal irritation or uterine manipulation; and (3) infectious complications (Schnider and Webster, 1965; Doll and associates, 1988; Pritchard and co-workers, 1985; Velard, 1984). The risk of teratogenicity of modern anesthetic agents appears to be negligible and not a threat to the fetus (Doll and associates, 1988; Barron, 1984). Uteroplacental insufficiency can generally be avoided with proper positioning of the patient with lateral tilt to displace the uterus from compressing the vena cava, by proper monitoring of maternal oxygenation, and by treatment as indicated with supplemental oxygen and blood and volume replacement (Pritchard and colleagues, 1985; Velard, 1984). Uterine irritability can be avoided by limiting uterine manipulation and the use of copious warm irrigation to remove peritoneal irritants (Schnider and Webster, 1965; Barron, 1984). Although somewhat controversial, the prophylactic use of tocolytic agents during and for 24–72 hours following abdominal surgery may decrease uterine irritability and premature labor. Infectious risks can be kept to a minimum with the appropriate use of antibiotics and careful surgical technique.

Pregnancy has several major effects on surgical intervention; the most obvious is the anatomic changes associated with the enlarged uterus, which can compromise exposure during intraabdominal surgery (Schnider and Webster, 1965). The pelvic vessels become markedly engorged as pregnancy advances and hemostasis may be difficult to achieve (Schnider and Webster, 1965). Pregnancy also increases the risk of thromboembolic complications (Laros and Alger, 1984; Hathaway and Bonner, 1978); all coagulation factors except XI and XIII are increased, fibrinolytic activity is decreased, and lower extremity venous blood flow is more static (Laros and Alger, 1984; Hathaway and Bonner, 1978). Therefore thromboembolic prophylaxis with mini-dose heparin or sequential compression hose are recommended.

GYNECOLOGIC MALIGNANCIES

Cervical Cancer

Carcinoma of the uterine cervix is the most frequently diagnosed cancer in pregnancy, complicating 1 of every 1240 pregnancies or 1 of every 34 women ever diagnosed with cervical cancer (Jolles, 1989). Women with cervical cancer during pregnancy are typically multigravidas in their mid-thirties. Since most pregnant women undergo routine pelvic exam and cervical cytology evaluation during the first trimester of pregnancy, the disease is often asymptomatic and diagnosed at an early stage (Economos and associates, 1993). Patients presenting with larger tumors or advanced disease most frequently complain of abnormal vaginal bleeding or vaginal discharge (Monk and Montz, 1992; Baltzer and colleagues, 1990; Hannigan, 1990; Zemlickis and co-workers, 1991; Hopkins and Morley, 1992). These symptoms are often attributed to pregnancy, and incomplete evaluations can lead to dangerous delays in diagnosis. The evaluation of a gravid patient with vaginal bleeding or discharge should always include a careful inspection of the cervix and further evaluation of any suspicious lesions (Chapter 31). Cervical biopsies performed during pregnancy, especially during the second and third trimester, can be technically difficult due to vaginal edema and redundancy and can be associated with heavy bleeding due to the increased vascularity of the pelvic viscera (Monk and Montz, 1992; Baltzer and colleagues, 1990; Hannigan, 1990; Zemlickis and co-workers, 1991; Hopkins and Morley, 1992). These factors necessitate careful planning of the procedure to include colposcopic direction of the biopsy in a setting where adequate lighting and exposure can be obtained. With very advanced disease, patients may present with lower extremity edema, pelvic pain, and weight loss. In these rare cases, pelvic exam will reveal an obvious cervical lesion, which frequently requires an examination under anesthesia in an operating room in order to safely obtain a biopsy specimen.

Once the diagnosis of cervical cancer is made, treatment decisions are based on stage of the disease and the patient's overall medical condition. The pelvic exam to determine if the tumor has invaded the parametrial tissue or extended to the pelvic sidewall remains the gold standard of clinical staging in cervical cancer. This examination may be much more difficult in the pregnant patient; cervical cyanosis, softening, effacement, and enlargement may make the identification and demarkation of cervical lesions more difficult (Monk and Montz, 1992; Baltzer and colleagues, 1990; Hannigan, 1990; Zemlickis and co-workers, 1991; Hopkins and Morley, 1992; Sivanesaratnam and associates, 1993). Late in pregnancy the firm fetal head, located deep in the pelvis, can make evaluation of parametrial involvement confusing. Proper staging also requires assessment of mechanical obstruction of the ureters. In the nonpregnant patient, this assessment is generally accomplished with an intravenous pyelogram or a computed tomographic scan of the abdomen and pelvis with contrast agents. To avoid fetal exposure to ionizing radiation, magnetic resonance imaging is a suitable substitute.

Gestational age of the pregnancy also has a significant impact on treatment options. When cervical cancer is diagnosed at or near the time of fetal maturity, treatment can often be delayed until after the delivery of the fetus (Baltzer and associates, 1990; Hannigan, 1990; Zemlickis and co-workers, 1991; Hopkins and Morley, 1992; Sivanesaratnam and colleagues, 1993). In these situations, treatment decisions can be made without having to consider the safety of the fetus. However, treatment of cervical cancer remote from fetal maturity often requires sacrificing the fetus in an effort to provide the woman lifesaving therapy.

Treatment

The treatment of stage Ia tumors with less than 3 mm of cervical invasion and no lympho-vascular space involvement diagnosed by a suitable cervical conization specimen may be expectant until the conclusion of the pregnancy, regardless of the gestational age of the fetus. In these patients, the mode of delivery of the fetus should be based on obstetric considerations only (Baltzer and associates, 1990; Hannigan, 1990; Zemlickis and co-workers, 1991; Hopkins and Morley, 1992; Sivanesaratnam and colleagues, 1993).

The management of all stage I tumors invading deeper than 3 mm and of stage IIa tumors requires radical surgical or radiation therapy (Baltzer and associates, 1990; Hannigan, 1990; Zemlickis and co-workers, 1991; Hopkins and Morley, 1992; Sivanesaratnam and colleagues, 1993). In these situations, the gestational age of the fetus is critical in determining whether to delay therapy until after delivery or to disregard the fetus and immediately institute curative therapy. Although the mother's wishes must dictate the timing of therapy, most oncologists are comfortable delaying therapy until fetal maturity and delivery when the pregnancy is at or beyond 24 weeks at the time cancer is diagnosed. Prior to 24 weeks, the majority of oncologists would prefer to initiate therapy immediately and sacrifice the fetus. This gestational age cutoff is based on the amount of time most oncologists feel it is safe to delay treatment without risking disease progression and worsening prognosis as well as recognition that fetal viability occurs at about 24 weeks. Most obstetricians and neonatologists would advise use of corticosteroids to accelerate fetal maturity with elective delivery after fetal lung maturity has been documented by amniocentesis (Monk and Montz, 1992; Baltzer and associates, 1990; Hannigan, 1990; Zemlickis and co-workers, 1991; Hopkins and Morley, 1992). This can usually be achieved by 33–34 weeks of gestational age.

Radiation therapy and surgery offer similar cure rates in stage I and IIa disease (Baltzer and associates, 1990; Hannigan, 1990; Zemlickis and co-workers, 1991; Hopkins and Morley, 1992; Sivanesaratnam and colleagues, 1993). Choice of therapy is based on the patient's general medical condition and her concerns regarding potential side effects of therapy. Young women with cervical cancer are at significant risk for sexual dysfunction with radiation treatment and accordingly often opt for surgical management. Prior to 20 weeks' gestation, radical hysterectomy with pelvic and periaortic lymphadenectomy can usually be performed with the fetus in situ. Radical surgery at later gestational ages requires hysterotomy and evacuation of the uterine contents due to the technical difficulties and decreased exposure from the enlarged uterus. The hysterotomy incision should be vertical and in the anterior fundus to avoid extension into the parametrial tissue and compromise of the surgical margins. When radical surgery is delayed until fetal maturity, the operation is generally performed following a classical cesarean section (Monk and Montz, 1992; Baltzer and associates, 1990; Hannigan, 1990; Zemlickis and co-workers, 1991; Hopkins and Morley, 1992; Sivanesaratnam and colleagues, 1993). The technique for this procedure is depicted in Figures 27–1 through 27–8.

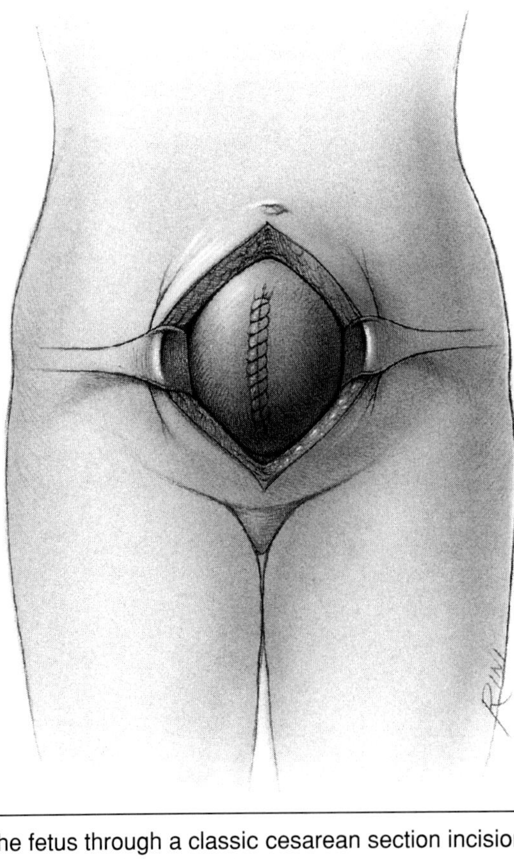

Figure 27–1. After delivery of the fetus through a classic cesarean section incision, the uterus is closed with a single running suture to increase exposure and decrease blood loss.

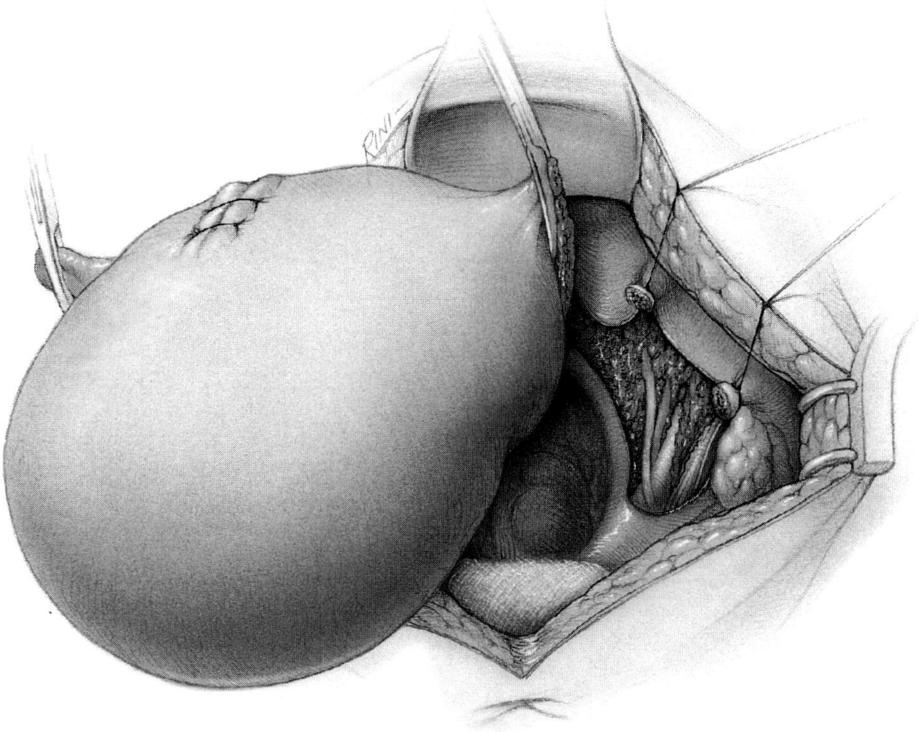

Figure 27–2. The round ligaments are then sacrificed close to the pelvic sidewall and the retroperitoneal spaces are opened. The ureters, pelvic vessels, and infundibulo-pelvic ligaments are clearly identified and the adnexa are separated from the uterus and reflected cephalad by incising the peritoneal to allow for their preservation. The ureter is then carefully dissected from its attachment to the medial leaf of the broad ligament using sharp dissection.

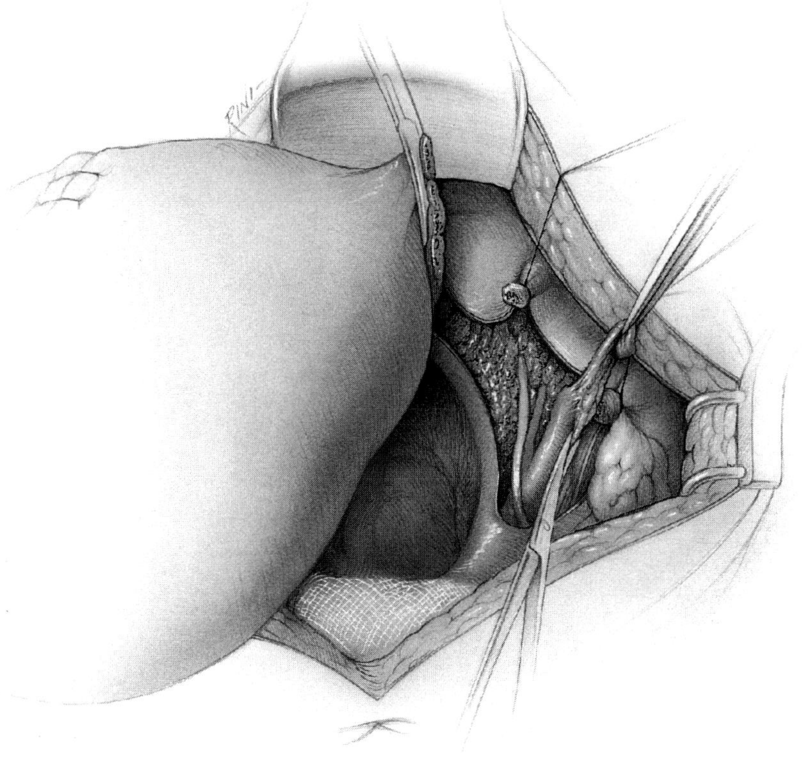

Figure 27–3. The pelvic lymphadenectomy is then accomplished. The borders of this dissection are the genital femoral nerve laterally, and the superior vesical artery medially (not shown), the obturator fossa in the caudad direction, and the bifurcation of the aorta in the cephalad direction.

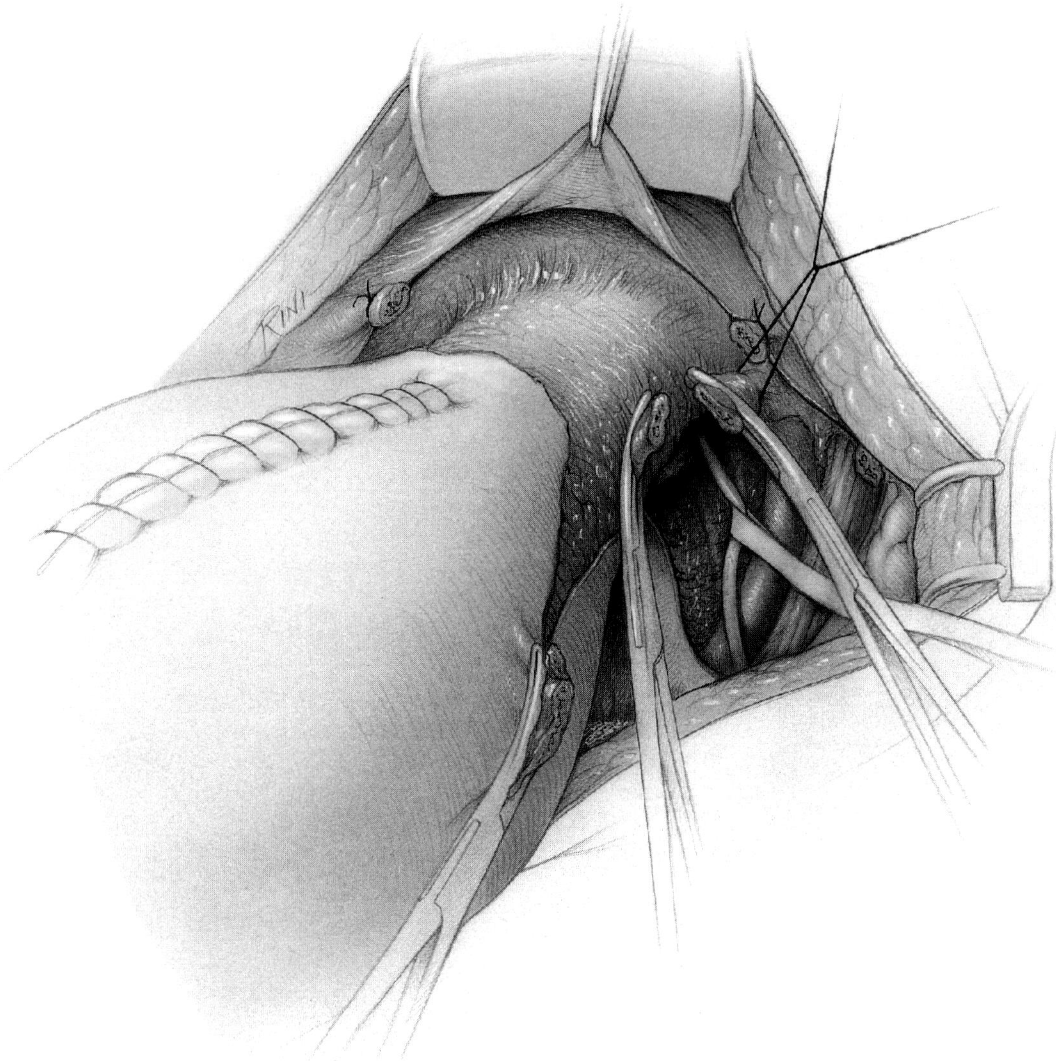

Figure 27–4. The bladder is sharply dissected free of its attachment to the lower uterine segment and the upper one third to one half of the vagina. The ureter is sharply dissected free and removed from the vesicouterine ligament. The uterine artery is identified and sacrificed at its origin. Each of these steps results in removal of far more parametrial tissue than occurs at the usual hysterectomy.

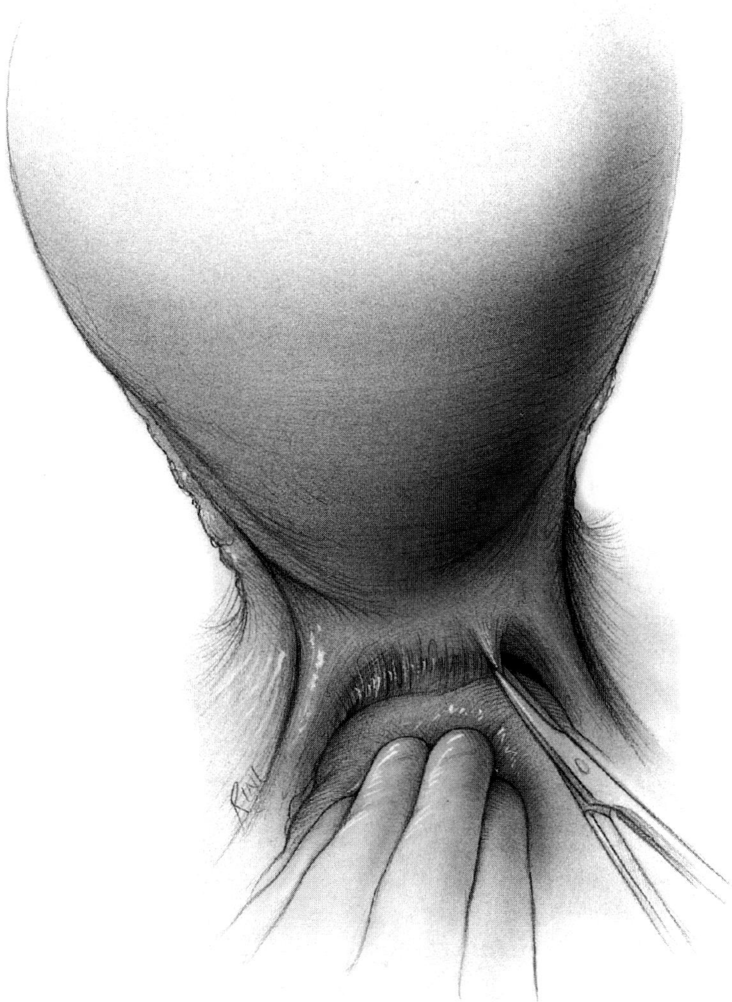

Figure 27–5. Posterior dissection involves separating the uterus and upper one third to one half of the vagina from its attachments to the rectum. Shown is initiation of sharp dissection of the posterior peritoneal reflection. This will allow the rectum to be either bluntly or sharply dissected off of the lower uterine segment and posterior vaginal wall and minimize the risk of injury to the rectum.

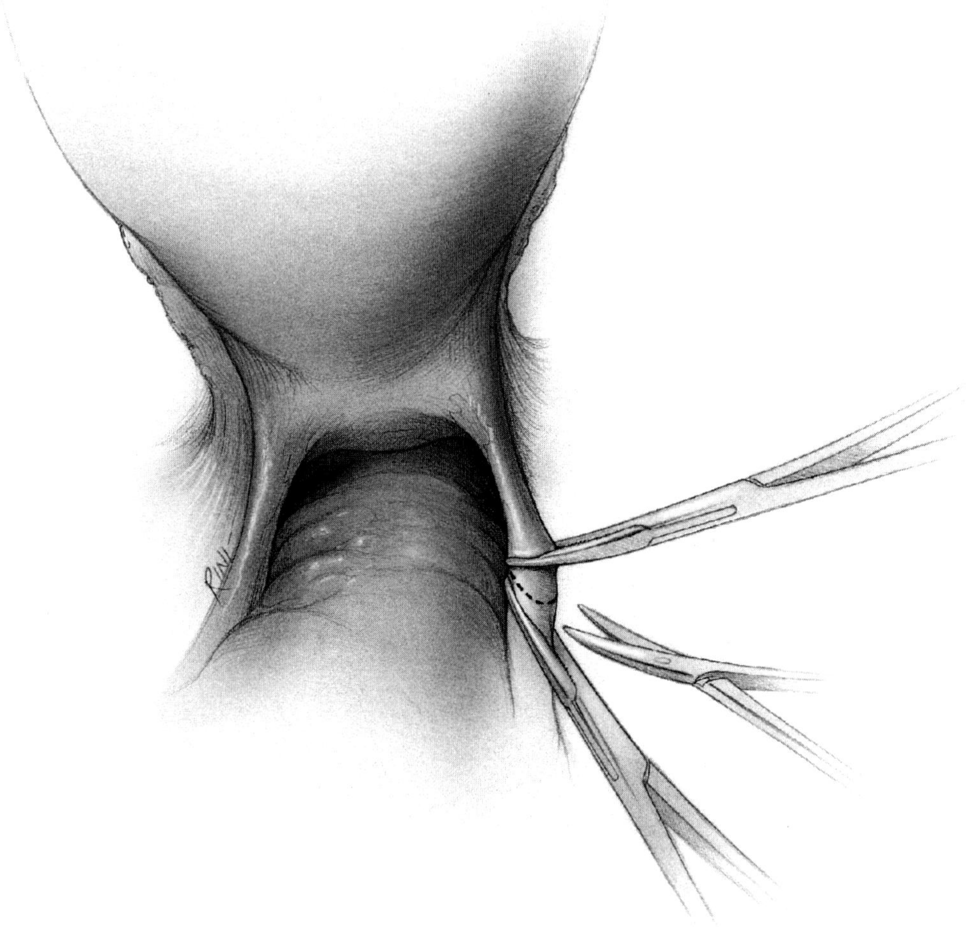

Figure 27–6. The uretero-sacral ligaments are transsected at their origin, well away from their uterine insertion site. Shown is use of a Heaney or Roger's type clamp to doubly clamp the utero-sacral ligament, following which it is severed between the clamps with Mayo scissors. The distal portion of the ligament is then secured with a transfixing suture.

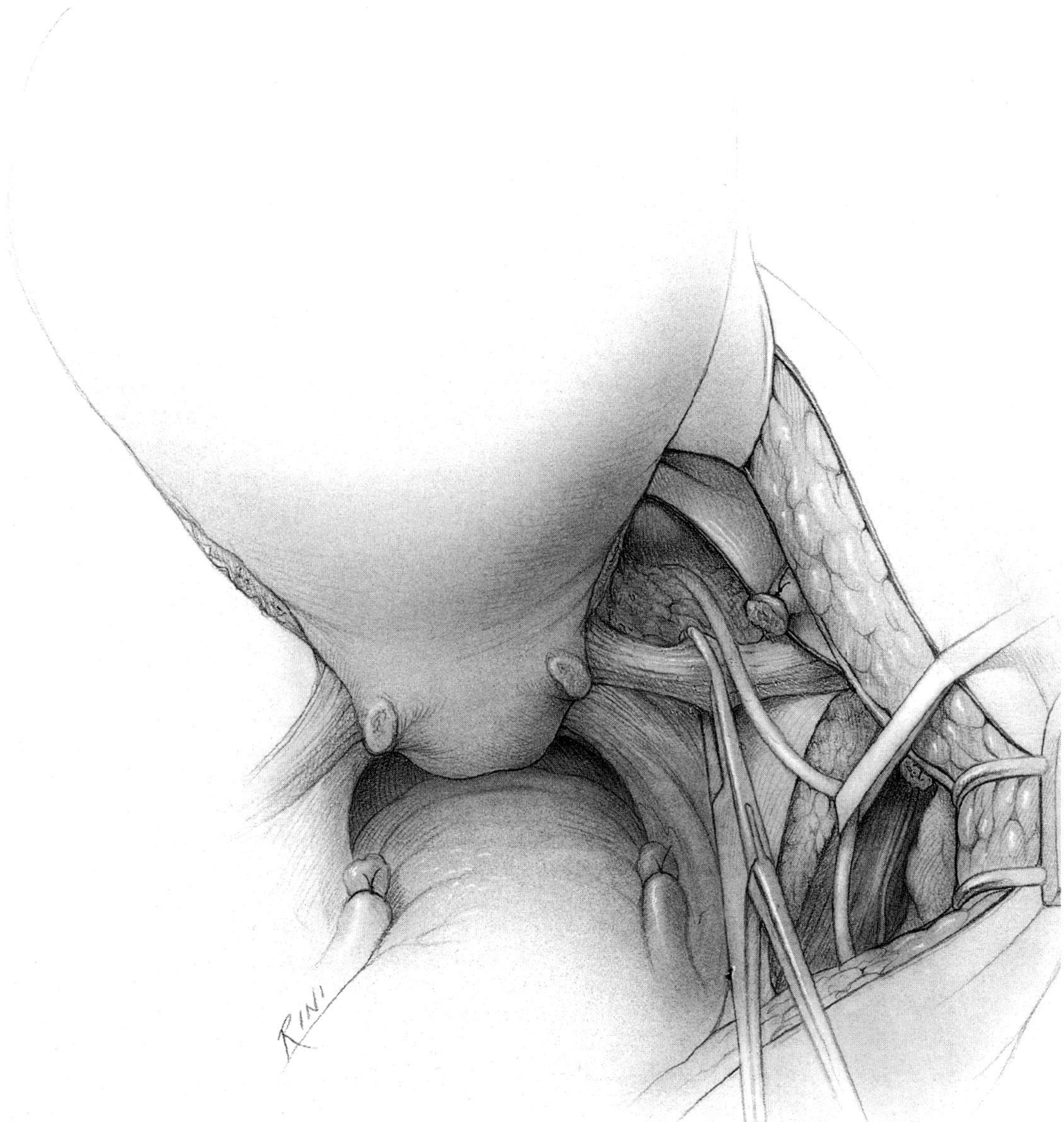

Figure 27–7. The cardinal ligaments are then transsected at their origin on the pelvic sidewall.

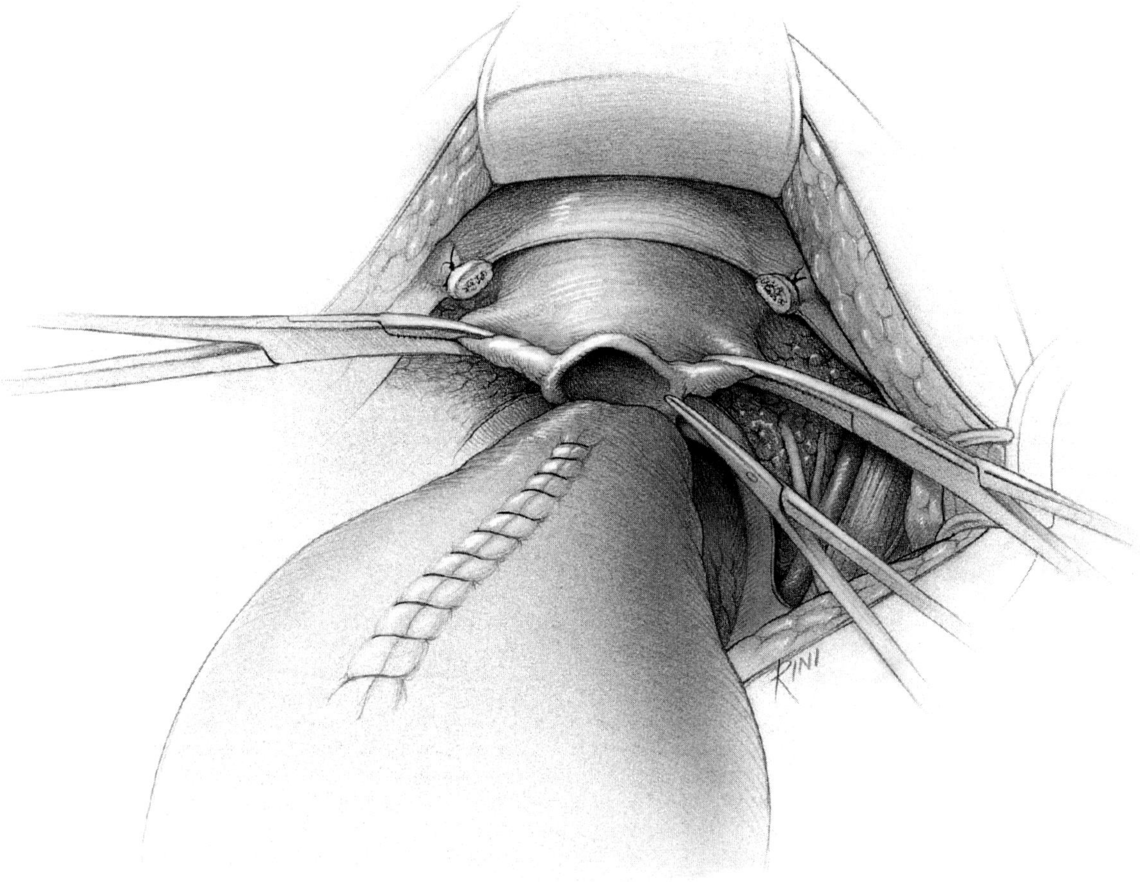

Figure 27–8. The radical hysterectomy is then completed by transecting the vagina at the juncture of the upper one third to lower two thirds. The vaginal cuff is then closed with a running, locking suture. Care should be taken to ensure that the cut vaginal mucosa is included throughout the closure. Visualization of the cut edge is often enhanced by use of Allis type clamps.

If the patient opts for radiation therapy, treatment can be instituted either prior to or after delivery of the fetus. When radiation therapy is begun with the fetus in situ, spontaneous abortion usually occurs before 4000 cGy is received to the pelvis by external beam (Baltzer and associates, 1990; Hannigan, 1990; Zemlickis and co-workers, 1991; Hopkins and Morley, 1992; Sivanesaratnam and colleagues, 1993). However, Creasman and associates (1970) reported that 27 percent of patients in their series required the surgical removal of the fetus after completing teletherapy (external beam). After completion of teletherapy, either brachytherapy or extended hysterectomy completes the treatment. If radiation therapy is delayed until fetal maturity, treatment can begin immediately after delivery of the fetus.

Although radical surgery may have an adjuvant role, the cornerstone of management in women with stage IIb or greater disease is radiation therapy. Timing of therapy is again related to the gestational age of the fetus and the overall prognosis of the patient. Patients with advanced disease and a poor prognosis may opt to delay palliative therapy until after fetal maturity and delivery. In patients with potentially curable disease the same considerations applied to stage I disease are used.

The mode of delivery of the fetus in patients with cervical cancer is controversial (Creasman and co-workers, 1970; Nisker and Allen, 1986). There have been no prospective trials addressing this issue and retrospective studies have been unable to identify any survival effect to the mother based on route of delivery (Monk and Montz, 1992; Baltzer and associates, 1990; Hannigan, 1990; Zemlickis and co-workers, 1991; Hopkins and Morley, 1992; Sivanesaratnam and colleagues, 1993). Still, theoretical concerns regarding dystocia, maternal hemorrhage, and the exportation of malignant cells have prompted some authors to recommend cesarean section for delivery. Several authors have reported the development of recurrent disease in the episiotomy scars of women who where delivered vaginally prior to treatment of their cervical cancer (Burgess and Waymont, 1987; Gordon and co-workers, 1989; Copeland and colleagues, 1987).

Stage for stage, the prognosis of cervical cancer does not appear to be altered by pregnancy. Retrospective reviews have been unable to demonstrate any effect of pregnancy on the prognosis of women with cervical cancer; however, the mode of therapy used and its timing dramatically impact fetal outcomes (Monk and Montz, 1992; Baltzer and associates, 1990; Hannigan, 1990; Zemlickis and co-workers, 1991; Hopkins and Morley, 1992; Sivanesaratnam and colleagues, 1993).

Ovarian Cancer

An adnexal mass complicates 1 of every 81–2500 pregnancies; however, ovarian cancer of any cell type is rarely associated with pregnancy and is seen in only 1 of every 12,000–25,000 pregnancies (Munell, 1963; Ghung and Birabaum, 1973). Similar to nonpregnant women of the same age, epithelial cell types predominate; however, germ cell tumors and sarcomas are also encountered in pregnancy (Munnell, 1963; Ghung and Birabaum, 1973; Halmo and associates, 1986; Booth, 1963; Yazigi and Driscoll, 1986; Creasman and colleagues, 1971). In contrast to the general population, where the majority of ovarian cancers are detected in advanced stages, most epithelial ovarian malignancies diagnosed during pregnancy are found at an early stage and are low grade or low malignant potential tumors (Jolles, 1989).

Early stage ovarian tumors are generally asymptomatic, incidental finding during routine pelvic exams, obstetric ultrasonography exams, or at cesarean section (Jolles, 1989; Munnell, 1963; Ghung and Birabaum, 1973; Halmo and associates, 1986; Booth, 1963; Yazigi and Driscoll, 1986; Creasman and colleagues, 1971; Jubb, 1963). Exceptions to this are tumors that may torse and/or rupture; these patients will often present with acute peritoneal signs. The germ cell tumors are the most likely cancers to present with torsion or rupture due to their rapid growth rates and the low density of their contents. Rarely will a pregnant patient with ovarian cancer present with the classical ovarian cancer symptoms of abdominal discomfort and dyspepsia (Jolles, 1989). Large ovarian neoplasms may present as a cause of dystocia during labor (Jacob and Stringer, 1990).

Definitive diagnosis of ovarian cancer is made histologically after surgical exploration. The indications, techniques, and timing of the evaluation of a pelvic mass in pregnancy are discussed in Chapter 22. Once the diagnosis of ovarian cancer is established, the surgical staging and treatment options for the pregnant patient are identical to those of the non-pregnant patient. The hallmarks of therapy include proper surgical staging and in epithelial tumors, aggressive cytoreductive surgery. Adjuvant chemotherapy is based on the cell type or grade of the tumor and the stage of disease. Although hysterectomy is often part of the surgical management of nonpregnant patients with ovarian cancer, the uterus itself is seldom heavily laden with tumor and there is no evidence that removal of the uterus improves survival. Therefore, leaving the pregnant uterus in situ should have no impact on patient survival as long as the principles of cytoreductive surgery are maintained. While chemotherapy can be administered without interrupting the pregnancy (Christman and associates, 1990), it is seldom required owing to the predominance of early stage tumors and tumors of low malignant potential in pregnancy (Halmo and colleagues, 1986). The specific indications and particular antineoplastic agents recommended for the various ovarian malignancies are beyond the scope of this chapter; however, these indications and treatment options are not affected by the pregnancy. Similarly, regardless of cell type, the prognosis for patients diagnosed with ovarian cancer is not affected by pregnancy (Munnell, 1963; Ghung and Birabaum, 1973; Halmo and colleagues, 1986; Booth, 1963; Yazigi and Driscoll, 1986; Creasman and associates, 1971; Jubb, 1963; Christman and co-workers, 1990; Malfetano and Goldkrand, 1990; Cashell and Cohen, 1991; Jung and associates, 1991; Rasmussen and co-workers, 1991; Powell and colleagues, 1993; Shaves and associates, 1990; King and co-workers, 1991; Henderson and colleagues, 1993).

Vulvar Cancer

Carcinoma of the vulva is most commonly diagnosed in women beyond their reproductive years. However, over the past several decades, the incidence of invasive vulvar lesions in women under the age of 40 has been increasing (Choo, 1982). Still, the diagnosis of vulvar cancer during pregnancy remains extremely rare, with less than 30 cases documented in the English literature (Barclay, 1974; Lutz and associates, 1977; Moore and co-workers, 1991; Del Priore and colleagues, 1992; Kuller and associates, 1990). Based on these limited data, pregnancy appears to have little impact on the diagnosis, treatment, or prognosis of women with vulvar cancer (Barclay, 1974; Lutz and associates, 1977; Moore and co-workers, 1991; Del Priore and colleagues, 1992; Kuller and associates, 1990).

Invasive lesions diagnosed during the first and second trimesters of pregnancy should be approached in the standard fashion with radical vulvectomy with or without inguinal lymphadenectomy based on the size of the lesion and the depth of tumor invasion. Pregnancy may continue in these patients and vaginal delivery should be possible if adequate healing of the surgical wounds has occurred. When invasive lesions are diagnosed during the last trimester of pregnancy, management usually consists of a wide local excision and delay of definitive surgical therapy until after the fetus has been delivered (Del Priore and associates, 1992). If adjuvant pelvic radiotherapy is required to treat nodal extension, it will have to be delayed until delivery if the patient elects to continue the pregnancy.

Vaginal Carcinoma

Primary squamous cell carcinomas of the vagina are rare and are generally diagnosed in postmenopausal women. There are fewer than 20 cases of squamous cell carcinoma of the vagina during pregnancy in the English literature (DiSaia and Creasman, 1993). Clear cell adenocarcinoma of the vagina is also a rare tumor; associated with in-utero exposure to diethylstilbestrol (DES) and generally seen in young women. Despite the early age at diagnosis of these tumors, fewer than 30 have been reported during pregnancy (DiSaia and Creasman, 1993). Sarcomas such as sarcoma botryoides have also been reported to occur during pregnancy, but are again extremely rare (DiSaia and Creasman, 1993).

Due to the rarity of primary vaginal carcinomas in pregnancy, few sound conclusions can be reached. In general, those tumors occurring in the upper half of the vagina should be approached in a manner similar to the approach in cervical cancer (DiSaia and Creasman, 1993; Collins and Barclay, 1972). In the first 24 weeks of pregnancy, radical radiation or surgical therapy should be employed without regard for the fetus. Patients with sarcoma botryoides require adjuvant chemotherapy (DiSaia and Creasman, 1993). Treatment of upper vaginal lesions diagnosed after the twenty-fourth week of gestation may be delayed until after fetal maturity and delivery depending upon the woman's decision. Lesions occurring in the lower half of the vagina should be treated in a manner similar to lesions of the vulva. Owing to anatomic considerations, radiation and chemotherapy play a more dominant role in the management of these lesions than does surgery (Collins and Barclay, 1972). There is no evidence that pregnancy affects the prognosis of patients with primary vaginal carcinoma (DiSaia and Creasman, 1993; Collins and Barclay, 1972).

Uterine Cancer

Adenocarcinoma of the endometrium concurrent with pregnancy has been reported but is extremely rare (Hoffman and associates, 1989; Karler and co-workers, 1972; Sandstrom and colleagues, 1979; Schumann, 1927; Suzuki and associates, 1984; Paulson and co-workers, 1990; Ojomo and associates, 1993). One well-documented case of endometrial carcinoma in pregnancy was reported by Suzuki and associates (1984). Ten other cases have also been cited since 1972 (Hoffman and co-workers, 1989; Karler and associates, 1972; Sandstrom and colleagues, 1979; Paulson and associates, 1990; Ojomo and co-workers, 1993); however, some authors have suggested that many of these cases may represent misdiagnosed Arias-Stella reaction. Uterine sarcomas have also been reported as incidental findings in surgical specimens after cesarean-hysterectomies.

Since the diagnosis of uterine cancer prior to the delivery of the fetus is unlikely, pregnancy has little impact on the treatment of the disease. As with the other gynecologic malignancies discussed, there is no evidence that pregnancy affects the prognosis of these tumors.

NONGYNECOLOGIC MALIGNANCIES

Breast Cancer

In the United States, carcinoma of the breast is the most frequently diagnosed malignancy in women. In pregnant women it is second in frequency, with cervical cancer being the most frequent (Gallenberg and Loprinzi, 1989). Breast cancer complicates approximately 1 in 3,000 pregnancies, and 2–5 percent of all breast cancers are diagnosed in pregnant women.

Malignancies of the breast rarely have symptoms. They are usually discovered by the patient or her health care provider during palpation of the breast (Gallenberg and Loprinzi, 1989; Allen and Nisker, 1988; Barnavon and Wallack, 1990; Saunders and Baum, 1993). In older women, screening mammography accounts for many of the diagnoses; however, screening mammography is not recommended for women in the reproductive years due to difficulties of interpretation in dense glandular breasts. The diagnosis of breast cancer in pregnant women is frequently delayed by 2–7 months (Gallenberg and Loprinzi, 1989; Allen and Nisker, 1988; Barnavon and Wallack, 1990; Saunders and Baum, 1993; Zemlickis and associates, 1992a; Petrek and colleagues, 1991; Tretli and co-workers, 1988; Theriault and associates, 1992; Clark, 1991b). This delay has been attributed to both the lack of physician aggressiveness in the evaluation of breast masses in pregnancy and the normal anatomic and physiologic changes of the breast that occur in pregnancy. Increases in the gland-to-stroma ratio with enlargement and engorgement of the pregnant breasts make the detection of small breast masses difficult. Therefore detection of the cancer in its early stage is less frequent than in the non-pregnant population. Owing to delayed detection, the rate of nodal metastasis is higher in the pregnant population than in their non-pregnant counterparts (Petrek and colleagues, 1991; Tretli and co-workers, 1988; Theriault and associates, 1992; Clark, 1991b).

The diagnostic tools used in evaluating suspicious breast masses are not altered by pregnancy. Physical exam is the mainstay for initial detection. Fine needle aspiration or biopsy of suspicious lesions should be performed without regard to pregnancy (Gupta and associates, 1993; Novotny and co-workers, 1991). Figure 27–9 is a positive fine needle aspirate from a pregnant patient with a breast mass (see Chapter 36).

Once diagnosed, the staging of breast cancer is the same as in nonpregnant women with the exception of the evaluation for bone metastasis. Although a bone scan is not absolutely contraindicated in pregnancy, it

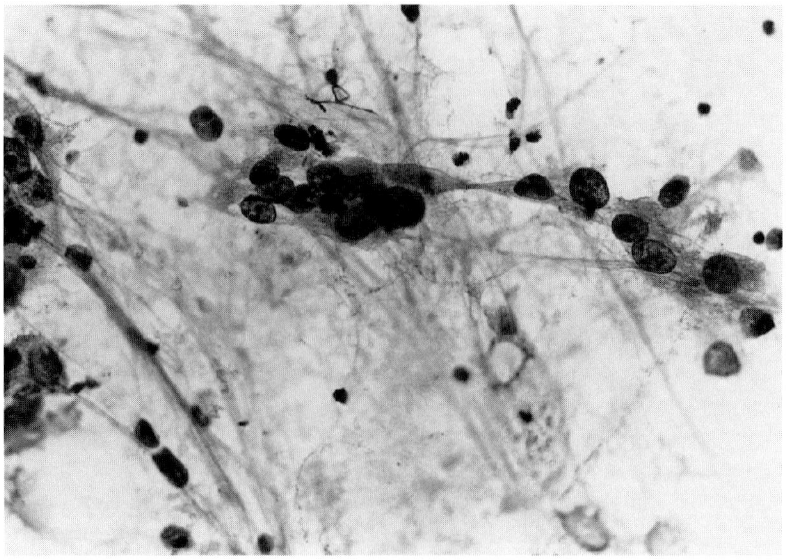

Figure 27–9. Fine-needle aspiration from a breast carcinoma. These specimens are characterized by cells with atypical nuclei, increased nuclear-cytoplasmic ratio, and a background that may contain numerous inflammatory cells or necrotic material. One of the most helpful diagnostic features is the presence of single atypical cells; benign lesions typically demonstrate cell clusters. (Photo courtesy of Christopher M. Zahn, MD.)

should be reserved for patients with symptoms or laboratory tests suggestive of bone involvement in order to minimize fetal exposure to radiation.

Treatment

The treatment of early stage breast cancer involves either modified radical mastectomy and axillary lymph node dissection or more conservative surgery with adjuvant radiation therapy for local and regional control of disease. Although both approaches offer a similar prognosis for the woman, the more radical surgical approach and avoidance of radiation exposure is generally recommended if the fetus is to remain in-utero during treatment. For control and prevention of distant disease, adjuvant cytotoxic chemotherapy is advocated regardless of lymph node status (Gallenberg and Loprinzi, 1989; Allen and Nisker, 1988; Barnavon and Wallack, 1990; Saunders and Baum, 1993; Willemse and associates, 1990). Although this treatment can be delivered with the fetus in utero with minimal risks, it is usually delayed until delivery. This may not be advisable if the cancer is diagnosed early in pregnancy. In such cases delaying chemotherapy until at least the second trimester is recommended. Hormonal therapy with agents such as tamoxifen is also used for many women with breast cancer (Gallenberg and Loprinzi, 1989; Allen and Nisker, 1988; Barnavon and Wallack, 1990; Saunders and Baum, 1993). Little is known about the effects of these agents on the fetus or the pregnancy; therefore it is generally recommended that they be withheld until after delivery.

Although patients diagnosed with breast cancer during pregnancy have a worse prognosis than their nonpregnant counterparts, this difference is attributable to the more advanced stage of disease at the time of diagnosis (Petrek, 1991; Tretli and associates, 1988; Theriault and associates, 1992; Clark, 1991b). In well-controlled studies where pregnant and nonpregnant patients were matched for age, stage, treatment, and histologic factors, pregnancy did not alter survival (Petrek, 1991; Tretli and associates, 1988; Theriault and associates, 1992; Clark, 1991b). Owing to theoretical concerns regarding the effects of placental hormones on breast cancer, therapeutic abortion was once recommended for all pregnant patients with breast cancer. Retrospective studies have been unable to demonstrate any survival improvement from this practice and abortion is no longer recommended.

The major effect of pregnancy on breast cancer is a delay in diagnosis. Pregnancy does not significantly alter the approach to diagnosis or treatment nor does it alter disease prognosis.

Malignant Melanoma

Malignant melanoma complicates from 0.14 to 2.8 per 1000 pregnancies. It is the third most common cancer diagnosed in pregnancy (Smith and Randal, 1969) and has the highest incidence of metastasis to the placenta and fetus (Potter, 1970).

The cornerstone of diagnosis is careful inspection of the skin and biopsy of all suspicious lesions. Pretreatment evaluation consists of histopathologic determination of the tumor thickness and melanoma type, palpation and radiographic evaluation of the draining lymph node chains, and search for distant metastases by chest radiography and computerized tomography or magnetic resonance imaging. All of these evaluations can be accomplished during pregnancy with the appropriate use of lead shields to decrease fetal exposure to radiation or substitution of nonionizing imaging sources such as MRI (Wong and Strassner, 1990).

The only effective therapy for malignant melanoma is surgical excision (Wong and Strassner, 1990). The use of cytotoxic drugs, hormonal agents, biologic response modifiers, or radiation appears to have little if any effect on these tumors, and their use is reserved primarily for palliation. Pregnancy does not alter these therapeutic considerations (Wong and Strassner, 1990).

The effect of pregnancy on the prognosis of patients with malignant melanoma is controversial (Wong and Strassner, 1990; Slingluff and associates, 1990, 1992; Pack and Schvnayel, 1951; Byrd and McGarity, 1954). The major prognostic indicators in malignant melanoma include tumor thickness, tumor type, location of tumor (extremities vs head, neck, or trunk), and the presence of lymph node metastasis. Many authors have suggested that pregnancy negatively influences prognosis (Slingluff and associates, 1990, 1992; Pack and Schvnayel, 1951; Byrd and McGarity, 1954). These authors have cited the theoretical concerns of increased levels of melanocyte-stimulating hormone and the increased skin pigmentation seen in pregnancy. Uncontrolled retrospective reviews have suggested that pregnant patients have a poorer survival than their nonpregnant counterparts (Pack and Schvnayel, 1951; Byrd and McGarity, 1954). One recent review, which was controlled for age only, reported shorter disease-free intervals and shorter time to lymph node metastasis in pregnant women, but could not demonstrate any difference in survival (Slingluff and associates, 1990, 1992). Most recent reviews have controlled for tumor thickness, tumor location, patient age, and stage of disease. These studies have not confirmed earlier studies and do not attribute any prognostic significance to pregnancy status (Wong and Strassner, 1990; George and associates, 1960; Elwood and Coldman, 1978; Houghton and co-workers, 1981).

Pregnancy has little impact on the diagnosis, treatment, or survival of women with malignant melanoma. Because of the unique characteristic of these tumors to metastasize to the products of conception, close inspection of the infant and the placenta is required at delivery.

Thyroid Cancer

Thyroid cancer in pregnancy is rare; however, thyroid cancer is one of the more common malignancies of women in their reproductive years (Hod and associates, 1989). Thyroid cancers usually present as an asymptomatic solitary nodule of the thyroid, which frequently demonstrates rapid growth. Although uniform enlargement of the thyroid gland is normal in pregnancy, development of asymmetry or the development of a solitary nodule should alert the clinician to the possibility of a thyroid malignancy (Hod and co-workers, 1989; Cunningham and Slaughter, 1970; Rosvoll and Winship, 1965). Other physical findings of concern include regional lymph node enlargement and/or fixation and rapid growth of the nodule.

The diagnosis of thyroid cancer is made either by fine needle aspiration or open biopsy of the thyroid nodule (Fukuda and associates, 1991). Figure 27–10 is from a positive fine needle aspirate in a pregnant patient with a thyroid nodule. Ultrasonography may be useful in locating and characterizing the thyroid nodule (Figure 27–11). Thyroid scanning, frequently used in the nonpregnant patient, is contraindicated during pregnancy as the radioactive isotope will readily cross the placenta and concentrate in the fetal thyroid (Hod and co-workers, 1989; Cunningham and Slaughter, 1970; Rosvoll and Winship, 1965).

Treatment of thyroid cancer is total or near-total thyroidectomy (Cunningham and Slaughter, 1970; Rosen and Walfish, 1985) and is not altered by pregnancy. In the presence of regional or distal metastasis additional therapy with either radioactive iodine or cytotoxic drugs such as cisplatin and adriamycin are required (Hod and associates, 1989; Rosvoll and Win-

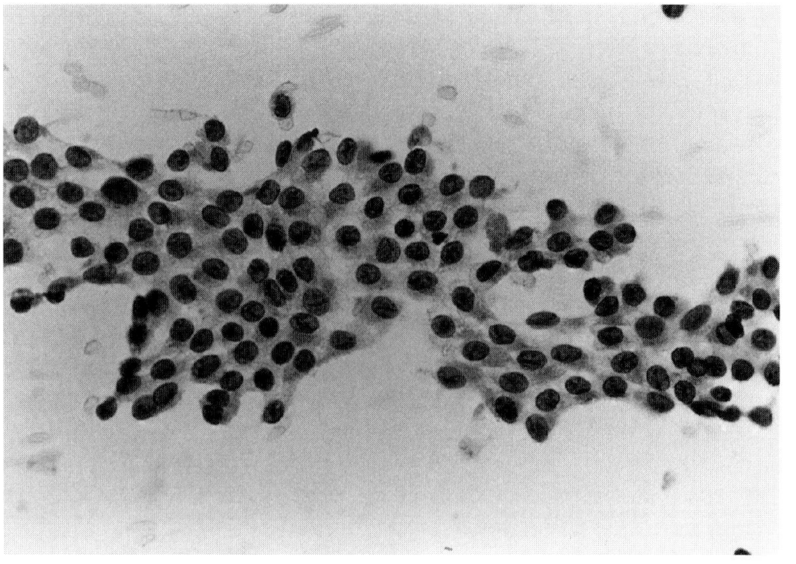

Figure 27–10. Fine-needle aspiration from a papillary thyroid carcinoma. These lesions typically contain papillary cell clusters. The characteristic diagnostic features are nuclear changes, which most commonly include nuclear inclusions or, as in this case, nuclear grooves. (Photo courtesy of Christopher M. Zahn, MD.)

ship, 1965). The use of radioactive iodine must be delayed until after delivery of the fetus or it will destroy the fetal thyroid gland.

Although many retrospective reviews have failed to demonstrate any negative effects from pregnancy prior to, during, or following the diagnosis of thyroid cancer, Rosen and Walfish (1986) reported that pregnancy increased the incidence of thyroid cancer as well as accelerated the growth of these neoplasms. Hod and associates (1989) expressed similar concerns in their review of thyroid cancer in pregnancy. At present, due to the rarity of this cancer in pregnancy, the true effect of pregnancy on the natural history of thyroid cancer remains unknown. However, the diagnostic and therapeutic principles used for the non-pregnant patient should be maintained in the pregnant patient with the exception of the use of radioactive isotopes.

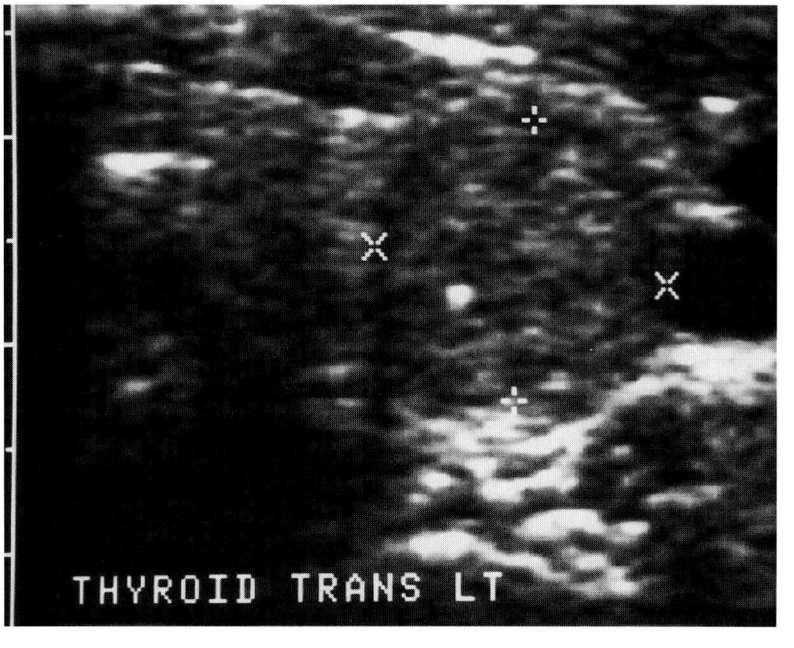

Figure 27–11. Sonograph of a malignant thyroid nodule. This nodule was palpated in a twenty-three-year-old, asymptomatic, pregnant woman at 16 weeks' gestation. Fine needle aspiration of this nodule revealed a papillary adenocarcinoma of the thyroid. Sonograph demonstrates a solid, well defined mass with areas of sonolucency and cystic changes as well as a single calcification. The presence of a surrounding halo; which is typically seen in a benign adenoma, is absent.

Digestive Tract Malignancies

Cancer of the colon or rectum complicates 1 of every 50,000–100,000 pregnancies (Bernstein and associates, 1993; Shushan and co-workers, 1992). Cancers of the stomach, small bowel, liver, and oral mucosa have also been reported but are extremely rare (Ueo and associates, 1991; Davis and Chen, 1991; Sommerville and colleagues, 1991; Woods and co-workers, 1992; Layton and colleagues, 1992). In the pregnant population, the majority of gastrointestinal tract malignancies occur in the rectum, below the peritoneal reflection (Bernstein and associates, 1993). Review of all colorectal cancers diagnosed during pregnancy reveals that approximately two-thirds of these cancers have been found in the rectum (Bernstein and associates, 1993; Shushan and co-workers, 1992). This contrasts with the nonpregnant population, in which only one-third of colorectal cancers are found in the rectum. There is no explanation for this difference.

Most early gastrointestinal tract malignancies are asymptomatic. In more advanced lesions rectal bleeding, constipation, abdominal pain, weight loss, nausea and vomiting, abdominal distention, and diarrhea may be present. Many of these symptoms are attributed to the pregnancy, thus delaying the diagnosis of malignancy (Bernstein and associates, 1993; Shushan and colleagues, 1992; Ueo and associates, 1991; Davis and Chen, 1991; Sommerville and colleagues, 1991; Woods and co-workers, 1992; Layton and colleagues, 1992). This accounts for the observations that gastrointestinal tract malignancies diagnosed during pregnancy are generally more advanced than those diagnosed in nonpregnant women. The majority of these malignancies are first detected at the time of rectal exam during pregnancy or early labor (Bernstein and co-workers, 1993). Definite diagnosis is generally made by endoscopically directed biopsy of suspicious mucosal lesions.

As with most solid tumors, curative therapy involves surgical resection of the tumor with clear margins (McClean and colleagues, 1955). When the tumor has spread to regional lymph nodes or distally, cure is seldom achieved (Bernstein and associates, 1993; Shushan and co-workers, 1992; McClean and colleagues, 1955). Because of these facts, pregnancy should not delay the surgical therapy of early disease unless fetal maturity is imminent. Pelvic tumors may create dystocia, in which case cesarean section followed by bowel resection may be appropriate (Mengert, 1935). If vaginal delivery is possible, delay of the cancer surgery for several days to allow involution of the uterus is preferred (Bernstein and associates, 1993). With advanced disease, the goal of therapy is palliation. In such cases surgical intervention prior to delivery should be restricted to diverting procedures to relieve bowel obstruction. Radiation and/or cytotoxic chemotherapy are so ineffective in these patients that their potential benefits do not justify the risks to the fetus. Because of the high incidence of ovarian metastasis in colon cancer, some surgeons recommend bilateral ovarian biopsies at the time of colon resection (Bernstein and associates, 1993). If ovarian metastasis are identified, bilateral salpingo-oophorectomy is performed. Other authors recommend oophorectomy for all low-lying colon tumors regardless of the presence of metastatic disease; however, there is no evidence that this practice improves survival (Bernstein and associates, 1993; Shushan and co-workers, 1992; Ueo and colleagues, 1991; Davis and Chen, 1991; Sommerville and associates, 1991; Woods and co-workers, 1992; Layton and colleagues, 1992; McClean, 1955; Mengert, 1935; O'Leary and Bebko, 1962; Green and associates, 1975).

The natural history of these tumors does not appear to be affected by pregnancy, and pregnancy rarely alters approaches to therapy (Bernstein and associates, 1993). The prognosis of patients with gastrointestinal tract malignancies does not appear to be different from that of the nonpregnant patient.

Leukemia

Leukemia complicates only 1 in 75,000 pregnancies (McClain, 1974). This low incidence can be partially explained by the high incidence of infertility in leukemia patients (McClain, 1974). The distribution between acute and chronic leukemia is approximately equal. Of the acute leukemias, the nonlymphocytic type predominates.

Acute leukemia is a rapidly progressive disease causing pancytopenia, bleeding, sepsis, bone pain, and splenomegaly. Untreated, death generally occurs within months of diagnosis. The chronic leukemias have a more indolent course with similar symptoms. Diagnosis is made by evaluation of peripheral blood smears and bone marrow aspiration.

The primary mode of therapy for all leukemias is multi-agent chemotherapy. In some instances, whole-brain or craniospinal radiation therapy may be required (Catarzarite and Ferguson, 1984; Sutcliffe and Chapman, 1986). Chemotherapy can be administered during pregnancy; however, craniospinal radiation results in unacceptably high radiation exposure to the fetus and must be delayed until after delivery. Although the use of multi-agent chemotherapy in the second and third trimesters of pregnancy has been accomplished without detrimental effects to the fetus, the use of these therapies in the first trimester is associated with a high rate of fetal anomalies (Catarizarite and Ferguson, 1984). In acute leukemia, where short delays in therapy can be associated with maternal death, treatment should be initiated emergently regardless of gestational age. When chemotherapy has been initiated in the first trimester, consideration of therapeutic abortion should be given after the mother's condition has been stabilized. In chronic leukemia, treatment can often be delayed until delivery or until the gestation has reached a safer age to begin chemotherapy.

The natural history and prognosis of leukemia does not appear to be altered by pregnancy (McClain, 1974; Catarzarite and Ferguson, 1984; Sutcliffe and Chapman, 1986; O'Dell, 1979). Leukemia is one of the few malignancies that has been found to metastasize to the products of conception (Potter and Schoeneman, 1970).

Lymphoma

The incidence of lymphoma in pregnancy is 1 in 1000–6000 pregnancies; the majority are of the Hodgkin's variety (Jacob and Stringer, 1990). The disease is frequently diagnosed during the evaluation of asymptomatic lymphadenopathy; however, symptoms of night sweats, fever, and weight loss may be present. The diagnosis requires histopathologic evaluation of a lymph node biopsy.

Although in the past staging of the disease required surgical exploration, modern imaging tests have all but eliminated such operations. In the pregnant patient, magnetic resonance imaging can generally provide all the pretreatment evaluation required. In non-Hodgkin's lymphomas, due to the lack of good salvage regimens, primary therapy with multi-agent chemotherapy and in some cases mantle or whole-nodal radiotherapy must be initiated without delay. In the first trimester this results in fetal loss, and in the latter trimesters it may result in significant fetal compromise. In Hodgkin's lymphoma, therapies can often be delayed until a more advanced fetal age or delivery is achieved. When only mantle radiotherapy is required, field modification and shielding will allow the therapy to be delivered with minimal risks to the fetus (Sutcliffe and Chapman, 1986; O'Dell, 1979; Sweet, 1976).

Lymphomas metastatic to the fetus and placenta have been reported; careful inspection of the placenta and the infant after delivery are important (Potter and Schoeneman, 1970; Pollack and associates, 1993). The prognosis of patients with lymphoma does not appear to be altered by pregnancy (Sutcliffe and Chapman, 1986; O'Dell, 1979; Sweet, 1976).

Pheochromocytoma

Although the association of pheochromocytoma and pregnancy is rare, the consequences of these two conditions occurring concurrently can be disastrous (Bakri and co-workers, 1992; Harper and associates, 1989). Owing to similarities in symptoms, the diagnosis of pheochromocytoma may be confused with preeclampsia. Failure to rapidly recognize and treat pheochromocytomas often results in maternal mortality secondary to hypertensive crises. These crises may be precipitated by labor, delivery, anesthesia, or even active fetal movement. The chronic sequelae of pheochromocytoma are manifested as intrauterine growth retardation due to uteroplacental insufficiency. Since the symptoms of pheochromocytoma are similar to those of preeclampsia, the key to diagnosis is a high index of suspicion, particularly for those patients with hypertension prior to 20 weeks' gestation and those with intermittent hypertension (Bakri and co-workers, 1992; Harper and associates, 1989).

The diagnosis of pheochromocytoma is made by the detection of elevated urinary catecholamines. Once the biochemical diagnosis has been made, tumor localization with the use of ultrasonography and magnetic resonance imaging should be performed.

Pharmacologic therapy should be initiated immediately after diagnosis with alpha-adrenergic blocking agents. Definitive surgical therapy depends upon gestational age. Prior to 24 weeks' gestation, the uterus is generally small enough to allow surgical exploration with localization and removal of the tumor. After 24 weeks' gestational age, delay until fetal maturity followed by cesarean section and tumor resection is recommended. In either case, alpha-adrenergic blockade is continued until after resection of the tumor and return of normal urinary catecholamine levels.

SUMMARY

Pregnancy has little to no effect on the natural history, treatment, or prognosis of most malignancies. Pregnancy can significantly alter the ability to diagnose cancers in a timely fashion and may alter therapy. In some circumstances effective treatment may not be compatible with fetal survival. The provider caring for pregnant women must always guard against the natural tendency to attribute maternal symptoms to discomforts of pregnancy. Investigation of these symptoms in a manner similar to the approach in the nonpregnant patient can potentially prevent untoward delays in diagnosis. Likewise, the evaluation of abnormal physical findings should not be delayed because of pregnancy. Once a cancer is diagnosed in pregnancy, a team approach using the skills of many disciplines is generally required to assist the patient through this very difficult physical and emotional time.

REFERENCES

Allen H, Nisker J. Cancer in pregnancy: an overview. In: Allen H, Nisker J, eds. Cancer in Pregnancy—Therapeutic Guidelines. Mount Kisco, NY: Futura, 1986.

Allen HH, Nisker JA. Cancer in pregnancy. Therapeutic guidelines. In: Allen HH, Nisker JA, eds. Cancer in Pregnancy: An Overview. Mount Kisco, NY: Futura, 1988.

Bakri YN, Ingemansson SE, Ali A, Pakrikh S. Pheochromocytoma and pregnancy. Acta Obstet Gynecol Scand 1992; 71:301.

Baltzer J, Regenbrecht ME, Kopcke W, Zander J. Carcinoma of the cervix and pregnancy. Int J Gynecol Obstet 1990; 31:317.

Barclay DL. Surgery of the vulva, perineum and vagina in pregnancy. In: Barber HRK, ed. Surgical Disease in Pregnancy. Philadelphia: Saunders, 1974; 310.

Barnavon Y, Wallack MK. Management of the pregnant patient with carcinoma of the breast. Gynecol and Obstet 1990; 171:347.

Barron W. The pregnant surgical patient: medical evaluation and management. Am Intern Med 1984; 101:683.

Beeley L. Adverse effects of drugs in the first trimester of pregnancy. Clin Obstet and Gynecol 1986; 13:177.

Bernstein MA, Madoff RD, Caushaj PF. Colon and rectal cancer in pregnancy. Dis Colon Rectum 1993; 36:172.

Blatt J, Mulvihill J, Ziegler J. Pregnancy outcomes following cancer chemotherapy. Am J Med. 1980; 69:828.

Booth RT. Ovarian tumors in pregnancy. Obstet Gynecol 1963; 21:189.

Brent R. Irradiation in pregnancy. In: Gerble A, Sciarra J, eds. Gynecology and Obstetrics. New York: Harper and Row, 1981.

Brill A, Forgotson E. Radiation and congenital malformations. Am J Obstet Gynecol 1964; 90:1149.

Burgess SP, Waymont B. Implantation of a cervical carcinoma in an episiotomy site: case report. Br J Obstet Gynaecol 1987; 94:598.

Byrd BF, McGarity WS. The effect of pregnancy on the clinical course of malignant melanoma. South Med J 1954; 47:196.

Cashell AW, Cohen ML. Masculinizing sclerosing stromal tumor of the ovary during pregnancy. Gynecol Oncol 1991; 43:281.

Catarzarite V, Ferguson J. Acute leukemia and pregnancy: a review of management and outcome 1972–1982. Obstet and Gynecol Surv 1984; 39:663.

Choo YC. Invasive squamous carcinoma of the vulva in young patients. Gynecol Oncol 1982; 13:158.

Christman JE, Teng NN, Lebovic GS, Sikic BI. Delivery of a normal infant following cisplatin, vinblastine, and bleomycin (PVB) chemotherapy for malignant teratoma of the ovary during pregnancy. Gynec Oncol 1990; 37:292.

Clark RM. Pregnancy-associated cancer. Cancer 1991a; 68:2490.

Clark RM. Prognosis of breast cancer associated with pregnancy. Br J of Med 1991b; 302:1401.

Collins CG, Barclay DC. Cancer of the vulva and cancer of the vagina in pregnancy. Clin Obstet Gynecol 1972; 6:927.

Committee on Biological Effects of Ionizing Radiation, National Research Council. Other somatic and fetal effects. In: Beir V. Effects of Exposure to Low Levels of Ionizing Radiaton, Washington, DC: National Academy Press, 1990.

Copeland LJ, Saul PB, Sneige N. Cervical adenocarcinoma: tumor implantation in the episiotomy sites of two patients. Gynecol Oncol 1987; 28:230.

Creasman W, Rutledge F, Fletcher G. Carcinoma of

the cervix associated with pregnancy. Obstet Gynecol 1970; 36:495.
Creasman WT, Rutledge F, Smith JP. Carcinoma of the ovary associated with pregnancy. Obstet Gynecol 1971; 38:111.
Cunningham MP, Slaughter DP. Surgical treatment of disease of the thyroid gland in pregnancy. Surg Gynecol Obstet 1970; 131:486.
Davis JL, Chen DM. Gastric carcinoma presenting as an exacerbation of ulcers during pregnancy. J Reprod Med 1991; 36:450.
Dekaben A. Abnormalities in children exposed to x-irradiation during various stages of gestation: tentative time-table of radiation injury to the human fetus. J Nucl Med 1968; 9:471.
Del Priore G, Schink JC, Lurain JR. A two-step approach to the treatment of invasive vulvar cancer in pregnancy. Int J Gynecol Obstet 1992; 39:335.
DiSaia PJ, Creasman WT. Clinical gynecologic oncology. 4th ed. St. Louis, MO: Mosby Year Book, 1993; 435.
Doll D, Ringenberg Q, Yarbro J. Management of cancer in pregnancy. Arch Intern Med 1988; 148:2058.
Doll DC, Ringenberg S, Yarbro JW. Antineoplastic agents and pregnancy. Semin Oncol 1989; 16:337.
Donegan W. Cancer and pregnancy. Cancer 1983; 33:194.
Economos K, Perez VN, Delke I, et al. Abnormal cervical cytology in pregnancy: a 17-year experience. Obstet Gynecol 1993; 81:915.
Elwood JM, Coldman AJ. Previous pregnancy and melanoma prognosis. Cancer 1978; 2:1000.
Farahmand SM, Marchetti DL, Asirwatham JE, Dewey MR. Ovarian endodermal sinus tumor associated with pregnancy: review of the literature. Gynecol Oncol 1991; 41:156.
Frederiksen MC, Casanova L, Schink JC. An elevated maternal serum α-fetoprotein leading to the diagnosis of an immature teratoma. Int J Gynecol Obstet 1991; 35:343.
Fukuda K, Hachisuga T, Sugimori H, Tsuzuku M. Papillary carcinoma of the thyroid occurring during pregnancy. Acta Cytol 1991; 35:725.
Gallenberg MM, Loprinzi CL. Breast cancer and pregnancy, Semin Oncol 1989; 16:369.
George PA, Fortner JG, Pack GT. Melanoma with pregnancy. Cancer 1960; 13:854.
Ghung A, Birabaum S. Ovarian cancer associated with pregnancy. Obstet Gynecol 1973; 41:211.
Goldberg I, Hod M, Katz I, et al. A case of hepatocellular carcinoma in pregnancy detected by routine screening of maternal alpha-feto-protein. Acta Obstet Gynecol Scand 1991; 70:241.
Gonsoulin W, Mason B, Carpenter RJ. Colon cancer in pregnancy with elevated maternal serum α-fetoprotein level at presentation. Am J Obstet Gynecol 1990; 163:1172.
Gordon AN, Jensen R, Jones HW III. Squamous carcinoma of the cervix complicating pregnancy: recurrence in episiotomy after vaginal delivery. Obstet Gynecol 1989; 73:850.
Green LK, Harris RE, Massey FM. Cancer of the colon during pregnancy: a review of the literature and report of a case associated with ulcerative colitis. Obstet Gynecol 1975; 46:480.
Gupta RK, McHutchison AGR, Dowle CS, Simpson JS. Fine-needle aspiration cytodiagnosis of breast masses in pregnant and lactating women and its impact on management. Diagn Cytopathol 1993; 9:156.
Hall EJ. Scientific view of low-level radiation risks. Radiographics 1991; 11:509.
Halmo S, Nisker J, Allen H. Primary ovarian cancer in pregnancy—therapeutic guidelines. Mount Kisco, NY: Futura, 1986; 269.
Hannigan EV. Cervical cancer in pregnancy. Clin Obstet Gynecol 1990; 33:837.
Harper MA, Murnaghan GA, Kennedy L, et al. Phaeochromocytoma in pregnancy. Five cases and a review of the literature. Br J Obstet Gynaecol 1989; 96:594.
Harvey E, Boice J, Honeyman M, et al. Prenatal x-ray exposure and childhood cancer in twins. N Engl J Med 1985; 312:541.
Hathaway W, Bonner JJ. Perinatal Coagulation. Philadelphia: Grune & Stratton, 1978.
Henderson CE, Elia G, Garfinkel D, et al. Platinum chemotherapy during pregnancy for serous cystadenocarcinoma of the ovary. Gynecol Oncol 1993; 49:92.
Hill CS, Clark RL, Wolf M. The effect of subsequent pregnancy on patients with thyroid carcinoma. Surg Gynecol Obstet 1966;122:1219.
Hod M, Sharony R, Friedman S, Ovadia J. Pregnancy and thyroid carcinoma: a review of incidence, course, and prognosis. Obstet Gynecol Surv 1989; 44:774.
Hoffman MS, Cavanagh D, Walter TS, et al. Adenocarcinoma of the endometrium and endometriod carcinoma of the ovary associated with pregnancy. Gynecol Oncol 1989; 32:82.
Hopkins MP, Morley GW. The prognosis and management of cervical cancer associated with pregnancy. Obstet Gynecol 1992; 80:9.
Houghton AN, Flannery J, Viola MV. Malignant melanoma of the skin occurring during pregnancy. Cancer 1981; 48:407.
Jacob JH, Stringer AC. Diagnosis and management of cancer during pregnancy. Semin Perinatol 1990; 14:79.
Johnson VP. Rare causes of elevated maternal serum α-fetoprotein. J Reprod Med 1992; 37:93.
Jolles CJ. Gynecologic cancer associated with pregnancy. Semin Oncol 1989; 16:417.
Jubb ED. Primary ovarian carcinoma in pregnancy. Am J Obstet Gynecol 1963; 85:345.
Jung MFK, Vadas G, Lotocki R, et al. Tubular

Krukenberg tumor in pregnancy with virilization. Gynecol Oncol 1991;41:81.

Kalter H, Warkany J. Congenital malformations. N Engl J Med 1983; 308:424.

Karler JR, Sterberg LB, Abbott JN. Carcinoma of the endometrium coexisting with pregnancy. Obstet Gynecol 1972; 40:334.

Kereiakes JG, Rosenstein M. Handbook of Radiation Doses in Nuclear Medicine and Diagnostic X-ray. Boca Raton, FL: CRC Press, 1980.

Kier R, McCarthy SM, Scoutt LM, et al. Pelvic masses in pregnancy: MR imaging. Radiology 1990; 176:709.

Kim DS, Moon H, Lee JA. Anticancer drugs during pregnancy: are we able to discard them? Am J Obstet Gynecol 1992; 166:265.

King LA, Nevin PC, Williams PP, Carson LF. Treatment of advanced epithelial ovarian carcinoma in pregnancy with cisplatin-based chemotherapy. Gynecol Oncol 1991; 41:78.

Kinlen L, Achejun F. Diagnostic irradiation, congenital malformations, and spontaneous abortion. Br J Radiol 1968; 41:648.

Kuller JA, Zucker PK, Peng TCC. Vulvar leiomyosarcoma in pregnancy, Am J Obstet Gynecol 1990; 162:164.

Laros R, Alger L. Thromboembolism in pregnancy. In: Depp R, Eschebach D, Sciarra J, eds. Gynecology and Obstetrics, Vol 3. New York: Harper & Row, 1984.

Layton SA, Rintoul M, Avery BS. Oral carcinoma in pregnancy. Br J. Oral Maxillofacial Surg 1992; 161.

Lutz MH, Underwood PB, Rozier JC, Putney FW. Genital malignancy in pregnancy. Am J Obstet Gynecol 1977; 129:536.

Malfetano JH, Goldkrand JW. Cis-platinum combination chemotherapy during pregnancy for advanced epithelial ovarian carcinoma. Obstet Gynecol 1990; 75:545.

McClain C. Leukemia in pregnancy. Clin Obstet Gynecol 1974; 17:185.

McClean DW, Arminski TW, Bradley GT. Management of primary carcinoma of the rectum diagnosed during pregnancy. Am J Surg 1955; 90:816.

Mengert WF. Dystocia due to carcinoma of the rectum and of the vagina. Am J Obstet Gynecol 1935; 26:451.

Mole R. Radiation effects on prenatal development and their radiologic significance. Br J Radiol 1979; 52:89.

Monk BJ, Montz FJ. Invasive cervical cancer complicating intrauterine pregnancy: treatment with radical hysterectomy. Obstet Gynecol 1992; 80:199.

Moore DH, Fowler WC, Currie JL, Walton LA. Squamous cell carcinoma of the vulva in pregnancy. Gyncol Oncol 1991; 41:74.

Moore JL, Martin JN. Cancer and pregnancy. Obstet Gynecol Clin North Am 1992; 19:815.

Munnell E. Primary ovarian cancer associated with pregnancy. Clin Obstet Gynecol 1963; 6:983.

Nisker J, Allen H. Carcinoma of the cervix in pregnancy; In: Allen H, Nisker J, eds. Cancer in Pregnancy—Therapeutic Guidelines. Mount Kisco, NY: Futura, 1986.

Novotny DB, Maygarden SJ, Shermer RW, Frable WJ. Fine needle aspiration of benign and malignant breast masses associated with pregnancy. Acta Cytol 1991; 35:676.

O'Dell R. Leukemia and lymphoma complicating pregnancy. Clin Obstet Gyncol 1979; 22:859.

O'Leary JA, Bebko FJ Jr. Rectal carcinoma and pregnancy. Am J Obstet Gynecol 1962; 84:459.

Ojomo EO, Ezimokhai M, Reale FR, Nwabineli NJ. Recurrent postpartum hemorrhage caused by endometrial carcinoma co-existing with endometrioid carcinoma of the ovary in a full term pregnancy. Br J Obstet Gynaecol 1993; 100:489.

Pack GT, Schvnayel IM. The prognosis for malignant melanoma in the pregnant woman. Cancer 1951; 4:321.

Paulson RJ, Sauer MV, Lobo RA. Pregnancy after in vitro fertilization in a patient with stage I endometrial carcinoma treated with progestins. Fertil Steril 1990; 54:735.

Petrek JA, Dukoff R, Rogatko A. Prognosis of pregnancy-associated breast cancer. Cancer 1991; 67:869.

Pollack RN, Sklarin NT, Rao S, Divon MY. Metastatic placental lymphoma associated with maternal human immunodeficiency virus infection. Obstet Gynecol 1993; 81:856.

Potter J, Schoeneman M. Metastasis of maternal cancer to the placenta and fetus. Cancer 1970; 25:380.

Powell JL, Johnson NA, Bailey CL, Otis CN. Management of advanced juvenile granulosa cell tumor of the ovary. Gynecol Oncol 1993; 48:119.

Pritchard J, MacDonald P, Gant N. Maternal adaption to pregnancy. In: Pritchard J, MacDonald P, Gant N, eds. Williams Obstetrics. 1st ed. Norwalk, CT: Appleton-Century-Crofts, 1985.

Rasmussen KL, Jensen ML, Nielsen KM, Velander G. Small cell carcinoma of the ovary diagnosed in early pregnancy. Acta Obstet Gynecol Scand 1991; 70:377.

Rosen BR, Walfish PG. Pregnancy and surgical thyroid disease. Surgery 1985; 98:1135.

Rosen BR, Walfish PG. Pregnancy as a predisposing factor in thyroid neoplasia. Arch Surg. 1986; 121:1287.

Rosvoll RV, Winship T. Thyroid carcinoma and pregnancy. Surg Gynecol Obstet 1965; 121:1038.

Sachs BP, Penzias AS, Brown DAJ, et al. Cancer-related maternal mortality in Massachusetts, 1954–1985. Gynecol Oncol 1990; 36:395.

Sandstrom RE, Welch WR, Green TH. Adenocarcinoma of the endometrium in pregnancy, Obstet Gynecol. 1979; 53(suppl):73.

Saunders CM, Baum M. Breast cancer and pregnancy: a review. J Soc Med 1993; 86:162.
Schlono P, Chung C, Myrianthopoulos N. Preconception radiation, intrauterine diagnostic radiation, and childhood neoplasia. J Natl Cancer Inst 1980; 65:681.
Schnider S, Webster G. Maternal and fetal hazards of surgery during pregnancy. Am J Obstet and Gynecol 1965; 92:891.
Schumann EA. Observations upon the coexistence of carcinoma fundus uteri and pregnancy. Trans Am Gynecol Soc 1927; 52:245.
Shaves M, Kamps RR, Laufman LR, Runowicz CD. A successful term pregnancy following the systemic and intraperitoneal administration of cisplatin chemotherapy. Gynecol Oncol 1990; 39:378.
Shushan A, Stemmer SM, Reubinoff BE, et al. Carcinoma of the colon during pregnancy. Obstet and Gynecol Surv. 1992; 47:222.
Sivanesaratnam V, Jayalakshmi P, Loo C. Surgical management of early invasive cancer of the cervix associated with pregnancy. Gynecol Oncol 1993; 48:68.
Slingluff CL Jr, Reintgen DS, Vollmer RT, Seigler HF. Malignant melanoma arising during pregnancy. Ann Surg 1990; 211:552.
Slingluff CL Jr, Seigler HF. Malignant melanoma and pregnancy. Ann Plast Surg 1992; 28:95.
Smith RS, Randal P. Melanoma during pregnancy. Obstet Gynecol 1969; 34:825.
Sommerville M, Koonings PP, Curtin JP, d'Ablaing G. Gastrointestinal signet ring carcinoma metastatic to the cervix during pregnancy. J Reprod Med 1991; 36:813.
Sutcliffe S, Chapman R. Lymphomas and leukemias. In Allen H, Nisker J, eds. Cancer in Pregnancy—Therapeutic Guidelines, Mount Kisco, NY: Futura, 1986; 135.
Sutcliffe S. Treatment of neoplastic disease during pregnancy: maternal and fetal effects. Clin Invest Med 1985; 8:333.
Suzuki A, Konishi I, Okamura H, Nakashima N. A case of grade II adenocarcinoma of the endometrium in pregnancy. Gynecol Oncol 1984; 18:261.
Sweet D, Kinzie J. Consequences of radiotherapy and antineoplastic therapy for the fetus. J Reprod Med 1976; 17:241.
Sweet D. Malignant lymphoma: implications during the reproductive years and pregnancy. J Reprod Med. 1976; 17:198.
Theriault RL, Stallings CB, Buzdar AU. Pregnancy and breast cancer: clinical and legal issues. Am J Clin Oncol 1992; 15:535.
Timothy A. Radiation and pregnancy. In: Allen H, Nisker J, eds. Cancer in Pregnancy—Therapeutic Guidelines. Mount Kisco, NY: Futura, 1986.
Tretli S, Kualheim G, Thoreson S, et al. Survival of breast cancer patients diagnosed during pregnancy or lactation. Br J Cancer 1988; 58:382.
Ueo H, Matsuoka H, Tamura S, et al. Prognosis in gastric cancer associated with pregnancy. World J Surg 1991; 15:293.
van der Zee AGJ, de Bruijn HWA, Bouma J, et al. Endodermal sinus tumor of the ovary during pregnancy. Am J Obstet Gynecol 1991; 164:504.
Velard K. Cardiorespiratory physiology of pregnancy. In: Depp R, Escherbach D, Sciarra J, eds. Gynecology and Obstetrics, Vol 3. New York: Harper and Row, 1984.
Willemse PHB, Van Der Sijde R, Sleijfer DTH. Combination chemotherapy and radiation for stage IV breast cancer during pregnancy. Gynecol Oncol. 1990; 36:281.
Wong DJ, Strassner HT. Melanoma in pregnancy. Clin Obstet Gynecol 1990; 33:782.
Woods JB, Martin JN Jr, Ingram FH, et al. Pregnancy complicated by carcinoma of the colon above the rectum. Am J Perinatol 1992; 9:102.
Yazigi R, Driscoll SG. Sarcoma complicating pregnancy. Gynecol Oncol. 1986; 25:125.
Zemlickis D, Lishner M, Degendorfer P, et al. Maternal and fetal outcome after invasive cervical cancer in pregnancy. J Clin Oncol. 1991; 9:1956.
Zemlickis D, Lishner M, Degendorfer P, et al. Maternal and fetal outcome after breast cancer in pregnancy. Am J Obstet Gynecol 1992; 166: 781.
Zemlickis D, Lishner M, Degendorfer P, et al. Fetal outcome after in utero exposure to cancer chemotherapy. Arch Intern Med 1992b; 152:573.

CHAPTER 28

Urologic and Gastrointestinal Injuries

Over the last 200 years the morbidity and maternal mortality associated with operative deliveries has been substantially reduced. In particular mortality rates associated with cesarean section have been reduced from nearly 100 percent prior to the turn of the century to about 120/100,000 cesarean births (Sachs and co-workers, 1988). As morbidity and mortality associated with abdominal delivery have decreased, there has been a shift from difficult operative vaginal deliveries to cesarean sections. With this change there has been a substantial reduction in the injuries to the lower urinary tract. The frequency of urologic injuries associated with cesarean section has been studied by a number of investigators. Eisenkop and colleagues (1982) reported their experiences at Los Angeles County/University of Southern California Medical Center over a 5-year period. The incidence of injuries to the bladder and ureter was 0.3 percent and 0.1 percent, respectively. Virtually all bowel injuries associated with childbirth are to the anal sphincter and lower rectum during vaginal deliveries. Bowel injuries during cesarean section are rare.

Risk factors associated with injuries to either the gastrointestinal or urinary tracts are listed in Table 28–1. Those factors that carry the greatest risk include emergent cesarean section, prior abdominal surgery, hemorrhage, and cesarean hysterectomy. Surgeons performing these operative procedures should be aware of risk factors for these injuries. Identification of the woman at risk will permit prompt recognition and repair of injuries to the gastrointestinal and urinary tracts, thus substantially reducing associated morbidity.

UROLOGIC INJURIES

The anatomic and physiologic changes that take place during pregnancy place the urinary tract at greater risk for injury during cesarean section. Elevation of the uterus results in bladder elevation, and uterine dextrorotation brings the left ureter more into the operative field. Furthermore, hydronephrosis characteristic of pregnancy, along with the marked dilation of vessels in the infundibulo-pelvic ligament, place the ureter at greater risk for injury during retroperitoneal dissections and isolation of the infundibulo-pelvic ligament. Great care must be taken during cesarean section to ensure that these structures are not injured. Intraoperative recognition of urinary tract injuries with immediate repair results in very little morbidity (Blandy and colleagues, 1991; Brubaker and Willbanks, 1991; Faricy and co-workers, 1978; Neuman and co-investigators, 1991).

TABLE 28–1. RISK FACTORS FOR UROLOGIC AND GASTROINTESTINAL INJURIES DURING CESAREAN SECTION DELIVERIES

Prior abdominal surgery
Prior pelvic or abdominal infection
Emergent delivery
Dysfunctional labor
Ruptured uterus
Hemorrhage
Cesarean hysterectomy
Malpresentation
Placenta previa
Distended bladder
Extraperitoneal cesarean section
Inadequate retraction or mobilization of bladder
Placenta accreta

From Barclay (1970), Bey and associates (1993), Mickal and colleagues (1969), Plauché and associates (1993), and Yancey and co-workers (1993).

Bladder Injuries

The bladder is the most common nonreproductive organ injured during obstetric events. Eisenkop and colleagues (1982) reported an incidence of cystotomy of 0.2 percent in primary cesarean sections and 0.6 percent of repeat cesarean sections. These injuries can be associated with either blunt or sharp dissection of the bladder flap, extensions of the uterine incision, or uterine rupture (Hsu and colleagues, 1992). Many of these injuries can be prevented with careful dissection and adequate development of the bladder flap prior to making the uterine incision. Fortunately, most injuries are to the dome of the bladder and usually do not involve the trigone. Intraoperative diagnosis can be confirmed by filling the bladder with dilute sterile milk. Once the injury is identified, care is taken to ensure that the injury does not involve the trigone or ureteral orifices. If these structures are clearly separate from the injury, then the cystotomy can be closed in two layers using 3-0 polyglycolic acid suture in a running fashion on the mucosa followed by a second layer of imbricating 2-0 polyglycolic acid suture in an interrupted fashion (Fig. 28–1). If the trigone is involved, great care should be taken not to disrupt the ureteral orifices. If the injury is very close to either ureter, then stents should be placed to maintain ureteral patency. Otherwise, the repair may compromise the ureteral orifices. If bladder lacerations involve one or both ureteral orifices such that proper repair without further ureteral injury or obstruction is impossible, then a ureteroneocystotomy should be performed.

Once the repair is complete, the bladder is filled passively with 250–300 mL of diluted sterile milk. Any site of extravasation is reinforced with imbricating sutures. Postoperatively, the bladder is drained either through a Foley or a suprapubic catheter for 7 days. Morbidity associated with intraoperative recognition of bladder injury and proper repair is negligible. Persistent extravasation of urine will lead to fistula formation. Prolonged drainage minimizes this risk.

Ureteral Injuries

The incidence of ureteral injury complicating cesarean delivery is 0.1 percent, and it is most commonly associated with extension of the uterine incision or attempted control of hemorrhage. The incidence rises to 0.2–0.6 percent when cesarean hysterectomy is performed (Barclay, 1970; Mickal and colleagues, 1969). Diagnosis is confirmed by injecting 5–10 mL of indigocarmine intravenously and observing the ureters for evidence of dye extravasation. It may be 10 minutes or more before the dye can be seen in the bladder or Foley, depending on urine production rate. If a cystotomy is performed, the dye should enter the bladder through both ureteral orifices almost simultaneously. Significant delay in the appearance of dye from one ureter relative to the other may signify a partial obstruction. An alternative to waiting for dye excretion is direct injection of indigocarmine into the ureter (O'Leary and O'Leary, 1968). Repair of ureteral injuries is dependent upon the type of injury and location.

Distal Ureteral Injuries. Crush injuries to the distal ureter and obstructions resulting from suture ligation or ureteral kinking may be alleviated with removal of the clamps or sutures causing the obstruction and placement of a ureteral stent. Stents can be placed either cystoscopically or through a cystotomy incision. Intraoperatively cystotomy is usually more convenient and should be performed in the dome of the bladder. A double-J, 7-French ureteral stent is placed over a guide wire. The guide wire is threaded retrograde through the ureteral orifice to the renal pelvis. The stent is passed up over the wire into the renal pelvis and the guide wire is

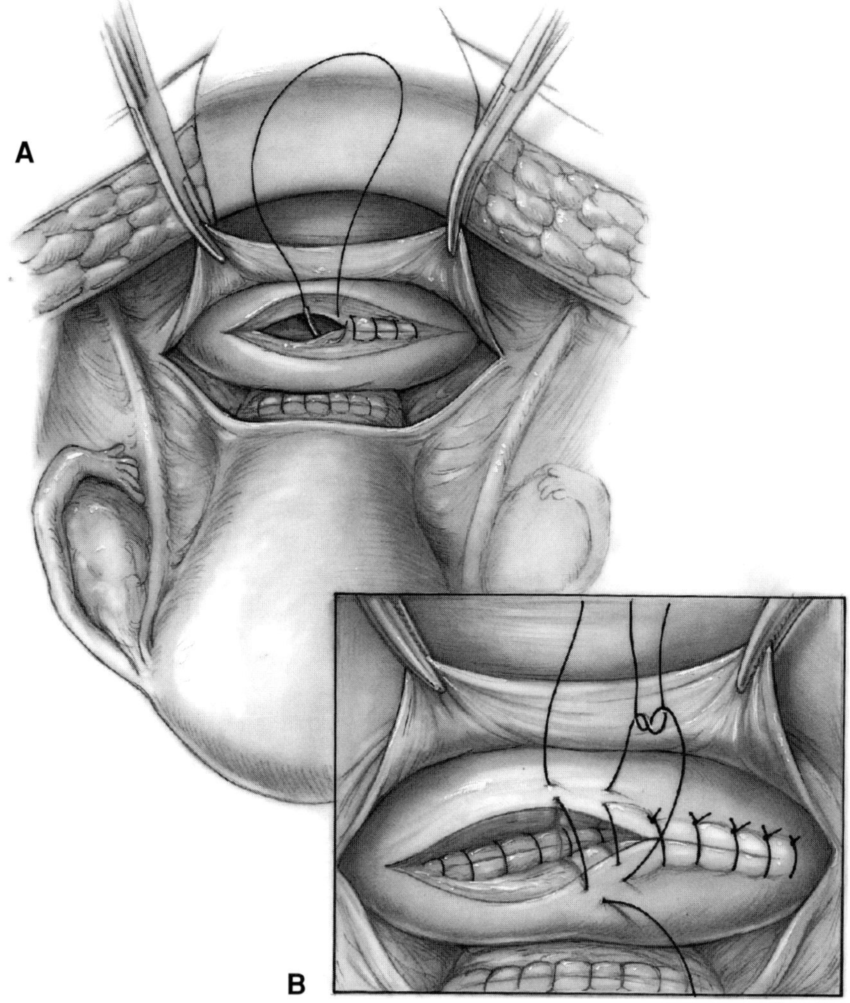

Figure 28–1. Cystotomy repair. **A.** The first layer is a continuous running mucosal suture with a 3-0 absorbable suture. **B.** The second layer is an imbricating interrupted layer of 2-0 absorbable sutures.

removed, allowing the stent to coil in the renal pelvis and the bladder. The cystotomy is then repaired as outlined above. An intraoperative abdominal x-ray will ensure proper placement. Postoperatively, the bladder is drained for 7 days and the ureteral stent can be removed in 3–6 weeks via the cystoscope. Prolonged bladder drainage is not necessary if the stents are placed cystoscopically. Women with injuries resulting in devascularization of the ureter, that is, crush injuries, should undergo intravenous pyelography before stent removal to ensure ureteral integrity.

Injuries to the distal third of the ureter are associated with extensions of the uterine incision and attempts to control blood loss. The left ureter is at greater risk because of its more anterior location with dextrorotation of the uterus during pregnancy. Partial or complete transection of the distal third of the ureter is handled by ureteroneocystostomy (Fig. 28–2). Vascularity of the distal ureter can be tenuous and result in impaired healing. Once the injury is identified, the distal portion of the ureter is ligated and the proximal portion is mobilized sufficiently to perform an anastomosis to the bladder without tension. A suture is placed through the distal portion of the ureter. A vertical cystotomy is performed in the dome of the bladder. A tonsil clamp is placed in the bladder and used to penetrate the bladder wall, the suture is passed to the tonsil clamp, and the ureter is pulled through the bladder wall and fixed to the bladder

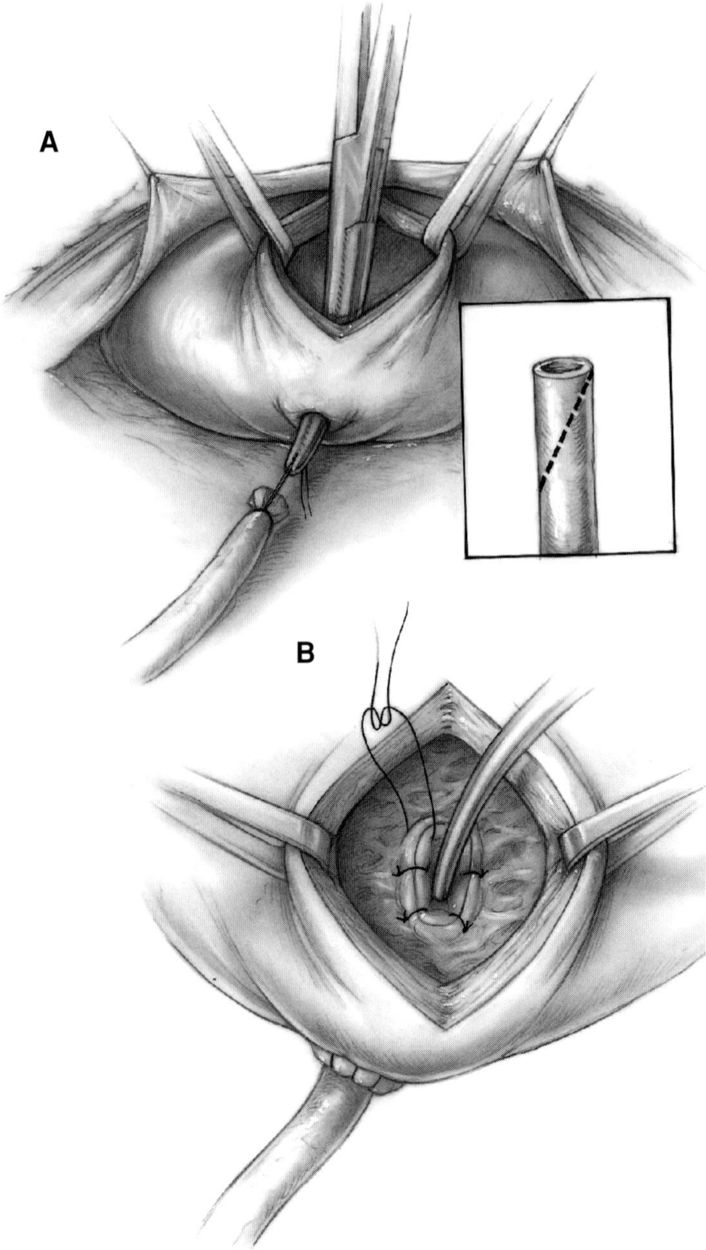

Figure 28–2. Ureteroneocystostomy. After the proximal segment of the transected ureter is mobilized, and the distal segment of ureter is ligated, a cystotomy is performed. **A.** A tonsil clamp is passed through the cystotomy and used to penetrate the wall of the bladder, and the ureter is grasped and pulled through the bladder wall. **B.** 2-0 absorbable sutures are placed on the bladder serosa to fix the ureter in place. The ureter is spatulated. It is then approximated to the bladder mucosa with 4-0 absorbable suture.

serosa with 2-0 polyglycolic acid suture. The ureter is spatulated with a 5-mm longitudinal incision in the distal end. The ureter is sewn to the bladder mucosa with 4-0 polyglycolic acid suture in an interrupted fashion to splay open the ureteral lumen. A ureteral stent is placed as previously described and the cystotomy closed.

Ureteral reflux may be decreased in women who are at risk of urinary infections by tunneling the ureter through the wall of the bladder (Harrow, 1968). This is done for approximately 1–2 cm prior to implanting the ureter into the bladder mucosa. Tunneling the ureter creates a flap valve, which decreases reflux and risk of ascending infections. If the anastomosis appears to be on tension, a psoas hitch is performed by sewing the bladder to the psoas fascia with 3-0 nonreactive permanent suture at a level high enough to provide relaxation of the anastomotic site. Permanent sutures should be placed while the bladder is open to ensure that permanent suture does not penetrate the bladder mucosa and thus provide a risk for stone formation. At the completion of the procedure, a one-way suction drain is placed in the pelvis below the anastomotic site to allow drainage of any urine that may extravasate. The bladder is drained for a minimum of 7 days postoperatively. An intravenous pyelogram is obtained between postoperative day 5 and 10. If there is no evidence of extravasation from bladder or ureter, the pelvic drains can be removed. The ureteral stent may be removed in 3–6 weeks.

Midpelvic Ureteral Injuries. Injuries to the ureter at or above the midpelvis most commonly occur during isolation or transection of the infundibulo-pelvic ligament and are best repaired by uretero-ureterostomy. This is performed by initially placing a ureteral stent. The stent may be placed through a cystotomy incision or the ureterotomy. Placement through the ureterostomy is performed first in a retrograde fashion through the proximal ureter; then the guide wire is removed, allowing the proximal portion of the ureteral stent to coil in the renal pelvis (Barone, 1993). The guide wire is passed through a small hole in the mid portion of the ureteral stent through the inferior portion of the stent and through the distal ureter into the bladder. The stent is advanced into the bladder and the guide wire is removed. The ureter should be spatulated by making a 5-mm longitudinal incision in the proximal and distal ureter. The ureter is approximated with 4-0 polyglycolic acid suture in an interrupted fashion taking care to ensure that the suture line is on an angle relative to the luminal direction of the ureter (Fig. 28–3). If the suture line is directly perpendicular to the lumen, contracture resulting from healing increases the risk of stenosis and obstruction. One-way suction drains should be placed adjacent to the ureter in case of leakage from the anastomosis. Postoperatively the bladder

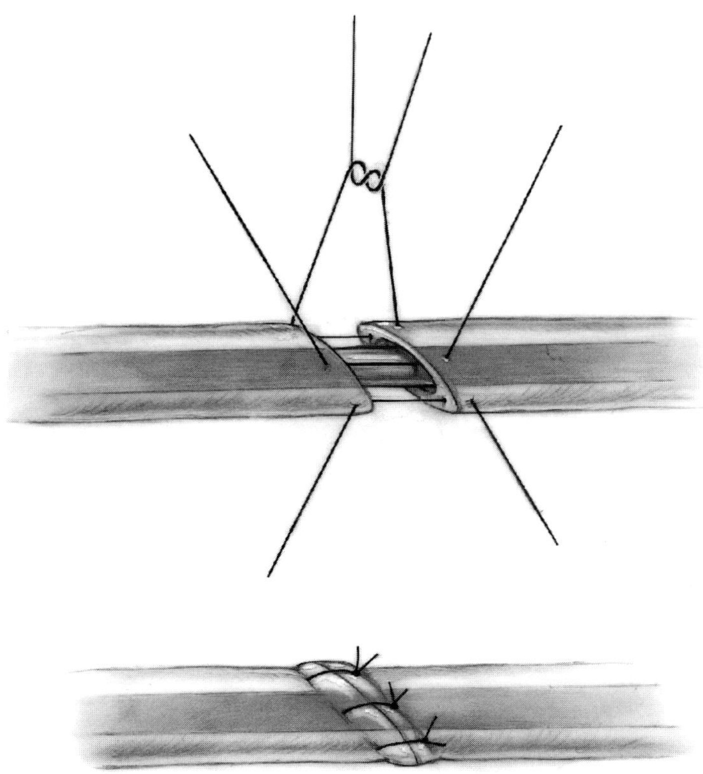

Figure 28–3. Ureteroureterostomy. Transected ureter with a ureteral stent in place, demonstrating spatulation of the proximal and distal ureter with 4-0 absorbable suture approximating the ureter on approximately 45 degree angle to the luminal direction.

is drained for 5–7 days if cystotomy was performed. The drains may be removed if there is less than 15 mL of drainage for 24 hours on 2 consecutive days or if there is no extravasation seen on intravenous pyelography done 7–10 days postoperatively. The ureteral stents should be left in place until the pyelogram is obtained to document patency and integrity of the anastomosis. The ureteral stent can be removed cystoscopically in 3–6 weeks.

In any ureteral repair, care is taken to minimize tension on the anastomotic site. Repair methods such as kidney mobilization, ileal conduit, or transureteroureterostomy are more difficult and carry considerable risks of complications. Therefore, consultation with a urologist should be obtained. Intraoperative consultation should also be considered if there is extensive retroperitoneal fibrosis resulting in difficulty in mobilization of the ureter or there is devascularization of the ureter resulting from retroperitoneal dissection.

Bowel Injuries

Injury to the gastrointestinal tract during cesarean section is uncommon and usually associated with prior abdominal surgery, history of pelvic or abdominal infections, or with cesarean hysterectomy. Diagnosis of bowel injuries is usually quite easy as there is extravasation of bowel contents onto the operative field. Methods of repair are dependent on size, location, and depth of injury. Serosal injuries seldom require repair. Larger serosal injuries may be repaired using 3-0 silk in an imbricating fashion with the suture placed parallel to the lumen of the bowel, with the suture line perpendicular to the luminal direction. These injuries do not require any particular modification in routine postoperative care.

Enterotomies in the small or large bowel that are less than or equal to half the circumference of the bowel can usually be repaired primarily. Injuries encountered prior to delivery of the infant may be marked with a long silk suture and isolated by wrapping the injured segment with a moist laparotomy pack and repaired after delivery. Fine silk sutures should be placed at the angles of the wound such that the direction of the wound is perpendicular to the luminal direction. The wound is repaired with 3-0 silk sutures in an imbricating fashion approximately 3–4 mm apart (Fig. 28–4). These sutures should be placed deep enough to include the muscularis and the lamina propria of the bowel. After repair, the bowel lumen is palpated to evaluate the luminal diameter, which should be at least 2 cm. The anastomotic site is inspected for leaks by placing luminal contents under mild pressure. If there is evidence of extravasation of bowel contents, the area should be reinforced with additional 3-0 silk sutures. Antimicrobial coverage is usually not necessary for small-bowel injuries. Women with large-bowel injuries are given broad-spectrum antimicrobials. Postoperatively, the woman should remain on bowel rest for at least 3 days, after which the diet can be advanced as tolerated.

Larger enterotomies or multiple enterotomies in proximity should be resected. Consultation with a general surgeon or gynecologic oncologist is usually recommended. Bowel resection is accomplished either manually or with intestinal staplers. Surgical staplers are preferable as there is improved blood supply to the anastomosis (Delgado, 1984). This provides for better healing and greater anastomotic luminal diameter, reducing the risk of stenosis and obstruction. Hand sewn end-to-end anastomoses are preferred if the staplers cannot be applied properly or when there is limited mobility of the bowel at the anastomotic site.

Stapler Repair. Intestinal resection and reanastomosis with staplers is usually quick and deceptively easy. Great care should be taken to ensure that the staplers are loaded and functional and properly placed and that no unintended tissue is included in the stapler. First, normal bowel proximal and distal to the injury is identified. A 1-cm defect in the mesentery immediately adjacent to the bowel is created with either blunt dissection or electrocautery. A GIA-60 stapler can be placed through this defect. The surgical stapler is applied such that the staple line is in the same plane as the mesentery. The antimesenteric border should be slightly shorter than the mesenteric side of the transected bowel. This will improve blood supply to the antimesenteric portion. The same procedure is performed distal to the injured bowel. The associated mesentery should be excised in a V-shape connecting the two enterotomies. The mesenteric vessels are

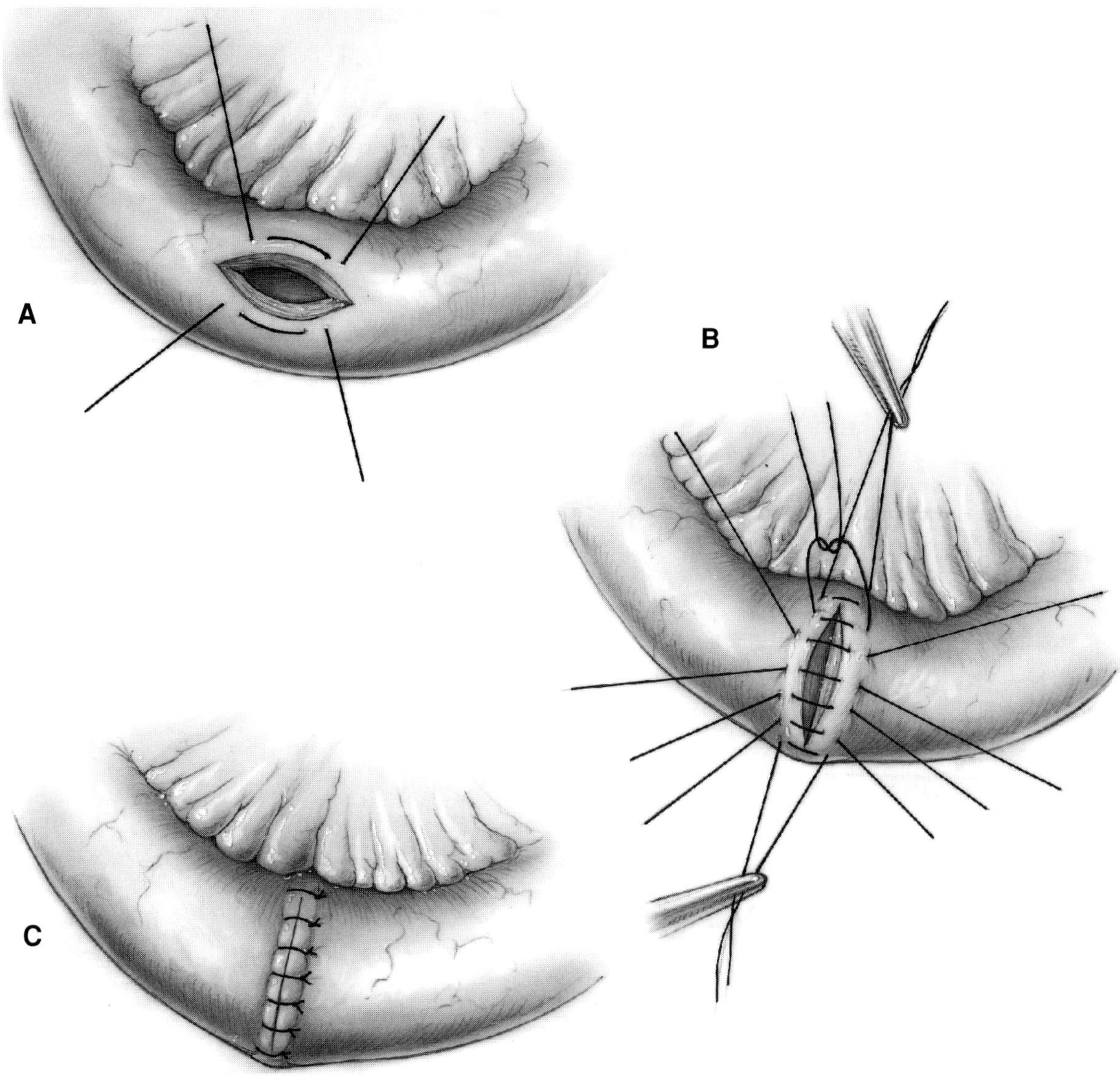

Figure 28–4. Enterotomy repair. **A.** Placement of traction sutures lateral to a longitudinal wound. **B.** Conversion of longitudinal wound to transverse wound with placement of imbricating sutures of 3-0 silk. **C.** Completed enterotomy repair.

ligated with 3-0 silk ties. The staple lines on the bowel are brought adjacent to one another and stay sutures with 3-0 silk placed on the antimesenteric edge to hold the two bowel segments together in parallel. A 1-cm incision is made on the antimesenteric portion of the staple line on both proximal and distal ends of the bowel. A GIA-60 stapler is inserted with one blade in the proximal bowel and one in the distal bowel. The stapler is then closed and fired.

GIA staplers are not intended to provide hemostasis; therefore, the suture line needs to be inspected prior to completing the anastomosis. Electrocautery or pressure may aid in achieving hemostasis. The bowel defect is placed on traction with either Allis clamps or stay sutures and closed with a TA-55 stapler. The defect in the mesentery is closed with 3-0 silk suture in an interrupted fashion to prevent internal hernias. Postoperatively, patients should remain at bowel rest for at least 3 days.

Nasogastric suction can be used if the woman has nausea; however, it is not routinely needed. Once adequate gastrointestinal motility returns, the diet is advanced as tolerated.

Manual Closure. In patients where the bowel is not sufficiently mobile to allow proper application of the surgical staplers, hand-sewn anastomoses are preferable. These are started much the same way as those described for intestinal staplers. A defect is created in the bowel mesentery at a site where there is healthy bowel remaining and requiring the least amount of resection possible. Intestinal clamps—Dennis or Allen clamps—may be applied to prevent spillage of gastrointestinal contents. The damaged section of bowel is resected and the open ends of the bowel are brought into proximity. A single-layer anastomosis can be started by placing traction sutures at the mesenteric and antimesenteric borders, which include both the proximal and distal bowel segment. This will maintain proper bowel alignment for the procedure. The crushed segment of bowel is partially excised. The internal or posterior suture line is placed using 3-0 or 2-0 permanent sutures in a horizontal mattress fashion at approximately 5-mm distances (Fig. 28–5). The intervening portion of the bowel can be oversewn with 3-0 or 2-0 permanent sutures in a figure-of-eight fashion. These sutures will provide a watertight seal and reduce the ridge created by the suture line (Barnes, 1974). Attention is then turned to the anterior suture line. This can be closed with Halsted sutures at approximately 5-mm intervals with Lembert sutures between the Halsted sutures. The middle sutures of the anterior and posterior suture line are left long to be used as traction sutures. Once the anterior and posterior rows of sutures are placed, the axis of traction is rotated 90 degrees. This will allow placement of the sutures at the mesenteric and the antimesenteric portions of the bowel, which are closed in the similar fashion. The mesentery is closed with 3-0 silk suture in an interrupted fashion. The anastomosis is examined for adequacy of luminal diameter and leaks. The abdomen is well irrigated at the completion of bowel surgery to minimize risk of infection. Postoperatively, patients should remain at bowel rest for at least 3 days, or preferably until their ileus resolves. This minimizes abdominal distention and pressure on the suture lines. Nasogastric suction is necessary only for those women who demonstrate persistent ileus that causes significant distention or nausea and vomiting.

Colon Injuries. Large-bowel injury incurred during cesarean section can be handled in much the same way as injuries to the small bowel, with one major difference. If there is evidence of ischemia, inflammation, or tension on the suture line, diverting colostomy must be considered. This ensures adequate healing of the injured bowel and minimizes the risk of spillage of fecal material into the peritoneal cavity. A loop colostomy is preferable because it is the simplest to close. The transverse colon is frequently sufficiently mobile to perform a loop colostomy. Occasionally, the descending colon is used. Mobilizing the descending colon to the splenic flexure requires incising the peritoneum of the pericolic recess from the pelvic brim to the spleen. The descending colon is retracted medially and the retroperitoneal areolar tissue is bluntly or sharply dissected. Once the bowel is adequately mobilized, a suitable location for the colostomy is selected and grasped with a Kocher clamp. Most commonly, a site in the left upper quadrant at or above the umbilicus and medial to the nipple line is used. This site will ensure that the appliance will be on a flat surface above the belt-line and easily visualized by the patient, allowing her to care for the colostomy. Once the Kocher clamp is applied, the skin is elevated and a scalpel is used to excise a circular portion of skin 3 cm in diameter. The incision is carried down in a circular fashion to the fascial level with electrocautery. The fascia is incised in either a vertical or circular fashion with a diameter of approximately 3 cm. Circular fascial incisions reduce stress points and risk of peristomal hernias. The peritoneum is entered. A suitable section of colon is identified that is sufficiently mobile to allow eversion of the loop colostomy. A defect in the mesentery just below the bowel is created. A half-inch Penrose drain can be placed through the mesenteric defect and used to deliver the colon loop through the colostomy wound.

The proximal and distal colon are fixed to the anterior abdominal wall with 2-0 silk suture. The primary abdominal wound can be closed. Once completed, the loop colostomy can either be opened and matured primarily or

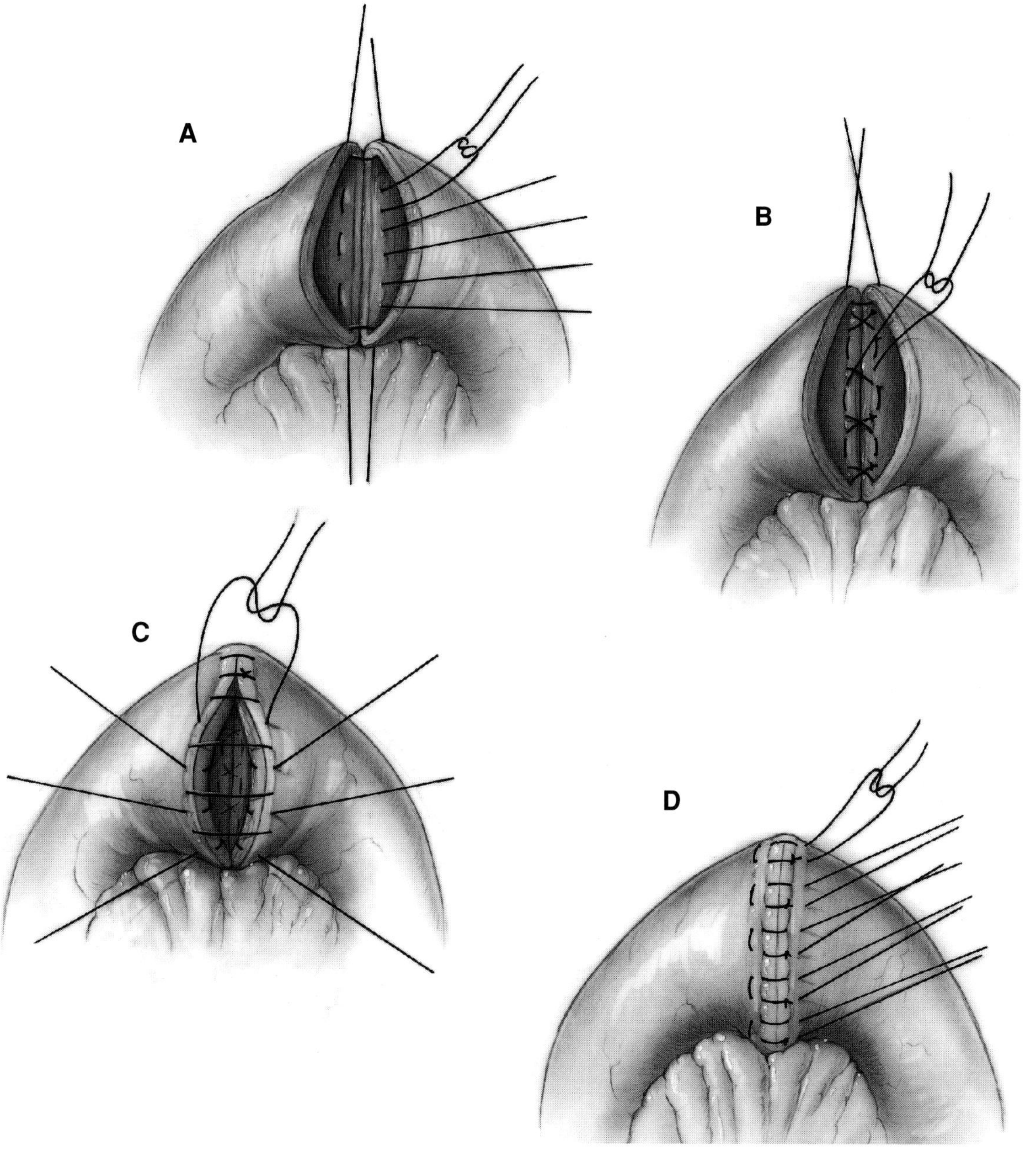

Figure 28–5. A. Intestinal lumens are approximated and the posterior anastomosis is performed with horizontal mattress sutures approximately 0.5 cm apart. **B.** Figure-of-eight sutures are placed between the horizontal mattress sutures to complete the posterior wall closure. **C.** The anterior wall is then closed with vertical Connell sutures. **D.** Halsted sutures are placed to complete the anastomosis of the anterior wall.

may be secured with a loop colostomy bar and opened on the first or second postoperative day with electrocautery. To mature the colostomy at the time of placement, a linear incision is made along the taeniae coli for approximately 3–4 cm. The bowel mucosa can be everted and sewn to the skin with 3-0 polyglycolic acid suture and an appliance applied. Postoperatively, consultation with an enterostomal therapist should be obtained to instruct the woman in proper care of her colostomy. The enterostomal therapist is a resource who is tremendously helpful and frequently overlooked. Early participation by the therapist helps alleviate patient fears and concerns, aids proper healing, and minimizes the risk for infection and postoperative complications. The diet is advanced as tolerated after colostomy and the colostomy bar can be removed on postoperative day 7–10.

The loop colostomy can be taken down in 3–6 months. A barium enema should be performed preoperatively to evaluate the anastomosis for stenosis and fistulas. The loop colostomy can be taken down by excising the mucocutaneous junction and the colostomy is mobilized. The mucocutaneous junction is excised from the colostomy to leave healthy bowel edges. The defect in the colon is approximated using TA-55 staplers or hand-sewn with 2-0 silk suture. The bowel is allowed to fall into the abdomen. The fascial defect is closed with permanent monofilament sutures. The skin wound should be packed for several days until healthy granulation tissue is apparent. Delayed closure minimizes the risk of infection. Postoperatively the patient remains at bowel rest for 1–2 days, and then the diet is advanced as tolerated. Intestinal motility is usually quick to return after colostomy closure.

SUMMARY

Urologic and gastrointestinal injuries are infrequent occurences during obstetrical surgical procedures. The most frequent injuries involve the urinary bladder and occur during cesarean section. When suspected the full extent of the injury should be defined, using sterile milk or instillation of dye if necessary. A layered repair without tension on the suture line should be performed, following which the repair should be tested to ensure that it is water-tight. The bladder should then be decompressed by catheterization to facilitate healing. Suspected injuries to the ureters should be completely evaluated intraoperatively, usually with the assistance of a urologist. Small bowel partial thickness injuries and full thickness injuries involving less than half the bowel circumference can usually be repaired primarily. Colon injuries and more extensive injuries to the small bowel justify consultation with a general surgeon.

REFERENCES

Barclay DL. Cesarean hysterectomy—Thirty years' experience. Obstet Gynecol 1970; 35:120.

Barnes JP. The techniques for end-to-end intestinal anastomosis. Surg Gynecol Obstet 1974; 138:433.

Barone JG, Vates TS, Vasselli AJ. A simple technique for intraoperatively stenting a transected ureter. Urology 1993; 149:535.

Bey MA, Pastorek JG II, Lu PY, et al. Comparison of morbidity in cesarean section hysterectomy versus cesarean section tubal ligation. Surg Gynecol Obstet 1993; 177:357.

Blandy JP, Bedenoch DF, Fowler CG, et al. Early repair of iatrogenic injury to the ureter or bladder after gynecological surgery. Urology 1991; 146:761.

Brubaker LT, Wilbanks GD. Urinary tract injuries in pelvic surgery. Surg Clin North Am 1991; 71:963.

Delgado G. The automatic staple versus the conventional gastrointestinal anastomosis in gynecological malignancies. Gynecol Oncol 1984; 18:293.

Eisenkop SM, Richman R, Platt LD, Paul RH. Urinary tract injury during cesarean section. Obstet Gynecol 1982; 60(5):591.

Faricy PO, Augspurger RR, Kaufman JM. Bladder injuries associated with cesarean section. Urology 1978; 120:762.

Harrow BR. A neglected maneuver for ureterovesical reimplantation following injury at gynecologic operations. Urology 1968; 100:280.

Hoch WH, Kursh ED, Persky L. Early, aggressive management of intraoperative ureteral injuries. Urology 1975; 114:530.

Hsu CD, Chen S, Feng TI, Johnson TR. Rupture of uterine scar with extensive maternal bladder laceration after cocaine abuse. Am J Obstet Gynecol 1992; 167:129.

Mickal A, Begneaud WP, Hawes TP, eds: Pitfalls and complications of cesarean section hysterectomy. Clin Obstet Gynecol 1969; 12:660.

Neuman M, Eidelman A, Langer R. Iatrogenic injuries to the ureter during gynecologic and obstetric operations. Surg Gynecol Obstet 1991; 173:268.

O'Leary JL, O'Leary JA. A simplified method of determining ureteral patency at operation. Am J Obstet Gynecol 1968; 101:271.

Plauché WC, Wycheck JG, Iannessa MJF, et al. Cesarean hysterectomy at Louisiana State University, 1975 through 1981. South Med J 1983; 76:1261.

Sachs BP, Yeh J, Acker D, et al. Cesarean section-related maternal mortality in Massachusetts, 1954–1985. Obstet Gynecol 1988; 71:385.

Yancey MK, Harlass FE, Benson, W, Brady K. The perioperative morbidity of scheduled cesarean hysterectomy. Obstet Gynecol 1993; 81:206.

CHAPTER 29

Diagnostic and Operative Laparoscopy

Acute surgical emergencies complicate between 0.5 and 1.0 percent of pregnancies (Barber and Graber, 1974; Barron, 1983). Pregnant women are susceptible to the same surgical maladies as their nonpregnant counterparts, and often even normal pregnancy is accompanied by a number of symptoms that may mimic the early phases of development of these acute abdominal surgical disorders. Laparoscopy often can provide the definitive diagnosis and may afford treatment for a number of these conditions, including acute appendicitis, acute cholecystitis, torsion or rupture of an adnexal mass such as a hemorrhagic corpus luteum, and perforation of a viscus such as might occur with peptic ulcer disease or colonic diverticular disease.

One of the diagnostic challenges of pregnancy is the nonlocalized or poorly localized nature of the pain, which is often found either diffusely throughout the abdomen or generalized to the lower abdomen. Awareness of the maternal physiologic and anatomic changes of pregnancy and how they may alter the clinical presentation of intraabdominal disease processes is of paramount importance. For instance, during pregnancy acute appendicitis may be difficult to differentiate from acute cholecystitis. Indeed, in the late third trimester, the appendix is usually displaced sufficiently cephalad so as to lie in juxtaposition with the gall bladder. Timely diagnosis and appropriate operative intervention are key management issues; the most serious error made in caring for pregnant women with intraabdominal disease processes is unnecessary delay in performance of surgery. Delay increases both maternal and fetal morbidity.

ADVANTAGES

Laparoscopy offers several advantages over traditional laparotomy (Soper and associates, 1994), including better and more complete visualization, especially with small incisions or in the obese patient in whom exposure is a problem. Although the incisions made for laparoscopy are often multiple, even in the aggregate, they and the resulting scar are smaller and less painful than those of laparotomy. Total operative time for laparoscopic procedures is less, and postoperative convalescence is reduced (Wolf, 1991; Azziz, 1989; and their colleagues). Other advantages include minimal use of post-operative analgesia and a reduced risk of atelectasis from postoperative hypoventilation. Patients are able to ingest a regular diet on the day of surgery and are usually discharged within 24 hours. Laparoscopy allows earlier ambulation, which decreases the risk of thromboembolic disease, particularly in pregnancy (Talbert, 1964). De novo adhesion formation is less likely, and brief hospital stays

TABLE 29–1. RELATIVE CONTRAINDICATION TO LAPAROSCOPY IN PREGNANCY

Access issues
Late second or third trimester
Advanced disease process, eg, walled-off abscess
Retrocecal location of appendix
Medical complications
Intraabdominal sepsis
Bleeding disorders
Ileus

may translate into considerable economic gains (Lundorff and co-workers, 1991; Levine, 1985; Chung and Broughan, 1992).

CONTRAINDICATIONS

Contraindications for a laparoscopic diagnosis and removal of either a diseased appendix or gallbladder during pregnancy are usually secondary to the patient's clinical status and gestational age. The gestational age at which the uterus would limit closed laparoscopic access to the abdominal cavity is of concern and remains controversial. Contraindications to endoscopic surgery include advanced disease, intraabdominal sepsis, retrocecal or walled-off perforated appendix, ileus, severe bleeding disorders, and late second or third trimester pregnancies. Neither absolute nor relative contraindications are fixed, but rather are subject to continuous updating as additional experience accumulates and is reported (Table 29–1).

PREGNANCY-SPECIFIC CONSIDERATIONS

Initial Evaluation

A thorough history and physical examination of the pregnant patient, both at initial presentation and often longitudinally across time, serve as the foundation for evaluation of apparent intraabdominal surgical problems (Hampton and associates, 1975). The antenatal history should emphasize medical complications (eg, cardiac disease, diabetes mellitus) and prior surgical procedures. Pertinent laboratory analysis should be performed, with results adjusted to reflect the normative values of pregnancy (Table 29–2). Preoperative assessment by ultrasound for fetal viability and lethal anomalies is desirable if time and resources allow. If there is vaginal bleeding, finding the source is given high priority, especially placental location and exclusion of placenta previa or abruptio.

Timing of Surgery

The optimal time for intraabdominal surgery is the early second trimester. This timing avoids the higher incidence of spontaneous abortion seen during the first trimester and the preterm labor seen more commonly in the late second and third trimesters. Operative field exposure is also excellent and not yet compromised by encroachment of the gravid uterus into the mid and upper abdominal quadrants with both displacement and crowding of the bowel and other intraabdominal contents.

Fetal Considerations

Anesthetic Risk

The intraabdominal process itself often represents a very real risk to the well-being of the pregnancy; however, the risk of the anesthetic, whether conduction or general, appears to be nil. Early reports that general anesthesia was associated with spontaneous abortion with first trimester exposure failed to control for the intraabdominal surgical disease process per se or for its severity (Knill-Jones and colleagues, 1975). If extensive uterine manipulation or upper abdominal exploration is anticipated, a general anesthetic is perferred both for its superior uterine relaxant properties and for maternal comfort and safety. Enflurane, isoflurane, and halothane all possess excellent myometrial muscle relaxant properties.

Teratogenic Risk

Carbon dioxide (CO_2) is the gas most often selected to establish a pneumoperitoneum for endoscopic procedures. Studies on the possible adverse effects of excessive exposure are few and do not adequately model the exposure seen with laparoscopy. Cardiac anomalies have been reported in pregnant rats exposed to 3 percent carbon dioxide and dental defects with exposures to as high as 30 percent ambient carbon dioxide (Haring, 1960: King and coworkers, 1962). Vertebral anomalies in the offspring of rabbits exposed to 8 percent ambient

TABLE 29–2. LABORATORY ALTERATIONS IN PREGNANCY

Laboratory Tests	Normal Values	
	Nonpregnant	*Pregnant*
Total protein (g/dL)	6.5–8.6	85% of NL
Total bilirubin (mg/dL)	0.1–1.2	Unchanged
Serum albumin (g/dL)	3.5–5.0	2.5–4.5
Blood urea nitrogen (mg/dL)	10–25	5-15
Serum creatinine (mg/dL)	0.8	0.6
Glucose (mg/dL)	70–110	65–100
Serum calcium (mEq/L)	4.6–5.5	4.2–5.2
Serum phosphate (mg/dL)	2.5–4.8	2.3–4.6
Alkaline phosphatase (IU/L)	35–48	35–150
Cholesterol (mg/dL)	120–290	177–345
Triglycerides (mg/dL)	33–166	130–400
Serum iron	50–110 μg/dL	30–100 μg/dL
Red blood cell count	$4.0–5.2 \times 10^{12}$/L	$3.8–4.4 \times 10^{12}$/L
White blood cell count	$5–10 \times 10^9$/L	$5–14 \times 10^9$/L
Hemoglobin (g/dL)	14 ± 2.0	> 11
Hematocrit (%)	36–41	33
Hemoglobin electrophoresis	> 98% A	Unchanged
	< 3.5%A_2	Unchanged
	< 2% F	Unchanged
Platelets (Plt/L)	$140–440 \times 10^9$	Unchanged
Reticulocyte count	0.5–1.0%	1.0–2.0%
Fibrinogen (mg/dL)	150–300	250–600
Bleeding time (Ivy)	1–5 min	Unchanged

NL = normal.

$C0_2$ for 1–2 days have also been reported (Shepard, 1986). Nitrous oxide administered over 1–2 days at 50 percent concentration has also been associated with increased spontaneous abortions, skeletal deformities, and small for gestational age babies (Pederson and Finster, 1979). However, even the most radical laparoscopic procedures are completed in less than 1 day.

Neonatal Morbidity/Mortality

Counseling patients regarding the potential perioperative increase in fetal morbidity and mortality should be based on institutional-specific outcomes data, if they are available. Prognosis for fetal survival and neonatal outcome requires accurate knowledge of gestational age and fetal weight (Phelan, 1990). Tocolysis may be a consideration for either elective or emergency cases whenever extensive uterine manipulation is likely to occur. Fetal heart rate (FHR) and uterine contraction monitoring can provide objective data not only preoperatively but intra- and postoperatively as well. The use of electronic monitoring should be determined by weighing the extent to which it might impede the surgical procedure against the benefits of therapeutic manipulations that monitoring might indicate. If the fetus is previable and tocolysis is not a consideration, simple documentation of FHR pre- and postoperatively will suffice. If the fetus is viable and a candidate for maximal tocolytic therapy, continuous monitoring of uterine activity might be in order. Similarly, administration of dexamethasone or betamethasone for induction of fetal maturation should be considered (NIH Consensus Panel, 1994). Studies have demonstrated that antenatal steroid treatment of preterm infants reduces the incidence of respiratory distress syndrome, intraventricular hemorrhage, and necrotizing enterocolitis (Liggins and Howie, 1972; Collaborative Group on Antenatal Steroid Therapy, 1981; NIH Consensus Panel, 1994).

Alterations of uteroplacental perfusion secondary to aorto-caval compression from supine hypotension or from increased intraabdominal pressure from gas insufflation at laparoscopy also may be heralded by alteration in the fetal heart rate tracing. Hemodynamic performance of the woman is maximized by the right or left lateral decubitus position. Accordingly, lateral tilt of the operating room table should be used. During endoscopy, the intraabdominal pressure increase seen with development of the pneumoperitoneum should be monitored carefully and limited to the amount necessary to allow adequate visualization and safety because increased intraabdominal pressure may compress the vena cava and elevate resistance to blood flow as well as decrease cardiac output.

PERIOPERATIVE MANAGEMENT

Perioperative management includes documentation and stabilization of vital signs, placement of intravenous lines, and assorted monitoring, which depending on circumstances may include ECG leads, pulse oximetry, and invasive or noninvasive blood pressure monitoring. Complete blood count, type, and screen (and cross-match if blood transfusion is a likely possibility) are also recommended. Serum electrolytes, liver enzymes, urinalysis and urine culture, clotting profile, plasma amylase, and plasma lipase may be indicated depending upon the clinical circumstances (Andres and associates, 1990). Alkaline phosphatase levels are normally elevated in pregnancy and therefore are nonspecific; however, transaminase levels remain in the normal range absent any disease process (Table 29–2).

Antibiotics

Broad-spectrum antibiotic coverage is indicated in many patients based upon clinical presentation alone. In these cases, the antimicrobials selected will depend on the preoperative working diagnosis. Patients without obvious infection but at risk for infection, such as insulin-dependent diabetics and women with heart disease, also should be treated with prophylactic broad-spectrum antibiotics perioperatively (Hemsell, 1991). Although rare, rheumatic heart disease remains the most common cause of "heart disease" worldwide. At-risk patients should receive antibiotics in an effort to prevent bacterial endocarditis. Ampicillin (2 g) plus gentamicin (1.5 mg/kg IV) 30–60 minutes prior to surgery and repeated twice at 8-hour intervals provides adequate coverage. In patients with peritonitis or a perforated viscus, gentamicin (1.0–1.5 mg/kg), clindamycin (1.6–2.5 g), and metronidazole (2.0 g) are recommended intravenously.

Prophylactic Heparin

Prophylactic low-dose heparin is recommended for the morbidly obese or bed confined patient. Depending upon patient size, 5000–8000 units of sodium heparin should be administered at least 1 hour prior to surgery and repeated at 12-hour intervals. Full heparinization may be considered for patients with prior documented pulmonary embolism and/or thrombophlebitis (Hyers and co-workers, 1986). When full heparinization is employed, serial determination of the activated partial thromboplastin time (aPTT) with a goal of approximately one and a half times the control value is used to adjust the heparin dose.

Assessment of Fetal–Maternal Hemorrhage

A Kleihauer-Bethke or similar test is recommended in cases with even minor trauma in order to detect any fetal to maternal bleeding (ACOG TB 148; ACOG TB 161). In the unsensitized Rh negative mother, 300 μg of Rh immune globulin should be administered following any invasive procedures such as abdominal surgery by either laparoscopy or laparotomy. The volume of blood required to produce sensitization is as little as 0.1 mL of Rh-positive erythrocytes (Bowman, 1989).

Anesthesia

Obstetric anesthesia is challenging and fraught with hazards; complications may result in significant maternal morbidity and mortality (Endler and colleagues, 1988). Each anesthetic option has its own unique maternal and fetal risks. The overall mortality rate due to anesthetic complications is approximately 0.6/100,000 live births and usually involves either loss of airway with general anesthetics (Rocke, 1992; May, 1989; Sachs, 1989; Endler, 1988; and their co-workers) or arrhythmias and/or hypotension and shock with conduction anesthesia (Marx, 1984; Marx and Berman, 1985).

General anesthesia is the preferred method for most obstetric surgical emergencies because of its speed and fewer concerns in the event the patient is hypovolemic. Mask anesthesia has no place in the obstetric patient; endotracheal intubation always should be used with general anesthesia to secure the airway. General anesthesia involves a rapid-sequence induction with sodium pentothal or Propofol-Diprivan followed by nitrous oxide (N_2O) and oxygen.

Many anesthesiologists prefer epidural or spinal anesthesia for early to mid second trimester surgery because it reduces the fetus's exposure to the anesthetic agents and other drugs. Although severe complications are rare, spinal and epidural blockade are occasionally associated with paraplegia and arachnoiditis. Post-epidural puncture headache and maternal hypotension from pharmacologic sympathectomy, generally defined as a systolic blood pressure less than 100 mm Hg, occur in 1.4–10 percent of patients (Parnass and Schmidt, 1990; Corke and Spielman, 1985).

Laparoscopy, at least in theory, significantly increases the pregnant patient's risk of aspirating gastric contents. Pregnancy-induced changes include delayed gastric emptying time, decreased esophageal smooth muscle tone, and incompetence of the lower esophageal-gastric sphincter (O'Sullivan and associates, 1987). While each of these physiologic alterations in isolation increases the risk of gastric aspiration during laparoscopy, the risk is accentuated by the pneumoperitoneum and associated increase in intraabdominal pressure.

Administering antacids shortly before induction of anesthesia has dramatically decreased mortality from obstetric anesthesia (Perissat and colleagues, 1990). The use of nonparticulate antacids such as 30 cc of 0.3*M* sodium citrate with citric acid (Bicitra) is suggested to neutralize the acidity of the gastric contents. Gibbs and Banner (1984) reported that Bicitra neutralizes gastric acid in nearly 90 percent of women undergoing cesarean section when prescribed 45 minutes preoperatively. Magnesium hydrochloride also is effective in neutralizing gastric acid but has a short duration of action and is particulate. (Particulate antacids themselves have been shown to cause pneumonitis if aspirated.) Cimetidine, while often given, requires a 60-minute interval when parenterally administered to effectively decrease gastric acidity. Risk of aspiration of gastric contents can be further reduced by nasogastric tube placement soon after induction of anesthesia with emptying of contents immediately upon nasogastric tube placement and prior to extubation.

Pregnant patients who are scheduled for diagnostic or operative laparoscopy should (1) receive nonparticulate antacids as prophylaxis against pulmonary aspiration; (2) undergo rapid-sequence anesthetic induction; (3) have the airway secured with a cuffed endotracheal tube; (4) have monitoring of both the SaO_2 by pulse oximetry, and end tidal CO_2 by capnography to assess adequacy of oxygenation and ventilation.

GENERAL ENDOSCOPIC ABDOMINAL SURGERY

As with any surgical procedure, qualified assistance is essential in order to properly prepare the patient and equipment before surgery, to minimize or prevent complications due to malfunctioning instruments, and to facilitate exposure. Ideally the assistant will be as capable as the surgeon in performing advanced endoscopic procedures.

Diagnostic laparoscopy facilitates the emergent assessment of suspicious intraabdominal signs or symptoms of many illnesses (Table 29–3). Laparoscopy has been particularly valuable in cases of questionable appendicitis: investigators report reductions of 20–40 percent in unnecessary appendectomies and the identification of other diseases requiring alternative therapy (Anteby, 1975; Leape, 1980; Deutsch, 1982; Patterson-Brown, 1986; Reiertsen, 1985; and their colleagues).

Technical limitations of laparoscopy include lessened depth perception, inability to directly palpate tissue, limitation of the number of instruments that can be used simultaneously, restriction of the angles available to approach the surgical field, and increased distance between the surgical field and the surgeons' hands. This increased distance intensifies motion, which makes fine movements more arduous. Laparoscopy has a complication rate of less than 3 percent and a mortality rate of 0.1/1000 procedures (Chamberlain, 1980). Table 29–4 lists the compilations associated with endoscopy. Laparotomy, the traditional approach to evaluate acute

TABLE 29–3. EMERGENT ASSESSMENT OF ABDOMINAL PAIN DURING PREGNANCY

Prior history of abdominal pain	
	Peptic ulcer disease
	Irritable bowel syndrome
	Hiatal hernia
	Pelvic inflammatory disease
Prior abdominal/pelvic surgery	
	Classical cesarean section
	Ectopic pregnancy
	Cholecystectomy
	Appendectomy
Pain characteristics	
	Type of pain
	Mode of onset
	Location
	Radiation
	Persistent
	Intermittent
	Duration
Associated signs and symptoms	
	Fever
	Fainting
	Loss of appetite
	Emesis
	Nausea
	Abdominal tenderness
	Hypotension

intraabdominal events, also has an excellent mortality of less than 0.1 percent (Perissat and associates, 1990).

In most cases not associated with pregnancy, the traditional approach to diagnostic laparoscopy is to proceed with an umbilical puncture for placement of the laparoscope and either one or two suprapubic punctures for the ancillary 5-mm trocar sleeves. During pregnancy, the technique is modified by placing the ancillary trocar sleeves above the umbilicus and away from the uterus. Awareness of the general location of the epigastric vessels as they course beneath the rectus muscle is important in order to avoid injuring them. For good intraabdominal visualization, a 10.5-mm cold light optic laparoscope with a 30 degree angle is recommended (Fig. 29–1). Patients are placed in the Trendelenburg position to establish optimal visualization of the pelvis. Other positions may better facilitate visualization of other structures; in the Trendelenburg position, for instance, the bowel may obscure the gallbladder.

Currently, there is no consensus as to the gestational age at which the uterus would limit laparoscopic access to the abdominal cavity. For closed-scope laparoscopy, 18–20 weeks generally is the upper limit of gestational age. The uterine fundus must be assessed in relation to the umbilicus; as gestational age advances, risk for injury increases. Accordingly, careful consideration of an "open laparoscopic technique" is appropriate to minimize trauma to the internal viscera. Open laparoscopy is especially useful and appropriate when adhesions, which increase the probability of visceral injury, are highly suspected (Hasson, 1974).

In creating a pneumoperitoneum, the Verres needle is most commonly used for

TABLE 29–4. ENDOSCOPIC COMPLICATIONS

Anesthesia Related	Procedure Related
Failed endotracheal intubation	Abdominal wall hematoma
Gastric aspiration	Bladder or bowel perforation
Cardiac arrythmias (SVT, PVC)	Vascular injury
Cardiac arrest	Peritonitis/sepsis
	Ureteral injuries
	Urinoma
	Urinary retention
	Vesicocutaneous fistula
	Pneumothorax
	Hypercarbia
	Hypotension

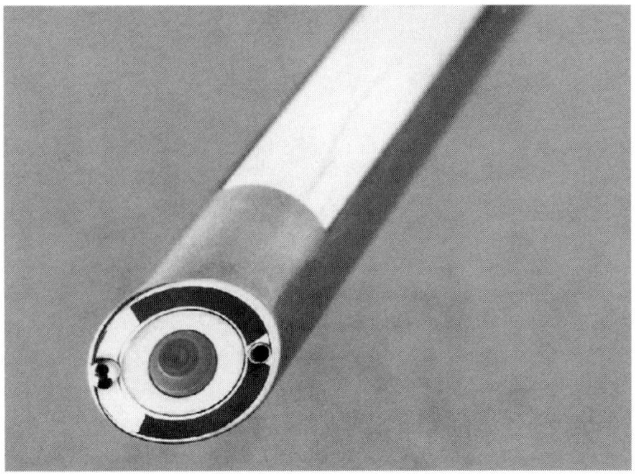

Figure 29–1. 10.5-mm cold light laparoscope with a 30 degree angle.

insufflation (Lukacs and Varees, 1976). This needle is spring-loaded with a blunt probe surrounded by a sharp beveled outer sleeve. Proper placement may be checked by obtaining a normal manometer reading or by free flow of normal saline through the needle into the peritoneal cavity. The filling procedure is performed up to a maximum intraabdominal pressure of 12–14 mm Hg or 3–6 L of gas, depending upon the volume of the woman's peritoneal cavity. Gas embolism has been reported when intraabdominal pressures greater than 20 mm Hg have been used to create a pneumoperitoneum (Shulman and Aronson, 1984).

Instilled intraabdominally, carbon dioxide rapidly forms carbonic acid on the parietal peritoneum, which can result in considerable discomfort or pain. Nitrous oxide (N_2O) for peritoneal insufflation will cause less irritation of the diaphragm. Because nitrous oxide is less irritating, it is preferred with local anesthesia; carbon dioxide is the gas of choice with general anesthesia.

The use of a sharp trocar for laparoscopic insertion is imperative. The insertion should be controlled by using appropriate force applied slowly with a slight twisting motion. Consistency of technique may minimize bowel and vascular injuries. Vascular gas embolism, although rare, has been reported (Yacoub and associates, 1982). Although these complications are relatively uncommon, delay in their identification may result in significant morbidity and mortality. Patients at high risk for adhesion formation, that is, those with previous bowel surgery or pelvic inflammatory disease, may be more appropriately managed with the open laparoscopic technique (Hasson, 1989). This procedure—sharp dissection of the skin, subcutaneous tissue, fascia, and peritoneum—allows direct insertion of the laparoscope sleeve with a blunt trocar. Ancillary trocars of 5 mm or larger then can be placed under direct visualization.

PROCEDURES

Laparoscopic Appendectomy

Appendiceal perforation occurs with an incidence of up to 60 percent in pregnant women in contrast to an incidence of 29 percent in the general population (NIH Consensus Conference, 1993). Therefore, early (aggressive) use of laparoscopy repeatedly has proven helpful in managing suspected appendicitis in the pregnant patient.

The technique used for a laparoscopic appendectomy requires first that the appendix be placed on traction with either a guiding suture located at the distal end of the appendix or with grasping forceps (Fig. 29–2). Second, blunt dissection into the avascular spaces of the mesoappendix with separate ligation or cauterization of the mesoappendiceal vessels is accomplished. The base of the vermiform appendix is then doubly ligated with pre-tied sutures or hemoclips (Figure 29–3). The mucosa of the appendiceal stump is then coagulated for desiccation. The appendix is removed through the 10- or 12-mm trocar sleeve. A purse string suture is placed with two needle holders prior to evaginating the appendiceal stump into the cecum (Fig. 29–4). Last, a Z-suture or second closing procedure may be performed to secure the purse string. The suture area is inspected for complete hemostasis, and the operation is terminated by removing the trocar sleeves under direct visualization with the endoscope. After deflation of the gas, the wound is closed with skin clips.

Laparoscopic appendectomy is within the purview of both obstetricians and general surgeons. In any given institution the individual who performs the operation should be designated based on skill and experience as opposed to specialty.

To date, there have been two small prospective randomized trials comparing open to laparoscopic appendectomy. In both series, the laparoscopic approach resulted in a shorter period of postoperative hospitalization, less pain, and fewer wound infections (McAnena, 1992; Attwood, 1992; and their associates). A series of 150 patients undergoing laparoscopic appendectomy reported by Schreiber (1990) included six pregnant patients at various stages of gestation. The overall complication rate for the 150 patients was 0.75 percent, but there were no complications among the pregnant patients. However, the series is too small to judge the efficacy of a laparoscopic approach to acute appendicitis in pregnancy.

While laparoscopic appendectomy during pregnancy is certainly feasible, laparoscopy's greatest value is diagnostic. The position of the appendix changes throughout gestation,

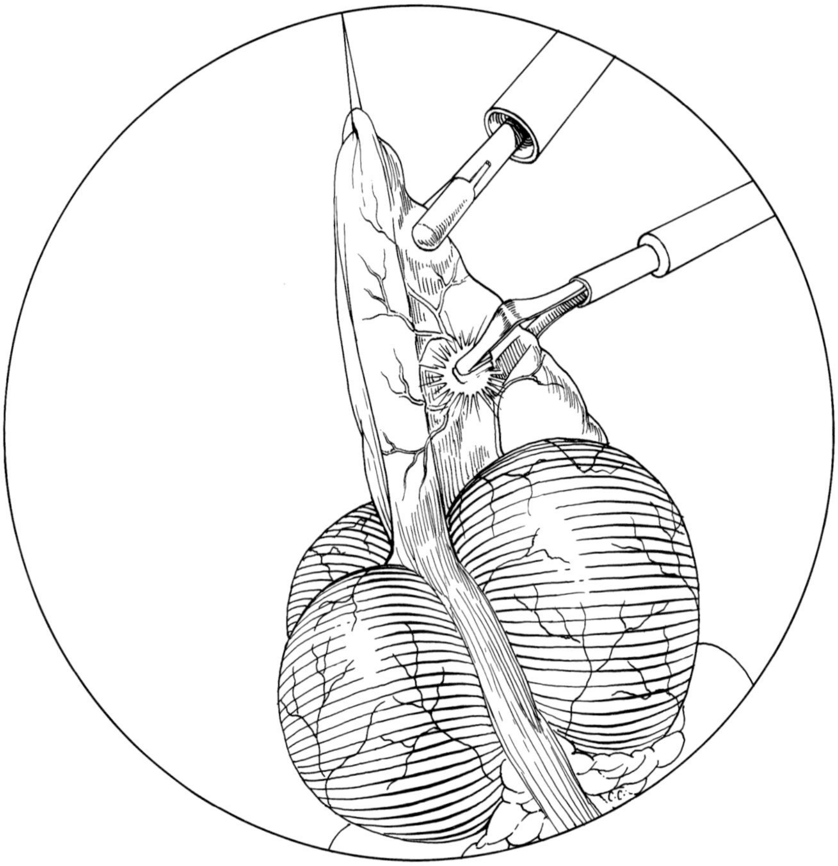

Figure 29–2. Guiding suture located at the distal end of the appendix. Also shown is cauterization of mesoappendiceal vessels.

thereby altering the location of signs and symptoms of acute appendicitis as pregnancy progresses.

Laparoscopic Cholecystectomy

Management of pregnant women with cholecystitis is basically conservative, with surgery rarely necessary. Indications for operative treatment include a lack of response to medical management, suspected perforation, peritonitis, or obstructive jaundice. Conservative treatment is less effective in the puerperium when acute cholecystitis is more frequent and severe. Therapeutic measures not usually recommended in pregnancy are endoscopic papillotomy with stone extraction, intrabiliary solvent infusion systems, medical dissolution with chenodeoxycholic acid, ursodiol, methylterbutylether, or monooctanoin.

Laparoscopic cholecystectomy is a relatively new operation that was first performed in France in 1987 and in the United States in 1988 (NIH Consensus Conference, 1993). In 1993 more than 85 percent of cholecystectomies in the United States were performed via this innovative procedure (Soper and associates, 1994). Most patients with symptomatic gallstones are candidates for laparoscopic cholecystectomy if they are able to tolerate general anesthesia and have no serious cardiopulmonary disease. Laparoscopic cholecystectomy has been accompanied by a 33 percent decrease in overall operative mortality per procedure compared to open cholecystectomy (Steiner and colleagues, 1994). As a rule, indications for laparoscopic cholecystectomy are similar to those for open cholecystectomy.

Ideally, first trimester patients should be treated conservatively until the second trimester, at which time a cholecystectomy may be performed electively. Laparoscopic cholecystectomy, and other laparoscopic procedures in general during the first trimester of pregnancy, is controversial because of the unknown effects of carbon dioxide pneumoperitoneum on the developing fetus (Baillie

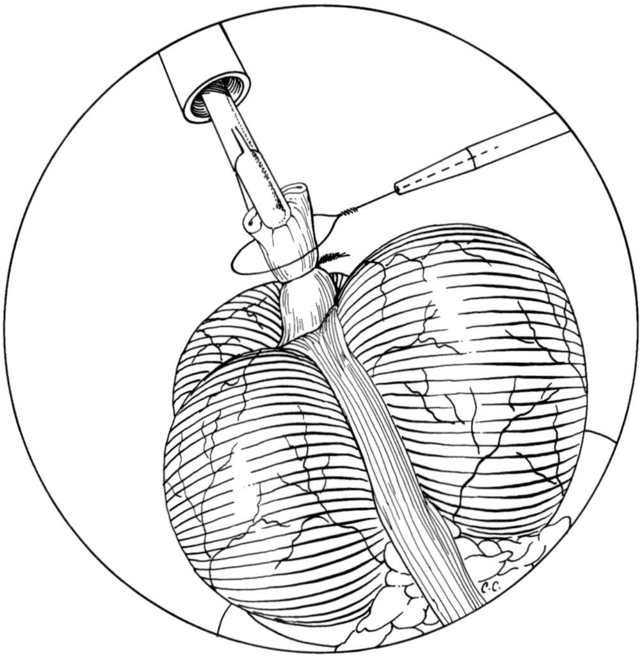

Figure 29–3. The base of the vermiform appendix is doubly ligated with pre-tied sutures or hemoclips. The second ligation can be performed either before or after the appendix has been severed and removed.

and co-workers, 1990). Carbon dioxide may cause fetal hypercarbia and respiratory acidosis (Ostman and associates, 1990). During the second trimester, patients needing surgical treatment are scheduled as soon as the acute cholecystitis subsides; third trimester patients are generally managed medically until the postpartum period. Any patient who does not improve with medical management should undergo surgical intervention regardless of gestational age.

Weber and co-workers (1991) reported the first laparoscopic cholecystectomy during pregnancy. Compared to laparotomy, the

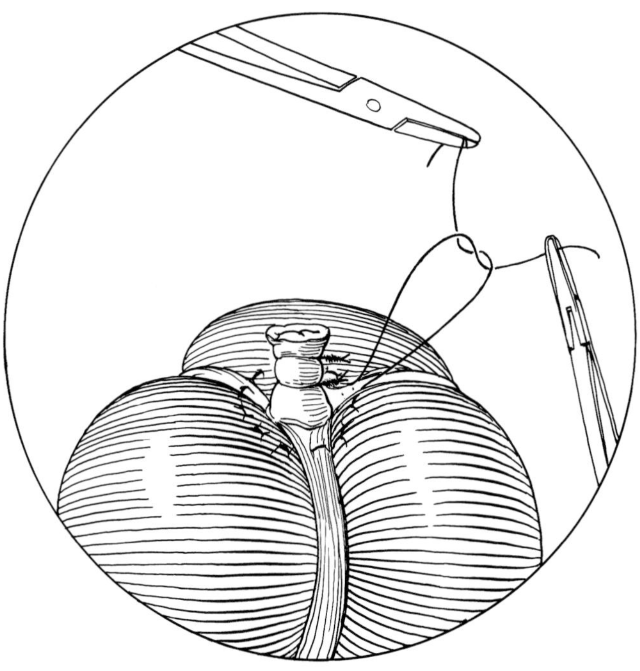

Figure 29–4. A purse string suture is placed with two needle holders prior to evaginating the appendiceal stump into the cecum.

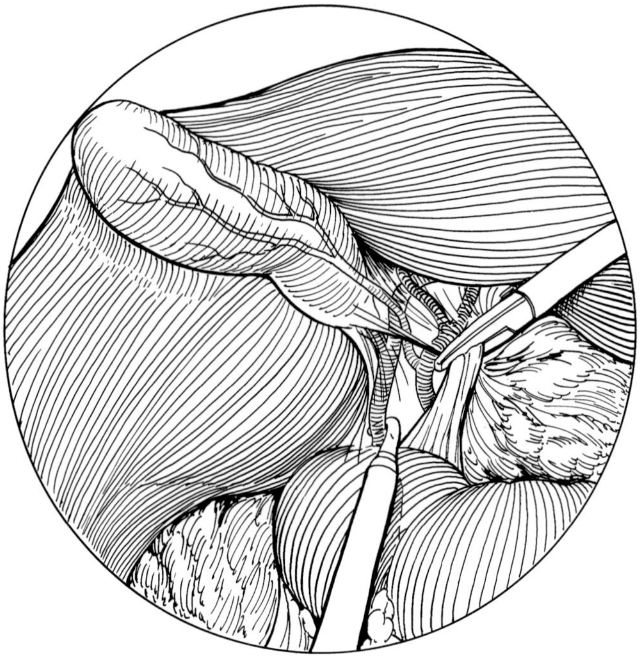

Figure 29–5. Anatomy for cholecystectomy demonstrating excellent visualization of cystic artery and hepatic, cystic, and common bile ducts.

recovery time was significantly shortened. Laparoscopic cholecystectomy requires sound knowledge of the relationship between the hepatoduodenal ligament, triangle of Calot, porta hepatica, cystic artery and duct, hepatic and common bile duct, and gallbladder (Fig. 29–5). Use of a 30-degree angled operative endoscope provides optimal circumferential visualization of the gallbladder and cystic duct. Lysing of any omental, colonic, and duodenal adhesions will aid in visualization and surgical field exposure. Dissection of the visceral peritoneum veil running from the ampulla to the hepatoduodenal ligament should next be accomplished (Fig. 29–6). The gallbladder is then grasped at its fundus

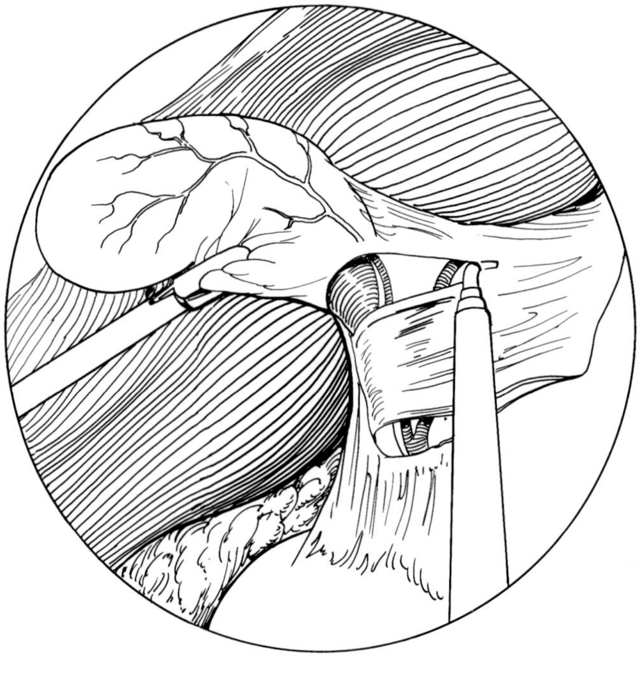

Figure 29–6. Dissection of the visceral peritoneum from ampulla to hepato duodenal ligament.

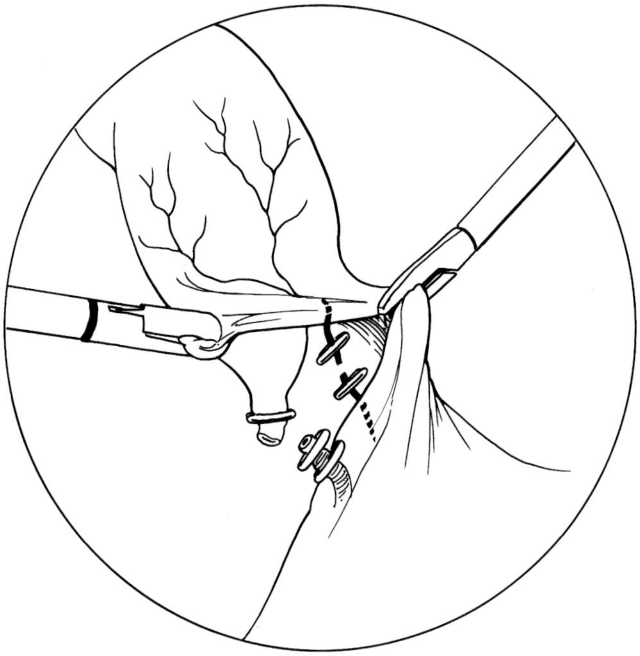

Figure 29–7. Cystic artery and duct having been exposed, they are clipped and transected through the laparoscope.

(Hartman's pouch) and retracted anteriorly, cephalad, and laterally to expose the hilar structures. Once identified and freely dissected, the cystic artery and cystic duct may be clipped and transected (Fig. 29–7). Identification of the cystic artery is important in order to avoid ligating the right hepatic artery. Similarly, attention to the junction between the cystic duct with the common bile duct is equally important. Dissection is continued to begin a surgical plane directly on the gallbladder wall in order to minimize bleeding. Vascular injuries may result in catastrophic hemorrhage and necessitate rapid conversion to an open laparotomy to avoid massive hemorrhage or exsanguination.

Sphincterotomy

The procedure of endoscopic sphincterotomy for extrahepatic biliary obstruction with gallstones during pregnancy has been reported by Baillie and co-workers (1990). Five patients, four of whom had acute cholangitis and one with gallstone pancreatitis, were treated by endoscopic sphincterotomy. All patients delivered at term. Successful endoscopic retrograde cholangiopancreatography (ERCP) and sphincterotomy for common duct stone extraction approaches 90–95 percent in expert hands.

POSTOPERATIVE MANAGEMENT

Labor Surveillance and Treatment

Continuous electronic fetal heart rate and uterine activity monitoring should be considered postoperatively in the context of gestational age and fetal viability. Surveillance of uterine activity augmented with cervical exams affords the best opportunity for timely diagnosis of premature labor. Premature labor may be arrested with either intravenous magnesium sulfate (4–6-g load and $\geq$ 2 g/hr for maintenance) or indomethacin (loading dose of 50–100 mg rectal suppository and 25 mg po q6h for maintenance $\times$ 48–72 hours) (Moise, 1993). Long-term use of intravenous betamimetics, such as terbutaline (Brethine) or ritodrine hydrochloride (Yutopar), is associated with significant metabolic and cardiovascular side effects; that is, hyperglycemia, hypokalemia, tachycardia, chest pain, pulmonary edema, shortness of breath, cardiac dysrhythmia, and electrocardiogram "ischemic" changes (Hankins, 1991; Hauth and associates, 1983; Benedetti, 1986). Short-term use of subcutaneous terbutaline in doses of 0.25 mg q20min for not more than three to four doses, or of a subcutaneous pump with both basal and bolus infusion, can be prescribed. Beta-sympathomimetic agents should not be used when there is active infection.

Pain Control

Plain acetaminophen often relieves minor postoperative discomfort. For more intense pain, acetaminophen plus codeine also should be considered (Briggs and co-workers, 1990). Long-term use of nonsteroidal antiinflammatory agents (NSAID) is relatively contraindicated during pregnancy and is not recommended (Kelley and associates, 1993; Keenan, 1992). However, NSAIDs may be substituted for or used to enhance pain relief with a narcotic for 24–36 hours. Narcotics offer excellent relief for severe pain. While narcotics are known to cause neonatal depression if administered within 1–2 hours of delivery, this is of little practical importance as imminent delivery is an unusual event in this setting.

Nausea and Vomiting

Postoperative nausea and vomiting are more common after laparoscopic procedures than after general surgical procedures (Bailey and co-workers, 1990). Emesis during pregnancy may be treated medically with droperidol (alpha butyrophenone—Class C), prochlorperazine, or metoclopramide (Tornetta, 1969; Pettit and colleagues, 1976). If vomiting is excessive or relentless, intravenous fluids should be administered to offset hypotension caused by the fluid loss. Narcotics should not be withheld because pain itself may cause nausea and vomiting. Effective nonmedical treatments of nausea and vomiting consist of reassurance, slow deliberate movements, warm blankets, and avoidance of pharyngeal suctioning.

SUMMARY

The literature pertaining to the ever expanding indications for operative laparoscopy consists predominately of descriptive studies; few randomized controlled trials have been performed. In 1988, the American Association of Gynecologic Laparoscopists reported a serious complication rate of 15/1000 procedures, and a mortality rate of 5.4/100,000 (Peterson and colleagues, 1990) (Table 29–4). Therefore, the obstetrician gynecologist must recognize his or her own limitations. Experience is increasing with the laparoscopic approach to the pregnant patient requiring appendectomy or cholecystectomy. This technique avoids increased morbidity, prolonged hospital stay, and recovery complications associated with the more traditional approach of laparotomy.

REFERENCES

American College of Obstetricians and Gynecologists. Management of isoimmunization in pregnancy. ACOG Technical Bulletin 148. Washington, DC: ACOG, 1990.

American College of Obstetricians and Gynecologists. Trauma during pregnancy. ACOG Technical Bulletin 161. Washington, DC: ACOG, 1991.

Andres RL, Piacquadio KM, Resnick R. A reappraisal of the need for autologous blood donation in the obstetric patient. Am J Obstet Gynecol 1990; 163:1551.

Anteby SO, Shenker JG, Polishuk WZ. The value of laparoscopy in acute pelvic pain. Ann Surg 1975; 181:484.

Attwood SEA, Hill ADK, Murphy PG, et al. A prospective randomized trial of laparoscopic versus open appendectomy. Surgery 1992; 112:497.

Azziz R, Steinkampf MP, Murphy A. Postoperative recuperation: relation to the extent of endoscopic surgery. Fertil Steril 1989; 51:1061.

Bailey PL, Streisand JB, Pace NL, et al. Transdermal scopolamine reduces nausea and vomiting after out-patient laparoscopy. Anesthesiology 1990; 72:977.

Baillie J, Cairns SR, Putman WS, Cotton PB. Endoscopic management of choledocholithiasis during pregnancy. Surg Obstet Gynecol 1990; 171:1.

Barber HRK, Graber EA. Surgical Disease in Pregnancy. Philadelphia: W. B. Saunders, 1974

Barcroft J. On anoxaemia. Lancet 1920; II:485.

Barron WM. The pregnant surgical patient: medical evaluation and management. Ann Intern Med 1984; 101:683.

Basso L, McCollum PT, Darling MR, et al. A study of cholelithiasis during pregnancy and its relationship with age, parity, menarche, breast-feeding, dysmenorrhea, oral contraception and a maternal history of cholelithiasis. Surg Obstet Gynecol 1992; 175:41,

Benedetti TJ. Life-threatening complications of betamimetic therapy for preterm labor inhibition. Clin Perinatol 1986; 13:843.

Bowman JM. Hemolytic disease (erythroblastosis fetalis). Maternal blood group immunization. In: Creasy RK, Resnick R, eds. Maternal–Fetal Medicine: Principle and Practice. 3rd ed. W.B. Saunders Company, Harcourt Brace Jovanovich, 1989.

Briggs GG, Freeman KR, Yaffe SJ. Drugs in Pregnancy and Lactation. A Reference Guide to Fetal and Neonatal Risk. 3rd ed. Baltimore: Williams & Wilkins, 1990:21a.

Chamberlain G. Gynaecological laparoscopy. Ann R Coll Surg Engl 1980; 62:113
Chung RS, Broughan TA. The phenomenal growth of laparoscopy cholecystectomy: a review. Cleve Clin J Med 1992; 59:186.
Collaborative Group on Antenatal Steroid Therapy. Effect of antenatal dexamethasone administration on the prevention of respiratory distress syndrome. Am J Obstet Gynecol 1981; 141:246.
Corke BC, Spielman FJ. Problems associated with epidural anesthesia in obstetrics. Obstet Gynecol 1985; 65:837.
de Swiet M. The respiratory system. In: Hytten F, Chamberlain G, eds. Clinical Physiology in Obstetrics. 2nd ed. Chap 3. London: Blackwell Scientific Publications, 1991:83.
Deutsch AA, Zelikovsky A, Reiss R. Laparoscopy in the prevention of unnecessary appendicectomies: a prospective study. Br J Surg 1982; 69:336.
Endler GC, Mariona FG, Sokol RJ, Stevenson LB. Anesthesia-related maternal mortality in Michigan. Am J Obstet Gynecol 1988; 159:187.
Gibbs CP, Banner TC. Effectiveness of Bicitra as a preoperative antacid. Anesthesiology 1984; 61:97.
Gilroy RJ, Mangura BT, Laviets MH. Rib cage and abdominal volume displacements during breathing in pregnancy. Am Rev Resp Dis 1988; 137:668.
Hampton JR, Harrison MJG, Mitchell JRA, et al. Relative contributions of history-taking, physical examination, and laboratory investigation to diagnosis and management of medical outpatients. Br Med J 1975; 2:486.
Hankins GDV. Complications of beta-sympathomimetic tocolytic agents. In: Critical Care Obstetrics. 2nd ed. Clark SL, Cotton DB, Hankins GDV, Phelan JP, eds. Boston: Blackwell Scientific, 1991:223.
Haring OM. Cardiac malformations in rats induced by exposure of the mother to carbon dioxide during pregnancy. Circ Res 1960; 8:1218.
Hasson, HM. Open laparoscopy. A report of 150 cases. Reprod Med 1974; 12:234.
Hasson HM. Open Laparoscopy in Operative Gynecological Endoscopy. In: Sanfilippo J, and Levine R, eds. New York: Springer-Verlag, 1989:57.
Hauth JC, Hankins GDV, Kuehl TJ, Pierson WP. Ritodrine hydrochloride infusion in pregnant baboons. I. Biophysical effects. Am J Obstet Gynecol 1983; 146:916.
Hemsell D. Prophylactic antibiotics in gynecologic and obstetric surgery. Rev Infect Dis 1991; 10(suppl):S821.
Hyers TM, Hull RD, Weg JG. Antithrombotic therapy for venous thromboembolic disease. Chest 1986; 89:26s.
Keenan, DL. The active management of postoperative pain. In: Thompson JD, Rock JA, eds. TeLinde's Operative Gynecology Updates. Vol. 1 No. 6, 1992.
Kelley MC, Hocking MP, Marchand CD, Sninsky CA. Ketorolac prevents postoperative small intestinal ileus in rats. Am J Surg 1993; 165.
King CTG, Wilk A, McClure FJ. Carbon dioxide induced acidosis in pregnant rats and caries susceptibility of their progeny. Proc Soc Exp Biol Med 1962; 11:486.
Knill-Jones RP, Newman BJ, Spence AA. Anesthetic practice and pregnancy. Lancet 1975; 2:807.
Leape LL, Ramenofsky ML. Laparoscopy for questionable appendicitis: can it reduce the negative appendectomy rate? Ann Surg. 1980; 191:410.
Levine RL. Economic impact of pelviscopic surgery. J Reprod Med 1985; 30:655.
Liggins GC, Howie RN. A controlled trial of antepartum glucocorticoid treatment for the prevention of respiratory distress syndrome in premature infants. Pediatrics 1972; 50:515.
Lukacs D, Verees E Jr. Szaz eve szuletett Verees Elemer. Orv Hetil 1976; 117:483.
Lundorff P, Hahlin M, Kallfelt B, et al. Adhesion formation after laparoscopic surgery in tubal pregnancy: a randomized trial versus laparotomy. Fertil Steril 1991; 55:911.
May WJ, Greiss GC Jr. Maternal mortality in North Carolina: a forty-year experience. Am J Obstet Gynecol 1989; 161:555.
Marx GF. Cardiotoxicity of local anesthetics—the plot thickens. Anesthesiology 1984; 60:3.
Marx GF, Berman JA. Anesthesia-related maternal mortality. Bull NY Acad Med 1985; 61:323.
McAnena OJ, Austin O, O'Connell PR, et al. Laparoscopic versus open appendicectomy: a prospective evaluation. Br J Surg 1992; 79:818.
Moise, KJ. Effect of advancing gestational age on the frequency of fetal ductal constriction in association with maternal indomethacin use. Am J Obstet Gynecol 1993; 168:1350.
NIH Consensus Conference. Gallstones and laparoscopic cholecystectomy. NIH Consensus Development Panel on Gallstones and Laparoscopic Cholecystectomy. JAMA 1993; 269.
NIH Consensus Statement. Effect of Corticosteroids for Fetal Maturation on Perinatal Outcomes. Vol 12, No 2, March 1994; Bethesda, Maryland.
Ostman PI, Pantle-Fisher FM, Faure EA, Glostew B. Vasculatory collapse during laparoscopy. J Clin Anesth 1990; 2:129.
O'Sullivan GM, Sutton AJ, Thompson SA, et al. Noninvasive measurement of gastric emptying in obstetric patients. Anesth Analg 1987; 66:505.
Parnass SM, Schmidt KJ. Adverse effects of spinal and epidural anaesthesia. Drug Safety 1990; 5:179.
Patterson-Brown S, Eckersley JR, Sim AJ, Dudley HA. Laparoscopy as an adjunct to decision making in the 'acute abdomen.' Br J Surg 1986; 73:1022.

Pederson H, Finster M. Anesthetic risk in the pregnant surgical patient. Anesthesiology 1979; 51:439.

Peoples JB. Cholecystectomy during pregnancy without fetal loss. Surg Gynecol Obstet 1992; 174:465.

Perissat J, Collet D, Belliard R. Gallstones: laparoscopic treatment-cholecystectomy, cholecystotomy and lithotripsy. Surg Endosc 1990; 4:1.

Peterson HB, Hulka JF, Phillips JM. American Association of Gynecologic Laparoscopists' 1988 membership survey on operative laparoscopy. J Reprod Med 1990; 35:587.

Pettit GP, Smith GA, McIlroy WL. Droperidol in obstetrics: a double-blind study. Milit Med 1976; 141:316.

Phelan JP. Fetal considerations in the critically ill obstetric patient. In: Clark SL, Cotton DB, Hankins GDV, Phelan JP, eds. Critical Care Obstetrics. 2nd ed. Boston: Blackwell Scientific, 1990:634.

Reiertsen O, Rosseland AR, Hoivik B, Solheim K. Laparoscopy in patients admitted for acute abdominal pain. Acta Chir Scand 1985; 151:521.

Rocke DA, Murray WB, Rout CC, Gouws E. Relative risk analysis of factors associated with difficult intubation in obstetric anesthesia. Anesthesiology 1992; 77:67.

Sachs BP, Oriol NE, Ostheimer GW, et al. Anesthetic-related maternal mortality, 1954 to 1985. J Clin Anesth 1989; 1:333.

Schreiber JH. Laparoscopic appendectomy in pregnancy. Surg Endosc 1990; 4:100.

Shepard TH. Catalog of Teratogenic Agents. Baltimore: Johns Hopkins University Press, 1986:262.

Shulman D, Aronson HB. Capnography in the early diagnosis of carbon dioxide embolism during laparoscopy. Can Anaesth Soc J 1984; 31:455.

Soper NJ, Brunt LM, Kerbl K. Laparoscopic general surgery. N Engl J Med 1994; 330:409.

Steiner CA, Bass EB, Talamini MA, et al. Surgical rates and operative mortality for open and laparoscopic cholecystectomy in Maryland. N Engl J Med 1994; 330:403.

Talbert LM, Langdell RD. Normal values of certain factors in the blood clotting mechanism in pregnancy. Am J Obstet Gynecol 1964; 90:44.

Tornetta FJ. Studies with the new antiemetic metoclopramide. Anesth Analg 1969; 48:198.

Weber AM, Bloom GP, Allan TR, Curry SL. Laparoscopic cholecystectomy during pregnancy. Obstet Gynecol 1991; 78:958.

Wolf BM, Gardiner B, Frey CF. Laparoscopic cholecystectomy: a remarkable development. JAMA 1991; 265:1573.

Woodhouse DR, Haylen B. Gallbladder disease complicating pregnancy. Aust NZ J Obstet Gynaecol 1985; 25:233.

Yacoub OF, Cardona I Jr, Coverler LA, Dodson MG. Carbon dioxide embolism during laparoscopy. Anesthesiology 1982; 57:533.

CHAPTER 30

Invasive Prenatal Diagnostic Procedures

The overall objective of prenatal diagnosis procedures is to obtain genetic, biochemical, and physiologic information about the fetus. The techniques described in this chapter—amniocentesis, chorionic villus sampling (CVS), and percutaneous umbilical blood sampling (PUBS)—allow detection of an ever-expanding list of inherited conditions. Ideally, perinatal centers should have the technical expertise to perform all of these procedures and to select the best procedure for each clinical situation. Of paramount importance is the ability to provide genetic counseling to patients about their various diagnostic options. These options and their risks and consequences should be communicated to patients in a nondirective, supportive way.

AMNIOCENTESIS

Amniocentesis was first used during the 1880s for decompression of polyhydramnios (Lambl, 1881; Schatz, 1992). In 1930 placental localization was achieved after the intraamniotic injection of contrast medium (Menees and associates, 1930). Aburel (1937) described the intraamniotic injection of hypertonic saline for termination of pregnancy. During the 1950s the role of amniocentesis and measurement of bilirubin concentration in monitoring Rhesus disease was reported (Bevis, 1950; Walker, 1957).

The application of amniocentesis for fetal chromosome analysis was also initiated in the 1950s. The number of human chromosomes was not known until 1956. The first reported application was for fetal sex determination (Fuchs and Riis, 1956). The feasibility of culturing and karyotyping amniotic fluid cells was demonstrated by Steele and Breg in 1966. The first prenatal diagnosis of an abnormal karyotype, a balanced translocation, was reported in 1967 (Jacobson and Barter, 1967). Trisomy 21 was first detected prenatally by Valenti and associates in 1968. During the same year the first diagnosis of the metabolic disorder galactosemia was reported (Nadler, 1968).

Indications for Amniocentesis

In the United States, it is considered standard practice to offer prenatal cytogenetic analysis to all women who will be 35 years of age or older at their expected time of delivery. The risk of numerical chromosomal abnormalities (aneuploidy) increases with advancing maternal age as a result of nondisjunction that occurs during maternal meiosis. Age 35 has been selected as a cutoff because, at this age, the risk of miscarriage associated with amniocentesis is equal to the risk of a fetal chromosome abnormality, approximately 1 in 200 (Hook and colleagues, 1983). The relationship between age and estimated risk of chromosomal abnormalities is demonstrated in Table 30–1 (Hook and colleagues, 1983; Hook , 1981).

Amniocentesis or chorionic villus sampling is indicated when there is a need to obtain fetal material for cytogenetic, biochemical, or DNA studies. The DNA abnormalities responsible for the etiology of many disorders are being increasingly identified. A list of common genetic conditions for which DNA-based prenatal diagnosis is available is given in Table 30–2 (D'Alton, 1994). As this list changes almost on a weekly basis, it is best to have contact with a medical genetics unit to get periodic updates on specific conditions.

The established screening test for fetal open spina bifida (OSB) is measurement of maternal serum α-fetoprotein (MSAFP) levels followed by amniocentesis in patients with elevated results (UK Collaborative Study, 1979). The ultrasound diagnosis of fetal OSB has been greatly enhanced by the recognition of associated abnormalities in the skull and brain. These abnormalities include cerebral ventriculomegaly, microcephaly, frontal bone scalloping (lemon sign), and obliteration of the cisterna magna with either an "absent" cerebellum or abnormal anterior curvature of the cerebellar hemispheres (banana sign) (Nicolaides and co-workers, 1986a). Van den Hof and colleagues (1990) have reported on the diagnosis of OSB in 130 fetuses among 1,561 patients at high risk for fetal neural tube defects who were referred for a detailed ultrasound examination. The examinations revealed associated abnormalities of the skull and brain in 129 of the 130 fetuses with OSB. As a result of this evidence of the high accuracy of ultrasound in the diagnosis of neural tube defects, the need for amniocentesis in the evaluation of an elevated MSAFP has been questioned.

In centers adept at diagnosing OSB sonographically, amniocentesis can be reserved for patients with suspicious ultrasound findings, large MSAFP elevations despite a normal scan, or inability to adequately visualize fetal anatomy. The American College of Obstetricians and Gynecologists (ACOG Technical Bulletin, 1991) now recommends amniocentesis in a woman with elevated MSAFP and correct dates; however, the bulletin is under revision at the time of this writing. Patients at increased risk for neural tube defects, that is, who have elevated MSAFP levels, who have a history of neural tube defects, or who are taking antifolate medications, should be referred to centers with sonologists experienced in diagnostic ultrasound. If ultrasound examination demonstrates a normal fetal spine, cranium, and cerebellum, the chance of an undetected spinal abnormality is low. Therefore amniocentesis, with a procedure-related risk of up to 1 percent, is probably unnecessary. Some centers have calculated a revised neural tube defect risk on the basis of the MSAFP value and a normal ultrasound examination at their particular center (Nadel, 1990; Richards, 1988; and their co-workers). For example, in our reference laboratory in a Caucasian patient with a priori risk for OSB of 1 in 1000, an MSAFP of 2.8 multiples of the median (MOM) gives a risk of 1 in 170. When an adequate ultrasound examination is performed by highly experienced ultrasonologists and is interpreted as a normal scan, this risk may be reduced by 95 percent, giving a reassigned risk of approximately 1 in 3400. In our center amniocentesis is reserved for cases in which there is incomplete visualization of the fetus (as a result of

TABLE 30–1. RELATION BETWEEN MATERNAL AGE AND THE ESTIMATED RATE OF CHROMOSOMAL ABNORMALITIES[a]

Age	Risk of Down Syndrome	Risk of Chromosomal Abnormality
20	1/1667	1/526
25	1/1250	1/476
30	1/952	1/385
35	1/385	1/202
36	1/295	1/162
37	1/227	1/129
38	1/175	1/102
39	1/137	1/82
40	1/106	1/65
41	1/82	1/51
42	1/64	1/40
43	1/50	1/32
44	1/38	1/25
45	1/30	1/20
46	1/23	1/16
47	1/18	1/13
48	1/14	1/10
49	1/11	1/7

[a]Ages are at the expected time of delivery.
Data have been modified from Hook (1981) and Hook and associates (1983). Reprinted with permission from D'Alton and DeCherney (1993).

TABLE 30–2. LIST OF CONDITIONS AMENABLE TO DNA ANALYSIS

Disorder	Mode of Inheritance	Chromosome
α_1-Antitrypsin deficiency	AR	14
α-Thalassemia	AR	16
Adult polycystic kidney disease (type 1)	AD	16
β-Thalassemia	AR	11
Congenital adrenal hyperplasia	AR	6
Cystic fibrosis	AR	7
DiGeorge syndrome	AD	22
Duchenne/Becker muscular dystrophy	XLR	X
Familial Alzheimer's disease	AD	21
Familial hypercholesterolemia	AD	19
Familial polyposis coli	AD	5
Fragile X syndrome	XLR	X
Gardner syndrome	AD	5
Hemoglobin SC	AR	11
Hemophilia A (factor IX deficiency)	XLR	X
Huntington's disease	AD	4
Marfan syndrome	AD	15
Multiple endocrine neoplasia, type I	AD	11
Multiple endocrine neoplasia, type, IIa	AD	10
Myotonic dystrophy	AD	19
Neurofibromatosis, type I	AD	17
Neurofibromatosis, type II	AD	22
Norrie's disease	XLR	X
Ornithine transcarbamylase deficiency	XLR	X
Phenylketonuria	AR	12
Retinoblastoma	AD	13
Sickle cell anemia	AR	11
Spinal muscular atrophy	AR/AD	5
Tay-Sachs disease	AR	5
Von Hippel-Lindau syndrome	AD	3
Wiskott-Aldrich syndrome	XLR	X

Reprinted with permission from D'Alton and associates (1994).

maternal obesity or fetal position), serum levels of MSAFP greater than 3.5 MOM in the presence of normal sonographic examination, or suspicious ultrasound findings.

The combined use of the maternal serum human chorionic gonadotropin level, unconjugated estriol level, α-fetoprotein (AFP) level, and maternal age can identify 60 percent of cases of Down syndrome, with a false positive rate of 6.6 percent (Haddow and associates, 1992). Individual estimates of patient risk are used, and amniocentesis is usually offered when risk is greater than 1 in 270. Although triple-marker screening is not the standard of care at present, it is likely to become standard practice. It is now routinely used in many programs.

Assessment of the severity of Rh disease and the need for fetal blood transfusion or early delivery has been traditionally based on amniocenteses and interpretation of the results of spectrophotometric estimation of amniotic fluid bilirubin (Liley, 1961). In the assessment of severe Rh sensitization in midtrimester, the only accurate method for predicting the severity of the disease is measurement of the hemoglobin concentration in samples obtained by percutaneous blood sampling (PUBS) (Nicolaides and associates, 1986b; 1988). (See section on PUBS.)

Premature delivery is one of the leading causes of perinatal death and chronic handicap. The association between intrauterine infection and premature labor, in the presence and absence of ruptured membranes, has stimulated research into amniocentesis for diagnosis of subclinical intrauterine infection (Romero and co-workers, 1989). If amniocentesis proves to be reliable in this diagnosis, the number of amniocenteses performed in preterm labor and premature rupture of membranes (PROM) will increase. At present, amniocentesis in preterm labor and PROM seems to be routinely used only in a few centers having a major research focus in this area. We reserve amniocentesis in preterm labor and PROM for those patients with suspicious clinical findings, that is, fetal tachycardia and/or leukocytosis.

Measurement of the amniotic fluid lecithin/sphingomyelin ratio (Gluck and associates, 1974) and phosphatidylglycerol level (Hallman and colleagues, 1976) is useful for the assessment of fetal lung maturity. However, the need for these tests has declined because of improved neonatal care and the introduction of better methods of ultrasound assessment of gestational age and fetal surveillance. Generally, elective preterm delivery should not be performed without a significant maternal or fetal indication; therefore assessment of fetal lung maturity adds little to the decision-making process.

Technique of Amniocentesis

Early attempts at genetic amniocentesis were made transvaginally. Subsequently, the transabdominal approach was adopted. During the 1960s amniocentesis was performed "blindly." During the 1970s and early 1980s, ultrasonography was used to identify a placenta-free area for entry into a pocket of amniotic fluid. This position was marked on the maternal abdomen, and after a variable length of time, the operator would "blindly" insert the needle.

In most centers amniocentesis is now performed with continuous ultrasound guidance. An ultrasound scan is first performed to determine the number of fetuses present, confirm gestational age and fetal viability, and document normal anatomy. The maternal abdomen is washed with antiseptic solution; it is unnecessary for the operator to scrub and gown. Continuously guided by ultrasound, a 22-gauge needle is introduced into the amniotic cavity (Fig. 30–1). Ultrasound examination may be performed with sector or linear-array transducers, and the procedure may be performed either free-hand or with needle guides (Lenke, 1985; Jeanty, 1983; and their co-workers). The free-hand technique allows easier manipulation of the needle if the position of the target is abruptly altered by a uterine contraction or fetal movement (Figure 30–2). The free-hand technique is easily adapted to all ultrasound-guided diagnostic or therapeutic procedures, for example, PUBS and thoracocentesis. The first 2 mL of aspirated amniotic fluid are discarded and the desired volume of amniotic fluid then withdrawn. Fetal heart rate and activity are documented immediately following the procedure.

Technique of Amniocentesis in Multifetal Gestations

Amniocentesis in multifetal pregnancy involves puncture of the first sac, withdrawal of amniotic fluid, injection of a dye, and then a new needle insertion to puncture the second sac (Elias and associates, 1980; Filkins and Russo, 1984). If the fluid aspirated after the second puncture is clear, then the operator knows it does not come from the first sac, which was injected with dye (Fig. 30–3).

A single-puncture method has been described in which the site of needle insertion is determined mainly by the position of the membrane separating the two sacs (Jeanty and associates, 1983). After entry into the first sac and aspiration of amniotic fluid, the needle is advanced through the dividing membrane into the second sac. In order to avoid contamination of the second sample with any amniotic fluid from the first sac still in the needle, the first 1 mL of fluid from the second sample is discarded. We do not favor this method, as it may cause iatrogenic rupture of

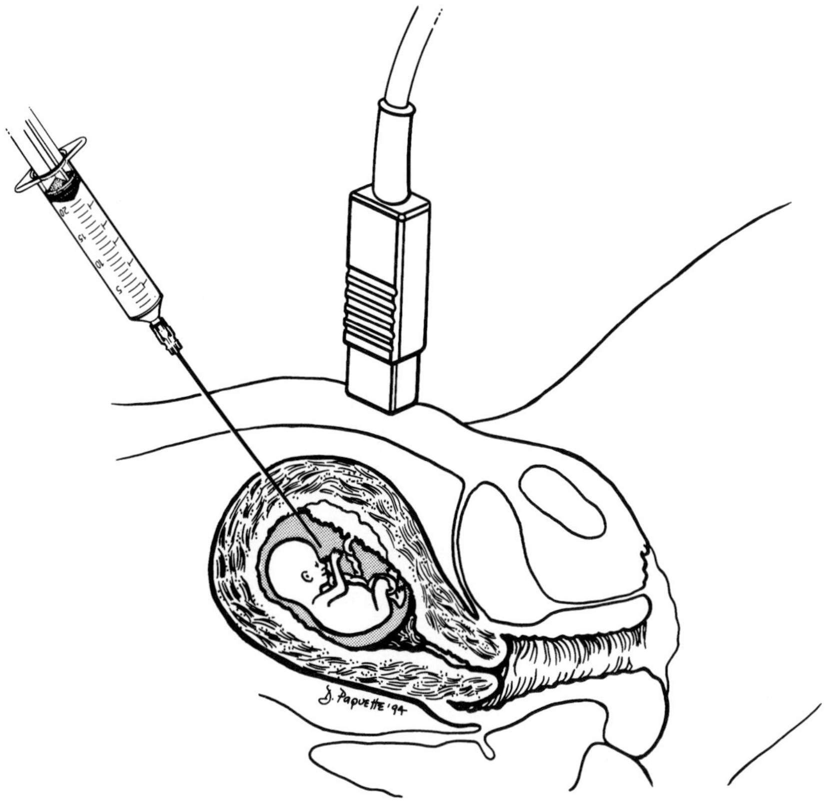

Figure 30–1. Diagrammatic representation of amniocentesis. Note sonographic direction to avoid placental puncture and to avoid direct fetal puncture. (Reprinted with permission from D'Alton and associates, 1994.)

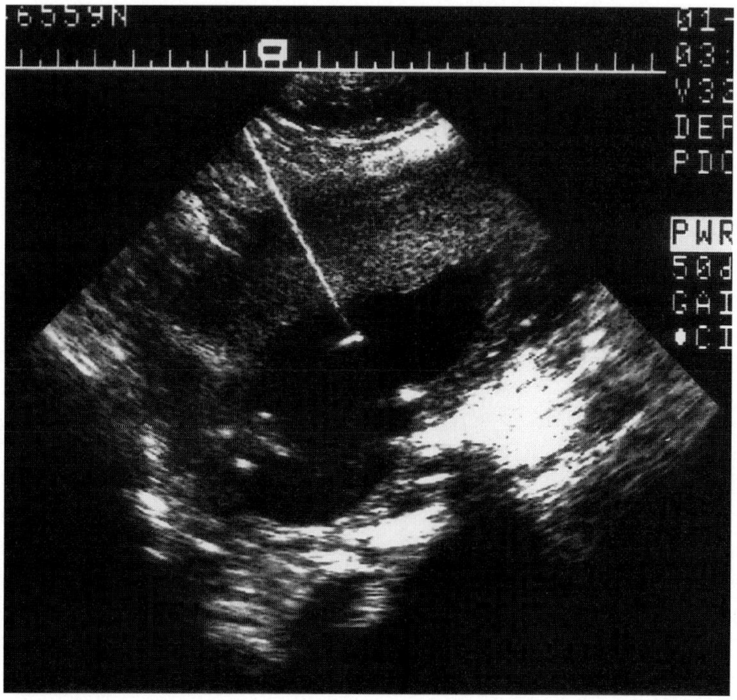

Figure 30–2. Ultrasound image of amniocentesis showing the highly reflective needle and the very bright image crested by the tip of the needle.

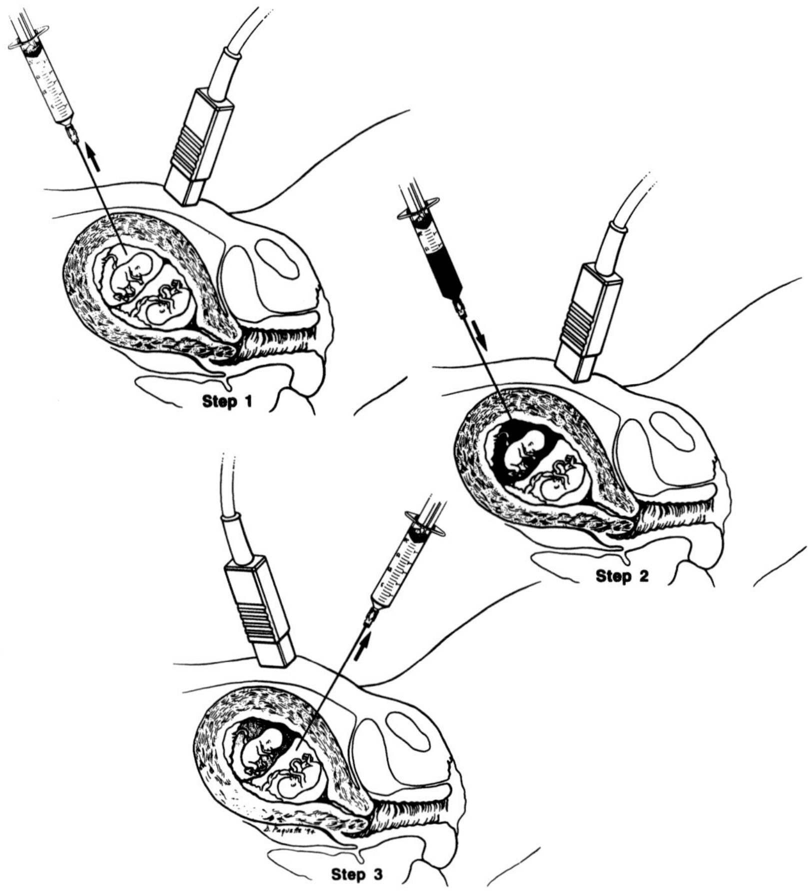

Figure 30–3. Diagrammatic representation of one method of performing amniocentesis in twins: Step 1. The fluid is aspirated from the first sac. Step 2. Indigo carmine is injected into the first sac. Step 3. Clear fluid is aspirated from the second sac.

the dividing membrane with creation of a monoamniotic sac and its attendant risk of cord entanglement.

Bahado-Singh and colleagues (1992) described a technique of amniocentesis in twins that entails identifying the separating membranes with a curvilinear or linear transducer. The first needle and transducer are left in place during the insertion of the second needle. Beekhuis and associates (1992) describes another technique using maternal hemoglobin as a dye marker to differentiate between the two sacs. Methylene blue is not recommended as a dye because it has been reported to cause hemolytic anemia or methemoglobinemia (Cowett and colleagues, 1976). An association between fetal intestinal atresia and the use of methylene blue dye for amniocentesis in twins has been reported (Nicolini and Monni, 1990; Van der Pol and associates, 1992). This association has not been demonstrated with indigo carmine (Cragan and co-workers, 1993).

Laboratory Considerations for Amniocentesis

Amniocyte culture failure occurs in less than 1 percent of cases. Chromosomal mosaicism, the presence of two or more cell lines with different karyotypes in a single person, occurs in approximately 0.5 percent of cases. This occurs as a result of postzygotic nondisjunction; however, the observation of multiple cell lines in a prenatal sample does not necessarily mean that the fetus has mosaicism. The most common type of mosaicism detected by amniocentesis is pseudomosaicism (Hsu and Perlis, 1984). This phenomenon should be suspected when an abnormality is evident in only one of several cultures of an amniotic fluid specimen. The abnormal cell lines arise during in vitro division; therefore they are not present in the fetus and are not clinically important. Contamination by maternal cells can be minimized by discarding the first few drops of aspirated amniotic fluid. True fetal mosaicism, diagnosed when the same abnormality is present on more than one cover slip, is rare (0.25 percent) but clinically important (Hsu and Perlis, 1984). The question of whether true mosa-icism is present is best resolved by karyotyping fetal lymphocytes obtained by PUBS (Gosden and associates, 1988), a method that provides results within 48 hours. Detailed ultrasound examination is also recommended to assess fetal growth and exclude the diagnosis of structural anomalies. If both ultrasound and fetal blood sampling results are normal, the parents can be reassured that the major chromosomal abnormalities have been excluded (Gosden and associates, 1988).

More than 100 abnormalities of lipid, mucopolysaccharide, amino acid, and carbohydrate metabolism are amenable to prenatal diagnosis from the study of cultured amniotic fluid cells. However, the substantially larger amount of tissue obtained by CVS than by amniocentesis makes CVS the preferred method of diagnosing this group of disorders.

Reported Use of Fluorescence in Situ Hybridization (FISH) in Prenatal Diagnosis

FISH permits determination of the number and location of specific DNA sequences in human cells, both in interphase nuclei and directly on metaphase chromosomes. The FISH procedure relies on the complementarity between the two strands of the DNA double helix. Probe DNA molecules are nonisotopically labeled by incorporation of a chemically modified neucleotide that is subsequently detected with a fluorescently tagged reporter molecule.

This technology detects aneuploidies caused by monosomies, free trisomies, trisomies associated with Robertsonian translocations, triploidy, and other numerical chromosomal abnormalities involving chromosomes 13, 18, 21, X, and Y. The technology was not designed to detect other cytogenetic abnormalities such as mosaics, translocations, or rare aneuploidies (Ward, 1993; Klinger, 1992; and their colleagues).

Ward and colleagues (1993) described the first large-scale application of interphase FISH for prenatal diagnosis. FISH was performed on physician request as an adjunct to cytogenetics in 4500 patients. Region-specific DNA probes to chromosomes 13, 18, 21, X, and Y were used to determine ploidy by analysis of signal number in hybridized nuclei. A sample was considered to be **euploid** when all autosomal probes generated two hybridization signals and when a normal sex chromosome pattern was observed in 80 percent or more of hybridized nuclei. A sample was considered to be **aneuploid** when 70 percent or more of hybridized nuclei displayed the same abnormal hybridization pattern for a specific probe. Of the attempted analyses, 90 percent met these criteria and were reported as "**informative**" to referring physicians within 48 hours.

The overall detection rate for aneuploidy was 73 percent (107/146). The accuracy of informative results for aneuploidies was described as being 93.9 percent (107/114). There were no false positives and seven false-negative autosomal aneuploidies. One false-positive sex chromosome aneuploidy has been reported (Benn, 1992; Ward, 1992; and their associates). The strict reporting criteria used to define and report samples as abnormal led to a lower detection rate of 73 percent for all aneuploidies. Ward and co-workers are now reevaluating these criteria; for example, if the criteria for reporting a sample as abnormal were changed to include all samples in which greater than 50 percent of hybridized nuclei were trisomic, the aneuploidy detection rate would improve to 82.9 percent (107 + 14/146). This change in the reporting criteria would have enhanced the detection rate without altering the false-positive or false-negative rates. In Ward's study for informative specimens, the sensitivity for identification of autosomal trisomy was 92.6 percent. This was less than anticipated on the basis of initial investigations by Klinger (1992) and Lebo (1992) and their associates. Undetected maternal cell contamination, increased background fluorescence as a result of excessive cellular debris, and autofluorescence of the microscope lens contributed to the observed false negatives, thereby decreasing the sensitivity.

The question of which populations should be studied with FISH is debatable. The study by Ward and colleagues provided the procedure to all patients who requested the analysis. Further study by Strovel and co-workers (1992) suggests only cells from patients whose risk of aneuploidy is 1 percent or greater (on the basis of maternal age, maternal serum findings, or ultrasonographic findings) should be analyzed. Retrospective analysis of 750 consecutive amniotic fluid samples obtained in their laboratory revealed that only 168, or 22 percent, of these cases had a risk of 1 percent or greater of being aneuploid. If FISH had only been performed on those 168 cases, 14 aneuploidies would have been detected whereas only five additional abnormalities would have been found in the other 582 cases. Therefore if the overall goal is to employ interphase FISH as an adjunct procedure, then a directed analysis optimizing its application by limiting the number of patients studied would yield the highest frequency of abnormalities.

FISH may be useful for rapid confirmation of potential numerical chromosomal aneuploidies when ultrasound examination reveals fetal abnormalities and may be an alternative to PUBS or placental biopsy.

Potential disadvantages of FISH include maternal anxiety after an uninformative result and the negative effect of receiving a disomic FISH result followed by the identification of a chromosome lesion not identified by the initial protocol (Ward and associates, 1993). At the present time there is a lack of laboratories availing themselves of this technology. In order for any technology to gain widespread acceptance, studies must be performed by multiple laboratories to validate its methodology and conclusions. Until the methodology has been used and established in several laboratories, it is not advisable to base pregnancy management decisions on FISH results alone. FISH clearly cannot yet be used as a totally independent procedure. Aneuploidies will only account for 50–70 percent of all abnormalities detected by standard cytogenetics. It is uncertain what information should be transmitted to the referring physician. The best use of the information is to prioritize existing cases suspected to be abnormal and at most provide preliminary results. All interphase FISH results must be followed by classical cytogenetic studies. Some authors feel that since the information obtained from the interphase FISH studies should not be used for pregnancy management, and should only be used in conjunction with classical cytogenetic studies, then the patient should not be asked to pay the cost of the test (Schwartz, 1993).

Complications of Amniocentesis

Fortunately, serious maternal complications such as septic shock are rare. Amnionitis occurs in 0.1 percent of cases (Turnbull and MacKenzie, 1983).

The development of rhesus isoimmunization (Golbus, 1979; Hill 1980; and their associates) can be avoided by prophylactic administration of anti-D immunoglobulin to Rh-negative women undergoing amniocentesis. Amniotic fluid leak or vaginal blood loss, noted by 2–3 percent of patients after amniocentesis, is usually self-limiting, although occasionally leakage of amniotic fluid persists throughout pregnancy (NICHD, 1976; Simpson and associates, 1981). A common finding is cramping for 1–2 hours and lower abdominal discomfort for up to 48 hours after the procedure.

The safety and accuracy of amniocentesis in midtrimester was documented in the mid 1970s by three collaborative studies performed in the United Kingdom, United States, and Canada (Medical Research Council, 1977; Working Party on Amniocentesis, 1978; NICHD, 1978). However, the only prospective, randomized, controlled trial is the Danish study, which reported on 4606 low-risk, healthy women, 25–34 years old, who were randomly allocated to a group having amniocentesis or to one having ultrasound examination (Tabor and co-workers, 1986). In this study, the total fetal loss rate in the patients having amniocentesis was 1.7 percent and in the controls 0.7 percent ($p<0.01$). The conclusions of this study were initially criticized because the study stated that an 18-gauge needle (which is associated with higher risks than smaller needles) was used. Tabor and colleagues (1988) subsequently reported that they had been mistaken in citing the use of an 18-gauge needle and had, in fact, used a 20-gauge needle for most of the procedures. The Danish study also demonstrated that there were significant associations between pregnancy loss and puncture of the placenta, high MSAFP, and discolored amniotic fluid (Tabor and associates, 1986).

Both the UK and Danish studies (Working Party on Amniocentesis, 1978; Tabor and co-workers, 1986) found an increase in respiratory distress syndrome and pneumonia in neonates from the amniocentesis groups. Other studies have not found this association. The UK study showed an increased incidence of talipes and dislocation of the hip in the amniocentesis group (Working Party on Amniocentesis, 1978). This finding has not been confirmed in several other studies.

Needle puncture of the fetus, reported in 0.1–3.0 percent of cases (Karp and Hayden, 1977; NICHD, 1978), has been suggested as the cause of exsanguination (Young and co-workers, 1977), intestinal atresia (Therkelsen and Rehder, 1981; Swift and associates, 1979), ileocutaneous fistula (Rickwood, 1977), gangrene of a fetal limb (Lamb, 1975), uniocular blindness (Merin and Beyth, 1980), porencephalic cysts (Youroukos and associates, 1980), patellar tendon disruption (Epley and co-workers, 1979), skin dimples (Broome and colleagues, 1976), and peripheral nerve damage (Karp and Hayden, 1977). Continuous use of ultrasound to guide the needle minimizes needle puncture of the fetus. Finegan and colleagues (1990) have reported an increased incidence of middle-ear abnormalities in children whose mothers had amniocentesis.

Complications of Amniocentesis in Multiple Gestation

Results of a large single center experience with 339 cases of multiple gestation undergoing prenatal diagnosis by amniocentesis revealed a spontaneous abortion rate (up to 28 weeks of gestation at 3.57%) compared with the singleton abortion rate of 0.60 percent (Anderson and associates, 1991). It is unclear how much of this increased risk is due to the normal biologic loss rate in twins. Unfortunately there are no reliable data for the spontaneous loss rate in multiple pregnancies from 16 to 28 weeks' gestation. Coleman and co-workers (1987) reported a spontaneous abortion rate of 5 percent in gestations in which the diagnosis of twins was made at 20.5 weeks. Patients with twins must also be counseled about the increased risk of having a karyotypically abnormal child. Several reports have noted an increase in chromosomal abnormalities in fetuses in multiple gestation (Lubs and Ruddle, 1970; Milunsky, 1979). Amniocentesis in twins does raise some very painful questions. Families need first to consider the possibility of a test showing that one of their twins is normal and the other, abnormal.

Early Amniocentesis (EA)

The introduction of first-trimester placental biopsy stimulated interest in the assessment of the feasibility of earlier amniocentesis. Experience with EA is accumulating; Table 30–3 presents the loss rates from four of the largest trials (Hanson, 1992; Assel, 1992; Penso, 1990; Henry, 1992; and their associates). EA cannot be assumed to be as safe as conventional amniocentesis. However, there is also a higher natural loss in pregnancies at 13–14 weeks' gestation than in those at 16–18 weeks' gestation, which may account for some of the increased loss rates for EA. The background loss rate of sonographically normal pregnancies before 14 weeks of gestation is reported to be approximately 2.1 percent (Liu, 1987; Wilson, 1984; Gilmore, 1985; and their colleagues).

The technique of EA is the same as for conventional amniocentesis. Incomplete fusion of the amnion and chorion is common before 14 weeks' gestation and, on occasion, aspiration of fluid may be hampered by tenting of the membranes. Amniocentesis can usually be completed by a more vigorous insertion of the needle. If not, the procedure may be rescheduled.

Laboratory Considerations for EA

Amniotic fluid samples obtained by EA are handled in the same manner as routine cases. Byrne and co-workers (1991) demonstrated successful amniotic fluid culture in 308 of 312 (98.7 percent) EA specimens and observed that although the total number of cells seen at 16–18 weeks' gestation was significantly greater than at 10–13 weeks' gestation, the number of viable cells was equivalent. The authors hypothesize that the cellular increase at 16–18 weeks' gestation is due to genitourinary tract exfoliated cells, most of which are not viable. Jorgensen and colleagues (1992) investigated the success rate of karyotyping in 132 EA specimens between 7 and 14 weeks' gestation. The authors found a marked difference in the success rate of karyotyping before week 11 (0 to 25%) compared with the success rate in week 11 (91%) and between weeks 12 and 14 (100%). Between 7 and 9 weeks' gestation the volume of amniotic fluid aspirated ranged from 0.5 to 6.5 mL, whereas between 10 and 12 weeks' gestation the volume varied from 2 to 24 mL. Culture success seems to correlate with increased fluid volume; the ideal volume of amniotic fluid to remove by EA remains unknown. Many centers have arbitrarily chosen a volume of 1 mL per gestational week.

One of the potential advantages of using EA rather than CVS is that biochemical testing for neural tube defects, which cannot be

TABLE 30–3. EARLY AMNIOCENTESIS AND FETAL LOSS RATE

Study (First Author)	Patients (*n*)	Total Loss Rate (%)	Spontaneous Loss Rate (%)	Gestational Age Distribution Early Amniocentesis (%)				
				<11	*11–11.8 wk*	*12–12.8 wk*	*13–13.8 wk*	*>14 wk*
Hanson (1992)	879	6.2	3.4	1.5	24.3	74.2	—	—
Assel (1992)	300	6.6	2.9	—	—	—	19.0	81.0
Penso (1990)	407	6.4	3.8	—	2.2	44.0	43.5	10.3
Henry (1992)	1805	1.6	0.6	—	0.8	10.7	23.6	64.9

Source: Reprinted with permission from D'Alton and associates (1994).

done on CVS samples, can be performed on these amniotic fluid samples. The usefulness, however, of measuring levels of acetylcholinesterase and AFP in the amniotic fluid obtained between 10 and 15 weeks' gestation is not yet clear. Crandall and co-workers (1989a, b) favorably reported on the usefulness of AFP and acetylcholinesterase measurements in amniotic fluid beyond 12 weeks' gestation. In contrast, Burton and associates (1989) found five false-positive results among 93 amniotic fluid samples obtained at 11–14 weeks' gestation compared with only one false-positive result among 951 samples obtained at 15–20 weeks' gestation. Wathen and colleagues (1991) studied 105 women undergoing amniocentesis between 8 and 13 weeks' gestation and observed that amniotic AFP levels were greatly elevated at 8 weeks' gestation, fell rapidly at 10 weeks' gestation, and rose slightly from 11 to 13 weeks' gestation. The volume of amniotic fluid was too small to be accurately sampled in 8 of 20 (40%) patients at 8 weeks' gestation. The rapidly changing levels of AFP from 8 to 11 weeks of pregnancy combined with the difficulties in sampling the amniotic cavity seem to make the determination of AF-AFP level of little use before 11 weeks.

Conclusions

Indications for amniocentesis have changed considerably over the years and are likely to evolve even further. The most common indication for amniocentesis is to obtain a fetal karyotype in women who will be 35 years of age or older at the time of delivery. Eventually, first-trimester amniocentesis may be performed more frequently than at present; however, a clearer definition of the risks of this procedure is necessary. The use of amniocentesis in the investigation of elevated MSAFP is declining. Maternal serum triple-marker biochemical screening of chromosomal defects is likely to become a routine antenatal test that may increase the number of second-trimester amniocenteses performed. For the assessment of fetal anemia in severe red blood cell isoimmunized pregnancies in the second trimester, amniocentesis is likely to be replaced by PUBS. Amniocentesis for lung maturity is likely to continue to decrease as ultrasound dating of pregnancy is commonly performed in many pregnancies, and premature deliveries are performed only for maternal or fetal indications. Amniocentesis as an aid to diagnosing infection with preterm labor and spontaneous rupture of membranes may increase in the short term.

CHORIONIC VILLUS SAMPLING (CVS)

The major drawback of conventional mid-second trimester amniocentesis for prenatal diagnosis is the delayed availability of the karyotype and the increased medical risks of performing a dilation and evacuation procedure late in the pregnancy. Furthermore, this delay inflicts a severe emotional burden on the patient, especially after the experience of feeling fetal movements. Chorionic villi as a source for fetal karyotyping during the tenth week of pregnancy was introduced experimentally by Hahnemann and Mohr (1969). The use of an endoscopic transvaginal approach was also evaluated by Hahnemann (1974). Clinical use of chorionic villi for fetal sex determination was described in 1975 by a Chinese group performing blind transvaginal aspiration without ultrasound examination (Tietung Hospital, 1975). CVS gained widespread acceptance and use only when ultrasound-guided technique for aspiration was introduced.

Technique of Transcervical CVS

Ultrasound examination immediately before the procedure confirms fetal heart activity, appropriate growth, and location of the placenta (Fig. 30–4). The position of the uterus and cervix is determined, and the anticipated catheter path is mentally mapped. If the uterus is severely anteverted, further filling of the urinary bladder will frequently straighten the uterine position. A uterine contraction may interfere with passage of the catheter, and a decision may be made to delay the procedure until the contraction dissipates. When the uterine condition and location are favorable, the patient is placed in the lithotomy position; and the vulva, vagina, and cervix are aseptically prepared with povidone-iodine (Betadine). A speculum is inserted, and the anterior lip of the cervix is grasped with a tenaculum to aid in manipulating the uterus. The distal 3–5 cm of the catheter is molded into a slightly curved shape and then gently passed through the cervix until a loss of resis-

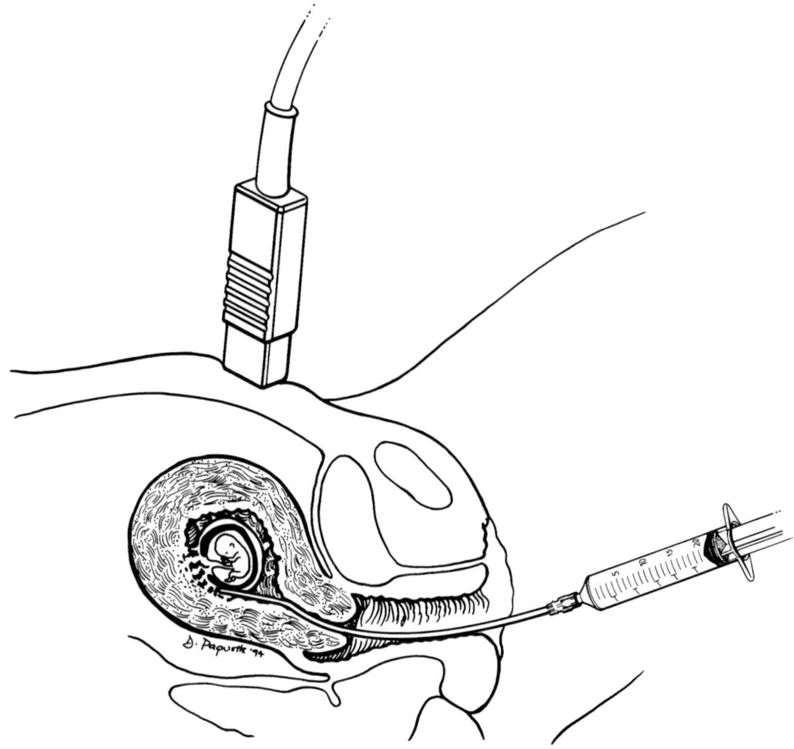

Figure 30–4. Diagrammatic representation of transcervical chorionic villus sampling. (Reprinted with permission from D'Alton and associates, 1994.)

tance is felt at the endocervix. The operator then waits until the sonologist visualizes the tip of the catheter.

The catheter is inserted parallel to the placenta and passed almost to its distal end (Fig. 30–5). The stylet is then removed and a 20-mL heparinized syringe containing nutrient medium is attached. Negative pressure is applied by means of the syringe. The catheter and attached syringe are pulled back slowly. The syringe is then visually inspected for villi, which are easily seen with the naked eye as white branching structures. Once an adequate sample is obtained, the patient is discharged and is told to contact her physician if she develops heavy bleeding, fever, or unusual vaginal discharge. A follow-up scan and MSAFP assay are performed at 16 weeks' gestation.

Technique of Transabdominal CVS

Continuous ultrasound is used to direct a 19- or 20-gauge spinal needle into the long axis of the placenta (Fig. 30–6). After removal of the stylet, villi are aspirated into a 20-mL syringe containing tissue culture media. Unlike transcervical CVS, transabdominal CVS can be performed throughout pregnancy and therefore constitutes an alternative to amniocentesis or PUBS if needed later in pregnancy. If oligohydramnios is present, transabdominal CVS may be the only approach available to determine fetal karyotype.

CVS in Multiple Gestations

Twin and triplet gestations have been sampled successfully using CVS, but there are inherent problems with the technique (Pergament, 1992; Brambati, 1991b; and their colleagues). Distinct placental sites must be identified and sampled individually. If there is any suspicion that two separate samples of placenta are not obtained, a backup amniocentesis should be offered if the fetal genders are concordant (Brambati and associates, 1991b).

Another potential difficulty with CVS in multiple gestations is the possible cross-contamination of samples when both placentae are on the same uterine wall (ie, both anterior or both posterior). In these cases, sampling the lower sac transcervically and the upper sac transabdominally minimizes the chance of contamination. When a biochemical diagnosis is required, the potential for misinterpretation is even greater because a small amount of normal tissue could significantly alter the test result. Therefore, unless individual samples can be guaranteed, amniocentesis should be resorted to.

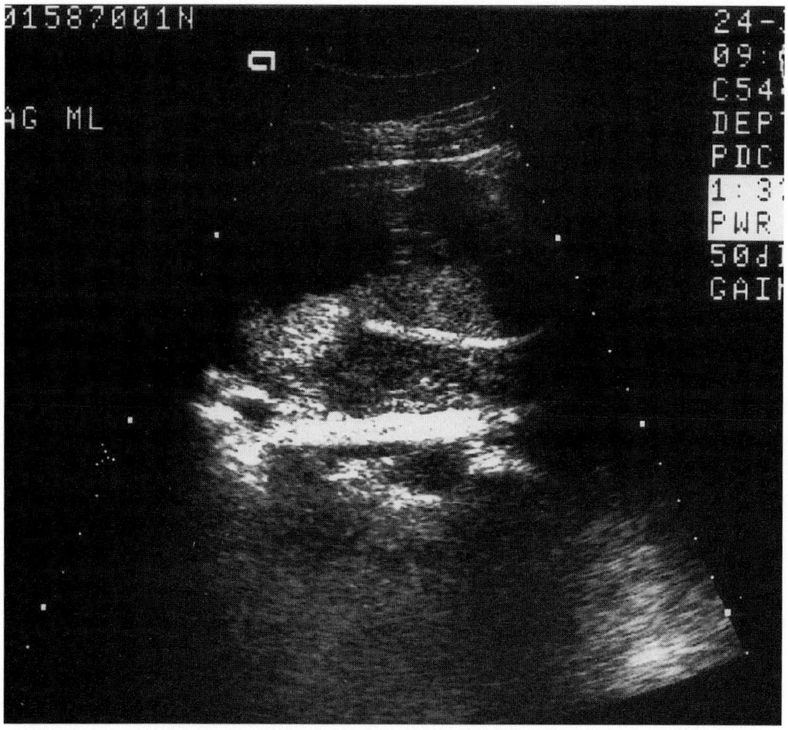

Figure 30–5. Ultrasound image of transcervical chorionic villus sampling demonstrating the catheter shown as the bright white line in the posterior placenta. (Reprinted with permission from D'Alton and associates, 1994.)

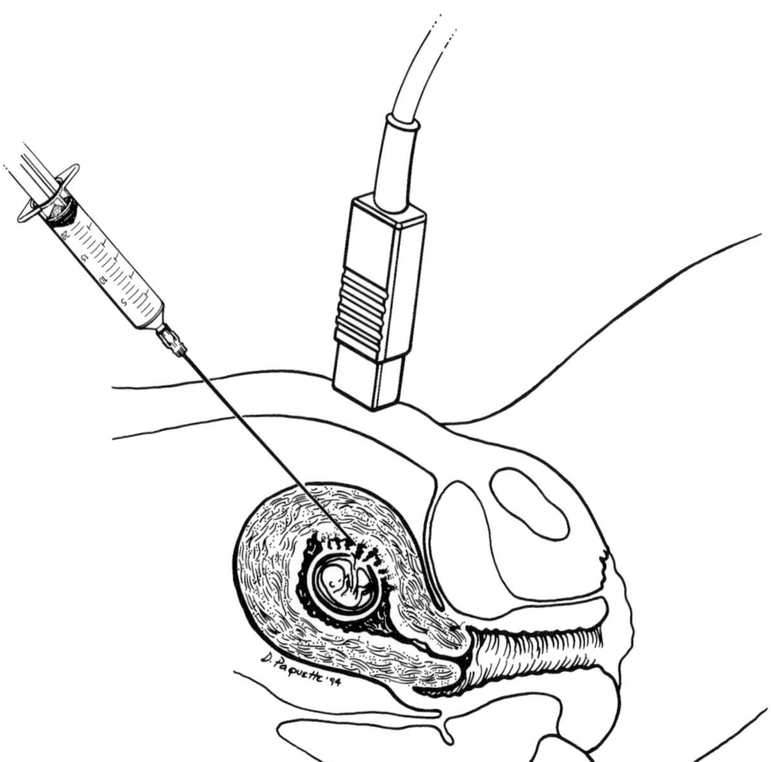

Figure 30–6. Diagrammatic representation of transabdominal chorionic villus sampling. (Reprinted with permission from D'Alton and associates, 1994.)

A detailed drawing of the locations of each placenta and fetus should be made at the time of the procedure. In the case of one abnormal result, this diagram will permit later identification of the affected fetus.

Laboratory Aspects of CVS

The average sample from a transcervical aspiration contains 15–30 mg of villous material. The villi identified in the syringe are carefully and aseptically transferred for confirmatory inspection and dissection under a microscope. Identification of this appropriate tissue is mandatory to minimize maternal decidual contamination. Clean, decidua-free villi are then transferred to Petri dishes for further preparation. Villi are processed for cytogenetic analysis in two ways: results of direct preparation are available within 3–4 days of the procedure; results of tissue culture are usually available within 6–8 days. Most laboratories wait to report both results simultaneously.

It is recommended that both the direct and culture methods be used with all samples. The direct method gives rapid results on cytotrophoblast and minimizes maternal decidual contamination. Tissue culture, which is subject to potential contamination from maternal cells, is a better means of identifying and evaluating discrepancies that may exist between the cytotrophoblast and the fetal state (Bianchi and co-workers, 1993).

Any biochemical diagnosis that can be made from amniotic fluid or cultured amniocytes can also be made from chorionic villi (Poenaru, 1987). In many cases the results are available more rapidly and efficiently when villi are used, sufficient enzyme being present to allow direct analysis rather than the products of tissue culture being required.

Pregnancy Loss Following CVS

The advantage of earlier diagnosis must be weighed against any increased risk of fetal loss that CVS may present. For statistical purposes, procedure-related spontaneous abortion has generally been defined as spontaneous miscarriage or diagnosed intrauterine fetal demise occurring until 28 completed weeks of gestation. Calculating such procedure-related losses is complicated by background pregnancy loss rates, since 2–5 percent of pregnancies viable at 7–12 weeks' gestation are either nonviable when rescanned at 8–20 weeks or will undergo spontaneous miscarriage before 28 weeks' gestation (Liu, 1987; Wilson, 1984; Gilmore, 1985; and their colleagues). The background spontaneous loss rate increases with maternal age and is therefore highest in the same age range in which women are likely to present for prenatal diagnosis (Wilson and associates, 1984; Gilmore and McNay, 1985).

Data evaluating the safety of CVS come primarily from three collaborative reports (Table 30–4). In 1989, the Canadian Collaborative CVS/Amniocentesis Clinical Trial Group reported its experience with a prospective randomized trial comparing the safety of CVS to that of amniocentesis. During the study period, patients across Canada were able to undergo CVS only in conjunction with the randomized protocol. The results of the Canadian group confirmed the safety of CVS as a first-trimester diagnostic procedure. There was a 7.6 percent fetal loss rate (spontaneous abortions, induced abortions, and late losses) in the CVS group, and a 7.0 percent loss rate in the amniocentesis group. An excess loss rate of 0.6 percent for CVS over amniocentesis was obtained, a difference that was not statisti-

TABLE 30–4. TOTAL PREGNANCY LOSS RATES OF CHORIONIC VILLUS SAMPLING (CVS) AND AMNIOCENTESIS (AC) IN THREE COLLABORATIVE TRIALS

Study	Eligible or Attempted (*n*)		Total Loss Rate (%)		CVS Excess Loss Rate (%)
	CVS	*AC*	*CVS*	*AC*	
Canadian Collaborative CVS/ Amniocentesis Clinical Trial Group (1989)	1191	1200	7.6	7.0	0.6
Rhoads and associates (1989)	2235	651	7.2	5.7	0.8[a]
MRC (1991)	1609	1592	13.6	9.0	4.6

[a]Corrected for difference in maternal age and gestational age.
Reprinted with permission from D'Alton and associates (1994).

cally significant. Surprisingly, there was a tendency toward losses beyond 28 weeks in the CVS group. No significant differences were noted between the two groups in the incidence of preterm birth or low birthweight. Maternal complications were equally uncommon in each group.

The US report involved a prospective, though nonrandomized, trial of 2235 women who chose either transcervical CVS or second-trimester amniocentesis (Rhoads and colleagues, 1989). An excess pregnancy loss rate of 0.8 percent in the CVS group over the amniocentesis group was calculated, which was not statistically significant. The rates of loss were lowest in cases in which relatively large amounts of tissue were obtained. Repeated catheter insertions was significantly associated with pregnancy loss. Cases requiring three or more catheter insertions had a 10.8 percent spontaneous abortion rate, compared with a rate of 2.9 percent in cases that required only one pass.

A prospective, randomized, collaborative comparison of more than 3200 pregnancies, sponsored by the European Medical Research Council, demonstrated that CVS may have a 4.6 percent greater pregnancy loss rate than amniocentesis (95% CI 1.6–7.5%) (MRC Working Party, 1991). This difference reflected more spontaneous deaths before 28 weeks' gestation (2.9%), more termination of pregnancy for chromosomal anomalies (1.0%), and more neonatal deaths (0.3%). In this study, villus sampling was performed by both the transcervical and transabdominal routes. The number of repeat procedures was significantly higher in the CVS group, compared with the amniocentesis group.

Exactly what factors contribute to the discrepant results between the European and North American studies remains uncertain. Variability in operator experience might account for part of this discrepancy. The United States trial consisted of 7 centers and the Canadian trial 11 centers. In the Medical Research Council Trial there were 31 participating centers contributing various numbers of cases and using different sampling and cytogenetic procedures. There were, on average, 325 cases per center in the United States study, 106 in the Canadian study, and 52 in the European trial. The pregnancy losses in the European series tended to occur before 20 weeks, compared with the Canadian study in which losses occurred significantly later. There is no apparent explanation for these findings.

Comparison of Transcervical and Transabdominal Approach to CVS

Brambati and associates (1991a) reported the results of a randomized trial of transabdominal versus transcervical CVS by a single operator in 1,194 patients. Over 110 cases deviated from the allocated procedure, and more than 80 percent of the deviations occurred in the transcervical arm of the trial. Moreover, the proportion of cases in which the operator chose to deviate from the allocated procedure increased in each of the 3 years of the study (4.6%, 9.7%, and 15.5%, respectively). More chorionic tissue was obtained by the transcervical method, but the proportion of cases in which less than 10 mg was obtained was similar in both groups. Bleeding was more common following transcervical CVS, whereas cramping was more common in the transabdominal group. No significant difference was detected in the overall fetal loss rate (transabdominal, 16.5% versus transcervical, 15.5%). The transabdominal technique required a significantly smaller proportion of repeat needle insertions (3.3% versus 0.3%), although this did not seem to affect pregnancy outcome. There were also no differences in birthweight, gestational age at delivery, or congenital malformations. The authors commented that a limitation of this study was the operator's eventual preference for the transabdominal approach. They conclude that the two techniques seem equally safe and effective, and the choice to perform one particular technique may largely depend on the operator's preference.

Jackson and co-workers (1992) conducted a randomized comparison of transcervical and transabdominal CVS at 7–12 weeks' gestation. Of 3,999 eligible patients, 94 percent in each arm of the study had the allocated procedure. Only one needle insertion was required in 94 percent of transabdominal CVS cases, and only one catheter pass was required in 90 percent of transcervical CVS procedures. The fetal loss rate, excluding elective terminations of pregnancy, was 3 percent in each group.

Smidt-Jensen and colleagues (1992) published their randomized comparison of routine amniocentesis, transabdominal CVS, and transcervical CVS in 3,706 low-risk patients. Patients were randomly assigned to one of the three procedures. The proportion of patients for whom a cytogenetic diagnosis was successfully obtained at the first attempt was 99.7 percent for amniocentesis, 98.1 percent for transabdominal CVS, and 96.0 percent for transcervical CVS ($p<0.0001$). Total fetal loss rates were 10.9 percent for transcervical CVS, 6.3 percent for transabdominal CVS, and 6.4 percent for amniocentesis, a statistically significant difference. A large difference between the transabdominal and transcervical CVS groups was noted in the proportion of postprocedural losses of cytogenically normal pregnancies (3.7% for transabdominal and 7.7% for transcervical CVS). The authors conclude that although transabdominal CVS and amniocentesis carry similar risks of fetal loss, transcervical CVS is associated with an overall higher rate of fetal loss, estimated to be in excess of 4.0 percent.

It is reasonable to speculate that the fetal loss rate will equilibrate in most centers once equivalent expertise is gained with either approach (Brambati and associates, 1987b). It is most reasonable to conclude that integration of both transcervical and transabdominal methods of CVS into any program offers the most practical and safe approach to first-trimester diagnosis.

Other Complications of CVS

Vaginal bleeding or spotting is relatively uncommon after transabdominal CVS procedures, occurring in 1 percent or less of cases (Rhoads and associates, 1989). Most centers report postprocedure bleeding in 7–10 percent of patients sampled by transcervical CVS. Minimal spotting is more common than bleeding and may occur in almost one-third of women sampled by the transcervical route (Rhoads and co-workers, 1989). A subchorionic hematoma may be visualized immediately after sampling in up to 4 percent of patients sampled transcervically (Brambati and associates, 1987b). The hematoma usually disappears before the sixteenth week of pregnancy and is usually not associated with adverse outcome.

There has been concern since the initial development of transcervical CVS that transvaginal passage of an instrument would introduce vaginal flora into the uterus, thereby increasing the risk of infection. Cultures have isolated bacteria in 30 percent of catheters used for CVS (Brambati, 1985, 1987a; Garden, 1985; McFadyen, 1985; Wass, 1985; and their colleagues). The reported incidence of post-CVS chorioamnionitis, however, is low and occurs following both transcervical and transabdominal procedures. In the United States collaborative trial, infection was suspected as a possible etiology of pregnancy loss in only 0.3 percent of cases (Rhoads and colleagues, 1989). Infection following transabdominal CVS has been demonstrated, at least in some cases, to result from bowel flora introduced by inadvertent puncture by the sampling needle. Early in the development of transcervical CVS, two life-threatening pelvic infections were reported (Barela, 1986; Blakemore, 1985; and their co-workers). A practice of using a new sterile catheter for each insertion has subsequently been universally adopted, and there have been no additional reports of serious infections resulting from the procedure.

Acute rupture of membranes within hours of the procedure can occur but is rare (Rhoads and associates, 1989); in 0.3 percent of cases rupture has been reported days to weeks after the procedure (Hogge and associates, 1986).

An acute rise in MSAFP after CVS has been consistently reported, implying a detectable degree of fetomaternal bleeding (Brambati, 1986; Shulman, 1990; Blakemore, 1986; and their colleagues). The MSAFP elevation is not related to the technique used to retrieve villi but seems to depend on the quantity of tissue aspirated (Shulman and Elias, 1990). Levels will return to normal ranges by 16–18 weeks of gestation, thus allowing serum screening to proceed according to usual prenatal protocols. All Rh-negative, nonsensitized women undergoing CVS should receive Rh_0D immune globulin subsequent to the procedure. Exacerbation of Rh immunization following CVS has been described. Existing Rh sensitization therefore represents a contraindication to the procedure (Moise and Carpenter, 1990).

Risk of Fetal Abnormality Following CVS

First reported by Firth and colleagues (1991), concern has been raised that CVS might cause severe limb deficiencies. Their series of 289 CVS pregnancies identified five infants with severe limb abnormalities; oromandibular-limb hypogenesis syndrome in four and a terminal transverse limb reduction defect in a fifth. The oromandibular-limb hypogenesis syndrome occurs with a birth prevalence of 1/175,000 live births (Hoyme and colleagues, 1982); therefore, the occurrence of this abnormality in more than 1 percent of CVS cases strongly suggested an association. In Firth's initial report, all the limb abnormalities followed transabdominal sampling performed at a relatively early gestational age: between 55 and 66 days' gestation. Burton and co-workers (1992) also reported transverse limb abnormalities after CVS. Apart from these two reports, most other series have found the incidence of limb reduction defects to be not significantly different from the expected rates. Using records of the experience of the eight centers participating in the United States collaborative evaluation of CVS, Mahoney (1991) reported no cases of oromandibular-limb hypogenesis syndrome and no increased incidence of transverse limb defects. Monni and co-workers (1991) reviewed their experience of CVS procedures performed before the 66th day of gestation. They identified 525 out of a total of more than 2700 procedures and reported no severe limb defects in the selected population. Two mild finger abnormalities were seen in their series. Defects have also been observed when CVS is performed after 66 days of gestation. Reports of limb abnormalities with CVS and population-based studies are summarized in Table 30–5.

A variety of mechanisms by which CVS could potentially lead to fetal malformation have been proposed. The occurrence of placental thrombosis with subsequent fetal embolization has been raised as one potential etiology. Inadvertent entry into the extraembryonic coelom with resulting amniotic bands has also been suggested. This seems unlikely because actual bands have not been observed in any cases. The most plausible mechanism is a form of vascular insult leading to underperfusion of the fetus (Brent, 1990). CVS could cause disruption of the vessels supplying the extracorporeal fetal circulation. This disruption would result in the release of vasoactive peptides, producing fetal vasospasm and hypoperfusion of the fetal peripheral circulation. Limb defects have been demonstrated in animal models after cocaine exposure (Brent, 1990; Webster and Brown-Woodman, 1990). Theoretically, an overly vigorous technique during the CVS procedure could lead to significant placental damage, with resulting vasospasm and hypovolemia.

Using transcervical embryoscopic visualization of the first-trimester embryo, Quintero and colleagues (1992) demonstrated the occurrence of fetal facial, head, and thoracic ecchymotic lesions following a traumatic CVS. Although these lesions consistently appeared following significant physical trauma to the placental site, the researchers were not able to produce them by the passage of a standard CVS catheter. Furthermore, these lesions were demonstrated only following the development of a subchorionic hematoma.

A workshop on CVS was convened by the National Institute of Child Health and Human Development (NICHD, 1993) and the American College of Obstetricians and Gynecologists at the National Institutes of Health in April, 1992. Some of those attending the workshop concluded that exposure to CVS may have caused limb defects, but others did not agree with this conclusion. All who attended agreed that the frequency of the syndrome of oromandibular-limb hypogenesis seemed to be more common among CVS-exposed infants. This may correlate with, but not be limited to, CVS performed earlier than 7 weeks' gestation. Further studies are needed to determine whether there are factors that correlate with CVS-associated limb defects. These may include gestational age at the time of the procedure, experience of the operator, and the size of the catheter or needle used to obtain the sample (NICHD, 1993).

Accuracy of CVS Cytogenetic Results

The overall incidence of chromosomal mosaicism in CVS specimens is estimated to be approximately 1 percent (Vejerslev and Mikkelsen, 1989). Generalized chromosomal mosaicism originates from a mutational event in the first or second postzygotic division, and all tissues of the fetus are affected (Kalousek and Dill, 1983). Confined placental mosaicism (CPM), defined as a dichotomy between the chromosomal constitution of placental and fetal tissues, results from mutations occurring in the trophoblast or extraembryonic mesoderm progenitor cells (Kalousek and associates, 1991). In most cases of mosaicism diagnosed by CVS, the cytogenetic abnormality is

TABLE 30–5. INCIDENCE OF LIMB-REDUCTION DEFECTS IN GROUPS UNDERGOING CHORIONIC VILLUS SAMPLING AND POPULATION-BASED STUDIES

Chorionic Villus Sampling Series

Study (First Author)	*55 to 66 Days*[a]	*Defect*	*>66 Days*[a]	*Defect*
Firth (1991)	5/289	1 Transverse limb-reduction defect, 4 combined limb-reduction defects with micrognathia or microglossia	0/250	—
Burton (1992)[b]	—	—	4/394	3 Finger-and-toe abnormalities, 1 finger abnormality
Monni (1991)	0/525	—	2/2227	2 Finger abnormalities
Mahoney(1991)[a]	1/1025	Longitudinal limb-reduction defect	6/8563	1 Longitudinal limb-reduction defect, 5 transverse limb-reduction defects (2 of the 5 were limited to fingers or toes)
Jackson (1991)[c]	1/2367	Bilateral aplasia of the thumbs	4/10,496	3 Transverse limb-reduction defects, 1 finger abnormality
Schloo (1992)	1/636	Microglossia and hypodactyly	3/2200	3 Finger abnormalities (2 of the 3 had a family history of limb defects)

Population-based Studies

Study (First Author)	*Defect*	*Incidence*
Froster-Iskenius (1989)	Combination of limb-reduction defects and micrognathia or microglossia	1/175,000
	Limb-reduction defects	1/1692
	Terminal longitudinal defects	1/2857
	Terminal transverse defects	1/6250
Froster (1992)	Hand	1/11,035
	Fingers	1/7016
	Foot	1/39,158
	Toes	1/43,354

[a]The number of days after the beginning of the last menstrual period at the time the procedure was performed.
[b]The number of procedures performed before 67 days was not reported.
[c]There was some overlap between the series studied by Mahoney and Jackson, et al.
Reprinted with permission from D'Alton and associates (1994).

confined to extraembryonic tissue (Vejerslev, 1989; Johnson, 1990; Breed, 1991; and their colleagues).

Initially, several studies reported a higher incidence of adverse perinatal outcome, including increased fetal loss rates and intrauterine growth retardation (IUGR) in pregnancies complicated by CPM (Kalousek, 1991; Johnson, 1990; and their co-workers). Kalousek and colleagues (1991) confirmed CPM in only one half of placentas studied after birth. IUGR was found only in cases of CPM confirmed in term placentae. Wapner and colleagues (1992) found a significantly higher rate of fetal loss (8.6%) among the 2.5 percent of patients with CPM, in comparison with patients with a normal karyotype (3.4%). Patients with pseudomosaicism had a pregnancy loss rate and perinatal outcome similar to that of the normal population. Issues that still need to be investigated are the exact contribution of CPM to IUGR, the significance of the specific chromosome involved in the mosaicism, and the significance of specific tissue sources (ie, direct cytotrophoblast preparations or mesenchymal tissue cultures) on pregnancy outcome. Counseling before CVS requires a discussion of the frequency and significance of CPM and the potential need for follow-up studies including ultrasound, amniocentesis, and PUBS (Miny and associates, 1991).

Conclusions

CVS is a viable alternative to second-trimester amniocentesis for prenatal diagnosis. Its immediate and long-term safety has been demonstrated; transcervical and transabdominal CVS are comparable regarding safety and efficiency. The techniques are complementary and offer the choice of early prenatal diagnosis to women who have the appropriate indications for the procedure.

PERCUTANEOUS UMBILICAL BLOOD SAMPLING (PUBS)

In 1983 Daffos and co-workers described a method of obtaining fetal blood using ultrasonographic guidance. This involved the passage of a 20-gauge spinal needle through the maternal abdomen into the umbilical cord. This technique, variously described as percutaneous umbilical blood sampling (PUBS), fetal blood sampling, cordocentesis, or funipuncture, offered considerable advantage over the fetoscopic methods previously used to obtain fetal blood.

Technique of PUBS

The main differences in the technique of fetal blood sampling are related to whether the operator uses a needle guide or uses a "free-hand" technique. A variety of needle guides that attach to the transducer can be used. The advantage to this approach is that the needle will be directed precisely to a specific target. The disadvantage is that if the fetus moves or the patient develops a contraction with the needle in the uterus, redirection of the tip may be difficult or impossible and will often require a repeat procedure. Because of these limitations we prefer the free-hand technique to the needle guide. Fetal vessels can be accessed within either the cord or the fetus itself. It is easier to enter the cord at the placental insertion site because it is anchored at this location (Figs. 30–7 and 30–8). Color Doppler imaging significantly enhances the ease of visualization of the cord insertion site and is especially useful when oligohydramnios is present. The hepatic vein is the most accessible vessel for blood sampling within the fetal body.

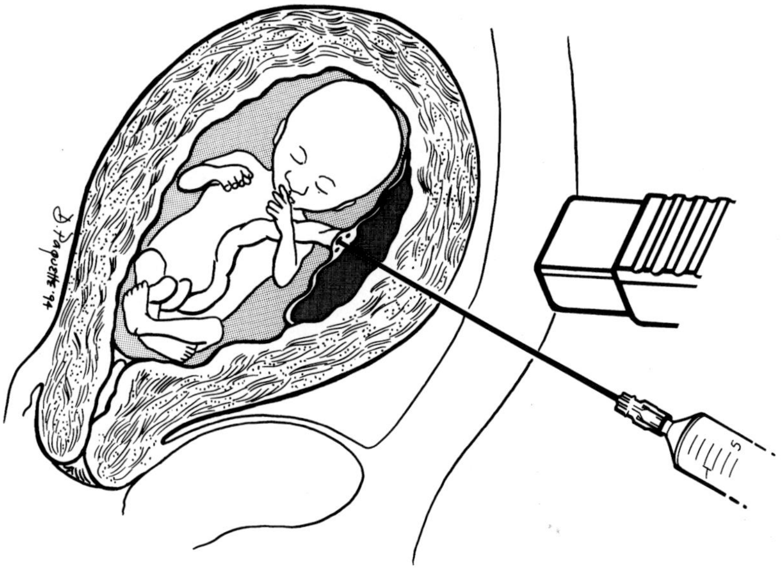

Figure 30–7. Diagrammatic representation of PUBS by ultrasound-guided insertion of the needle into the umbilical vein. Shown is transplacental passage into umbilical vein at the cord-placenta interface.

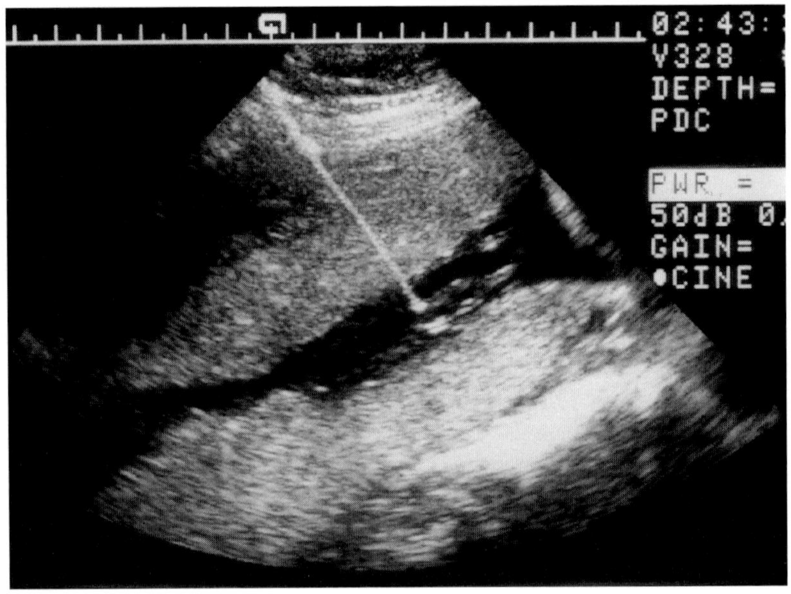

Figure 30–8. Ultrasound image of PUBS demonstrating the needle above the umbilical vein. (Reprinted with permission from D'Alton and associates, 1994.)

Once a sample of blood has been aspirated, it is essential to verify that it is fetal in origin. The most definitive way to establish this is to compare the mean corpuscular volume (MCV) of the red cells to that of a sample of maternal blood; this comparison is easily performed on small aliquots of blood by a standard channeling instrument. It is preferable to have this instrument in the procedure room. Fetal red blood cells are considerably larger than those of an adult and therefore afford rapid differentiation. Alternatively, one can inject a small amount of sterile saline, and if the needle is in the umbilical vein, the microbubbles created by the injection will be seen to move toward the fetus. Forestier and colleagues (1988) recommend performing studies on the aspirated blood that include a complete blood count with differential analysis and determination of anti-I and anti-i cold agglutinin, B-subunit of hCG, factors IX and VIIIC, and AFP levels. It is not our practice to perform all of these studies; we simply compare the fetal and maternal MCV determinations from a Coulter counter in the procedure room.

Success Rates and Safety

The rate of fetal loss after PUBS is approximately 2 percent higher than the background risk for that particular fetus (Daffos and associates, 1985; Shulman and Elias, 1990). Because many of the fetuses studied have severe congenital malformations, the background loss rate is high in comparison with that of the generally lower risk population that undergoes CVS and amniocentesis.

The North American PUBS registry, which is maintained in the United States at Pennsylvania Hospital in Philadelphia, collects data from 16 centers in the United States and Canada. Information on 7462 diagnostic procedures performed on 6023 patients is available (Ludomirsky, 1993). The most common needle used for procedures is a 22-gauge spinal needle. Fetal loss is defined as intrauterine fetal death within 14 days of the procedure. Fetal loss rate is calculated to be 1.12 percent per procedure and 1.33 percent per patient. There were 84 pregnancies that were considered to be lost as a direct consequence of the fetal blood sampling. The major causes for fetal loss are chorioamnionitis, rupture of membranes, bleeding from the puncture site, severe bradycardia, and thrombosis. The range of losses for participating centers varies from 1 percent to 6.7 percent; this range reflects operator experience. These figures are subjective, relying on the operator's impression that a pregnancy loss was directly related to the procedure itself and not to the underlying fetal condition that necessitated the procedure. As many of these fetuses were quite compromised at the time of the PUBS, it is certainly possible that an in utero death following the procedure might have been entirely unrelated. On the other hand, this assessment is subjective, because it could be responsible for an underestimation of the true loss rates for PUBS.

The authors suggest that the intrahepatic vein is an alternative site of sampling or transfusion when access is difficult or failure occurs at the placental cord insertion site. Nicolini and colleagues (1990a) have described their experience with 214 fetal blood sampling procedures performed from the fetal hepatic vein and report success rates of 91 percent and 90 percent for diagnostic and therapeutic procedures, respectively. Fetal loss rates comparable to those for blood sampling procedures performed at the placental cord insertion site were reported. Because PUBS entails a substantially greater risk of pregnancy loss than amniocentesis, it should be reserved for situations in which rapid diagnosis is essential or in which diagnostic information cannot be obtained by safer means (D'Alton and DeCherney, 1993).

Indications for PUBS

Approximately two-thirds of the cases of diagnostic fetal blood sampling procedures reported to the PUBS registry were performed either to determine a rapid karyotype or to evaluate hematologic status in pregnancies at risk for red blood cell isoimmunization (Ludomirsky, 1993). One-third of the procedures were performed to rule out fetal infection or to evaluate nonimmune hydrops, fetal acid-base status, twin-to-twin transfusion syndrome, or fetal platelet count.

Chromosome Analysis

The ultrasonographic detection of fetal morphologic malformations is now the most common indication for rapid fetal karyotyping in the United States (Table 30–6). With PUBS, fetal karyotypes are usually available from fetal white blood cells within 48–72 hours. The main advantage cited for PUBS is the rapid availability of the results that it affords. Its disadvantage is that it entails a greater risk of pregnancy loss than does amniocentesis. We recommend PUBS only when rapid diagnosis is essential or when diagnostic information cannot be obtained by a safer means (D'Alton and associates, 1993a); amniocentesis with the FISH technique for the rapid assay of chromosomes 21, 18, 13, X, and Y is preferred (D'Alton and associates, 1993b). An exception is the case in which the amniotic fluid is blood stained, as FISH is then uninformative. We then proceed to PUBS and a placental biopsy if rapid karyotyping is essential. Karyotyping fetal white blood cells is also indicated for mosaicism detected in material obtained from amniotic fluid or chorionic villi. Although most cases of mosaicism found in chorionic villi can be effectively ruled out by amniocentesis, there have been reports of trisomy 21 mosaicism in which the chorionic villus culture revealed two cell lines, the amniotic fluid culture was entirely normal, yet true mosaicism was demonstrated in fetal blood (Ledbetter and co-workers, 1990).

DNA Analysis

Most inherited hematologic disorders can now be diagnosed by the study of fetal DNA obtained from amniocytes or chorionic villi. Therefore, the antenatal detection of most

TABLE 30–6. INDICATIONS FOR PUBS

Most Frequent	Less Frequent
Rapid karyotyping	Nonimmune hydrops fetalis
when ultrasound detects anatomic malformation	Fetal platelet assessment
when mosaicism is reported from amniotic fluid or CVS specimens	Fetal infection
Fetal red cell isoimmunization	Fetal acid-base status
	Diagnosis of twin–twin transfusion
	Hemoglobinopathies
	Coagulation factor deficiencies
	Immunologic deficiencies

Reprinted with permission from D'Alton and associates (1994).

congenital coagulopathies, hemoglobinopathies, white blood cell disorders, and immune disorders does not usually require direct analysis of fetal blood specimens. In some of these cases, family studies are uninformative and PUBS is necessary for diagnosis. This is now the exception rather than the rule.

Fetal Anemia

Assessment of fetal anemia in cases of red blood cell isoimmunization is most accurate with direct measurement of fetal blood. Since Liley's study in 1961, the degree of fetal anemia in Rh isoimmunized pregnancies has usually been assessed by serial amniocenteses and studies of ΔOD 450 values as a function of gestational age. These values reflect the amount of bilirubin pigment in the amniotic fluid and, as such, are an indirect indicator of the degree of fetal hemolysis. All the data in Liley's original paper, however, were collected at 28 weeks' gestation or later, and extrapolation of the lines dividing the zones in the original graph to earlier gestational ages may not be appropriate (Nicolaides and co-workers, 1986b). Nicolaides found that the ΔOD 450 values accurately reflected the degree of fetal anemia in the third trimester but not in the second trimester when amniotic fluid ΔOD 450 values were compared with fetal hematocrits. Furthermore, there was no pattern to the inaccuracies; in some cases, high ΔOD 450 values inappropriately suggested the need for transfusion, and in other cases, low values were found in fetuses with significant anemia. Therefore, in severely affected cases of Rh isoimmunization before 28 weeks' gestation, determination of the fetal hemoglobin level is the most accurate and reliable way to determine the fetal status and the optimal timing of a transfusion.

Fetal blood sampling for determination of fetal anemia in red cell isoimmunization is the second most common reason for this procedure. It accounts for 23 percent of all cases reported to the PUBS registry (Ludomirsky, 1993). Fetal blood may also be obtained in cases of red blood cell isoimmunization to determine the antigen status of the fetus when the father is heterozygous for the discordant antigen. A single invasive procedure can rule out the disease, and no further diagnostic testing will be necessary. For fetal Rhesus D blood type determination, techniques such as amniocentesis and maternal blood sampling may eventually replace PUBS (Bennett, 1993; Lo, 1993; and their associates).

Fetal Thrombocytopenia

Women with idiopathic thrombocytopenic purpura (ITP) have up to a 15 percent chance of delivering a neonate with significant depression of its platelet count. The risk of significant neonatal bleeding, specifically intracranial hemorrhage, is rare. Nevertheless, some reports advocate delivery by cesarean section if the fetal platelet count is lower than 50,000/mm^3 in order to avoid the trauma that may result from labor. There are no data to show, however, that cesarean section offers an advantage over vaginal delivery. The fetal platelet count can be determined by scalp sampling during labor. This method may not be an accurate reflection of the fetal platelet count and may be falsely low secondary to platelet clumping, or to dilution from amniotic fluid or scalp edema. Furthermore, to allow fetal scalp sampling the patient must be in labor with the cervix dilated, the fetal head engaged, and the membranes ruptured. Additionally, there may not be sufficient time for scalp sampling in women with precipitous labor.

In cases of fetal thrombocytopenia, the timing of intracranial hemorrhage is unclear. It is possible that it may occur early in labor before scalp sampling is technically feasible. An alternative approach is to perform PUBS in women with ITP at term, before the onset of labor. Most studies have determined that PUBS at term reliably predicts the cord platelet count at the time of delivery (Moise, 1988; Scioscia, 1988; Garmel, 1994; Leonardi, 1995; and their co-workers). It is unclear if cesarean section in the 10–15 percent of cases with documented fetal thrombocytopenia will prevent intracranial hemorrhage. We have found documentation of the fetal platelet count before delivery to be helpful in choosing the site of delivery (Garmel and associates, 1994). If the fetal platelet count is normal, the patient can deliver at a community hospital. The small percentage of patients carrying severely thrombocytopenic fetuses can deliver at a tertiary care center, allowing immediate treatment of the newborn. In one series of 41 mothers with ITP there were six fetuses with a platelet count of lower than 50,000/mm^3. All of these patients were delivered by cesarean section. In all cases neonatal therapy with steroids and intravenous gamma globulin was required (Garmel and co-workers, 1994).

Alloimmune thrombocytopenia is the platelet equivalent of Rh disease. In this disorder, the mother makes antibodies to antigens on the fetal platelets, and transplacental passage of these antibodies results in fetal thrombocytopenia. This disorder is associated with a much more marked depression of the fetal platelet count than is found in ITP. Unlike ITP, intracranial hemorrhage may occur in utero long before the onset of labor. Because severe thrombocytopenia and intracranial hemorrhage have been documented as early as 20 weeks' gestation in this disorder, prolonged antenatal therapy is necessary to protect the fetus against the possibility of spontaneous bleeding. Since platelets have a life span of only 5–7 days, repeated in utero transfusions would be required if this were the chosen therapeutic option. Most fetuses with alloimmune thrombocytopenia will respond to intravenous gamma globulin at a dose of 1 g/kg administered intravenously once a week to the mother (Bussel, 1988; Lynch, 1992; and their colleagues).

The risk of PUBS is higher in patients with alloimmune thrombocytopenia than for the general population. In these cases, the blood sampling should be performed in a facility with access to rapid automated platelet counts at the time of the procedure, and a count should be determined before the sampling needle is withdrawn. A concentrate of washed maternal platelets should be available. If the fetal platelet count is found to be lower than $40,000/mm^3$ to $50,000/mm^3$, a transfusion of maternal platelet concentrate can then be given.

Infectious Disease Diagnosis

Evaluation for fetal infection is the third most common indication for fetal blood sampling in the PUBS registry (8% of all cases). Daffos and colleagues (1988) reported on more than 700 pregnancies exposed to *Toxoplasma gondii* infection and demonstrated that 95 percent were not infected. Although sampling has been performed for *T. gondii* in the United States, screening for toxoplasma is not offered routinely to pregnant women; therefore, it is performed rarely. Direct isolation of the organism from fetal blood or amniotic fluid is the most reliable evidence of fetal infection. Technical difficulties and the length of time necessary for culture of the organism often make this approach impractical. Another method is to evaluate the fetal antibody response. Production of specific IgM antibodies is gestational-age dependent and also seems to depend on the organism involved. Almost 100 percent of fetuses with congenital rubella infection produce specific IgM antibodies after 22 weeks (Daffos and associates, 1984), whereas only 15 percent of those infected with *T. gondii* tested between 24 and 29 weeks produce specific IgM antibodies against the parasite (Daffos and co-workers, 1988). Therefore, although detection of specific IgM antibodies in fetal blood is reliable evidence of fetal infection, their absence does not rule it out. Nonspecific evidence of infection includes fetal thrombocytopenia, erythroblastosis, leukocytosis, eosinophilia, and elevated levels of gamma-glutamyltransferase, lactic dehydrogenase, interferon, and total IgM antibodies (Raymond, 1990; Lebon, 1985; and their colleagues).

In recent years PCR analysis has been highly reliable in detecting cytomegalovirus in amniotic fluid. Preliminary data suggest that PCR analysis of amniotic fluid is both highly sensitive and specific for the toxoplasma organism, affording a diagnosis in a few hours (Grover and associates, 1990). It is likely that amniocentesis and molecular techniques will replace PUBS for the confirmation of fetal infection.

Fetal Physiological Status

Because cord pH at the time of delivery is a well-accepted indicator of neonatal status, it was hoped that fetal blood sampling for blood gasses would also accurately predict the fetal condition. Theoretically, PUBS could prove to be useful when more conventional forms of fetal assessment (nonstress testing, biophysical profile) were either equivocal or conflicting. Nicolaides and co-workers (1989) found significantly more hypoxemia, hypercapnia, hyperlactic-acidemia, and acidosis when 196 growth-restricted fetuses were compared with 208 who were appropriate in size for gestational age. Nicolini and colleagues (1990b), however, found that acid-base determination did not predict perinatal outcome in a group of growth-restricted fetuses. In their study, 26 growth-restricted fetuses with normal anatomy and karyotypes and absent end-diastolic flow on Doppler examination of the umbilical artery were compared with 20 similar fetuses, with end-diastolic flow evident on Doppler examination. The perinatal mortality was 65.4 percent in the first group and 0 in the latter. Significant differences in fetal blood values of Po_2, Pco_2, base equivalents, and nucleated red cell counts were demonstrable between the groups. These measurements did not, however, discriminate between surviving fetuses and those who died perinatally. The values in fetuses who survived were similar to those in fetuses who died in the perinatal period. The authors concluded that PUBS has a limited role in monitoring fetal well-being. Appreciable fetal acidosis and hypoxia are found only when the umbilical artery Doppler waveform and the fetal heart rate pattern are abnormal (Nicolini, 1990b; Pardi, 1993; and their associates). Doppler velocimetry of the umbilical artery seems to be a much more powerful predictor than PUBS of the compromised IUGR fetus. Furthermore, there is a much higher incidence of fetal distress, necessitating emergency cesarean section when PUBS is performed in IUGR fetuses (Ludomirsky, 1993). Because of this, amniocentesis is the preferred technique when determination of fetal karyotype is indicated in the workup of the growth-restricted fetus.

Fetal Therapy

The greatest success achieved with intravascular therapy to date has been the treatment of fetal anemia. Platelet transfusions have been administered to severely thrombocytopenic fetuses in utero. This has been done as a single procedure immediately before delivery in order to avoid the necessity of performing an elective cesarean section and has also been done on serial occasions for the management of alloimmune thrombocytopenia.

Several fetal conditions have been treated through administration of therapeutic agents to the mother. An example of this form of fetal therapy is the treatment of fetal arrhythmias with various antiarrhythmic agents (Dumesic and associates, 1982). In some cases, however, the drugs must be given directly into the fetal circulation because they cross the placenta poorly, if at all. For example, maternally administered digoxin is not always effective in treating supraventricular tachycardia in hydropic fetuses because transplacental passage of the drug is suboptimal in the presence of fetal congestive heart failure (Weiner and Thompson, 1988).

Animal data suggest that in utero stem cell transplantation is feasible provided it is done early in fetal life but that the chances of rejection increase as pregnancy progresses (Crombleholme and co-workers, 1991). Chimeras have been successfully created in utero and maintained after birth in various species without immunosuppression (Flake and colleagues, 1986). In humans, antenatal stem cell transplantation has thus far been reported in only a few cases. Access to the fetal circulation allows the potential for this type of therapeutic strategy to be attempted during fetal life.

Conclusions

Access to the fetal circulation has led to important contributions to the understanding of fetal physiology and disease states. PUBS has an overall fetal loss rate of 2 percent. There is now a decline in the indications for fetal sampling because of advances in molecular and cytogenetic techniques, which allow for diagnosis from amniotic fluid and chorionic villi. Performance of less invasive procedures that provide the same information is encouraged. PUBS should be reserved for those situations in which diagnostic information cannot be obtained by safer methods. However, it is possible that over the next decade we will witness more use of PUBS for intrauterine therapy, such as for stem cell transplantation.

Summary

Midtrimester amniocentesis created the field of prenatal diagnosis and has become the standard to which all other methods are compared. It remains the procedure of choice when fetal safety is the primary consideration. Earlier prenatal diagnostic methods have increasing appeal for many patients. The most studied of these methods is CVS. Both transcervical and transabdominal techniques are comparably effective; individual operator experience and placental location are usually the criteria for choice. Experience with early amniocentesis is accumulating; however, assessment of its safety awaits more clarification by randomized controlled trials. Advances in molecular techniques have led to a declining number of reasons for using PUBS. It is now rarely the chosen procedure for determining fetal karyotype. It is, however, the most direct method of evaluating the severity of Rh sensitization and is the preferred method in severe cases. PUBS is likely to be used more frequently for fetal therapy than for karyotyping over the next decade. Helping the patient select the most appropriate diagnostic procedure for each indication is a role of crucial importance for the obstetrician and genetic counselor.

REFERENCES

Aburel ME. Le declenchement du travail par injections intraamniotique de serum sale hypertonique. Gynecol Obstet 1937; 36:398.

ACOG Technical Bulletin. Alpha-fetoprotein. April 1991; 154:3.

Anderson RL, Goldberg JD, Golbus MS. Prenatal diagnosis in multiple gestation: 20 years' experience with amniocentesis. Prenat Diagn 1991; 11:263.

Assel BG, Lewis SM, Dickerman LH, et al. Single-operator comparison of early and mid-second trimester amniocentesis. Obstet Gynecol 1992; 79:940.

Bahado-Singh R, Schmitt R, Hobbins JC. New technique for genetic amniocentesis in twins. Obstet Gynecol 1992; 70:304.

Barela AI, Kleinman GE, Golditch IM, et al. Septic shock with renal failure after chorionic villus sampling. Am J Obstet Gynecol 1986; 154:1100.

Beekhuis JR, DeBruijn HWA, Van Lith JMN, et al. Second trimester amniocentesis in twins. Br J Obstet Gynaecol 1992; 99:126.

Benn P, Ciarleglio L, Lettieri L, et al. A rapid (but wrong) prenatal diagnosis. N Engl J Med 1992; 326:1638.

Bennett PR, Le Van Kim C, Colin Y, et al. Prenatal determination of fetal RhD type by DNA amplification. N Engl J Med 1993; 329:607.

Bevis DCA. Composition of liquor amnii in haemolytic disease of the newborn. Lancet 1950; 2:443.

Bianchi DW, Wilkins-Haug LE, Enders AC, et al. Origin of extraembryonic mesoderm in experimental animals: relevance to chorionic mosaicism in humans. Am J Med Gene 1993; 46:542.

Blakemore KJ, Mahoney MJ, Hobbins JC. Infection and chorionic villus sampling. Lancet 1985; 2:339.

Blakemore KJ, Baumgarten A, Schoenfeld-Dimaio M, et al. Rise in maternal serum alpha-fetoprotein concentration after chorionic villus sampling and the possibility of isoimmunization. Am J Obstet Gynecol 1986; 155:988.

Brambati B, Terzian E, Tognoni G. Randomized clinical trial of transabdominal versus transcervical chorionic villus sampling methods. Prenat Diagn 1991a; 11:285.

Brambati B, Tului L, Lanzani A, et al. First-trimester genetic diagnosis in multiple pregnancy: principles and potential pitfalls. Prenat Diagn 1991b; 11:767.

Brambati B, Matarrelli M, Varotto F. Septic complications after chorionic villus sampling. Lancet 1987a; 1:1212.

Brambati B, Oldrini A, Ferrazzi E, et al. Chorionic villus sampling: an analysis of the obstetric experience of 1000 cases. Prenat Diagn 1987b; 7:157.

Brambati B, Guercilena S, Bonacchi I, et al. Feto-maternal transfusion after chorionic villus sampling: clinical implications. Hum Reprod 1986; 27:37.

Brambati B, Varotto F. Infection and chorionic villus sampling. Lancet 1985; 2:609.

Breed ASPM, Mantingh A, Vosters R, et al. Follow-up and pregnancy outcome after a diagnosis of mosaicism in CVS. Prenat Diagn 1991; 11:577.

Brent RL. Relationship between uterine vascular clamping, vascular disruption syndrome and cocaine teratology. Teratology 1990; 41:757.

Broome DL, Wilson MG, Weiss B, et al. Needle puncture of fetus: a complication of second-trimester amniocentesis. Am J Obstet Gynecol 1976; 126:247.

Burton BK, Schulz CJ, Burd LI. Limb anomalies associated with chorionic villus sampling. Obstet Gynecol 1992; 79:726.

Burton BK, Nason LM, DeHenati MJ. False positive acetylcholinesterase with early amniocentesis. Obstet Gynecol 1989; 74:607.

Bussel J, Berkowitz RL, McFarland JG, et al. Antenatal treatment of neonatal alloimmune thrombocytopenia. N Engl J Med 1988; 319:1374.

Byrne D, Azar G, Nicolaides K. Why cell culture is successful after early amniocentesis. Fetal Diagn Ther 1991; 6:84.

Canadian Collaborative CVS/Amniocentesis Clinical Trial Group. Multicentre randomized clinical trial of chorion villus sampling and amniocentesis. Lancet 1989; 1:1.

Coleman BG, Grumbach K, Aarger PH, et al. Twin gestations: monitoring of complications and anomalies with US. Radiology 1987; 165:449.

Cowett R, Hakanson D, Kocon R, et al. Untoward neonatal effect of intraamniotic administration of methylene blue. Obstet Gynecol 1976; 48(suppl): 745.

Cragan JD, Martin ML, Khoury MJ. Dye use during amniocentesis and birth defects (Letter). Lancet 1993;341:1352.

Crandall BF, Hanson FW, Tennant F. Acetylcholinesterase (ACHE) electrophoresis and early amniocentesis (Abstract 1010). Am J Hum Genet 1989a; 4(suppl):A257.

Crandall BF, Hanson FW, Tennant F, et al. Alpha-fetoprotein levels in amniotic fluid between 11 and 15 weeks. Am J Obstet Gynecol 1989b; 160:1204.

Crombleholme TM, Langer JC, Harrison MR, et al. Transplantation of fetal cells. Am J Obstet Gynecol 1991; 164:218.

D'Alton ME, DeCherney AH. Prenatal diagnosis. N Engl J Med 1993a; 328:114.

D'Alton ME, Corelli M, Ward B. Utilization of fluorescence in situ hybridization (FISH) for rapid aneuploidy detection in a perinatal diagnosis center. Am J Obstet Gynecol (SPO abstract) 1993b; 168:399.

D'Alton ME, Craigo S, Bianchi D. Prenatal diagnosis procedures. Cur Prob Ob/Gyn Fertil 1994a; 17:41.

D'Alton ME. Prenatal diagnostic procedures. Part 1—Diagnosis and treatment of fetal disease. Semin Perinatal 1994b; 18:140.

Daffos F, Capella-Pavlovsky M, Forestier F. Fetal blood sampling during pregnancy with use of a needle guided by ultrasound: a study of 606 consecutive cases. Am J Obstet Gynecol 1985; 153:655.

Daffos F, Capella-Pavlovsky M, Forestier F. Fetal blood sampling via the umbilical cord using a needle guided by ultrasound. Prenat Diagn 1983; 3:271.

Daffos F, Forestier F, Capella-Pavlovsky M, et al. Prenatal management of 746 pregnancies at risk for congenital toxoplasmosis. N Engl J Med 1988; 318:271.

Daffos F, Forestier F, Grangeot-Keros L, et al. Prenatal diagnosis of congenital rubella. Lancet 1984; 2:1.

Dumesic DA, Silverman NH, Tobias S, et al. Transplacental cardioversion of fetal supraventricular tachycardia with procainamide. N Engl J Med 1982; 307:1128.

Elias S, Gerbie AB, Simpson JL, et al. Genetic amniocentesis in twin gestations. Am J Obstet Gynecol 1980; 138:169.

Epley SL, Hanson JW, Cruikshank DP. Fetal injury with midtrimester diagnostic amniocentesis. Obstet Gynecol 1979; 53:77.

Filkins K, Russo J. Genetic amniocentesis in multiple gestations. Prenat Diagn 1984; 4:223.

Finegan JAK, Quarrington BJ, Hughes HE, et al. Child outcome following mid-trimester amniocentesis: development, behaviour, and physical status at age 4 years. Br J Obstet Gynaecol 1990; 97:32.

Firth HV, Boyd PA, Chamberlain P, et al. Severe limb abnormalities after chorion villus sampling at 56–66 days gestation. Lancet 1991; 337:762.

Flake AW, Harrison MR, Adzick NS, et al. Transplantation of fetal hematopoietic stem cells in utero: the creation of hematopoietic chimeras. Science 1986; 233:776.

Forestier F, Cox WL, Daffos F, et al. The assessment of fetal blood samples. Am J Obstet Gynecol 1988; 158:1184.

Froster UG, Baird PA. Limb-reduction defects and chorionic villus sampling. Lancet 1992;339:66.

Froster-Iskenius UG, Baird PA. Limb reduction defects in over one million consecutive livebirths. Teratology 1989; 39:127.

Fuchs F, Riis P. Antenatal sex determination. Nature 1956; 177:330.

Garden AS, Reid G, Benzie RJ. Chorionic villus sampling. Lancet 1985; 1:1270.

Garmel S, Craigo S, Morin L, et al. The management of immune thrombocytopenic purpura with percutaneous umbilical blood sampling (Abstract). Am J Obstet Gynecol 1994; 170(1, part 2):335.

Gilmore DH, McNay MB. Spontaneous fetal loss rate in early pregnancy. Lancet 1985; 2:107.

Gluck L, Kulovich MV, Borer RC, et al. The interpretation and significance of the lecithin/sphingomyelin ratio in amniotic fluid. Am J Obstet Gynecol 1974; 109:142.

Golbus MS, Loughman WD, Epstein CJ. Prenatal genetic diagnosis in 3000 amniocenteses. N Engl J Med 1979; 300:157.

Gosden C, Nicolaides KH, Rodeck CH. Fetal blood sampling in investigation of chromosome mosaicism in amniotic fluid cell culture. Lancet 1988; 1:613.

Grover CM, Thulliez P, Remington JS, et al. Rapid prenatal diagnosis of congenital toxoplasma infection by using polymerase chain reaction and amniotic fluid. J Clin Microbiol 1990; 28:2297.

Haddow JE, Palomaki GE, Knight GJ, et al. Prenatal screening for Down's syndrome with use of maternal serum markers. N Engl J Med 1992; 327:588.

Hahnemann N. Early prenatal diagnosis; a study of biopsy techniques and cell culturing from extraembryonic membranes. Clin Genet 1974; 6:294.

Hahnemann N, Mohr J. Antenatal foetal diagnosis in genetic disease. Bull Eur Soc Hum Genet 1969; 3:47.

Hallman M, Kulovich M, Kirkpatrick E, et al. Phosphatidylinositol and phosphatidylglycerol in amniotic fluid: indices of lung maturity. Am J Obstet Gynecol 1976; 125:613.

Hanson FW, Tennant FR, Hune S, et al. Early amniocentesis: outcome, risks, and technical problems at ≤ 12.8 weeks. Am J Obstet Gynecol 1992; 166:1707.

Henry GP, Miller WA. Early amniocentesis. J Reprod Med 1992; 37:396.

Hill LM, Platt LD, Kellogg B. Rh-sensitization after genetic amniocentesis. Obstet Gynecol 1980; 56:459.

Hogge WA, Schonberg SA, Golbus MS. Chorionic villus sampling: experience of the first 1000 cases. Am J Obstet Gynecol 1986; 154:1249.

Hook EB, Cross PK, Schreinemachers DM. Chromosomal abnormality rates at amniocentesis and in live-born infants. JAMA 1983; 249:2034.

Hook EB. Rates of chromosome abnormalities at different maternal ages. Obstet Gynecol 1981; 58:282.

Hoyme HF, Jones KL, Van Allen MI, et al. Vascular pathogenesis of transverse limb reduction defects. J Pediatr 1982; 101:839.

Hsu LYF, Perlis T. United States survey on chromosome mosaicism and pseudomosaicism in prenatal diagnosis. Prenat Diagn 1984; 4:97.

Jackson LG, Zachary JM, Fowler SE, et al. A randomized comparison of transcervical and transabdominal chorionic villus sampling. N Engl J Med 1992; 327:594.

Jackson LG, Wapner RJ, Brambati B. Limb abnormalities and chorionic villus sampling. Lancet 1991; 337:1423.

Jacobson CB, Barter RH. Intrauterine diagnosis and management of genetic defects. Am J Obstet Gynecol 1967; 99:795.

Jeanty P, Rodesch F, Romero R, et al. How to improve your amniocentesis technique. Am J Obstet Gynecol 1983; 146:593.

Johnson A, Wapner RJ, Davis GH, et al. Mosaicism in chorionic villus sampling: an association with poor perinatal outcome. Obstet Gynecol 1990; 75:573.

Jorgensen FS, Bang J, Lind AM, et al. Genetic amniocentesis at 7–14 weeks of gestation. Prenat Diagn 1992; 12:277.

Kalousek DK, Howard-Peebles PN, Olson SB, et al. Confirmation of CVS mosaicism in term placentae and high frequency of intrauterine growth retardation association with confined placental mosaicism. Prenat Diagn 1991; 11:743.

Kalousek D, Dill F. Chromosomal mosaicism confined to the placenta in human conceptions. Science 1983; 221:665.

Karp, LE, Hayden PW. Fetal puncture during midtrimester amniocentesis. Obstet Gynecol 1977; 49:115.

Klinger K, Landes G, Shook D, et al. Rapid detection of chromosome aneuploidies in uncultured amniocytes by using fluorescence in situ hybridization (FISH). Am J Hum Genet 1992; 51:55.

Lamb MP. Gangrene of a fetal limb due to amniocentesis. Br J Obstet Gynaecol 1975; 82:829.

Lambl D. Ein seltener Fall von Hydramnios. Zentrabl Gynaskol 1881; 5:329.

Lebo RV, Flandermeyer RR, Diukman R, et al. Prenatal diagnosis with repetitive in situ hybridization probes. Am J Med Genet 1992; 43:848.

Lebon P, Daffos F, Checoury A, et al. Presence of an acid-labile alpha-interferon in sera from fetuses and children with congenital rubella. J Clin Microbiol 1985; 21:775.

Ledbetter DH, Martin AO, Verlinsky Y, et al. Cytogenetic results of chorionic villus sampling: high success rate and diagnostic accuracy in the United States collaborative study. Am J Obstet Gynecol 1990; 162:495.

Lenke RR, Cyr DR, Mack LA. Midtrimester genetic amniocentesis with simultaneous ultrasound guidance. J Clin Ultrasound 1985; 13:371.

Leonardi MR, Berry SM, Wolfe HM, et al. Determination of fetal platelet counts in pregnancies complicated by ITP. Am J Obstet Gynecol 1995; 172:281.

Liley AW. Liquor amnii analysis in the management of the pregnancy complicated by rhesus isoimmunization. Am J Obstet Gynecol 1961; 82:1359.

Liu DTV, Jeavons B, Preston C, et al. A prospective study of spontaneous miscarriage in ultrasonically normal pregnancies and relevance to chorion villus sampling. Prenat Diagn 1987; 7:223.

Lo YM, Bowell PJ, Selinger M, et al. Prenatal determination of fetal RhD status by analysis of peripheral blood of rhesus negative mothers. Lancet 1993; 341:1147.

Lubs HA, Ruddle FH. Chromosomal abnormalities in the human population: estimation of rates based on New Haven newborn study. Science 1970; 169:495.

Ludomirsky A. Intrauterine fetal blood sampling—a multicenter registry; evaluation of 7462 procedures between 1987–1991 (Abstract). Am J Obstet Gynecol 1993; 168:318.

Lynch L, Bussel JB, McFarland JG, et al. Antenatal treatment of alloimmune thrombocytopenia. Obstet Gynecol 1992; 80:67.

Mahoney J. Limb abnormalities and chorionic villus sampling. Lancet 1991; 337:1422.

McFadyen IR, Taylor-Robinson D, Furr PM, et al. Infections and chorionic villus sampling. Lancet 1985; 2:610.

Medical Research Council. Diagnosis of Genetic Disease by Amniocentesis During the Second Trimester of Pregnancy. Ottawa: MRC, 1977.

Menees TD, Miller JD, Holly LE. Amniography: preliminary report. Am J Roentgenol Radium Ther 1930; 24:363.

Merin MD, Beyth Y. Uniocular congenital blindness as a complication of midtrimester amniocentesis. Am J Ophthalmol 1980; 89:299.

Milunsky A. Genetic Disorders and the Fetus: Diagnosis, Prevention, and Treatment. New York: Plenum Press, 1979.

Miny P, Hammer P, Gerlach B, et al. Mosaicism and accuracy of prenatal cytogenetic diagnoses after chorionic villus sampling and placental biopsies. Prenat Diagn 1991; 11:581.

Moise KJ, Carpenter RJ. Increased severity of fetal hemolytic disease with known Rhesus alloimmunization after first trimester transcervical chorionic villus biopsy. Fetal Diagn Ther 1990; 5:76.

Moise KJ, Carpenter RJ, Cotton DB, et al. Percutaneous umbilical cord blood sampling in the evaluation of fetal platelet counts in pregnant patients with autoimmune thrombocytopenic purpura. Obstet Gynecol 1988; 72:346.

Monni G, Ibba RM, Lai R, et al. Limb-reduction defects and chorion villus sampling. Lancet 1991; 337:1091.

MRC Working Party on the Evaluation of Chorion Villus Sampling. Medical Research Council European Trial of Chorion Villus Sampling. Lancet 1991; 337:1491.

Nadel AS, Green JK, Holmes LB, et al. Absence of need for amniocentesis in patients with elevated levels of maternal serum alpha-fetoprotein and normal ultrasonographic examinations. N Engl J Med 1990; 323:557.

Nadler HL. Antenatal detection of hereditary disorders. Pediatrics 1968; 42:912.

NICHD Amniocentesis Registry. The Safety and Accuracy of Mid-Trimester Amniocentesis. DHEW Publication No. (NIH) 78-190. Washington, DC: Department of Health, Education and Welfare, 1978.

NICHD Amniocentesis Registry. Midtrimester amniocentesis for prenatal diagnosis: Safety and accuracy. JAMA 1976; 236:1471.

NICHD Workshop on Chorionic Villus Sampling and Limb and Other Defects, October 20, 1992. Teratology 1993; 48:7.

Nicolaides KH, Gabbe SG, Campbell S, et al. Ultrasound screening for spina bifida: cranial and cerebellar signs. Lancet 1986a; 2:72.

Nicolaides KH, Rodeck CH, Mibashan RS, et al. Have Liley charts outlived their usefulness? Am J Obstet Gynecol 1986b; 155:90.

Nicolaides KH, Economides DL, Soothill PW. Blood gases, pH, and lactate in appropriate- and small-for-gestational-age fetuses. Am J Obstet Gynecol 1989; 161:996.

Nicolaides KH, Clewell WH, Mibashan RS, et al. Fetal haemoglobin measurement in the assessment of red cell isoimmunization. Lancet 1988; 1:1073.

Nicolini U, Nicolaides P, Nicholas M, et al. Fetal blood sampling from the intrahepatic vein: analysis of safety and clinical experience with 214 procedures. Obstet Gynecol 1990a; 76:47.

Nicolini U, Nicolaides P, Fisk NM, et al. Limited role of fetal blood sampling in prediction of outcome in intrauterine growth retardation. Lancet 1990b; 2:768.

Nicolini U, Monni G. Intestinal obstruction in babies exposed in utero to methylene blue. Lancet 1990; 336:1258.

Pardi G, Cetin I, Marconi AM, et al. Diagnostic value of blood sampling in fetuses with growth retardation. N Engl J Med 1993; 328:692.

Penso CA, Sandstrom MM, Garber MF, et al. Early amniocentesis: report of 407 cases with neonatal follow-up. Obstet Gynecol 1990; 76:1032.

Pergament E, Schulman JD, Copeland K, et al. The risk and efficacy of chorionic villus sampling in multiple gestations. Prenat Diagn 1992; 12:377.

Poenaru L. First trimester prenatal diagnosis of metabolic diseases: a survey in countries from the European community. Prenat Diagn 1987; 7:333.

Quintero R, Romero R, Mahoney MJ, et al. Fetal haemorrhagic lesions after chorionic villus sampling. Lancet 1992; 339:193.

Raymond J, Poissonnier MH, Thulliez PH, et al. Presence of gamma interferon in human acute and congenital toxoplasmosis. J Clin Microbiol 1990; 28:1434.

Rhoads GG, Jackson LG, Schlesselman SE, et al. The safety and efficacy of chorionic villus sampling for early prenatal diagnosis of cytogenetic abnormalities. N Engl J Med 1989; 320:609.

Richards DS, Seeds JW, Katz VL, et al. Elevated maternal serum alpha-fetoprotein with normal ultrasound: Is amniocentesis always appropriate? A review of 26,069 screened patients. Obstet Gynecol 1988; 71:203.

Rickwood AMK. A case of ileal atresia and ileocutaneous fistula caused by amniocentesis. J Pediatr 1977; 91:312.

Romero R, Sirtori M, Oyarzun E, et al. Infection and labor. V. Prevalence, microbiology and clinical significance of intraamniotic infection in women with preterm labor and intact membranes. Am J Obstet Gynecol 1989; 161:817.

Schatz F. Eine besondere Art von ein seitiger Oligohydramnie bei Zwillingen. Arch Gynecol 1992; 65:329.

Schloo R, Miny P, Holzgreve W, et al. Distal limb deficiency following chorionic villus sampling? Am J Med Genet 1992; 42:404.

Schwartz S. Efficacy and applicability of interphase fluorescence in situ hybridization for prenatal diagnosis; invited editorial. Am J Hum Genet 1993; 52:851.

Scioscia AL, Grannum PAT, Copel JA, et al. The use of percutaneous umbilical blood sampling in immune thrombocytopenic purpura. Am J Obstet Gynecol 1988; 159:1066.

Shulman LP, Meyers CM, Simpson JL, et al. Fetomaternal transfusion depends on amount of chorionic villi aspirated but not on method of chorionic villus sampling. Am J Obstet Gynecol 1990; 162:1185.

Shulman LP, Elias S. Percutaneous umbilical blood sampling, fetal skin sampling, and fetal liver biopsy. Semin Perinatal 1990; 14:456.

Simpson JL, Socol ML, Aladjem S, et al. Normal fetal growth despite persistent amniotic fluid leakage after genetic amniocentesis. Prenat Diagn 1981; 1:277.

Smidt-Jensen S, Permin M, Philip J, et al. Randomised comparison of amniocentesis and transabdominal and transcervical chorionic villus sampling. Lancet 1992; 340:1237.

Spencer JW, Cox DN. Emotional responses of pregnant women to chorionic villi sampling or amniocentesis. Am J Obstet Gynecol 1987; 157:1155.

Steele MW, Breg WR, Jr. Chromosome analysis of human amniotic fluid cells. Lancet 1966; 1:383.

Strovel JW, Lee KD, Punzalan C, et al. Prenatal diagnosis by direct analysis of uncultured amniotic fluid cells using interphase fluorescence in situ hybridization (FISH). Am J Hum Genet 1992(suppl); S1:A12.

Swift PGF, Driscoll IB, Vowles KDJ. Neonatal small bowel obstruction associated with amniocentesis. Br Med J 1979; 1:720.

Tabor A, Philip J, Bang J, et al. Needle size and risk of miscarriage after amniocentesis. Lancet 1988; 1:183-184.

Tabor A, Philip J, Madsen M, et al. Randomised controlled trial of genetic amniocentesis in 4606 low-risk women. Lancet 1986; 1:1287.

Therkelsen AJ, Rehder, H. Intestinal atresia caused by second trimester amniocentesis: case report. Br J Obstet Gynaecol 1981; 88:559.

Tietung Hospital of Anshan Iron and Steel Co., Anshan, China, Dept. of Ob/Gyn. Fetal sex prediction by sex chromatin of chorionic villi cells during early pregnancy. Chin Med J 1975; 1:117.

Turnbull AC, MacKenzie IZ. Second-trimester amniocentesis and termination of pregnancy. Br Med Bull 1983; 39:315.

UK Collaborative Study on Alpha-Fetoprotein in Relation to Neural Tube Defects. Amniotic fluid alpha-fetoprotein measurements in antenatal diagnosis of anencephaly and open spina bifida in early pregnancy. Lancet 1979; 2:652.

Valenti C, Schutta EJ, Kehaty T. Prenatal diagnosis of Down's syndrome. Lancet 1968; 2:220.

Van den Hof MC, Nicolaides KH, Campbell J, et al. Evaluation of the lemon and banana signs in 130 fetuses with open spina bifida. Am J Obstet Gynecol 1990; 162:322.

Van der Pol JG, Volf H, Boer K, et al. Jejunal atresia related to the use of methylene blue in genetic amniocentesis in twins. Br J Obstet Gynaecol 1992; 99:141.

Vejerslev LO, Mikkelsen M. The European collaborative study on mosaicism in chorionic villus sampling: data from 1986 to 1987. Prenat Diagn 1989; 9:575.

Walker A. Liquor amnii studies in the prediction of haemolytic disease of the newborn. Br Med J 1957; 2:376.

Wapner RJ, Simpson JL, Golbus MS, et al. Chorionic mosaicism: association with fetal loss but not with adverse perinatal outcome. Prenat Diagn 1992; 12:347.

Ward BE, Gersen SL, Klinger KW. A rapid (but wrong) prenatal diagnosis: integrated genetics replies. N Engl J Med 1992; 326:1639.

Ward BE, Gersen SL, Carelli MP, et al. Rapid prenatal diagnosis of chromosomal aneuploidies by fluorescence in situ hybridization: clinical experience with 4,500 specimens. Am J Hum Genet 1993; 52:854.

Wass D, Bennett MJ. Infection and chorionic villus sampling. Lancet 1985; 2:338.

Wathen NC, Cass PL, Campbell DJ, et al. Early amniocentesis: alphafetoprotein levels in amniotic fluid, extraembryonic coelomic fluid and maternal serum between 8 and 13 weeks. Br J Obstet Gynaecol 1991; 98:866.

Webster W, Brown-Woodman T. Cocaine as a cause of congenital malformations of vascular origin: experimental evidence in the rat. Teratology 1990; 41:689.

Weiner CP, Thompson MIB. Direct treatment of fetal supraventricular tachycardia after failed transplacental therapy. Am J Obstet Gynecol 1988; 158:570.

Wilson RD, Kendrick V, Wittman BK, et al. Risk of spontaneous abortion in ultrasonically normal pregnancies (Letter). Lancet 1984; 2:920.

Working Party on Amniocentesis. An assessment of hazards of amniocentesis. Br J Obstet Gynaecol 1978; 85:1.

Young PE, Matson MR, Jones OW. Fetal exsanguination and other vascular injuries from midtrimester genetic amniocentesis. Am J Obstet Gynecol 1977; 129:21.

Youroukos S, Papadelis F, Matsaniotis N. Porencephalic cysts after amniocentesis. Arch Dis Child 1980; 55:814.

CHAPTER 31

Operative Procedures on the Cervix

EMBRYOLOGY, ANATOMY, AND PHYSIOLOGIC CHANGES OF PREGNANCY

Like the uterine corpus, the cervix is formed as the paramesonephric ducts fuse beginning around 6 weeks' gestation (Langman, 1981). By 11 weeks, the cervix can be seen as a fusiform thickening of mesenchyme at the juncture of the upper vagina and uterine corpus. While the exact source of the ectocervical and endocervical epithelium has been debated, most believe this to be of Müllerian origin rather than an extension of the urogenital sinus invagination.

The major blood supply of the cervix is derived from the internal iliac system as a descending limb of the uterine artery known as the cervicovaginal branch. This artery runs laterally on each side of the cervix in the cardinal ligaments. Lymphatic drainage is primarily through the hypogastric, obturator, external iliac, and presacral nodes. Nerves supplying the cervix pass through Frankenhauser's plexus above and posterior to the cervix and through the second, third, and fourth sacral nerves (Cunningham and coauthors, 1993).

Early in pregnancy, the lower uterine segment becomes softened such that the cervix can be readily distinguished from the body of the uterus on bimanual exam (Hegar's sign). Along with the vaginal walls, the surface of the cervix appears more blue secondary to increased vascularity (Chadwick's sign). As pregnancy progresses, the squamocolumnar junction appears to move outward on the vaginal portio of the cervix, resulting in a physiologic eversion of the endocervical mucosa. The increased blood supply and eversion of the glandular epithelium render the cervix friable and prone to bleed with relatively minor trauma such as occurs with a simple smear taken for cytology.

The stroma of the cervix differs from that of the uterine corpus; there is a relative lack of smooth muscle compared to the amount of collagenous and elastic tissue. The well-described softening of the cervix in pregnancy is likely due to changes in the biochemistry of this fibrous tissue. Using cervical biopsy specimens, Rechberger and colleagues (1988) have shown that when compared to the nonpregnant state, cervical tissue from pregnant subjects demonstrates a decrease in mechanical strength, a 50 percent reduction in the amounts of hydroxyproline and sulfated glycosaminoglycans, a lesser reduction in hyaluronic acid, and increases in collagen extractability and collagenolytic activity.

Finally, in addition to changes in the appearance and consistency of the cervix, slight dilation of the os is normal by the third trimester of pregnancy even in nulliparous women. Schaffner and Schanzer (1966) examined the cervices of 299 women between 28 and 32 weeks' gestation and found that one third were already dilated to 2–3 cm. Furthermore, the rates of prematurity and preterm rupture of the membranes in this group of patients were not higher than for those in the nondilated group. Other investigators have documented similar findings. Floyd (1961) noted cervical dilation of more than 1 cm by 24 weeks' gestation in 15 percent of primigravidas and 72 percent of multigravidas. Yet none of these patients delivered before 36 completed weeks' gestation.

ETIOLOGY OF INCOMPETENT CERVIX

While some have suggested that use of the term *cervical incompetence* may cause unnecessary feelings of guilt in women suffering such a pregnancy loss, the term remains ubiquitous in obstetric practice. Lash and Lash (1950) first used the term *cervical incompetence* while describing repetitive abortion presenting as ". . . sudden rupture of the bag of waters followed by a rapid and relatively painless extrusion of the products of conception."

Estimates of the incidence of cervical incompetence vary widely. Toaff and associates (1977) reported an incidence of 1 in 54 pregnancies, while Little and Tenney (1963) reported a rate closer to 1 of every 2000 pregnancies. In their monograph, Shortle and Jewelewicz (1989) suggested that cervical incompetence accounts for 8–15 percent of all habitual abortions.

Cousins (1980) has classified the etiology of cervical incompetence as either acquired (traumatic) or congenital. Acquired cervical incompetence may be the result of extensive cervical conization, rapid or excessive cervical dilation during abortion, or secondary to obstetric lacerations suffered at the time of vaginal delivery. Congenital cervical incompetence may be idiopathic or may be secondary to Müllerian anomalies, in utero exposure to diethylstilbestrol (DES), or an abnormally muscular cervix.

Cold-knife Conization

Reports are divided as to whether cold-knife conization of the cervix is a risk factor for development of cervical incompetence. Lee (1978), Moinian and Andersch (1982), and others have reported higher rates of second trimester pregnancy loss in patients with a history of cervical conization. On the contrary, Buller and Jones (1982) and Weber and Obel (1979) reported no increased rate of midtrimester pregnancy loss. Similarly, McLaren and colleagues (1974) found no increased risk of cervical incompetence among 50 patients who had "extensive" cone biopsies. Whether conization results in the subsequent development of cervical incompetence most likely depends on the extent of the cone biopsy. Leiman and associates (1980) reported that rates of second-trimester loss and preterm delivery were increased when the cone specimen exceeded 2 cm in height or 4 cm^3 in total volume.

Some of the conflict in the literature may be explained by differences in the types of pregnancy outcomes reported. In a cohort study, Kristensen and colleagues (1993) demonstrated an increase in preterm birth after cervical conization compared to controls without a history of conization [odds ratio 4.13, 95 percent confidence interval (CI) 2.53–6.75, $p < .001$]. Interestingly, they also demonstrated that women with subsequent cervical conization had a higher rate of preterm birth in previous pregnancies (odds ratio 1.78, 95 percent CI 1.07–2.97, $p < .05$), suggesting that conization was not the only factor affecting the increased rate of preterm delivery in this group of women. When comparing the rates of preterm delivery between women with a prior history of conization with that of women with a subsequent conization, the authors again found the procedure to be a significant risk factor (odds ratio 2.26, 95 percent CI 1.07–4.75, $p < .05$). These authors did not stratify by gestational age at the time of delivery, nor by whether the preterm delivery resulted from cervical incompetence or from preterm labor. As discussed later, cervical cerclage plays no role in the prevention of preterm labor. Thus while multiple studies may show an increased risk of preterm delivery in patients with a history of cervical conization, this does not equate with the need for prophylactic cerclage. Coustan (1993) suggests that the most reasonable approach to the pregnant patient with a prior history of cone biopsy is expectant management with weekly or biweekly cervical exams beginning around 16 weeks' gestation.

Large Loop Excision of the Cervical Transformation Zone (LLETZ)

Diathermy loop excision, or LLETZ, has gained popularity as a means to both diagnose and treat cervical intraepithelial neoplasia. Reports of subsequent pregnancy outcome in patients who have undergone LLETZ are of concern. Although Keijser and associates (1992) concluded that the procedure does not affect subsequent fertility and pregnancy outcome, of 96 pregnancies reported in their retrospective study, 7 ended in preterm delivery and 8 in abortion. Importantly, these 15 cases were not characterized sufficiently to determine whether any or all were secondary to cervical incompetence. With a retrospective case control study of 40 pregnancies occurring after LLETZ, Blomfield and colleagues (1993) reported that the procedure was associated with a lower mean birthweight, more preterm deliveries, and more admissions to a neonatal intensive care unit. Despite absolute differences in LLETZ versus controls in the number of preterm deliveries (17.5% vs 11.3%, $p = .34$) and neonatal intensive care unit admissions (10 % vs 5%, p not reported), only the difference in birthweights was statistically significant (2877 g vs. 3208 g, $p = .03$). A major weakness of the study was the exclusion of pregnancy losses prior to 20 weeks' gestation, the gestational range at which cervical incompetence classically presents. Until larger well-controlled studies are published, patients with a prior history of a LLETZ procedure should be followed carefully for the development of cervical incompetence in a manner similar to women who have undergone cervical conization.

Induced Abortion

Similar to cervical conization, the literature does not support prophylactic cerclage for women with a prior history of induced abortion. While some authors (Johnstone and associates, 1974; Caspi and colleagues, 1983) suggest that dilation of the cervix for abortion results in persistent abnormalities of the uterine cervix, large retrospective series do not confirm an increased rate of cervical incompetence after first-trimester induced abortion (Daling and Emannel, 1977; Schultz and colleagues, 1983).

DES Exposure

Singer and Hochman (1978) were the first to report a case of cervical incompetence in a woman exposed to diethylstilbestrol (DES) in utero. Since that time, several authors (Goldstein, 1978; Cousins and associates, 1980) have reported increased rates of second-trimester pregnancy loss and cervical incompetence among women exposed to DES in utero. In a review article, Cousins (1980) was careful not to recommend prophylactic cerclage to all DES-exposed women, cautioning that prospective, controlled studies with larger samples needed to be conducted. To date, such a randomized, controlled trial to address this issue has not been published.

In the largest series yet reported, Kaufman and colleagues (1984) reviewed the pregnancy outcomes of 327 women enrolled in the Diethylstilbestrol-Adenosis Project (DESAD), reporting no improvement in pregnancy outcomes among 17 women treated with cerclage compared to non-treated controls. The authors concluded that prophylactic cerclage was not indicated for the pregnant DES-exposed woman. In a smaller prospective study, conducted over a 5-year period, Ludmir and associates (1987) enrolled 63 DES-exposed pregnant patients in a standardized protocol whereby women with a prior history of second-trimester loss or a hypoplastic cervix on initial examination underwent prophylactic cervical cerclage. The control group was followed expectantly, with cerclage placed emergently if needed. Of the control group, 44 percent received an emergency cerclage for demonstrated cervical change. Because so many controls required emergency cerclage, and because all five perinatal deaths occurred in the group managed expectantly, the authors suggested that strong consideration should be given to placing an early prophylactic cerclage in DES-exposed women. The study was not randomized, and the rate of cervical incompetence among DES-exposed controls was much higher than the 3.6–11 percent reported by other authors (Mangan and associates, 1982; Herbst and colleagues, 1980).

Other investigators have achieved excellent clinical results with expectant management of DES-exposed patients using ultrasound or physical examination to monitor for cervical incompetence. Levine and Berkowitz (1993) reported the pregnancy outcomes among 50 DES-exposed women with 120 pregnancies managed expectantly. In their series, one woman required cerclage for a classic history of cervical incompetence while one other required cerclage for acute cervical change in the second trimester. Patients with cervical dilation after 25 weeks were managed with bed rest. Of 94 pregnancies surviving the first trimester, 92 percent resulted in the discharge of a viable infant while 78 percent reached term. The rates of preterm labor and preterm rupture of the membranes were 6.5 percent and 3.8 percent, respectively. Among 27 pregnancies in DES-exposed women managed expectantly with serial ultrasound, Michaels and associates (1989) reported that five cerclages were placed for demonstrated cervical change. Importantly, however, these authors reported no perinatal deaths and no deliveries before 36 weeks' gestation. In light of these reports, the most reasonable approach to pregnant women with a history of DES exposure, like those with a prior cone biopsy, appears to be expectant management with careful surveillance for the development of cervical incompetence.

DIAGNOSIS OF INCOMPETENT CERVIX

The diagnosis of cervical incompetence is most easily made by eliciting a "classic history." Cousins (1980) described this as repetitive, acute, painless, second-trimester evacuation of the uterus without associated bleeding or contractions. In practice, most patients do not present with this history. More commonly they are seen with histories of pregnancy loss that do not fit this classic picture. Symptoms and signs that may accompany cervical incompetence include urinary frequency, lower abdominal pressure, a bearing-down sensation, bloody show, or a watery discharge (Toaff and Toaff, 1974). Additionally, menstrual like cramps and a pattern of uterine irritability or frequent small-amplitude contractions may occur as the membranes protrude, distend the cervix, and activate the Ferguson reflex. Consequently, during pregnancy the diagnosis of cervical incompetence is not always straightforward. Another presentation of cervical incompetence is the incidental discovery of an abnormally short or dilated cervix during prenatal ultrasound. Riley and coauthors (1992) identified a shortened (< 3 cm) cervix or funneling of the membranes into an open internal os in 31 women undergoing prenatal ultrasound for a variety of indications not necessarily related to preterm labor or cervical incompetence. Of these, 19 (61%) went on to manifest preterm labor, cervical incompetence, or preterm birth. Other conditions that may present with herniated membranes and/or a dilated cervix, but for which cerclage would be contraindicated, include preterm labor, infection, preterm rupture of the membranes, and possibly abruptio placenta.

TREATMENT OF CERVICAL INCOMPETENCE

Preconception cerclage is associated with infertility rates as high as 50 percent (Harger, 1983). Consequently, most authors advocate placement after conception and usually after the first trimester in hopes of avoiding unnecessary procedures in patients destined to spontaneously abort. A basic ultrasound examination should be performed to confirm fetal viability and to exclude obvious lethal congenital anomalies. Finally, if there are indications for prenatal genetic diagnosis, one may consider early chromosome diagnosis via chorionic villus biopsy or early amniocentesis. While there are no data to support the use of perioperative antibiotics or tocolytics for placement of a prophylactic cerclage (Chap. 38), many authors achieving higher success rates with emergent procedures use these medications liberally (Barth and colleagues, 1990; Novy and associates, 1990).

In a monograph reviewing the world's literature, Shortle and Jewelewicz (1989) found over 35 different procedures for treatment of the incompetent cervix. Techniques reported as treatments of incompetent cervix include such diverse therapies as electrocautery of the internal os, scarification with benzoin and talc, pessaries, intravaginal balloon devices, and various hormones. However, the majority of procedures in use today are modifications of one of three different surgical procedures: the Shirodkar (1955), McDonald (1957), or transabdominal cervicoisthmic cerclage (Benson and Durfee, 1965).

Shirodkar Technique

V. N. Shirodkar first presented his procedure for the treatment of cervical incompetence at a film festival in Paris in 1950. Numerous modifications to Shirodkar's original technique have been reported. Most notably, the suture materials have changed, progressing from the original human fascia lata to synthetic woven surgical tape with attached atraumatic needles. The procedure as performed by the authors is as follows.

After induction of general or adequate regional anesthesia, the patient is placed in the dorsal lithotomy position in moderate Trendelenburg. If the membranes are not protruding, a gentle surgical prep of the perineum and vagina is performed. A weighted speculum and right angle retractors are used to facilitate exposure. The cervix is then grasped with two or three DeLee cervical tenacula or sponge forceps. Next, with moderate traction on the tenacula, the angle formed by the cardinal ligament and the lateral margin of the cervix is palpated to establish the distance that the bladder must be mobilized in order to place the suture at the level of the internal os. The mucosa is then incised horizontally over the anterior lip of the cervix at the reflection of the bladder similar to when beginning a vaginal hysterectomy (Fig. 31–1). Occasionally, sharp dissection may be required to initiate the correct plane; however, the bladder can usually be advanced with gentle pressure from a gloved finger (Fig. 31–2). This is continued until the surgeon can palpate the lower uterine segment ballooning out ahead of the dissecting finger; this corresponds to the level of the internal os. A vertical incision is then made over the posterior aspect of the cervix with care taken not to enter the pouch of Douglas. Again with a gloved finger, the reflection of the pouch of Douglas can be advanced with gentle pressure. Next, one jaw of a curved Allis clamp is placed in the posterior mucosal incision and the other jaw of the clamp is placed in the anterior incision on one side of the cervix. The clamp should be placed as high on the cervix as possible to make maximal use of the dissection. With slight pressure against the cervix, the clamp is closed parallel to the axis of the vagina, thereby effectively bunching the paracervical vasculature within the clamp (Fig. 31–3). A 5-mm Mersilene tape with attached atraumatic needles (Ethicon) is then driven from posterior to anterior just distal to the clamp and above the insertion of the cardinal ligaments (Fig. 31–4). Because the braided Mersilene tape may act with a sawing effect when pulled through edematous tissue, we lubricate the tape with a sterile gel lubricant and use the doubly loaded suture so that less tape has to be pulled completely around the cervix. The needle should pass just beneath the end of the Allis clamp so as not to travel too deeply, thereby minimizing the risk of rupture of the fetal membranes. After assuring that the tape lies flat against the cervix posteriorly, the suture is tied anteriorly such that the external os will admit only a fingertip and the internal os is closed (Fig. 31–5). While some (Coustan, 1993) prefer to place the knot posteriorly to avoid the possibility of erosion into the bladder, we place the knot anteriorly to allow easier removal at term when the posteriorly placed knot may be difficult to expose. The mucosal incisions are closed over the tape with small absorbable suture only if active bleeding is noted (Fig. 31–6). The cut free ends of the tape are left exposed to facilitate later removal. In general, at 37 weeks the cerclage is either removed or cut and left in situ to spontaneously dislodge during labor.

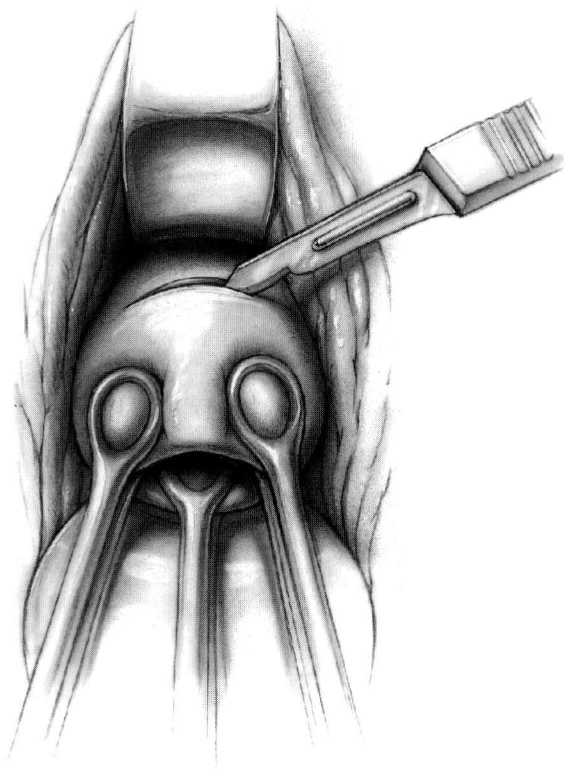

Figure 31–1. Modified Shirodkar cerclage. Note the placement of the DeLee cervical tenacula and the location of the initial transverse incision in the anterior cervicovaginal mucosa just distal to the bladder reflection.

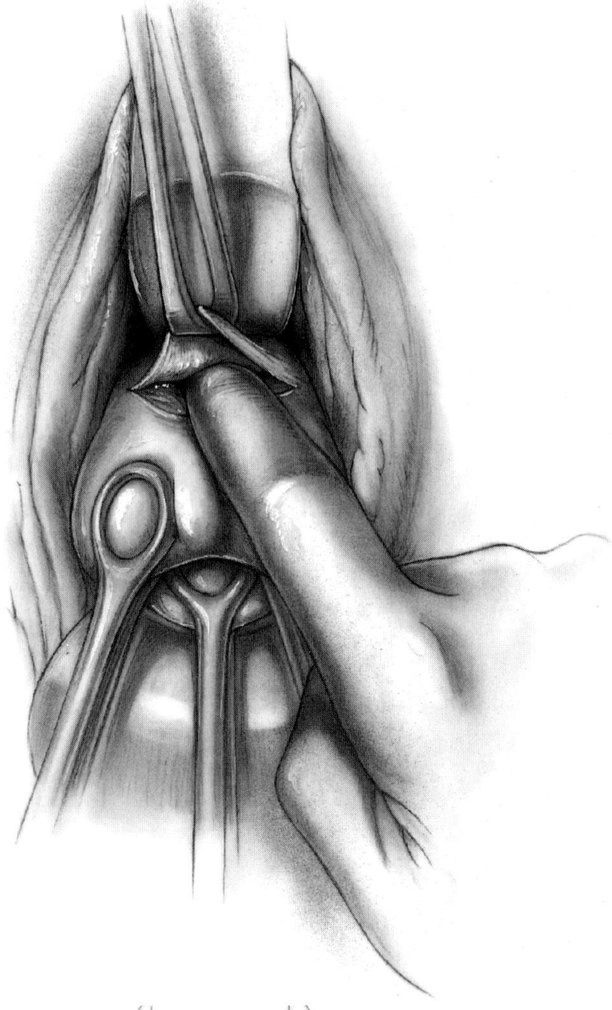

Figure 31–2. Modified Shirodkar cerclage. Allis clamps are used to lift the reflection of the bladder flap. With a gloved finger, gentle pressure will advance the plane of dissection to the level of the lower uterine segment. Sharp dissection may occasionally be required.

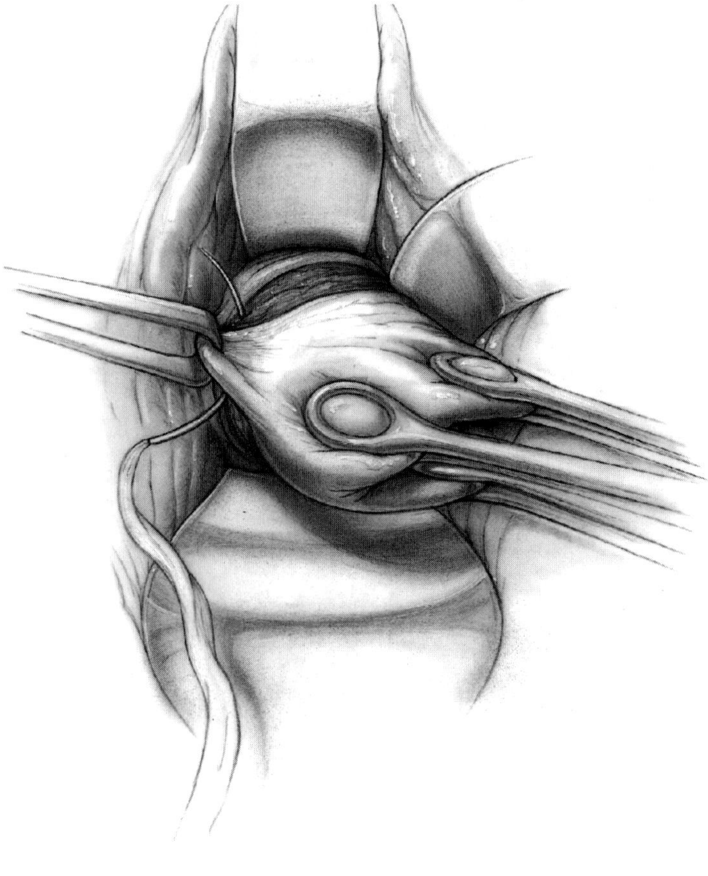

Figure 31–3. Modified Shirodkar cerclage. An Allis clamp is opened, one arm then placed into the anterior mucosal incision, the other into the posterior incision. With gentle pressure against the cervix, the clamp is closed, effectively bunching the paracervical tissue and vasculature within the clamp.

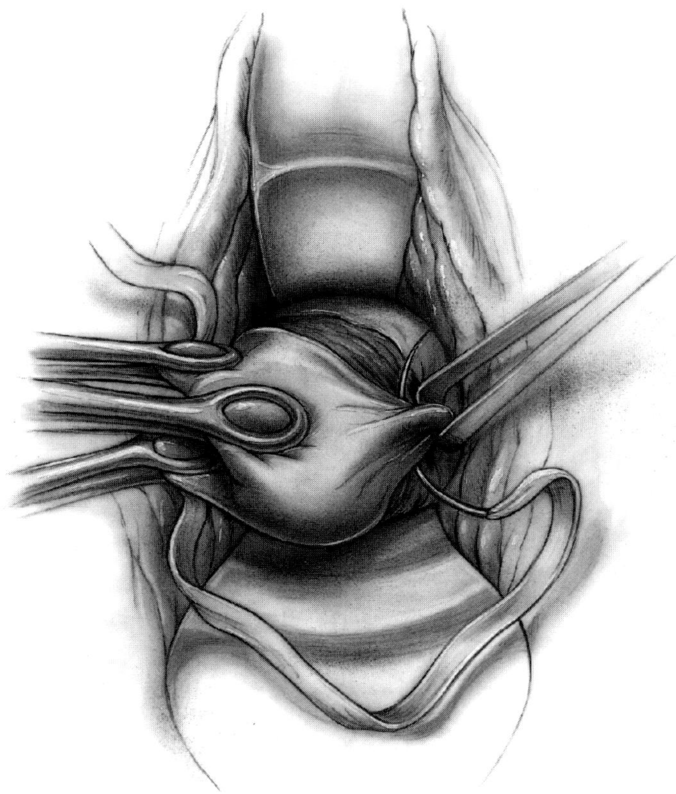

Figure 31–4. Modified Shirodkar cerclage. From posterior to anterior, the 5 mm Mersilene tape loaded on a CT-1 needle is passed through the cervical stroma just beneath the Allis clamp on each side of the cervix. If placed correctly, the Mersilene tape will then be above the cervical insertion of the cardinal ligaments.

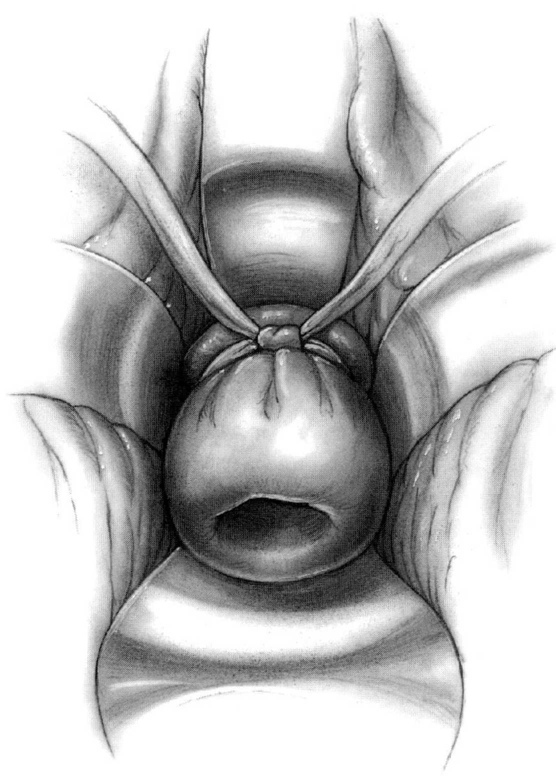

Figure 31–5. Modified Shirodkar cerclage. After assuring that the tape lies flat posteriorly, a single overhand knot is thrown and cinched down until the internal cervical os will not admit a fingertip. Five or six additional throws are then placed in the Mersilene knot.

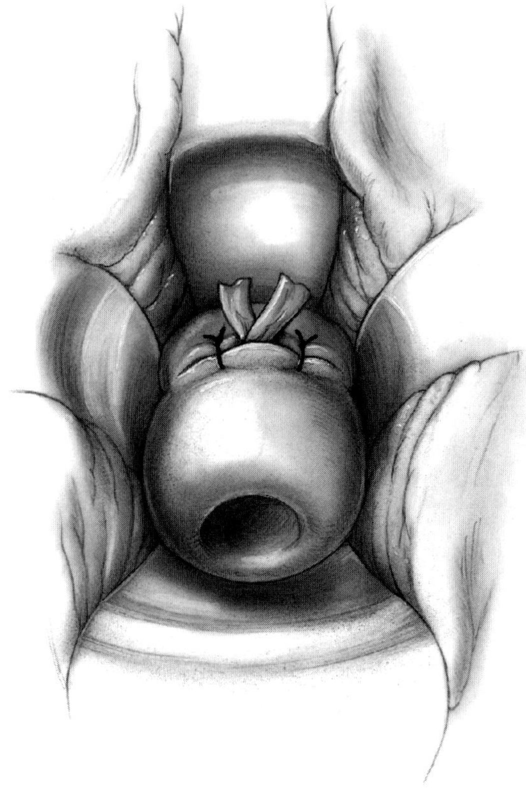

Figure 31–6. Modified Shirodkar cerclage. The cut free ends are left exposed to facilitate removal at term. If bleeding, the mucosal incisions may be closed with an absorbable suture.

McDonald Cerclage

In 1951 Ian McDonald encountered a woman whose cervix was 3 cm dilated with membranes protruding into the vagina. Under general anesthesia, he reduced the membranes and encircled the cervix with catgut suture, thus preventing the imminent delivery. After three more such procedures conducted at 2-week intervals, the patient delivered a viable 2000-g infant at 34 weeks' gestation. Using more permanent suture material, McDonald performed a series of these procedures, which he published after learning of Shirodkar's work (McDonald, 1957; McDonald, 1987).

For placement of a McDonald cerclage, the patient is prepared and positioned in the manner described above. However, should clinical conditions prevent the use of regional or general anesthesia, the McDonald cerclage may be placed with local or paracervical infiltration or with a pudendal block (McCulloch, 1993). While possible, we do not recommend this approach.

After grasping the cervix with DeLee or sponge forceps, the level of the bladder reflection is noted anteriorly by gently moving the cervix back and forth. Just distal to the vesicocervical reflection, a suture is used to encircle the cervix in four or five bites in a purse string fashion (Fig. 31–7). The suture should be large and nonabsorbable such as the double swedged 5-mm Mersilene tape or 0 Ethibond loaded on a free needle. The cerclage should be placed well posteriorly, as close to the uterosacral ligaments as possible without traversing the cul-de-sac. Each bite is placed deep enough to include cervical stromal tissue with care taken not to enter the endocervical canal. The knot is usually placed anteriorly with the cut free ends left long enough to allow easy removal later in pregnancy.

Transabdominal Cervicoisthmic Cerclage

Transabdominal cervicoisthmic cerclage was first advocated by Benson and Durfee (1965) for patients who were deemed poor candidates for a vaginal procedure. They defined such patients as those with (1) an obvious congenitally short or extensively amputated cervix; (2) marked scarring of the cervix; (3) deeply notched multiple cervical defects; (4) unhealed, penetrating, forniceal lacerations; or (5) subacute cervicitis. The indications for transabdominal cervicoisthmic cerclage today

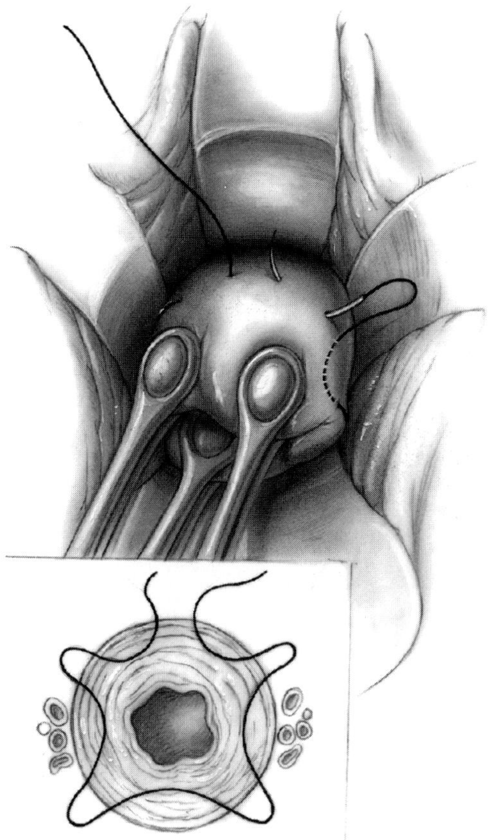

Figure 31–7. McDonald cerclage. Without mucosal incisions, the stitch is used to encircle the cervix in four to six bites. Anteriorly, the suture is placed as close to the cervicovesical reflection as possible. Posteriorly, the bites are taken as high as possible without traversing the pouch of Douglas. As shown in the schematic inset, the needle is guided into the cervical stroma beneath the lateral vasculature with care to avoid the endocervical canal.

are limited and remain controversial. Rust (1991) suggests that the procedure should be limited to women who have a marked cervical deformity and have failed a previously well-placed transvaginal cerclage. He cautioned that the validity of placing a transabdominal cervicoisthmic cerclage for the sole indication of a Müellerian anomaly or a history of DES exposure remains to be established. Similar to most other therapies for cervical incompetence, the success rate when compared to each patient's prior obstetric history seems impressive. Summarizing all of the published series to date, Novy (1991) noted an improvement in pregnancy salvage rate from 21 percent to 89 percent with the use of transabdominal cerclage. No prospective or randomized series of this procedure have been published.

Because exposure becomes increasingly difficult in the second trimester, placement is best accomplished before 12 completed weeks of gestation. The abdomen is entered via a low vertical or Pfannenstiel incision and the bowel is packed away superiorly. The peritoneal reflection is incised and the bladder advanced as during an abdominal hysterectomy. As the procedure is usually performed in women who have failed multiple prior vaginally placed cervical cerclages, marked scarring of the bladder to the lower uterine segment and cervix has been a nearly constant finding. The bladder flap is developed sharply with Metzenbaum scissors and blunt dissection is avoided to prevent incidental cystotomy. This process is carried only to the level of the uterine isthmus to minimize bleeding beneath the bladder flap (Fig. 31–8). With firm upward traction on the uterine fundus to facilitate exposure, the uterine artery is palpated by the first assistant, then bunched laterally to protect the vessels as the needle is positioned (Fig. 31–9). As with the Shirodkar, we use a lubricated 5-mm Mersilene tape doubly loaded with two CT-1 needles. The needle is passed from anterior to posterior on each side with the needle traversing the lateral cervicouterine stroma rather than the paracervical and parametrial vascular space. Use of DeLee ovum forceps posteriorly as a splint through which the needle can be driven with countertraction, as well as the suture advanced against countertraction, minimizes manipula-

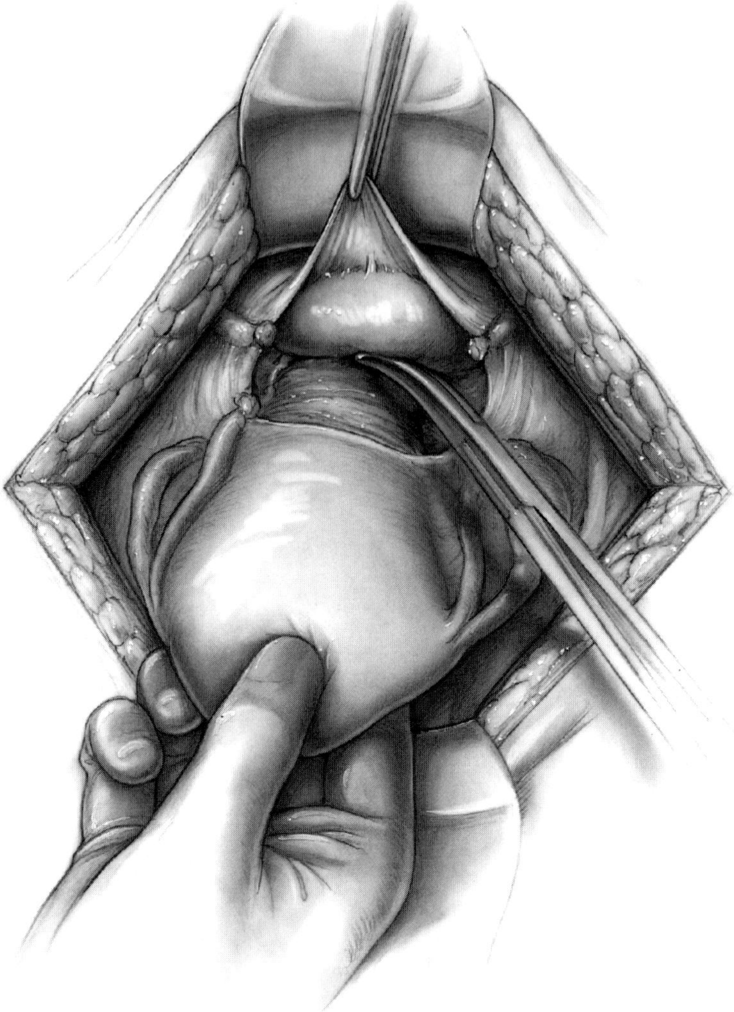

Figure 31–8. Transabdominal cervicoisthmic cerclage. After laparotomy, the anterior uterine visceral peritoneum in incised and a bladder flap is created with blunt and sharp dissection. This is carried only to the level of the uterine isthmus.

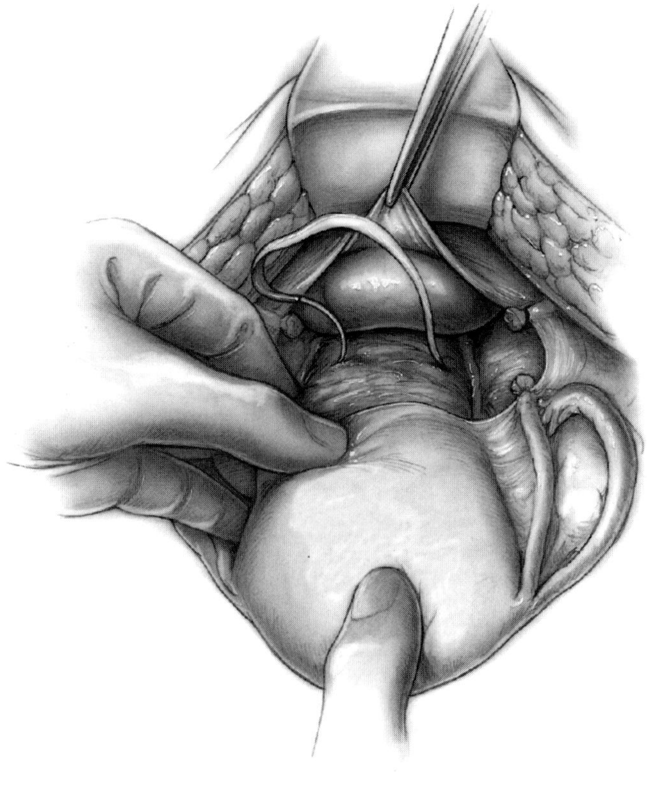

Figure 31–9. Transabdominal cervicoisthmic cerclage. First assistant elevates the uterus with right hand and protects the parametrial vessels between fingers of the other hand. With direct visualization the suture is then passed from anterior to posterior through the lateral aspect of the uterine isthmic stroma on each side.

tion of the uterus and its contents. The cerclage is tied posteriorly with a single square knot over the posterior visceral peritoneal surface (Fig 31–10). The cut free ends are sutured to the band using small permanent suture such as 00 or 000 prolene. Finally, the bladder flap is replaced over the cerclage with absorbable suture.

While this may be the procedure of choice in a select few women with cervical incompetence, several disadvantages are readily apparent. Not only is laparotomy required for placement, but a second laparotomy and hysterotomy are required for delivery as the band cannot usually be removed vaginally. Furthermore, should a miscarriage or intrauterine demise occur, hysterotomy may be needed to empty the uterus. Novy (1991), however, has reported the successful evacuation of the products of conception after a 13-week demise without removing the Mersilene band. Other disadvantages include the risk of hemorrhage from the dilated parametrial vessels, potential compromise of uterine vascular supply, and a high procedure-related fetal loss rate of 5 percent (Marx, 1989). In light of the recognized complications of transabdominal cerclage, Ludmir and associates (1991) have demonstrated that transvaginal cerclage with continuous ultrasound guidance for cases of severe cervical hypoplasia may obviate the need for an abdominal approach.

Emergency Cerclage

In the past, clinicians have been reluctant to offer cervical cerclage when the amnionic membranes are protruding through a widely dilated cervix. Early attempts to salvage such cases with cervical cerclage were associated with success rates less than 50 percent

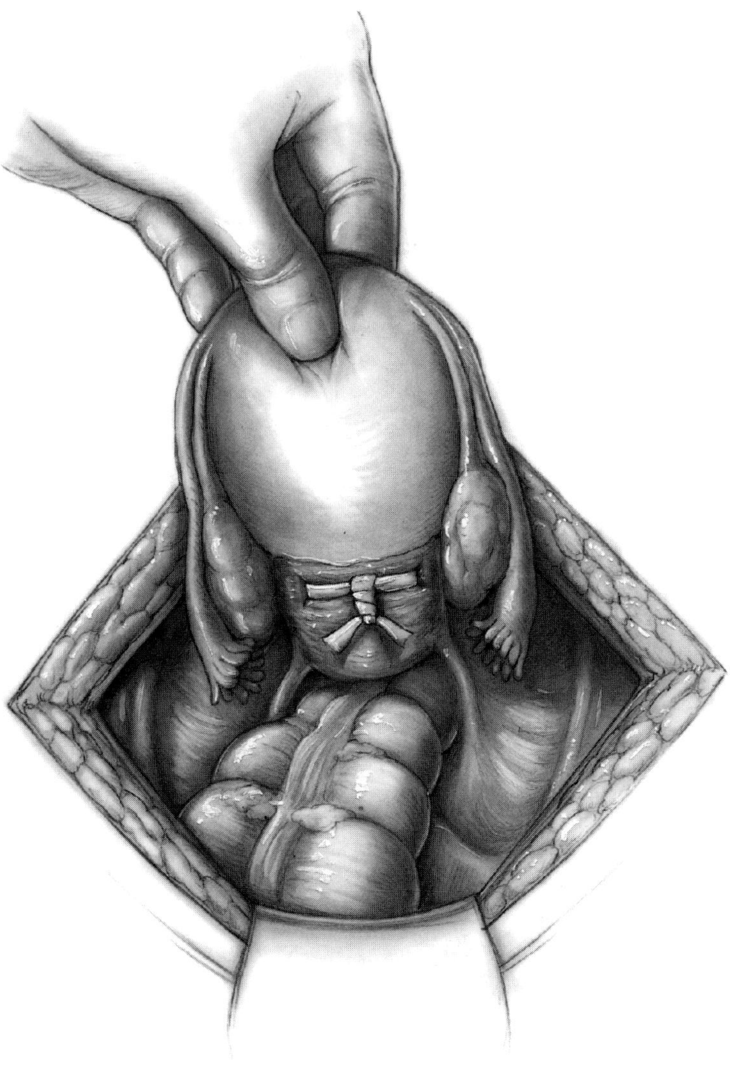

Figure 31–10. Transabdominal cervicoisthmic cerclage. A single square knot is tied posteriorly and the cut free ends are sutured to the Mersilene band. Unless the rectum must be mobilized to expose the posterior uterine isthmus, no posterior serosal incision is required.

(Harger and associates, 1983; McDonald, 1987). Recently, however, several groups (Barth and colleagues, 1990; Novy and associates, 1990; Mitra and colleagues, 1992) have reported salvage rates in excess of 70 percent even when the cervix is widely dilated with herniated membranes. Methods used to replace bulging membranes have included (1) reduction of the membranes with a large Foley catheter placed gently through the os (Holman, 1973); (2) amniocentesis to reduce tension (Goodlin, 1979); (3) stay sutures to stretch the cervix safely beyond the membranes (Olatunbosun and Dyck, 1981), and more recently, (4) distention of the bladder with 1–1.5 L of normal saline, thereby elevating the lower uterine segment and drawing the membranes back through the os (Sheerer and associates, 1987). While the efficacy of antibiotics or tocolytics in the setting have not been established, reports with higher success rates have employed aggressive tocolysis, antibiotic coverage, and if necessary, amniocentesis. In the setting of bulging membranes, some authors (Evans and colleagues, 1992) have emphasized the use of indomethacin with its dual value as a tocolytic agent as well as its recognized dose-dependent reduction in amnionic fluid volume.

CONTRAINDICATIONS TO CERVICAL CERCLAGE

Contraindications to cervical cerclage include active bleeding, preterm labor, ruptured membranes, chorioamnionitis, hydramnios, or the confident diagnosis of a lethal fetal anomaly. Additionally, most authors agree that, beyond 26 weeks' gestation, cervical cerclage should not be offered as neonatal survival at this gestational age now exceeds 50 percent (Gilstrap and associates, 1985; Copper and associates, 1993). Patients presenting with cervical incompetence beyond 25 weeks' gestation have been managed with prolonged bed rest without cervical cerclage with remarkable success (Levine and Berkowitz, 1993).

COMPLICATIONS OF CERCLAGE

Complications reported after cerclage include preterm rupture of the membranes, chorioamnionitis, suture displacement, preterm labor, cervical lacerations, and cesarean section when the cerclage cannot be removed (Harger, 1980). Less common maternal complications include damage to the surrounding organs such as the bladder and urethra (Ben-Baruch and associates, 1980; Bates and Cropley, 1977). Estimates of the frequency of each of these must be extrapolated from retrospective series and, consequently, are fraught with biases. Nonetheless, Newton and Newton (1988) suggest a procedure-related fetal loss rate of 2–4 percent with the majority due to chorioamnionitis (60%) or preterm delivery (26%).

Rupture of Membranes

Preterm rupture of the membranes may occur at the time of placement or much later in gestation. While most would agree that the former constitutes a surgical failure and requires immediate removal of the cerclage, optimal management of delayed rupture of membranes is less well-defined. Those who recommend removal of the cerclage do so for fear of infectious complications. Using a protocol in which all cerclages were removed on admission, Yeast and Garite (1988) detected no difference in neonatal or maternal infectious morbidity when patients with a cerclage in place at the time of preterm rupture of the membranes were compared to gestational age–matched controls with ruptured membranes and no cerclage. However, this study excluded patients with amnionitis, labor, or fetal distress on presentation, a group that probably contained significant infectious morbidity. Dubouloz and colleagues (1980) compared infectious morbidity among 75 patients who had a cerclage for incompetent cervix with 68 gestational age matched controls. Of seven perinatal deaths in the cerclage group, five were due to sepsis. In contrast, there was only one perinatal death among the controls. Maternal febrile morbidity, whether due to chorioamnionitis or postpartum metritis, was increased fivefold over controls. Likewise, Kuhn and Pepperell (1977) reported three neonatal deaths after 32 weeks' gestational age and two cases of maternal septic shock among 71 patients with a cerclage and ruptured membranes. Maternal deaths have been reported secondary to sepsis when cerclage was complicated by premature rupture of the membranes (Dunn and associates, 1959; Lipshitz, 1975). In a series from Boston, Goldman and colleagues (1990) reported the maternal and neonatal outcomes of 46 pregnancies with a cerclage and preterm rupture of the membranes managed without immediate removal. In contrast to previous reports, these authors found no increase in maternal or neonatal infectious morbidity when compared to gestational age–matched controls. Among the 71 patients reported by Kuhn and Pepperell (1977), 40 had the cerclage removed immediately while 31 were managed conservatively until spontaneous labor ensued. Interestingly, while infection was common (38%), immediate removal of the cerclage did not decrease the risk of sepsis. On the other hand, among women at less than 29 weeks' gestation, retention of the suture was associated with significant prolongation of the pregnancy. Although vigilance for infection should remain high, preterm rupture of the membranes in a patient with a cerclage does not mandate its immediate removal.

Suture Displacement

Another complication that presents a difficult management decision is suture displacement. Estimates from previous publications suggest that 5–13 percent of cerclages will pull through and allow subsequent dilation of the cervix (Aarnoudse and Huisjes, 1979; Newton and Newton 1988). The clinician and patient must then decide between delivery, a second cerclage, or conservative management with bed rest. While the efficacy of "rescue cerclage" has not been established, there are anecdotal reports of salvage with a second operation. Stromme and associates (1960) were able to prolong pregnancy another 30 days in 3 of 4 pregnancies when the initial cerclage had failed before 25 weeks' gestation. Two additional groups (Aaroundse and Huisjes, 1979; Schulman and Farmakides, 1985) have reported small series of successful surgical treatment of failed therapeutic cerclage.

Intrapartum Complications

The presence of a cervical cerclage may complicate labor and delivery. Cervical lacerations occur in 3–13 percent of patients while cervical dystocia secondary to scarring complicates another 5 percent (Newton and Newton, 1988). Whether this dystocia is responsible for the increased cesarean section rate seen with cerclage patients is not clear. Some feel that cerclage's only contribution to increased use of cesarean section is the inability to remove it during active labor (Harger and associates, 1983). Removal of a cerclage in labor may require a regional anesthetic to achieve adequate visualization. Finally, emphasizing the need to remove the cerclage, Peters and colleagues (1979) reported three cases of uterine rupture associated with active labor before removal of a Shirodkar cerclage could be performed.

If a cesarean section is planned for other reasons, the woman desires future fertility, and the cerclage is completely buried beneath the mucosa, some would allow the suture to remain in place thus obviating the need for another procedure in the subsequent gestation. However, once childbearing is complete, the cerclage should be removed. Erosion of the permanent suture through the cervix and nearby structures has resulted in large bladder calculi, hemorrhagic ulceration of the trigone, and vesicovaginal and ureterovaginal fistulas requiring a subsequent repair (Bates and Cropley, 1977; Ben-Baruch and colleagues, 1980; Ehrenpreis and associates, 1986; Hortenstine and Witherington, 1987).

EFFICACY OF CERVICAL CERCLAGE

Most reports that claim to show an improvement in pregnancy outcome with cerclage have done so by comparing salvage rates before and after the procedure using each patient as her own historical control. In their review of the world's literature, Shortle and Jewelewicz (1989) reported improvement in pregnancy success rates from 21 to 76 percent with the Shirodkar procedure, from 23 to 74 percent with McDonald's cerclage, and from 24 to 86 percent with transabdominal cervicoisthmic cerclage. While this may initially seem impressive, several authors have reported that the chances of a successful pregnancy outcome in patients with two or more consecutive losses can be as high as 79–85 percent without cerclage (Bakketeig and associates, 1979; Harger, 1980; Carr-Hill and Hall, 1985).

Realizing that pregnancy salvage rates may be high with or without therapy, and that such therapy has the potential for significant morbidity, the need for randomized controlled trials becomes readily apparent. Only four prospective, randomized controlled trials have been conducted that compare outcomes with and without cervical cerclage. First, Dor and colleagues (1982) randomized 50 twin pregnancies to either prophylactic cerclage at 13 weeks or to no therapy. They detected no improvement in preterm delivery or neonatal death rates, and concluded that prophylactic cervical cerclage was of no benefit in twin pregnancy. Next, Rush and associates (1984) studied the effect of cerclage on pregnancy outcome in patients determined to be at high risk for preterm delivery by randomizing 194 such women to either cerclage or to no treatment. Defining high-risk patients as those with a history of two or more deliveries prior to 37 weeks or one between 14 and 36 weeks, the authors found no evidence that cerclage prolonged gestation or improved survival. Furthermore, patients randomized to cerclage had significantly longer hospital stays, and although the differences were not statistically significant, they received tocolytic drugs more frequently and experienced more febrile morbidity.

Using a complex scoring system to determine the risk of preterm delivery, Lazar and colleagues (1984) randomized 506 patients at "moderate" risk to either cervical cerclage or a control group. Again, no difference was detected in preterm birth or neonatal death rates. Significantly, the cerclage group spent more time in the hospital and received more tocolytic agents. Moreover, although not statistically significant, the cerclage group had more preterm deliveries and more cesarean sections.

The largest prospective randomized controlled trial of cervical cerclage was conducted by the Medical Research Council/Royal College of Obstetricians and Gynaecologists at the National Perinatal Epidemiology Unit in Oxford (MacNaughton and associates, 1993). Between 1981 and 1988 the authors enrolled and randomized 1318 women to treatment with or without cerclage. The study included women whose obstetricians were unsure as to whether a cerclage should be placed. The majority of patients had either previous preterm deliveries, first- or second-trimester miscarriages, or previous cervical surgery. Patients who had classic histories for cervical incompetence or an examination diagnostic of incompetence were excluded. The authors demonstrated a small but significant reduction in the number of deliveries before 33 completed weeks' gestation from 17 percent in the controls to 13 percent in the cerclage group (odds ratio 0.72; 95% CI 0.53–0.97, p = .03). Subgroup analysis, which should be interpreted with caution, suggested that the difference was largely due to a reduction in the number of pregnancies lost in a manner consistent with classic cervical incompetence. Like the previously discussed randomized controlled trials, this study confirmed an increase in obstetric interventions such as hospitalization, use of tocolytic medications, inductions of labor, and cesarean sections. Additionally, patients in the cerclage group suffered twice the rate of puerperal fever (6%) when compared to controls (3%)(odds ratio 2.12; 95% CI 1.08–4.16; p = .03). Nonetheless, the authors confidently concluded that "on the balance, cervical cerclage should be offered to women at high risk, such as those with a history of three or more pregnancies ending before 37 weeks gestation." This conclusion should be interpreted with caution in that "three or more pregnancies ending before 37 weeks" was not the original criterion for enrollment in the study.

In light of the marginal benefits of cervical cerclage, and increased incidences of obstetric interventions and infectious morbidity, one must conclude that prophylactic cerclage should be offered only to those women with classic histories of cervical incompetence in previous pregnancies. Emergency cerclages may be offered to women whose clinical presentations are consistent with cervical incompetence in their current pregnancies. Other patients with questionable histories and risk factors should be followed conservatively but carefully with serial pelvic or ultrasound examinations.

BIOPSY OF THE CERVIX IN PREGNANCY

The prevalences of preinvasive and invasive diseases of the cervix are no different in pregnancy than in similar nonpregnant reproductive-age women. In the largest series yet published, Boutselis (1972) reported rates of 0.14 and 0.07 for preinvasive and invasive cervical disease, respectively. Consistent with an observed increase in the rate of abnormal Papanicolaou (Pap) smears in both pregnant and nonpregnant women in recent years, Hannigan (1990) reported that 10 percent of all prenatal patients enrolled at the University of Texas Medical Branch at Galveston had abnormal Pap smears. Low-grade abnormalities, with or without koilocytosis, accounted for the vast majority of these (86%) with high-grade lesions less common (14%). Others (Lurain and Gallup, 1979; Kohan and associates, 1980) have reported cervical intraepithelial neoplasia (CIN) rates of less than 2 percent and emphasize that one cannot extrapolate prevalence estimates from one population to another.

Whether cervical intraepithelial lesions behave differently in pregnancy compared to similar lesions in nonpregnant patients remains the subject of controversy (Schneider and colleagues, 1987; Garry and Jones, 1985). On the other hand, pregnancy-induced physiologic changes in the cervix clearly alter its appearance and probably affect the collection of cytologic specimens. Kohan and associates (1980) described the colposcopic changes associated with pregnancy to include (1) epithelial hyperplasia and glandular hypertrophy; (2) edema and vasocongestion which change the sharpness of borders between CIN and squamous metaplasia; (3) erosions and ulcerations secondary to increased mucus production with bursting of Nabothian cysts; (4) decidualization of the stroma surrounding endocervical glands; and finally (5) an increase in pseudopolyps and ulcerations in areas of decidual change. Kost and colleagues (1993) demonstrated that endocervical cells are commonly absent in cytologic specimens taken from pregnant women. The authors suggested this to be a normal phenomenon in pregnancy and, with follow-up, demonstrated that repeat testing and evaluation may be safely deferred until postpartum in patients whose only abnormality was a lack of endocervical cells.

The goal of routine cervical cytology screening in pregnancy is the detection of invasive and preinvasive disease at an early stage. Even though pregnancy has no influence on the prognosis of invasive carcinoma of the cervix (Baltzer and colleagues, 1990), prompt evaluation of an abnormal cervical cytology specimen is imperative to avoid a delay in diagnosis and therapy. As discussed elsewhere in this text (see Chap. 27), the treatment of invasive cancer of the cervix varies depending on gestational age and the patient's desire for continuation of pregnancy. In this regard, most authors now advocate a general philosophy of expectant management after a confident exclusion of invasive disease (Berman and Disia, 1994; Hannigan, 1990). Despite widespread acceptance of this general approach, opinions vary as to which procedures should be used for a "confident exclusion of invasive disease."

Before colposcopy gained widespread acceptance, aggressive use of cone biopsy was advocated for diagnosis even in pregnant patients (Greene and Peckham, 1958; Mussey and Decker, 1967; Curlin, 1968; Crisp and associates, 1968; Bolognese and Corson, 1969). These reports and others demonstrated that cone biopsy was more accurate than the policy of multiple random punch biopsies that antedated colposcopy. As experience grew, the risks of cervical conization during pregnancy became apparent. Fetal loss rates associated with the procedure ranged from 6.3 to 27.9 percent (Averette and colleagues, 1970; Fowler and associates, 1980; Hannigan and colleagues, 1982). Hannignan and colleagues (1982) reported excessive intraoperative blood loss in 40 of 448 (8.9%) patients and delayed hemorrhage in another 15 of 411 (3.7%). These authors reported blood loss in excess of 500 mL in 12.4 percent of procedures. Hemorrhage was significant enough to require transfusion, readmission, or reoperation in 6.2 percent. They and others (Mikuta and associates, 1968; Averette and colleagues, 1970) noted a greater propensity toward excessive hemorrhage when cone biopsy was performed in the third trimester. Even with attempts at shallow conization, pregnant patients remained at increased risk for significant hemorrhage (Crisp and associates, 1968). In addition to procedure-related pregnancy loss and significant hemorrhage, multiple authors (Crisp and associates, 1968; Boutselis, 1972; Fowler and colleagues, 1980; Hannigan and associates, 1982) have demonstrated increased rates of residual disease in histologic specimens obtained from patients who had previously undergone cervical conization during pregnancy. Boutselis (1972) documented residual disease in 37 percent, 45 percent, and 75 percent of patients undergoing conization in the first, second, and third trimesters, respectively.

Recognizing these complications, other authors (Ortiz and Newton, 1971; Stafl and Mattingly, 1973; Lurain and Gallup, 1979; Kohan and associates, 1980; Hannigan and colleagues, 1982) have reported that competent use of colposcopy and colposcopically directed biopsies dramatically reduced the need for cone biopsy in pregnancy without compromising diagnostic accuracy. Complications of colposcopically directed cervical biopsies are rare. Combining the experiences from four large series (Lurain and Gallup, 1979; Fowler and colleagues, 1980; Kohan and associates, 1980; Benedet and coauthors, 1987), the risk of significant hemorrhage from a cervical biopsy during pregnancy is estimated at 1 percent. Specifically, only 4 of 379 patients experienced hemorrhage severe enough to warrant placing a hemostatic suture. On the other hand, although a specific number was not mentioned, Averette and colleagues (1970) noted that several patients lost more than 500 mL of blood after cervical punch biopsy in their outpatient clinic.

Several authors have suggested avoiding even cervical biopsy during pregnancy unless there is a colposcopic or cytologic suspicion of invasive disease (DePetrillo and co-workers, 1975; Talebian and associates, 1976; McDonnell and colleagues, 1981; Hellberg and associates, 1987; Benedet and colleagues, 1987; Economos and co-authors, 1993). The success of this approach depends on the reliability of colposcopic diagnosis. The literature is replete with warnings that cervical biopsy should only be omitted by an expert colposcopist. Realizing that approximately 10 percent of microinvasive cancers will have normal colposcopic examinations (Sugimori and associates, 1979), omission of colposcopically directed cervical biopsies will result in false-negative diagnoses. While several authors have reported cases in which microinvasive disease was missed until a postpartum evaluation (McDonnell and co-authors, 1981; Hellberg and associates, 1987), the report of Benedet and colleagues (1987) is of particular concern. These authors reported initially encouraging results (Benedet and associates, 1977) which led them to adopt a policy whereby cervical biopsies were performed only for confirmation of invasive disease seen on colposcopy or for cases in which the colposcopic examination was uninterpretable. Publishing their results 10 years later, the authors disclosed that while following this protocol, 5 of 9 invasive cancers during pregnancy were missed. Noting that no invasive cancers would have been missed if this approach had been limited to women less than 30 years of age, the authors continued to advocate a conservative approach to cervical biopsies during pregnancy. However, realizing that this study was conducted by experienced colposcopists, those physicians and patients electing to omit cervical biopsies in pregnancy must be willing to accept a small, but potentially serious, false-negative rate for the detection of invasive disease.

Economos and associates (1993) suggest that colposcopically directed cervical biopsies should be performed for the following indications: (1) colposcopic evidence of invasion or CIN III; (2) discordance between colposcopic findings and cervical cytology; (3) patients electing pregnancy termination, and finally (4) for patients whose reliability or capability for adequate follow-up examination is in doubt. Several options are available to the clinician faced with an inadequate colposcopic exam due to inability to fully visualize the squamocolumnar junction or the full extent of an identified lesion. In recognition of the progressive eversion of the cervical glandular epithelium with advancing gestational age, Economos and colleagues (1993) advocate repeat examinations at 4-week intervals in hopes that this will facilitate visualization. In their series, all patients had an adequate colposcopic exam by 20 weeks' gestation. Nevertheless, as the gestational age approaches 20–24 weeks, options regarding diagnosis and therapy of invasive cervical disease become limited. In this setting, additional options include use of an endocervical speculum or sponge forceps to visualize the endocervix. While endocervical curettage has been performed during pregnancy (Jafari and Sansquiri, 1978), most authors do not advocate this approach for fear of disrupting the fetal membranes.

Cervical Punch Biopsy Technique

In general, the technique of cervical biopsy during pregnancy should not be different from that used in nonpregnant patients. Small, sharp biopsy forceps (Kevorkian) should be used. Recognizing the technical difficulties of adequate exposure of the cervix during pregnancy, Lurain and Gallup (1979) noted the utility of skin hooks to help isolate the area of planned biopsy. Silver nitrate sticks, ferric subsulfate (Monsel's) solution, a generous supply of large cotton swabs, and suture material should be available in anticipation of bleeding from the pregnant cervix.

Cervical Cone Biopsy

With modern cytology and histology services available, most authors agree that the indications for cone biopsy of the cervix during pregnancy are (1) suspected microinvasion on colposcopy or colposcopically directed biopsy or (2) persistent cytologic evidence of invasive disease not explained by colposcopy and cervical biopsy (Hannigan, 1990; Economos and associates, 1993; Berman and DiSaia, 1994). Adenocarcinoma in situ is another indication for cone biopsy in pregnancy, as invasive adenocarcinoma cannot be adequately excluded on cervical biopsy alone (Lurain and Gallup, 1979; Drew, 1984). Neither failure to visualize the complete squamocolumnar junction nor the inability to fully visualize an identified lesion mandate cone biopsy in pregnancy in the absence of cytologic evidence of invasive disease. Further, because cone biopsy is associated with such high rates of residual disease, it is not considered a primary treatment option. Cone biopsy has been associated with complications in all three trimesters; therefore the timing of the cone biopsy should be based upon whenever indications are encountered, with some flexibility to allow for patient preferences and proximity to the expected delivery. Generally we would avoid a cone biopsy during the last 4–6 weeks of pregnancy.

Cervical Cone Biopsy Technique

After an adequate level of regional anesthesia is achieved, the patient is placed in the dorsal lithotomy position with left lateral tilt if in the second or third trimester. A long, weighted speculum is placed into the vagina and smooth retractors are used to expose the cervix. Schiller's solution is poured into the vaginal vault, thereby covering the vaginal portio of the cervix. After a brief time, the solution is removed with surgical suction with care taken to avoid abrasion of the cervical epithelium with the suction tip. A sharp, single-tooth tenaculum is affixed to the anterior lip of the cervix to facilitate manipulation and exposure. Using a figure-of-eight technique, No. 1 absorbable sutures are placed at the 3 and 9 o'clock positions for hemostasis. The needles are left on the suture for later use. The tenaculum is removed, and the long free ends of the hemostatic sutures are used for gentle traction. A dilute pharmacologic vasoconstrictor is then injected into the cervical stroma in a circumferential fashion in an amount sufficient to effect blanching of the cervix. Curlin (1968) administered 1–1.5 mL of vasopressin (10 units in 80 cc normal saline) in each of 4 quadrants of the cervix and reported an average estimated blood loss of less than 100 mL in 27 patients subjected to cone biopsy in pregnancy. Local anesthetics with dilute epinephrine (1 to 100,000) are readily available and may be used as an alternative to vasopressin. Interestingly, most of the cases of serious hemorrhage noted in Averett's series (1970) occurred prior to the use of infiltration with vasoconstricting agents.

Initially introduced by Crisp and associates (1968), most authors advocate the use of a "shallow" cone specimen in pregnancy. This type of cone biopsy is performed to a depth of less than 7 mm below the squamocolumnar junction. Berman and DiSaia (1994) recommend a "coin" biopsy (Fig. 31–11) rather than a traditional cone biopsy when performed during pregnancy. In general, the shape and size of the cone specimen should be tailored to the indication for which the procedure is being performed. Thus, as seen in the figure, while a shallow or "coin" specimen might be appropriate to rule out frank invasion in a patient with cervical biopsies showing microinvasion, a deeper, conical specimen may be more suitable for the patient with adenocarcinoma in situ or persistently unexplained malignant cytology thought to be from the endocervix.

After the cone biopsy specimen has been removed and labeled for the pathologist, if necessary, electrocautery is used to achieve hemostasis. To further assure short-term hemostasis, the ends of the stay sutures, with needles still attached, are used to encircle the cervix just as for a McDonald cerclage. One or two passes are made through the anterior and posterior cervical stroma as deemed necessary. If performed at a point in pregnancy when preterm labor is of concern, postoperatively patients are monitored on labor and delivery for the development of uterine activity, with tocolytic medications used as indicated.

Recognizing the tendency of clinicians to compromise the size of cone biopsy specimens in pregnant women for fear of hemorrhage or pregnancy loss, Goldberg and associates (1991) have reported their initial experience with a procedure combining conization with placement of a traditional McDonald cerclage. The authors imply that the technique allows conization during pregnancy without limiting

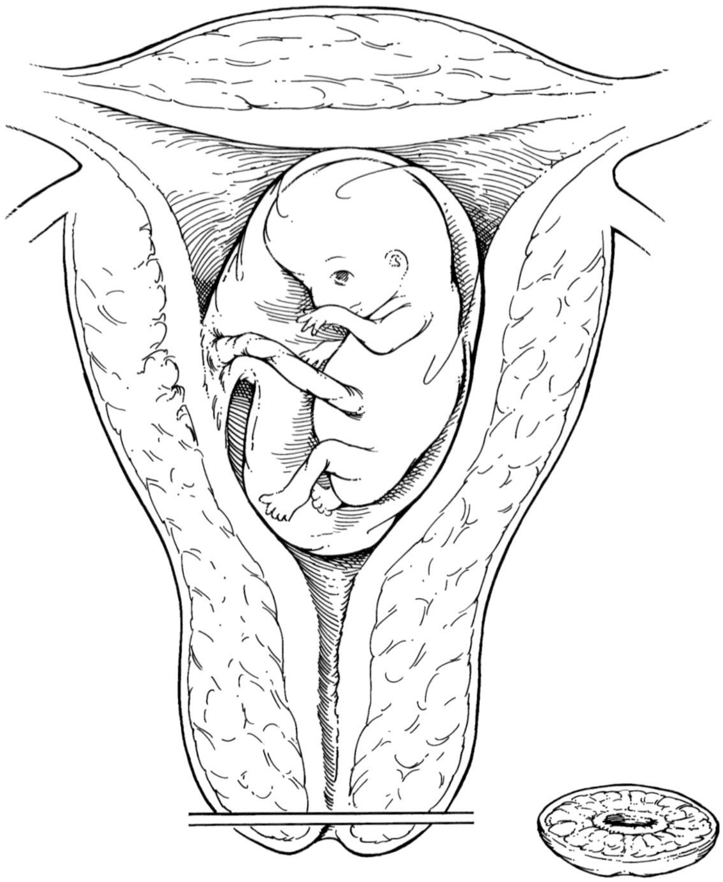

Figure 31–11. Modified cone biopsy of the cervix during pregnancy. Figure shows a "coin" biopsy advocated by Berman and DiSaia (1994). While such a shallow specimen may be appropriate to rule out invasion in a lesion that is completely visualized and does not involve the endocervix, such a biopsy would prove inadequate for adenocarcinoma in situ or suspected endocervical disease.

the specimen size and therefore its diagnostic value. No hemorrhage or pregnancy loss was reported in 17 patients treated. While encouraging, and perhaps applicable to patients with suspected invasive endocervical disease requiring deep cone biopsy, the study was small and retrospective. However, because the need for extensive conization during pregnancy is rare, significantly larger series are unlikely to be published. While the authors recommend this technique for all pregnant patients undergoing cone biopsy, in light of the well-documented increase in infectious morbidity associated with prophylactic cerclage placed for other reasons, this procedure should be considered only for the exceptional case requiring extensive resection.

Electrosurgical large loop excision of the transformation zone (LLETZ) has recently gained popularity as an effective method for the outpatient diagnosis and treatment of cervical intraepithelial neoplasia (Bloss, 1993). As discussed previously, several authors have described pregnancy outcomes in patients with a prior history of a LLETZ procedure (Keijser and colleagues, 1992; Blomfield and associates, 1993). However, use of this technology during an ongoing pregnancy has yet to be reported, and manufacturers of the equipment list pregnancy as a contraindication to the procedure. Nonetheless, Berman and DiSaia (1994) suggest that this procedure may prove especially suited to obtaining a specimen from the pregnant woman who requires a shallow cone biopsy.

MASSIVE CERVICAL CONDYLOMATA ACUMINATA DURING PREGNANCY

Condyloma acuminata is a commonly encountered sexually transmitted disease easily recognized as genital warts on the perineum, vagina, and cervix. The disease is a manifestation of infection with a human papillomavirus (HPV), usually serotype 6 or 11. While the vertical transmission of HPV has been documented from mother to infant in the form of laryngeal papillomatosis, the epidemiology of this occurrence does not support a policy of prophylactic cesarean section for its prevention (CDC, 1989). On the other hand, during pregnancy condylomata acuminata may become so extensive as to preclude vaginal delivery for maternal indications. Obstructed labor, poor episiotomy healing, and massive hemorrhage secondary to lacerations through irregular tissue planes have all been reported in conjunction with condyloma acuminata during pregnancy (Wilson, 1973; Snyder and associates, 1990). In an often cited series, Benschine (1941) reported a maternal death secondary to uncontrollable hemorrhage associated with massive vaginal and vulvar condylomata acuminata.

Treatment of condylomata acuminata is usually accomplished with topical application of podophyllum resin in a benzoin base. However, podophyllum toxin is an antimitotic agent and, as such, is considered contraindicated during pregnancy by some authors (Gibbs and Sweet, 1994). Others have suggested that, after the first trimester, judicious use of podophyllum for the treatment of smaller external lesions may be associated with less risk than procedures that, alternatively, would require the use of anesthesia (Ross, 1982; Snyder and Hankins, 1990). A more acceptable option during pregnancy is the application of a 50–85 percent solution of trichloroacetic acid. Trichloroacetic acid acts by precipitating intracellular proteins and is not absorbed systemically (see Chap. 19). Schwartz and colleagues (1988) have reported a clinical success rate over 95 percent for the treatment of genital condylomata during pregnancy with a combination of trichloroacetic acid and laser therapy.

For cases with extensive lesions and for those that have failed medical therapy, a number of options are available, including electrocautery, surgical resection, cryotherapy, and laser ablation. Electrocautery and surgical resection of cervical lesions, while easily performed in the nonpregnant patient, are complicated by the increased edema and vascularity of the cervix when attempted during pregnancy. Recognizing the difficulty of these procedures during pregnancy, Bergman and associates (1987) reported their experience with cryotherapy for bulky cervical condylomata in 28 pregnant women. Using serial treatments if necessary, these authors treated women with massive (average 14 cm^2, range 7–23 cm^2) lesions and reported no adverse maternal or neonatal sequelae. Laser ablation of genital tract condylomata during pregnancy has been reported by several groups (Ferenczy, 1984; Schwartz and associates, 1988; Hankins and colleagues, 1989). While none of these series contained more than a few patients with cervical lesions, the report by Hankins and colleagues is particularly worrisome and deserves additional comment. They described the case of a woman with a large cervical lesion treated at 36 weeks' gestation with laser ablation. More than two and a half hours into the operation and with only 60 percent of the lesion treated, the authors decided to stop in favor of a staged procedure. The surgeons had encountered a purulent discharge and multiple abscesses as the lesions were vaporized. Less than 8 hours after the surgery, the patient developed clinical chorioamnionitis with intact membranes manifest by fever and uterine tenderness. Delivered by cesarean section with Apgar scores of 8 and 8 at 1 and 5 minutes, respectively, the infant developed immediate respiratory distress and septic shock syndrome thought secondary to congenital pneumonia. The infant survived but required 2 days of dobutamine for blood pressure support as well as prolonged antibiotic therapy. Importantly, preoperative cervical cultures for group B beta-hemolytic streptococcus, gonorrhea, and chlamydia had all returned negative. Largely due to this case, we have elected not to treat bulky cervical lesions in the latter part of pregnancy, preferring instead to accomplish delivery by cesarean section with plans to reevaluate the cervical lesions at the postpartum visit.

DÜHRSSEN'S INCISIONS

In all but the most extreme circumstances, the safety of modern-day cesarean section has rendered Dührssen's incisions obsolete. Condemned as early as 1790 by Baudelocque, incision of the incompletely dilated cervix was popularized by Alfred Dührssen of Berlin in 1890 as a means to expedite delivery (DeLee, 1940). In the seventh edition of his text, DeLee writes, "several deaths have occurred from hemorrhage, and if the tissues are incised before obliteration [effacement] of the cervix is complete, the wounds are likely to tear further during extraction and open up the broad ligaments, even the peritoneal cavity." Modern indications for Dührssen's incisions are few and primarily limited to entrapment of the aftercoming head during precipitous vaginal breech delivery of a preterm infant. In this setting, such incisions may prove lifesaving for the infant. Another indication may be to allow an instrumental delivery for the occurrence of umbilical cord prolapse when funic replacement or immediate cesarean section is not possible.

Before Dührssen's incisions are performed, the cervix should be completely effaced and at least 6 cm dilated. Placenta previa is considered a contraindication. As described by Nicholson J. Eastman (1950), the procedure is performed as follows (Fig. 31–12): "Sponge forceps are applied to the cervix at 2, 6, and 10 o'clock; that is, at the sites where incisions are to be made. Once the first incision has been made, the remaining rim of cervix tends to retract and becomes more difficult to reach, unless held by a clamp. Although the two extra forceps are somewhat in the way when the first incision is made, experience shows that this practice is worth the trouble if the operation is to be a thorough one." Duncan Reid (1962) noted that the incisions should be carried nearly to the cervicovaginal junction and that while the 6 o'clock incision may be required on some occasions, the two anterior incisions will usually suffice. Most authors stress the critical importance of adequate exposure and recommend the use of vaginal sidewall retractors. When the after-coming head of a precipitously delivered preterm infant is

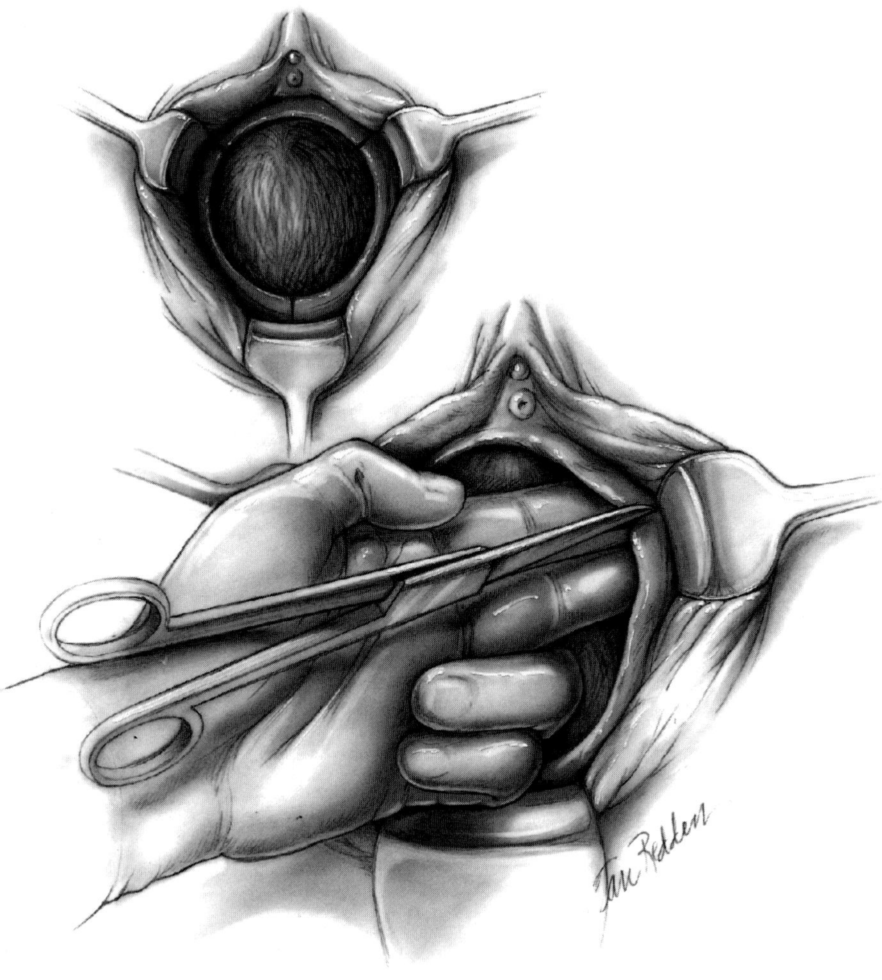

Figure 31–12. Dührssen's incisions. Figure shows location of two anterior incisions and the placement of DeLee cervical tenacula or sponge forceps. The 6 o'clock incision is made only if necessary.

entrapped, direct exposure and placement of ring forceps may be impossible. In this circumstance, the operator should place one or two fingers inside the cervix along the infant's neck and head. Bandage scissors with a blunt tip are introduced along the surgeon's fingers and an incision is made at the 2 o'clock position. The procedure may be repeated at 10 o'clock, and then, 6 o'clock if necessary. After a careful examination to rule out extension beyond the vaginal vault, the incisions are repaired with a running, interlocking chromic suture in the same manner as for a spontaneous cervical laceration (see Chap. 14).

SUMMARY

Prophylactic cerclage should be offered only to women with a classic history of pregnancy loss due to cervical incompetence. Women considered to have an increased risk for incompetent cervix, such as those exposed to DES or with cervical trauma, should be followed conservatively. Therapeutic cerclage then may be offered to those who develop cervical change demonstrated on serial physical exam or ultrasound. No single cerclage procedure has proven to be superior to others; and the choice depends largely on the surgeon's experience and training. Cone biopsy of the cervix, rarely indicated during pregnancy, is recommend only for suspected microinvasion on colposcopy or colposcopically directed biopsy, or persistent cytological evidence of invasive disease not explained by colposcopy and cervical biopsy. Massive condyloma involving the cervix and lower genital tract may be treated with trichloracetic acid during pregnancy. In general, if medical therapy fails and bulky cervical condyloma persist into the third trimester, consideration should be given to cesarean delivery. Finally, although discredited under most circumstances, Dührssen's incisions, may prove life saving for cervical entrapment for the aftercoming head during precipitous breech delivery of a preterm infant.

REFERENCES

Aarnoudse JG, Huisjes HJ. Complications of cerclage. Acta Obstet Gynecol Scand 1979; 58:225.

Averette HE, Nasser N, Yankow SL, Little WA. Cervical conization in pregnancy. Analysis of 180 operations. Am J Obstet Gynecol 1970; 106:543

Bakketeig LS, Hoffman HJ, Harley EE. The tendency to repeat gestational age and birthweight in successive births. Am J Obstet Gynecol 1979; 135:1086.

Baltzer J, Regenbrecht ME, Kopcke W, Zander T. Carcinoma of the cervix and pregnancy. Int J Gynaecol Obstet 1990; 31:317.

Barth WH Jr, Yeomans ER, Hankins GDV. Emergent cerclage. Surg Gynecol Obstet 1990; 170:323.

Bates JL, Cropley T. Complication of cervical cerclage. Lancet 1977; 2:1035.

Ben Baruch G, Rabinovitch O, Madjar I, et al. Ureterovaginal fistula: a rare complication of cervical cerclage. Isr J Med Sci 1980; 16:400.

Benedet JL, Boyes DA, Nichols TM, Millner A. Colposcopic evaluation of pregnant patients with abnormal cervical smears. Br J Obstet Gynaecol 1977; 84:517.

Benedet JL, Selke PA, Nickerson KG. Colposcopic evaluation of abnormal Papanicolaou smears in pregnancy. Am J Obstet Gynecol 1987; 157:932.

Benschine FW. Massive condylomata acuminata of the vulva complicating labor. Am J Obstet Gynecol 1941; 42:338.

Benson RC, Durfee RB. Transabdominal cervicouterine cerclage during pregnancy for the treatment of cervical incompetency. Obstet Gynecol 1965; 25:145.

Bergman A, Matsunaga J, Bhatia NN. Cervical cryotherapy for condylomata acuminata during pregnancy. Obstet Gynecol 1987; 69:47.

Berman ML, DiSaia PJ. Pelvic malignancies, gestational trophoblastic neoplasia, and nonpelvic malignancies. In Creasy RK, Resnik R, eds. Maternal-Fetal Medicine—Principles and Practice. Philadelphia: Saunders, 1994:1112.

Blomfield PI, Buxton J, Dunn J, Luesley DM. Pregnancy outcome after large loop excision of the cervical transformation zone. Am J Obstet Gynecol 1993; 169:620.

Bloss JD. The use of electrosurgical techniques in the management of premalignant diseases of the vulva, vagina, and cervix: An excisional rather than an ablative approach. Am J Obstet Gynecol 1993; 169:1081.

Bolognese RJ, Corson SL. Cervical conization in pregnancy. Surg Gynecol Obstet 1969; 128:1244.

Boutselis JG. Intraepithelial carcinoma of the cervix associated with pregnancy. Obstet Gynecol 1972; 40:657.

Buller RE, Jones HW. Pregnancy following cervical conization. Am J Obstet Gynecol 1982; 142:506.

Carr-Hill RA, Hall MH. The repetition of spontaneous preterm labour. Br J Obstet Gynaecol 1985; 92:921.

Caspi E, Schneider D, Sadovsky G, et al. Diameter of cervical internal os after early abortion by laminaria or rigid dilation. Am J Obstet Gynecol 1983; 146:106.

Centers for Disease Control. 1989 Sexually transmitted diseases treatment and guidelines. MMWR 38(suppl 1), September 1, 1989.

Copper RL, Goldenberg RL, Creasy RK, et al. A multicenter study of preterm birth weight and gestational age-specific neonatal mortality. Am J Obstet Gynecol 1993; 168:78.

Cousins L. Cervical incompetence, 1980: a time for reappraisal. Clin Obstet Gynecol 1980; 23:467.

Cousins L, Karp W, Lacey C, Lucas WE. Reproductive outcome of women exposed to diethylstilbestrol in utero. Obstet Gynecol 1980; 56:70.

Coustan DR. Cervical cerclage. In: Nichols DH, ed. Gynecologic and Obstetric Surgery. St. Louis: Mosby, 1993:1031.

Crisp WE, Shalauta H, Bennett WA. Shallow conization of the cervix. Obstet Gynecol 1968; 31:755.

Cunningham FG, Macdonald PC, Gant NF, et al. Williams Obstetrics, 19th ed. Norwalk, CT: Appleton & Lange, 1993:73.

Curlin JP. Conization of the cervix during pregnancy. J Ark Med Soc 1968; 65:184.

Daling JR, Emannel I. Induced abortion and subsequent outcome of pregnancy in a series of American women. New Engl J Med 1977; 297:1241.

DeLee JB. The Principles and Practice of Obstetrics, 7th ed. Philadelphia: Saunders, 1940.

DePetrillo AD, Townsend DE, Morrow CP, et al. Colposcopic evaluation of the abnormal Papanicolaou test in pregnancy. Am J Obstet Gynecol 1975; 121:441.

Dor J, Shalev J, Mashiach S, et al. Elective cervical suture of twin pregnancies diagnosed ultrasonically in the first trimester following induced ovulation. Gynecol Obstet Invest 1982; 13:55.

Drew NC. Adenocarcinoma-in-situ of the cervix uteri associated with cervical intraepithelial neoplasia in pregnancy. Case report. Br J Obstet Gynaecol 1984; 91:498.

Dubouloz P, Maye D, Beguin F. Cerclage et infections: Etude clinique et therapeutique. J Gyn Obst Biol Reprod 1980; 9:671.

Dunn LJ, Robinson JC, Steer CM. Maternal death following suture of incompetent cervix during pregnancy. Am J Obstet Gynecol 1959; 78:335.

Eastman NJ. Williams Obstetrics, 10th ed. New York: Appleton-Century-Crofts, 1950.

Economos K, Veridiano NP, Delke I, et al. Abnormal cervical cytology in pregnancy: a 17-year experience. Obstet Gynecol 1993; 81:915.

Ehrenpreis MD, Alarcon JA, Firfer R. Case profile: Large bladder calculus post cervical cerclage. Urology 1986; 27:366.

Evans DJ, Kofinas AD, King K. Intraoperative amniocentesis and indomethacin treatment in the management of an immature pregnancy with completely dilated cervix. Obstet Gynecol 1992; 79:881.

Ferenczy A. Treating genital condyloma during pregnancy with the carbon dioxide laser. Am J Obstet Gynecol 1984; 148:9.

Floyd WS. Cervical dilation in the mid-trimester of pregnancy. Obstet Gynecol 1961; 18:3880.

Fowler WC Jr, Walton LA, Edelman DA. Cervical intraepithelial neoplasia during pregnancy. South Med J 1980; 73:1180.

Garry R, Jones R. Relationship between cervical condylomata, pregnancy and subclinical papillomavirus infection. J Reprod Med 1985; 30:393.

Gibbs RS, Sweet RL. Maternal and fetal infections. Clinical disorders. In: Creasy RK, Resnik R, eds. Maternal–Fetal Medicine—Principles and Practice. Philadelphia: Saunders, 1994:639.

Gilstrap LC, Hauth JC, Bell RE, et al. Survival and shortterm morbidity of the premature neonate. Obstet Gynecol 1985; 65:37.

Goldberg GL, Altaras MM, Bloch B. Instruments and methods: Cone cerclage in pregnancy. Obstet Gynecol 1991; 77:315.

Goldman JM, Greene MF, Tuomala RE: Outcome of expectant management in preterm premature rupture of the membranes with cervical cerclage in place [abstract 139]. Tenth Annual Meeting, Society of Perinatal Obstetricians, Houston, TX, 1990.

Goldstein DP. Incompetent cervix in offspring exposed to diethylstilbestrol in utero. Obstet Gynecol 1978; 52:73s.

Goodlin RC. Cervical incompetence, hourglass membranes, and amniocentesis. Obstet Gynecol 1979; 54:748.

Greene RR, Peckham BM. Preinvasive cancer of the cervix and pregnancy. Am J Obstet Gynecol 1958; 75:551.

Hankins GDV, Hammond TL, Snyder RR, Gilstrap LC III. Use of laser vaporization for management of extensive genital tract condyloma acuminata during pregnancy. J Infect Dis 1989; 159:1001.

Hannigan EV. Cervical cancer in pregnancy. Clin Obstet Gynecol 1990; 33:837.

Hannigan EV, Whitehouse HH III, Atkinson WD, Becker SN. Cone biopsy during pregnancy. Obstet Gynecol 1982; 60:450.

Harger JH. Comparison of success and morbidity in cervical cerclage procedures. Obstet Gynecol 1980; 53:543.

Harger JH. Cervical cerclage: patient selection, morbidity, and success rates. Clin Perinatol 1983; 10:321.

Harger JH, Archer DF, et al. Etiology of recurrent pregnancy losses and outcome of subsequent pregnancies. Obstet Gynecol 1983; 62:574.

Hellberg D, Axelsson O, Gad A, Nilsson S. Conservative management of the abnormal smear during

pregnancy. A long-term follow-up. Acta Obstet Gynecol Scand 1987; 66:195.
Herbst AL, Hubby MM, Blough RR, Azizi F. A comparison of pregnancy experience in DES-exposed and DES-unexposed daughters. J Reprod Med 1980; 24:62.
Holman MR. An aid for cervical cerclage. Obstet Gynecol 1973; 42:468.
Hortenstine JS, Witherington R. Ulcer of the trigone: A late complication of cervical cerclage. J Urol 1987; 137:109.
Jafari K, Sansguiri R. Role of endocervical curettage in colposcopy. Am J Obstet Gynecol 1978; 131:83.
Johnstone FD, Boyd IE, McCarthy TG. The diameter of the uterine isthmus during the menstrual cycle, pregnancy, and the puerperium. J Obstet Gynecol Br Commum 1974; 81:558.
Kaufman RH, Noller K, Adam E, et al. Upper genital tract abnormalities and pregnancy outcome in diethylstibestrol-exposed progeny. Am J Obstet Gynecol 1984; 148:973.
Keijser KGG, Kenemans P, van der Zanden P, et al. Diathermy loop excision in the management of cervical intraepithelial neoplasia: Diagnosis and treatment in one procedure. Am J Obstet Gynecol 1992; 166:1281.
Kohan S, Beckman EM, Bigelow B, et al. The role of colposcopy in the management of cervical intraepithelial neoplasia during pregnancy and postpartum. J Reprod Med 1980; 25:279.
Kost ER, Snyder RR, Schwartz LE, Hankins GDV. The "less than optimal" cytology: Importance in obstetric patients and in a routine gynecologic population. Obstet Gynecol 1993; 81:127.
Kristensen J, Langhoff-Roos J, Kristensen FB. Increased risk of preterm birth in women with cervical conization. Am J Obstet Gynecol 1993; 81:1005.
Kuhn RJP, Pepperell RJ. Cervical ligation: A review of 242 pregnancies. Aust NZ J Obstet Gynaec 1977; 17:79.
Langman J. Medical embryology. 4th ed. Baltimore: Williams & Wilkins, 1981.
Lash AF, Lash SR. Habitual abortion: The incompetent internal os of the cervix. Am J Obstet Gynecol 1950; 59:68.
Lazar P, Gueguen S, Dreyfus J, et al. Multicentered controlled trial of cervical cerclage in women at moderate risk of preterm delivery. Br J Obstet Gynaecol 1984; 91:731.
Lee NH. The effect of cone biopsy on subsequent pregnancy outcome. Gynecol Oncol 1978; 6:1.
Leiman G, Harrison NA, Rubin A. Pregnancy following conization of the cervix: Complications related to cone size. Am J Obstet Gynecol 1980; 136:14.
Levine RU, Berkowitz KM. Conservative management and pregnancy outcome in diethylstilbestrol-exposed women with and without gross genital tract abnormalities. Am J Obstet Gynecol 1993; 169:1125.
Lipshitz J. Cerclage in the treatment of incompetent cervix. S Afr Med J 1975; 49:2013.
Little B, Tenney B Jr. Incompetent cervical os. Clin Obstet Gynecol 1963; 6:423.
Ludmir J, Jackson GM, Samuels P. Transvaginal cerclage under ultrasound guidance in cases of severe cervical hypoplasia. Obstet Gynecol 1991; 78:1067.
Ludmir J, Landon MB, Gabbe SG, et al. Management of the diethylstilbestrol-exposed pregnant patient: A prospective study. Am J Obstet Gynecol 1987; 157:665.
Lurain JR, Gallup DG. Management of abnormal Papanicolaou smears in pregnancy. Obstet Gynecol 1979; 53:484.
MacNaughton MC, Chalmers IG, Dubowitz V, et al. Final report of the Medical Research Council/Royal College of Obstetricians and Gynaecologists Multicentre Randomized Trial of Cervical Cerclage. Br J Obstet Gynaecol 1993; 100:516.
Mangan CE, Borow L, Burnett-Rubin MM, et al. Pregnancy outcome in 98 women exposed to diethylstilbestrol in utero, their mothers, and unexposed siblings. Obstet Gynecol 1982; 59:315.
Marx PD. Transabdominal cervicoisthmic cerclage: A review. Obstet Gynecol Survey 1989; 44:518.
McCulloch B, Bergen S, Pielet B, et al. McDonald cerclage under pudendal nerve block. Am J Obstet Gynecol 1993; 168:499.
McDonald IA. Suture of the cervix for inevitable miscarriage. J Obstet Gynecol Brit Comm 1957; 64:346.
McDonald IA. Cervical incompetence as a cause of spontaneous abortion. In: Bennet MJ, Edmonds DK, eds. Spontaneous and Recurrent Abortion. London: Blackwell Scientific, 1987:168
McDonnell JM, Mylotte MJ, Gustafson RC. Colposcopy in pregnancy. A twelve year review. Br J Obstet Gynaecol 1981; 88:414.
McLaren HC, Jordan JA, Glover M, Atwood ME. Pregnancy after cone biopsy of the cervix. J Obstet Gynaecol Br Commun 1974; 81:383.
Michaels WH, Thompson HO, Schreiber FR, et al. Ultrasound surveillance of the cervix during pregnancy in diethylstilbestrol exposed offspring. Obstet Gynecol 1989; 73:230.
Mikuta JJ, Enterline HT, Braun TE Jr. Carcinoma in situ of the cervix associated with pregnancy. A clinical-pathological review. JAMA 1968; 204:105.
Mitra AG, Katz VL, Bowes WA Jr, Carmichael S. Emergency cerclages: a review of 40 consecutive procedures. Am J Perinatol 1992; 9:142.
Moinian M, Andersch B. Does cervix conization increase the risk of complications in subsequent pregnancies? Acta Obstet Gynecol Scand 1982; 61:461.
Mussey E, Decker DG. Intraepithelial carcinoma of

the cervix in association with pregnancy. Am J Obstet Gynecol 1967; 97:30.

Newton M, Newton ER. Complications of obstetric operations. In: Complications of Gynecologic and Obstetric Management. Philadelphia: Saunders, 1988:229.

Novy MJ. Transabdominal cervicoisthmic cerclage: A reappraisal 25 years after its introduction. Am J Obstet Gynecol 1991; 164:1635.

Novy MJ, Haymond J, Nichols M. Shirodkar cerclage in a multifactorial approach to the patient with advanced cervical changes. Am J Obstet Gynecol 1990; 162:1412.

Olatunbosun OA, Dyck F. Cervical cerclage operation for a dilated cervix. Obstet Gynecol 1981; 57:166.

Ortiz R, Newton M. Colposcopy in the management of abnormal cervical smears in pregnancy. Am J Obstet Gynecol 1971; 109:46.

Peters WA, Thiagarajah S, Harbert GM. Cervical cerclage: Twenty years experience. South Med J 1979; 72:933.

Rechberger T, Ulbjerg N, Oxlund H. Connective tissue changes in the cervix during normal pregnancy and pregnancy complicated by cervical incompetence. Obstet Gynecol 1988; 71:563.

Reid DE: A Textbook of Obstetrics. Philadelphia: Saunders, 1962.

Riley L, Frigoletto FD Jr, Benacerraf BR. The implications of sonographically identified cervical changes in patients not necessarily at risk for preterm birth. J Ultrasound Med 1992; 11:75.

Ross SM. Sexually transmitted diseases in pregnancy. Clin Obstet Gynecol 1982; 9:565.

Rush RW, Isaacs S, McPherson K, et al. A randomized controlled trial of cervical cerclage in women at high risk of spontaneous preterm delivery. Br J Obstet Gynaecol 1984; 91:724.

Rust L. Discussion (Novy MJ. Transabdominal cervicoisthmic cerclage: A reappraisal 25 years after its introduction. Am J Obstet 1991; 164:1635) Am J Obstet Gynecol 1991; 164:1641.

Schneider A, Hotz M, Gissman L. Increased prevalence of human papillomaviruses in the lower genital tract of pregnant women. Int J Cancer 1987; 40:198.

Schulman H, Farmakides G. Surgical approach to failed cervical cerclage: A report of three cases. J Reprod Med 1985; 30:626.

Schultz KF, Grimes DA, Cates W Jr. Measures to prevent cervical injury during suction curettage abortion. Lancet 1983; 1:1182.

Schwartz DB, Greenberg MD, Daoud Y, Reid R. Genital condylomas in pregnancy: Use of trichloroacetic acid and laser therapy. Am J Obstet Gynecol 1988; 158:1407.

Sheerer LJ, Lam F, Katz M. A new technique for cervical cerclage in the presence of prolapsed fetal membranes [abstract 144]. In Abstracts of the Seventh Annual Meeting, Society of Perinatal Obstetricians, Lake Buena Vista, 1987:144.

Shirodkar VN. A new method of operative treatment for habitual abortion in the second trimester of pregnancy. Antiseptic 1955; 52:299.

Shortle B, Jewelewicz R. Clinical Aspects of Cervical Incompetence. Chicago: Yearbook Medical Publishers, 1989:3.

Singer MS, Hochman M. Incompetent cervix in a hormone-exposed offspring. Obstet Gynecol 1978; 51:625.

Snyder RR, Hammond TL, Hankins GDV. Human papillomavirus associated with poor healing of episiotomy repairs. Obstet Gynecol 1990; 76:664.

Snyder RR, Hankins GDV. Human papillomavirus infection during pregnancy. In: Gilstrap LC III, Faro S, eds. Infection in Pregnancy. New York: Alan R. Liss, 1990:193.

Stafl A, Mattingly RF. Colposcopic diagnosis of cervical neoplasia. Obstet Gynecol 1973; 41:168.

Stromme WB, Wagner RM, Reed SC. Surgical management of the incompetent cervix. Obstet Gynecl 1960; 15:635.

Sugimori H, Matsuyama T, Kashimura Y, et al. Colposcopic findings in microinvasive carcinoma of the uterine cervix. Obstet Gynecol Surv 1979; 34:804.

Talebian F, Krumholz BA, Shayan A, Mann LI. Colposcopic evaluation of patients with abnormal cytologic smears during pregnancy. Obstet Gynecol 1976; 47:693.

Toaff R, Toaff ME. Diagnosis of impending late abortion. Obstet Gynecol 1974; 43:756.

Toaff R, Toaff ME, Ballas, Ophir A. Cervical incompetence: Diagnostic and therapeutic concepts. Israel J Med Sci 1977; 13:39.

Weber T, Obel E. Pregnancy complications following conization of the uterine cervix. Acta Obstet Gynecol Scand 1979; 58:259.

Wilson J. Extensive vulval condylomata acuminata necessitating cesarean section. Aust NZ J Obstet Gynaecol 1973; 13:121.

Yeast JD, Garite TR. The role of cervical cerclage in the management of preterm premature rupture of the membranes. Am J Obstet Gynecol 1988; 158:106.

CHAPTER 32

Cervical Ripening

Cervical ripening refers to a prelabor change in the physical and biochemical configuration of collagen fiber in the uterine cervix, which allows for greater compliance during labor. In the past, the cervix was believed to play a passive role in parturition, with dilation and effacement occurring only in response to uterine contractions. Now cervical ripening is recognized as an active process associated with biochemical and histologic changes in which the cervix changes shape and consistency. The cervix is considered to be ripe when it most closely assumes the characteristics of a term cervix that is about to enter spontaneous labor.

The development and maturation of the cervix and myometrium are regulated by the same factors and proceed together throughout gestation. The effect of pregnancy on the human cervix has been well described by Danforth and associates (1974). The cervix is firm in the first trimester; 50 percent of its dry weight is tightly aligned and bound collagen and 20 percent is smooth muscle. The remainder is ground substance produced by fibroblasts and composed of elastin and glycosaminoglycans (chondroitin, dermatan sulfates, hyaluronidase). As pregnancy progresses, the collagen fibers become disrupted because concentrations of hyaluronidase, which weakly binds collagen, increase from 6 to 33 percent, while concentrations of dermatan and chondroitin sulfates, which bind collagen more tightly, decrease. In addition, the concentration of collagenase and elastase enzymes increase, leading to a gradual breakdown in the structure of collagen and reduction of collagen content. The vascularity and water content of the cervix also increase with advancing gestation. All of these histologic changes are influenced by prostaglandins, estrogen/progesterone, relaxin, and leukotrienes.

The duration of any induction of labor is affected primarily by parity and cervical status rather than baseline uterine sensitivity to oxytocin. In most pregnancies, some degree of cervical ripening is evidenced near term and generally precedes spontaneous labor. However, the cervix is often unripe or unfavorable at earlier gestational ages and in a significant number of pregnancies thought to be postdate.

In 1964, Bishop and Edward described a scoring system for multiparous patients (Table 32–1) that indicated that a cervical score exceeding 8 was predictive of a vaginal delivery regardless of whether labor was induced or spontaneous (Bishop and Edward, 1964). A Technical Bulletin of the American College of Obstetricians and Gynecologists (ACOG) later suggested that a cervical score of at least 6 was considered favorable and likely to result in successful labor induction without need of a cervical ripening agent (ACOG, 1991b). Induction of labor with a lower cervical score has been associated with a higher risk of a failed induction, prolonged labor, and cesarean delivery (Brindley and Sokol, 1988).

When the cervix is found to be unripe or unfavorable, and induction of labor is indi-

TABLE 32–1. BISHOP SCORING SYSTEM

Score	Dilation (cm)	Effacement (%)	Station	Consistency	Position
0	Closed	0–30	–3	Firm	Posterior
1	1–2	40–50	–2	Medium	Mid-Position
2	3-4	60–70	–1, 0	Soft	Anterior
3	5	80–100	+1, +2		

cated, various hormonal and mechanical methods can be used to affect cervical change. This chapter focuses on these methods—their indications, technical applications, means of monitoring, and limitations.

INDICATIONS FOR CERVICAL RIPENING

Voluntary pregnancy termination is an option up to 23 weeks, 6 days in most states. Induction beyond this period must be based on either a fetal or maternal indication or both. Induction is indicated when the benefits to the mother and/or fetus outweigh those of continuing the pregnancy. Indications and contraindications for cervical ripening and induction of labor include those listed in Table 32–2. Absolute contraindications to cervical ripening are few because certain clinical situations (eg, active herpes infection and the presence of fetal death) will still warrant induction of labor.

Induction of labor should be preceded by evaluation of fetal status and documentation of the cervical examination. Fetal lung maturity should be considered when intervention is planned before term or at an unknown gestational age (ACOG, 1991) (Table 32–3). The site of cervical ripening and labor induction should include facilities that allow fetal monitoring and immediate cesarean delivery. An explanation to the patient of the need to use a cervical ripening agent should be documented in the chart, although written informed consent is unnecessary.

TABLE 32–2. INDICATIONS AND CONTRAINDICATIONS FOR CERVICAL RIPENING

Potential Indications
- Pregnancy-induced hypertension
- Premature rupture of membranes
- Chorioamnionitis
- Suspected fetal jeopardy (eg, severe fetal growth retardation, abnormal heart rate pattern, isoimmunization)
- Maternal medical problems (eg, diabetes mellitus, renal disease, chronic pulmonary disease)
- Fetal death
- Logistic factors (eg, risk of rapid labor, distance from hospital, psychosocial indications)
- Postdate pregnancy

Contraindications
- Placenta or vasa previa
- Transverse fetal lie
- Prolapsed umbilical cord
- Prior classical uterine incision
- Active genital herpes infection

Proceed with Caution
- Multifetal gestation
- Hydramnios
- Maternal cardiac disease
- Grand multiparity
- Breech presentation
- Presenting part above the pelvic inlet

TABLE 23–3. CRITERIA OF ASSUMED FETAL MATURITY

1. Fetal heart tones have been documented for 20 weeks by nonelectronic fetoscope or for 30 weeks by Doppler.
2. 36 weeks have passed since a positive serum or urine human chorionic gonadotropin pregnancy test was performed by a reliable laboratory.
3. Ultrasound measurement of the crown-rump length, obtained at 6–11 weeks, supports a gestational age of 39 weeks.
4. Ultrasound at 12–20 weeks confirms the gestational age of 39 weeks determined by clinical history and physical examination.

ACOG (1991a).

TYPES OF RIPENING METHODS

Prostaglandins

Prostaglandins consist of 20 carbon compounds synthesized in all cells (Craft, 1972; Ueland and Conrad, 1983). Exogenous prostaglandins have been administered orally, intravenously, and extra-amniotically to ripen the cervix or induce labor (Beazley, 1970; Ulmsten, 1982; Calder, 1977; and their associates). Each of these routes has significant drawbacks. The application of prostaglandins near the target organ has been shown to increase efficacy while decreasing maternal systemic effects and uterine hyperstimulation (Brindley and Sokol, 1988). Prostaglandin F_2 is not available as a cervical ripening agent because it requires ten times the equivalent dose of PGE_2 for equal efficacy which, in turn, results in more systemic side effects. PGE_2 has thus become the prostaglandin of choice for cervical ripening.

Cervical changes described in physiologic cervical ripening and spontaneous labor are reproduced with exogenous PGE_2. A dissolution of collagen, increase in glucose glycosaminoglycans, and increase in fibroblast activity have been described in early gestation in humans and late pregnancy in rabbits (Danforth, 1974; Uldbjerg, 1981; Rayburn, 1994; and their colleagues). Although these ripening effects may occur without contractions, PGE_2 is known to enhance myometrial sensitivity to oxytocin (Huszar and Walsh, 1991; Calder and Greer, 1991; Anderson and Turnbull, 1968; Wikland and co-workers, 1984; Gillespie, 1972). Prostaglandins have been reported to accelerate gap junction formation leading to more coordinated uterine contractions. Myometrial strips taken from the fundus during spontaneous labor have been reported to be stimulated with PGE_2 while smooth muscle of the lower uterine segment and cervix are inhibited by PGE_2 (Wikland and associates, 1984; Gillespie, 1972; Takahashi and colleagues, 1980; Liggins, 1978).

Most clinical protocols have used either 0.5 mg of PGE_2 blended in an inert base of triacetin for intracervical instillation or 2–5 mg (usually 2.5 or 3.0 mg) in methylcellulose for intravaginal application (Nimrod, 1984; Wingerup, 1983; Noah, 1987; Thiery, 1984; Owen, 1991; and their co-workers). These different doses have not been well evaluated in a controlled manner. An increase in dose of prostaglandin gel does not increase the overall likelihood of vaginal delivery but may reduce the subsequent requirement for oxytocin while increasing the chance of both spontaneous labor and uterine hyperstimulation.

Figure 32–1 illustrates how the standard 2–3 mL volume is placed in the cervical canal up to the internal os or alternatively at the posterior vaginal fornix next to the external cervical os. A speculum is necessary to adequately visualize the external cervical os. The cervix should be swabbed to remove any excess secretions beforehand. Caution should be taken not to administer the gel above the cervical os because this increases the risk of uterine hyperstimulation. The patient should remain supine for 15–30 minutes following gel installation to minimize leakage of the medication. Careful fetal heart rate monitoring is recommended for from 30 minutes to 2 hours after instillation (ACOG, 1993).

The United States Food and Drug Administration (FDA) has approved a PGE_2 gel preparation for cervical ripening for women at or near term who have a medical or obstetric indication for induction of labor. The gel contains 0.5 mg of dinoprostone (a form of PGE_2) in a syringe containing 2.5 mL of triacetin gel. At least 6 hours should elapse before either the dose is repeated or intravenous oxytocin is administered. The manufacturer recommends a maximum cumulative dose of 1.5 mg of dinoprostone (7.5 mL gel) in any 24-hour period. This low dose when applied intracervically offers the advantage of initiating minimal uterine activity while sometimes ripening even the most unfavorable cervix.

Regardless of the PGE_2 preparation applied, the cumulative experience with more than 5000 pregnancies in over 70 prospective clinical trials supports the belief that PGE_2 is superior to placebo or no therapy in enhancing cervical effacement and dilation. A low dose of PGE_2 has been reported to significantly increase the Bishop score of the cervix, enhance the chance of successful initial induction of labor, decrease the incidence of prolonged labor, and reduce the total and maximal doses of oxytocin (Owen, 1991; Rayburn, 1989; Williams, 1985; Sawai, 1991; Mainprize, 1987; Prins, 1986; Bernstein, 1991; and their associates). Approximately half of treated women will enter into labor, and half of nulliparous and more than half of multiparous

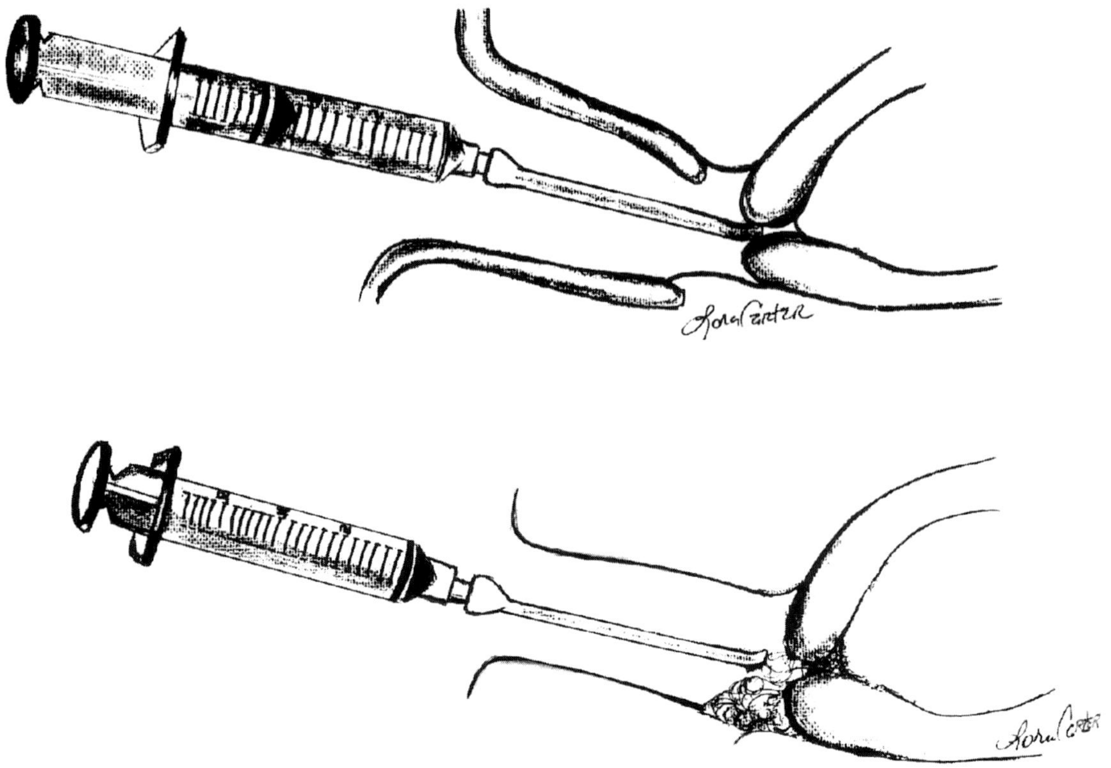

Figure 32–1. The standard 2–3 mL volume is placed in the cervical canal at the level of the internal cervical os (top) or alternatively at the posterior vaginal fornix next to the external cervical os (bottom).

patients will deliver in 24 hours (Rayburn, 1989). A metanalysis of 1811 patients who received a single application of at least 5 mg of PGE_2 gel intravaginally or 0.5 mg intracervically found no decrease in the overall cesarean delivery rate (Owen and co-workers, 1991). However, general reduction in cesarean delivery rates is difficult to prove without large patient enrollments.

A sustained-release vaginal pessary containing 10 mg of PGE_2 has been shown in clinical investigations to be effective in ripening the term cervix, initiating labor, and reducing the need for cesarean delivery for a failed induction (Rayburn and associates, 1992). The use of small doses (0.5 mg) of a PGE_1 analogue has been described in investigational protocols involving pregnancy termination (Rodger and Baird, 1987). Because of concerns regarding hyperstimulation, such preparations are currently appropriate only for investigational use.

Prostaglandin E_2 is available as a 20-mg suppository (Prostin, Upjohn, Kalamazoo, MI) for evacuation of products of conception after 12 weeks' gestation for missed abortions, hydatidiform moles, and stillbirths up to 28 weeks' gestation. These suppositories are placed in the upper vagina every 3–5 hours until the products of conception are expelled. The average time from beginning therapy until delivery is 16 hours, and 85 percent of cases deliver within 24 hours (Rayburn and colleagues, 1982). The time interval from beginning therapy until delivery is less for multiparous patients during the second half of gestation.

Less experience with pregnancy termination has been described with 15 methyl PGF_{2a}. An intramuscular injection of a 0.25 mg dose is necessary every 2–3 hours. The PGF_{2a} preparation has fewer side effects, but cervical ripening is less and tears may be more frequent.

Maternal systemic effects occur infrequently when low doses of PGE_2 are applied topically. Reported systemic effects include fever, vomiting, and diarrhea, all of which are usually negligible. Upjohn Pharmaceuticals has expressed caution about use of any PGE_2 product in cases of glaucoma, severe hepatic or renal impairment, and asthma. However, bronchial constriction or significant blood pressure changes have not been reported after low doses of PGE_2, and asthma is not a contraindication for its use. Indeed, PGE_2 has been described as an alternative to betamimetic agents for the *treatment* of asthma (Moncada and co-workers, 1980).

Neonatal outcomes following prostaglandin cervical ripening compare favorably with those of oxytocin induction. There is no delayed closure of the ductus arteriosus (Danford and co-workers, 1993). Infant follow-up at 2 and 6 months of age has shown no unusual sequelae from the use of PGE_2 gel.

Mechanical Dilators

Mechanical or osmotic dilators have been used for cervical ripening in early and late gestation. The basis of action of these methods is dilation of the cervical canal and promotion of endogenous prostaglandin release. Commercially available products include laminaria tents and artificial laminaria known as Lamicel and Dilipan. The use of extra-amniotic Foley catheters to dilate the cervical canal has been described but has had limited clinical experience (Atad and associates, 1991; Lewis, 1983).

Laminaria tents have been used for several decades (Roberts and co-workers, 1986; Cross and Pitkin, 1978). Laminaria tents are made from the seaweed *Laminaria japonicum.* Lamicel is made from magnesium sulfate impregnated on a polyvinyl polymer sponge, and Dilipan is a hydrogel polymer (Sanchez-Ramos, 1992; Blumenthal, 1991; Johnson, 1985; and their colleagues). Refinements in product design have largely eliminated problems with infection and fragmentation. All three dilators are hydrophilic and expand by osmosis from their original size. Maximal expansion is achieved with laminaria tents by 8 hours, Lamicel by 4 hours, and Dilipan by 4 hours. The more rapid expansion of Dilipan, and by extrapolation Lamisel, is associated with greater pelvic discomfort (Blumenthal and Ramanauskas, 1991).

The FDA has approved the use of osmotic dilators in conjunction with pregnancy termination. The use of these devices prior to mechanical dilatation may reduce the risk of cervical tears. Late in pregnancy, osmotic dilators also may be effective for preinduction cervical ripening, but much less experience has been reported with these agents than with PGE_2. In some cases, these dilators may enhance cervical dilation after a trial of topical PGE_2 has successfully softened the cervix.

Osmotic dilators usually are placed in the cervical canal as shown in Figure 32–2 within 12–16 hours of performing a pregnancy termination. As many dilators as possible (between 1 and 8, usually 2 to 4) are inserted in the cervical canal without rupturing the membranes. Alternately the swollen dilators may be removed after 8–10 hours and a second set (usually an increased number) placed within the cervix for an additional 10–12 hours prior to the procedure. Evidence from controlled trials supports the contention that these methods increase Bishop scores and thus make an amniotomy easier to perform. Evidence is lacking that subsequent labor induction is easier or more successful than with prostaglandins.

Estradiol

Extra-amniotic instillation of estradiol has been found to increase the production of cervical enzymes responsible for collagen breakdown. Uterine stimulation has not been apparent, and conflicting evidence has been reported as to whether cases pretreated with estradiol are more easily induced or have changes in their cervical scores. One placebo-controlled study indicated that estrogen significantly increased the Bishop score while reducing the time interval from instillation to delivery (Pedersen and colleagues, 1981).

Relaxin

This polypeptide hormone is similar in structure to insulin and is produced in the ovary and decidua. Investigators have demonstrated that Relaxin affects cervical distensibility in both the rat and pig models by increasing cervical water content and remodeling collagen through effects on cervical fibroblasts (MacLennan and associates, 1986). One placebo-controlled study in humans revealed that a 1–2-mg dose of Relaxin significantly increased the Bishop score, increased the incidence of labor before scheduled induction, and shortened the duration of labor (MacLennan and co-workers, 1986). Relaxin is not commercially available in the United States, and randomized trials have not conclusively shown

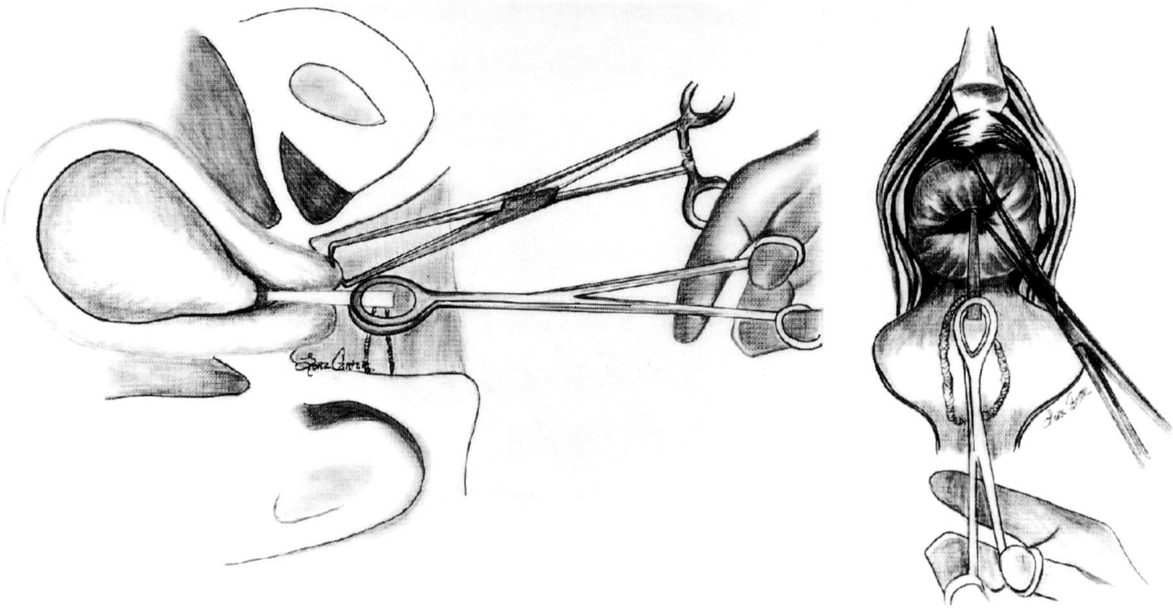

Figure 32–2. Placement of osmotic dilators. The cervix is directly visualized, and the anterior cervical lip is grasped with a tooth tenaculum. With an ovum forceps, as many osmotic dilators as can be advanced are passed into the cervix. Vaginal packing often helps to retain the position of the laminaria within the endocervical canal.

relaxin to be effective in cervical ripening. If Relaxin becomes available for study, large randomized trials will be necessary to assess its efficacy.

RU486

Mifepristone (RU486) is a steroid compound that antagonizes progesterone at the receptor level to mature and dilate the pregnant cervix and increase uterine activity. The drug has been used outside the United States for several obstetric indications including uterine evacuation in cases of fetal death or desired pregnancy termination anytime during pregnancy. When compared with a placebo, RU486 has been shown to shorten spontaneous labor and reduce the need for oxytocin as well as the interval between onset of labor and delivery (Frydman and colleagues, 1992). This compound is anticipated to become available for use in the United States.

Stripping of Amniotic Membranes

Introduction of a finger through the internal cervical os to separate amniotic membranes from the lower uterine segment is known as stripping. An attempt to induce labor by stripping the membranes is common practice, although its reported efficacy and safety are limited (McColgin and co-workers, 1990). In most cases the cervix is favorable when this procedure is performed and does not require an additional cervical ripening agent. Membrane stripping may be associated with a decreased incidence of postdate pregnancies (McColgin and associates, 1990). Risks and benefits of this technique have not been conclusively determined.

Nipple Stimulation

Nipple stimulation prompts a release of oxytocin by the posterior pituitary. Contractions are often recorded through this neural reflex. Two studies have reported nipple stimulation to be a method of cervical ripening (Elliot and Flaherty, 1983; Salmon and associates, 1986). One controlled study demonstrated that regular nipple stimulation for 3 hours per day over a 3-day period at term resulted in a significant change in Bishop score and an increased rate of spontaneous labor. Information was unavailable on the ease of induction, and concern was raised by the authors about the possibility of uterine hyperstimulation.

Amniotomy

Artificial rupture of the membranes is a nonpharmacologic method of enhancing labor, particularly once the cervix is ripened. At term, labor usually commences within 12 hours of membrane rupture (Brindley and Sokol, 1988). Evidence indicates that amniotomy alone is often inadequate to induce effective contractions, and most studies examining amniotomy involve patients already in early labor. The weight of evidence suggests that oxytocin infusion is more effective in achieving delivery within a reasonable time when it is combined with amniotomy than when it is used alone (Mitchell and colleagues, 1977; Bakos and Backstrom, 1987).

Amniotomy is best performed when the cervix is 3 cm dilated and the presenting fetal part is applied to the cervix. Care should be taken during amniotomy to palpate for umbilical cord and avoid dislodging the fetal head. Rupture of membranes with an assistant applying fundal pressure may reduce the risk of cord prolapse. The fetal heart rate should be recorded before and immediately after the procedure.

Amniotomy is generally performed with a plastic hook such as an amnio hook or similar instrument introduced blindly into the cervical canal with the examining finger (Fig. 32–3). The practitioner's fingers should remain in the vagina to assess the quantity and quality of amniotic fluid as well as to ensure that the umbilical cord does not prolapse (frequency of 0.1–0.4/1000 patients). Alternatively, if use of a fetal scalp electrode is planned, it can be attached directly through the fetal membranes. Invariably egress of amniotic fluid will follow over the next several minutes. Following amniotomy, it may be possible to decrease the rate of any oxytocin being infused.

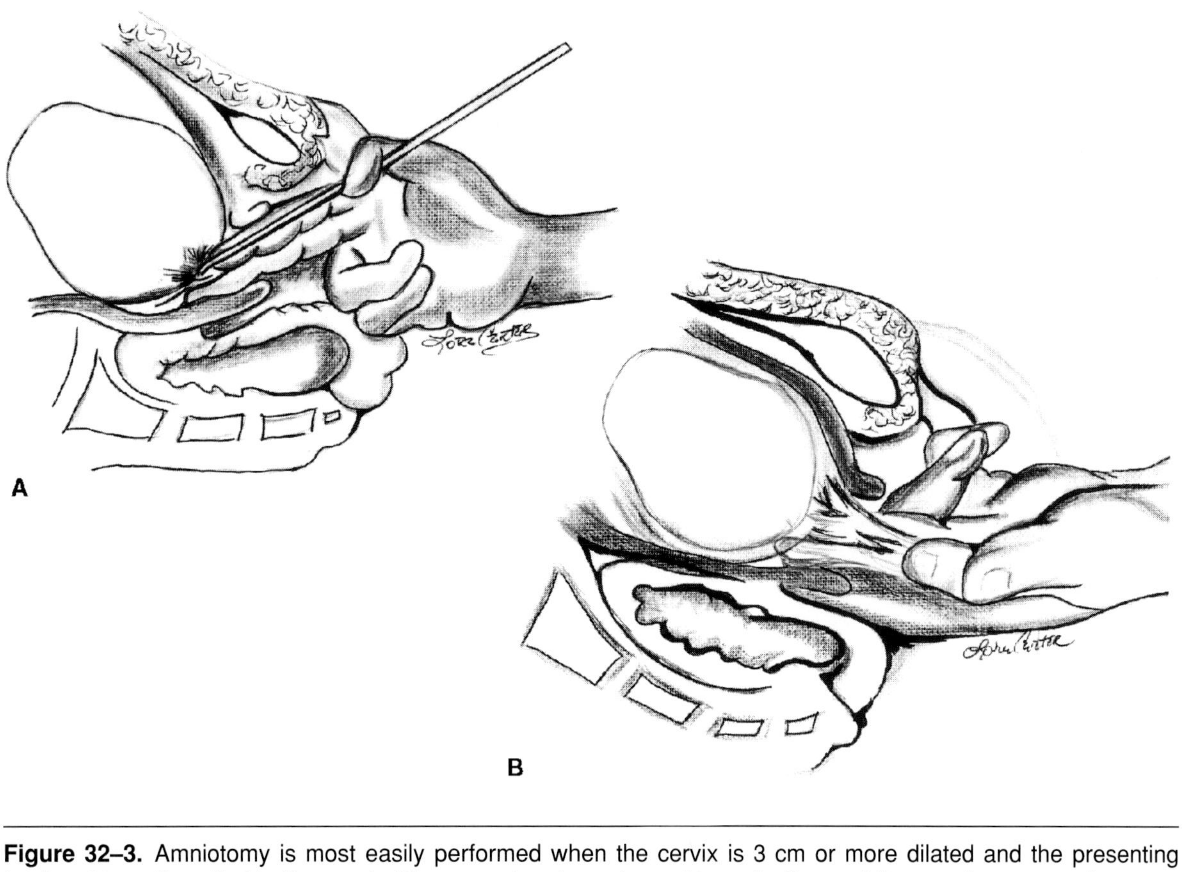

Figure 32–3. Amniotomy is most easily performed when the cervix is 3 cm or more dilated and the presenting fetal part is well applied to the cervix. The procedure is performed by palpation and the membranes can be punctured with either a plastic hook device (**A**) or by direct application of a fetal scalp electrode. When the puncture is small, it can be enlarged by blunt finger dissection (**B**).

Oxytocin

Oxytocin is synthesized in the hypothalamus, chorion, and decidua (Dawood and colleagues, 1978a,b, 1979; Fuchs, 1985; Fuchs and associates, 1991). Myometrial and decidual oxytocin receptors increase throughout gestation, reaching a maximum in early labor (Fuchs, 1985, 1991; Dawood, 1979; and their co-workers). This increase in receptor concentration results in a 100-fold increase in myometrial sensitivity to oxytocin in labor. Activation of these receptors in the decidua has been shown to stimulate prostaglandin production, which in turn stimulates myometrial gap junction formation. The individual's response to oxytocin infusion depends on the degree of preexisting uterine activity, uterine sensitivity, and cervical status. These factors relate both to individual biologic differences and to the duration of pregnancy. The human uterus becomes increasingly sensitive to oxytocin as gestation advances. Maternal serum levels of oxytocin also increase steadily throughout gestation. In parturition, there appears to be a pulsatile release of oxytocin every 30 minutes, with the amplitude of the pulsation increasing in the first and second stages of labor (Dawood, 1978a,b; Fuchs, 1982, 1984, 1981a,b; and their associates).

The effective dose of oxytocin is a function of both plasma clearance and myometrial sensitivity. These findings vary widely between patients and can therefore be unpredictable. The plasma half-life of exogenous oxytocin is between 15 and 20 minutes, resulting in steady-state plasma concentrations by 40–60 minutes after any given infusion level is begun (Brindley and Sokol, 1988). Oxytocin is primarily cleared by enzymatic inactivation (Fuchs and co-workers, 1981a,b).

After other cervical ripening methods, oxytocin therapy should proceed with caution. Oxytocin is most often infused as a dilute intravenous solution (10 or 20 U/1000 mL) of a balanced electrolyte solution. The minimum infusion rate that results in a myometrial response is 0.5 mU/minute (Calderyo-Barcia and Poseiro, 1960; Keirse and Chalmers, 1989; Theobald and associates, 1969). To avoid bolus infusion, oxytocin should be administered via a controlled infusion device and piggy backed through a main intravenous line close to the venous puncture site. A uterine response generally occurs within 3–5 minutes of intravenous administration (Calderyo-Barcia, 1960, 1968; Kruse, 1986; Seitchik, 1984, 1987; and their colleagues).

A number of oxytocin infusion rates and dosage intervals are acceptable. No single infusion rate or range of rates is dictated by standard of care, for either induction or augmentation of labor. The avoidance of prolonged hyperstimulation is, however, important regardless of the oxytocin concentration or infusion rate selected.

Continuous infusion shows first-order saturation kinetics with a progressive linear stepwise increase with each incremental increase in the infusion rate (Seitchik and associates, 1984, 1987). A steady-state concentration of oxytocin is reached 20–40 minutes after initiating or altering the infusion rate. When the rate is increased at intervals of less than 30 minutes, the frequency of either uterine hyperstimulation or a nonreassuring fetal heart rate pattern increases. Accordingly, dosage increases at intervals of less than 30 minutes should be made with close surveillance.

Minimal effective uterine activity has been described as three contractions in a 10-minute period with each contraction averaging greater than 25 mm Hg above the baseline (Brindley and Sokol, 1988). However, adequate labor describes a wide range of uterine activity. The amplitude of each contraction should vary from 25 to 75 mm Hg, and the total duration of contractions in a 10-minute window should last over 2–5 minutes to achieve 95–395 Montevideo units (MU). Hauth and co-workers demonstrated that 200 MU should generally be achieved prior to consideration of cesarean section for active phase arrest (Hauth and colleagues, 1986, 1991).

Cervical dilatation of 1 cm/hour is another guide for adequacy of oxytocin. Further increases in the dose of oxytocin after achieving a cervical dilation rate of at least 1 cm/hour in the active phase of labor or maximal uterine activity is generally unnecessary. In some cases, the dose may be reduced as the cervix continues to dilate.

MONITORING PROTOCOL

Cervical ripening is most beneficial when the Bishop score is 4 or less. Any patient given PGE_2 should be afebrile and not have unexplained vaginal bleeding or an allergy to prostaglandins. Other prerequisites include a reassuring fetal heart rate tracing or biophysical profile of 8 or 10. The woman also should not be in spontaneous labor. PGE_2 must not be used simultaneously with oxytocin (Rayburn, 1989; Miller and co-workers, 1991).

Any method to ripen the cervix should initially be undertaken either at or near the labor and delivery suite, where careful uterine activity and fetal heart rate can be monitored. Outpatient cervical ripening offers more convenience at a potentially lower cost, but further study is needed to evaluate safety and proper patient selection. As cervical ripening is undertaken, the patient should remain recumbent for a minimum of 30 minutes. Transfer, ambulation, or discharge may occur after 1–2 hours in the absence of regular contractions or a nonreassuring fetal heart rate pattern (ACOG, 1993).

Contractions during cervical ripening are usually irregular, infrequent, and similar to those in early spontaneous labor. The wide variation in contraction patterns is explained by differences in individual responsiveness, parity, dosage rate and absorption, and initial Bishop score. Contractions usually become apparent in the first hour, peak in the first 4 hours, and persist in approximately half (25–76%) of all cases (Miller and associates, 1991). If regular uterine contractions persist, uterine and fetal monitoring should be considered.

COMPLICATIONS OF CERVICAL RIPENING

The most common complications with any cervical ripening agent are uterine hyperstimulation and failure to change the cervical status (Seitchik, 1987; Egarter and co-workers, 1991). Uterine hyperstimulation may present in two manners: (1) tachysystole, that is, more than 5 contractions in 10 minutes, and (2) hypertonus with contractions lasting 2 minutes or more. Hyperstimulation is a concern in the presence of either a nonreassuring fetal heart rate pattern (repetitive decelerations or bradycardia) or unusual and persistent maternal discomfort. All ripening agents have the propensity for initiating labor and uterine hyperstimulation. For PGE_2 the reported rates are 1 percent for intracervical gel (0.5 mg) and 3–5 percent for intravaginal gel (2–5 mg) (Egarter and associates, 1991). Hyperstimulation occurs more often in the presence of a predosing Bishop score of more than 4 or preexisting labor and often begins within the first hour after gel application. Hyperstimulation may be reversed by removing the agent and irrigating of the cervix and vagina. A beta-adrenergic drug (terbutaline 250 μg intravenously or subcutaneously) or magnesium sulfate (4 g IV) may be given with no adverse effects except transient tachycardia. Rapid resolution of the worrisome hyperstimulation can be expected in 98 percent of cases without apparent untoward intrapartum effects (Rayburn, 1989; Miller, 1991; Egarter, 1991; and their co-workers).

Failure of cervical ripening and a committed induction attempt is especially common for indicated preterm deliveries. Response increases gradually during gestation until becoming relatively stable after 33 weeks. Studies to evaluate prostaglandin and oxytocin requirements prior to 33 weeks are few and difficult to interpret, because the reason for induction may have involved several variables that in and of themselves would alter uterine sensitivity. When delivery is indicated but not urgent, serial or sequential use of cervical ripening agents may be appropriate.

SUMMARY

Cervical ripening is an important aspect of clinical obstetrics. Primary techniques in widespread use include mechanical (laminaria) or medical (oxytocin, prostaglandin gels) treatments. The urgency with which cervical ripening needs to be accomplished sequentially over several days will significantly influence the provider's choice. Even when time is limited, repeated application of prostaglandin gel or repeated insertion of laminaria often proves superior to one-at-a-time procedures.

REFERENCES

American College of Obstetricians and Gynecologists. Fetal maturity assessment prior to elective repeat cesarean delivery. Committee Opinion No. 98. ACOG, Washington, DC: 1991a.

American College of Obstetricians and Gynecologists. Induction and Augmentation of Labor.

Technical Bulletin No. 157. Washington, DC: ACOG, 1991b.
American College of Obstetricians and Gynecologists. Prostaglandin E_2 gel for cervical Ripening. Committee Opinion No. 123. Washington, DC: ACOG, 1993.
Anderson ABM, Turnbull AC. Spontaneous contractility and oxytocin sensitivity of the human uterus in midpregnancy. J Obstet Gynaecol Br Commonw 1968;75:271.
Atad J, Bernstein J, Calderon I, et al. Nonpharmaceutical ripening of the unfavorable cervix and induction of labor by novel double balloon device. Obstet Gynecol 1991;77:146.
Bakos O, Backstrom T. Induction of labor: a prospective, randomized study into amniotomy and oxytocin as induction methods in a total unselected population. Acta Obstet Gynecol Scand 1987;66:537.
Beazley JM, Dewhurst CJ, Gillespie A. The induction of labor with prostaglandin E_2. J Obstet Gynaecol Br Commonw 1970;77:193.
Bernstein P. Prostaglandin E_2 gel for cervical ripening and labour induction: a multicentre placebo-controlled trial. Can Med Assoc J 1991; 145:1249.
Bishop EH, Edward H. Pelvic scoring for elective induction. Obstet Gynecol 1964;24:266.
Blumenthal PD, Ramanauskas R. Randomized trial of Dilipan and Laminaria as cervical ripening agents before induction of labor. Obstet Gynecol 1991;75:365.
Brindley BA, Sokol RJ. Induction and augmentation of labor: basis and methods for current practice. Obstet Gynecol Surv 1988;43:730.
Calder AA, Embrey MP, Tait T. Ripening of the cervix with extra-amniotic prostaglandins E_2 in viscous gel before induction of labor. Br J Obstet Gynaecol 1977;84:264.
Calder AA, Greer IA. Pharmacological modulation of cervical compliance in the first and second trimesters of pregnancy. Semin Perinatol 1991;15:162.
Calderyo-Barcia R, Poseiro JJ. Physiology of the uterine contraction. Clin Obstet Gynecol 1960;3:386.
Calderyro-Barcia R, Theobald GW. Sensitivity of the pregnant human myometrium to oxytocin. Am J Obstet Gynecol 1968;102:1181.
Craft, I. Amniotomy and oral prostaglandin E2 titration for induction of labour. Br Med J 1972;2:191.
Cross W, Pitkin RM. Laminaria as an adjunct in induction of labor. Obstet Gynecol 1978;51:606.
Danford D, Miller A, Felix G, et al. Effect of low-dose intravaginal doses of prostaglandin E_2 on the closure time of the ductus arteriosus in term newborns. J Pediatr 1993;122:632.
Danforth DN, Veis A, Breen M, et al. The effect of pregnancy and labor on the human cervix: changes in collagen, glycoproteins, and glycosaminoglycans. Am J Obstet Gynecol 1974;120:641.
Dawood MY, Raghaven KS, Pociask C, Fuchs F. Oxytocin in human pregnancy and parturition. Obstet Gynecol 1978a;51:138.
Dawood MY, Wang CF, Gupta R, Fuchs F. Fetal contribution to oxytocin in human labor. Obstet Gynecol 1978b;52:205.
Dawood MY, Ylikorkala O, Trivedi D, Fuchs F. Oxytocin in maternal circulation and amniotic fluid during pregnancy. J Clin Endocrinol Metab 1979;49:429.
Egarter CH, Husslein PW, Rayburn WF. Uterine hyperstimulation after low-dose prostaglandin E2 therapy: tocolytic treatment in 181 cases. Am J Obstet Gynecol 1991;163:794.
Elliot JP, Flaherty JF. The use of breast stimulation to ripen the cervix in term pregnancies. Am J Obstet Gynecol 1983;145:553.
Frydman R, Lelaidier C, Baton-Saint-Mleux C, et al. Labor induction in women at term with mifepristone (RU486): a double-blind, randomized, placebo-controlled study. Obstet Gynecol 1992;80:972.
Fuchs A, Goeschen K, Husslein P, et al. Oxytocin and the initiation of human parturition. III. Plasma concentrations of oxytocin and 13,14-dehydro-14-keto-prostaglandin F2-alpha in spontaneous and oxytocin-induced labor at term. Am J Obstet Gynecol 1981a;141:694.
Fuchs AR, Fuchs F, Husslein P, Soloff MS. Oxytocin receptors in the human uterus during pregnancy and parturition. Am J Obstet Gynecol 1984; 150:734.
Fuchs AR, Fuchs F, Soloff MS, Fenstrom MJ. Oxytocin receptors and human parturition: a dual role for oxytocin in the initiation of labor. Science 1982;215:1396.
Fuchs AR, Husslein P, Fuchs F. Oxytocin and the initiation of human parturition. II. Stimulation of prostaglandin production in human decidua by oxytocin. Am J Obstet Gynecol 1981b; 141:694.
Fuchs AR, Romero R, Keefe D, et al. Oxytocin secretion and human parturition: pulse frequency and duration increase during spontaneous labor in women. Am J Obstet Gynecol 1991;165:1515.
Fuchs F. Role of maternal and fetal oxytocin in human parturition. In Amico JA, Robinson AG, eds. Oxytocin: Clinical and Laboratory Studies. Amsterdam: Elsevier Science Publishers BV (Biomedical Division), 1985:236.
Gillespie A. Prostaglandin-oxytocin enhancement and potentiation and their clinical applications. Br Med J 1972;1:150.
Hauth JC, Hankins GDV, Gilstrap LC, et al. Uterine contraction pressures with oxytocin induction/augmentation. Obstet Gynecol 1986; 68:305.

Hauth JC, Hankins GDV, Gilstrap LC. Uterine contraction pressures achieved in parturients with active phase arrest. Obstet Gynecol 1991;78:344.
Huszar GB, Walsh MP. Relationship between myometrial and cervical functions in pregnancy and labor. Semin Perinatol 1991;15:97.
Johnson IR, Macpherson MBA, Welch CC, Filshie GM. A comparison of Lamicel and prostaglandin E2 vaginal gel for cervical ripening before induction of labor. Am J Obstet Gynecol 1985;151:604.
Keirse MJNC, Chalmers I. Methods for inducting labour. In: Chalmers I, Enkin M, Keirse MJNC, eds. Effective Care in Pregnancy and Childbirth. Oxford: Oxford University Press, 1989:1057.
Kruse J. Oxytocin: pharmacology and clinical application. J Fam Prac 1986;23:473.
Lewis GJ. Cervical ripening before induction of labor with prostaglandin E2 pessaries or a Foley's catheter. Obstet Gynecol 1983;3:173.
Liggins GC. Ripening and cervix. Sem Perinatol 1978;2:261.
MacLennan AH, Green RC, Grant P, Nicolson R. Ripening of the human cervix and induction of labor with intracervical purified porcine relaxin. Obstet Gynecol 1986;68:598.
Mainprize T, Nimrod C, Dodd G, Persaud D. Clinical utility of multiple-dose administration of prostaglandin E2 gel. Am J Obstet Gynecol 1987;156:341.
McColgin SW, Hampton HL, McCaul JF, et al. Stripping membranes at term: can it safely reduce the incidence of post-term pregnancies? Obstet Gynecol 1990;76:678.
Miller AM, Rayburn WF, Smith CV. Patterns of uterine activity after intravaginal prostaglandin E2 during preinduction cervical ripening. Am J Obstet Gynecol 1991;165:1006.
Mitchell MD, Flint APF, Bibby J, et al. Rapid increases in plasma prostaglandin concentrations after vaginal examination and amniotomy. Br Med J 1977;2:1183.
Moncada S, Flower RJ, Vane JR: Prostaglandins. In: Goodman AGG, Gilman LS, Goodman A, eds. Prostacyclin and Thromboxane A2 in the Pharmacologic Basis of Therapeutics. New York: 1980:678.
Nimrod C, Currie J, Yee J, et al. Cervical ripening and labor induction with intracervical triacetin base prostaglandin E2 gel: a placebo-controlled study. Obstet Gynecol 1984;64:476.
Noah ML, Decoster JM, Fraser TJ, Orr JD. Preinduction cervical softening with endocervical PGE_2 gel. A multi-center trial. Acta Obstet Gynecol Scand 1987;66:3.
Owen J, Winkler CL, Harris BA, et al. A randomized, double-blind trial of prostaglandin E_2 gel for cervical ripening and meta-analysis. Am J Obstet Gynecol 1991;165:991.
Pedersen S, Moller-Pedersen J, Aegidus J. Comparison of oestradiol and prostaglandin E_2 vaginal gel for ripening the unfavourable cervix. Br Med J 1981;282:1395.
Prins RP, Neilson DR, Bolton RN, et al. Preinduction cervical ripening with sequential use of prostaglandin E_2 gel. Am J Obstet Gynecol 1986;154:1275.
Rayburn W, Lightfoot S, Newland J, et al. A model for investigating microscopic changes induced by prostaglandin E_2 in the term cervix. J Matern Fetal Invest (in press).
Rayburn W, Wapner R, Barss V, et al. Intravaginal controlled-release PGE_2 pessary for cervical ripening and initiation of labor. Obstet Gynecol 1992;79:443.
Rayburn WF, Motley ME, Stempel LE. Antepartum prediction of the postmature infant. Obstet Gynecol 1982;60:148.
Rayburn WF. Prostaglandin E_2 gel for cervical ripening and induction of labor: a critical analysis. Am J Obstet Gynecol 1989;160:529.
Roberts WE, North DH, Speed JE, et al. Comparative study of prostaglandin, laminaria, and minidose oxytocin for ripening of the unfavorable cervix prior to the induction of labor. J Perinatol 1986;6:16.
Rodger MW, Baird DT. Induction of therapeutic abortion in early pregnancy with Mifepristone in combination with prostaglandin pessary. Lancet 1987;2:1415.
Salmon YM, Kee WH, Tan SL, Jen SW. Cervical ripening by breast stimulation. Obstet Gynecol 1986;67:21.
Sanchez-Ramos L, Kaunitz AM, Connor PM. Hygroscopic cervical dilators and prostaglandin E_2 gel for preinduction cervical ripening: a randomized, prospective comparison. J Reprod Med 1992;37:355.
Sawai S, Williams M, O'Brien W, et al. Sequential outpatient application of intravaginal prostaglandin E_2 gel in the management of postdates pregnancy. Obstet Gynecol 1991;78:19.
Seitchik J, Amico J, Robinson AG, Castillo M. Oxytocin augmentation of dysfunctional labor. IV. Oxytocin pharmacokinetics. Am J Obstet Gynecol 1984;150:225.
Seitchik J. The management of functional dystocia in the first stage of labor. Clin Obstet Gynecol 1987;30:42.
Takahashi D, Diamond F, Bieniarz J, et al. Uterine contractility and oxytocin sensitivity in preterm, term, and postterm pregnancy. Am J Obstet Gynecol 1980;136:774.
Theobald GW, Robards MF, Suter PEN. Changes in myometrial sensitivity to oxytocin in man during the last six weeks of pregnancy. Br J Obstet Gynaecol 1969;76:385.
Thiery M, DeCoster JM, Parewijck W, et al. Endocervical prostaglandin E2 gel for preinduction cervical softening. Prostaglandins 1984;27:429.
Ueland K, Conrad JT. Characteristics of oral

prostaglandin E_2-induced labor. Clin Obstet Gynecol 1983;26:87.

Uldbjerg N, Ekman G, Malmstron A, et al. Biochemical and morphological changes of human cervix after local application of prostaglandin E2 in pregnancy. Lancet 1981;2:267.

Ulmsten U, Wingerup L, Belfrage P, et al. Intracervical application of prostaglandin gel for induction of term labor. Obstet Gynecol 1982;59:336.

Wikland M, Lindblom B, Wiquist N. Myometrial response to prostaglandins during labor. Gynecol Obstet Invest 1984;17:131.

Williams JK, Wilkerson WG, O'Brien WF, Knuppel RA. Use of prostaglandin E_2 topical cervical gel in high-risk patient: a critical analysis. Obstet Gynecol 1985;66:769.

Wingerup L, Ekman G, Ulmsten U. Local application of prostaglandin E_2 in a gel. A new technique to ripen the cervix during pregnancy. Acta Obstet Gynecol Scand 1983;113(suppl):131.

CHAPTER 33

Pregnancy Termination: First and Second Trimesters

Although controversy has always surrounded the issue of induced abortion, anthropologists have found evidence of its existence in all known cultures, whether primitive or modern (Sheeran, 1987; McFarland, 1993). Nationally, the estimated 1.5 million legal induced abortions each year comprise the most frequently performed gynecologic procedure and pose a major challenge when considering the need for safe and appropriate surgical management. The intent of this chapter is to provide information about (1) trends in abortion services; (2) the epidemiology of legal induced abortion, and mortality associated with it in the United States; (3) an overview of the surgical management of induced abortion; and (4) details about legal abortion–related complications and their management.

ABORTION SERVICES

Legal induced abortions in the United States are provided in various health care settings including hospitals, free-standing surgical centers, abortion clinics, and private physicians' offices. Legalization of abortion following the *Roe* v *Wade* decision in 1973 did not lead to the availability of services in all areas. Throughout the 1970s the number of facilities providing abortion services increased, reaching 2908 in 1982. The number of facilities declined to 2618 in 1987 and to 2582 in 1988 (Henshaw and Van Vort, 1990). This decline occurred entirely among hospitals and in nonmetropolitan counties. In 1977, 1654 hospitals offered abortion services; this number fell to 1405 in 1982, to 1191 in 1985, and to 1040 in 1988 (Henshaw and Van Vort, 1990). While abortion facilities have generally been concentrated in urban areas, this concentration has been more pronounced in recent years. In 1988, 90 percent of all abortion facilities and providers were in metropolitan counties (Henshaw and Van Vort, 1990). As a result of traditional surgical facilities (hospitals) not rising to meet the challenge for these large numbers of procedures, a new institution, the free-standing abortion clinic, came into existence. In 1973, slightly more than half of all abortions were performed in hospitals; by 1988, the proportion of abortions performed in hospitals declined to 10 percent, while the proportion performed in free-standing clinics increased each year, from 46 percent in 1973 to 86 percent in 1988 (Henshaw and Van Vort, 1990). While providing the majority of abortion services in the United States, and usually maintaining high medical standards (NAF standards of care), these clinics are able to provide excellent service at a cost far below other kinds of surgical care. Moreover, most clinics also provide on-site contraceptive counseling and supplies, and include patient follow-up as part of the usual fee. In 1989, the average woman having a first trimester non-hospital abortion paid $251; an abortion at 10 weeks' gestation in a hospital cost an average of $1757. Charges were higher in facilities with small abortion caseloads. Charges for abortions at 16 weeks averaged $509 in abortion clinics, compared with $1539 in hospitals for dilation and evacuations (D&E), and $2246 for labor induction procedures (Henshaw, 1991).

Because clinics are concentrated in metropolitan counties, women seeking abortion often face many obstacles. The Alan Guttmacher Institute estimates that 9 percent of non-hospital abortion patients must travel more than 100 miles, and 18 percent travel 50–100 miles for abortion services (Henshaw, 1991). Other obstacles facing women seeking abortion services include: only 43 percent of abortion facilities offer abortion services beyond 12 weeks' gestation; approximately one-third of non-hospital facilities do not treat women who are HIV positive. Women who need special services such as Rh immune globulin administration, general anesthesia, or HIV testing usually pay extra for these services (Henshaw, 1991).

Another barrier facing women desiring abortion services has occurred as a result of declining availability of hospital-based procedures. As fewer residency training programs (mostly hospital-based) in family practice and obstetrics and gynecology have provided exposure for their trainees to abortion services, fewer providers completing training have become familiar with and competent in performing the basic procedures (Darney and associates, 1987; Grimes, 1992b; Henshaw and co-workers, 1987). This trend has been heightened by a concomitant decrease in interest among resident physicians in training programs that do provide abortion services. (Westhoff and associates, 1993). The 1995 mandate by the Residency Review Committee for Obstetrics and Gynecology that requires residency programs to provide training in abortion services is intended to reverse these trends.

The unstable legal climate related to abortion during the 1980s and early 1990s may have been a decisive factor in the decline of provider willingness to provide abortion services. Though physicians frequently favor unlimited access to safe legal abortion (Westfall and co-workers, 1991), their lack of desire to participate in programs and learn to perform abortions may be due, in part, to a reluctance to spend training time learning a procedure that has the potential for becoming severely restricted or illegal.

The personal risks associated with providing abortion services are undoubtedly a part of the residents' decision making. Continued harassment and repeated attacks on providers during the last several years, and the fact that abortion providers were murdered in Florida and Massachusetts in 1993 and 1994, attest to the lack of safety furnished those who choose to perform abortions. In 1985, of 1250 abortion facilities that provided services to 83 percent of all women in the United States seeking abortion, 73 percent were the victims of at least one illegal activity; only 6 percent were subjected solely to picketing. The national rates of violence between 1977 and 1988 were 3.7/100 abortion providers, and 7.2/100 non-hospital abortion facilities—far higher than the rates of complications for those individuals undergoing the procedure (Forrest and Henshaw, 1987; Grimes and colleagues, 1991). Indeed, the dwindling number of physician providers willing to perform abortion services has prompted the American College of Obstetricians and Gynecologists to endorse the training of nurse practitioners and nurse midwifes for the provision of abortions. Thus, the most powerful limitation to a woman's access to abortion in the years to come may be the dearth of providers. It would be a tragedy if the decline continued until there were obvious public health consequences, such as increases in illegal procedures, and the associated increase in morbidity and mortality known to accompany them.

LEGAL ABORTION EPIDEMIOLOGY AND MORTALITY

Numbers, Ratios, and Rates

The numbers and characteristics of women obtaining legal abortions in the United States have been monitored and published by the Centers for Disease Control and Prevention, Atlanta, Georgia (CDC), since 1969. In addition, numbers of induced abortions in the United States are monitored and reported by the Alan Guttmacher Institute (AGI), New York City. AGI also reports information about abortion services collected through periodic surveys of abortion providers. Since 1972, the CDC has also conducted ongoing surveillance of abortion-related deaths.

By 1973, the year of the *Roe* v *Wade* decision, CDC was receiving data from all 52 targeted reporting areas (50 states, New York City, and the District of Columbia). In 1985, central health agencies reported data for 44 areas; hospitals and other medical facilities reported data in the remaining 8 areas (Lawson, 1989a). However, because abortion reporting laws vary in different states, and because some abortion providers may not report or may under-report the numbers of abortions to central health agencies, the numbers of abortions reported to the CDC may be less than the total numbers of abortions performed in the United States. AGI is the only other organization that collects national abortion statistics. AGI's numbers are based on a direct survey of abortion providers throughout the United States (AGI, 1988). However, unlike the CDC, AGI does not collect information on the characteristics of women obtaining abortions. AGI has consistently reported an average of 20 percent more abortions than has the CDC (Atrash and co-workers, 1990).

From 1973 through 1990, 21,424,281 legal abortions were reported to CDC. The number of legal abortions reported to CDC increased from 615,831 in 1973 to 1,429,577 in 1990. The abortion ratio (number of abortions per 1000 live births) increased from 196 in 1973 to its highest value of 364 in 1984, then decreased to 344 in 1990. The abortion rate (number of abortions per 100,000 females of reproductive age) increased from 14 in 1973 to its highest value of 25 in 1980 and then was stable at an annual rate of 23–24 for the period 1981–1990 (Lawson and associates, 1989b; CDC, 1992) (Table 33–1).

General Characteristics

During the initial 18-year period (1973–1990) when legal induced abortions were available nationwide, women obtaining abortions were mostly young, white, unmarried, of low parity, and had their abortion performed by suction

TABLE 33–1. REPORTED NUMBERS OF LEGAL ABORTIONS, ABORTION RATIOS, ABORTION RATES, AND PERCENT DISTRIBUTION OF WOMEN WHO OBTAINED LEGAL ABORTIONS BY SELECTED CHARACTERISTICS—UNITED STATES, 1973 AND 1990

Characteristic	1973	1990	Characteristic	1973	1990
Number	615,831	1,429,577	Marital Status		
Ratio[a]	196	344	Married	27.4	21.0
Rate[b]	14	24	Unmarried	72.6	79.0
Residence			Age		
In-state	74.8	91.7	≤19	32.7	22.3
Out-of-state	25.2	8.3	20–24	32.0	33.2
Race			≥25	35.5	44.5
White	72.5	64.5	Number of Live Births		
Other	27.5	35.5	0	48.6	49.2
Weeks of Gestation			1	18.8	24.4
≤8	36.1	51.2	2	14.2	16.9
9–10	29.4	25.4	3	8.7	6.1
11–12	17.9	11.8	≥4	9.7	3.4
13–15	6.9	6.5	Type of Procedure		
16–20	8.0	4.1	Curettage	88.4	98.8
≥21	1.7	1.0	*Suction*	*74.9*	*96.0*
			Sharp	*13.5*	*2.8*
			Instillation	10.4	0.8
			Other	1.3	0.4

[a]Per 1000 live births.
[b]Per 1000 women aged 15–44 years.
From Lawson and associates (1989b) and CDC (1992).

curettage at 12 weeks of gestation or earlier. Although the overall picture did not change significantly, some changes have occurred in the characteristics of women who obtained these abortions (Table 33–1).

Compared with 1973, in 1990, a higher proportion of women obtaining legal abortions were older. In 1973, approximately one-third (32.7%) of the women undergoing abortion were teenagers at the time of the procedure, one-third (32.0%) were 20–24 years of age, and one-third (35.3%) were ≥25 years (Lawson and co-workers, 1989a). By 1990, the proportion of teenaged women dropped to 22.3 percent, whereas the proportion of women ages 20–24 years increased to 33.2 percent, and the proportion aged ≥25 years increased to 44.5 percent (Table 33–1).

In 1973, 72.5 percent of all women obtaining abortions were white; 27.5 percent were of black and other minority races. By 1990, the proportion of white women decreased to 64.5 percent, whereas the proportion of women of black and other minority races increased to 35.5 percent. In 1973, 27.4 percent of all women obtaining abortions were married; by 1990, married women represented only 21.0 percent of the total (Table 33–1).

In 1973, 48.6 percent of all women seeking abortions had no previous live births. This proportion increased to 58.8 percent in 1980, and dropped again to 49.2 percent in 1990. The proportion of women with one or two previous live births also increased, whereas the proportion of women with three or more previous live births decreased from 18.4 percent in 1973 to 7.6 percent in 1985 and then increased again to 9.5 percent in 1990 (Lawson and associates, 1989b; CDC, 1992) (Table 33–1).

From 1973 through 1990, the procedures used to perform abortions also changed. Curettage was used for abortions in 88.4 percent of the cases in 1973, compared with 98.8 percent in 1990. The proportion of instillation (labor induction) procedures for pregnancy termination decreased from 10.4 percent in 1973 to 0.8 percent in 1990, and the use of hysterectomy, hysterotomy, and other procedures for pregnancy termination (such as vaginal suppositories and intramuscular injections) became negligible (Table 33–1).

In 1990, more women obtained abortions during the first trimester (88.4%) than did women in 1973 (83.4%). The major change was in abortions performed at ≤8 weeks' gestation. The proportion of all abortions performed at ≤8 weeks increased from 36.1 percent in 1973 to 51.2 percent in 1990, whereas the proportion of abortions performed at all other gestational ages decreased (Table 33–1).

In a survey of a nationally representative sample of US abortion patients in 1987, AGI found that half of all abortion patients were practicing contraception during the month in which they conceived, and a substantial proportion of those who were not doing so had stopped using a method only a few months before becoming pregnant (Henshaw and Silverman, 1988). Young, poor, black, Hispanic, and less educated women were less likely to be using a contraceptive at the time of conception (Henshaw and Silverman, 1988). The survey also found that women who profess no religion had a higher abortion rate than women who report some religious affiliation. Unmarried, co-habitating women were nine times as likely as married women living with their husbands to have an abortion (Henshaw and Silverman, 1988). Other characteristics associated with above-average likelihood of abortion included current school enrollment, current employment, low income, Medicaid coverage, intention to have no more children, and residence in a metropolitan county (Henshaw and Silverman, 1988).

Most women in AGI's 1987 survey reported several factors contributing to their decision to obtain an abortion. The majority (76%) reported that having a baby would interfere with work, school, or other responsibilities, and for 16 percent of women, this was the main reason for having an abortion. Sixty-eight percent of women reported that they could not afford a child (the main reason for abortion for 21% of women). Fifty-one percent said they did not want to be single parents or they had problems with their relationship (the main reason for abortion for 12% of women). Other reasons for obtaining abortion reported by women included: not ready for responsibility (31%, main reason for abortion for 21%), does not want others to know she is pregnant (31%, main reason for 1%), not mature or too young to have a child (30%, main reason for 11%), has all the children she wanted or has all grown-up children (26%, main reason for 8%), husband or partner wants her to have abortion (23%, main reason for 1%), fetus has possible health problems (13%, main reason for 3%), woman has health problems (7%, main reason for 3%), woman's parents want her to have abortion (7%, main reason for a negligible number), and woman was victim of rape or incest (1%, main reason for 1%) (Torres and Forrest, 1988).

Women having abortions at ≥16 weeks' gestation reported several factors that contributed to their delay in seeking abortion services. Most commonly (71%), women attributed their delay to not having realized they were pregnant or not knowing soon enough the actual gestation of their pregnancy or to trouble arranging for the abortion, usually because they needed time to raise money (48%). Other common contributing factors were that the woman was afraid to tell her partner or parents (33%) and the woman took time to decide to have an abortion (24%) (Torres and Forest, 1988).

ABORTION MORTALITY

Abortion-related mortality has been monitored by the CDC since 1972. From 1972 through 1987, 240 legal abortion-related deaths were identified and investigated by the CDC (Lawson and colleagues, 1994).

The annual number of legal abortion-related deaths identified by the CDC decreased from 24 deaths in 1972 to 6 in 1987. The mortality rate decreased from 4.1/100,000 abortions in 1972 to 0.4 in 1987 (Lawson and associates, 1994) (Table 33–2). The main factors that contribute to an increased risk of abortion-related death are: age, race, parity, gestational age, and type of procedure (Lawson and co-workers, 1994) (Table 33–3).

During the period 1972 through 1987, teenaged women had the lowest risk of abortion-related death, 1.0 deaths/100,000 procedures. The risk of death increased with increasing age and was highest for women 40 years or older at 3.1 deaths/100,000 procedures (Table 33–3).

Black and other minority women had a significantly higher risk (2.5 times higher) of death from legal abortion than did white women. The risk of death increased with increasing parity; however, only women who had given birth three or more times had a statistically significant increased risk of abortion-related death (2.8 times higher than nulliparous women) (Table 33–3).

There were marked increases in the risks of death at more advanced gestational ages. Compared with women having abortions during the first 8 weeks of gestation (0.4 deaths/100,000 procedures), the risk of death rose significantly by factors of 2.1–31.5, with

TABLE 33–2. ABORTION-RELATED DEATHS REPORTED TO CDC, BY TYPE OF ABORTION, UNITED STATES, 1972–1987

Year	Induced		Spontaneous	Unknown	Total	CFR[a]
	Legal	*Illegal*				
1972	24	39	25	2	90	4.1
1973	25	19	10	3	57	4.1
1974	26	6	21	1	54	3.4
1975	29	4	14	1	48	3.4
1976	11	2	13	1	27	1.1
1977	17	4	16	0	37	1.6
1978	9	7	9	0	25	0.8
1979	22	0	10	0	32	1.8
1980	9	1	7	2	19	0.7
1981	8	1	3	0	12	0.6
1982	11	1	6	0	18	0.8
1983	11	1	7	0	19	0.9
1984	12	0	6	0	18	0.9
1985	10	1	8	1	20	0.8
1986	10	0	5	2	17	0.8
1987	6	2	12	0	20	0.4
Total	240	88	172	13	513	1.3

[a]Case fatality rates calculated as deaths associated with legal induced abortion per 100,000 legal abortions.

TABLE 33–3. LEGAL ABORTIONS, DEATHS, CASE-FATALITY RATES AND RELATIVE RISKS BY SELECTED CATEGORIES, UNITED STATES, 1972–1987

	Deaths	Abortions	Rate[a]	Relative Risk (95% CI)
Race				
White	111	12,158,687	0.9	Referent
Black & Other	129	5,654,834	2.3	2.5 (1.9–3.2)
Age group				
≤19	54	5,147,112	1.0	Referent
20–24	81	6,104,795	1.3	1.3 (0.9–1.8)
25–29	44	3,523,831	1.2	1.2 (0.8–1.8)
30–34	30	1,854,937	1.6	1.5 (1.0–2.4)
35–39	22	894,737	2.5	2.3 (1.4–3.8)
≥40	9	288,112	3.1	3.0 (1.5–6.0)
Parity[b]				
0	86	9,721,464	0.9	Referent
1	41	3,634,748	1.1	1.3 (0.9–1.9)
2	29	2,570,826	1.1	1.3 (0.8–1.9)
≥3	47	1,886,483	2.5	2.8 (2.0–4.0)
Gestational age[c]				
≤8 weeks	33	8,673,759	0.4	Referent
9–10 weeks	39	4,847,321	0.8	2.1 (1.3–3.3)
11–12 weeks	33	2,360,768	1.4	3.7 (2.3–5.8)
13–15 weeks	28	962,185	2.9	7.7 (5.0–11.7)
16–20 weeks	74	794,093	9.3	24.5 (18.6–32.3)
≥21 weeks	21	175,395	12.0	31.5 (22.2–44.5)
Procedure[d]				
Curettage[e]	80	14,721,443	0.5	Referent
D&E[f]	40	1,076,202	3.7	6.8 (4.9–9.5)
Instillation	38	536,541	7.1	13.0 (9.7–17.5)
Hyst/Hyst[g]	10	19,381	51.6	95.0 (69.6–129.5)
Other	5	257,363	1.9	3.6 (1.5–8.3)
Totals	240	17,813,521	1.3	

[a]Legal abortion deaths per 100,000 abortions.
[b]Denominators for calculating rates by parity use previous live birth data from abortion surveillance; excludes deaths with unknown parity.
[c]Excludes deaths with unknown gestation.
[d]Figures for 1972–73 excluded because data necessary to calculate rates by procedures were not collected; excludes deaths with unknown procedure.
[e]Suction and sharp curettage.
[f]Dilatation and evacuation.
[g]Hysterectomy/hysterotomy.

increasing gestational age (Table 33–3) (Lawson and associates, 1994).

Abortions performed by suction or sharp curettage during the first trimester were associated with the lowest mortality rate of 0.5/100,000 procedures. Compared with curettage procedures, the risk of death was significantly higher for abortions performed by D&E after 12 weeks of gestation (6.8 times higher), for instillation procedures (13.0 times higher) and for hysterectomy/hysterotomy procedures (95 times higher) (Lawson and coworkers, 1994) (Table 33–3).

Embolism, infection, hemorrhage, and anesthesia complications contributed equally to mortality related to legal abortion, together accounting for 82 percent of all legal abortion-related deaths. However, the leading causes of death have changed over the 16 years of abortion mortality surveillance. During the time period 1972–1976, the two leading causes of legal abortion-related death were infection and embolism, whereas during the time period 1983–1987, anesthesia complications emerged as the leading cause of such deaths (Lawson, 1994) (Fig. 33–1).

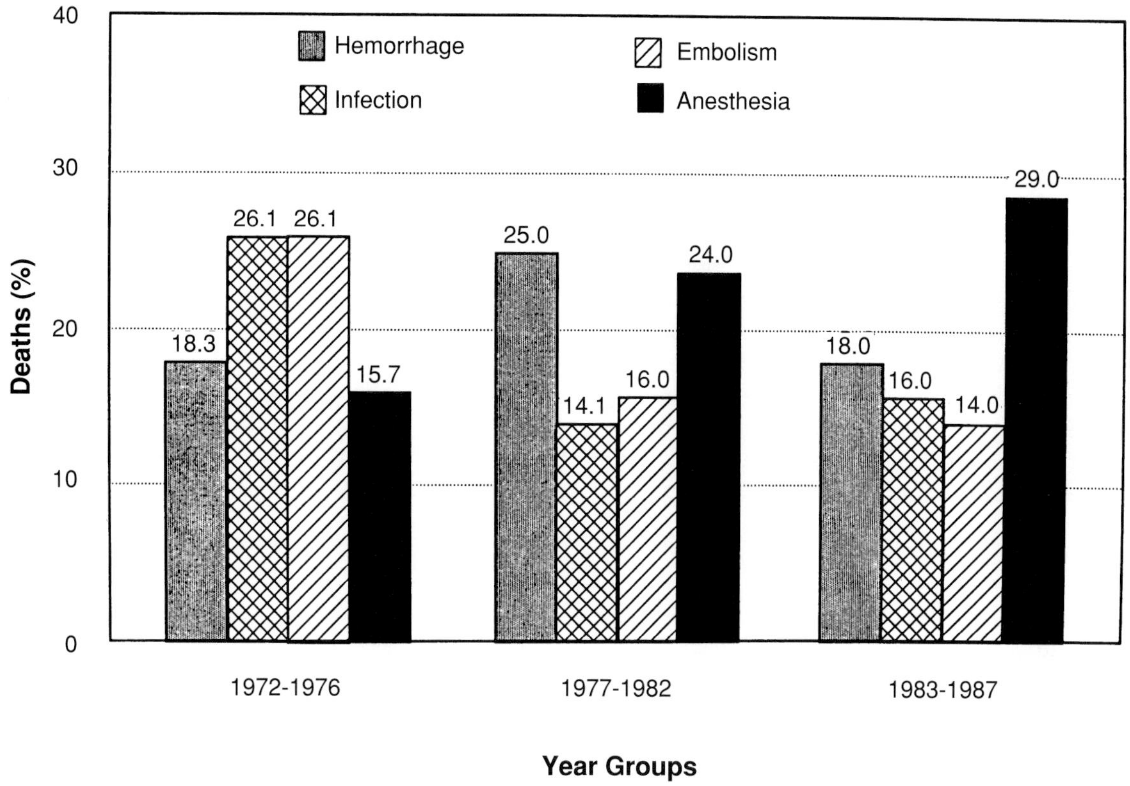

Figure 33–1. Mortality trends for legal abortion, United States, by cause of death, 1972–1976, 1977–1982, 1983–1987.

SURGICAL MANAGEMENT OF INDUCED ABORTION

An elective induced abortion is a procedure intended to terminate an intrauterine pregnancy prior to fetal viability (CDC, 1978). Some abortions are done to treat or prevent medical complications of pregnancy, when rape or incest is an issue, or when fetal reduction is desired for multiple pregnancies induced by fertility drugs (see Chap. 34). However, most abortions are a result of a complex interaction of several factors including personal health and social issues. The most frequent indication for an abortion today is that a woman requests that it be done. Henry P. David noted that "for many women and couples the personal decision to terminate an unwanted pregnancy is seldom easy and often agonizing" (David, 1982). He further noted that "the attitudes of professionals providing care are central to the objective provision of services," and that "for many providers, the issue of abortion represents both an ethical and moral dilemma between a personal commitment to save lives and a woman's decision to terminate her unwanted pregnancy. The role conflict between serving as a medical implementor of a woman's decision and the more traditional orientation of medical decision maker is perhaps a greater divisive influence in the abortion debate than are more widely discussed moral and ethical issues" (David, 1982).

Counseling

Although most women requesting abortion have already considered their options and have made a decision, doubts frequently linger and conflicts with family and significant others may remain. Moreover, some women will have obvious psychiatric problems or ambivalence based on religious issues surrounding abortion. Therefore every woman considering terminating her pregnancy needs and deserves time with an objective, informed and nonjudgmental person (physician, nurse, counselor) to once again review, not only options available, but methods and risks associated with the various procedures. In addition it is important to have consultants readily available (psychiatrists, clergy) should the desire or need arise (Burgess, 1976; Ivey, 1975; Beresford, 1978; Bracken, 1977). Many women have little difficulty with their decision, but others may have feelings of ambivalence, and therefore the counselor should review the following concerns with her: (1) current life situation and view of her partner; (2) own feelings about childbearing and abortion; (3) plans for the future including childbearing and contraception.

Pretreatment Evaluation

In addition to discussing the above-noted decisions, it is important to discuss in as descriptively and detailed a manner as possible the steps of the procedure. Although such questions only rarely occur, it is helpful to be prepared to make some general statements about the fetus to the woman should she request it.

It is essential that appropriate informed consent be obtained. Although this has been an important standard of practice for many years, increasing concerns about risk management for clinics and individual providers has mandated that it be performed. Moreover, it inherently makes sense to provide easy-to-read and understandable materials and discuss the procedure with the woman so that she understands in detail (1) the method to be used, (2) all reasonable alternatives, and (3) both short- and long-term risks of the procedure. It is important to point out the major risks: bleeding, infection, uterine perforation, incomplete abortion, continued pregnancy, and death. In addition it is important to point out any conditions associated with future pregnancies that may occur as a result of multiple induced abortions. The woman should then sign a document that is witnessed by an impartial person in the clinic or other health facility. It is essential that detailed written documentation of all consultations between patient and provider be placed in the medical record.

Medical History

A complete medical history should be taken, with particular emphasis on accurately recording last normal menstrual period (LNMP), history of prior pregnancies, use of and timing of contraceptives, allergies, smoking status, and current use of medications or abuse of alcohol or illegal drugs.

Physical Exam

A general physical exam including assessment of vital signs, heart, lungs, breasts, abdomen, and extremities is important. It is essential that careful examination of the pelvis be performed with emphasis on assessing uterine size and position. If mild discrepancy exists between the estimation of gestational age by exam and LNMP, other historical indicators such as irregular bleeding or irregular use of contraceptives should be considered in attempting to accurately ascertain the actual gestational age. If serious discrepancy exists (>2 weeks), or if uterine malformations, leiomyomata, multiple or abnormal gestations are suspected, ultrasonographic evaluation of the pelvis, the uterus, and its contents should be performed.

Laboratory

Laboratory studies should be individualized depending on the assessment of the patient, but the minimum should include a highly sensitive urine pregnancy test, determination of the hematocrit, Rh factor status, and a urinalysis. If indicated, PAP smears and cultures for gonorrhea and chlamydia should also be performed. Prophylaxis against potential Rh sensitization of Rh-negative women with Rh immune globulin is indicated. Virtually 100 percent of these women can be protected by a single dose of Rh immune globulin (300 μg IM) prior to their discharge from the abortion facility.

METHODS

Until recently, all methods of abortion could be divided into two basic groups, surgical evacuation and labor induction. Today, a third important category has come onto the horizon: oral or parenteral anti-progestational agents. Surgical evacuation includes suction (vacuum) curettage, sharp curettage, D&E (usually defined as transcervical evacuation beyond 12 completed weeks of gestation), hysterotomy, and hysterectomy. Labor-induction methods include abortifacients introduced either intrauterine or systemically. Anti-progestational agents include Mifepristone (RU486) and methotrexate. Several aides such as laminaria tents and other osmotic dilators, as well as oxytocin, and the prostaglandins play a role in provision of abortion services (see Chap. 32).

A particular provider or clinic should determine which procedures to offer to women and whether to limit services to standard first-trimester vacuum curettage or include midtrimester curettage and midtrimester labor-induction procedures. Midtrimester abortion services dictate special considerations: (1) labor-induction methods usually require hospital services, and both the labor induction and midtrimester curettage methods unquestionably require greater surgical skills; (2) there is need for greater cervical dilation, achieved by overnight insertion of laminaria tents or other osmotic dilators; (3) there is the necessity for at least one extra visit and more extensive patient instruction; and (4) the patient is at greater risk of complications than with first-trimester curettage. The use of anti-progestational agents deserves special consideration and will be discussed later.

Surgical Abortion

First-trimester Dilation and Vacuum Curettage

Early suction curettage is often termed menstrual regulation, menstrual extraction, or minisuction. These simple, safe procedures are most often performed between 40 and 50 days of gestation with small flexible cannulae (4–6 mm), and frequently require neither anesthesia nor cervical dilation (Laufe, 1977; Stubblefield 1986) (Fig. 33–2). Two main concerns of using this method include performing the procedure on nonpregnant women, and failing to abort the pregnancy. Although the terms *menstrual regulation* and *extraction* may imply that the procedures are done without performing a pregnancy test, the authors

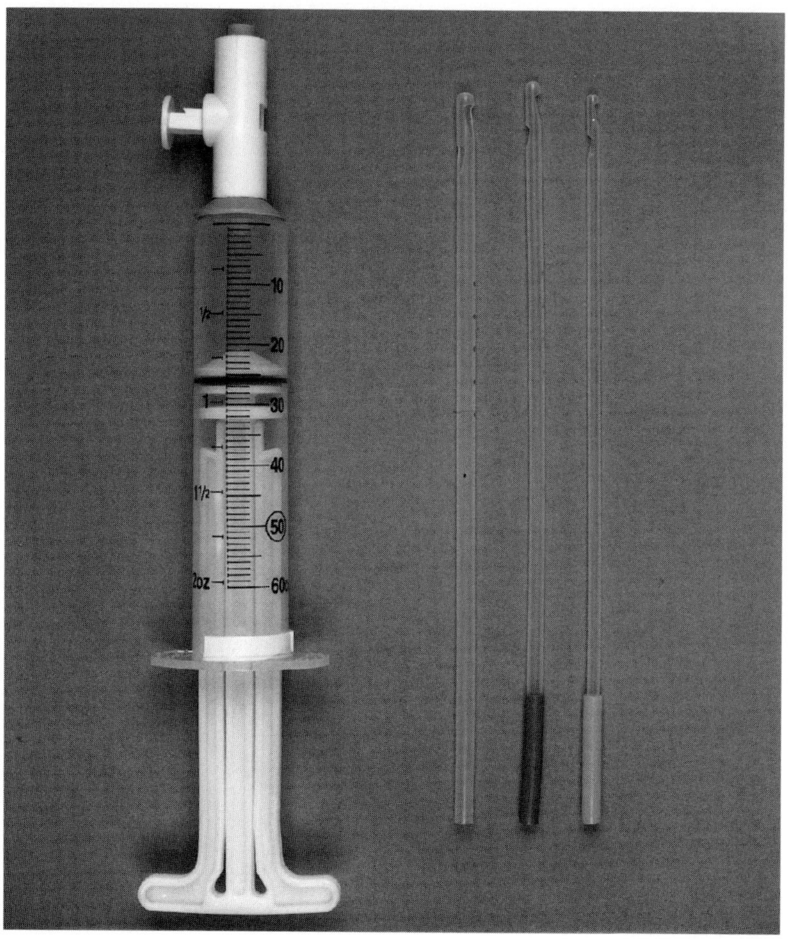

Figure 33–2. Karman cannulae, self-locking syringe with pinch valve used for early abortion. (Photograph courtesy of IPAS, Carrboro, NC.)

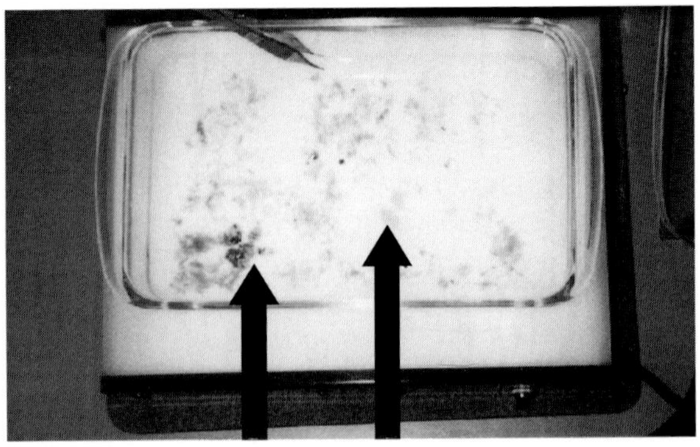

Figure 33–3. Products of conception at 6 week's gestation in water seen with back lighting. Placental tissue seen in lower left section of dish. (Photo courtesy of Dr. Lewis Koplik, Albuquerque, NM.)

strongly discourage such an approach. Examination of tissue and adequate patient follow-up will decrease the chances of failing to timely diagnose a continuing pregnancy (Kaunitz and associates, 1985) (Fig. 33–3).

The most widely used technique for first-trimester pregnancy termination in the United States is vacuum curettage with mechanical dilation, using tapered cervical dilators such as Hanks or Pratt dilators, or the Denniston plastic autoclavable Pratt-design cervical dilators (Fig. 33–4). Many providers recommend and use osmotic dilators such as laminaria tents (dried seaweed—the *japonicum* species is preferred over *digitata* because it remains firm when swollen with water) or synthetic dilators (Lamicel or Dilapan). For most first-trimester procedures, only

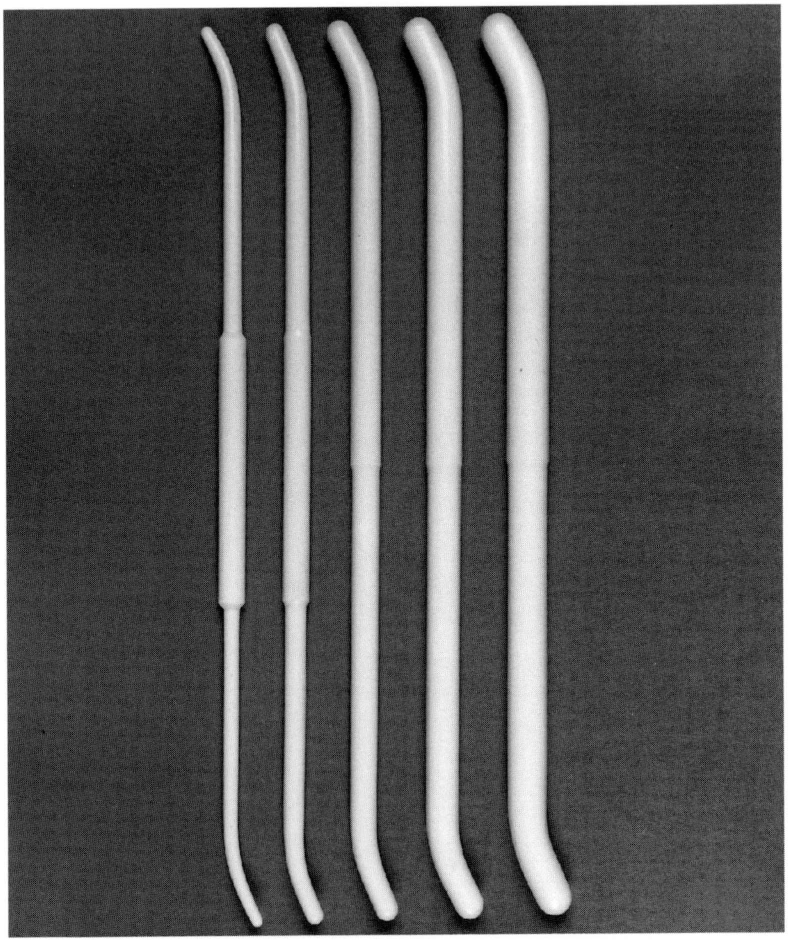

Figure 33–4. Denniston dilators. (Photograph courtesy of IPAS, Carrboro, NC.)

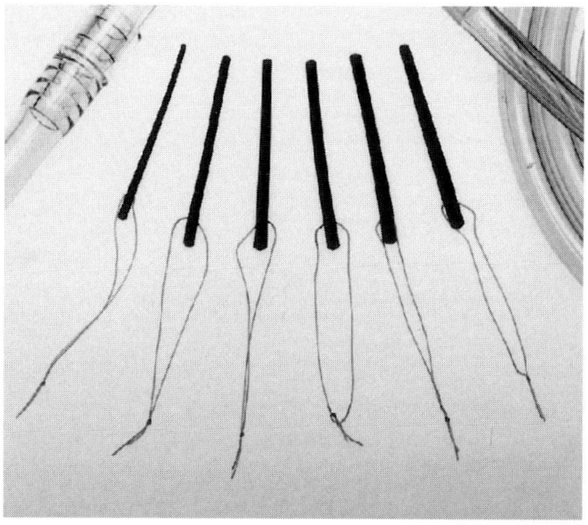

Figure 33–5. Photograph of *Laminaria japonica* tent. Laminaria tents are available in sizes ranging from 2 mm to 6 mm. (Courtesy of Berkeley Medevices, Inc., Berkeley, CA.)

one osmotic dilator is necessary for adequate dilation. Adequate cervical dilation can be attained within 4 hours of laminaria placement (Figs. 33–5 and 33–6). Although an intravenous infusion is not necessary during the procedure, it may be advisable to place a heparin lock in case there is a need to give the woman volume support at a later time. The use of premedication can be offered as an option. Some clinicians suggest the use of intravenous fentanyl, 0.1 mg or butorphanol 2 mg or midazolam 1–2.5 mg with atropine 0.4 mg to provide both analgesia and protection from the vaso-vagal reactions occasionally associated with manipulation of the cervix. Appropriately counseled patients, whose anxiety has been diminished, usually reject the use of any premedication. Once the patient is properly positioned on the examination or operating table and sufficiently comfortable, and with the perineum adequately exposed, the provider, using unsterile protective gloves should perform a careful bimanual examination to assess uterine size (estimated gestational age) and position. Previously placed hydrophilic dilators may be removed at this time and assessed for effectiveness in terms of their expansion and cervical dilitation. After putting on sterile gloves, the cervix should be exposed with a sterile speculum (Figs. 33–7 and 33–8). Although sterile instruments should be used, to prevent contamination throughout the procedure, a "no touch" technique, avoiding contact with the distal ends of all instruments, should be used. To reduce the risk of contamination, the paracervical area should first be swabbed with a povidone-iodine solution or another substance, such as chlorhexidine gluconate, if the patient is allergic to iodine. Using a 22-gauge spinal needle attached to a 20-cc glass or plastic disposable syringe, 1–2 mL of either 1 percent chlorprocaine or 1 percent lidocaine should be injected superficially into the anterior lip of the cervix at 12:00. A single-toothed tenaculum or long Allis clamp should then be applied to the anterior lip of the cervix to provide for the slight traction necessary to straighten the cervical canal. A long Allis clamp reduces the risk of cervical bleeding upon removal of the clamp

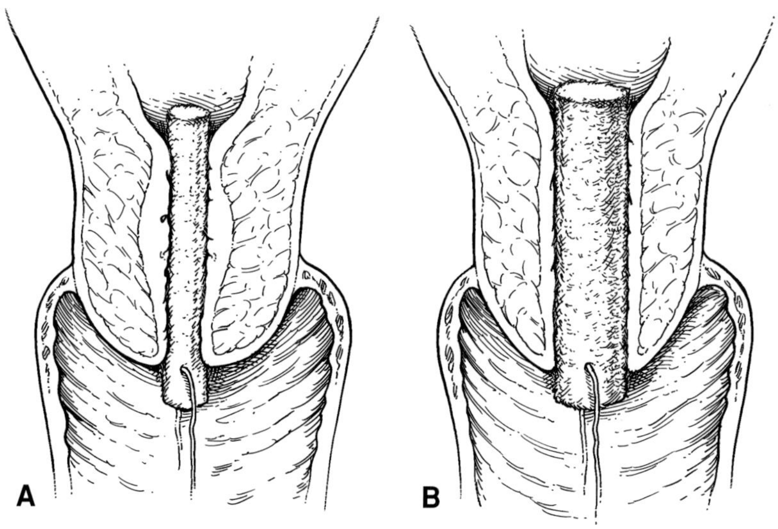

Figure 33–6. Insertion of laminaria prior to suction curettage. **A.** Laminaria immediately after being appropriately placed with its upper end just through the internal os. **B.** The swollen laminaria and dilated, softened cervix about 8 hours later.

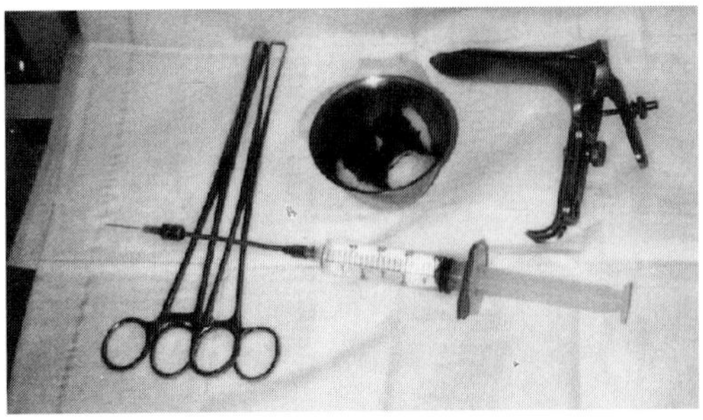

Figure 33–7. Perineal tray in preparation for performing abortion procedure. (Photo courtesy of Dr. Lewis Koplik, Albuquerque, NM.)

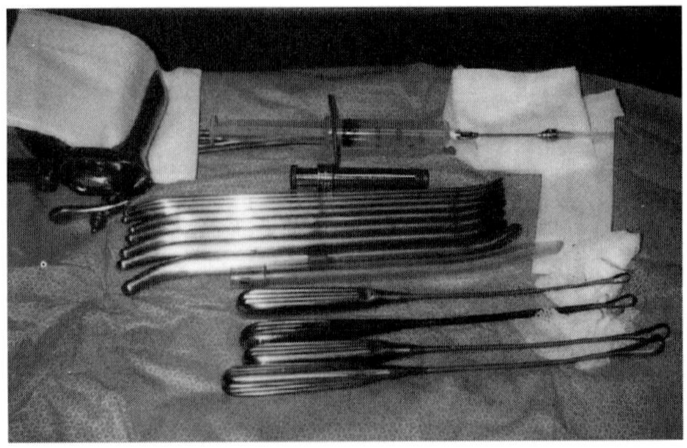

Figure 33–8. Instrument setup for performing D&E at 14 weeks' gestation. Tray includes graduated Pratt dilators, curettes, and a 14-mm curved plastic cannula. (Photo courtesy of Dr. Lewis Koplik, Albuquerque, NM.)

and has minimal subjective discomfort associated with its use. A paracervical block is next performed using the same agents and syringe–needle combination as above. Depending on the patient's weight, the dose used should vary between 4 and 8 mL per side. The local anesthetic should be injected slowly near the cervicovaginal junction at 4 and 8 o'clock, taking care to aspirate the syringe prior to each injection to avoid intravascular injection of the anesthetic agent. The injection should raise a wheal in the adjacent area. After waiting 2–3 minutes to obtain maximal effect from the local anesthetic, either a curved rigid plastic cannula or a flexible Karman cannula should be selected and gently inserted into the cervical canal, passed through the internal os, and into the uterine cavity (Fig. 33–9). The size of the cannula used should depend on the gestational age measured in weeks. If rigid cannulae are used, the size of the cannula in millimeters should equal the gestational age through 12 weeks. If flexible cannulae are preferred, a 5-mm Karman cannula may be used

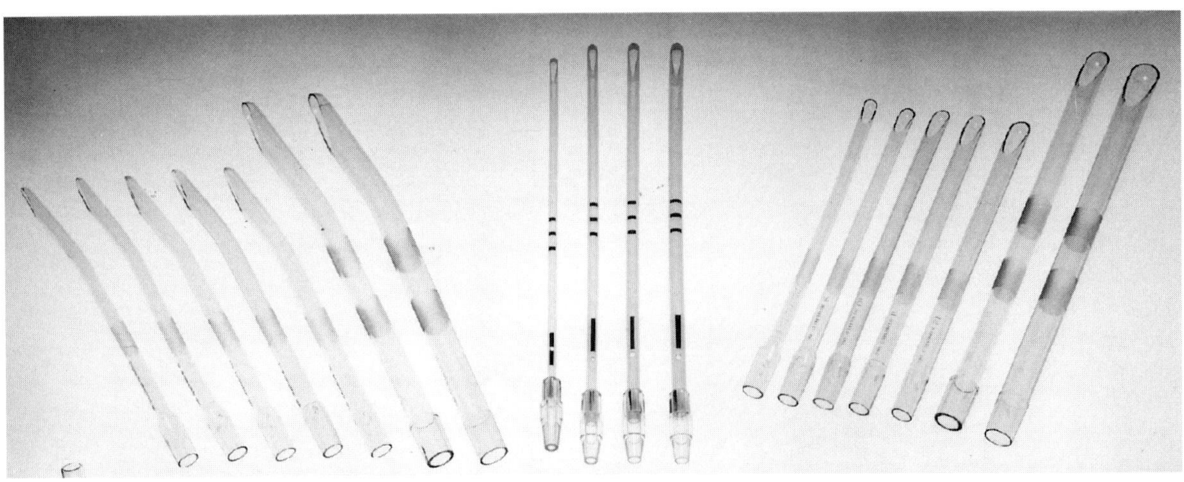

Figure 33–9. Plastic cannulae of various sizes for performing suction curettage. Left, rigid curved-tip cannulae. Center, flexible Karman-type cannulae. Right, rigid straight-tipped cannulae. (Courtesy of Berkeley Medevices, Inc., Berkeley, CA.)

to 7 weeks; 6 mm to 10 weeks; 7 mm to 11 weeks; and 8 mm to 12 weeks. If with gentle pressure there does not appear to be adequate dilatation of the cervical canal, which is more apt to occur if rigid cannulae are used, either with or without osmotic dilators, tapered dilators like the Pratts or Dennistons should be used to achieve further dilation of the cervix (Fig. 33–10). If flexible cannulae are used, little if any dilation is usually necessary. Once inserted, the cannula should be attached to a suction control handle and tubing that is connected to a high-performance surgical suction machine such as those available from Cabot-Berkeley Company (Fig. 33–11). The amount of suction used will depend on atmospheric pressure, but should ideally be in the green or safe zone of the suction machine's pressure gauge. Once appropriate placement of the cannula into the lower uterine segment is achieved (Fig. 33–12), the suction apparatus should be turned on and the contents of the uterus evacuated using either (1) a rotating motion of the inserted rigid cannula or (2) a gentle in and out and rotating movement of the flexible cannula, taking care to only rotate the cannula on the out movement to prevent avulsing the tip of the flexible cannula. This is continued until the uterus begins to involute around the cannula, signaling the completion of evacuation (Fig. 33–13). At this point, the cannula should be completely removed from the uterus to observe for bleeding. If little bleeding is observed, the operator may feel assured that the procedure is complete. If bleeding is subjectively heavy, gentle reinsertion of the cannula and reaspiration until the side walls of the uterus seem to firmly adhere to the cannula should be performed. Sharp curettage is optional in these procedures. Some individuals suggest that it is essential to perform sharp curettage to be assured that

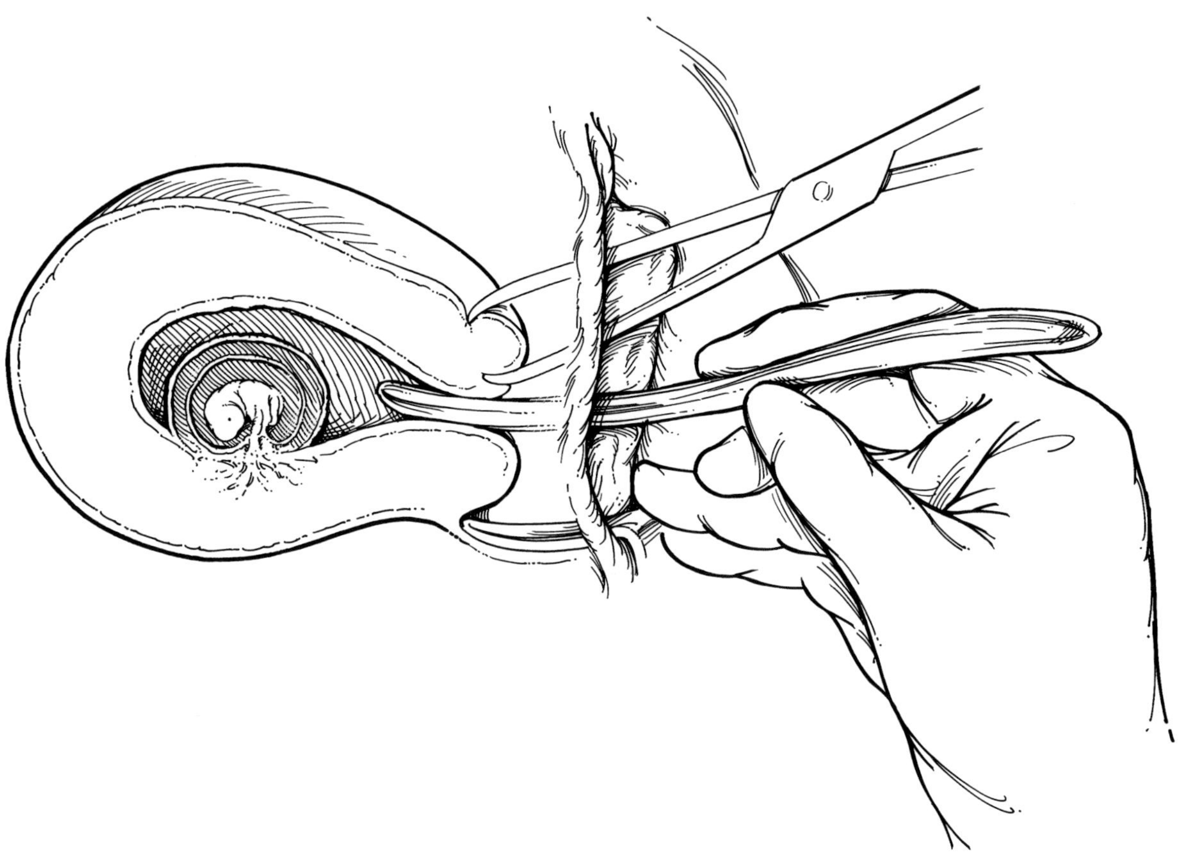

Figure 33–10. Dilation of the cervix with a Pratt dilator. Note that the fourth and fifth fingers rest against the perineum and buttocks, lateral to the introitus. This maneuver provides a measure of safety from exerting overzealous pressure on the cervix, a potential cause of uterine perforation.

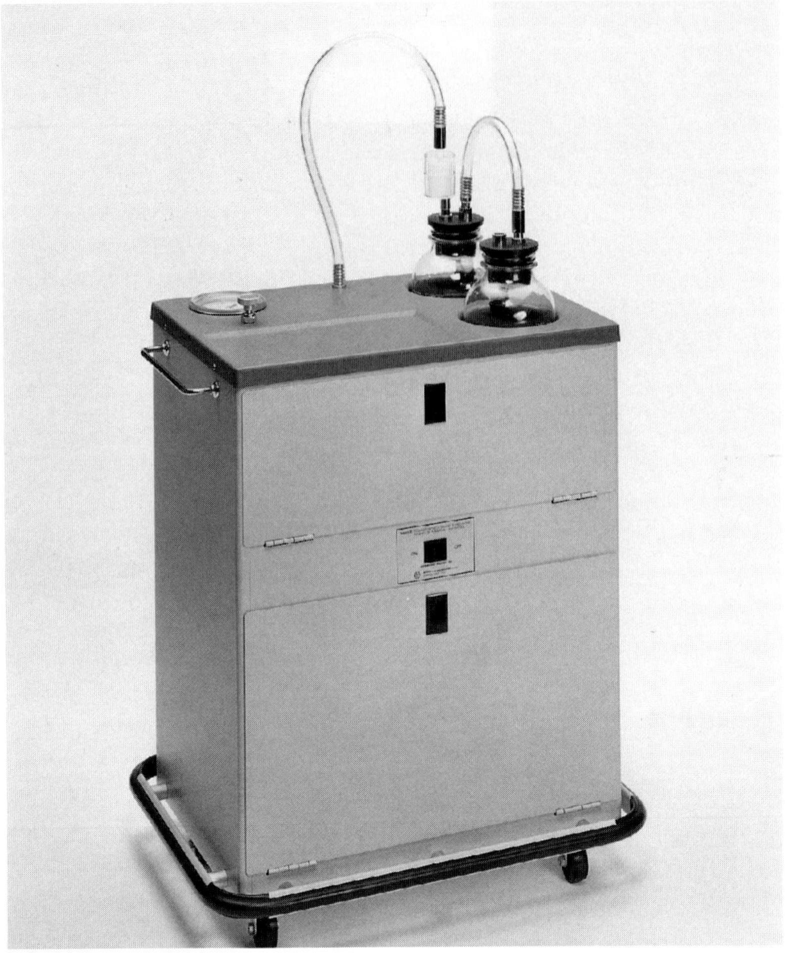

Figure 33–11. An example of an efficient surgical vacuum aspirator. (Courtesy of Berkeley Medevices, Inc., Berkeley, CA.)

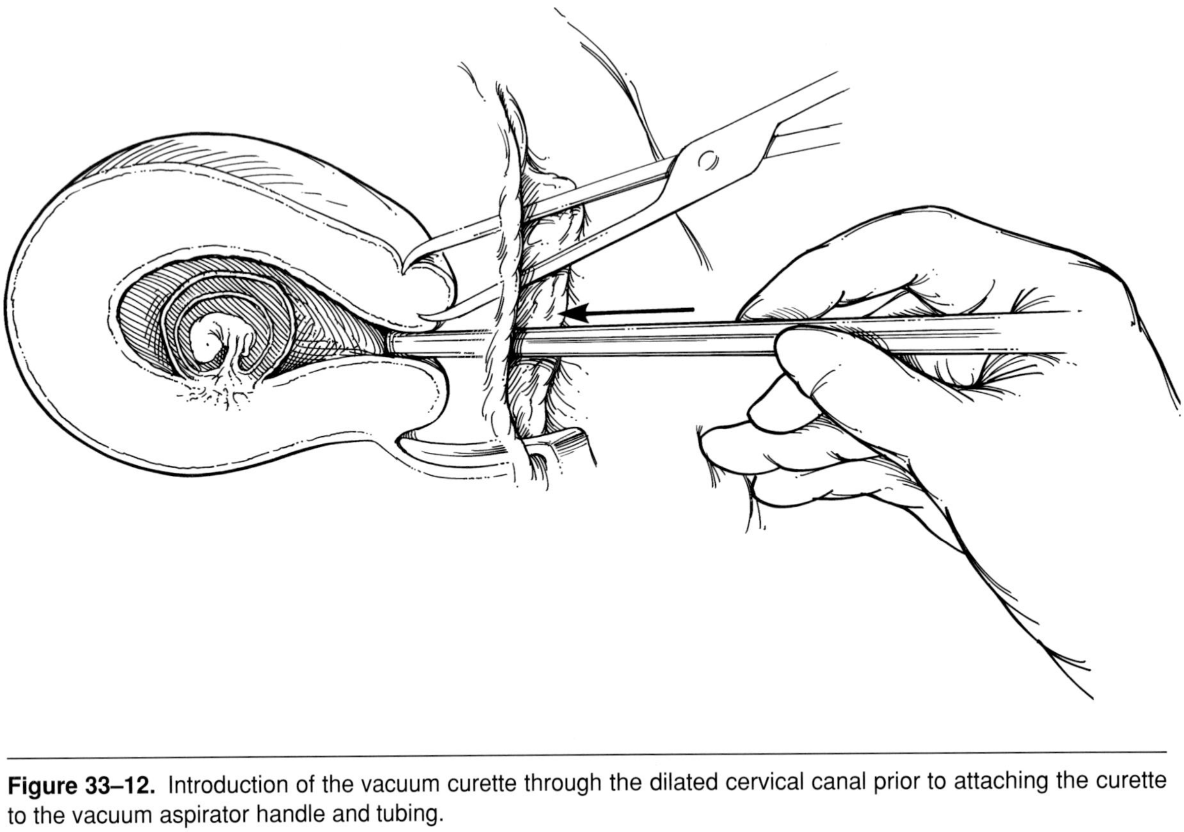

Figure 33–12. Introduction of the vacuum curette through the dilated cervical canal prior to attaching the curette to the vacuum aspirator handle and tubing.

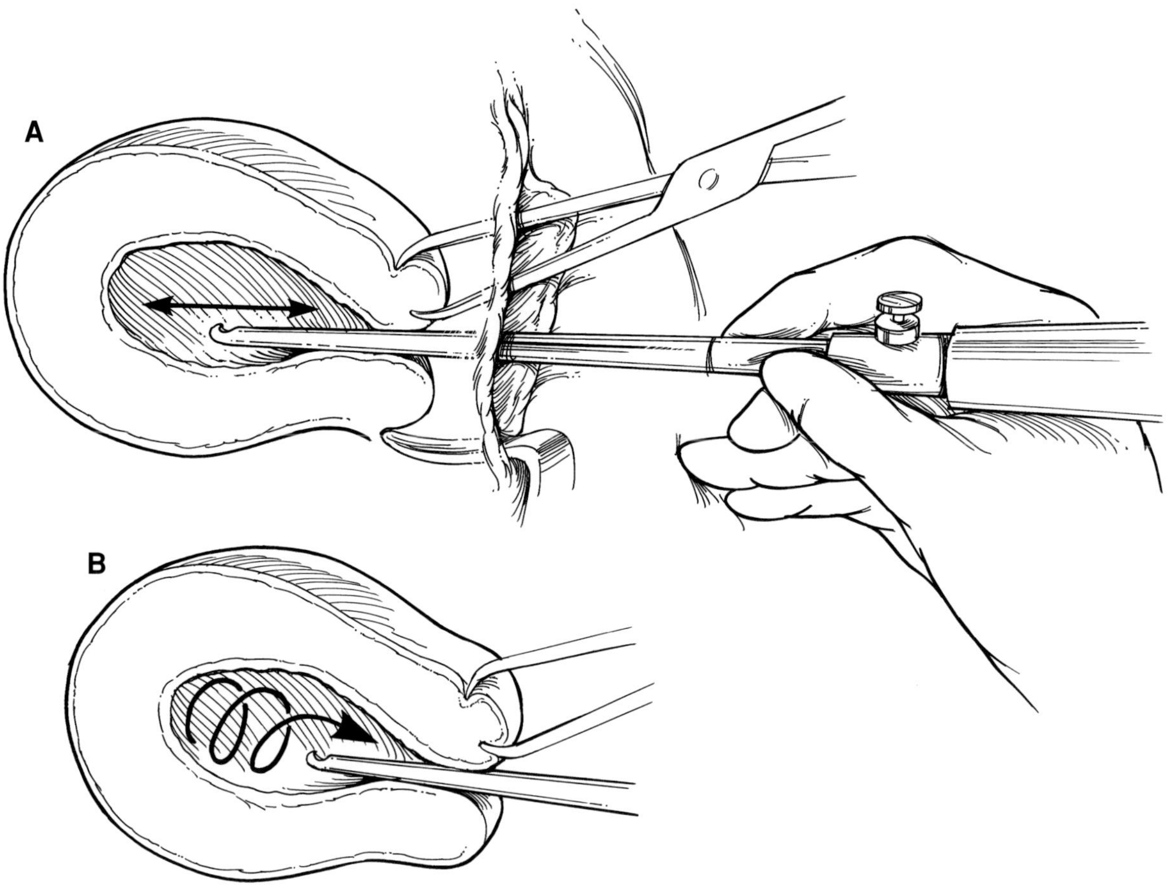

Figure 33–13. Uterine aspiration. **A.** The cannula is inserted just beyond the internal os. **B.** The products of conception are evacuated by rotary motion of the cannula.

the products of conception have been adequately removed; this procedure has the potential of increasing the amount of intraoperative bleeding (Darney, 1987). Once bleeding is minimal, all instruments should be removed and a gentle bimanual examination be performed to assess the size and firmness of the uterus and its involution. If the uterus seems boggy and enlarged, products of conception may remain in the uterus. If firm, however, the operator can be assured that the procedure has been adequately completed. In some facilities, methergine 0.2 mg IM or 2.0 mg PO is given routinely either just before, during, or after the procedure to assist in firm contraction of the uterus and thus reduce the risk of heavy postprocedure bleeding.

Once the procedure has been completed, the tissue collected via a gauze bag attached in one of the suction machine's collection bottles should be rinsed in saline or water and examined for the presence of trophoblastic, fetal, and decidual tissue (Fig. 33–14). Prior to 9 completed weeks at least trophoblastic tissue, including placenta and sac, should be observed. Both fetal and trophoblastic tissue should be observed beyond 9 weeks EGA in order to ensure that the procedure is complete (Grimes and associates, 1992). If products of conception are not identified grossly, histologic examination should be performed so that an ectopic pregnancy will not escape detection.

Perioperative Antibiotics. There is currently sufficient evidence to suggest that in most women, the use of either prophylactic antibiotics or a short postoperative therapeutic course of antibiotics is protective against postoperative infection. Wide-spectrum antibiotics such as the tetracyclines or doxycyclines are ideal for this purpose (Grimes, 1992;

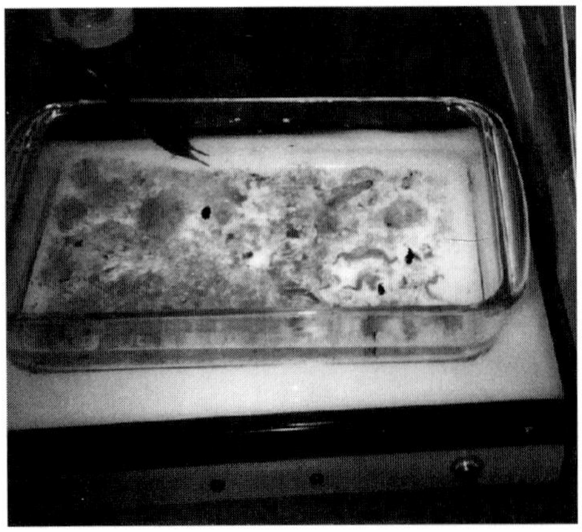

Figure 33–14. Products of conception at 9 weeks' gestation in water seen with back lighting. Placental and fetal tissue is observed in the dish. (Photo courtesy of Dr. Lewis Koplik, Albuquerque, NM.)

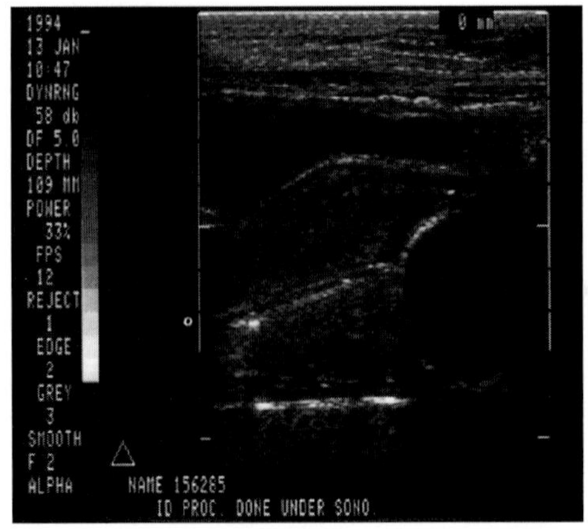

Figure 33–15. Ultrasonographic image during midtrimester D&E procedure. Bierer forceps with blades open grasping tissue within the uterus. (Courtesy of Reproductive Health Services, St. Louis, MO.)

Hodgson, 1975; Schulz, 1984; Sonne-Holme, 1981; Levallois, 1988; and their colleagues). Any woman at risk of developing subacute bacterial endocarditis should receive preoperative antibiotic prophylaxis.

Midtrimester Vacuum Aspiration

The majority of midtrimester abortions are performed using the D&E technique. Technologic advances such as use of real-time ultrasound during the procedure has made D&E both safer and easier to perform (Darney, 1983) (Fig. 33–15). Large studies have demonstrated that D&E, in terms of morbidity and mortality, is safer than other methods from 13 to 16 weeks' gestation. However, that benefit is less clear at later gestational ages when comparing D&E with labor-induction methods.

Although midtrimester D&E abortions are performed in a similar manner to those during the first 12 weeks of gestation, certain issues need special attention. For instance, D&E requires considerably more cervical dilation and an instrument is needed to assist evacuation of more advanced pregnancies.

Osmotic dilators are used in virtually all procedures performed beyond 13 completed weeks of gestation. Their use decreases the risk of cervical laceration and uterine perforation. Depending on the gestational age at the time of the procedure, 2 or more days of progressive dilation of the cervix using osmotic dilators may be necessary (Hern, 1984). Overnight use of multiple laminaria tents can result in as much as 15–20 mm of cervical dilation without excessive risk or discomfort to the patient. Two centimeters or more of dilation may be necessary if grasping forceps such as the Sopher or Bierer are contemplated during the procedure.

Prior to beginning the procedure, it is advisable that an intravenous line be established and that oxytocin be available for IV administration of fluids (40–100 units/L) postevacuation. As the difficulty of the procedure increases with advancing gestational age, so do the advantages of the preoperative medications previously mentioned. A paracervical block should be administered; the only difference from that associated with first-trimester abortion is that the operator may wish to add vasopressin at a ratio of 5 units/15 mL of anesthetic agent to help reduce the risk of bleeding. Patients with a history of hypertension or vascular disease should not receive vasopressin because inadvertent intravascular injection can result in serious complications.

The cervix should be grasped anteriorly with either an atraumatic tenaculum or other instrument and the adequacy of cervical dilation tested by gently inserting the grasping forceps or dilators through the cervical os, taking care not to rupture the fetal membranes. If cervical dilation is inadequate, consideration may be given to reinserting additional osmotic dilators and delaying the procedure for 6–24 hours. If dilation is deemed adequate, a plastic cannula should be passed through the dilated cervix into the uterine cavity to rupture the amniotic sac and to then evacuate as much amniotic fluid as possible. This procedure may reduce the risk of amniotic fluid embolus. A 14–15-week pregnancy may be evacuated with a 14-mm cannula; a ≥16-week pregnancy with a 16-mm cannula. Once amniotic fluid has been removed, the suction cannula should also be removed. The removal of placenta and fetus should be accomplished, under direct ultrasound observation, using Bierer, Sopher, or similar forceps as necessary. Once the forceps are introduced into the uterine cavity, they should be widely opened and the anterior blade placed between the uterine wall and the products of conception. The forceps are then closed and if POC is felt between the blades, traction using a slight rotating motion should be used as the forceps are withdrawn from the uterus. Using this technique the fetus and placenta are removed from the uterus. Simultaneous use of real-time ultrasound during the procedure greatly facilitates the safe maneuvering of instruments within the uterus and the complete removal of the intrauterine contents. Ultrasound guidance also has the advantage of possibly reducing the pain associated with the procedure by limiting the necessity to pass the cannula or forceps high into the uterus. Furthermore, real-time visualization of the procedure reduces the risk of uterine perforation. Once evacuation appears complete, sharp curettage of the uterine cavity should be performed. It is very important to examine all tissue to assure that the evacuation is complete. Adequate placental tissue for gestational age plus all fetal parts should be identified, particularly the calvarium. The calvarium is the fetal part most frequently missed. If not accounted for, ultrasound-directed grasping forceps or a sharp curette will aid its safe removal. Once the procedure is completed, the woman should be observed for 2–4 hours for any untoward symptoms or signs prior to discharge.

Hysterotomy and Hysterectomy

Hysterotomy and hysterectomy should no longer be considered primary methods of induced abortion. The risks of complications and death far outweigh any benefits to be derived from these methods except in those rare situations where a true indication for hysterectomy exists.

Labor-induction Abortions

Although recent CDC and AGI data suggest that the majority of midtrimester abortions in the United States are now performed by D&E, there is no clear evidence that at later gestational ages (beyond 18 weeks) there is less risk in performing D&E versus one of several labor-induction methods. The provider or patient may choose one of the labor-induction methods of abortion beyond 18 weeks' gestation, as is common with late genetic terminations. One disadvantage of this approach is the need for hospitalization for part or all of the procedure.

In 1993, Hern and colleagues reported 10 years of experience in performing outpatient midtrimester abortions for women with complicated advanced pregnancies (fetal anomalies, diagnosed genetic disorders, or fetal death) (Hern and associates, 1993). Their objective was to determine the safety of providing such services. Gestational lengths ranged from 15 to 34 menstrual weeks, and fetal diagnoses included various chromosomal abnormalities, malformations, and death. At less than 20 weeks' gestation, D&E following serial multiple laminaria treatment of the cervix was used; after 20 menstrual weeks the technique included serial multiple laminaria placement and either instillation of intraamniotic hyperosmolar urea or induction of fetal death by injection of digoxin and/or hyperosmolar urea into the fetus, followed by artificial rupture of membranes, induction of labor, and assisted expulsion or instrumental extraction of the fetus. They had only one serious complication; a cervical laceration. Based on the finding that the complication rates were not significantly related to gestation length, they concluded that outpatient abortion could be performed safely in most cases of fetal disorder, including death, through 34 menstrual weeks under proper conditions. Nevertheless, a great proportion of these terminations still require hospitalization.

The agents used for labor-induction abortions can be grouped into two categories: hypertonic solutions and uterotonic agents. The first group consists largely of saline and urea while the second group is dominated by various prostaglandins.

Hypertonic Saline/Urea

The use of intraamniotic hypertonic saline solution for midtrimester abortion is mainly of historical significance. Although still used for late procedures, there are serious risks that are specifically associated with this method, including disseminated intravascular coagulopathy, renal failure, and cardiovascular and pulmonary collapse. Moreover, when used alone, the mean time from instillation of the hypertonic saline to abortion is 33–35 hours, considerably longer than other currently used methods (Kerenyi and co-workers, 1973). With intravenous oxytocin, the mean time for the procedure is reduced by approximately one third (Berger and Edelman, 1975). Although the method of action is largely unknown, the fetal death attributed to the hypertonic saline is hypothetically the stimulus for labor induction. Ivanisevic and Djelmis, in Zagreb, reported in 1990 that after intraamniotic instillation of 20 percent saline solution in 12 women between 16 and 18 weeks' gestation, there was a statistically significant increase in the levels of PGE_2 and $PGF_{2\alpha}$ in both amniotic fluid and maternal plasma. These findings suggest that the release of primary prostaglandins is important in the chain of events initiating labor and maturation of the cervix in abortions induced with intraamniotic instillation of hypertonic NaCl solution (Ivanisevic and Djelmis, 1990).

Hypertonic urea solution has also been used. This agent has the advantage of not being as risky as saline but has the disadvantage of causing higher mean instillation-to-abortion intervals. Binkin and associates compared saline to urea combined with $PGF_{2\alpha}$ and found that the latter method offered a shorter instillation-to-abortion time and fewer serious complications (Binkin and associates, 1983).

The technique for intraamniotic instillation differs little from diagnostic amniocentesis. Using sterile technique, direct real-time ultrasound-assisted introduction of the trochar into the amniotic sac is achieved. Once adequate flow of amniotic fluid is established, no additional fluid removal is necessary. Gravity feed of the instilled agent (urea or saline) is preferred over syringe introduction.

Prostaglandins

The most common agents currently used for labor induction are the prostaglandins, primarily in the form of prostaglandin E_2 suppositories. Although these substances could theoretically be used for first trimester abortion, their use is too time consuming to be practical when compared to the effectiveness of vacuum curettage. Once the cervix is adequately prepared by insertion of osmotic dilators, a 20-mg prostaglandin E_2 suppository is inserted high into the vagina, adjacent to the cervix, and then repeated every 3–4 hours. This method has the advantage of simplicity and a mean time to abortion of approximately 13.5 hours. Although intramuscular 15-methyl $PGF_{2\alpha}$ is available for induction of labor, its use, either alone or in conjunction with intraamniotic urea, offers no advantage over the PGE_2 suppositories.

The prostaglandins have several disadvantages, not the least of which are their noxious side effects. Up to one half of women develop fever, and there is a high frequency of nausea, vomiting, and diarrhea. Moreover, when used alone it may not be feticidal, necessitating the use of additional drugs such as intraamniotic digoxin. Prophylactic use of medications such as antipyretics, antidiarrheal agents, and antinauseants are helpful but not uniformally effective. The most effective means of reducing symptoms is the use of fewer doses of the medication, which can often be accomplished by preparing the cervix with serial placement of osmotic dilators.

Although there is a higher risk of serious complications with labor-induction methods of abortion than with D&Es, the risks can be minimized by close patient observation. Preventing untoward outcomes by active management of ineffective labor is essential. The rate of serious complications rises significantly as the induction-to-abortion time increases. If failed abortion appears imminent, steps need to be taken, including use of intramuscular 15M-$PGF_{2\alpha}$ or PGE_2 suppositories to augment labor. If the operator has the appropriate skills, it may be easiest to effect a D&E. It is reported that D&E is more easily performed after initial labor induction than as a primary procedure since the cervix is usually well dilated and the uterus contracted with the fetus and placenta located in the lower uterine segment. If a D&E can be successfully accomplished, the woman can be spared the necessity of having a hysterotomy with all the additional risks associated with an abdominal operation and anesthesia. It is reasonable to suggest that most of the morbidity associated with the labor-induction methods can be prevented or minimized by meticulous attention to the details of caring for these patients.

Induction Abortion

Historically, a number of substances of plant origin have been reported to be of value as abortifacients. The Chinese reported success with use of certain herbal medications for induction of abortions (Chen and Lols, 1982). In recent years certain medications including antimetabolites and antiprogesterones have entered the spotlight. These substances offer the prospect of having medical abortifacients available that are effective, easy to administer, and inexpensive.

Methotrexate

Methotrexate is one of these medications. It is an antimetabolite that has been available for many years for the treatment of neoplastic diseases such as choriocarcinoma, for severe psoriasis, and for adult rheumatoid arthritis. Its mechanism of action is the inhibition of dehydrofolic acid reductase, interfering with DNA synthesis, repair, and cellular replication. As a result, actively proliferating tissues such as certain malignant cells, as well as fetal and trophoblastic cells, are particularly susceptible to the drug. There have been a number of reports of the use of this drug in the medical treatment of early unruptured ectopic pregnancy with good success (Stovall and associates, 1991; Stovall and Ling, 1993), although there have not been well-designed randomized clinical trials into the effectiveness and side effects of such treatment. Nevertheless, there is some evidence that the anticellular effects of the medication, in seemingly low doses, offer the possibility of medical induction of abortion in the future, hopefully with minimal maternal risk. In a recent study, the use of intramuscular methotrexate, in conjunction with a prostaglandin analogue, successfully effected abortion in the majority of study subjects (n = 10), all of whom were less than 8 weeks pregnant (Creinin and Darney, 1993). Although this technique must still be considered investigational, there is promise that it will become an effective and safe method to medically induce abortion.

Antiprogesterones

The first of the antiprogesterones to gain importance is mifepristone (RU486), a derivative of norethindrone, a progestin frequently used in oral contraceptives. RU486 has an α-side chain and an 11-β ring substitution that determines its antagonist action. The substance is mainly a competitive progesterone antagonist acting at the level of progesterone and glucocorticoid receptors in target tissues. During the normal menstrual cycle and in early pregnancy, RU486 probably acts primarily on the endometrium. During late pregnancy, the compound has significant effects on the myometrium, including the induction of gap junctions between myometrial cells, required for muscle contractility during labor. The usc of RU486 has helped to demonstrate that progesterone is required for maintenance of the late stages of pregnancy in women (Garfield and Baulieu, 1987). Its availability for study or clinical use in the United States has been hampered by antiabortion sentiment and a political climate that strongly supported the views of the antiabortion movement. In 1993, the Clinton Administration overturned a previously imposed ban on the study of RU486 in the United States and at the time of this writing a committee of experts to the Institute of Medicine has urged extensive research on mifepristone and similar drugs to assess their efficacy, toxicity, and long-term safety and to evaluate their usefulness for contraception and pregnancy termination and for a variety of reproductive and nonreproductive conditions. In a report entitled "Clinical Applications of Mifepristone (RU-486) and Other Antiprogestins," they feature 20 recommendations regarding the evaluation of antiprogestins and spell out a range of potential uses. Included are the reproduction-related applications of abortifacient and contraceptive, as well as their potential for treating endometriosis, uterine leiomyomata, and benign brain tumors known as meningiomas (Donaldson and associates, 1993).

Numerous clinical studies of RU486, conducted in 15 countries, have shown that the drug is very effective in inducing abortion if administered orally shortly after conception. Although successful induction of abortion occurs in >90 percent of women whose last normal menstrual periods occurred within the previous 6 weeks, it is ineffective in later pregnancies. It is hypothesized that after 7 weeks' gestation, the failure of RU486 may relate to its inability to successfully compete for progesterone receptors with the enormously high levels of progesterone then being produced by the placenta (Van Look, 1988; Couzinet, 1986; Grimes, 1988; Cervest, 1985; and their colleagues). When RU486 is used in combination with one of the prostaglandin analogues, induction of abortion occurs in 95–99 percent of cases (Avrech, 1991; Swahn, 1990; Rodger, 1989; Wu, 1992; Aubeny, 1991; and their co-workers). Moreover, the results of a recent randomized clinical trial (n = 16 women) conducted to evaluate RU486 as a "menstrual regulator" suggest that the drug should be useful for inducing menstrual bleeding in women with menses delayed up to 10 days. In this study half of the women in each treatment group proved to be pregnant. Seven of eight who received mifepristone were not pregnant at 2-week follow-up, while four of eight who received the placebo were (p = .15). Mifepristone may thus hold promise for "menstrual regulation" for women who do not have access to medical confirmation of pregnancy or who choose not to have this determination made (Grimes and associates, 1992).

RU486 is currently not available in the United States; however, if future reported side effects are no more serious than those already seen, it may be a good alternative to early suction curettage. Its most important advantage is that it is not a surgical procedure but offers effectiveness comparable to suction curettage prior to 7 weeks' gestation, particularly if administered with a prostaglandin analogue (Kaunitz and co-workers, 1985).

THE EPIDEMIOLOGY OF ABORTION MORBIDITY

Although legal abortion in the United States has been documented in several large studies to be a safe procedure, there are inherent risks. Complications can range from minor to potentially life-threatening. The complications of abortion can be categorized into immediate and late. The immediate category can be subdivided into early (intraoperative or immediately postoperative) and delayed.

Incidence rates of abortion complications in the United States were obtained from three large multicenter prospective studies—the Joint Programs for the Study of Abortion (JPSA). These studies were conducted to examine the early and delayed complications of legal induced abortion and the risk factors associated with legal abortion morbidity. JPSA-I (1970–1971) was conducted by the Population Council and sponsored by CDC; JPSA-II (1971–1974) and JPSA-III (1975–1978) were conducted by CDC. These studies involved 237,733 legal abortions performed at participating hospitals and free-standing clinics. In all three studies, institutions were requested to obtain follow-up information on patients 2–6 weeks after the procedure. Most of what is known today about complications of induced abortion is a result of these three studies.

Postabortion complications reported to JPSA were comprehensive, including 31 categories in JPSA-I and 100 categories in both JPSA-II and JPSA-III. Included were complaints ranging from minor (eg, breast engorgement and vomiting after anesthesia) to major complications (eg, uterine perforation, hemorrhage, and pelvic infection). The total complication rate refers to the percentage of women who sustained one or more complications of any variety or severity; the major complication rate denotes the percentage of women sustaining one or more of 15 complications including: cardiac arrest; convulsion; death; endotoxic shock; fever for 3 or more days; hemorrhage necessitating blood transfusion; hypernatremia; injury to the bladder, ureter, or intestines; pelvic infection with 2 or more days of fever and a peak of at least 40° C or with hospitalization for ≥11 days; pneumonia; psychiatric hospitalization for ≥11 days; pulmonary embolism or infarction; thrombophlebitis; major surgical treatment of complications; and wound disruption after hysterotomy or hysterectomy (Tietze and Lewit, 1972; Grimes and associates, 1977b). A broader category of "serious complications" was defined for JPSA-III and includes: fever of ≥38° C for 3 or more days; unintended major surgical procedure; transfusion; and death (Buehler and associates, 1985). The JPSA studies found the rates of total complications of abortion procedures to range from 9.6 percent in JPSA-I to 14.8 percent in JPSA-III; major complication rates were less than 1 percent (Buehler and co-workers, 1985) (Table 33–4). The risk of developing major complications from legal abortion decreased greatly during the 1970s. In JPSA-I (1970–1971), women without preexisting medical conditions obtaining legal abortions had a major complications rate of 1.0/100 abortions; in JPSA-II (1971–1974), the major complication rate

TABLE 33–4. COMPLICATION RATES PER 100 PROCEDURES BY GESTATION AND METHOD OF ABORTION

Gestation /Method	Total Complication Rate			Major Complication Rate		
	JPSA-I	*JPSA-II*	*JPSA-III*	*JPSA-I*	*JPSA-II*	*JPSA-III*
Gestation (weeks)						
≤ 6	5.2	7.2	7.9	0.9	0.4	0.10
7–8	4.2	4.7	8.5	0.4	0.3	0.07
9–10	4.8	5.6	9.2	0.6	0.4	0.09
11–12	6.8	8.2	10.4	1.0	0.8	0.11
13–14	15.9	17.0	14.3	2.1	1.4	0.26
15–16	24.0	33.1	28.2	2.5	1.9	0.83
17–20	24.0	39.9	45.6	2.2	2.2	1.26
≥ 21	22.8	36.1	33.2	2.1	2.3	1.44
Method						
Suction	4.7	5.0	9.0	0.5	0.4	0.08
D&E	6.7	10.6	11.6	0.6	0.9	0.35
Saline	23.8	42.7[a]	34.2	1.8	1.9[a]	1.93
Prostaglandin	NR	NR	58.6	NR	NR	0.87
Hysterotomy	37.3	49.4	NR	8.1	14.9	NR
Hysterectomy	51.0	52.9	NR	15.4	16.1	NR
Total	9.6	12.3	14.8	1.0	0.8	0.29

[a]Rates are for all instillation procedures combined.
NR, Not reported.
From JPSA-I: Tietze and Lewit (1972); JPSA-II: Cates and Grimes (1981); Grimes and co-workers (1977d). Rates for JPSA-III are unpublished.

dropped to 0.8 percent and in JPSA-III (1975–1978), the rate decreased to 0.29/100 abortions (Tietze, 1972; Grimes, 1977d; Cates, 1981; and their colleagues) (Table 33–4). The only other recently published large study of abortion complications is by Hakim-Elahi and associates (1990). This report included data on 170,000 first-trimester abortions performed in three free-standing clinics in New York City from 1971 to 1987. Hakim-Elahi reported a total complication rate of 0.9 percent and a major complication rate of 0.07 percent (Hakim-Elahi and co-workers, 1990). Other recent estimates of abortion complication rates are available from the National Abortion Federation (NAF). Data compiled by NAF for 1988 on 68,828 patients with follow-up indicate that about 0.5 percent of patients needed hospitalization because of an abortion complication (Gold, 1990).

Risk Factors

All three JPSA studies identified gestational age and type of procedure as the major risk factors for abortion morbidity. In all three studies, the risk of both total and major complications increased steadily with increasing gestational age. Total and major complication rates were lowest among women obtaining abortions at ≤8 weeks of gestation. The rates were two times higher for abortions performed at 13–14 weeks and 4–10 times higher for abortions performed after 15 weeks of gestation. Complication rates were lowest among women whose abortions were performed using curettage procedures. Compared with curettage procedures, the risk of complications was 6 times higher for abortions performed using labor-induction procedures and more than 10 times higher for abortions performed by hysterectomy or hysterotomy (Tietze, 1972; Grimes, 1977d; Cates, 1981; and their colleagues) (Table 33–4). Moreover, for midtrimester abortions, it was found that intra-amniotic instillation of prostaglandin ($PGF_{2\alpha}$) was associated with the highest complication rate, saline instillation had a lower complication rate, and D&E had the lowest rate of complication (Grimes and co-workers, 1977a; CDC, 1977). It is important to note, however, that the effects of delays in seeking abortion and the method chosen to perform an abortion are not independent, as suction curettage (the safest procedure) is unlikely to be used at later gestational ages.

Complication rates vary by age, race, parity, and number of previous spontaneous and induced abortions. However, unlike other pregnancy-related complications, the complications of induced abortions for black women were similar to white women. For Hispanic women, the risk was similar to white women during the first 12 weeks but was 1.74 times higher during the mid-trimester. During the first 12 weeks of gestation, very little difference in risk of complications was noticed for women of different age groups. However, after 12 weeks' gestation, there was an increase in risk for older women (Buehler and associates, 1985).

There was some increased risk of abortion complications among women who had previous pregnancies. Women with one or more previous induced abortion had slightly more than a 50 percent increased risk of complications prior to 12 completed weeks' gestation, but no increased risk after 12 weeks. Women with one or more previous deliveries had a 34 percent increased risk of complications across all gestational ages, whereas no increased risk of complications was observed among women with a history of a spontaneous abortion (Buehler and co-workers, 1985).

Other risk factors for abortion complications include type of anesthesia, method of cervical dilation, and the degree of training of the person performing the abortion. The use of general anesthesia for suction curettage abortion during the first trimester was not associated with a significantly higher complication rate than the use of local anesthesia. However, different types of complications were associated with the two types of anesthesia: general anesthesia was associated with higher rates of uterine hemorrhage, uterine perforation, intraabdominal hemorrhage, and cervical trauma, whereas local anesthesia was associated with higher rates of fever and convulsions (CDC, 1978; Grimes and associates, 1979). Higher rates of cervical injury and uterine perforation were found when using rigid dilators for cervical dilatation, and when the abortion was performed by a resident in training (CDC, 1985; Schulz, 1983; Grimes, 1984; and their co-workers). A study in Italy of 10,000 abortions performed between 1982 and 1986 found that the overall risk of complications following abortion is nearly doubled if a general anesthetic is used rather than a local anesthetic (Osborn and colleagues, 1990). The use of general anesthesia increased the risk of hemorrhage 4.6 times, the risk of injury 1.3 times, and the risk of other complications 1.6 times.

Abortion Complications and Their Management

As noted above, two of the most important determinants of the likelihood of complications are gestational age at the time of abortion and the method used. The immediate complications include hemorrhage, uterine perforation, cervical injury, and acute hematometra.

Immediate Complications

Hemorrhage. Excessive bleeding is fairly uncommon, but rises in incidence with increasing gestational age. Because of definitional problems (researchers defining hemorrhage as blood loss ranging between 100 and 1000 mL) and the imprecision in estimating volumes of blood loss, the reported incidence of hemorrhage has varied from 0.05 to 4.9/100 abortions (Cates, 1979; Hakim-Elahi, 1990; and their colleagues). Blood loss increases with the use of general anesthesia, especially those agents that produce uterine relaxation (CDC, 1978; Grimes, 1979; Osborn, 1990; and their associates). The best index of significant blood loss is the need for blood transfusion. The transfusion rate associated with suction curettage was reported at 0.06/100 abortions (Cates and co-workers, 1979). The rate was higher for abortions performed later in pregnancy and varied by method of abortion: 0.26 for D&E, 0.32 for urea-prostaglandin, and 1.72 for saline instillation (Kafrissen, 1984; Binkin, 1983; and their colleagues).

The two main causes of hemorrhage are uterine hypotonus and retained products of conception. Visualization of the cervix and bimanual pelvic examination are essential in attempting to distinguish between these two major causes. With uterine atony the examination shows a soft, nontender uterus along with a steady trickle of blood. Gentle uterine massage and parenteral uterotonics (oxytocin, methylergonovine, 15-methyl prostaglandin-$F_{2\alpha}$) should cause the uterus to contract and involute. Bleeding that does not respond to the above measures or heavier, brighter bleeding suggests the presence of retained products of conception. If retained products are suspected, management is repeat vacuum aspiration of the uterus. Real-time ultrasound can be useful in localizing retained products of conception and assisting in their successful removal. If these measures do not control the bleeding, other reasons for the hemorrhage must be considered, including cervical laceration, uterine wall perforation, and rarely, a clotting disorder.

Uterine Perforation. The incidence of uterine perforation has consistently been reported at 0.2/100 abortions (Cates and associates, 1979). However, the real incidence may be much higher because of asymptomatic and unsuspected perforations. Kaali and colleagues (1989) reported eight uterine perforations among 6408 women undergoing first trimester abortions, for an incidence rate of 0.13/100 procedures. However, among 706 women who underwent first-trimester abortions at the same time as laparoscopic sterilization, the authors found 14 perforations. Twelve of these were unsuspected but discovered during laparoscopy, for an incidence of 2.0/100 procedures (Kaali and associates, 1989). Several factors have been identified as being associated with an increased risk of uterine perforation. A curettage procedure performed by a resident rather than by an attending physician increases the risk of uterine perforation more than fivefold, whereas cervical dilation by laminaria decreases the risk by approximately 80 percent (Grimes and associates, 1984a). The risk of perforation increases significantly with advancing gestational age; multiparous women have three times the risk of nulliparous women (Grimes and co-workers, 1984a).

Perforations can occasionally cause significant intraabdominal bleeding. Although the risk of perforation is increased in procedures performed during the midtrimester, significant intraabdominal bleeding does not appear to increase with advancing gestational age at the time of the procedure (Grimes and associates, 1977b). While perforations most commonly occur in the mid-fundal region (Kaali and co-workers, 1989), the most serious ones occur laterally in the area of the lower uterine segment. Perforations in this area can result in serious bleeding from uterine artery injury. If a fundal perforation is identified intraoperatively, the procedure can frequently be completed under direct real-time ultrasound observation and guidance. Close postoperative patient observation for at least 2 hours should reveal whether any serious bleeding will occur. Although most perforations do not require treatment, if signs and symptoms of serious (>400 cc) intraabdominal hemorrhage (increased abdominal pain, altered vital signs, or changes in the hematocrit) are present, an exploratory laparotomy may be indicated, with definitive measures taken to correct any observed injury.

Another serious hazard of perforation is injury to various intraabdominal structures. Perforations with sounds or dilators are less likely to damage abdominal contents (Grimes, 1992a; Castadot, 1986). These injuries are more likely due to perforations caused by sharp or suction curettes, particularly those of large bore as used for midtrimester D&Es. Prevention of perforation entails careful evaluation of the patient, appropriate operator skill, and use of osmotic dilators, particularly at later gestations.

Cervical Lacerations. Cervical tears may occur during dilation of the cervix, from traumatic removal of fetal tissue or as a result of a tenaculum or other cervical stabilizer tearing through tissue. Reported rates of cervical injury range from 0.01 to 1.6/100 abortions (Cates, 1979; Schulz, 1983; Hakim-Elahi, 1990; and their colleagues). The lowest rates were noted for suction curettage (0.18–0.96), with higher rates reported for D&E at 13–20 weeks (1.16/100). The cervical injury rate for labor induction procedures was 0.55/100 abortions. Women with a previous abortion have a reduced risk of cervical injury, whereas women under age 17 were reported to have an increased risk. Although there is risk of serious injury, particularly at the time of mechanical dilation, such complications are uncommon. If minor, lacerations can be treated with applied pressure or with simple suture of the tear. Suture ligature using absorbable material at the cervicovaginal junctions at 3:00 and 9:00 will frequently include the descending cervical branch of the uterine artery and stop serious bleeding. Ultimately, if a site for the bleeding is not found, exploratory laparotomy is indicated. Effective prevention of cervical injuries include use of local anesthesia, osmotic dilators for gentle cervical dilation, and an atraumatic instrument to stabilize the cervix such as a Bierer tenaculum or a long

Allis clamp (Schulz and co-workers, 1983; Grimes, 1992a).

Hematometra. The so-called postabortion syndrome or postabortal hematometra may occur within minutes to several hours after a procedure, particularly among patients undergoing late first-trimester or early second-trimester suction curettage or D&E. The incidence of this condition has been reported to be 5/1000 induced abortions (Sands and co-workers, 1974). These women will subjectively have little visible bleeding, but have severe lower abdominal cramping pain. This crampiness is often accompanied by diaphoresis and syncopal episodes, both of which are vasovagal in origin. When examined, they will have an enlarged, tense, and tender uterus, and on speculum exam may have a few small dark clots in either the vagina or the cervical os. Treatment is prompt evacuation of the clotted material from the uterus and the use of methylergonovine to help contract the uterus. This provides almost instant pain relief. If vasovagal symptoms of bradycardia, hypotension, nausea, faintness, or diaphoresis are severe, atropine (0.4 mg IM or IV) may be indicated.

Vasovagal Symptoms

Vasovagal symptoms may also occur during an abortion procedure as a result of cervical stimulation or occasionally following paracervical block. The symptoms of syncope and the bradycardia usually clear within minutes. Although not recommended in all cases, prevention of this sometimes frightening complication is by use of atropine preoperatively.

Delayed Complications

Incomplete Abortion. Retained products of conception is one of the most important causes of abortion morbidity and may result in infection, bleeding, or both. It is usually manifested by continued vaginal bleeding of a greater than expected degree several days or even weeks after the procedure, often accompanied by cramping lower abdominal and back pain. The incidence after D&E is reported to be less than 1 percent, whereas that associated with instillation procedures may be as high as 36/100 procedures (Burkman, 1984; Grimes, 1977b; Hakim-Elahi, 1990; and their colleagues).

When a woman suspected of having this condition is examined, bleeding from the cervix will often be present; however, the os will only rarely be dilated. Bimanual pelvic exam will frequently show uterine tenderness and usually softening and enlargement. Ultrasound may help document the presence of tissue within the uterus. The suggested treatment is vacuum reaspiration using a cannula with a smaller diameter than that used initially for the procedure, followed by a therapeutic course of broad-spectrum antibiotics such as doxycycline 100 mg b.i.d. for 5–7 days.

Infection. Infection after induced abortion most frequently is secondary to retained products of conception. However, endometritis or pelvic peritonitis may occur in the absence of retained tissue, particularly among women who have a preexisting gonococcal or chlamydia infection. Definitions vary, but if specified as temperature of ≥38° C for 1 or more days, rates reported following suction curettage are 0.75 percent, for D&E 1.5 percent, and for instillation 5.0 percent (Kafrissen, 1984; Binkin, 1983; and their colleagues). Women are at increased risk of postabortal infection if their abortion is performed late in pregnancy, if labor induction methods are used instead of D&E, or if local rather than general anesthesia is used for suction curettage (CDC, 1978; Grimes and co-workers, 1979a).

Symptoms and signs often include lower abdominal pain and fever as well as increased bleeding and lower abdominal cramps, especially if retained tissue is present. On examination a firm, small, but tender uterus usually suggests infection with absence of retained tissue. If the uterus is softened, and slightly enlarged as well as tender, there may be infection with retained tissue present. Ultrasound is useful to determine whether reaspiration as well as antibiotics are indicated or whether the woman can be treated with antibiotics alone. In either case, a regimen combining parenteral and oral antibiotics is suggested, using broad-spectrum antibiotics like ceftriaxone 250 mg IM for one dose followed by a 10-day course of doxycycline 100 mg b.i.d. If clinical indicators are more severe, that is, fever >38° C, nausea, vomiting, or signs of severe peritoneal irritation are present, the patient should be hospitalized for observation and treatment with intravenous fluids and a standard course of antibiotics for pelvic inflammatory disease. Studies have indicated that the organisms responsible for postabortal infection are similar to those for other gynecologic infections (Heistberger, 1988). The most frequent isolates reported are group B (beta)-hemolytic streptococci, *Bacteroides* species, *Neisseria gonorrhea, E. coli,* and *Staphylococcus aureus* (Burkman and associates, 1977a). The risk of postabortal infections can be minimized by pre-procedure gonorrhea and chlamydia treatment, if indicated (Burkman, 1976; Moller, 1982; and their co-workers), treatment of cervicitis, complete emptying of the uterus, and antibiotic prophylaxis (Grimes, 1984b; Sonne-Holm, 1981; and their colleagues).

Continuing Pregnancy. Failure to interrupt an intrauterine pregnancy is a rare occurrence following an elective induced abortion (0.1–0.3%) (CDC, 1985). It is more often a problem associated with attempted interruption of an earlier pregnancy but can occur even when chorionic villi are confirmed histologically following a routine induced-abortion procedure. Occasionally, a continuing pregnancy will occur if twin pregnancies are not initially identified and are incompletely aspirated. Such procedures are purposefully conducted when fetal reduction is desired to enhance fetal outcomes among infertile women whose pregnancies have been assisted with fertility drugs. The best way to prevent this occurrence in the majority of instances is to carefully examine tissue following the procedure to verify placental and fetal tissue. It is also good practice to perform a careful 2-week postoperative pelvic examination on each woman who has undergone an elective abortion procedure.

Other Complications. Several other complications of abortion have been reported, such as venous thrombophlebitis, pulmonary embolism, severe coagulopathies like disseminated intravascular coagulation (DIC), anesthesia complications, hypernatremia, water intoxication, and a liveborn fetus. For the most part, however, good population-based data are not available to assess the attributable risk of these conditions. Only abortion mortality data attest to the severity of these rare complications.

The incidence of thromboembolism, air embolism, and amniotic fluid embolism during and after abortion is not known. However, amniotic fluid embolism has been identified as an important complication of induced abortion (Grimes and Cates, 1977).

Coagulation defects, previously believed to be associated only with hypertonic saline, now appear to be associated with other hypertonic abortifacients, as well as late D&E procedures—implying that the syndrome may not be restricted to labor induction methods (Burkman and associates, 1977b; Grundy and Craven, 1976; Koplik, 1977). This condition occurs at a rate of 0.3/100 saline abortions (Grimes and co-workers, 1977c); oxytocin administration appears to increase the risk of coagulopathy fivefold during saline abortion (Cohen and Ballard, 1974). The incidence of coagulopathies among women who received intraamniotic urea augmented by oxytocin or prostaglandin $F_{2\alpha}$ was 0.12/100 abortions (Burkman and associates, 1977b).

Hypernatremia is a very rare, but overemphasized, complication of saline abortion. Only two cases of hypernatremia were reported among over 24,000 saline abortions in the first two phases of JPSA, yielding an incidence of less than 1/10,000 abortions (Grimes and co-workers, 1977c; Tietze and Lewit, 1972).

Water intoxication is usually iatrogenic and therefore an entirely preventable complication of abortion. Most women who have developed water intoxication have been given a high-dose oxytocin infusion mixed in electrolyte-free solutions over long time periods. Administering oxytocin in buffered saline solutions will reduce the risk of water intoxication, as has been demonstrated in animal studies (Lauersen and Birnbaum, 1975).

The incidence of liveborn fetuses following induced abortions has been reported to be 1.7/1000 procedures after saline instillation procedures and hysterotomies (Pakter and Nelson, 1972; Stroh and Hinman, 1976). The two factors contributing most to the likelihood of producing a viable liveborn are the choice of abortion technique and gestational age. Postabortal live births increase with advancing gestation (Stroh and Hinman, 1976). Prior to wide use of ultrasound, the provider's underestimation of the length of gestation contributed substantially to this problem.

Whereas hypertonic saline solutions are feticidal, and the time of fetal death in utero is related to the concentration of sodium chloride in the amniotic fluid (Stroh and Hinman, 1976), prostaglandin $F_{2\alpha}$ is not. As a result, fetuses aborted by prostaglandin are more likely to be alive and to have a better prospect for long-term survival (Grimes, 1979).

Late Complications

A variety of adverse reproductive health outcomes have been ascribed anecdotally to legal induced abortion. They include sterility, menstrual disorders, and psychiatric conditions as well as an increase in the incidence of premature births, tubal ectopic pregnancies, stillbirths, birth defects, and spontaneous abortion in subsequent pregnancies. Because the number of induced abortions performed every year is very large, even a minor increase of risk associated with induced abortion would have a significant public health implication.

Although some reproductive complications may be associated with previous induced abortions, the recent scientific literature agrees that most induced abortions have little, if any, physical impact on the woman. Many of the published studies have serious limitations; some were conducted in countries where abortion has not been legalized, such as Greece, Israel, and Taiwan, whereas others failed to control adequately for factors known to contribute to the immediate and long-term complications of induced abortion. Such factors include the patients' demographic profile and medical risk factors, the surgeons' experience and skill, type of anesthesia, type and amount of cervical dilation, type and size of instrumentation, length of operative procedure, type of abortifacient selected, type of facility or service, use of prophylactic antibiotics, and concurrent sterilization (Hogue and associates, 1982, 1983; Cates, 1979; Atrash and Hogue, 1990).

Moreover, several methodologic problems arise in examining the risk of adverse pregnancy outcomes following an induced abortion. The most important considerations include the choice of an appropriate comparison group, the number of previous induced abortions, the type of procedure used to perform the abortion, and the gestational age at the time of abortion (Atrash and Hogue, 1990).

The choice of an appropriate comparison group has been a subject of dispute. A woman who becomes pregnant after an induced abortion with her first pregnancy (gravida 2 para 0) is unlike a woman who is pregnant for the first time (gravida 1 para 0) and also unlike a woman who is pregnant for the second time but whose first pregnancy was carried to term (gravida 2 para 1). Yet there is no perfect comparison group, and women who are pregnant after an induced abortion have been compared with women who are pregnant for the first time and with women who are pregnant for the second time and whose first pregnancy resulted in a live birth (Atrash and Hogue, 1990).

Although a history of previous induced abortion has been shown to contribute to an increased risk of late effects of abortion (Atrash and Hogue, 1990), very few studies have considered the number of previous abortions when looking at the risk of adverse pregnancy outcomes. The type of procedure used to terminate a pregnancy has also been found to be an important contributing factor to the increased risk of adverse pregnancy outcomes in future pregnancies. Yet many reports have not examined the risk of late effects by type of procedure. Furthermore, because both gestational age and type of procedure have been determined to be independent risk factors for immediate short-term complications of induced abortion (Grimes, 1979), and because most studies failed to control for gestational age when reporting procedure-specific complications, it is not possible to determine whether the increased risk of adverse pregnancy outcomes among women whose pregnancies were terminated by D&E procedures during the midtrimester results from the gestational age at the time of the procedure or the method.

Secondary Infertility. A review of the world literature concluded that induced abortion is not associated with an increased incidence of secondary infertility (Atrash and Hogue, 1990). The most recent prospective studies on the association between induced abortion and secondary infertility were published in 1984, 1985, and 1993 (WHO, 1984; Stubblefield, 1984; Daling, 1985; Cramer, 1985; Frank, 1993; and their colleagues). All five studies concluded that there is no significant effect of induced abortion on secondary infertility. Furthermore, in two studies (Hogue, 1978; Stubblefield, 1984; and their co-workers), fertility was found to be greater among women following their abortions as indicated by significantly shorter interpregnancy intervals. In Stubblefield's report, the indication of greater fecundity was evident only for women who had three or more previous induced abortions. Because women who experience an unwanted pregnancy are likely to be among the more fertile group of women (Hogue and associates, 1978), finding shorter interpregnancy intervals among this group is not surprising.

Ectopic Pregnancy. The temporal association between a dramatic increase in the numbers of induced abortions and the numbers of ectopic pregnancies in the United States (Lawson and associates, 1989a; CDC, 1992) raises a question of whether a portion of the ectopic pregnancy increase could be associated with prior induced abortion. Studies evaluating this issue have yielded inconsistent results, have often been carried out in settings with dissimilar practices, or have used methodology or samples that are inadequate to evaluate critical issues. Available evidence does not support an overall etiologic relationship between legal induced abortion and subsequent ectopic pregnancy (Hogue and co-workers, 1982; Atrash and Hogue, 1990). However, only a few, small case-control studies have attempted to evaluate this relationship. The strongest associations between induced abortion and ectopic pregnancy were observed in studies with small numbers of ectopic pregnancy cases, studies that failed to control for important risk factors, and studies conducted in countries where abortion was illegal (Sawazaki and Tanaka, 1966; Shinagawa and Nagayama, 1969; Panayotou and associates, 1972; Dziewulska, 1973; Hren and associates, 1974). Other studies reported a significant increase in the incidence of ectopic pregnancy after abortions that were complicated by infection or retained products of conception (Chung and co-workers, 1982). If there is an etiologic relationship, it is likely mediated through infection (either preexisting and untreated or postabortion infection). Because infection is a relatively rare complication of induced abortion, small case-control studies could miss this subset of susceptible women.

Spontaneous Abortion. Because it is very difficult to detect first-trimester spontaneous abortions, most studies of first-trimester spontaneous abortion following induced abortion have been seriously flawed (Hogue and colleagues, 1982). As a result, most of our current knowledge pertains to the incidence of midtrimester spontaneous abortion following induced abortion.

Most studies have concluded that vacuum aspiration, commonly used to terminate pregnancies during the first trimester, carries no increased risk of spontaneous abortion, whereas D&E, during the midtrimester, is associated with a significantly increased risk of spontaneous abortion (Atrash and Hogue, 1990).

Premature Delivery. Independent of the type of procedure, the relative risk of premature delivery was higher among women having induced abortion when compared with gravida 2 para 1 women, than when compared with gravida 1 para 0 women, although in neither case were the differences statistically significant (Atrash and Hogue, 1990). This observation suggests that women whose first pregnancy was terminated by induced abortion have a higher risk of low birthweight than women who carried their first pregnancy to term; and therefore, induced abortion is not protective of the well-known risk of low birthweight for firstborn offspring.

Low Birthweight. Overall, studies have shown no significantly increased risk of low birthweight following abortions performed using vacuum aspiration. However, D&E has been found in most reports to be associated with an increased risk of low birthweight (Hogue and associates, 1982; Atrash and Hogue, 1990). Similar to the risk of premature delivery, the reported relative risk of low birthweight was higher when women with abortions induced by vacuum aspiration were compared with gravida 2 para 1 women than when they were compared with gravida 1 para 0 women (Atrash and Hogue, 1990). Similarly, the relative risk of low birthweight following D&E procedures were higher in comparison to parous women than in comparison to nulliparous women (Atrash and Hogue, 1990).

Psychologic Effects. Numerous researchers have attempted to determine the extent to which abortion results in psychologic problems. Some reported that a large number of women having an abortion experience severe emotional problems subsequently, as a result of the procedure. Some consider what has been called "postabortion syndrome" to be a form of posttraumatic stress disorder, even though abortion does not meet the American Psychiatric Association's definition of trauma (Gold, 1990).

After reviewing more than 250 studies of the psychologic outcomes of abortion, former Surgeon General C. Everett Koop concluded in 1989 that most research in this area has serious flaws and cannot support the contention that abortion is dangerous to women's mental health (Congressional Record, Mar. 21, 1989, p. E908, in Gold, 1990).

Other Late Complications. Placenta previa has been studied as a possible late sequela of induced abortion. One case-control study reported a 10-fold higher risk (Barrett and coworkers, 1981). However, a later study, which accounted for the potential confounding risk factors of gravidity and age, in a predominantly black population, found the relative risk to be 1.1 and not statistically significant (Grimes and Techman, 1984). In a prospective cohort study, Frank and colleagues (1987) conducted a 10-year follow-up of 6418 women who had an induced abortion and 8059 women who had an unplanned pregnancy but did not terminate the pregnancy. Pregnancies occurred among 729 women in the case group and 1754 women in the control group. The researchers reported that prior induced abortion had no material effect on the rate of pregnancy-related morbidity (including hemorrhage before labor, mental illness, preeclampsia, hemorrhage in labor, feto-pelvic disproportion, trauma at delivery, forceps delivery, cesarean section, and fetal distress). However, the incidence of anemia of pregnancy was found to be significantly reduced, whereas the incidence of urinary tract infection was significantly increased.

SUMMARY

Since abortion is among the most frequent outcomes of human conception, it deserves careful consideration, in terms of provider attention to the needs of women and careful monitoring for serious complications. Only through maintaining access to safe skilled abortion services in the United States can we ensure that women will not face the risk of serious complications and death from the absence of or inadequate performance of these procedures. Training providers to perform these procedures and providing them with the necessary protection from forces that desire to endanger their lives is necessary, while additional strides are made to develop contraceptives that are safe and widely accepted.

REFERENCES

The Alan Guttmacher Institute (AGI). Stanely Henshaw S, Van Vort J, eds. Abortion services in the United States, each state and metropolitan area, 1984–1985. New York: AGI, 1988.

Atrash HK, Lawson H, Smith JC. Legal abortion in the United States: trends and mortality. Contemporary Ob/Gyn 1990; 35:58.

Atrash HK, Hogue CJR. The effect of pregnancy termination on future reproduction. In: Bygdeman M, ed. Medical Induction of Abortion, Baillaire's Clinics in Obstetrics and Gynecology. Vol 4. 1990: 391.

Avrech OM, Golan A, Weinraub Z, et al. Mifepristone (RU486) alone or in combination with a prostaglandin analogue for termination of early pregnancy: a review. Fertil Steril 1991; Sept.

Aubeny E. RU486 combined with PG analogs in voluntary termination of pregnancy. Adv Contraception 1991; Dec.

Barrett JM, Boehm FH, Killam AP. Induced abortion: a risk factor for placenta previa. Am J Obstet Gynec 1981; 141:769.

Berger GS, Edelman DA. Oxytocin administration, instillation to abortion time, and morbidity associated with saline instillation. Am J Obstet Gynecol 121:941, 1975.

Beresford T. Short term relationship counseling. Baltimore, Planned Parenthood of Maryland, 1978.

Binkin NJ, Schulz KF, Grimes DA, Cates W Jr. Urea-prostaglandin versus hypertonic saline for instillation abortion. Am J Obstet Gynecol 1983; 146:947.

Bracken MB. Psychosomatic aspects of abortion: implications for counseling. J Reprod Med 1977; 19:265.

Buehler JW, Schulz KF, Grimes DA, Hogue CJR. The risk of serious complications from induced abortion: do personal characteristics make a difference? Am J Obstet Gynecol 1985; 153:14.

Burgess L, Churchirillo L. A Resource Manual for Abortion Counselors. Franconia, NH: Preterm Institute, 1976.

Burkman RT, Tonascia JA, Atienza MF, King TM. Untreated endocervical gonorrhea and endometritis following elective abortion. Am J Obstet Gynecol 1976; 126:648.

Burkman RT, Atienza MF, King TM. Culture and treatment results in endometritis following elective abortion. Am J Obstet Gynecol 1977a; 128:556.

Burkman RT, Bell WR, Atienza MF, King TM (1977b). Coagulopathy with midtrimester induced abortion: association with hyperosmolar urea administration. Am J Obstet Gynecol 1977b; 127:533.

Burkman RT, King TM. Second trimester termination of pregnancy. In: Symonds EM, Zuspan FP, eds. Clinical and Diagnostic Procedures in Obstetrics and Gynecology. Part B: Gynecology. New York: Marcel Dekker, 1984: 241.

Castadot RG. Pregnancy termination: techniques, risks, and complications and their management. Fertil Steril 1986; 45:5.

Cates W Jr. Late effects of induced abortion: hypothesis or knowledge? J Reprod Med 1979; 22:207.

Cates W Jr, Schulz KF, Grimes DA, Tyler CW Jr. Short-term complications of uterine evacuation techniques for abortion at 12 weeks' gestation or earlier. In: Zatuchni GI, Sciarra JJ, Speidel JJ, eds. Pregnancy Termination Procedures, Safety and New Developments. Hagerstown, MD: Harper & Row, 1979: 127.

Cates W Jr, Grimes DA. Morbidity and mortality of abortion in the United States. In: Hodgson SE, ed. Abortion and Sterilization: Medical and Social Aspects. London: Academic Press, 1981: 155.

Centers for Disease Control (CDC). Abortion Surveillance 1975. Atlanta: CDC, 1977.

Centers for Disease Control (CDC). Abortion Surveillance 1976. Atlanta: CDC, 1978.

Centers for Disease Control (CDC). Abortion Surveillance 1981. Atlanta: CDC, 1985.

Centers for Disease Control and Prevention (CDC). Abortion surveillance—United States, 1990. Morbid Mortal Weekly Rev 1992; 41:936.

Cervest AM, Haspels AA. Preliminary results with the anti-progestational compound RU486 for interruption of early pregnancy. Fertil Steril 1985; 44:627.

Chen P, Lols A. Population and birth planning in the People's Republic of China. Popul Rep J 1982; 10:J-594.

Chung CS, Smith RG, Steinhoff PG, et al. Induced abortion and ectopic pregnancy in subsequent pregnancies. Am J Epidemiol 1982; 115:879.

Cohen E, Ballard CA. Consumptive coagulopathy associated with intraamniotic saline instillation and the effect of intravenous oxytocin. Obstet Gynecol 1974; 43:300.

Couzinet B, et al. Termination of early pregnancy by progesterone antagonist RU486 (Mifepristone). N Engl J Med 1986; 315:1565.

Cramer DW, Schiff I, Schoenbaum SC, et al. Tubal infertility and the intrauterine device. N Engl J Med 1985; 312:941.

Creinin MD, Darney PD. Methotrexate and misoprostol for early abortion. Contraception 1993; 48:339.

Daling JR, Weiss NS, Voigt L, et al. Tubal infertility in relation to prior induced abortion. Fertil Steril 1985; 43:389.

Darney PD, Landy U, MacPherson S, Sweet RL. Abortion training in U.S. obstetrics and gynecology residency programs. Fam Plann Perspect 1987; 19:158.

Darney PD. Midtrimester abortion under ultrasound guidance. Proceedings of a Post Graduate Course, National Abortion Federation, Tampa, FL, Jan. 31, 1983.

Darney PD. First trimester uterine evacuation technique. In: Darney PD, ed. Handbook of Office and Ambulatory Gynecologic Surgery. Oradell, NJ: Medical Economics Books, 1987: 132.

David HP. Induced abortion: psychosocial aspects. In: Sciarra JJ, Zatuchni GI, Daly MJ, eds. Gynecology and Obstetrics, Vol. 6. Hagerstown, MD: Harper & Row, 1982: 7.

Donaldson M, Dorflinger L, Brown S, Benet L, eds. Clinical Applications of Mifepristone (RU-486) and Other Antiprogestins—Institute of Medicine Report. Washington, DC: National Academy Press, 1993.

Dziewulska W. Abortion in the past versus the fate of the subsequent pregnancy. Ginekologia Polska 1973; 44:1003.

Forrest JD, Henshaw SK. The harassment of U.S. abortion providers. Fam Plann Perspect 1987; 19:9.

Frank PI, Kay CR, Scott LM, et al. Pregnancy following induced abortion: maternal morbidity, congenital abnormalities and neonatal death. Royal College of General Practitioners/Royal College of Obstetricians and Gynaecologists Joint Study. Br J Obstet Gynaecol 1987; 94:836.

Frank PI, McNamee R, Hannaford PC, et al. The effect of induced abortion on subsequent fertility. Br J Obstet Gynecol 1993; 100:575.

Garfield RE, Baulieu EE. The antiprogesterone steroid RU 486: a short pharmacological and clinical review, with emphasis on the interruption of pregnancy. Clin Endocrinol Metab 1987; Feb.

Gold, RB. Abortion and Women's Health: A Turning Point for America. New York: The Alan Guttmacher Institute, 1990.

Grimes DA. Complications from legally induced abortion: a review. Obstet Gynecol Surv 1979; 34:177.

Grimes DA. Surgical management of abortion. In: Thompson JD, Rock JA, eds. Te Linde's Operative Gynecology. 7th ed. Philadelphia: J.B. Lippincott, 1992a: 317.

Grimes DA. Clinicians who provide abortions: the thinning ranks. Obstet Gynecol 1992b; 80:719.

Grimes DA, Cates Jr. Fatal amniotic fluid embolism during induced abortion 1972–1975. South Med J 1997; 70:1325.

Grimes DA, Techman T. Legal abortion and placenta previa. Am J Obstet Gynecol 1984; 149:501.

Grimes DA, Schulz KF, Cates W Jr, Tyler CW Jr. Methods of midtrimester abortion: which is safest? Int J Gynaecol Obstet 1977a; 15:184.

Grimes DA, Schulz KF, Cates W Jr, Tyler CW Jr. Midtrimester abortion by dilatation and evacuation. N Engl J Med 1979b; 296:1141.

Grimes DA, Schulz KF, Cates W Jr, Tyler CW Jr. Midtrimester abortion by intraamniotic prostaglandin: safer than saline? Obstet Gynecol 1977c; 49:612.

Grimes DA, Schulz KF, Cates W Jr, Tyler CW. The Joint Program for the Study of Abortion/CDC: a preliminary analysis. In: Hern W, Andrikopoulos B, eds. Abortion in the Seventies. New York: National Abortion Federation, 1977d: 41.

Grimes DA, Schulz KF, Cates W Jr, Tyler CW Jr. Local versus general anesthesia: which is safer for performing suction curettage abortions? Am J Obstet Gynecol 1979; 135:1030.

Grimes DA, Schulz KF, Cates W Jr. Prevention of perforation during curettage abortion. JAMA 1984a; 251:2108.

Grimes DA, Schulz KF, Cates W Jr. Prophylactic antibiotics for curettage abortion. Am J Obstet Gynecol 1984b; 150:689.

Grimes DA, et al. Early abortion with a single dose of the antiprogestin RU486. Am J Obstet Gynecol 1988; 158:1307.

Grimes DA, Mishell DR Jr, David HP. A randomized clinical trial of mifepristone (RU486) for induction of delayed menses: efficacy and acceptability. Contraception 1992; Jul.

Grimes DA, Forrest JD, Kirckman AL, Radford B. An epidemic of anbtiabortion violence in the United States. Am J Obstet Gynecol 1991; 165:1263.

Grundy MFB, Craven ER. Consumption coagulopathy after intraamniotic urea. Br Med J 1976; 2:677.

Hakim-Elahi E, Tovell HMM, Burnhill MS. Complications of first-trimester abortion: a report of 170,000 cases. Obstet Gynecol 1990; 76:129.

Henshaw SK. Accessibility of abortion services in the United States. Fam Plan Perspect 1991; 23:246.

Henshaw SK, Silverman J. The characteristics and prior contraceptive use of U.S. abortion patients. Fam Plan Perspect 1988; 20:158.

Henshaw SK, Van Vort J. Abortion services in the United States, 1987 and 1988. Fam Plan Perspect 1990; 22:102.

Henshaw SK, Forrest JD, Van Vort J. Abortion services in the United States, 1984 and 1985. Fam Plann Perspect 1987; 19:63.

Heistberger L. Pelvic inflammatory disease following induced first trimester abortion. Dan Med Bull 1988; 35:64.

Hern WM. Abortion Practice. J.B. Lippincott, Philadelphia: 1984.

Hern WM, Zen C, Ferguson KA, et al. Outpatient abortion for fetal anomaly and fetal death from 15–34 weeks' gestation: techniques and clinical management. Obstet Gynecol 1993; 81:301.

Hodgson JE, Major B, Portman K, et al. Prophylactic use of tetracycline for first trimester abortions. Obstet Gynecol 1975; 45:574.

Hogue CJ, Schoenfelder JR, Gesler WM, et al. The interactive effects of induced abortion, inter-pregnancy interval, and contraceptive use on subsequent pregnancy outcome. Am J Epidemiol 1978; 107:15.

Hogue CJR, Cates W Jr, Tietze C. The effects of induced abortion on subsequent reproduction. Epidemiol Rev 1982; 4:66.

Hogue CJR, Cates W Jr, Tietze C. Impact of vacuum aspiration abortion on future childbearing: a review. Fam Plann Perspect 1983; 15:119.

Hren M, Tomazevic T, Seigel D. Ectopic pregnancy. In: Andolsck L, ed. The Ljubljana Abortion Study, 1971–1973. Bethesda, MD: Center for Population Research, National Institutes of Health, 1974: 34.

Ivanisevic M, Djelmis J. Amniotic fluid and maternal plasma prostaglandins in hypertonic saline-induced abortion. Int J Gynaecol Obstet 1990; 31(4): 355.

Ivey AE. Microcounselling: Innovations in Interviewing Training, Springfield, IL: Charles C Thomas, 1975.

Kaali SG, Szigetvari IA, Bartfai GS (1989). The frequency and management of uterine perforations during first-trimester abortions. Am J Obstet Gynecol 1989; 161:406.

Kafrissen ME, Schulz KF, Grimes DA, Cates W Jr. Midtrimester abortion, intrauterine instillation of hyperosmolar urea and prostaglandin $F_{2\alpha}$ versus dilatation and evacuation. JAMA 1984; 251:916.

Kaunitz AM, Rovira EZ, Grimes DA, et al. Abortions that fail. Obstet Gynecol 1985; 66:533.

Kerenyi TD, Mandelaman N, Sherman DH. Five thousand consecutive saline abortions. Am J Obstet Gynecol 1973; 116:593.

Koplik L. Disseminated intravascular coagulation after a dilatation and evacuation abortion at 16 weeks' gestation. Presented at the Annual Meeting of the National Abortion Federation, Denver, CO, October 3, 1977.

Lauersen NH, Birnbaum S. Water intoxication associated with oxytocin administration during saline-induced abortion. Am J Obstet Gynecol 1975; 121:2.

Laufe LE. The menstrual regulation procedure. Stud Fam Plann 1977; 8:253.
Lawson HW, Atrash HK, Saftlas AF, Finch EL. Ectopic pregnancy in the United States, 1970–1986. MMWR Surv Sum 1989a; 38(SS-2):1.
Lawson HW, Atrash HK, Saftlas AF, et al. Abortion surveillance, United States, 1984–1985. MMWR Surv Sum 1989b; 38(SS-2):11.
Lawson HW, Frye A, Atrash HK, et al. Abortion mortality, United States, 1972–1987. In press.
Levallois P, Rioux JE. Prophylactic antibiotics for suction curettage abortion: results of a clinical controlled trial. Am J Obstet Gynecol 1988; 158:100.
McFarland DR. Induced abortion: an historical overview. Gynecol Health 1993; 7:25.
Moller BR, Ahrons S, Laurin J, Mardh P. Pelvic infection after elective abortion associated with *Chlamydia trachomatis.* Obstet Gynecol 1982; 59:210.
Osborn JF, Arisi E, Spinelli A, Stazi MA. General anesthesia, a risk factor for complication following induced abortion? Eur J Epidemiol 1990; 6:416.
Pakter J, Nelson FG. Effects of a liberalized abortion law in New York City. Mt Sinai J Med 1972; 39:535.
Panayotou PP, Kaskarelis DB, Miettinen OS, et al. Induced abortion and ectopic pregnancy. Am J Obstet Gynecol 1972; 114:507.
Rodger MW, Logan AF, Baird DT. Induction of early abortion with mifepristone (RU486) and two different doses of prostaglandin pessary (gemeprost). Contraception 1989; May.
Sands RX, Burnill MS, Hakim-Kelahi E. Post-abortal uterine atony. Obstet Gynecol 1974; 43:595.
Sawazaki C, Tanaka S. The relationship between artificial abortion and extrauterine pregnancy. In: Koya Y, ed. Harmful Effects of Induced Abortion. Tokyo: Family Planning Association of Japan, 1966: 49.
Schulz KF, Grimes DA, Cates W Jr. Measures to prevent cervical injury during suction curettage abortion. Lancet 1983; 1:1182.
Schulz KF, Grimes DA, Park T, Flock M. Prophylactic antibiotics to prevent febrile complications of curettage abortion. Paper presented at 8th Annual Meeting of the National Abortion Federation, Los Angeles, CA, May 15, 1984.
Sheeran PJ. Women, Society, the State and Abortion: A Structuralist Analysis. New York: Praeger, 1987.
Shinagawa S, Nagayama M. Cervical pregnancy as a possible sequela of induced abortion. Report of 19 cases. Am J Obstet Gynecol 1969; 105:282.
Sonne-Holm S, Heisterberg L, Hebjorn S, et al. Prophylactic antibiotics in first-trimester abortions: a clinical controlled trial. Am J Obstet Gynecol 1981; 139:693.
Stewart GK, Goldstein SP. Medical and surgical complications of therapeutic abortion. Obstet Gynecol 1972; 51:318.
Stovall TG, Ling FW. Single-dose methrotrexate: an expanded clinical trial. Am J Obstet Gynecol 1993; 168:1759.
Stovall TG, Ling FW, Gray LA. Single-dose methotrexate for treatment of ectopic pregnancy. Obstet Gynecol 1991; 77:754.
Stroh G, Hinman AR. Reported live births following induced abortion: two and one-half years' experience in Upstate New York. Am J Obstet Gynecol 1976; 126:8390.
Stubblefield PG. Pregnancy termination. In: Gabbe SG, Niebyl JR, Simpson JL, eds. Obstetrics. Normal and Problem Pregnancies. New York: Churchill Livingstone, 1986:1051.
Stubblefield PG, Monson RR, Schoenbaum SC, et al. Fertility after induced abortion: a prospective follow-up study. Obstet Gynecol 1984; 63:186.
Swahn ML, Gottlieb C, Green K, Bygdeman M. Oral administration of RU 486 and 9 methylene PGE_2 for termination of early pregnancy. Contraception, 1990; May.
Tietze C, Lewit S. Joint program for the study of abortion (JPSA): early medical complications of legal abortion. Stud Fam Plann 1972; 3:97.
Torres A, Forrest JD. Why do women have abortions? Fam Plan Perspect 1988; 20:169.
Van Look PFA. Postovulatory methods of fertility regulation. Research in Human Reproduction; Biennial Report 1986–87, Geneva: WHO, 1988: 153.
Westfall JM, Kallail KJ, Walling AD. Abortion attitudes and practices of family and general practice physicians. J Fam Pract 1991; 33:47.
Westhoff C, Marks F, Rosenfield A. Residency training in contraception, sterilization and abortion. Obstet Gynecol 1993; 81:311.
World Health Organization Task Force on Sequelae of Abortion, Special Programme of Research, Development and Research Training in Human Reproduction. Secondary infertility following induced abortion. Stud Fam Plann 1984; 15:291.
Wu S, Gao J, Wu Y, et al. Clinical trial on termination of early pregnancy with RU486 in combination with prostaglandin. Contraception, 1992; Sept.

CHAPTER 34

Multifetal Pregnancy Reduction

As a by-product of successful assisted reproductive technology, substantial numbers of women have conceived three or more fetuses over the past several years. These pregnancies are at increased risk for a variety of problems, but preterm delivery poses the greatest threat to the fetus. The chance of delivering prematurely is directly proportional to the number of fetuses present, that is, as a group, triplets deliver earlier than twins, quadruplets earlier than triplets, and so on. This suggests that the preterm labor in these patients is a consequence of factors that might be favorably affected by simply reducing the number of fetuses present. The procedure referred to as multifetal pregnancy reduction (MPR) was designed to achieve that objective. The intent of this chapter is to present the rationale for performing this procedure, describe technical aspects of how it is accomplished, review its success, and briefly discuss some attending ethical issues.

Before proceeding, however, a brief discussion of nomenclature is in order. The predecessor of fetal reduction procedures was the termination of an anomalous twin in utero within the time frame that an elective abortion could be performed. This type of procedure, whether performed in a twin pregnancy or one with more fetuses, has become known as a selective termination. The term is appropriate because when one fetus in a multifetal pregnancy is known to be abnormal it is "selected" for termination, and that selection is in fact the reason for doing the procedure. In the original series of fetal reductions performed in the first trimester the authors referred to the procedure as "selective abortion" (Dumez and Oury, 1986), but this simply meant that some apparently normal fetuses were chosen to be terminated while others were left undisturbed. In these procedures the determining factor in the selection process is physical accessibility as opposed to anything intrinsic to the fetuses themselves. Selection in this context is clearly very different from that which occurs when one twin is abnormal. Unfortunately, some authors failed to recognize this distinction, and early descriptions of the first trimester procedures refer to them as "selective reductions." In an editorial written in 1990, Berkowitz and Lynch describe a situation in which a national television network planned to promote a program about this procedure by asking the viewer how he or she would feel if it were necessary for them to decide which fetus "they would kill" if they were confronted with a high-order multifetal pregnancy. The implication was that someone, perhaps the patient, has to make a kind of "Sophie's choice" in selecting which fetuses should be reduced. As a result of this experience, it was suggested that the first trimester procedures described in this chapter be differentiated from selective terminations by referring to them as multifetal pregnancy reductions. The term *multifetal pregnancy reduction* says what it means and does not imply anything else. Reading of the recent literature indicates that this concept has been accepted, and it has been adopted in the most recent committee opinion on the subject (Committee on Ethics, 1991).

NATURAL HISTORY OF MULTIFETAL GESTATIONS

Four series published between 1988 and 1990 present natural history data on 332 sets of triplets (Australian In-Vitro Fertilization Collaborative Group, 1988; Lipitz, 1989; Newman, 1989; Gonen, 1990; and their associates). In these reports delivery occurred at less than 37 weeks in 86–100 percent of cases, at less than 32 weeks in 20–39 percent of cases, and between 24 and 28 weeks in 3–10 percent of cases. The last interval is of greatest concern, of course, because of the increased possibility that surviving fetuses born at that time may suffer irreversible damage as a consequence of their severe prematurity. The mean age of delivery for all infants in these series was 33 weeks, which is precisely the same as that of 110 sets of triplet neonates described in three earlier publications with cases going back as far as 1946 (Itzkowic, 1979; Holcberg and associates, 1982; Syrop and Varner, 1985).

Recent publications have made the issue somewhat more confusing. Porreco and coworkers (1991) prospectively compared 13 women with triplets who underwent MPR to twins with 11 patients whose triplet pregnancies were followed expectantly. The mean gestational ages at delivery were 35.5 and 35.7 weeks, and the mean birthweights were 2227 and 2239 g, respectively. Furthermore, neonatal and maternal complications as well as neonatal hospital days were not statistically different in the two groups. On the other hand, Macones and colleagues (1993) compared 14 nonreduced triplet pregnancies with 47 triplet pregnancies reduced to twins and 63 nonreduced twin gestations and found statistically significant different mean ages at delivery (31.2, 35.6, and 34.8 weeks, respectively), mean birthweights (1592, 2217, and 2292 g, respectively), and perinatal mortality rates per 1000 live births (210, 30, and 40, respectively). Sassoon and colleagues (1990) compared 15 unreduced triplet and twin pregnancies that were matched for maternal age, race, type of medical insurance, delivery mode, parity, and history of previous preterm delivery. These authors found that the women with triplets had significantly higher preterm delivery rates (87 vs 26.7%), and neonatal hospital stays (29 vs 8.5 days), with lower mean birthweights (1720 vs 2475 g), and mean gestational ages at delivery (33 vs 36.6 weeks). However, no significant differences in maternal morbidity or major neonatal complications were noted. Finally, Vohra and associates (1994) have compared 19 unreduced triplet pregnancies with 38 matched twin controls and found that the former had statistically significant increases in preterm labor (63 vs 18%), maternal antepartum admissions (84 vs 37%), mean antepartum stay per patient (17 vs 3 days), Neonatal Intensive Care Unit admissions (63 vs 40%), and mean neonatal stay (15 vs 9 days), with significantly lower gestational age at delivery (34.2 vs 36.4 weeks), and mean birth weights (1947 vs 2411 g). No differences in major neonatal complications were detected, but the financial costs of caring for the triplet pregnancies were approximately 3.4 times higher than that for the twins due to more frequent and longer maternal hospitalizations, greater number of admissions to the NICU, and longer neonatal stays.

Much less data is available for quadruplets. Four series (Gonen, 1990; Vervliet, 1989; Lipitz, 1990; Collins, 1990; and their associates) reporting the outcome of a total of 89 sets of quadruplets indicate that 98 percent delivered earlier than 37 weeks, 57 percent at less than 32 weeks, and 22 percent between 24 and 28 weeks. Virtually nothing but case reports describe the outcome of pregnancies with five or more fetuses, but presumably the perinatal outcome in those cases is considerably worse than for quadruplets.

While controversy certainly exists about the benefits of offering MPR to patients with triplets, there is very little doubt that the risks of delivering extremely premature infants for patients carrying four or more fetuses are excessively high.

TECHNICAL ASPECTS

In 1986 Dumez and Oury published a series of 15 multifetal pregnancies reduced to four singletons, 10 sets of twins, and one set of triplets. The technique employed consisted of transcervical aspiration of one or more sacs under ultrasound guidance. At the time the report was written nine women had delivered successfully, four pregnancies were ongoing, and two patients had lost their entire pregnancy. Anomalous twins had been selectively terminated prior to that time by a variety of techniques (Aberg, 1978; Kerenyi, 1981;

Wittman, 1986; Beck, 1980; Rodeck, 1982; Antsaklis, 1984; Philip, 1985; and their colleagues), but this was the first description of procedures performed on presumably normal fetuses in order to reduce the potential for preterm delivery. In 1988 Berkowitz and associates published the first series of transabdominal multifetal pregnancy reductions. In this collection of 12 patients the first three procedures were performed by transcervical aspiration, but the third patient experienced intractable bleeding during the procedure and it was necessary to terminate her entire pregnancy at that time. As a result of that experience a technique was adopted in which a small quantity of potassium chloride is injected into the fetal thorax through a needle introduced transabdominally under ultrasonic guidance (Fig. 34–1). The following year Itskovitz and co-workers (1989) described a modification of this technique in which the needle is introduced transvaginally.

In the past few years several relatively large series have been published describing the pregnancy outcome of patients undergoing multifetal pregnancy reduction (Lynch, 1990; Wapner, 1990; Boulot, 1990; Timor-Tritsch, 1993; and their colleagues). The transcervical method seems to have been universally abandoned, and while some authors favor the transvaginal technique, the majority use the transabdominal approach.

Transabdominal Approach

Each woman referred for MPR undergoes an initial ultrasound examination to verify the number and crown–rump lengths of all viable fetuses present. Following this the couple are counseled extensively about the risks and possible benefits of multifetal pregnancy reduction. This session occurs at least 1 day prior to the procedure in order to give each couple some time to consider the issues that were discussed and to ask and receive answers to all of their questions. The procedure is done in an outpatient setting with an intravenous infusion of 5 percent dextrose in water started on admission to the ultrasonography room. A single dose of cefazolin 1 g is administered intravenously unless the patient is allergic to that medication. An ultrasound examination is then performed to locate the position of each

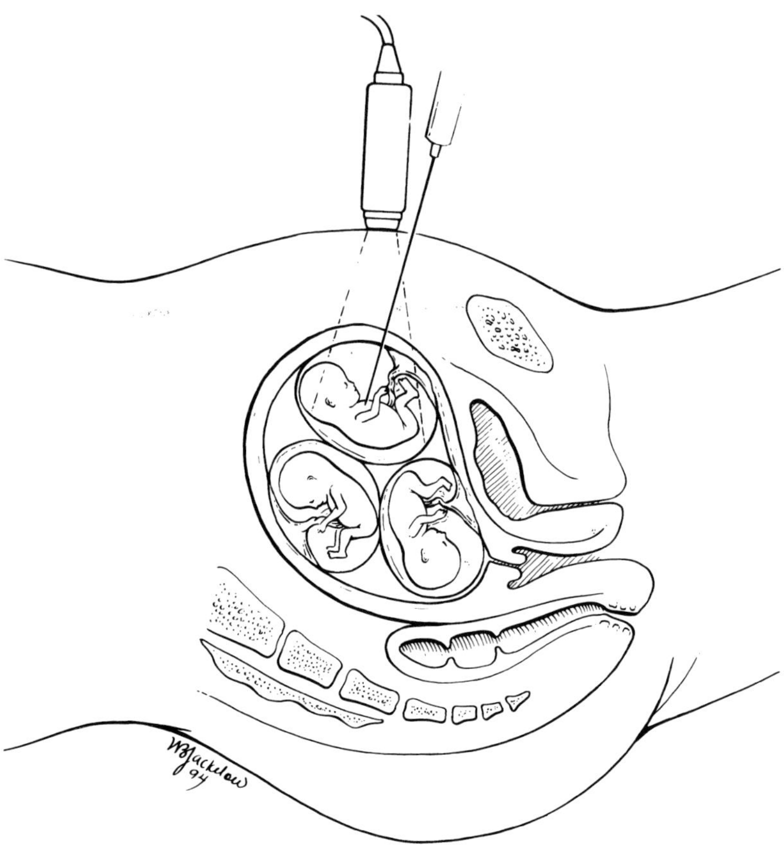

Figure 34–1. A needle is introduced transabdominally under ultrasound guidance into the fetal thorax and a small quantitiy of potassium chloride is injected.

fetus, reverify viability and crown–rump lengths, look for morphologic abnormalities, and evaluate the thickness of the membranes separating all of the sacs. Following this the operator and assistant scrub and gown. The ultrasound transducer is placed in a sterile sheath. The maternal abdomen is prepped, draped, and covered with sterile scanning gel over the anticipated needle entry site(s). A 22-guage 9-cm needle is used for each insertion, unless longer needles are necessary. No needle is ever reinserted into the maternal abdomen once it has been removed to minimize the risk of infecting the pregnancy. Whenever possible the fetus in the lowest sac is left alone unless it has an obvious anomaly, has an abnormally small crown–rump length, or appears to be a member of a monochorionic set of twins. A needle is then introduced under direct ultrasonic guidance into the fetus to be terminated, and 2–3 mEq of potassium chloride is injected (Fig. 34–1). If cardiac activity persists, additional potassium chloride is administered. The needle is left in place for 3 minutes after asystole has been observed in order to reduce the chances of a resumption of cardiac activity. The procedure is repeated for every fetus undergoing feticide. When six or more fetuses are present, the reductions are usually done in two or three sessions separated by 1-week intervals. After completion of each procedure, the patient is rescanned to be certain that the fetuses that were left alone have heart rates within the normal range and that those who were injected show no evidence of cardiac activity. After an hour or more of sitting in a waiting area a final scan is performed prior to sending the patient home. The woman is advised to limit her activities for the following 48 hours and to report any episodes of significant bleeding, loss of fluid, or contractions, as well as signs of early infection. Follow-up ultrasound examination 2 weeks later is recommended.

In a series of 200 completed cases from New York's Mount Sinai Hospital, 89.5 percent were done between 11 weeks and the end of the twelfth week (Berkowitz and associates, 1993). The other 21 cases were performed outside this range but later than 9 weeks 4 days and prior to 13 weeks 3 days. There were several reasons for choosing this narrow interval. While it is technically feasible to do the procedure earlier, it is more difficult to accomplish with a smaller fetus. Secondly, by waiting until 11 weeks there is a greater opportunity to see a morphologic abnormality or evidence of diminished growth. Thirdly, there is a greater potential for spontaneous death in utero of one or more fetuses to occur than if the procedure is done earlier. Finally, if one waits more than 12 completed weeks, the advantages of further delay must be weighed against the increased fetal mass of the larger dead fetuses that will be left when the procedure is completed.

In the Mount Sinai series the average duration of the procedure was 6.6 minutes per fetus, with a range of 2–30 minutes. It should be noted that in most cases this included 3 minutes of observing asystole with the needle still in place. In 76 percent of the cases the duration was 7 minutes or less per fetus. The average amount of potassium chloride administered was 3.6 mEq per fetus, with a range of 2–10 mEq. In 93 percent of the cases the amount of potassium chloride used was 5 mEq per fetus or less.

Transvaginal Approach

The transvaginal approach uses a needle guide or automated spring loaded device which attaches to a transvaginal ultrasound transducer (Fig. 34–2). With this approach the procedure can be done considerably earlier in gestation, but that would reduce the chances of detecting a morphologically abnormal fetus. As a consequence, in the largest study of transvaginal procedures published to date the authors chose to perform the procedures after 9.5 weeks (Timor-Tritsch and co-workers, 1993). Another theoretical concern is that the sac over the internal os is the easiest to reach with the transvaginal approach, but death of the fetus in that sac could predispose the patient to ruptured membranes later in the pregnancy. The results of the series by Timor-Tritsch and associates (1993), however, suggest that this has not proved to be not an important clinical problem. Finally, the risk of introducing infection may be greater when the vaginal route is used. In the aforementioned study there were three clinically apparent infections following 134 procedures. Two of those infections responded to antibiotic therapy, but the third pregnancy had to be terminated. There were no infections in the Mount Sinai series, but currently there are not enough data to definitively resolve this question. Advantages of the vaginal approach

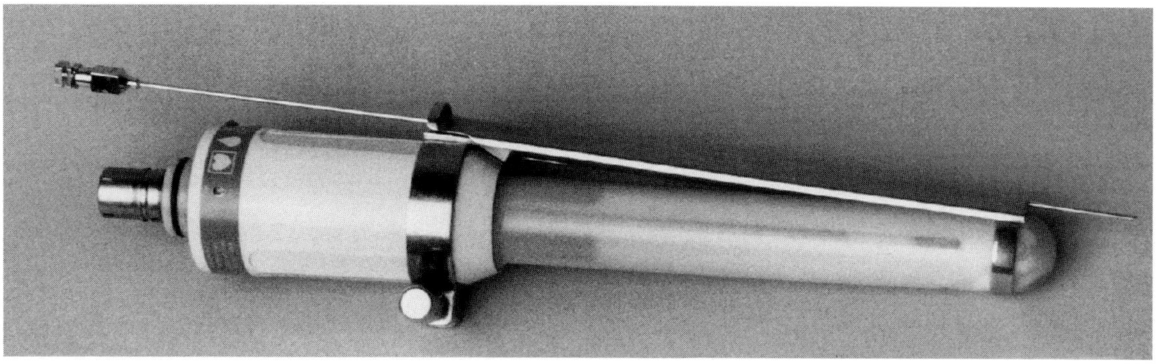

Figure 34–2. A needle guide or automated spring-loaded device attaches to a transvaginal ultrasound transducer.

include the fact that it is much easier to employ in obese women as well as in those with substantial abdominal scarring.

Similar to the transabdominal approach, it is recommended that a vaginal prep be performed with betadine soap and paint solutions immediately prior to the procedure. Use of a single-dose broad-specturm antibiotic is also recommended.

MPR SERIES OUTCOMES

In the Mount Sinai series 88 women had triplets, 89 had quadruplets, 16 had quintuplets, and 7 had from 6 to 9 fetuses at the time of the procedure (Berkowitz and co-workers, 1993). These 200 cases were reduced to 189 sets of twins, 5 sets of triplets, and 6 singletons. No reductions to singletons were performed unless there was a medical reason to believe that the patient might be at increased risk to have a poor outcome with a twin gestation. There were no cases of chorioamnionitis or any other significant maternal adverse sequelae to the procedure. While most patients were not followed with serial clotting profiles, there were no clinically evident cases of disseminated intravascular coagulation as a consequence of carrying the retained dead fetuses.

One or more liveborn infants were delivered after 24 weeks' gestation by 181 women in this series, and 19 (9.5%) lost their entire pregnancies at or before 24 weeks. For all those who delivered after 24 weeks, the mean gestational age was 35.7 weeks. Fifty-five percent were delivered at or later than 36 weeks, 36 percent from 32 to 36 weeks, 6 percent from 28 to 32 weeks, and 3 percent from 24 to 28 weeks. The mean gestational age at delivery varied inversely with the number of presenting fetuses from 36.1 weeks for triplets to 33.8 weeks for 6 or more fetuses. These figures were almost identical when those 174 women whose pregnancies were reduced to twins and who were delivered after 24 weeks were considered separately.

A collaborative report combining the results of 463 transabdominal MPR procedures performed by six groups in the United States and Europe included 18 women with twins, 175 with triplets, 193 with quadruplets, 52 with quintuplets, and 25 with six or more fetuses at the time of the procedure (Evans and colleagues, 1993). These pregnancies were reduced to 26 sets of triplets, 380 sets of twins, and 57 singletons. Some of the reductions to singletons were done for purely elective reasons. One or more liveborn infants were delivered after 24 weeks by 83.8 percent of the women in the collaborative study and 16.2 percent lost their entire pregnancies at or before 24 weeks. For those who delivered after 24 weeks, 83.5 percent gave birth at 33 weeks gestation or later, 9.4 percent between 29 and 32 weeks, and 7.1 percent between 25 and 28 weeks. Nineteen of the 75 pregnancy losses before 24 weeks occurred within 4 weeks of the procedure, and the remaining 56 were lost after that time.

It is difficult to determine a precise procedure-related loss rate for multifetal pregnancy reduction. While the complete pregnancy loss rates prior to 24 weeks were 9.5 percent and 16.2 percent for the Mount Sinai and collaborative study, respectively, 84 percent and 75 percent of these abortions occurred more than 4 weeks after the procedure had been performed. As the duration of time between the procedure and the loss increases, the relationship between these two events becomes more suspect. Many series have indicated that women who conceive following ovulation induction, with or without assisted reproductive technology, have a higher rate of spontaneous abortion than those who become pregnant without these forms of therapy (Australian In Vitro Fertilisation Collaborative Group, 1985; Cohen, 1988; Saunders, 1989; Hill, 1990; Wennerholm, 1991; and their co-workers). This may be due in part to the older age of the treated patients, the underlying cause of their inability to conceive, or the infertility therapy itself. There is no doubt that whenever a needle is placed into a pregnant uterus the risk of pregnancy loss is increased, but when experienced operators perform MPR, data suggest that the risk of the procedure is considerably less than 5 percent and may be comparable to that of fetal blood sampling.

The published data suggest that MPR is capable of achieving its objective of reducing the risk of early preterm delivery for women with multifetal pregnancies. The mean gestational age at delivery of the neonates in the Mount Sinai series is almost identical to that expected for twins. It is interesting to note, however, that as the number of presenting fetuses increases there is a proportional increase in the rate of pregnancy loss and decrease in the gestational age at delivery.

Some major morphologic anomalies can be detected with ultrasound at the time of the MPR procedure, but most karyotypic abnormalities will not be discovered unless chorionic villus sampling or early amniocentesis is performed. The use of either of those invasive procedures, however, would increase the risks of pregnancy loss, as well as possibly delay the time at which the reduction was performed. Furthermore, the safety of amnioncentesis performed before 12 weeks' gestation has not been established. Finally, definitive identification of the source of each villus sample may be extremely difficult, especially if more than three fetuses are present. One could simplify the process by only testing those fetuses chosen to be left alive at the end of the procedure, but these might be difficult to identify following the delay necessary to perform the studies. In any case, attempts to diagnose karyotypic abnormalities before the reduction procedure will certainly add some additional risk, delay, and expense. Therefore, it might be reasonable to individualize cases and to only offer preprocedure genetic testing to those women with a significantly increased chance of having a chromosomally abnormal fetus or Mendelian disorder by virtue of their age or history.

The decision to undergo an MPR procedure is not easy for couples considering this option. In virtually all cases they are infertility patients who have expended considerable time, effort, and money to become pregnant. In order to determine if there were persistent psychologic sequelae, a psychologist contacted the first 100 women who had undergone MPR procedures at Mount Sinai (Schreiner-Engel and associates, 1993). Ninety-one of these patients, one of whom had undergone seperate procedures in each of two different pregnancies, agreed to participate in a 45 minute structured telephone interview. The interviews were conducted in 1992, which was 2–6 years after the procedures had been performed. Eighty-two of the pregnancies had resulted in the birth of one or more healthy babies, and the other 10 had ended in miscarriage. Although nearly all the women deeply regreted having to undergo the procedure, 93 percent of the former group and 70 percent of the latter stated that they would make the same decision again. In the vast majority of cases the primary rationale for making the decision was stated to be the couple's perception of the need to sacrifice the lives of some fetuses in order to preserve the viability and health of the remaining few. Almost all of the women found the decision process and ensuing procedure to be extremely stressful and emotionally painful. Nevertheless, the successful achievement of their goals to mainatin a pregnancy and give birth to healthy infants enabled most of them to reconcile their grief reaction to the fetal loss(es), bond normally to the remaining fetuses, and have few persistent negative feelings. Mild feelings of guilt and anger, and moderate sadness about the MPR, persisted for many patients. A small subsample of women continued to react to their fetal reduction with considerable emotional distress, although not at the level of clinical significance. The women who had the most intense lingering feelings were more likely to be younger and more religious, to have initially conceived larger numbers of fetuses, and to have viewed their multifetal pregnancy more often on ultrasound. It should be noted that the mean number of ultrasound exams these women had undergone before being scanned in our unit was 3.8, and 18 percent had been scanned between 6 and 15 times. Frequent ultrasound visualizations of the multifetal gestation were strongly associated with increased longing for and recurrent thoughts about the reduced fetuses, and with more intense and persistent feelings of sadness after the procedure.

SUMMARY

The ethical issues associated with multifetal pregnancy reduction are troublesome. Is it justifiable to lower the number of fetuses in the uterus in order to reduce an unspecified risk to all the fetuses? It could be argued that in a society where abortion is available on demand, a multifetal pregnancy reduction procedure requires no additional rationale. It should be remembered, however, that women who conceive multiple fetuses as a result of treatment for infertility are particularly anxious to have children, and the elective termination of a healthy fetus is almost never something they have contemplated before achieving their goal of becoming pregnant. The medical justification for performing MPR is philosophically akin to the "life boat analogy", that is, that some drowning passengers can legitimately be denied access to an overcrowded lifeboat if bringing them aboard will cause it to sink and result in the loss of additional lives. In the case of women carrying multifetal pregnancies this translates into the argument that "innocent" fetal lives can be sacrificed in order to increase the chances of survival, or decrease the risk of serious morbidity, in the survivors of the procedure. If one ignores social and economic issues and concentrates only on those of medical relevance, it is clear that the risk of very early preterm delivery with its associated increase in perinatal mortality or severe morbidity is effectively reduced by MPR in women carrying four or more fetuses. The data are not as convincing for triplets, but until larger series describing the outcome of these pregnancies managed in modern obstetric and neonatal units are available, this will remain a gray area. Most obstetricians feel that MPR cannot be justified for medical indications in twin pregnancies unless there are special factors mitigating against successful outcome in a particular case, that is, a woman with a bicornuate uterus or a history of early preterm delivery of a singleton.

For those who accept the notion that abortion on demand justifies a reduction in number for nonmedical reasons, there is no reason to deny a woman with two or more fetuses a reduction to one. It should be remembered, however, that the procedure does have the potential of causing a miscarriage, and therefore the couple must be counseled not to consider undergoing a reduction unless they are prepared for the possibility of loosing the entire pregnancy as a consequence.

Obviously, reduction is far from an ideal solution to the problems associated with multifetal pregnancies. It would be much better to avoid the problem by effectively monitoring patients receiving ovulatory stimulants and minimizing the number of embryos transferred in in-vitro fertilization/embryo transfer programs. It is understood that even in the most skilled hands, the creation of multifetal pregnancies cannot be entirely eliminated in patients receiving therapy for their infertility with existing modalities. Nevertheless, it should be possible to substantially reduce the number of cases of triplets currently being seen, and to virtually eliminate those with four or more fetuses if concientious attention is paid to appropriate monitoring. When, however, three or more fetuses have been conceived, the experience to date suggests that MPR is a relatively safe and effective option to consider for patients whose only choices in the past were either to accept the risk of extreme prematurity or terminate their entire pregnancy.

REFERENCES

Aberg A, Mittelman F, Cantz M, et al. Cardiac puncture of fetus with Hurler's disease avoiding abortion of unaffected co-twin. Lancet 1978; 2:990.

Antsaklis A, Politis J, Karagiannopoulos C, et al. Selective survival of only the healthy fetus following prenatal diagnosis of thalassaemia major in binovular twin gestation. Prenat Diagn 1984; 4:289.

Australian In Vitro Fertilisation Collaborative Group. High incidence of preterm births and early losses in pregnancy after in vitro fertilisation. Br Med J 1985; 291:1160.

Australian In-Vitro Fertilization Collaborative Group. In-vitro fertilization pregnancies in Australia and New Zealand, 1979–1985. Med J Austr 1988; 148:429.

Beck L, Terinde R, Dolff M. Zwillingsschwangerschaft mit freier Trisomie 21 eines kindes: Sectio parva mit entfernung des kranken and spatere geburt des gesundes kindes. Geburtshilfe Frauenheilkunde 1980; 40:397.

Berkowitz RL, Lynch L, Chitkara U, et al. Selective reduction of multifetal pregnancies in the first trimester. N Engl J Med 1988; 318:1043.

Berkowitz RL, Lynch L. Selective reduction: an unfortunate misnomer. Obstet Gynecol 1990; 75:873.

Berkowitz RL, Lynch L, Lapinski R, Bergh P. First-trimester transabdominal multifetal pregnancy reduction: a report of two hundred completed cases. Am J Obstet Gynecol 1993; 169:17.

Boulot P, Hedon B, Pelliccia G, et al. Obstetrical results after embryonic reductions performed on 34 multiple pregnancies. Hum Reprod 1990; 5:1009.

Cohen J, Mayaux MJ, Guihard-Moscato ML. Pregnancy outcomes after in vitro fertilization. A collaborative study on 2342 pregnancies. Ann NY Acad Sci 1988; 541:1.

Collins MS, Bleyl JA. Seventy-one quadruplet pregnancies: management and outcome. Am J Obstet Gynecol 1990; 162:1384.

Committee on Ethics. Multifetal pregnancy reduction and selective fetal termination. ACOG Committee Opinion 1991; 94:1.

Dumez Y, Oury JF. Method for first trimester selective abortion in multiple pregnancy. Contr Gynecol Obstet 1986; 15:50.

Evans MI, Dommergues M, Wapner RJ, et al. Efficacy of transabdominal multifetal pregnancy reduction: collaborative experience among the world's largest centers. Obstet Gynecol 1993; 82:61.

Gonen R, Heyman E, Asztalos EV, et al. The outcome of triplet, quadruplet, and quintuplet pregnancies managed in a perinatal unit: obstetric, neonatal, and follow-up data. Am J Obstet Gynecol 1990; 162:454.

Hill GA, Bryan S, Herbert CM, et al. Complications of pregnancy in infertile couples: routine treatment versus assisted reproduction. Obstet Gynecol 1990; 75:790.

Holcberg G, Biale Y, Lewenthal H, Insler V. Outcome of pregnancy in 31 triplet gestations. Obstet Gynecol 1982; 59:472.

Itskovitz J, Boldes R, Thaler I, et al. Transvaginal ultrasonography-guided aspiration of gestational sacs for selective abortion in multiple pregnancy. Am J Obstet Gynecol 1989; 160:215.

Itzkowic D. A survey of 59 triplet pregnancies. Br J Obstet Gynaecol. 1979; 86:23.

Kerenyi TD, Chitkara U. Selective birth in twin pregnancy with discordancy for Down's syndrome. N Engl J Med 1981; 304:1525.

Lipitz S, Reichman B, Paret G, et al. The improving outcome of triplet pregnancies. Am J Obstet Gynecol 1989; 161:1279.

Lipitz S, Frenkel Y, Watts C, et al. High-order multifetal gestation—management and outcome. Obstet Gynecol 1990; 76:215.

Lynch L, Berkowitz RL, Chitkara U, Alvarez M. First-trimester transabdominal multifetal pregnancy reduction: a report of 85 cases. Obstet Gynecol 1990; 75:735.

Macones GA, Schemmer G, Weinblatt V, Wapner RJ. Comparison of perinatal outcome of triplet pregnancies undergoing fetal reduction to non reduced multifetal gestations. SPO Abstract. Am J Obstet Gynecol 1993; 168:381.

Newman RB, Hamer C, Miller MC. Outpatient triplet management: a contemporary review. Am J Obstet Gynecol 1989; 161:547.

Philip J, Bang J. Prenatal diagnosis in multiple gestations and selective termination of pregnancy. In: Filkins K, Russo JF, eds. Human Prenatal Diagnosis. New York: Marcel Dekker, 1985:159.

Porreco RP, Burke S, Hendrix ML. Multifetal reduction of triplets and pregnancy outcome. Obstet Gynecol 1991; 78:335.

Rodeck CH, Mibashan RS, Abramowics J, Campbell S. Selective feticide of the affected twin by fetoscopic air embolization. Prenat Diagn 1982; 2:189.

Sassoon DA, Castro LC, Davis JL, Hobel CJ. Perinatal outcome in triplet versus twin gestations. Obstet Gynecol 1990; 75:817.

Saunders DM, Lancaster P. The wider perinatal significance of the Australian in vitro fertilization data collection program. Am J Perinatol 1989; 6:252.

Schreiner-Engel P, Walther VN, Mindes J, et al. Psychological impact of multifetal pregnancy reduction (MPR) on bereavement and attachment behaviors. Scientific Abstract. The American Fertility Society, 49th annual meeting, Palais des Congres, October, 1993.

Syrop CH, Varner MW. Triplet gestation: maternal and neonatal implications. Acta Genet Med Gemellol 1985; 34:81.

Timor-Tritsch IE, Peisner DB, Monteagudo A, et al. Multifetal pregnancy reduction by transvaginal puncture: evaluation of the technique used in 134 cases. Am J Obstet Gynecol 1993; 168:799.

Vervliet J, De Cleyn K, Renier M, et al. Management and outcome of 21 triplet and quadruplet pregnancies. Eur J Obstet Gynecol Reproduc Biol 1989; 33:61.

Vohra N, Lynch L, Lapinski R, et al. Triplet versus twin pregnancies: perinatal outcome and financial costs. Scientific Abstract. The Society of Perinatal Obstetricians, Las Vegas, NV, January 1994.

Wapner RJ, Davis GH, Johnson A, et al. Selective reduction of multifetal pregnancies. Lancet 1990; 335:90.

Wennerholm UB, Janson PO, Wennergren M, Kjellmer I. Pregnancy complications and short-term follow-up of infants born after in vitro fertilization and embryo transfer (IVF/ET). Acta Obstet Gynecol Scand 1991; 70:564.

Wittman BK, Farquharson DF, Thomas WDS, et al. The role of feticide in the management of severe twin transfusion syndrome. Am J Obstet Gynecol 1986; 155:1023.

CHAPTER 35

Trauma

Injury or trauma can be defined as physical harm or bodily damage as a result of mechanical, thermal, chemical, or other environmental energy. Trauma may be sustained at any point during life from in utero to the very elderly, but unlike many serious disease states, mortality from trauma is usually in the young. Recognition of this is evidenced by the emphasis placed on the statistic **potential years of life lost (PYLL)** in trauma epidemiology.

According to the World Health Organization (1989), trauma is the fifth leading cause of death worldwide, accounting for approximately 800,000 deaths each year. Throughout the developed world, approximately 180,000 people die each year in motor vehicle crashes, making it the most frequent cause of death from unintentional injury. In the United States, there were nearly 50,000 vehicular deaths in 1988, equivalent to approximately 20 deaths for each 100,000 persons. This is the fifth highest among countries reporting per capita statistics. However, when corrected for actual miles driven, the United States has one of the lowest recorded mileage fatality rates, 1.6 deaths per million miles driven.

The overall death rate of women due to unintentional injury is 24/100,000 population; motor vehicle crashes, suicide, and homicide account for over 95 percent of these. Overall, females are more likely than males to be involved in auto accidents, viz, 143 female drivers versus 95 male drivers per 10 million miles driven per National Safety Council data. Considerable geographic variation exists in both death rates and cause of death due to trauma. Death from motor vehicle crashes is encountered at much higher rates in areas of low population density, for example, Manhattan versus Esmarelda County, Nevada—2.5 versus 558 per 100,000, respectively. Conversely, firearm deaths and homicides are higher in the West and South, particularly in areas of low income and high population density (Baker and colleagues, 1988). Fetal loss due to trauma is difficult to quantify as there are no compiled statistics on pregnancy loss from trauma, and in individual cases, the relationship of trauma to pregnancy loss is not always clear.

The provision of modern trauma service relies on the cooperative effort of a variety of care providers. When the trauma victim is pregnant, the obstetrician becomes a vital member of the multidisciplinary trauma team. Often, particularly in cases of minor trauma, the obstetrician is the central figure in providing care. It is the obstetrician who has the special skills and knowledge relevant to pregnancy that best serve the interest of the woman and her fetus. All trauma centers should have a protocol for incorporating an obstetrician into the trauma team, and likewise, obstetricians should be prepared to assist the trauma team when the victim is pregnant.

PHYSIOLOGIC CHANGES OF PREGNANCY

Crucial to resuscitation of the pregnant trauma victim is an understanding of both fetal and maternal physiology, particularly the physiologic response to stress and hypovolemia. Fundamental differences in the physiologic response to trauma occur as a result of pregnancy, and obstetric expertise is an invaluable asset to the trauma team. An overview of some of these changes during pregnancy is shown in Table 35–1.

Fetal Physiology

Several factors are important in determining the impact of a traumatic event on pregnancy outcome. These include gestational age, type and severity of trauma, and the extent of disruption of normal maternal and fetal physiology (Pearlman and associates, 1990a). In the first week of conception, the non-implanted embryo is relatively resistant to noxious stimuli. Even during the first trimester, the uterus resides safely within the confines of the bony pelvis and is protected to a large degree from direct uterine trauma. However, at any gestational age after implantation, maternal hypovolemic shock may have a significant impact on the developing embryo/fetus. Blood flow to the uterine vessels cannot autoregulate, that is, uterine blood flow is maximal in the normal physiologic state. Maternal hypovolemia may result in vasoconstriction in many vascular beds, including those of the uterus. Even in the absence of uterine artery vasoconstriction, decreases in maternal blood pressure may result in decreased uterine blood flow. These facts underlie the importance of maintaining adequate maternal blood volume as a first step in fetal resuscitation. The third-trimester fetus can adapt to decreased uterine blood flow and oxygen delivery by diverting blood distribution to the heart, brain, and adrenal glands (Wilkening and Meschia, 1983). Furthermore, because fetal hemoglobin has a greater affinity for oxygen than adult hemoglobin, fetal oxygen consumption does not decrease until the oxygen delivery is reduced by 50 percent (Iwamoto, 1989).

Blunt or penetrating trauma to the fetus may result in rupture of the amnionic membranes. In the second trimester, rupture of membranes without reaccumulation of fluid may result in pulmonary hypoplasia or orthopedic deformity. In addition, infection may develop with ruptured membranes at any gestational age. Injury to the placenta may result in separation or laceration leading to fetal anemia, hypoxemia, or hypovolemia (Dahmus, 1993; Goodwin, 1990; Pearlman, 1990b; Williams, 1990; and their associates).

Maternal Anatomic and Physiologic Changes

Nearly every maternal organ system undergoes anatomic or physiologic changes during pregnancy. The description that follows emphasizes the importance of some of these changes in managing the pregnant trauma victim, particularly as these differences impact on the usual practice of trauma management.

A major concern for trauma victims is internal hemorrhage and hypovolemia. The

TABLE 35–1. ANATOMIC AND PHYSIOLOGIC CHANGES OF PREGNANCY

Cardiovascular	
Cardiac output	Increases 1–1.5 L/min
Blood pressure	Decreases 5–15 mm Hg in mid-pregnancy
Heart rate	Increases 5–15 bpm
Supine positioning	May decrease cardiac output 30% in some women
Hematologic	
Blood volume	Increases 40–50% during 13–32 weeks
Hemoglobin	Decreases 1–2 g/dL as plasma volume increases more than red cell mass
Gastrointestinal	
Intestines	Displaced into upper abdomen in later gestation
Gastric emptying time	Increases
Urinary	
Bladder	Displaced cephalad becoming an abdominal organ after first trimester
Ureters	Dilated (right more than left)
Reproductive	
Uterine size	Increases to 36-cm, 1000-g organ
Uterine blood flow	Increases from 60 mL/min to 600 mL/min

sentinel findings are changes in vital signs, typically hypotension and tachycardia. Consideration is given to the normal decrease in systemic vascular resistance resulting in a decrease in blood pressure of 10–15 mm Hg and an increased pulse rate of 5–15 bpm, particularly in the second trimester. These changes can be accentuated if the woman is placed in the supine position—for example, strapped to a long board in order to secure the maternal spine. The resultant potential decrease in venous return from the lower extremities can reduce central venous volume and result in a diminished cardiac output of up to 30 percent. Simple manual displacement of the uterus to the left or placement of a rolled towel under the backboard while assuring the spine remains secure will alleviate most of this effect.

Blood volume increases by a mean of 50 percent in the singleton gestation. This is usually maximal by 28–32 weeks. Red cell mass increases to a lesser degree than does plasma volume, resulting in a slightly decreased hemoglobin and hematocrit concentration. Iron-deficiency anemia is also common during pregnancy, and together with the so-called physiologic anemia, hemoglobin concentration may be in the 9–11 g/dL range. These hematologic changes have two potential implications in the management of the trauma victim: (1) anemia may be confused with active bleeding and hypovolemia and (2) blood volume estimates should be modified upward during fluid resuscitation.

The two major pregnancy-induced changes in the gastrointestinal tract that have implications for trauma management are cephalad displacement of the bowel and decreased bowel motility resulting in increased transit time. Compartmentalization of bowel upward serves to protect it during lower abdominal trauma, but increases the risk of injury when there is penetrating trauma to the upper abdomen in later pregnancy. Complex injuries to the small bowel can be encountered with multiple entry and exit wounds as a result of its being crowded and compacted into the upper abdomen. Decreased gastric motility results in prolonged gastric emptying time, thereby increasing the risk of aspiration. Rebound tenderness and guarding are less usually apparent in advanced gestation; thus, clinical diagnosis of hemoperitoneum is less reliable. This is likely due to stretching of the abdominal musculature and peritoneum.

Dramatic increases in uterine blood flow, from 60 to 600 mL/min, may result in rapid exsanguination if there is avulsion of the uterine vessels or rupture of the uterus. Retroperitoneal hemorrhage is also a common complication of pelvic fracture due to remarkably hypertrophied vasculature. Enlargement of the uterus makes it susceptible to direct abdominal trauma. Injury to the uterus itself (uterine rupture), adjacent organs (bladder rupture), or uterine contents (abruptio placentae or direct fetal injury) are possible. While some of these are typically seen with direct and violent trauma, for example, uterine rupture, others may occur with minimal maternal trauma, for example, abruptio placentae.

BLUNT ABDOMINAL TRAUMA

Motor vehicle crashes are the most common cause of blunt abdominal trauma during pregnancy. These are followed by falls, direct assaults to the abdomen, and miscellaneous causes (Pearlman and associates, 1990b). While some investigations have implied that changes in the center of gravity due to pregnancy result in increased clumsiness and propensity to injury, there is no evidence that the frequency or severity of trauma is greater during pregnancy (Buchsbaum, 1968; Crosby, 1983, 1986; Pearlman and colleagues, 1990a). However, due to anatomic and physiologic changes discussed above, certain patterns of injury have been noted. For example, an increased incidence of spleen rupture and retroperitoneal hemorrhage is reported during pregnancy, whereas bowel injuries may occur less frequently (Buchsbaum, 1967; Pepperell and associates, 1977; Rothenberger and coworkers, 1978). Battering is probably underestimated as a cause of trauma during pregnancy, with more than 8 percent of otherwise healthy inner-city women reported being physically abused during pregnancy. An additional 20 percent reported abuse prior to the pregnancy or were threatened with abuse during the pregnancy (Helton and colleagues, 1987).

While maternal death is uncommon during pregnancy, trauma is frequently the most commonly cited cause of death during pregnancy (Fildes and associates, 1992; Varner, 1989). In the setting of blunt trauma, head injury and hemorrhagic shock are equal contributors to over 85 percent of all maternal mortality (Crosby and Costiloe, 1971).

Fetal well-being is a major concern whenever a pregnant woman has been injured. The fetus can be harmed by a variety of mechanisms that include direct fetal injury, abruptio placentae, or massive fetomaternal hemorrhage. While fetal injuries are more frequent following severe trauma, minor trauma (Fig. 35–1) occurs so much more frequently that most fetal losses follow relatively minor accidents (Dahmus, 1993; Goodwin, 1990; Pearlman, 1990b; Williams, 1990; and their colleagues). According to Crosby and Costiloe (1971), the most frequent cause of fetal death was maternal death. This was certainly true with severe motor vehicle accidents from the 1960s when only two-point driver and passenger restraints were available and when seat belts were infrequently used. Since then, numerous series have demonstrated that most fetal deaths occur in association with relatively minor maternal injuries (Agran and associates, 1987; Fries and Hankins, 1989; Lane, 1989; Stafford and colleagues, 1988). It is again emphasized that this is due to the high ratio of minor to life-threatening injuries, though it is clear on a case-by-case analysis that severe injury more commonly results in fetal loss (Pearlman and colleagues, 1990b; Rothenberger and colleagues, 1978).

In four reports of fetal and neonatal deaths due to trauma, 57 deaths were recorded (Agran, 1987; Hoff, 1991; Lane, 1989; Pepperell, 1977; and their colleagues). Only six of these were associated with maternal deaths. Of the other 51 deaths, over half were associated with minor maternal injury—often considered trivial. Over two-thirds of the fetal deaths were due to abruptio placentae, and there was direct fetal injury in 25 percent (Fig. 35–2). There was a disproportionate number—over 90 percent—of fetal losses due to abruptio placentae in the minor injury group, suggesting that even minor degrees of uterine deformation may result in abruptio placentae.

Complications

Abruptio Placentae

Premature placental separation is the most common cause of fetal/neonatal loss resulting from trauma during pregnancy. The mechanism of this injury has been well described by Crosby and colleagues (1968) in their study of seat belts in pregnant baboons. Using high-speed cameras and intrauterine pressure catheters, they demonstrated that there are two times during an accident when the intrauterine environment is at risk for injury (Fig. 35–3). In a front-facing decelerative event—for example, a restrained woman in a car hitting a tree at 25 mph—the body is thrown suddenly forward. The uterus within the abdominal cavity is also thrown forward. During the initial phase of deceleration, (0–0.06 sec), there is an increase in intrauterine pressure to about 500 mm Hg. This corresponds to a time period when the body is compressed downward into the seat. It may also result from the uterus being thrown forward against the anterior abdominal wall. There is

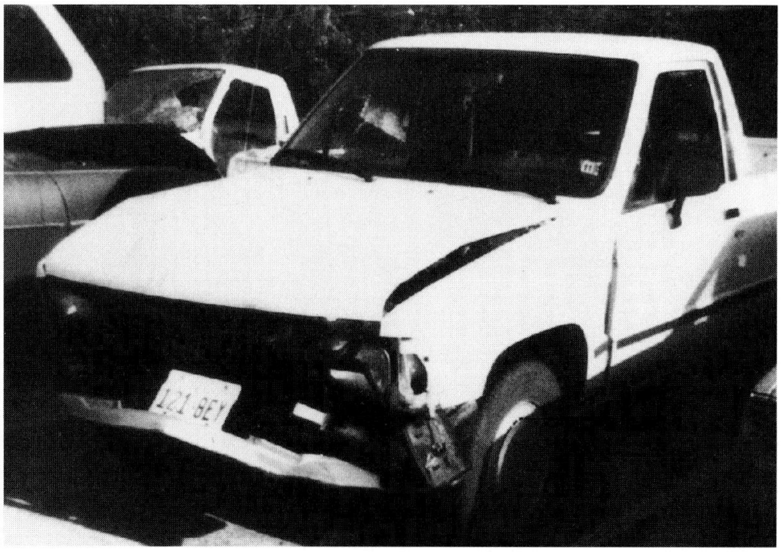

Figure 35–1. Motor vehicle accident with relatively minor damage to the vehicle and no evidence of maternal trauma, yet death of the fetus due to intracranial and intrahepatic hemorrhage.

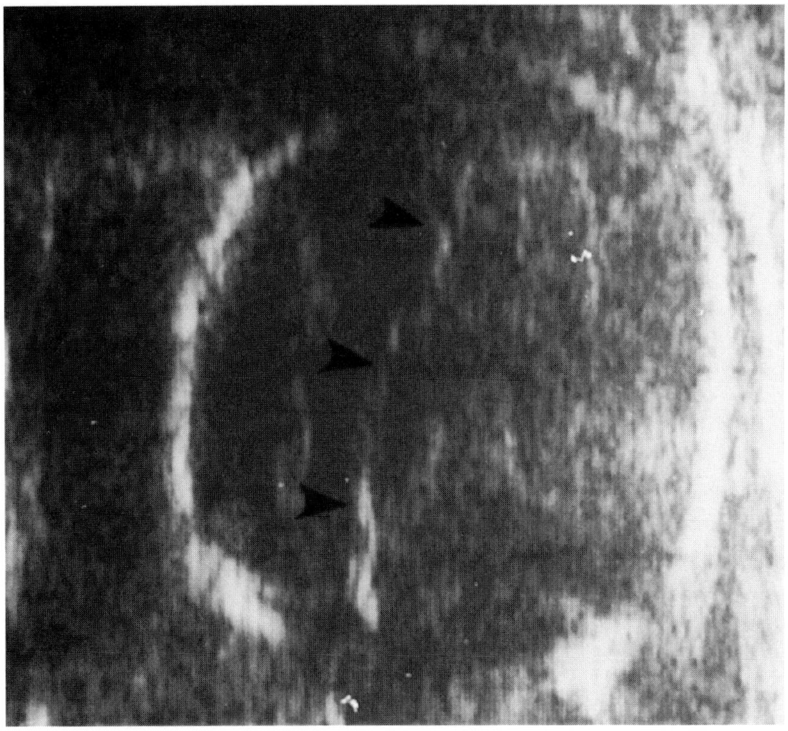

Figure 35–2. Ultrasound of the head of the fetus involved in the accident shown in Figure 35–1 demonstrating a midline shift (arrows point to falx) and large intracranial hemorrhage. The fetus also demonstrated repetitive variable decelerations on electronic heart rate monitoring.

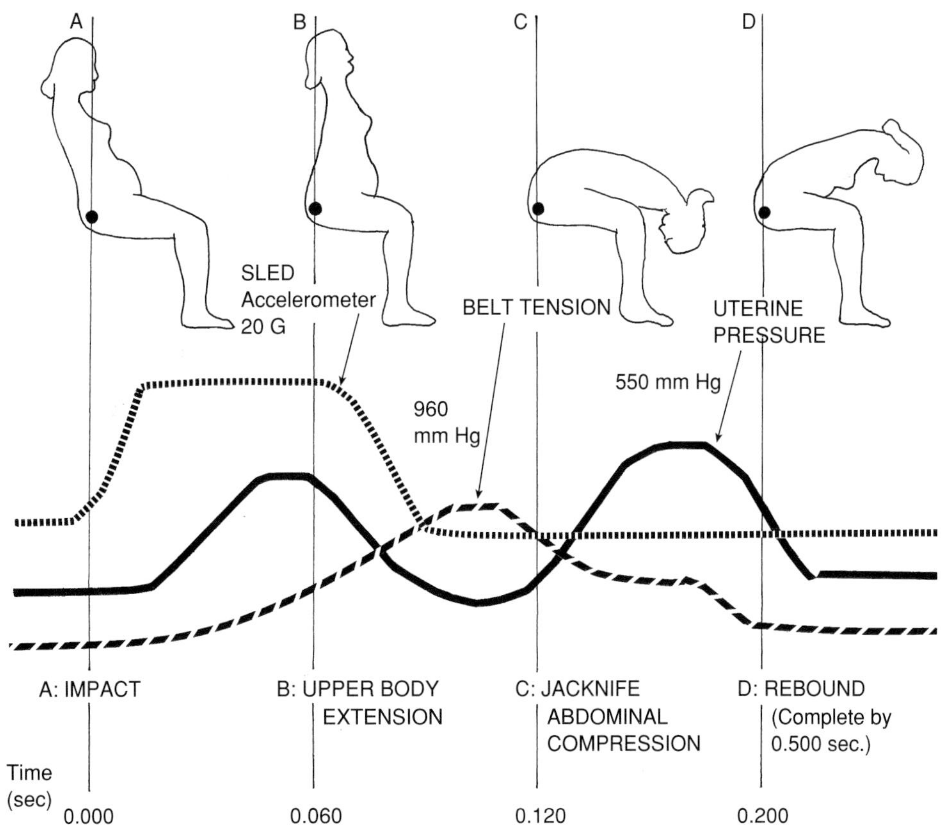

Figure 35–3. Impact sequence. Relationship between body motion, uterine pressure, and belt tension. (Modified from Crosby and associates, 1968, with permission.)

a second increase in intrauterine pressure with a two-point restraint, whereby the uterus is compressed by the hyperflexed torso (Fig. 35–3). With a three-point restraint, there were similar increases in intrauterine pressure at the time in which the body was compressed against the shoulder harness. The effect of air bags, which have become standard on many vehicles sold in the United States, has not been tested during pregnancy. Current studies on the effects of various restraint systems during pregnancy are being conducted jointly by the University of Michigan and General Motors Corporation.

Abruptio placentae complicates 1–5 percent of minor trauma cases compared with 20–50 percent following major injuries (Pearlman and Tintinalli, 1991). The physical characteristics of the uterine and placental tissues appear to play an important role in the pathogenesis of abruptio placentae due to trauma. Deformation of the relatively elastic myometrium can result in a shearing effect of the inelastic placenta away from the decidua basalis (Fig. 35–4). The placenta does not have to be implanted anteriorly, as the original impact sets up a wave within the uterus, causing initial elongation and narrowing of the uterus, followed by shortening and widening. As these deforming forces affect the entire uterus, any placental location is at risk for separation following impact. In some circumstances, abruptio placentae develops without direct uterine impact. For example, we have managed two cases of abruptio placentae that developed following hard falls directly on the buttocks. Presumably, the fall resulted in transmission of this energy to setting up a waveform within the uterus.

Uterine Rupture

Uterine rupture resulting from trauma is an infrequent event, reported in about 0.6 percent of all trauma during pregnancy (Pearl-

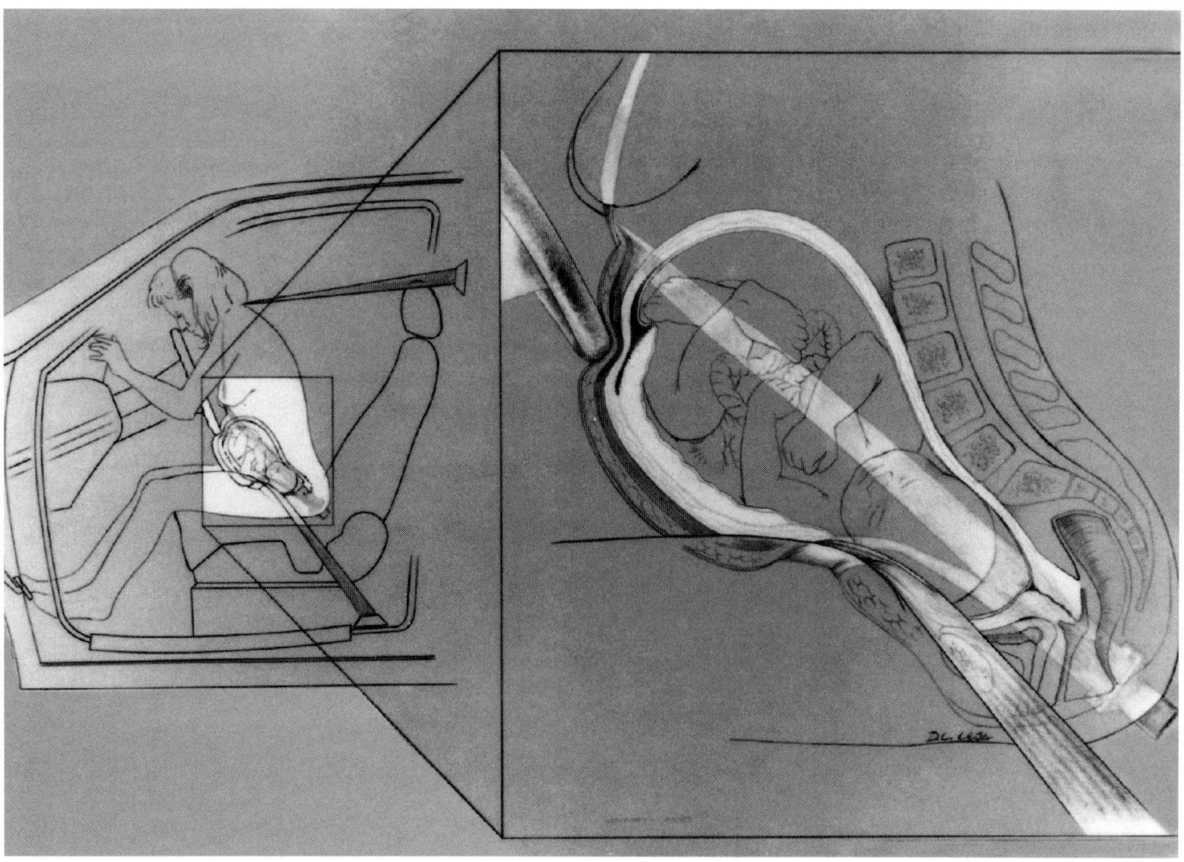

Figure 35–4. Illustration of woman striking a steering wheel with deformation of the uterus and separation of the placenta from the decidua basalis.

man and colleagues, 1990a). Unlike abruptio placentae, uterine rupture is associated with direct and intense uterine impact (Buchsbaum, 1968; Handel, 1978; Weinstein and Pallais, 1968). Factors that predispose to uterine rupture during labor—for example, prior uterine scar, multiple gestation, and hydramnios—also predispose to traumatic rupture. Importantly, traumatic uterine rupture also occurs in the absence of any predisposing factors. Even in the presence of a uterine scar, traumatic uterine rupture has been described remote from the uterine scar (Weinstein and Pallais, 1968).

During early pregnancy, the uterus is relatively resistant to direct injury. This is so even in the face of intense direct abdominal injury unless the pelvic ring collapses as a result of fracture (Crosby and Costiloe, 1971). After the first trimester, the uterus becomes an abdominal organ and is susceptible to direct trauma. Direct uterine trauma may result in (1) complete disruption of the myometrial wall with or without extrusion of the fetus, placenta, or umbilical cord into the abdominal cavity; (2) avulsion of the uterine vasculature with intraperitoneal or retroperitoneal hemorrhage; (3) less than full thickness injury to the myometrial wall, for example, serosal hemorrhage or abrasions; or (4) complete uterine avulsion, which has been described as a result of an improperly placed lap belt (McCormick, 1968).

Prompt diagnosis of uterine rupture is essential to reduce the risk of maternal and fetal mortality. Initial clues to substantial uterine injury may include either hypertension or hypotension and tachycardia suggesting hypovolemia. **Normal vital signs do not preclude the possibility of uterine rupture.** This is due, in part, to the expanded maternal blood volume. Galle and Anderson (1979) described an avulsion injury of the uterine vein with rapid development of maternal hypotension and tachycardia despite normal vital signs documented just minutes before. Their first warning of any abnormality was late fetal heart rate decelerations followed by fetal bradycardia.

Most cases of uterine rupture involve the fundus. While other locations of full-thickness ruptures have been described, over 75 percent of reported cases involve the fundus. Under these circumstances, clinical findings may provide several clues to the diagnosis. Signs of peritoneal irritation such as guarding, rigidity, distention, and rebound tenderness may be present. Unfortunately, these findings are less reliable during pregnancy because of gradual stretching of the parietal peritoneum or rectus diastasis. The fundus may be difficult to palpate if there is significant disruption. An abnormal lie may be suggested by Leopold's maneuver if the fetus has been extruded from the uterus. Absence of fetal heart tones is also a clue to uterine rupture, though abruptio placentae causes fetal demise much more frequently than uterine rupture.

If uterine rupture is suspected based on the circumstances of the accident or by clinical findings, several adjunctive tests are useful to assist in the diagnosis. Abdominal x-ray may demonstrate an abnormal fetal lie in the case of an extruded fetus, or there may be free air in the peritoneal cavity. Sonography may also be helpful in instances of uterine rupture with partial or complete extrusion of the fetus. Peritoneal lavage has been shown to be both safe and accurate in diagnosing intraabdominal hemorrhage at any gestational age (Rothenberger and colleagues, 1977). Of course, none of these findings are diagnostic of uterine rupture, and laparotomy is often necessary to confirm the diagnosis and provide definitive treatment.

Other methods used to detect intraabdominal or retroperitoneal bleeding include computerized tomography (CT) and magnetic resonance imaging (MRI). The accuracy of ultrasound in diagnosing intraperitoneal hemorrhage during pregnancy has not been established, but this may be particularly problematic in late gestation. Similarly, while there are case reports of intraperitoneal and retroperitoneal hemorrhage diagnosed during pregnancy with computed tomography or magnetic resonance imaging, the sensitivity and specificity of these techniques are unknown. The theoretical risk of fetal radiation exposure with abdomino-pelvic tomography is discussed in Chapter 21. Fetal dosimetry studies suggest an x-irradiation exposure of 2–5 rads during a complete study of the maternal abdomen and pelvis.

Early case reports of traumatic uterine rupture suggested that total or subtotal hysterectomy should be performed in most cases; only rarely would repair of the laceration be feasible. More recent experiences suggest that in the absence of life-threatening hemorrhage or "significant" uterine vascular injury, salvage of the uterus is possible even with extensive laceration. Smith and colleagues (1994) described two cases of extensive uterine fundal lacerations that were primarily repaired. In both cases subsequent pregnancy was satisfactory, although one of these women developed a subclinical uterine dehiscence. Repair follows the same principles previously outlined in Chapter 18. If the uterus is repaired primarily following uterine rupture, cesarean delivery should be planned for subsequent pregnancies.

Fetomaternal Hemorrhage

There have been three prospectively controlled studies that clearly establish that fetomaternal hemorrhage is increased three- to fourfold in women who have suffered trauma during pregnancy compared with matched controls (Goodwin and Breen, 1990; Pearlman and colleagues, 1990b; Rose and co-workers, 1985). Additionally, women with fetomaternal hemorrhage following trauma had significantly larger volume bleeds than did matched controls. Such bleeding can be fatal to the fetus. Neither severity of trauma nor mechanism of injury seem to be related to the incidence of fetomaternal hemorrhage. Interestingly, both anterior placental location and uterine tenderness are associated with a twofold increased risk. In two of these three studies, the presence of hemorrhage was not predictive of adverse fetal outcome.

The use of the Kleihauer-Betke or a similar assay for determining the estimated volume of hemorrhage has been advocated particularly in D-negative women so that adequate D-immune globulin prophylaxis can be administered (American College of Obstetricians and Gynecologists, 1991). The role of a routine Kleihauer-Betke test following trauma in predicting adverse outcome, including abruptio placentae and fetal death, is not clear. In two studies, abruptio placentae and fetal death were predicted with much greater accuracy using fetal monitoring than laboratory tests (Goodwin and Breen, 1990; Pearlman and coworkers, 1990b).

Pelvic Fractures

While the discussion of specific maternal injuries is generally beyond the scope of this chapter, pelvic fractures deserve special mention because they are fairly common, are associated with significant morbidity and mortality, and may cause problems at the time of delivery. There frequently is bleeding into the retroperitoneal space with pelvic fractures and this can extend into the broad ligament, simulating a uterine vascular injury (Pearlman and Tintinalli, 1988). Retroperitoneal bleeding can cause hypovolemic shock with or without concomitant intraperitoneal bleeding. This is especially true during pregnancy, as the hypertrophied pelvic vasculature can undergo extensive disruption with a pelvic fracture. If there has been disruption of the bladder or urethra, gross hematuria may be seen. Disruption of the urethra may create difficulty in passing a urinary catheter.

In general, pelvic fracture does not preclude an attempt at vaginal delivery. Numerous authors have demonstrated safe vaginal delivery even in the presence of a slightly displaced pelvic fracture. However, the presence of a large healing callus or a severely dislocated or unstable pelvic fracture may contraindicate vaginal delivery. This latter circumstance is encountered in a minority of pelvic fractures, perhaps as few as 10 percent.

Outcome

A number of investigators have retrospectively evaluated the predictive value of different trauma scoring systems, for example, injury severity scoring, abbreviated injury scores, trauma score, Champion trauma score, and Glasgow coma score (Drost, 1990; George, 1992; Hoff, 1991; Kissinger, 1991; and their colleagues). These trauma scoring systems combine various anatomic and physiologic characteristics, which are scored based on the severity of derangement, and an additive score is given. While many claim that one or more of these scoring systems allow prediction of fetal outcome, none have been tested in a prospective, clinically relevant design. Conversely, the use of continuous fetal heart rate monitoring following trauma has been shown in various prospective study designs to predict adverse fetal outcome (Dahmus and Sibai, 1993; Goodwin and Breen, 1990; Pearlman and associates, 1990b; Williams and colleagues, 1990). If no immediate adverse outcome results from trauma—usually abruptio placentae, ruptured membranes, or fetal death—then pregnancy outcome generally appears to be good (Pearlman and colleagues, 1990b). This is not, however, universally true, as attested to by the cranial computed tomograph shown in Figure 35–5. Despite the fact that this mother sustained only minor trauma, the 31-week breech fetus sustained considerable direct trauma from the shoulder restraint with resultant hemiplegia.

Management

The best interests of both mother and fetus are served by concentrating initial efforts on evaluation and stabilization of the mother. Initial steps include maintenance of a patent airway, oxygenation, volume replacement, and optimizing venous return by displacing the pregnant uterus. Volume replacement is critically important during pregnancy, as uteroplacental perfusion is directly related to intravascular volume. The increased plasma volume of pregnancy—up to 50 percent in singletons—must be considered when calculating fluid replacement (Mighty, 1994).

If possible, the injured pregnant woman who is at more than 20 weeks' gestation should be kept in the lateral decubitus position. If this is not possible due to suspected back or neck injuries, the uterus should be displaced to the left. This can be accomplished with a 6-inch towel rolled and placed under the hip or backboard. Alternatively, an individual can be assigned to manually deflect the uterus.

Military anti-shock trousers (MAST) have been commonly used in hypovolemic shock in an attempt to displace pooled blood from the lower extremities into the circulating volume. Appropriate use of these trousers can improve blood pressure, increase preload and systemic vascular resistance, and control abdominal and pelvic hemorrhage. There is little or no published experience with the use of this device during pregnancy, and inflating the abdominal component could, in theory, compress the uterus against the vena cava and further decrease preload (Pearlman and colleagues, 1990a).

Once the maternal vital signs have been stabilized and the extent of maternal injury has been determined, the fetal heart rate should be determined. The obstetric evaluation and care of the fetus are dependent to a large degree on gestational age. Newborns frequently survive intact beyond 26 weeks, and occasionally before that. Continuous monitoring of uterine activity and fetal heart rate should be initiated routinely following trauma after midpregnancy. Even if attempts are not made to salvage the fetus, such monitoring adds another "vital sign" of maternal stability.

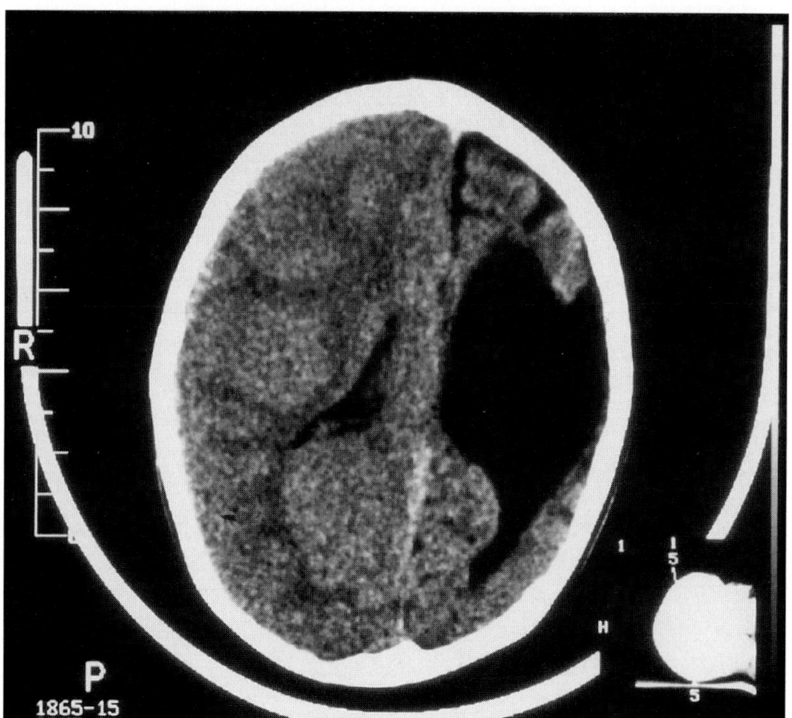

Figure 35–5. Cranial computed tomograph demonstrating a large defect of the brain in the distribution of the right middle cerebral artery. The fetus was in breech presentation and the shoulder restraint would have been in close proximity to the left parietal bone. At delivery, some 10 weeks after the accident, one-third of the placental surface area had also infarcted.

The prediction of abruptio placentae following trauma is best made using both components of cardiotocographic monitoring. Continuous fetal heart rate monitoring is useful to detect sudden fetal decompensation, as can occur with placental separation or intraabdominal hemorrhage. While bradycardia can be detected with either continuous monitoring or intermittent auscultation, more subtle signs of fetal hypoxia such as persistent late decelerations or loss of beat-to-beat variability are more easily detected by continuous monitoring (Fig. 35–6). Monitoring of uterine activity appears to be the most sensitive method of detecting abruptio placentae. In three separate studies, continuous electronic monitoring for short periods of time permitted detection of all cases of abruptio placentae. The most consistent finding of abruptio placentae was frequent uterine activity (Goodwin and Breen, 1990; Pearlman and colleagues, 1990b; Williams and co-workers, 1990).

The American College of Obstetricians and Gynecologists (1991) recommends that following trauma of any severity, pregnant women beyond 22–24 weeks' gestation should be routinely monitored for a minimum of 4 hours. Monitoring should begin as soon as feasible following maternal stabilization. In women with four or more uterine contractions in any 1 hour during this period, the monitoring period is extended to 24 hours. While nearly all women who subsequently develop abruptio placentae will have contractions during the monitoring period, so will many others who do not suffer abruptio placentae. Typically, women with abruptio placentae continue to have uterine contractions and will often develop other signs such as vaginal bleeding, uterine tenderness, changes in the fetal heart tracing, hypertonic contractions, or uterine pain. In the others, the frequency of contractions typically decreases over time. A small number of women continue to have contractions and go into labor without evidence of abruptio placentae. This latter scenario is uncommon and difficult to differentiate from the woman with abruptio placentae (Pearlman and colleagues, 1990b). For this reason, most investigators do not recommend tocolysis for uterine contractions following trauma. The use of β-mimetics is particularly problematic in this setting because they induce tachycardia and decrease systemic blood pressure

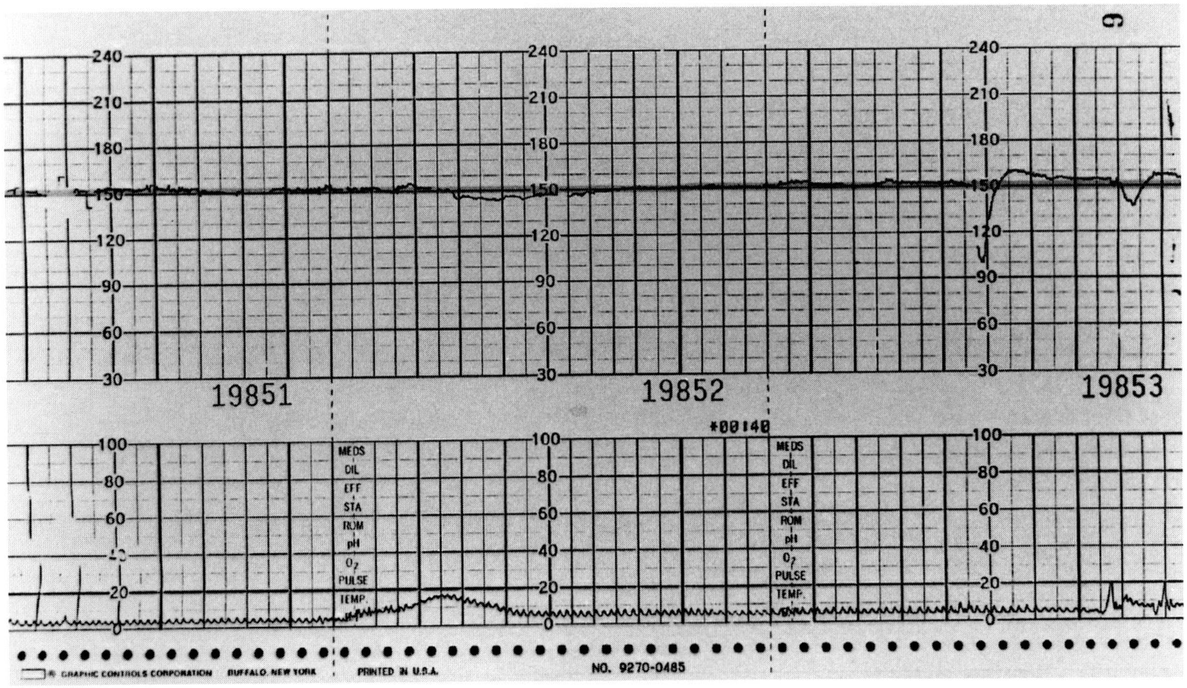

Figure 35–6. Fetal heart rate tracing of fetus shown in Figure 35–5. Note the virtual absence of beat-to-beat variability despite the fact that this is an external fetal monitor. Also shown is a subtle late and variable type decelerations.

findings hard to differentiate from hypovolemia. If tocolytics are to be used, then magnesium sulfate is preferred.

Continuous electronic fetal heart rate and uterine activity monitoring are superior to ultrasound in diagnosing abruptio placentae (Goodwin and Breen, 1990; Pearlman and associates, 1990b;). Ultrasonic evaluation is useful in the setting of trauma to establish gestational age, determine fetal well-being if monitoring is equivocal, estimate amnionic fluid volume if ruptured membranes are suspected, or confirm fetal death. An algorithm useful in the management of blunt abdominal trauma is provided in Figure 35–7.

PENETRATING TRAUMA

Penetrating trauma complicating pregnancy is encountered much less frequently than blunt trauma. The majority of penetrating trauma is from bullets from handguns—some of which are self-inflicted—and stab wounds. Swords, animal horns, cannon balls, sickles, shrapnel from mines, and even a barbecue fork injury have been reported! Numerous case series of penetrating trauma during pregnancy have been published, dating back to the 1800s. Two important observations can be made from reviewing the management of penetrating trauma during pregnancy in the late nineteenth and early twentieth century. First, observation of women with penetrating abdominal wounds—the typical management in this era—resulted in very low mortality rates—less than 10 percent—compared with penetrating wounds suffered in nonpregnant patients, which generally exceeded 50 percent at that time. Second, since 1912, no cases of maternal mortality due to penetrating uterine trauma have been reported.

There have been a number of case series of penetrating abdominal wounds reported. As shown in Table 35–2, there is disparate risk for the woman and her fetus following penetrating trauma. This is true for at least two reasons. First, the likelihood of injury to an intraabdominal organ is directly proportional to the size of that organ. In late pregnancy, the uterus occupies a large proportion of the intraabdominal volume, placing the uterus and its contents at significant risk for injury. Second, the mass of the myometrium, amnionic fluid, fetus, and placenta acts as a "shield" against injury of maternal intraabdominal organs. A projectile penetrating the abdominal cavity and uterus transfers energy to the tissues through which it is passing. The loss of kinetic energy to the surrounding tissue slows the velocity of the bullet, with the bullet often coming to rest within the uterus. This is demonstrated in clinical series with injuries isolated to the uterus in more than two-thirds of cases (Table 35–2). Thus, when the uterus is injured by penetrating wounds, the fetus is more likely than the mother to be injured (Fig. 35–8).

As the uterus enlarges, the abdominal viscera are forced upward, occupying a smaller volume in the upper abdomen. While the uterus does "protect" abdominal viscera by diminishing missile velocity and displacing the viscera, penetrating wounds that enter or exit above the uterus can create very complex wounds, with the possibility of multiple entry and exit wounds in the bowel. High-velocity projectiles can penetrate through the entire uterus, causing serious injury to organs posterior to the uterus, for example, the aorta and sigmoid colon.

Essentially there are three decisions to be made in the management of penetrating wounds during pregnancy: (1) whether to perform exploratory laparotomy, (2) whether to deliver the fetus, and (3) if delivery is planned, the mode of delivery.

The first decision—whether to explore—is easy if there is obvious hypovolemia and hemoperitoneum, but it is usually more difficult because many of these women are hemodynamically stable. Most authors agree that pregnant women who suffer gunshot wounds to the abdomen should be explored (Franger and colleagues, 1989; Kirshon and associates, 1988). As a bullet enters the abdominal cavity, it can be deflected by abdominal structures. This can dramatically alter its path, making it impossible to accurately predict the course of the bullet once it has entered the body. As the bullet is deflected, it tends to tumble, which creates more extensive damage to internal organs than the small entry wound might suggest. In addition, high-velocity projectiles create shock waves, and temporary cavitation can damage tissue well outside the actual projectile path. While extrauterine injuries are not particularly common with penetrating trauma, when they do occur most result from gunshot

STABILIZATION

- Maintain airway and oxygenation
- Deflect uterus to left
- Maintain circulatory volume
- Secure cervical spine if head or neck injury suspected

↓

COMPLETE EXAMINATION

- Control external hemorrhage
- Identify/stabilize serious injuries
- Examine uterus
- Pelvic examination to identify ruptured membranes or vaginal bleeding
- Obtain initial blood work (including Kleihauer-Betke test)
- Obstetrical consultation

↓

FETAL EVALUATION

↙ ↘

$\leq$20 weeks → Document

$\geq$20 weeks → Initiate monitoring

↓

Presence of:

- More than 4 uterine contractions in any one hour ($\geq$20 weeks)
- Rupture of amnionic membranes
- Vaginal bleeding
- Serious maternal injury
- Fetal tachycardia; late decelerations; non-reactive NST

↙ ↘

Yes

Hospitalize; continue monitor if $>$20 weeks

No

Other definitive treatment (may be done concomitant with monitoring):

- Suture lacerations
- Necessary x-rays
- Anti-D globulin if indicated
- Tetanus toxoid if indicated

↓

Discharge with follow-up and instructions

Figure 35–7. Algorithm for management of trauma during pregnancy.

TABLE 35–2. PENETRATING TRAUMA DURING PREGNANCY

		Percent with:			
Series	***N***	*Extrauterine Injuries*	*Maternal Mortality*	*Fetal Injuries*	*Perinatal Mortality*
Kobak and Hurwitz (1954)	33	24	9 (all before 1912)	70	70
Martinez and Garcia (1964)	45	27	6.6 (all before 1912)	75	71
Buchsbaum (1968)	16	38	0	59	71
Buchsbaum (1975)	9	33	0	89	66
Buchsbaum (1979)	16	19	0	59	41

wounds. For these reasons, we recommend that gunshot injuries to the abdomen during pregnancy be explored.

Knife wounds to the uterus are much less likely to result in extrauterine injuries, and overall their prognosis is much better compared with gunshot wounds. The decision to perform laparotomy in the pregnant woman with an abdominal stab wound must be individualized (Kuhlmann and Cruikshank, 1994). Stab wounds to the upper abdomen are more likely to cause visceral injury than lower abdominal stab wounds, and exploration is necessary in most cases of upper abdominal wounds. While stab wounds to the lower abdomen have been successfully managed without laparotomy, several considerations must be addressed (Grubb, 1992). In nonpregnant patients, stab wounds do not penetrate the peritoneum in about a third of cases. Unless a large extraperitoneal vessel is lacerated, for example, the inferior epigastric artery, these extraperitoneal wounds generally do not need exploration. However, distention and attenuation of the abdominal wall during pregnancy may make it more susceptible to peritoneal penetration. A fistulogram of the wound can be performed to determine if there has been peritoneal penetration. Demonstration of spillage into the gastrointestinal or urinary tract require surgical intervention. An intravenous pyelogram or retrograde cystourethrogram are useful adjuncts if injury to the urethra or bladder is suspected. Amniocentesis has been suggested to determine if there is blood or bacteria within the amnionic fluid. However, the presence of bloody amnionic fluid alone is not an indication for delivery, particularly for the very immature fetus. Likewise, growth of a few colonies of bacteria from the amnionic fluid in the clinically uninfected uterus does not mandate delivery.

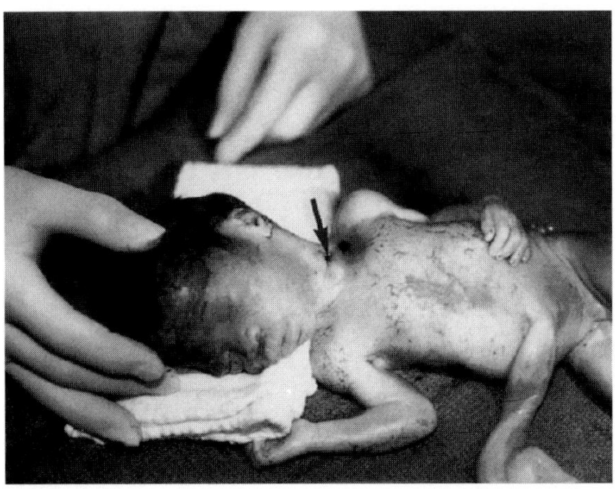

Figure 35–8. This 25-week fetus was killed by a gunshot wound to the neck. The .22 caliber bullet entered the uterine fundus anteriorly and lodged posteriorly in the lower uterine segment just beneath the serosa. (From Cunningham, 1993, with permission. Photograph courtesy of Dr. R. Santos.)

The uterine vessels are lateral and somewhat posteriorly placed during pregnancy, making them unlikely to be injured by stab wounds. However, longer blades or lateral abdominal wall entry may lacerate uterine vessels. Because of the increased blood flow to the uterus—600 mL/minute at term—evidence of hypovolemia is usually quickly evident if there is uterine vascular injury. If there is any question as to whether there is significant intraperitoneal bleeding, peritoneal lavage is a simple and accurate method of establishing whether there is a hemoperitoneum (Rothenberger and colleagues, 1977). If the uterus has been penetrated, there is significant risk for fetal injury. It is very difficult to assess the extent of fetal injury unless the fetus has died. The decision to intervene in a pregnancy where uterine perforation is known or suspected can be difficult. There is little reason to intervene if the fetus is not viable, unless the uterus must be emptied to adequately explore or repair maternal injuries. While some authors have proceeded with cesarean section when uterine stab wounds were found at exploration, most of the fetal wounds were either superficial or of such severity that immediate delivery would not have had impact on outcome. Finally, tetanus prophylaxis should be administered to pregnant women who suffer penetrating injuries.

THERMAL INJURY

As many as 8 percent of burn patients admitted to hospitals are pregnant (Amy and coworkers, 1985; Smith and colleagues, 1983). The physiologic changes of pregnancy are particularly important in these women, as fluid management and the hypermetabolic state following thermal injuries are often quite complicated. Fluid shifts and electrolyte disturbances are common, and special attention must be paid to these. The hypermetabolic state increases caloric demand, and glucose monitoring is critical to prevent maternal hypoglycemia and associated fetal complications. In addition, burn patients are more likely to develop hypernatremia and to lose intravascular volume and protein. Because of these, careful attention to assessment of intravascular volume is necessary by frequent measurement of vital signs, urine output, and central filling pressures (Kuhlmann and Cruikshank, 1994).

Respiratory injury frequently complicates burn injury and may result in both maternal hypoxemia and elevated carboxyhemoglobin levels. These may develop even in the absence of obvious thermal injury. Because fetal hemoglobin has a higher affinity for carbon monoxide than adult hemoglobin, smoke inhalation may be more dangerous to the fetus than to the mother.

Prior series reporting outcome of thermal injury during pregnancy emphasize the strong correlation between percent of body surface area involvement and pregnancy outcome (Matthews, 1982). If thermal injury exceeded 60 percent of body surface area, 80 percent of these women died compared with less than 3 percent maternal deaths if less than 40 percent is burned. Given these dismal outcome statistics in severely burned women, if body surface area burn injury exceeds 50–60 percent, strong consideration should be given to delivery within 24 hours if the fetus is alive and of viable gestational age. Fetal survival likewise depends on the extent of injury. In the study by Rode and colleagues (1990), if the maternal body surface injury exceeded 50 percent, then fetal survival was approximately 10 percent. This compared with 80 percent fetal survival when maternal injury was less than 50 percent. Obstetric indications should dictate the route of delivery in burn victims, and under most circumstances, vaginal delivery is preferred in these critically ill women.

Sepsis is a common complication in the burn patient and may predispose the pregnant woman to preterm labor. Phospholipase A_2 causes release of arachidonic acid from membrane-bound phospholipids and the subsequent production of prostaglandin. Direct tissue injury may also result in release of prostaglandin E_2. Some physicians use tocolytics in burn patients with less than 50 percent injury, but this should be done with caution. The use of β-mimetics can be very dangerous in pregnant burn victims because fluid disturbances, direct respiratory injury, hypoproteinemia, and infection all predispose to pulmonary edema. For these reasons, magnesium sulfate would be the tocolytic of choice in these women. Careful monitoring of serum magnesium level and urine output are necessary.

ELECTRICAL INJURY

The damage created by these uncommon injuries depends in large part on the entry and exit points of the current. If the current path is from the upper body to the lower extremity, the uterus and its contents are subject to injury. This is true due to the low resistance of the amnionic fluid and placenta. Serious maternal injury frequently results from cardiac dysrhythmias or respiratory arrest and are most likely if the thorax is part of the current path.

Human experiences with electrical injury during pregnancy are limited. Pierce and associates (1986) summarized 11 cases of lightning injuries during pregnancy. Remarkably, there were no maternal deaths, and fetal deaths occurred immediately with no described long-term problems in fetal survivors of the immediate event. This experience is contrasted by a report of six pregnancies complicated by electrical injury (Leiberman and co-workers, 1986). Though all the mothers survived, there were two immediate fetal deaths, one delayed fetal death complicated by growth retardation and oligohydramnios, and two of the three other livebirths were complicated by oligohydramnios. While the experience is limited, serial ultrasound monitoring of amnionic fluid volume seems prudent following electrical injury in which the fetus survives.

SEXUAL ASSAULT

According to the Federal Bureau of Investigation (United States Department of Justice, 1988), the incidence of sexual assault has increased fourfold compared with other crimes in the United States. It generally is held that only 10–20 percent of sexual assaults are reported. Until recently, there has been limited published experiences of rape in pregnancy.

Satin and co-workers (1991) reviewed over 5700 sexual assaults that were committed in Dallas County over 6 years and found that 2 percent of the victims were pregnant. Perhaps surprisingly, associated physical trauma was less common than in nonpregnant rape victims, and only a third of assaults took place beyond 20 weeks' gestation. From a forensic standpoint, evidence collection was not altered because of pregnancy. As stressed by Hampton, 1995, psychologic counselling for the rape victim and her family cannot be overemphasized.

SUMMARY

Trauma is seen with increasing frequency in all segments of society, including pregnant women. Blunt trauma is far more frequent in pregnant women than is penetrating trauma. The first priority is to stabilize the mother; only then is attention directed towards the pregnancy. With blunt trauma, abruptio placenta should be considered. The diagnosis is often apparent, but may be subtle and present as nothing more than an abnormal fetal heart rate pattern and uterine irritability. Sonography is not reliable for either diagnosing or excluding placental abruption. With penetrating trauma—especially to the abdomen—surgical exploration often is required. In cases involving penetrating trauma to the lower abdomen, fetal prognosis is considerably worse than the prognosis for the mother.

REFERENCES

American College of Obstetricians and Gynecologists. Trauma during pregnancy. Technical Bulletin No. 161, 1991.

Agran PF, Dunkle DE, Winn DG, Kent D. Fetal death in motor vehicle accidents. Ann Emerg Med 1987; 16:1355.

Amy BW, McManus WF, Goodwin CW, et al. Thermal injury in the pregnant patient. Surg Gynecol Obstet 1985; 161:209.

Baker SP, Whitfield RA, O'Neill B. County mapping of injury mortality. J Trauma 1988; 28:741.

Buchsbaum HJ. Splenic rupture in pregnancy. Obstet Gynecol Surv 1967; 22:381.

Buchsbaum HJ. Accidental injury complicating pregnancy. Am J Obstet Gynecol 1968; 101:752.

Buchsbaum HJ. Diagnosis and management of abdominal gunshot wounds during pregnancy. J Trauma 1975; 15:425.

Buchsbaum HJ. Penetrating injury of the abdomen. In: Buchsbaum HJ, ed. Trauma in Pregnancy. Philadelphia: Saunders, 1979:82.

Crosby WM. Traumatic injuries during pregnancy. Clin Obstet Gynecol 1983; 4:902.

Crosby WM. Trauma in the pregnant patient. Conn Med 1986; 4:251.

Crosby WM, Costiloe JP. Safety of lap-belt restraint for pregnant victims of automobile collisions. N Engl J Med 1971; 284:632.

Crosby WM, Snyder RG, Snow CC, Hanson PG. Impact injuries in pregnancy. Am J Obstet Gynecol 1968; 101:100.

Dahmus MA, Sibai BM. Blunt abdominal trauma: are there any predictive factors for abruptio placentae or maternal-fetal distress? Am J Obstet Gynecol 1993; 169:1054.

Drost TF, Rosemurgy AS, Sherman HF, et al. Major trauma in pregnant women: maternal/fetal outcome. J Trauma 1990; 30:574.

Fildes J, Reed L, Jones N, et al. Trauma: the leading cause of maternal death. J Trauma 1992; 32:643.

Franger AL, Buchsbaum HJ, Peaceman AM. Abdominal gunshot wounds in pregnancy. Am J Obstet Gynecol 1989; 160:1124.

Fries MH, Hankins GDV. Motor vehicle accident associated with minimal maternal trauma but subsequent fetal demise. Ann Emerg Med 1989; 18:301.

Galle PC, Anderson SG. A case of automobile trauma during pregnancy. Obstet Gynecol 1979; 54:467.

George ER, Vanderkwaak T, Scholten DJ. Factors influencing pregnancy outcome after trauma. Am Surg 1992; 58:594.

Goodwin TM, Breen MT. Pregnancy outcome and fetomaternal hemorrhage after noncatastrophic trauma. Am J Obstet Gynecol 1990; 162:665.

Grubb DK. Nonsurgical management of penetrating uterine trauma in pregnancy: a case report. Am J Obstet Gynecol 1992; 166:583.

Hampton HL. Care of the woman who has been raped. N Engl J Med 1995; 332:234.

Handel CK. Case report of uterine rupture after an automobile accident. J Reprod Med 1978; 20:90.

Helton AS, McFarlane J, Anderson ET. Battered and pregnant: a prevalence study. Am J Public Health 1987; 77:1337.

Hoff WS, D'Amelio LF, Tinkoff GH, et al. Maternal predictors of fetal demise in trauma during pregnancy. Surg Gynecol Obstet 1991; 172:175.

Iwamoto HS. Cardiovascular responses to reduced oxygen delivery: studies in fetal sheep at 0.55–0.7 gestation. In: Gluckman P, Johnson BM, Nathanielsz P, eds. Advances in Fetal Physiology. Ithaca, NY: Perinatology Press, 1989:43.

Kirshon B, Young R, Gordon AN. Conservative management of abdominal gunshot wound in a pregnant woman. Am J Perinatol 1988; 5:232.

Kissinger DP, Rozycki GS, Morris JA, et al. Trauma in pregnancy: Predicting pregnancy outcome. Arch Surg 1991; 126:1079.

Kobak AJ, Hurwitz CH. Gunshot wounds of the pregnant uterus. Obstet Gynecol 1954; 4:383.

Kuhlmann RS, Cruikshank DP. Maternal trauma during pregnancy. Clin Obstet Gynecol 1994; 37:274.

Lane PL. Traumatic fetal deaths. J Emerg Med 1989; 7:433.

Leiberman JR, Mazor M, Molcho J, et al. Electrical accidents during pregnancy. Obstet Gynecol 1986; 67:861.

Matthews RN. Obstetric implications of burns in pregnancy. Br J Obstet Gynecol 1982; 89:603.

McCormick RD. Seat belt injury: case of complete transection of pregnant uterus. J AOA 1968; 67:1139.

McNabney WK, Smith EI. Penetrating wounds of the gravid uterus. J Trauma 1973; 12:1024.

Meizner I, Potashnik G. Shrapnel penetration in pregnancy resulting in fetal death. Isr J Med Sci 1988; 24:431.

Mighty H. Trauma in pregnancy. Crit Care Clin 1994; 10:623.

Pearlman MD, Tintinalli JE. Trauma in pregnancy [Clinical Conference]. Ann Emerg Med 1988; 17:829.

Pearlman MD, Tintinalli JE. Evaluation and treatment of the gravida and fetus following trauma during pregnancy. Obstet Gynecol Clin North Am 1991; 18:371.

Pearlman MD, Tintinalli JE, Lorenz RP. Blunt trauma during pregnancy. N Engl J Med 1990a; 323:1609.

Pearlman MD, Tintinalli JE, Lorenz RP. A prospective controlled study of outcome after trauma during pregnancy. Am J Obstet Gynecol 1990b; 162:1502.

Pepperell RJ, Rubinstein E, MacIsaac IA. Motorcar accidents during pregnancy. Med J Aust 1977; 1:203.

Pierce MR, Henderson RA, Mitchell JM. Cardiopulmonary arrest secondary to lightning injury in a pregnant woman. Ann Emerg Med 1986; 15:597.

Pierson R, Mihalovits H, Thomas L, Beatty R. Penetrating abdominal wounds in pregnancy. Ann Emerg Med 1986; 15:144.

Rode H, Miller AJ, Cywes S, et al. Thermal injury in pregnancy—the neglected tragedy. S Afr Med J 1990; 77:346.

Rose PG, Strohm PL, Zuspan FP. Fetomaternal hemorrhage following trauma. Am J Obstet Gynecol 1985; 153:844.

Rothenberger DA, Quattlebaum FW, Zabel J, Fischer RP. Diagnostic peritoneal lavage for blunt trauma in pregnant women. Am J Obstet Gynecol 1977; 129:479.

Rothenberger D, Quattlebaum FW, Perry JF, et al. Blunt maternal trauma: a review of 103 cases. J Trauma 1987; 18:173.

Satin AJ, Hemsell DL, Stone IC Jr, et al. Sexual assault in pregnancy. Obstet Gynecol 1991; 77:710.

Smith A, LeMire WA, Hurd WW, Pearlman MD. Repair of the traumatically ruptured gravid uterus: a report of two cases resulting in subsequent viable pregnancies. J Reprod Med (in press).

Smith BK, Rayburn WF, Feller I. Burns and pregnancy. Clin Perinatol 1983; 10:383.

Stafford PA, Biddinger PW, Zumwalt RE. Lethal intrauterine fetal trauma. Am J Obstet Gynecol 1988; 159:485.

Trauma in Pregnancy in Advanced Trauma Life Support. Amer Coll Surg 1985.

United States Department of Justice, Federal Bureau of Investigation. Uniform crime reports for the United States. Washington DC: United States Government Printing Office, 1988:46.

Varner MW. Maternal mortality in Iowa from 1952 to 1986. Surg Gynecol Obstet 1989; 168:555.

Weinstein EC, Pallais V. Rupture of the pregnant uterus from blunt trauma. J Trauma 1968; 8:1111.

World Health Organization. Geneva: World Health Statistics, 1989.

Wilkening RB, Meschia F. Fetal oxygen uptake, oxygenation, and acid-base balance as a function of uterine blood flow. Am J Physiol 1983; 244:H749.

Williams JK, McClain L, Rosemurgy AS, Colorado NM. Evaluation of blunt abdominal trauma in the third trimester of pregnancy: maternal and fetal considerations. Obstet Gynecol 1990; 75:33.

CHAPTER 36

Breast Disease During Pregnancy and Lactation

The breasts normally undergo remarkable physiologic changes during pregnancy and lactation. As in the nonpregnant woman, numerous diseases may affect the breasts, ranging from physiologic and/or anatomic abnormalities to neoplasms. There are also some abnormal conditions unique to pregnancy and lactation. Finally, as a result of normal physiologic changes, some diseases, particularly malignant neoplasms, may be more difficult to diagnose. Knowledge of the normal anatomy and physiology of the breast during pregnancy and lactation is essential to further understanding of disease conditions, diagnostic methods and their interpretation, and therapeutic options.

NORMAL ANATOMY AND PHYSIOLOGY

Nonpregnant

The breast is a modified sweat gland underlying subcutaneous tissue and skin. The main functional unit consists of a single gland composed of two major parts, the terminal duct–lobular unit and a large duct system (Fig. 36–1). The terminal duct–lobular unit is formed by a lobule and terminal ductule. This connects with the large duct system, which is a series of increasingly larger ducts leading from the terminal ducts to a collecting duct, which empties into the nipple. Division of breast tissue into these two components also reflects disease processes that affect the breast. Conditions such as fibrocystic changes, ductal hyperplasias, and carcinomas affect the terminal duct–lobular unit, whereas the large duct system is the site of duct ectasias and papillomas (Appozardi, 1979; Wellings and associates, 1975).

The lobules and ducts consist primarily of a two-cell type epithelium. The *luminal epithelium* consists mainly of secretory and absorptive cells; for histopathologic and functional purposes, these cells may be considered as a single entity. Underlying the luminal epithelium is a network of *myoepithelial cells,* which function as contractile elements that assist in the secretory process.

Functional breast changes are largely under hormonal control and may therefore demonstrate a variety of macro- and microscopic changes under normal conditions. The prepubertal breast is largely inactive, containing small lobules and infrequent ducts. Hormonal changes during puberty result in growth and differentiation. Although estrogen provides the major influence, full differentiation of breast tissue requires an interplay of a variety of hormones, including prolactin, progesterone, insulin, cortisol, thyroxine, and growth hormone (Fig. 36–2A) (Topper, 1970).

During the reproductive years, the breast exhibits changes that vary according to the

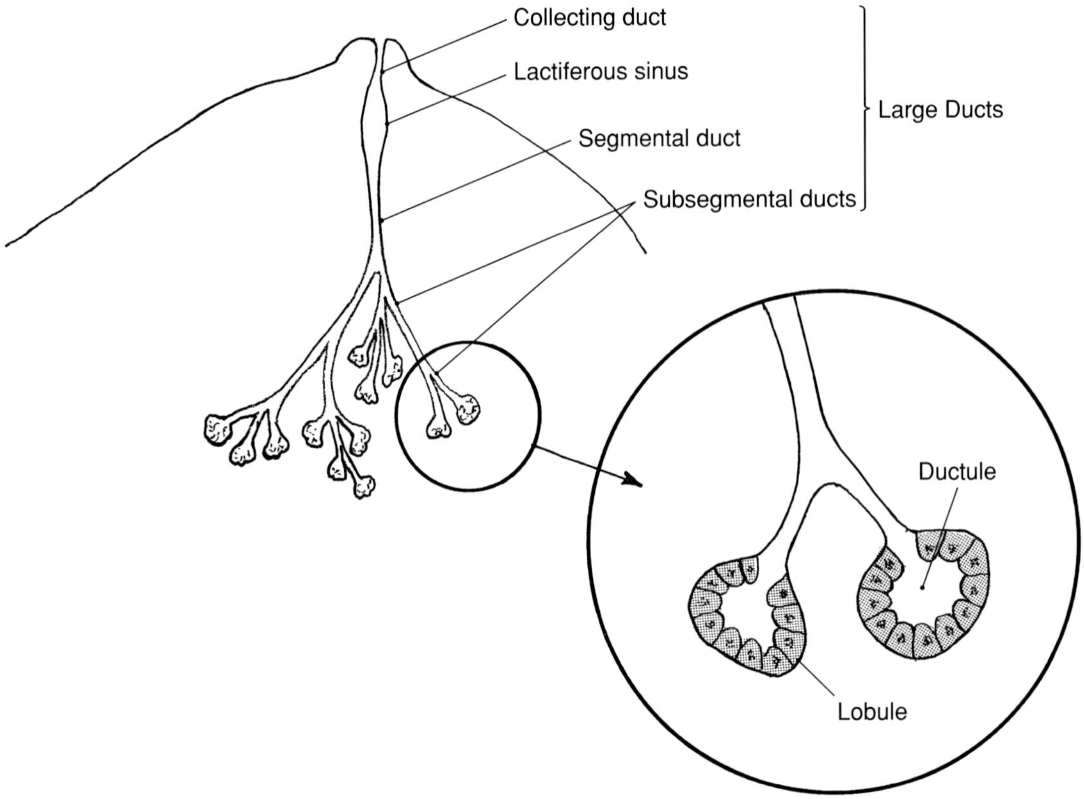

Figure 36–1. Schematic illustration of the terminal duct–lobular unit (TDLU) of the breast.

menstrual cycle. In simple terms, estrogen primarily stimulates epithelial proliferation in the ductal portion of the glands, and progesterone influences growth of the lobule (Speroff and associates, 1989). Hormonal manipulation during reproductive years has effects on the breast as it would other hormonally dependent female organs.

The breast may undergo involution during postmenopausal years, although this is dependent on exogenous administration or endogenous conversion of sex hormones. Both the epithelium and stroma become inactive; the epithelium atrophies and the stroma may be replaced by dense fibrous connective tissue (Fig. 36–2B). Histologic preparations usually demonstrate minimal lobular tissue. The lobules may undergo microcystic change; however, these are not fibrocystic changes because of lack of proliferation.

Pregnancy and Lactational Changes

The breasts undergo marked physiologic and micro-anatomic changes during pregnancy and lactation. The physiology of lactation requires a complex interplay of hormones already described as being involved in differentiation of the breast, at, however, significantly altered levels. Additionally, there is the contribution of oxytocin, and to some extent, human placental lactogen. A full description of these changes is beyond the scope of this chapter.

During pregnancy, numerous secretory glands develop from gland buds and there is proliferation of all cell types (Joshi and colleagues, 1986). In contrast to nonpregnancy, in which stroma predominates over glands, the breast during pregnancy is characterized by many more glands and progressively decreasing stroma (Cotran and associates, 1989). The epithelial cells develop secretory vacuoles, which contain lipid, becoming most predominant in the third trimester. Some apocrine secretion is apparent as the vacuoles develop; however, significant secretions are not present until lactation (Fig. 36–3).

With hyperplasia, the breasts increase in size. Blood vessels and lymphatic channels proliferate in pregnancy, and there is increased stromal edema (Gupta and associates, 1993). As subsequently detailed, these changes may lead to difficulty in diagnosing breast lesions.

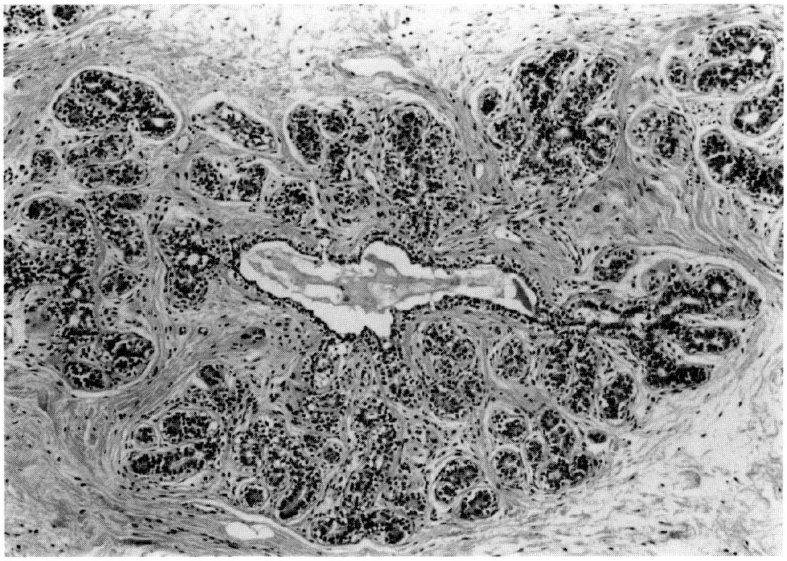

A

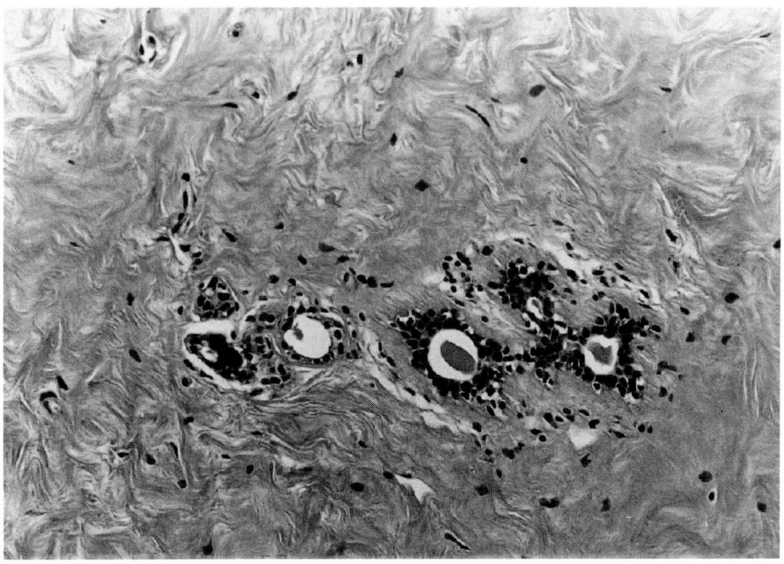

B

Figure 36–2. A. Normal functional breast tissue. The breast is affected by hormonal influence. Estrogen primarily stimulates ductal epithelial proliferation; progesterone stimulates growth of the lobule. For clinical and histopathologic purposes, distinction between the proliferative and secretory phases is not usually necessary. **B.** Postmenopausal atrophy. With the lack of hormonal stimulation, atrophic ducts are the main component present.

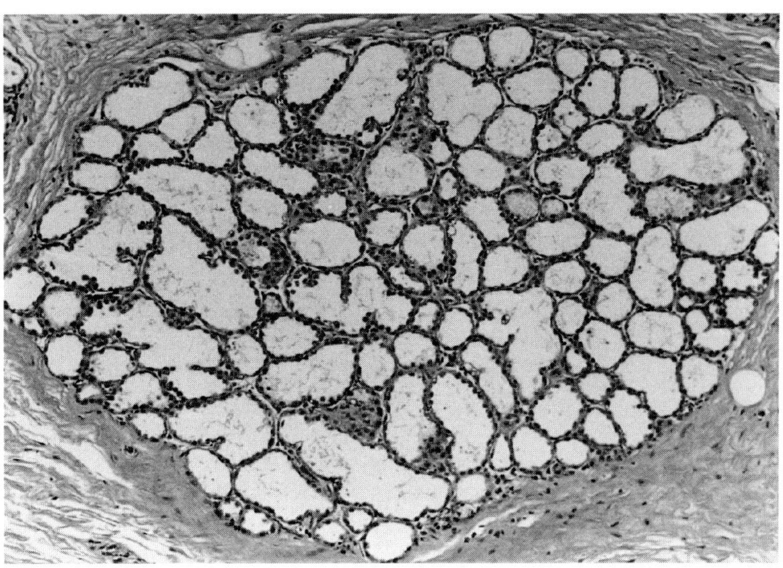

Figure 36–3. A section from a lactating adenoma, which in this area demonstrates lactational changes that may be seen in a normal breast tissue during pregnancy and lactation. Note the marked increase in lobular glandular tissue, secretory changes, and decreased stroma in the lobule.

These physiologic changes, particularly edema, increased density, and increased fat, make interpretation of mammography difficult during pregnancy (Donegan, 1988; Gallenberg and Loprinzi, 1989; Lichter and Lippman, 1988).

Mammary Hyperplasia

While the breasts normally increase in size during pregnancy and lactation, massive enlargement occasionally occurs (Eben and colleagues, 1993). This is due to normal but extreme hyperplasia of glands and stroma. Abnormal enlargement usually starts in the first trimester, and often complicates subsequent pregnancies (Beischer and co-workers, 1989). Many different treatment regimens have been used, including testosterone, stilbestrol, corticosteroids, and progesterone (Eben and colleagues, 1993). In nearly all cases, reduction mammoplasty or mastectomy was eventually required to relieve symptoms. More recently, bromocriptine has been used with successful outcomes following doses of 5–7.5 mg/day in divided doses, although doses as high as 20 mg daily have been reported (Hedberg and associates, 1979; Turkalj and colleagues, 1982). Bromocriptine appears to be well tolerated by the fetus, although there are reports of fetal growth retardation (Briggs and associates, 1990). Although many of these bromocriptine-treated women also required subsequent surgery, some have been treated successfully with bromocriptine alone (Eben and colleagues, 1993).

INFLAMMATORY BREAST LESIONS

Mastitis

Breast infection may complicate the puerperium in up to 2 percent of women (Stehman, 1990). Although this common disorder usually responds quickly to therapy, it can also lead to significant maternal morbidity if an abscess develops. The diagnosis is not always straightforward; for example, engorgement may confuse the clinical picture. Occasionally, the reproductive-age woman will present with an inflammatory breast cancer.

The woman with mastitis typically presents 2–3 weeks postpartum complaining of flu-like symptoms, decreased milk secretion, and a swollen, tender area in one breast. Most infections occur within the first 5 weeks of delivery, but may be seen up to 10 months postpartum (Niebyl and associates, 1978). It is not unusual for fever as high as 40°C to occur. On examination there is erythema, heat, induration, tenderness, and edema in a relatively well-defined area corresponding to a breast lobule. Axillary nodes may be enlarged and there usually is leukocytosis with a left shift.

By contrast, breast engorgement is almost always bilateral with generalized involvement. The woman with exquisite tenderness secondary to mastitis may also have engorgement because she has discontinued breast feeding, but physical findings usually indicate an infection.

Stehman (1990) emphasizes that the best feature to differentiate mastitis from inflammatory breast carcinoma is knowledge of prior breast findings. With normal findings antepartum, a neoplastic process is much less likely, although breast cancer can first become apparent during lactation. Among 103 nonnursing women with inflammatory breast cancer, the mean interval between the first symptom and diagnosis of cancer was 45 days (Bozzetti and colleagues, 1981). These women present with mastitis-like findings with unilateral erythema, heat, and induration; but the process is usually more diffuse. Additionally, the skin is thickened or demonstrates *peau d' orange* changes due to tumor involvement of skin lymphatics. There may also be purplish discoloration and satellite nodules. This very lethal form of breast cancer is currently managed by prompt institution of preoperative chemotherapy with follow-on radiation therapy and/or surgery (Jones and Jones, 1990). Biopsy should not be delayed if either a clinical suspicion of inflammatory carcinoma exists or if a woman with mastitis fails to respond to conventional antibiotic therapy. Mammography provides less than optimal information in the lactating breast and is usually not helpful to diagnose inflammatory carcinoma.

Epidemiology

Contrary to older reports, primiparous women are not more predisposed to mastitis (Devereux, 1970). Older literature describes **epidemic mastitis** and **nonepidemic** or **sporadic mastitis.** The epidemic variety was largely staphylococcal and associated with simultaneous manifestations in clusters of hospitalized or recently discharged mothers and infants with the same strains of organisms. In the last 20 years, there have been few reports of such epidemics; however, no explanation is clearly apparent. Because epidemic mastitis was invariably associated with streptococcal or staphylococcal outbreaks in nurseries, improved measures to limit nosocomial infections, as well as earlier discharge may explain why this is seen infrequently today.

Gibberd (1953) concluded that the epidemic variety was secondary to infection of the entire lactiferous system, as opposed to cellulitis involving primarily the breast parenchyma characteristic of the sporadic variety. Because it is the milk and ductal system that is infected in the epidemic variety, the entry point would necessarily be the nipple duct opening; therefore, if bacteria enter several ducts, nonadjacent lobes could be involved as well as the contralateral breast.

The sporadic or nonepidemic variety of mastitis is more likely encountered today. It is best characterized as a mammary cellulitis involving periglandular connective tissue. It usually remains confined to a single pyramidal-shaped breast lobule as demarcated by the normal divisions created by Cooper's ligaments.

There are no known risk factors for the development of mastitis; however, fissured and chaffed nipples have been implicated. It is reasonable to assume that breaks in protective barriers might predispose to bacterial infection by direct entry into the ducts and periductal lymphatics. On the other hand, the majority of women who are nursing have nipple fissures at some time and do not get infected, just as many women without fissures develop mastitis. Because milk is a good culture medium, it can be hypothesized that anything causing milk stasis may predispose to infection with pathogenic bacteria. Stasis may develop from simple engorgement with its attendant edema and decreased egress of milk from ducts secondary to surrounding tissue pressure. Plugging of terminal ducts by epithelial debris can also result in stasis similar to a galactocele.

Microbiology

Exposure to various bacteria occurs from skin colonization, nosocomial bacteria, and the infant's skin, nose, and oropharynx. The most common organism isolated in acute sporadic puerperal mastitis is *Staphylococcus aureus,* ranging from 40 to 90 percent (Niebyl and coworkers, 1978; Schwartz, 1982; Thomsen and co-workers, 1985). In recent years, with improved microbiologic detection methods, a variety of other pathogens have been found to include anaerobic bacteria, coagulase-negative staphylococci, group A and group B streptococci, *Hemophilus influenzae* and *parainfluenzae, Escherichia coli, Streptococcus faecalis, Klebsiella pneumoniae, Enterobacter cloacae, Serratia marcescens,* and *Pseudomonas picetti.*

Because sporadic mastitis is primarily a subcutaneous cellulitis, it is not surprising that the causative organism is not always cultured from milk. Some therefore recommend routine culturing of the infant. Niebyl and colleagues (1978), however, reported no correlation with bacteriologic cultures from milk and infant nasopharyngeal cultures. Only one infant had *S. aureus* and this organism was not found in the mother's milk. In contrast, Wysham and co-investigators (1957) found that similar organisms were cultured from the infant and the mother in all of their cases. Matheson and co-workers (1988a) reported a case of recurrent mastitis secondary to reinfection with *S. aureus* from the infant's skin and nostrils.

Some have questioned the utility of routine cultures of breast milk. Moreover, the clinical significance of a positive culture is also controversial. The frequent presence of coagulase-negative staphylococci in milk from nursing women is confusing because these bacteria are normal skin flora. However, staphylococcal species are predominant findings in women with mastitis. Because of their frequent isolation from women with mastitis, along with recognition that these organisms are pathogens in bovine mastitis, Thomsen and colleagues (1985) designed an investigation to examine the pathogenicity of *S. epidermis* and *S. saprophyticus.* These human isolates were inoculated into the mammary glands of lactating mice and the glands examined histopathologically. Although no clinical evidence of mastitis was found, 80–90 percent of glands had histologic changes of mastitis. While all lesions healed spontaneously in the mice within a week, several abscesses developed. Using an immunofluorescence technique, these same investigators found the universal presence of antibody-coated bacteria in the milk of women with signs of mastitis (Thomsen, 1982). The only organism identified in 25 percent of these women was coagulase-negative staphylococci.

Contradicting the hypothesis that coagulase-negative staphylococci are pathogens in mastitis was the finding that similar distributions of presumed nonpathogenic bacteria were isolated from the affected as well as the unaffected breast (Matheson and colleagues, 1988a). These investigators also obtained cultures of milk from 100 healthy nursing mothers and the frequency of coagulase-negative staphylococci was similar to that found in women with signs and symptoms of mastitis.

If culture is felt to be indicated, it should be done prior to instituting antimicrobial therapy. The nipple and areola are cleaned with an antiseptic solution, allowed to dry, then cultures taken of manually expressed milk. Initial samples are discarded to avoid the possibility of the cleansing preparation interfering with the cultures. Aerobic and anaerobic cultures are recommended.

Attempts to develop quantitative parameters for the diagnosis of mastitis have been reported (Thomsen and associates, 1983). These investigators determined leukocyte counts per milliliter of milk and performed quantitative microbiologic cultivation. These parameters were then employed prospectively to stratify women to different randomized treatment arms, including antibiotic therapy; there was, however, considerable variation in clinical course. Therefore, it was concluded that there was no discernible advantage to the prompt institution of antibiotic therapy in a patient with presumed, but still subclinical, mastitis (Thomsen and colleagues, 1984).

TABLE 36–1. CONSERVATIVE CLINICAL APPROACH TO PRESUMED MASTITIS

1. Examination
2. Culture milk from affected breast (controversial)
3. Consider culture of infants' nose, throat, skin (especially if recurrent mastitis) or notify pediatricians that mother is being treated for mastitis
4. Complete blood count
5. Antibiotic therapy for 10 days
    - Dicloxacillin 250 mg orally every 6 hours
    - Amoxicillin/clavulinate 250–500 mg orally every 8 hours

   For penicillin-allergic patients:
    - Erythromycin 500 mg orally every 6 hours
6. Analgesics
7. Continued nursing—gentle pumping if necessary
8. Hot or cold packs for symptomatic comfort
9. Continued surveillance for abscess
    - Lack of response to therapy within 48–72 hours
    - Development of mass

Treatment

Timely institution of antimicrobial therapy is important in the management of acute puerperal mastitis. Devereux (1970) reported a 10 percent incidence of abscess formation in 71 cases of mastitis in 53 women treated with antibiotics. Antibiotic therapy was delayed for longer than 24 hours in 9 of these women, and 6 subsequently developed abscesses. Early therapy in 20 women with clinical findings consistent with mastitis resulted in prompt resolution of symptoms and no abscess formation in the series reported by Niebyl and coinvestigators (1978).

Table 36–1 outlines a conservative approach to the management of the woman with presumed mastitis. Because of the high frequency with which *S. aureus* is isolated in association with clinical mastitis, most investigators recommend initial therapy with a penicillinase-resistant penicillin such as dicloxacillin. Amoxicillin/clavulinate offers similar *S. aureus* coverage plus broader spectrum coverage for other organisms including anaerobes, but its increased cost is probably not justifiable. For penicillin-allergic women who are hospitalized, vancomycin is given intravenously. If hospitalization is not necessary, then the drug of choice is erythromycin, which achieves concentrations in breast milk that are 50–100 percent of serum concentrations (Graham, 1992).

Nursing

Continuation of nursing is important for treatment of mastitis. Many mothers are concerned about passing infection to their infant, but no untoward effects have been reported (Matheson and colleagues, 1988b; Niebyl and associates, 1978; Thomsen and co-investigators, 1984). Indeed, as previously discussed, many of these infections probably originate from colonization of the nursing neonate. Using restriction fragment length polymorphism (RFLP) of total DNA and of ribosomal DNA, Bingen and colleagues (1992) reported five cases of maternal transmission of *Streptococcus agalactiae* to their neonates via breast milk. All the mothers had postpartum mastitis caused by this organism. One infant was found to be colonized with *S. agalactiae* and four others developed late-onset (5–19 days) infection with meningitis (one case), arthritis (one case), and urinary infection (two cases). The late onset likely excluded acquisition via the maternal genital tract at birth or nosocomial transmission. Although they definitively provided evidence that the maternal milk and infant strains of *S. agalactiae* were identical, it was not possible to prove the original source of the infection.

Because antibiotics cross into breast milk, there may be benefit to providing simultaneous treatment of both mother and infant. There is evidence of increased concentration of phenoxymethyl penicillin in the milk of women with mastitis in contrast to healthy controls (Matheson and colleagues, 1988b). Possible mechanisms for this increased drug concentration include increased blood flow, increased concentration of binding proteins entering the milk, and pH changes. There was also a slight but significant increase in the inflamed breast compared with the contralateral breast.

The importance of continued breastfeeding was demonstrated by Marshall and colleagues (1975). They reported that the only three abscesses that developed in 65 women with mastitis were among 15 women who chose to wean their infants. Thomsen and coworkers (1984) observed that vigorous milk expression was sufficient treatment alone in half of women with proven mastitis. Early therapy and continued lactation was successful in avoiding abscess formation in all 20 women in the series by Niebyl and co-investigators (1978).

If the infected breast is too tender to allow suckling, gentle pumping until nursing can be resumed is the best recommendation. Sometimes the infant will not nurse on the inflamed breast. This is probably not related to any changes in the taste of the milk, but is secondary to engorgement and edema, which can make the areola harder to grip. Pumping can alleviate this. If nursing can continue bilaterally, it is best to begin suckling on the uninvolved breast. This allows letdown to commence before moving to the more tender breast.

Problems with cracked and fissured nipples are most common during the first several weeks of breastfeeding, when the incidence of mastitis is also highest. Several randomized studies have failed to demonstrate that any antepartum "nipple preparation" technique or treatment such as nipple rolling, expression of colostrum, or various creams and ointment can alleviate this universal problem (Brown and Hurlock, 1975). There are some hygienic measures that can help lessen nipple soreness once suckling has begun. The most important is cleansing the nipple with clean water after each feeding (Niebyl and colleagues, 1978). Encrusted milk can cause significant inflammation and irritation and agents such as soaps and alcohol should be avoided. Additionally, mothers should be instructed on the duration of nursing at each nipple and on proper release of the infant's grip on the areola and nipple by inserting a finger into the corner of the infant's mouth. Once fissured, and especially if a coexisting mastitis is present, nipples should be air dried and a nipple shield employed to avoid chaffing by clothing.

Engorgement can be caused by either failure to empty the entire breast or from blockage of a single excretory duct from inspissated milk and epithelial debris. Such blockage can appear as a segmental process, but as stated earlier, erythema and fever will be lacking. Nursing should obviously be continued to prevent diffuse engorgement. This alone will usually result in spontaneous clearance of the obstruction. Direct pressure with manual expression on the engorged segment, as well as mechanical pumping, may also be helpful. Local warm, wet compresses or prone soaks in a hot tub have also been suggested to soften the breast tissue (Neibyl and co-investigators, 1978). The most important caveat is to avoid the archaic remedy of binders or discontinuation of breastfeeding.

Breast Abscess

Abscesses can be difficult to detect clinically because they tend to be confined within the normal architectural segments created by Cooper's ligaments. Thus, the abscess extends or burrows into the underlying breast parenchyma in a pyramidal fashion, and it appears much smaller (Schwartz, 1982). Confinement and associated edema and induration can make evaluation of fluctuance very difficult. Surrounding tissue reaction decreases tissue perfusion and interferes with antibiotic penetration to the abscess cavity. Primary clinical suspicion for an abscess is either failure of mastitis to promptly respond to initial therapy within 48–72 hours or a palpable mass on initial presentation. Because physical examination can be difficult, imaging with ultrasound using a high-frequency transducer can be helpful to identify an abscess. If doubt remains, aspiration is performed and purulent exudate can be sent for culture and Gram stain. For difficult diagnostic situations there may be a place for magnetic resonance or computed tomographic imaging.

An abscess requires prompt drainage under general anesthesia. Vigorous finger dissection of the loculations caused by parenchymal ligaments is necessary for adequate treatment. The wound should be packed open. If cancer is suspected, a small portion of breast tissue can be sent for histopathology. Radial skin incisions and counterincisions to afford dependent drainage are entities of the past (Stehman, 1990). The incision should correspond to skin lines to achieve a good cosmetic result. This often can be done via a circumareolar incision. Even though the wound will be left to heal via secondary intention, excellent cosmetic results can be achieved as long as drainage has been effected prior to massive tissue necrosis and extension throughout multiple breast lobules. After drainage, frequent dressing changes are employed and antibiotics continued until all evidence of cellulitis and inflammation has subsided.

Breast abscesses are primarily ominous threats to breast integrity and only rarely cause sepsis (Schwartz, 1982). Considerable disfigurement can result if an abscess is not treated early or adequately and spontaneous drainage occurs. Demey and co-workers (1989) reported a case of toxic shock syndrome (TSS) developing in a woman with mastitis 8 days postpartum. Although no mass was seen in imaging during the acute process, computerized tomography done for other reasons 3 weeks later disclosed a breast abscess. This was aspirated but subsequently developed a second abscess 3 months later. Surgical drainage was accomplished with removal of 500 mL of purulent exudate.

Unusual Forms of Mastitis

Antepartum Mastitis

There are rare reports of antepartum bacterial mastitis and most are in late pregnancy (Wong and associates, 1986). Presentation, clinical findings, and treatment are identical to that of puerperal mastitis. One of the two women reported by Wong and co-workers (1986) remained febrile and symptomatic for 120 hours after intravenous methicillin had been started. No abscess was ever found with multiple diagnostic techniques. The other patient experienced resolution of symptoms and fever by 4 days.

Tuberculous Mastitis

Although exceedingly rare in the United States, tuberculous mastitis can pose a diagnostic dilemma and may easily be confused with carcinoma. Women at particular risk are from endemic areas such as India, Africa, or Asia. Alagaratnam (1981) reported 16 women from Hong Kong, of whom one was pregnant and three were lactating. They presented with a tender abscess or persistent, firm mass. Axillary adenopathy was present in half of the patients and a fourth had evidence of active tuberculosis elsewhere. Another condition that raises suspicion of a tuberculous process is a recurrent abscess that has failed appropriate drainage or one with multiple draining sinus tracts. Diagnosis can be made by biopsy, revealing typical caseating granulomas and Langhans' type giant cells or by culture. Differential diagnoses include cancer, abscess, and nonspecific granulomatous mastitis. Most of these tuberculous lesions can be treated by simple excision of the abscess. Simple mastectomy is necessary when the majority of the breast has been destroyed. Antituberculosis drug therapy is given for 18 months.

Granulomatous Mastitis

An uncommon granulomatous lesion clinically mimicking breast cancer has been described over the last two decades. This lesion is unique to parous, reproductive-age women. Although a few have been observed in lactating women, there is not a consistent history of breastfeeding. In one series of seven women, all were within 6 years of a gestational event (Fletcher and associates, 1982). Another case was reported in a woman who was 24-weeks pregnant (Macansh and co-workers, 1990). Patients typically present with an enlarging breast mass and axillary nodes which are not usually enlarged or tender. Most were treated by excisional biopsy because of the clinical impression of carcinoma. Macansh and colleagues (1990) described a woman who was diagnosed using fine-needle aspiration and successfully managed with close observation.

Histopathologically, there is an inflammatory reaction consisting of noncaseating epithelioid granulomas. Foreign body giant cells and microabscesses are usually identified. Occasionally multiple granulomas are present, but they are invariably confined to one lobular unit. These lesions can be distinguished from tuberculous granulomas by negative culture, lack of acid-fast bacilli, and noncaseation. The entity is also distinct from plasma cell mastitis, which has an absolute predominance of plasma cells. Accompanying ductule dilatation and inflammation, squamous metaplasia, and foreign body giant cells surrounding keratinaceous material suggest that damage to ductule epithelium is from infection or trauma or is chemically induced by secretory material (Fletcher and colleagues, 1982).

While the precise etiology is unclear, older literature suggested that the histologic similarity to granulomatous thyroiditis and orchitis was evidence for an antigen–antibody reaction. Autoimmune hypotheses are further supported by the association with erythema nodosum and resolution with steroid therapy (Adams and associates, 1987; Fletcher and coworkers, 1982). These latter investigators found a high incidence of postexcision wound infection in 3 of 5 women, and one developed a recurrent mass requiring re-excision. This lends support to an unidentified infectious agent.

BREAST MASSES AND CARCINOMA

Noninfectious breast masses occur relatively infrequently in pregnancy. Because most benign and malignant conditions are indistinguishable, it is difficult to separately describe these, so they will be considered simultaneously. Any of the various benign and malignant conditions that develop in the nonpregnant breast can be found in pregnancy. Although early investigators suggested there was a predominance of specific conditions during pregnancy or lactation, more recent studies have shown that the distribution of general disease categories is similar to that of nonpregnant women.

Histologic subtypes of carcinoma are similar in frequency to those in nonpregnant women, although scirrhous carcinomas is more frequent in pregnancy-associated cancer (Ishida and co-workers, 1992; King and associates, 1985). Some abnormalities that are seen much more frequently in the pregnant or lactating woman include galactoceles, lactating adenomas, and fibroadenomas with lactational change (Table 36–2). Awareness of these pregnancy-related benign conditions is important because false-positive diagnoses may be made on cytologic preparations (Finley and co-investigators, 1989; Novotny and associates, 1991). Importantly, the presence of benign changes does not exclude a malignant process; for example, lobular hyperplasia or mastitis has been reported associated with breast cancer in up to a third of cases (Byrd and colleagues, 1962).

Incidence

Before interpreting reported incidence and prognostic information concerning breast cancer in pregnancy, it is important to be aware that the definition of "pregnancy-associated breast cancer" varies among studies. Some include women in whom breast cancer arises during pregnancy, in some breast cancer predated pregnancy, or in others breast cancer was diagnosed after pregnancy for up to 2 years. In some series, breast cancer diagnosed postpartum is referred to as "lactational-associated." The average age of women with pregnancy-associated breast cancer is 35. The youngest reported was 16 years old, and the youngest with disseminated disease was 18 years old.

Although the lifetime incidence of breast cancer in all women is 1 in 9, the actual inci-

TABLE 36–2. CAUSE OF BREAST MASSES IN 214 PREGNANT AND LACTATING WOMEN

Pathologic Findings	Incidence	(%)
Benign pregnancy/ lactational changes[a]	103	(48)
Cystic change (includes galactocele)	26	(12)
Fibroadenoma with lactational change	36	(16)
Lactating adenoma	2	(1)
Inflammatory conditions	34	(16)
Carcinoma	4	(4)

[a]Includes lobar hyperplasia.
Gupta and colleagues (1993).

dence varies widely by age category according to Survival, Epidemiology and End-Results (SEER) data from the National Cancer Institute (Hankey and colleagues, 1991). They cite incidences that range from 1 in 19,600 in women age 25, to 1 in 622 at age 35, to 1 in 93 at age 45. The incidence then increases significantly in women over 50 and approaches 1 in 30 at age 55 to 1 in 24 by age 60.

The incidence reported for pregnancy-associated breast cancer is about 10–40/100,000, with approximately 1–3 percent of all breast cancers discovered in pregnant or lactating women (Donegan, 1983; Saunders and Baum, 1993; Thierault and colleagues, 1992; Wallack and co-investigators, 1983). As shown in Table 36–3, the incidence of pregnancy-associated breast cancer is significantly higher in the childbearing age group, approaching 15 percent. The incidence in premenopausal women may be increasing, and thus, there may be an increase in pregnancy-associated malignancies (Gloeckler and co-investigators, 1987; Saunders and Baum, 1993).

Investigators have also examined the effect of pregnancy on the incidence of subsequent breast cancer, with controversial findings. Lambe and associates (1994) reported a case-control study of over 12,000 patients, finding that uniparous women had a transiently increased relative risk of developing breast cancer compared to nulliparous or biparous women, particularly if the first delivery occurred at an age greater than 30. After time, this relative increase actually dropped to a relative risk lower than that of nulliparous women. In contrast, Cummings and colleagues (1994), in a case control study involving 2300 patients found no difference in the incidence of breast carcinoma for any time period after pregnancy when compared to controls.

Natural History and Clinical Assessment

Early investigators concluded that breast cancer in pregnancy was a more aggressive disease with a poor prognosis. Since these earlier reports, numerous studies have demonstrated that survival is similar to nonpregnant women, although there is a significant increase in the proportion of those presenting with advanced-stage disease compared with nonpregnant women. Thus, while pregnancy-associated breast cancer is not a more aggressive disease, pregnant women often experience delayed diagnosis that results in presentation at a more advanced stage. For example, Clark and Chua (1989) reported that 46 of 154 (30%) pregnant women and 25 of 96 (26%) lactating patients experienced a delay of greater than 12 months. Delay in diagnosis is reported to range from 2 to 15 months and is significant when compared with diagnosis and institution of therapy in nonpregnant women (Ishida and co-workers, 1992; Zemlickis and associates, 1992). Delays of 3–6 months have been associated with decreased survival; longer delays have been associated with an increased proportion of women with lymph node metastases at diagnosis (Piliphsen, 1984; Bottles, 1985; Donegan, 1983; Parente, 1988; Vernon, 1985, and all their associates).

Montgomery (1961) reported that while 90 percent of 70 pregnant women detected their own cancer, the physician was responsible for diagnostic delay in 60 percent. Bunker and Peters (1963) reported that more than half their patients had a delay from detection to diagnosis of more than 6 months. In another study, more than half of women diagnosed postpartum had a breast mass that was followed clinically during pregnancy (Petrek and associates, 1991).

TABLE 36–3. INCIDENCE OF PREGNANCY-ASSOCIATED BREAST CANCER IN REPRODUCTIVE-AGE WOMEN

Investigators	Age Criteria	Number of Women	Pregnant or Lactating (%)
Applewhite and associates (1973)	<45	655	7
Treves and Holleb (1958)	<35	549	14
Horsley and co-workers (1969)	<35	67	10
Nugent and O'Connell (1985)	25–40	176	11

Diagnostic delay is attributed to physiologic changes as well as physician reluctance to use diagnostic tests or initiate therapy. In many cases a lump is interpreted as consistent with physiologic change, and as a result evaluation of a questionable mass may be postponed until postpartum. Masses may become artifactually small due to enlargement of the normal breast, giving the erroneous impression the mass is resolving (Lichter and Lippman, 1988). There may be a reluctance to perform a biopsy because of potential hemorrhage, increased risk of infection, and development of milk fistula (Donegan, 1988). Finally, there may be a reluctance to initiate therapy because of potentially harmful fetal effects.

The most important tenet, therefore, is to avoid delay in diagnosis and/or treatment just because a woman is pregnant. This includes avoiding delay in evaluation of self-diagnosed masses or symptoms. Breast self-examination has been shown to be associated with a more favorable stage at presentation and with reduced mortality (Foster and associates, 1992). If there is a low suspicion of malignancy, masses may be observed for a short time (2–4 weeks), and if persistent, they should be further evaluated (Barnavon and Wallack, 1990). Breast cancer is the number one reason for "failure to diagnose" suits among obstetrician/gynecologists (Fiorica, 1992). Because there is a much higher frequency of patient–physician contact during antepartum care, Hoover (1990) expresses surprise at this observation.

Clinical Presentation

Benign and malignant lesions of the breast usually will present as a mass. Cancers may also be associated with skin changes including thickening, retraction, or fixation; solid masses; surrounding erythema or edema; or persistent crusting of the nipple (Barnavon and Wallack, 1990; Fiorica, 1992). Serosanguineous or bloody nipple discharge is also worrisome, although its most common cause is an intraductal papilloma. Milk rejection by the nursing infant has been reported associated with cancer, but this obviously is a subjective association (Goldsmith, 1974).

The woman may present with evidence of metastases that include palpably enlarged or knotted axillary lymph nodes, bone pain, pathologic fractures, effusions, or functional visceral abnormalities such as from metastatic disease to the ovaries or gastrointestinal tract. Evans and associates (1992) described a woman who presented with type B lactic acidosis due to metastatic breast cancer at 37 weeks' gestation.

Evaluation

The mainstay of breast mass evaluation involves needle aspiration and/or biopsy. As previously emphasized, clinical findings alone should not be used to "follow" a lesion for an extended period. Moreover, masses should not be disregarded until the postpartum evaluation. Drawbacks to mammography in pregnancy and lactation have been addressed. The precise role of sonography to evaluate breast masses in these women has not been elucidated. While the evaluation of cystic masses may be aided by ultrasound, fine-needle aspiration has been used more commonly and provides the potential for cytopathologic diagnosis rather than a radiologic impression.

Mammography

The same physiologic changes that compromise clinical detection also affect mammography interpretation, which requires contrast analysis. Contrast is significantly reduced during pregnancy and lactation due to increased water content and breast density (Gallenberg and Loprinzi, 1989; Thierault and associates, 1992). The false-negative rate in nonpregnant women ranges from 10 to 15 percent, but may be higher in pregnant or lactating women (Fiorica, 1992; Lichter and Lippman, 1988). In one series, mammograms were considered negative in 75 percent of pregnant or lactating women subsequently diagnosed with breast cancer (Max and Klamer, 1983). Therefore, mammography during pregnancy or lactation has minimal clinical utility.

Mammography has a very small radiation risk for the fetus. The average fetal dose with abdominal shielding is approximately 100 mrad (Barnavon and Wallack, 1990). Not surprisingly, in a series of 368 pregnant women, no adverse effects from mammography were identified in their offspring (Rickert and Rajan, 1974).

Fine-needle Aspiration (FNA)

The use of breast mass needle aspiration has been validated extensively in nonpregnant women. Aspiration may be performed for both cystic and solid lesions, and aspirates from solid lesions potentially contain small tissue fragments. Over the past decade, many investigators have described characteristics from breast lesion aspirates in pregnant and lactating women (Bottles and Taylor, 1985; Finley, 1989; Grenko, 1990; Gupta, 1993; Kline, 1981; Macansh, 1990; Novotny, 1991; and their coinvestigators).

The technique of fine-needle aspiration has been well described. A 10- or 20-mL syringe usually is used. It may be held in a Franzen single-hand grip syringe holder for stability and consistency of attempts. Needles recommended range from 20 to 23 gauge. Multiple passes are usually performed, maintaining negative pressure consistently. The material is rapidly expirated onto slides and spread evenly to provide a thin preparation. Air-dried smears are stained with the Diff-Quik method (modified Wright stain) and alcohol-fixed smears are usually stained by the Papanicolaou method. Cell blocks may be prepared if any solid material is present. In contrast to cytologic smears, these tissue fragment preparations are similar to histologic biopsy specimens.

While detailed description of features from breast aspirates is beyond the scope of this chapter, familiarity with some cytologic features as well as differences between aspirates from pregnant and nonpregnant women is important. The cytopathologist must be given the appropriate clinical history regarding pregnancy status. In nonpregnant women, common lesions tend to have fairly uniform cytologic appearances, as described by Koss and Zajicek (1992). For example, fibroadenomas are typically characterized by aspirates containing large sheets or fragments of uniform, bland epithelial cells with a background of dissociated stromal or myoepithelial cells (Fig. 36–4). In contrast, other benign breast lesions typically contain only a few cells. Cystic lesions, such as those seen in fibrocystic changes, are often hypocellular, and when cells are present, they are usually bland epithelial cells or apocrine cells. By contrast, carcinomas are usually characterized by very cellular specimens, forming irregular tissue fragments and sometimes appearing discohesive and often as single cells (Fig. 36–5). Nuclear atypia is often present and is characterized by an increased nuclear/cytoplasmic ratio and hyperchromasia; multiple large nucleoli are often seen. Presence of isolated single atypical cells containing multiple large nucleoli are considered key features for the cytologic diagnosis of breast cancer (Koss and Zajicek, 1992).

Breast lesions in pregnancy may have different cytologic features. For example, nonlactating adenomas are characterized by uniform cells with occasional vacuoles and a background of occasional myoepithelial cells. Lactational changes in these adenomas may involve lobular proliferation, mitotic activity, and secretions (Fig. 36–6). Nuclear features have been shown to vary significantly in some studies, while others have identified nuclear

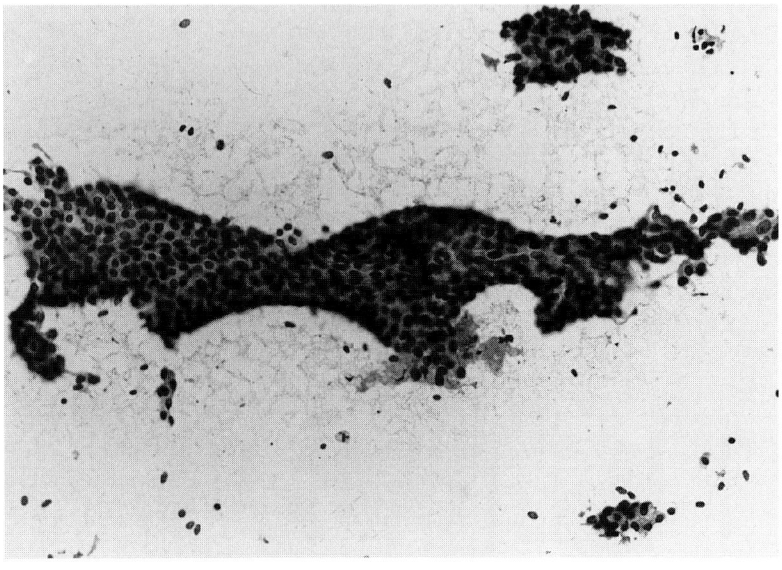

Figure 36–4. Fine-needle aspiration specimen from a fibroadenoma. The cellular specimen is highly organized with monotonous nuclear features and apparent myoepithelial cells. (Photo courtesy of Kevin McCabe, MD.)

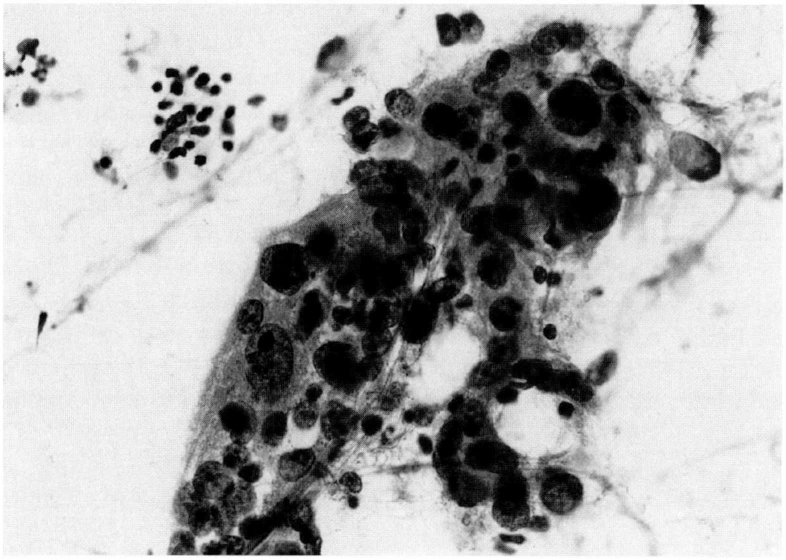

Figure 36–5. Fine-needle aspiration specimen from a mammary carcinoma. Note the nuclear pleomorphism, "dirty" background, and cellular discohesion. (Photo courtesy of Kevin McCabe, MD.)

features to be fairly uniform and not significantly different from lesions in nonpregnant women. Nuclei from lactating adenomas may show marked size variability and prominent irregular nucleoli, varying degrees of chromaticity, and focal cellular discohesion with single cells (Finley and colleagues, 1989; Novotny co-workers, 1991). The degree of atypia may increase proportionate to gestational age. These lactational features, however, are nearly the same as those described as cytologic features of carcinoma in nonpregnant women, particularly single cells and prominent nucleoli. Masses with these lactational nuclear changes all proved to be benign based on subsequent biopsy or clinical follow-up. Therefore, the risk of false-positive malignant diagnosis is significant. Prominent nucleoli and cellular discohesion have been cited as the primary cause of these erroneous diagnoses (Kline, 1981).

Even with worrisome nuclear changes, other factors associated with cancer can be used to distinguish lactational change from carcinoma. In general, aspirates from carcinomas tend to demonstrate greater degrees of hyperchromasia and discohesion, abnormally shaped nuclear membranes, anisocyto-

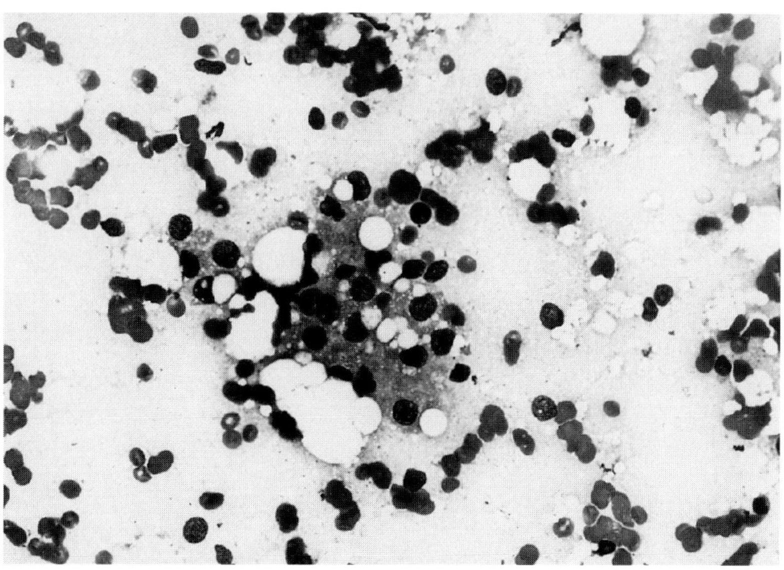

Figure 36–6. Fine-needle aspiration specimen from a lactating adenoma. Although the nuclei may focally appear pleomorphic, the background demonstrates lipid secretions. (Photo courtesy of Kevin McCabe, MD.)

sis, abnormal mitotic figures, angulated nucleoli, and a background of inflammation and/or necrosis (Finley and colleagues, 1989; Gupta and associates, 1993; Novotny and co-workers, 1991). Cell blocks may prove useful in helping to distinguish lactational features from carcinoma due to the presence of small tissue fragments. These fragments typically form lobules or intact acini in lactational change, but are very irregular with no intact structure in carcinoma. A "dirty" background with inflammation and necrosis is also helpful for distinguishing carcinoma, whereas the background in lactational change often contains lipid or secretions.

Although mainly described for lactating adenomas, similar lactational cellular changes may also be seen in other pregnancy-associated lesions, such as galactoceles, fibroadenomas with lactational change, or in juvenile fibroadenomas. A characteristic of all these lesions is the presence of protein/lipid and foam cells in the background, which is not seen in aspirates from carcinomas (Novotny and co-investigators, 1991).

There are clinical features that help to distinguish benign from malignant lesions, although these are not solely adequate. Some of these features are outlined in Table 36–4. Although the combination of clinical features and fine-needle aspiration are often satisfactory, if there is any doubt, then biopsy is done.

TABLE 36–4. CLINICOPATHOLOGIC FEATURES OF BENIGN AND MALIGNANT BREAST LESIONS

Galactocele
Cloudy fluid
Immediate regression following aspiration
Abundant protein/lipid secretions
Numerous foam cells
Lactating adenoma
Mass develops *during* pregnancy
Intact lobules/acini
Protein/lipid secretions
Scant stroma
Fibroadenoma with lactational change
Mass develops *prior* to pregnancy
Minimal secretions
Epithelial sheets
Stroma increased
Carcinoma
Cellular material
Necrosis
Little secretion
Cellular dispersion/discohesion

The sensitivity of fine-needle aspiration in nonpregnant or nonlactating women has been reported to range from 65 to 95 percent, with a specificity of 95 percent (Abele and co-investigators, 1983; Canter and colleagues, 1983; Toma and co-workers, 1985). It is difficult, however, to elucidate sensitivity and specificity in pregnant and lactating women because disease is uncommon. Gupta and colleagues (1993) published their 10-year experience with aspirations performed on almost 10,000 women. Of these, 214 women were pregnant or lactating and 201 specimens were interpreted as benign, and in subsequent follow-up none developed cancer. Eight cases were diagnosed as carcinoma by cytology; four cases were considered nondiagnostic; and in only one case was the cytologic specimen suspicious for carcinoma, and this was confirmed on biopsy.

Biopsy

Breast biopsy obviously provides more tissue for diagnosis. The use of anesthesia in an operating room setting is usually necessary. Although breast biopsy in pregnancy is generally safe, there are risks of anesthesia, increased bleeding, and infection (Niefert, 1992). Biopsy is often done to sample a palpable mass. Stereotactic biopsies (needle localization) are often performed in nonpregnant women, usually for abnormalities detected by mammography. Because most pregnant women present with a palpable mass, and because mammography provides less than optimal evaluation, stereotactic biopsies are not often performed.

The cytologic feature of biopsies in malignancy and lactational change are the same as the features described for fine-needle aspiration. Biopsy provides larger tissue fragments, thus allowing for analysis of architecture to assist in diagnosis of difficult lesions. Biopsies should be performed if any question remains after fine-needle aspiration, and may be indicated if there are clinical signs of malignancy, such as skin changes, suspicious lymph nodes, or evidence of metastases.

Receptors

Estrogen and progesterone receptor (ER/PR) status is often determined in breast cancer specimens. With receptor-positive tumors, 50–80 percent of patients will respond to hormonal therapy; however, only up to 15 percent of patients with receptor-negative tumors respond to hormonal therapy, and generally they have a worse prognosis (Danforth, 1992; Lichter and Lippman, 1988; Maloisel and associates, 1990). Receptor status also varies according to age. Premenopausal women generally have less estrogen-receptor positive tumors; however, progesterone-receptor positivity is increased compared with all women with breast cancer (Danforth, 1992; Nugent and O'Connell, 1985; Wallack and associates, 1983).

In studies in which receptor status was determined in pregnancy or lactational-associated breast cancer, pregnant women generally had a significantly lower rate of receptor positivity compared with nonpregnant counterparts. Originally, low receptor positivity was thought to contribute to the generally poor prognosis in these women; however, in contrast to nonpregnant patients, their prognosis is not altered by hormonal-altering procedures such as castration. Thus, the role of receptor status in prognosis with pregnancy-associated breast cancer is unknown. However, receptor negativity in pregnancy-associated breast cancer may be artifactual. High levels of circulating estrogen may result in an underestimate of receptor content by saturating available receptors, resulting in their down-regulation (Barnavon and Wallack, 1990; Elledge and associates, 1993; Hoover, 1990). Therefore, other methods for analyzing receptor status have been used, including monoclonal anti-estrogen receptor antibody analysis and removing unbound estrogen followed by exchange assays to detect cytosol and nuclear-occupied estrogen receptors (Barnavon and Wallack, 1990; Hoover, 1990). Elledge and associates (1993) studied receptor determination using ligand-binding assay, immunohistochemical staining, and assays of two estrogen receptor related proteins, pS2 and Hsp-27. They reported that estrogen-receptor positive tumors were found less often in pregnant or lactating women than in those nonpregnant, although half of these patients were positive for pS2 and Hsp-27. Progesterone-receptor positive tumors were nearly equivalent. Overall receptor positivity was the same in pregnant women—67 percent—as in those nonpregnant. Obviously larger studies are necessary to determine the potential utility of these newer techniques.

Other receptors have been identified in breast tissue. These include receptors for glucocorticoids, androgens, mineralocorticoids, vitamin D, Her-2-neu (erb B-2), as well as others. Most of these are used in research with estrogen and progesterone receptors used for therapy and prognosis (Danforth, 1991). Prolactin receptors are also present in breast tissue and have been identified in 20–50 percent of breast cancers. Increased prolactin receptors have been described in estrogen-receptor negative tumors (L'Hermite and associates 1984, 1987; Welsch and Nagasawa, 1977).

Staging

Various staging criteria have been used in the past. The system now most often used for breast cancer involves the TNM classification (Table 36–5). Staging is important for pregnant or lactating women; however, there is hesitation to

TABLE 36–5. TNM SYSTEM FOR BREAST CANCER STAGING

T Criteria (tumor)

- T_0 in situ
- T_1 ≤ 2 cm
- T_2 $> 2 < 5$ cm
- T_3 > 5 cm
- T_4 any size with extension to chest wall or skin

N Criteria (nodes)

- N_0 ipsilateral axillary nodes negative
- N_1 palpable, movable ipsilateral axillary nodes
  - a. not considered to contain tumor
  - b. considered to contain tumor
- N_2 palpable, fixed ipsilateral axillary nodes
- N_3 palpable ipsilateral regional nodes (clavicular) with tumor or arm edema

M Criteria (metastases)

- M_0 no distant metastases
- M_1 distant metastases—includes skin beyond breast area

Staging:	*T*	*N*	*M*
I:	T1	N_0 or N_{1a}	M_0
II:	T_0	N_{1b}	M_0
	T_1	N_{1b}	M_0
	T_2	N_0, N_{1a}, or N_{1b}	M_0
III:	T_1 or T_2	N_2	M_0
	T_3	N_0, N_1, or N_2	M_0
IV:	T_4	any N	M_0
	any T	N_3	any M
	any T	any N	M_1

perform procedures involving radiation. In nonpregnant women, procedures include bone scan, liver scan, and computed tomography, depending on clinical indications. Unquestionably, some of these have significant radiation doses for the fetus. In general, however, most diagnostic studies may be done with minimal fetal risk. For example, bone scanning provides approximately 100 mrad exposure, abdominal radiographs 40 mrad, and chest radiographs 8 mrad (Hoover, 1990). Thus, most diagnostic studies result in inconsequential exposure and they should not be withheld if indicated.

Bone scanning is recommended for patients with bone pain. It is preferable to skeletal survey radiographs because it provides more information with less radiation (Gallenberg and Loprinzi, 1989; Saunders and Baum, 1993). In the absence of bone pain, bone scanning is indicated if alkaline phosphatase is elevated; however, pregnancy itself causes such elevations. Because bone scans in nonpregnant women are rarely positive in Stage I or II disease, they are considered unnecessary for pregnant women with early disease (Hoover, 1990).

Therapy

It is important that therapy be initiated when indicated; hence, there is usually no reason to postpone treatment until postpartum, particularly surgical treatment. Some have suggested that if disease is discovered late in pregnancy, therapy can be postponed until postpartum as long as this is not prolonged (Bunker and Peters, 1963). There have also been recommendations to delay therapy until after delivery because the prognosis of women treated in the second and third trimesters—although worse than for treatment in the first trimester—was the same if therapy was delayed until after delivery (Clark and Chua, 1989; Donegan, 1988; Ishida and associates, 1992; Peters, 1968; White, 1955a,b). These differences in survival by trimester are based on small retrospective series in which patients often were not staged (Donegan, 1988). Most studies have found no difference in survival when stratified according to trimester (Donegan, 1988; Thierault and coworkers, 1992; Zemlickis and associates, 1992).

Surgery

As with nonpregnant women, surgery is the mainstay of breast cancer treatment, particularly early stage disease. Modified radical mastectomy with axillary dissection is the primary definitive surgery performed in pregnant women with Stage I and II disease (Gallenberg and Loprinzi, 1989; Hoover, 1990; Lichter and Lippman, 1988). In advanced stages, chemotherapy and radiation have a dominant role; however, surgery may still be an option for advanced tumors, particularly if there is response to chemotherapy or radiation (Bush and McCredie, 1986).

In nonpregnant women, conservative breast-sparing surgery using lumpectomy with or without axillary dissection is often done for early stage lesions (Fisher and associates, 1985; Lichter and Lippman, 1988). Without adjuvant radiation therapy, 30 percent of these will develop local recurrence; however, if the recurrence is treated with modified radical mastectomy, survival is not decreased compared with women treated primarily with mastectomy (Fisher and co-workers, 1985). Therefore, adjuvant radiation therapy is often used with conservative surgery. This approach has not been studied in pregnant women and it may be inappropriate to extrapolate to pregnancy-associated breast cancer. Importantly, as subsequently discussed, radiation therapy may carry significant fetal risk. Thus, lumpectomy with adjuvant radiation is not considered an appropriate option for pregnant women unless delivery is soon accomplished and radiation is given postpartum. If the woman is remote from term and strongly desires a conservative approach, lumpectomy with local radiation boost may be employed with limited fetal radiation exposure, and whole breast irradiation is delayed until after delivery (Lichter and Lippman, 1988; Hoover, 1990).

In lactating women, therapeutic decisions are easier. They are offered the same surgical options as nonpregnant patients. Bromocriptine may be used preoperatively to reduce the size and vascularity of the breast in lactating women (Bush and McCredie, 1986; Saunders and Baum, 1993).

Anesthesia Issues

Consideration of surgical options for either diagnosis or therapy must include anesthesia concerns for the woman and her fetus. These are addressed in Chapter 21.

Radiation

Radiotherapy may be used as adjunct treatment after primary surgery, either in conjunction with lumpectomy or after modified radical mastectomy for nodal metastases (Hoover, 1990). Although adjuvant radiation is being studied for node-negative patients as well, the benefits are still undetermined. Radiation therapy is also used as primary treatment in advanced disease, often in conjunction with chemotherapy.

Radiation dose to the fetus is a significant concern. Fetal exposure from most diagnostic radiation procedures is usually inconsequential. In contrast, therapeutic radiation doses are considerably higher, with a typical course totaling 5000 rads. These higher doses result in a significant fetal risk. Fetal dose is calculated based on a number of factors. As shown in Table 36–6, the dose to the fetus varies according to gestational age. Therefore, in late pregnancy, fetal dose may be as high as 100 rads (Lichter and Lippman, 1988). In other studies, a dose of 5000 rads resulted in fetal doses of 10–30 rads in early pregnancy, but up to 200 rads in late pregnancy (Petrek, 1991; van der Vange and van Dongen, 1991).

Knowledge of the potential fetal effects of a calculated dose is necessary for effective counselling. Much of the data regarding radiation effects are from animal studies, and there is limited human data. The main concerns are anomalies, post-embryonic effects, and long-term potential neoplastic effects (Sweet and Kinzie, 1976). Radiation effects, like the dose, are related to gestational age. In general, a significant exposure during implantation phase (day 0–10) is associated with an "all or none" response. Exposure during organogenesis (days 11-56) may result in anomalies. From 16 to 20 weeks' gestation, effects include mental retardation or fetal growth retardation. Beyond 20 weeks, while the fetus is fairly resistant to radiation effects, growth retardation, microcephaly, cataracts, and mental retardation can result from higher doses (Debakan, 1968; Hall, 1978; Sanders and Baum, 1993).

TABLE 36–6. FETAL RADIATION DOSE BASED ON UTERINE SIZE

	Percent Total Radiation Dose	
Fundus Location	*Breast Only*	*Breast and Regional Nodes*
Pelvis	1	1.5
Midabdomen	3	4
Term	7	11

Adapted from Clark and Chua (1989).

For these reasons, it is recommended that adjuvant radiation therapy be delayed until after pregnancy. In selected cases, early delivery may be considered weighing the maternal risks of delayed therapy and the fetal risks from preterm delivery. In advanced disease, early initiation of therapy is important if there is any chance for response, and radiation is often used. In this setting, the woman is counselled as to fetal risks, and decisions must be made regarding pregnancy termination.

Chemotherapy

Like radiation, chemotherapy may be used as adjunctive therapy or as primary treatment for advanced disease. Adjunctive therapy for early stage disease is usually reserved for women with nodal metastases. Chemotherapy in this setting has been associated with increased disease-free survival and overall survival (Barnavon and Wallack, 1990; Bonadonna and Valagussa, 1981; Thierault and co-workers, 1992). This is an important consideration in pregnant or lactating women because many of these have positive nodes and adjunctive chemotherapy is often recommended. Tamoxifen is also used, particularly in hormone-receptor positive tumors, but it is being studied as a possible adjunct in all breast cancer patients. Tamoxifen has weak estrogenic activity and potential fetal effects must be considered. It is classified as Pregnancy Category D. Gonadotropin-releasing hormone (GnRH) agonists have also been used in hormone-receptor positive breast cancers; however, these have not been evaluated in pregnancy (Hoover, 1990).

Chemotherapy is given primarily in advanced disease, including preoperatively to reduce tumor size. Chemotherapy may also be used as palliative treatment. Multiple agents are used in this setting and several combinations have been used. Some of these include doxorubicin, 5-fluorouracil, cyclophosphamide, vincristine, and methotrexate (Dreicer and Love, 1991; Maloisel and colleagues, 1990; Thierault and co-investigators, 1992; Willemse and co-workers, 1990).

Appropriate counselling regarding chemotherapy includes possible fetal effects. Most information regarding chemotherapy during pregnancy involves hematopoietic malignancies, although there are some reports of breast cancer antineoplastics. Fetal effects of chemotherapy, like radiation, are largely related to gestational age at exposure. When fetuses are exposed in the first trimester, the risk of anomalies is significant when all agents are considered and ranges from 10 to 25 percent (Doll and colleagues, 1988; Mulvihill and coworkers, 1987; Nicholson, 1968; Schapira and Chadley, 1984). If aminopterin is eliminated, the risk of anomalies is markedly reduced and ranges from 4 to 8 percent (Murray and coworkers, 1984; Sweet and Kinzie, 1976).

Other agents such as 5-fluorouracil, busulfan, methotrexate, and alkylating agents have been associated with anomalies if given in the first trimester; however, these are isolated reports or small series. Moreover, radiation was also used in some of these women (Loprinzi, 1991; Stephens and associates, 1980; Willemse and co-workers, 1990). The reduced rate of anomalies when aminopterin is excluded and the controversial risk of anomalies with most of the other agents have led some to suggest that chemotherapy may be given safely in the first trimester, although most recommend waiting beyond this period.

Chemotherapy after the first trimester is generally well-tolerated, with a risk of fetal anomalies of less than 2 percent (Danforth, 1991; Garber, 1989; Nicholson, 1968; Sutcliffe, 1985; Willemse and co-workers, 1990). Other potential risks are preterm labor and low birthweight (Krepart and Lotocki, 1986; Zemlickis and associates, 1992). Women in these latter reports were not analyzed regarding separate obstetric risk factors, and it is difficult to ascertain whether these complications are related to chemotherapy or to other factors.

Finally, low birthweight and preterm delivery have been reported in up to 40 percent of women who conceive within one year following chemotherapy (Mulvihill and associates, 1987). In a 15-year follow-up study of infants born to four couples who conceived during chemotherapy, no anomalies were identified, although three-fourths demonstrated failure-to-thrive (Gulati and co-workers, 1986). In this same study, 14 pregnancies were conceived after completion of therapy; two had anomalies (one trisomy) and the 12 who were normal had no developmental delay. Green and colleagues (1991) studied several agents and found no single anomaly associated with a specific agent, nor was there any relation between the number of agents used and anomalies. Interestingly, infants born to women treated with actinomycin D had a 10 percent incidence of cardiac defects, compared with a 0.6 percent in the control group. Other studies have not substantiated this relationship (Li and Jaffe, 1974; Pastorfide and Goldstein, 1973; Rustin and associates, 1984).

Therapeutic Abortion

Based upon early impressions that pregnancy-associated breast cancer was a more aggressive disease, pregnancy termination was considered necessary to possibly improve prognosis (Adair, 1953; Holleb and Farrow, 1962). Subsequently, a large number of studies have shown no prognostic benefit of elective pregnancy termination. Interestingly, in their series of 109 women, Clark and Chua (1989) showed that those undergoing elective abortion actually had decreased survival compared with those continuing to term. There is some suggestion that for advanced stage disease, elimination of a high estrogenic state, viz, pregnancy, may result in palliation (Donegan, 1988). Conversely, these same studies, although often not stratified according to stage, failed to demonstrate benefit from pregnancy termination in advanced disease (Hubay and associates, 1978).

Failure of pregnancy termination to improve prognosis initially seemed reasonable, because most pregnancy-associated breast cancers were thought to be receptor-negative. As discussed, receptor negativity may be artifactual and thus may have only a partial role in determining prognosis. Thus, elective termination provides no prognostic benefit for either early or advanced disease, although termination may be an option when early pregnancy chemotherapy or radiation therapy is planned.

Castration

Similar to the original suspicion that pregnancy termination might improve prognosis, oophorectomy was originally thought to improve prognosis. Subsequently, several studies have not documented improved survival from oophorectomy (Donegan, 1988; Hoover, 1990; Saunders and Baum, 1993). The same concerns regarding receptor status addressed for pregnancy termination applies to issues of castration. Conventional wisdom is that oophorectomy provides no benefits for prognosis for either early or advanced stage disease.

Prognosis

Node Status

The most important factor in breast cancer prognosis is stage, which is affected by node status (Danforth, 1991; Petrek and associates, 1991). Pregnant women present more often with advanced stages due to delay in diagnosis, which is also reflected in the observation that node positivity is more common. The incidence of lymph node metastases for pregnancy-associated breast cancer generally ranges from 50 to 90 percent (Table 36–7). By contrast, nonpregnant women have an average node positivity of 45–50 percent (Lichter and Lippman, 1988; Petrek and associates, 1991).

The high rate of node positivity in women with pregnancy-associated breast cancer supports the performance of lymph node dissection even in clinically early stage or small tumors. Additionally, the incidence of skip metastases to axillary lymph nodes, while sparing pectoral nodes, is 10–40 percent (Bush and McCredie, 1986). There are theories suggesting that the increased vascularity and lymphatic drainage in the pregnant or lactating breast leads to a higher risk of node positivity; however, nodal metastases are also likely a reflection of delay in diagnosis (Holleb and Farrow, 1962). Finally, the number of lymph nodes involved with metastases seems to be important in prognosis. In Stage I or II, 5-year survival in patients with one to three positive nodes was about 60 percent; however, this dropped to 30 percent if four or more positive nodes were found (Henderson and Canellos, 1980).

Women with pregnancy-associated breast cancer often present with larger primary tumors than nonpregnant counterparts (Ishida and co-workers, 1992). In one series, tumors less than 2 cm in diameter were much less common in pregnant than nonpregnant patients (Petrek and colleagues, 1991). Larger tumors therefore also contribute to advanced stage.

TABLE 36–7. FREQUENCY OF AXILLARY LYMPH NODE METASTASES WITH PREGNANCY-ASSOCIATED BREAST CANCER

Study	Number	Percent
Harrington (1937)	92	85
White and White (1956)	37	68
Holleb and Farrow (1962)	133	72
Miller (1962)	45	67
Peters and Meakin (1965)	60	65
Earley and colleagues (1969)	46	50
Haagensen (1971)	48	55
Applewhite and associates (1973)	48	69
Cheek (1973)	33	75
Clark and Reid (1978)	201	82
Donegan (1979a,b)	50	71
Maier (1979)	71	50
Deemarsky and Neishtadt (1981)	100	67
King and co-workers (1985)	63	62
Ribeiro and co-investigators (1986)	121	72
Greene and Leis (1989)	65	59
Petrek and associates (1991)	56	61
Ishida and colleagues (1992)	192	58
Totals	1461	67

Survival

There are several studies examining prognosis, measured as survival, of pregnancy-associated breast cancer. Comparison is difficult because of issues summarized by Saunders and Baum (1993) and van der Vange and van Dongen (1991). For example, definitions vary, and therefore tumors included as "pregnancy-associated" varies considerably. Lactating and pregnant women are often included together in this category, yet therapy may be different. Studies vary as to which therapeutic regimens were used, and obviously the response to therapy may differ. Operative criteria vary; thus, some cases considered operable in one series may be considered inoperable in others. Some studies did not address prognosis of women considered inoperable. Also, operative procedures and the use of pre- or postoperative adjunctive therapy are often not consistently reported. Staging criteria and the use of diagnostic measures to define stage vary. Some studies match patients by stage to a control group of nonpregnant women, while others use separate studies of nonpregnant women as "controls."

Historically, pregnancy-associated breast cancer was considered very aggressive. Indeed, it was described as "excessively malignant" by Gross in 1880. Kilgore (1929) demonstrated a 5-year survival of only 17 percent.

Haagenson and Stout (1943) similarly demonstrated a dismal survival despite surgery, and concluded that pregnancy-associated breast cancer was incurable. Harrington (1937) found that although prognosis for women with positive nodes was poor—5 percent 5-year survival—those with negative nodes had a good survival rate—60 percent. Despite Harrington's findings, earlier conclusions prevailed and little was done for these patients. As more favorable results accrued, opinions shifted. Haagenson (1967) subsequently reported a 32 percent 5-year survival which led him to suggest surgery as an option. By then, other reports emerged that also demonstrated improved survival with pregnancy-associated breast cancer, particularly those with negative nodes. Wallack and colleagues (1983) reviewed 23 series of pregnancy-associated breast cancer reported from 1923 to 1979. Node-negative patients had a 5-year survival of 30–100 percent and 10-year survival of 22–50 percent. Node-positive patients, however, had only a 0–42 percent 5-year survival and 0–22 percent 10-year survival.

Although these more recent studies suggest a better prognosis, the prevailing impression was that pregnancy-associated breast cancer still had a worse prognosis compared with nonpregnant patients. There were a number of studies done to compare cancer in pregnant and lactating women with nonpregnant women. In some of these, in which patients were matched according to age and stage, prognosis was similar (Table 36–8). Importantly, women with negative nodes had 5-year survival approaching 75–100 percent (Byrd and colleagues, 1962; Hochman and Schreiber, 1953; King and co-workers, 1985; Peete and associates, 1966). One study demonstrated similar 5-year survival for pregnant versus nonpregnant women matched by node status; however, 10-year survival was worse for node-positive pregnant women (Petrek and colleagues, 1991).

Thus, data regarding prognosis for pregnancy-associated breast cancer is controversial and difficult to analyze. In general, these women have a similar prognosis to that of nonpregnant women when accordingly matched. This similarity is the main argument suggesting that pregnancy itself does not portend a worse prognosis, but rather pregnant women are more likely to present with node metastases and advanced stage. Thus, delay in diagnosis is the critical variable leading to presentation with advanced stage.

Subsequent Pregnancy

It is estimated that 10–15 percent of women will have one or more pregnancies after completing therapy, and that 70 percent are within the first 5 years (Cooper and Butterfield, 1970; Donegan, 1977; Hassey, 1988; Peters, 1968; Rissanen, 1968). Because receptor status and response to hormonal therapy in nonpregnant patients is important, there is concern that subsequent pregnancy after therapy may affect prognosis or stimulate a recurrence.

Literature regarding breast cancer and subsequent pregnancy is summarized in Table 36–9. Generally, women who subsequently became pregnant had a good prognosis. They had a 5-year survival of 71 percent, which was comparable to Stage I and II patients who did not become pregnant. Those with negative nodes had a 5-year survival of 85 percent and

TABLE 36–8. SURVIVAL WITH PREGNANCY-ASSOCIATED BREAST CANCER ACCORDING TO STAGE

		Survival (Percent)			
Study	Number	*Stage I 5yr/10yr*	*Stage II 5yr/10yr*	*Stage III 5yr/10yr*	*Stage IV 5yr/10yr*
Peters (1968)	187	60 —	39 —	18 —	0 —
Rissanen (1968)	33	80 / 80	80 / 77	15 / 22	0 0
King and colleagues (1985)	63	73 —	52 —	25 —	8 —
Ribiero and co-workers (1986)	88	90 / 90	37 / 21	15 / 10	0 0
Nugent and O'Connell (1986)	19	100 / —	50 —	0 —	— —
Greene and Leis (1989)	65	71[a]/49[a]		20 / 0	0 —

[a]*Combined Stage I and II.

TABLE 36–9. SURVIVAL WITH PREGNANCY-ASSOCIATED BREAST CANCER AND SUBSEQUENT PREGNANCY

Study	Number	Survival (%)					
		Overall 5-year	Overall 10-year	5-year		10-year	
				Node(-)	*Node(+)*	*Node(-)*	*Node(+)*
Harrington (1937)	107	—	—	98.5	64	92	50
Westberg (1946)	45	—	—	96	50	75	22
Holleb and Farrow (1962)	52	52	—	—	—	64	38
Bunker and Peters (1963)	31	77	—	—	—	—	—
Peters and Meakin (1965)	63	71	55	—	—	—	—
Rissanen (1969)	53	77	70	—	—	—	—
Cooper and Butterfield (1970)	32	75	—	95	46	—	—
Clark and Reid (1978)	109	79	65	—	—	—	—
Harvey and colleagues (1981)	41	—	—	—	—	80	79
Mignot and co-workers (1986)	68	—	71	—	—	—	—
Ribiero and associates (1986)	57	69	53	—	—	64	26
Ariel and Kempner (1989)	46	—	—	—	—	77	56

Modified from Danforth (1991).

those with positive nodes had a 50 percent 5-year survival, similar to survival rates of those not becoming pregnant. In another series, 10-year survival was the same for women with positive nodes whether becoming pregnant or not (Ariel and Kempner, 1989). Mean survival for Stage I patients was 90 percent, again similar to women not becoming pregnant (Danforth, 1991). The number of subsequent pregnancies did not have any effect and multiple subsequent pregnancies did not alter prognosis compared with a single pregnancy (Clark and Reid, 1978; Cooper and Butterfield, 1970; Rissanen, 1969).

Conversely, others concluded there was improved survival in women subsequently becoming pregnant (Cooper and Butterfield, 1970; Peters, 1962; Rissanen, 1969). This led to speculation that subsequent pregnancy may have a cancer-suppressing effect (Barnavon and Wallack, 1990; Saunders and Baum, 1993). It is more likely that there is a selection bias in patients with subsequent pregnancies and that those conceiving post-therapy had surpassed the usual period of developing a recurrence by the time of conception. The timing of conception may be important. Clark and Reid (1978) found that women who conceived less than 6 months after completing therapy had a poorer prognosis (5-year survival of 55%) compared with those conceiving from 6 months to 2 years after therapy (5-year survival of 30%). Likewise, Peters and Meakin (1965) reported that women becoming pregnant within 1 year of therapy had a much worse prognosis compared with those waiting more than 1 year. In contrast, Harvey and colleagues (1985) showed no detrimental effect from subsequent pregnancy even with early conception.

Pragmatically, because the risk of cancer recurrence is highest in the first 2–3 years, it is recommended that women defer subsequent pregnancy until at least this time (Barnavon and Wallack, 1990; Danforth, 1991; Donegan, 1988; van der Vange and van Dongen, 1991).

Breastfeeding After Diagnosis and Therapy

The ability of the woman to breastfeed after diagnosis and therapy of breast cancer is important. Effects of both surgery and adjunctive treatment must be considered. These have been summarized by Niefert (1992). Breast surgery during pregnancy or lactation may result in hemorrhage because of increased vascularity, infection, or milk fistulae. Biopsy may also affect breastfeeding depending on the location. If biopsy is performed in the periareolar area, milk ducts may be severed and emptying impaired. Additionally, innervation may be affected and cause reduced duct emptying (Day, 1986; Niefert, 1992). Breast-sparing procedures such as lumpectomy may also have similar incisional effects, and lactation may be affected by the overall amount of tissue removed.

Radiation therapy may result in lobular atrophy, ductal shrinkage, and periductal fibrosis (Findlay and associates, 1988; Rostom and O'Cathail, 1986; Ulmer, 1988; Varsos and Yahalom, 1991). As a result, breast tissue does not undergo normal lactational changes, resulting in little or no milk production. If the radiation was primarily unilateral, the contralateral breast may be unaffected; however, this is difficult to predict because there is significant variation in radiation dose and technique.

There is little information on effects of chemotherapy on breastfeeding. There are possible neonatal effects of some antineoplastic agents. For example, methotrexate and cyclophosphamide attain reasonable levels in breast milk and have been associated with neonatal neutropenia (Beely, 1981; Sutcliffe, 1985).

Fetal Effects of Breast Cancer

Low birthweight and preterm labor have been reported in pregnancies complicated by breast cancer. Whether these effects are related to therapy or to the disease itself is unclear. Potter and Schoeneman (1970) reviewed 24 cases of cancer metastatic to the placenta or fetus. Seven of eight cases had fetal metastases; seven were from malignant melanoma and another was from a lymphosarcoma. Those cases with breast cancer metastatic to the placenta had no fetal metastases, and all resulted in normal neonates.

Fertility and Hormonal Status After Therapy

As discussed previously, subsequent pregnancies do not have an adverse impact on prognosis in women with a history of breast cancer as long as conception is delayed for 2–3 years after therapy. Important concerns include the need for contraception as well as estrogen deficiency and premature menopause.

Cytotoxic drugs have been associated with diminished ovarian function and subsequent amenorrhea, vaginal atrophy, and infertility (Gulati and co-workers, 1986; Schilsky and colleagues, 1980, 1981; Sutton and associates, 1990). Decreased sexual function, decreased libido, and menopausal symptoms have also been reported. The proportion of women experiencing these effects is variable. In the series reported by Schilsky and colleagues (1981) of women receiving MOPP chemotherapy—nitrogen mustard, vincristine, procarbazine, and prednisone—almost half developed persistent amenorrhea. Interestingly, 90 percent of the amenorrheic patients were older than 25, and of those under 25, 80 percent eventually had recurrence of regular menses. In another series, amenorrhea persisted in only 10 percent (Sutton and co-workers, 1990), while in women less than 35 years of age, half maintained normal menstrual function after therapy (Hortobagyi and colleagues, 1986). Drugs associated with these effects are alkylating agents such as busulfan and cyclophosphamide; these have been associated with ovarian failure in up to half of treated patients (Uldall and colleagues, 1972; Warne and co-investigators, 1973).

Symptoms result from ovarian failure. Serum levels of follicle-stimulating hormone (FSH) and luteinizing-hormone (LH) approach those of perimenopausal or menopausal patients (Chapman and co-investigators, 1979a,b; Schilsky and associates, 1980). Histopathologic examination of ovaries from symptomatic women demonstrate fibrosis and follicle destruction (Miller and co-workers, 1971; Sobrinho and co-investigators, 1971). The severity of these changes correlates with the number of drugs used and duration of therapy (Himelstein-Braw and colleagues, 1978; Nicosia and co-workers, 1985). These findings are consistent with effects seen in males in which testes have decreased germinal epithelial lining of seminiferous tubules, aplasia, and resultant oligo- or azoospermia (Schilsky and co-workers, 1980).

Thus, ovarian failure is a significant risk, and it is apparent that its magnitude and persistence are related to age. Ovarian dysfunction may be reversible with reversibility related to age, drug, dose, and duration. Importantly, ovarian failure is not an all-or-none response; some women may experience partial failure and milder effects (Chapman and associates, 1979a,b).

Conversely, partial ovarian failure may progress with time to complete and irreversible failure. Therefore, although young women may have less sustained ovarian effects that may be reversible, they must be informed that these effects may vary over the long-term and could potentially worsen.

The ovary is sensitive to effects of radiation. While usually not in the field of effect for typical breast radiation protocols, the ovary potentially receives some exposure. This is particularly true if radiation therapy is given for metastatic disease to the pelvis and/or abdomen. Even low-dose radiation (500–600 rads) may induce follicular degeneration, fibrosis, and vascular changes (Fisher and Cheung, 1984; Gronroos and associates, 1982). The stroma appears to be more resistant than the follicles (Janson and co-workers, 1981). As a result of these changes, a significant number of women with radiotherapy exposure to the ovaries will experience ovarian failure (Stillman and co-investigators, 1981).

SUMMARY

A number of conditions seen in the non-pregnant breast also may affect the breast in pregnant or lactating women. Some such as puerperal mastitis are unique to the postpartum period. Breast cancer in pregnant or lactating women may be increasing in incidence as more women delay childbearing. Unfortunately, delayed diagnosis and therapy are common in pregnant women because normal anatomic and physiologic changes of the breast often mask potential malignancies. In addition, because physicians hesitate to use diagnostic tools and therapeutic modalities in pregnant women, these women present more often with advanced stage disease. Pregnant and lactating women with breast cancer have a similar prognosis to non-pregnant women with the same stage of disease, and they should be managed similarly. Management should include counseling regarding the effects of various therapies on pregnancy, breast feeding, and future fertility. A multidisciplinary team approach to management is likely to optimize outcome for both mother and fetus.

REFERENCES

Abele JS, Miller TR, Goodson WH, et al. Fine needle aspiration of palpable breast masses. Arch Surg 1983; 118:859.

Adair EA. Cancer of the breast. Surg Clin North Am 1953; 33:313.

Adams DH, Hubscher SG, Scott DGI. Granulomatous mastitis: a rare cause of erythema nodosum. Postgrad Med J 1987; 63:581.

Alagaratnam TT. Uncommon forms of mastitis. Aust NZ J Surg 1981; 51:45.

Applewhite RR, Smith LR, DiVincenti F. Carcinoma of the breast associated with pregnancy and lactation. Am Surg 1973; 39:101.

Appozardi JG. Problems in breast pathology. In: Bennington JL, ed. Major Problems in Pathology. Vol. 11. Philadelphia: Saunders, 1979.

Ariel IM, Kempner R. The prognosis of patients who become pregnant after mastectomy for breast cancer. Int Surg 1989; 74:185.

Barnavon Y, Wallack MK. Management of the pregnant patient with carcinoma of the breast. Surg Gynecol Obstet 1990; 171:347.

Beely L. Drugs and breast feeding. Clin Obstet Gynecol 1981; 8:291.

Beischer NA, Hueston JH, Pepperell RJ. Massive hypertrophy of the breasts in pregnancy: report of 3 cases and review of the literature, 'never think you have seen everything.' Obstet Gynecol Surv 1989; 44:234.

Bingen E, Denamur E, Lanbert-Zechovsky N, et al. Analysis of DNA restriction fragment length polymorphism extends the evidence for breast milk transmission in streptococcus agalactiae late-onset neonatal infection. J Infect Dis 1992; 165:569.

Bonadonna G, Valagussa P. Dose-response effect of adjuvant chemotherapy for breast cancer. N Engl J Med 1981; 304:10.

Bottles K, Taylor RN. Diagnosis of breast masses in pregnant and lactating women by aspiration cytology. Obstet Gynecol 1985; 66:765.

Bozzetti FJ, DeLena M, Salvadori B. Inflammatory cancer of the breast: an analysis of 114 cases. J Surg Oncol 1981; 18:355.

Briggs G, Freeman R, Summer YJ, eds. Drugs in Pregnancy and Lactation. Baltimore: Williams & Wilkins, 1990:68.

Bunker ML, Peters MV. Breast cancer associated with pregnancy or lactation. Am J Obstet Gynecol 1963; 85:312.

Brown MS, Hurlock JT. Preparation of the breast for breastfeeding. Nurs Res 1975; 24:448.

Bush H, McCredie JA. Carcinoma of the breast during pregnancy and lactation. In: Allen HH, Nisker JA, eds. Cancer in Pregnancy. Therapeutic Guidelines. Mount Kisco, NY: Futura, 1986:91.

Byrd BF, Bayer DS, Robertson JC, Stephenson JE Jr. Treatment of breast tumors associated with pregnancy and lactation. Ann Surg 1962; 155:940.

Canter JW, Oliver GC, Zaloudek CJ. Surgical diseases of the breast during pregnancy. Clin Obstet Gynecol 1983; 26:853.

Chapman RM, Sutcliffe SB, Malpas JS. Cytoxic-induced ovarian failure in women with Hodgkin's disease. I. Hormone function. JAMA 1979a; 242:1877.

Chapman RM, Sutcliffe SB, Malpas JS. Cytoxic-induced ovarian failure in Hodgkin's disease. II. Effects on sexual function. JAMA 1979b; 242:1882.

Cheek JH. Cancer of the breast in pregnancy and lactation. Am J Surg 1973; 126:729.

Clark RM, Chua T. Breast cancer and pregnancy: the ultimate challenge. Clin Oncol 1989; 1:11.

Clark RM, Reid J. Carcinoma of the breast in pregnancy and lactation. Int J Radiat Oncol Biol Phys 1978; 4:693.

Cooper DR, Butterfield J. Pregnancy subsequent to mastectomy for cancer of the breast. Ann Surg 1970; 171:429.

Cotran RS, Kumar V, Robbins SL, eds. Robbins Pathologic Basis of Disease. Philadelphia: Saunders, 1989:1181.

Cummings P, Stanford JL, Daling JR, et al. Risk of breast cancer in relation to the interval since last full term pregnancy. Br Med J 1994; 308:1672.

Danforth DN. How subsequent pregnancy affects outcome in women with a prior breast cancer. Oncology 1991; 5:23.

Danforth DN Jr. Hormone receptors in malignancy. Crit Rev Oncol Hematol 1992; 12:91.

Day TW. Unilateral failure of lactation after breast biopsy. J Fam Pract 1986; 23:161.

Debakan A. Abnormalities in children exposed to x-irradiation during various stage of gestation. I. Tentative time-table of radiation injury to the human fetus. J Nucl Med 1968; 9:471.

Deemarsky LJ, Neishtadt EL. Breast cancer and pregnancy. Breast 1981; 7:717.

Demey HE, Hautekeete ML, Buytaert P, Bossaert LL. Mastitis and toxic shock syndrome. A case report. Acta Obstet Gynecol Scand 1989; 68:87.

Devereux WP. Acute puerperal mastitis. Am J Obstet Gynecol 1970; 108:78.

Doll DC, Rigenberg QS, Yarbo JW. Management of cancer during pregnancy. Arch Intern Med 1988; 14:2058.

Donegan WL. Mammary carcinoma and pregnancy. Major Probl Clin Surg 1967; 5:170.

Donegan WL. Breast Cancer and pregnancy. Obstet Gynecol 1977; 50:244.

Donegan WL. Mammary carcinoma and pregnancy. Major Probl Clin Surg 1979a; 5:448.

Donegan WL. Mammary carcinoma and pregnancy. In: Donegan WL, Spratt JS, eds. Cancer of the Breast. 2nd ed. Philadelphia: Saunders, 1979b: 448.

Donegan WL. Cancer and pregnancy. Cancer 1983; 33:194.

Donegan WL. Mammary carcinoma in pregnancy. In: Donegan WL, Spratt JS, eds. Cancer of the Breast. 3rd ed. Philadelphia: Saunders, 1988:679.

Dreicer R, Love RR. High total dose 5-fluorouracil treatment during pregnancy. Wis Med J 1991; 90:582.

Early TK, Gallagher JQ, Chapman KE. Carcinoma of the breast in women under 30 years of age. Am J Surg 1969; 118:832.

Eben F, Cameron MD, Lowy C. Successful treatment of mammary hyperplasia in pregnancy with bromocriptine. Br J Obstet Gynecol 1993; 100:95.

Elledge RM, Ciocca DR, Langone G, McGuire WL. Estrogen receptor, progesterone receptor, and Her-2-neu protein in breast cancer from pregnant patients. Cancer 1993; 71:2499.

Evans TRJ, Stein RC, Ford HT, et al. Lactic acidosis. A presentation of metastatic breast cancer arising in pregnancy. Cancer 1992; 69:453.

Findlay PA, Gorrle CR, E'Angelo T, Glatstein E. Lactation after breast radiation. Int J Radiat Oncol Biol Phys 1988; 15:511.

Finley JL, Silverman JF, Lannin DR. Fine-needle aspiration cytology of breast masses in pregnant and lactating women. Diagn Cytopathol 1989; 5:255.

Fiorica JV. Breast disease. Curr Opinion Obstet Gynecol 1992; 4:897.

Fisher B, Bauer M, Margolese R, et al. Five-year results of a randomized clinical trial comparing total mastectomy and segmental mastectomy with or without radiation in the treatment of breast cancer. N Engl J Med 1985; 312:665.

Fisher B, Cheung AYC. Delayed effects of radiation therapy with or without chemotherapy on ovarian function in women with Hodgkin's disease. Acta Radiol Oncol 1984; 23:43.

Fletcher A, Magrath IM, Riddell RH, Talbot IC. Granulomatous mastitis: a report of seven cases. J Clin Pathol 1982; 35:941.

Foster RS, Worden JK, Costanza MC, Solomon LJ. Clinical breast examination and breast self-examination: past and present effect on breast cancer survival. Cancer 1992; 69:2001.

Gallenberg MM, Loprinzi CL. Breast cancer and pregnancy. Semin Oncol 1989; 16:369.

Garber JE. Long-term follow-up of children exposed in utero to antineoplastic agents. Semin Oncol 1989; 16:437.

Gibberd GF. Sporadic and epidemic puerperal breast infections. Am J Obstet Gynecol 1953; 65:1038.

Gloeckler Ries LA, Hankey BF, Edwards BK, eds. Cancer Statistics Review 1973–1987. NCI and US Department of Health and Human Services, Section II:II. I–II.49, 1987.

Goldsmith HS. Milk rejection as a sign of breast cancer. Am J Surg 1974; 127:280.

Graham EM. Erythromycin. Obstet Gynecol Clin North Am 1992; 19:539.

Green DM, Zevon MA, Lowrie G, et al. Congenital anomalies in children of patients who received chemotherapy for cancer in childhood and adolescence. N Engl J Med 1991; 325:141.

Greene FL, Leis HP. Management of breast cancer in pregnancy: a thirty-five year multiinstitutional experience (abstract). Proc Annu Meet Am Soc Clin Oncol 1989; 8:A94.

Grenko RT, Lee KP, Lee KR. Fine needle aspiration cytology of lactating adenoma of the breast. A comparative light microscopic and morphometric study. Acta Cytol 1990; 34:21.

Gronroos M, Klemi P, Piiroinen O, et al. Ovarian function during and after curative intracavitary high-dose irradiation: steroidal output and morphology. Eur J Gynecol Reprod Biol 1982; 14:13.

Guinee VF, Olsson H, Möller T, et al. Effect of pregnancy for young women with breast cancer. Lancet 1994; 343:1587.

Gulati SC, Vega R, Gee T, et al. Growth and development of children born to patients after cancer therapy. Cancer Invest 1986; 4:197.

Gupta RK, McHutchison GR, Dowle CS, Simpson JS. Fine-needle aspiration cytodiagnosis of breast masses in pregnant and lactating women and its impact on management. Diagn Cytopathol 1993; 9:156.

Haagensen CD. Cancer of the breast in pregnancy and during lactation. Am J Obstet Gynecol 1967; 98:141.

Haagensen CD. Diseases of the Breast. Philadelphia: Saunders, 1971:662.

Haagensen CD, Stout AP. Carcinoma of the breast, criteria for operability. Ann Surg 1943; 118: 859.

Hall EJ. Radiobiology for the Radiobiologist. New York: Harper & Row, 1978:397.

Hankey BF, Brinton LA, Kessler LG, Abrams J. Section IV: Breast. In: Miller BA, Reis LAG, Hankey BF, eds. SEER Cancer Statistics Review, 1973–90. Bethesda, MD: US Department of Health and Human Services, Public Health Service, National Institutes of Health, National Cancer Institute, 1991: IV.1-IV.24: DHHS publication No. (NIH)93-2789.

Harrington SW. Carcinoma of the breast. Ann Surg 1937; 106:690.

Harvey JC, Rosen PP, Ashikari H, et al. The effect of pregnancy on the prognosis of carcinoma of the breast following radical mastectomy. Surg Gynecol Obstet 1981; 153:723.

Harvey EB, Boice JD Jr, Honeyman M, Flannery JT. Prenatal x-ray exposure and childhood cancer in twins. N Engl J Med 1985; 312:541.

Hassey KM. Pregnancy and parenthood after treatment for breast cancer. Oncol Nurs Forum 1988; 15:439.

Hedberg K, Karlsson K, Lindstedt G. Gigantomastia during pregnancy: effect of a dopamine agonist. Am J Obstet Gynecol 1979; 133: 928.

Henderson IC, Canellos GP. Cancer of the breast. The past decade (first of two parts). N Engl J Med 1980; 302:17.

Himelstein-Braw R, Peters H, Faber M. Morphologic studies of the ovaries of leukaemic children. Br J Cancer 1978; 38:82.

Hochman A, Schreiber H. Pregnancy and cancer of the breast. Obstet Gynecol 1953; 2:268.

Holleb AI, Farrow JH. The relation of carcinoma of the breast and pregnancy in 238 patients. Surg Gynecol Obstet 1962; 115:65.

Hoover HC. Breast cancer during pregnancy and lactation. Surg Clin North Am 1990; 70:1151.

Horsley JS, Alrich EM, Creighton BW. Carcinoma of the breast in women 35 years of age or younger. Ann Surg 1969; 169:839.

Hortobagyi GN, Busdar AU, Marcus CE, Smith TL. Immediate and long-term toxicity of adjuvant chemotherapy regimens containing doxorubicin in trials at M.D. Anderson Hospital and Tumor Institute. Natl Cancer Inst Monogr 1986; 1:105.

Hubay CA, Barry FM, Murr CC. Pregnancy and breast cancer. Surg Clin North Am 1978; 58:819.

Ishida T, Yoko T, Kasumi F, et al. Clinicopathologic characteristics and prognosis of breast cancer patients associated with pregnancy and lactation. Analysis of case-control study in Japan. Jpn J Cancer Res 1992; 83:1143.

Janson PO, Jansson I, Skryten A, et al. Ovarian endocrine function in young women undergoing radiotherapy for carcinoma of the cervix. Gynecol Oncol 1981; 11:218.

Jones RC, Jones SE. Treatment of advanced malignant lesions including inflammatory cancer. In: Hindle WH, ed. Breast Disease for Gynecologists. Norwalk, CT: Appleton & Lange, 1990:215.

Joshi K, Ellis JTB, Perusinghe N, et al. Cell proliferation in the human mammary epithelium. Differential contribution by epithelial and myoepithelial cells. Am J Pathol 1986; 124:199.

Kilgore AS. Tumors and tumor-like lesions of the breast in association with pregnancy and lactation. Arch Surg 1929; 18:2079.

Kim Y, Pomper J, Goldberg ME. Anesthetic management of the pregnant patient with carcinoma of the breast. J Clin Anesth 1993; 5:76.

King RM, Walsh JS, Martin JK, Coulam CB. Carcinoma of the breast associated with pregnancy. Surg Gynecol Obstet 1985; 160:228.

Kline TS. Masquerades of malignancy. A review of 4,241 aspirates from the breast. Acta Cytol 1981; 25:263.

Koss LG, Zajicek J. Aspiration biopsy. In Koss LG, ed. Diagnostic Cytology and Its Histopathologic Bases. 4th ed. Philadelphia: Lippincott, 1992:1293.

Krepart GR, Lotocki RJ. Chemotherapy during pregnancy. In: Allen HH, Nisker JA, ed. Cancer in Pregnancy. Mount Kisco, NY: Futura, 1986:69.

Lambe M, Hsieh CC, Trichopoulos D, et al. Transient increase in the risk of breast cancer after giving birth. N Engl J Med 1994; 331:5.

L'Hermite-Baleriaux M, Casteels S, Vokaer S, et al. Prolactin and prolactin receptors in human breast disease. In: Bresciani F, Lippman ME, King RJB, Namer M, eds. Progress in Cancer Research and Therapy. Vol. 31. New York: Raven Press, 1984:325.

L'Hermite-Baleriaux M, Casteels S, L'Hermite M.

Prolactive receptors in breast cancer: importance of the membrane preparation. In: Klijn JGM, Paridaens R, Foekens JA, ed. Hormonal Manipulation of Cancer: Peptides, Growth Factors, and New (Anti) Steroidal Agents. New York: Raven Press, 1987:157.

Li FP, Jaffe JN. Progeny of childhood-cancer survivors. Lancet 1974; 2:707.

Lichter AS, Lippman ME. Special situations in the treatment of breast cancer. In: Lippman ME, Lichter AS, Danforth DN, eds. Diagnosis and Management of Breast Cancer. Philadelphia: Saunders, 1988:414.

Loprinzi CL. Pregnancy poses tough questions for cancer treatment (interview). J Natl Cancer Inst 1991; 83:900.

Macansh S, Greenberg M, Barraclough B, Pacey F. Fine needle aspiration cytology of granulomatous mastitis. Review of a case and review of the literature. Acta Cytol 1990; 34:38.

Maier WP. Carcinoma of the breast in pregnancy and lactation. Breast 1979; 4:12.

Maloisel F, Dufour P, Bergerat JP, et al. Results of initial doxorubicin, 5-fluorouracil, and cyclophosphamide combination chemotherapy for inflammatory carcinoma of the breast. Cancer 1990; 65:851.

Marshall BR, Hepper JK, Zubiel CC. Sporadic puerperal mastitis—an infection that need not interrupt lactation. JAMA 1975; 233:1377.

Matheson I, Aursnes I, Horgen M, et al. Bacteriological findings and clinical symptoms in relation to clinical outcome in puerperal mastitis. Acta Obstet Gynecol Scand 1988a; 67:723.

Matheson I, Samseth M, Lobert R, et al. Mild transfer of phenoxymethylpenicillin during puerperal mastitis. Br J Clin Pharmacol 1988b; 25:33.

Max MH, Klamer TW. Pregnancy and breast cancer. South Med J 1983; 76:1088.

Mignot L, Morvan F, Sarrazin D, et al. Breast carcinoma and subsequent pregnancy. Proc Annu Meet Am Soc Clin Oncol 1986; 5:557.

Miller HK. Cancer of the breast during pregnancy and lactation. Am J Obstet Gynecol 1962; 83:607.

Miller JJ III, Williams GF, Leissring JC. Multiple late complications of therapy with cyclophosphamide, including ovarian destruction. AM J Med 1971; 5:530.

Montgomery TL. Detection and disposal of breast cancer in pregnancy. Am J Obstet Gynecol 1961; 81:926.

Mulvihill JJ, McKeen EA, Rosner F, Zarrabi MH. Pregnancy outcome in cancer patients. Experience in a large cooperative group. Cancer 1987; 60:1143.

Murray CL, Reichert JA, Anderson J, Twiggs LB. Multinodal cancer therapy for breast cancer in the first trimester of pregnancy. JAMA 1984; 352:2607.

Nicholson HO. Cytotoxic drugs in pregnancy. Review of reported cases. J Obstet Gynaecol Br Commonw 1968; 75:307.

Nicosia SU, Matus-Ridley M, Meadows AT. Gonadal effects of cancer therapy in girls. Cancer 1985; 55:2364.

Niebyl JR, Spence MR, Parmley TH. Sporadic (nonepidemic) puerperal mastitis. J Reprod Med 1978; 20:97.

Niefert M. Breastfeeding after breast surgical procedure on breast cancer. NAACOGS Clin Issues Perinatol Women's Health Nurs 1992; 3:673.

Novotny DB, Maygarden SJ, Shermer RW, Frable WJ. Fine needle aspiration of benign and malignant breast masses associated with pregnancy. Acta Cytol 1991; 35:676.

Nugent P, O'Connell TX. Breast cancer and pregnancy. Arch Surg 1985; 120:1221.

Parente JT, Amsel M, Lerner R, Chinea F. Breast cancer associated with pregnancy. Obstet Gynecol 1988; 71:861.

Pastorfide GB, Goldstein DP. Pregnancy after hydatidiform mole. Obstet Gynecol 1973; 42:67.

Peete CH, Honeycutt HC, Cherney WB. Cancer of the breast in pregnancy. NC Med J 1966; 27:514.

Peters MV. Carcinoma of the breast associated with pregnancy. Radiology 1962; 78:58.

Peters MV. The effect of pregnancy in breast cancer. In: Forrest AP, Kunkler PB, eds. Prognostic Factors in Breast Cancer. Baltimore: Williams & Wilkins, 1968:65.

Peters MV, Meakin JW. The influence of pregnancy in carcinoma of the breast. Prog Clin Cancer 1965; 1:471.

Petrek JA. Pregnancy-associated breast cancer. Semin Surg Oncol 1991; 7:306.

Petrek JA, Dukoff R, Rogatko A. Prognosis of pregnancy-associated breast cancer. Cancer 1991; 67:869.

Piliphsen SJ, Gerardi J, Bretsky S, Robbins GF. The significance of delay in treating patients with potentially curable breast carcinoma. Breast 1984; 10:16.

Potter JF, Schoeneman M. Metastasis of maternal cancer to the placenta and fetus. Cancer 1970; 25:380.

Ribeiro GG, Jones DA, Jones M. Carcinoma of the breast associated with pregnancy. Br J Surg 1986; 73:607.

Rickert R, Rajan S. Localized breast infarcts associated with pregnancy. Arch Pathol 1974; 97:159.

Rissanen PM. Carcinoma of the breast during pregnancy and lactation. Br J Cancer 1968; 22:663.

Rissanen PM. Pregnancy following treatment of mammary carcinoma. Acta Radiol Ther Phys Biol 1969; 8:415.

Rostom AY, O'Cathail S. Failure of lactation following radiotherapy for breast cancer. Lancet 1986; 1:163.

Rustin GJS, Booth M, Dent J, et al. Pregnancy

after cytotoxic chemotherapy for gestational trophoblastic tumors. Br Med J 1984; 288:103.

Saunders CM, Baum M. Breast cancer and pregnancy: a review. J R Soc Med 1993; 86:162.

Schapira DV, Chadley AE. Successful pregnancy, following continuous treatment with combination chemotherapy before conception and throughout pregnancy. Cancer 1984; 54:800.

Schilsky RL, Lewis BJ, Sherins RJ, Young RC. Gonadal dysfunction in patients receiving chemotherapy for cancer. Ann Intern Med 1980; 93:109.

Schilsky RL, Sherins RJ, Hubbard SM, et al. Long-term follow-up of ovarian function in women treated with MOPP chemotherapy for Hodgkin's disease. Am J Med 1981; 71:552.

Schlanger H, Ben Yosef R, Baras M, Catane R. The effect of pregnancy at diagnosis on the prognosis in breast cancer. Presented at the European Association for Cancer Research Tenth Biennial Meeting, Galway, Ireland; September 10–13, 1989.

Schwartz GF. Benign neoplasms and "inflammations" of the breast. Clin Obstet Gyncol 1982; 25:373.

Sobrinho LG, Levine RA, De Conti RC. Amenorrhea in patients with Hodgkin's disease treated with antineoplastic agents. Am J Obstet Gynecol 1971; 109:135.

Speroff L, Glass RH, Kase NG, eds. Clinical Gynecologic Endocrinology and Infertility. 4th ed. Baltimore: Williams & Wilkins, 1989:284.

Stehman FB. Infections and inflammations of the breast. In: Hindle WH, ed. Breast Disease for Gynecologists. Norwalk, CT: Appleton & Lange, 1990:151.

Stephens JD, Golbus MS, Miller TR, et al. Multiple congenital anomalies in a fetus exposed to 5-fluorouracil during the first trimester. Am J Obstet Gynecol 1980; 137:747.

Stillman RJ, Schinfield JS, Schiff I, et al. Ovarian failure in long-term survivors of childhood malignancy. Am J Obstet Gynecol 1981; 139:62.

Sutcliffe SB. Treatment of neoplastic disease during pregnancy. Maternal and fetal effects. Clin Invest Med 1985; 8:33.

Sutton R, Buzdar AU, Hortobagyi GN. Pregnancy and offspring after adjuvant chemotherapy in breast cancer patients. Cancer 1990; 65:847.

Sweet DL, Kinzie J. Consequence of radiotherapy and anti-neoplastic therapy for the fetus. J Reprod Med 1976; 17:241.

Thierault RL, Stallings CB, Buzdar AU. Pregnancy and breast cancer: clinical and legal issues. Am J Clin Oncol 1992; 15:535.

Thomsen AC, Espersen T, Maigaard S. Course and treatment of milk stasis, noninfectious inflammation of the breast, and infectious mastitis in nursing women. Am J Obstet Gynecol 1984; 149:492.

Thomsen AC, Hansen KB, Moller BR. Leukocyte counts and microbiologic cultivation in the diagnosis of puerperal mastitis. Am J Obstet Gynecol 1983; 146:938.

Thomsen AC. Infectious mastitis and occurrence of antibody-coated bacteria in milk. Communications in Brief 1982; 144:350.

Thomsen AC, Morgensen SC, Jepsen FL. Experimental mastitis in mice induced by coagulase-negative staphylococci isolated from cases of mastitis in nursing women. Acta Obstet Gynecol Scand 1985; 64:163.

Toma S, Nicola G, Bruzzi P. Single needle aspiration in the diagnostic evaluation of breast lumps. Breast 1985; 11:25.

Topper YJ. Multiple hormone interactions in the development of the mammary gland in vitro. Recent Prog Horm Res 1970; 26:287.

Tretli S, Kvalheim G, Thoresen S, Host H. Survival of breast cancer patients diagnosed during pregnancy or lactation. Br J Cancer 1988; 58:382.

Treves N, Holleb AI. A report of 549 cases of breast cancer in women 35 years of age or younger. Surg Gynecol Obstet 1958; 107:271.

Turkalj I, Braun P, Krupp P. Surveillance of bromocriptine in pregnancy. JAMA 1982; 247:1589.

Uldall PR, Kerr DNS, Tacchi D. Sterility and cyclophosphamide. Lancet 1972; 1:693.

Ulmer JU. Lactation after conserving therapy of breast cancer? Int J Radiat Oncol Biol Phys 1988; 15:512.

van de Vijver MJ, Peterse JL, Mooi WJ, et al. Neu-protein overexpression in breast cancer. N Engl J Med 1988; 319:1239.

van der Vange N, van Dongen JA. Breast cancer and pregnancy. Eur J Surg Oncol 1991; 17:1.

Varsos G, Yahalom J. Lactation following conservation surgery and radiotherapy for breast cancer. J Surg Oncol 1991; 46:141.

Vernon SW, Tilley BC, Neale AV, Steinfeldt L. Ethnicity, survival, and delay in seeking treatment for symptoms of breast cancer. Cancer 1985; 55:1563.

Wallack MK, Wolf JA Jr, Bedwinek J, et al. Gestational carcinoma of the female breast. Curr Probl Cancer 1982; 7:1.

Warne GL, Fairley KF, Hobbs JB, Martin FIR. Cyclophosphamide-induced ovarian failure. N Engl J Med 1973; 289:1159.

Wellings SR, Jensen HM, Marcum RG. An atlas of subgross pathology of the human breast with special reference to possible precancerous lesions. J Natl Cancer Inst 1975; 55:231.

Welsch CW, Nagasawa H. Prolactin and murine mammary tumorigenesis, a review. Cancer Res 1977; 37:951.

Westberg SV. Prognosis of breast cancer for pregnant and nursing women. Acta Obstet Gynecol Scand 1946; 25(suppl 4):1.

White TT. Prognosis of breast cancer for pregnant and nursing women: analysis of 1413 cases. Surg Gynecol Obstet 1955a; 100:661.

White TT. Carcinoma of the breast in the pregnant and the nursing patient. Am J Obstet Gynecol 1955b; 69:1277.

White TT, White WC. Breast cancer and pregnancy. Report of 49 cases followed 5 years. Ann Surg 1956; 144:384.

Willemse PHB, Vander Sijde R, Sleijfer DT. Combination chemotherapy and radiation for Stage IV breast cancer during pregnancy. Gynecol Oncol 1990; 36:281.

Wong MK, Smith CV, Phelan JP. Antepartum mastitis: a report of two cases. J Reprod Med 1986; 31:511.

Wysham DN, Mulhern ME, Navarre GC, et al. Staphylococcal infections in an obstetrical unit. II: Epidemiologic study of puerperal mastitis. N Engl J Med 1957; 257:304.

Zemlickis D, Lisher M, Degendorfer P, et al. Maternal and fetal outcome after breast cancer in pregnancy. Am J Obstet Gynecol 1992; 166:781.

CHAPTER 37

Gestational Trophoblastic Diseases

Gestational trophoblastic diseases comprise a spectrum of neoplastic and hyperplastic disorders derived from the trophoblastic cells of the human placenta. These disorders are unique by virtue of the fact that they develop from an allograft, the abnormal conceptus, and secrete a marker, human chorionic gonadotropin (hCG). This marker provides a sensitive and specific means to detect and monitor these potentially fatal disorders (Miller and colleagues, 1989). While the potentially fatal forms of these diseases require chemotherapy for cure, surgery is occasionally necessary to achieve that goal.

DEFINITIONS

Gestational trophoblastic diseases, as defined by the World Health Organization (WHO, 1983), refer to both the benign and malignant manifestations of these proliferative trophoblastic disorders. Included are the hydatidiform mole, invasive mole, gestational choriocarcinoma, and placental site trophoblastic tumor. Hydatidiform mole is a general term that includes two distinct entities: the complete hydatidiform mole and the partial hydatidiform mole. A complete hydatidiform mole is an abnormal conceptus with loss of villus vascularity and without an embryo or fetus. Gross hydropic swelling and central cistern formation, plus pronounced cytotrophoblastic and syncytiotrophoblastic hyperplasia, are characteristic findings. A partial hydatidiform mole is an abnormal conceptus with persistent embryonic or fetal elements and a "mosaic" placenta with normal-appearing villi alternating with areas of focal villus swelling and trophoblastic hyperplasia. An invasive mole is a hydatidiform mole that has invaded the myometrium or metastasized. It usually regresses spontaneously, although disease progression may be seen. Gestational choriocarcinoma is a malignant neoplasm of cytotrophoblastic and syncytiotrophoblastic elements without villus formation. Placental site trophoblastic tumor is composed mainly of cytotrophoblastic intermediate cells arising from the placental implantation site. Gestational trophoblastic tumors are those gestational trophoblastic diseases that can progress clinically, invade tissues and organs, metastasize, and are fatal if left untreated. Gestational trophoblastic tumors include the invasive mole, choriocarcinoma, and placental site trophoblastic tumor. This term has replaced gestational trophoblastic neoplasia, since invasive mole is not considered a true neoplasm (WHO, 1983).

HYDATIDIFORM MOLE

The term *hydatidiform mole* represents at least two separate clinical entities with distinct genetic, pathologic, and clinical features.

Pathogenesis

Complete Hydatidiform Mole

The most common type of hydatidiform mole is the complete mole. It is thought to arise by fertilization of an abnormal ovum by a single haploid 23,X sperm that undergoes endoreduplication, resulting in a completely homozygous paternally derived genome of 46,XX. The fate of the maternal genome is unknown, but it is probably lost before fertilization. The androgenetically derived cells of these total allografts grow by normal mitosis, cytokinesis, and polyploidization and undergo enlargement through endomitosis and endoreduplication (Sarto and associates, 1984). The fetal precursor elements either fail to develop or die before organogenesis. The villi develop, lose their vascularity, and vesiculate, leading to central villus cistern formation and characteristic hydropic swelling. This process is accompanied by hyperplasia of the syncytial and cytotrophoblastic elements, which invade the endometrial blood vessels (Fig. 37–1). These changes can be identified after 4 weeks of development. As the tissue mass grows, the uterus enlarges and hemorrhage and necrosis may ensue, resulting in the gross finding of fresh blood, clots, vesicles of up to 2 cm, and varying amounts of adherent decidua.

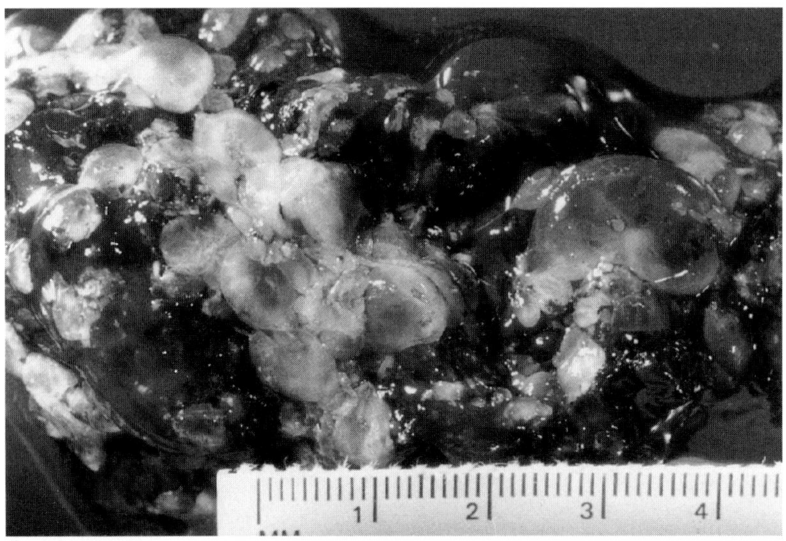

A

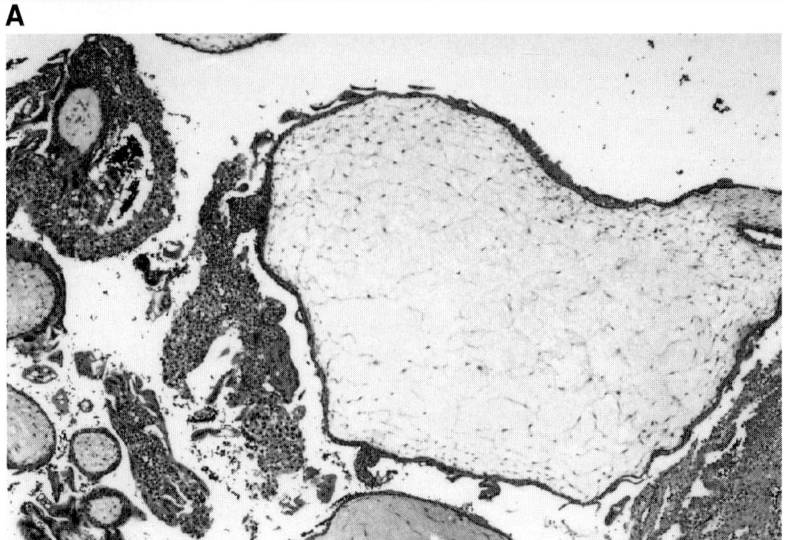

B

Figure 37–1 A. Complete hydatidiform mole showing hydropic villi ranging in size from several millimeters to almost 2 cm. **B.** A large (>2 cm) hydropic, avascular villus with adjacent trophoblastic proliferation is seen in complete hydatidiform mole (40x). (Courtesy of Julianne S. Sandstad, MD.)

Partial Hydatidiform Mole

The partial hydatidiform mole results from the fertilization of a presumed normal haploid 23,X ovum by two haploid sperm (dispermy) or by a single diploid sperm. The resulting diandric conceptus can have a triploid genome of 69,XXX, 69,XXY, or 69,XYY (Watson and coworkers, 1987). The fertilization of a diploid ovum by a haploid sperm results in an abnormal digynic triploid conceptus. In the partial hydatidiform mole, the fetus usually dies at or before 8–9 weeks' gestation and only rarely survives to delivery. Careful scrutiny of pathologic specimens will detect fetal remnants or membranes. The placenta develops as a mosaic of normal-appearing villi and those that resemble the hydropic changes seen in complete hydatidiform mole, characterized by scalloping of the villus outline. Trophoblastic hyperplasia is focal and mainly involves the syncytial cells, with prominent stromal trophoblastic inclusions (Fig. 37–2). Careful cytogenetic and histopathologic evaluation of the concomitant mole and fetus will allow differentiation of the true partial mole from the rare dizygotic twins of complete hydatidiform mole and diploid fetus (Block and Merrill, 1982; Teng and Ballon, 1984).

Human Chorionic Gonadotropin

The key to the diagnosis and treatment of gestational trophoblastic diseases is the identification of the specific marker, human chorionic gonadotropin. hCG is produced by the trophoblastic cells of normal placentas and of gestational trophoblastic diseases. A mitotically active cytotrophoblast differentiates by fusion to form the mitotically inactive but functionally active syncytiotrophoblast. The syncytiotrophoblast secretes hCG, although the hormone may also be found in the cytotrophoblast (Lurain, 1986). It has been estimated that 1000 trophoblastic cells are required to produce a serum hCG level of 0.03–0.5 mIU/mL, which is below the sensitivity of currently available clinical assays. Very early in normal human gestation, the doubling time for hCG is 1½–2 days.

Successful management of gestational trophoblastic disease requires the use of a sensitive, specific, and accurate assay of hCG that can detect the hormonal elaboration of the smallest number of viable trophoblast cells. Such an assay should be able to discriminate hCG from other glycoproteins (especially LH), produce comparable results over the course of months to years, and provide an accurate reflection of the disease status of the patient (Brewer and associates, 1979).

The development of a β-subunit-specific radioimmunoassay (RIA) permitted accurate hCG testing even in the presence of LH. RIA uses the binding of a specific antibody to radioactively labeled and unlabeled hCG. The bound complex is then precipitated by a second antibody and measured to a sensitivity of 1 mIU/mL. Although this assay appears to be ideal for monitoring serum levels of hCG in patients with gestational trophoblastic disease, limitations to the sensitivity and specificity of the technique remain (Wu, 1983;

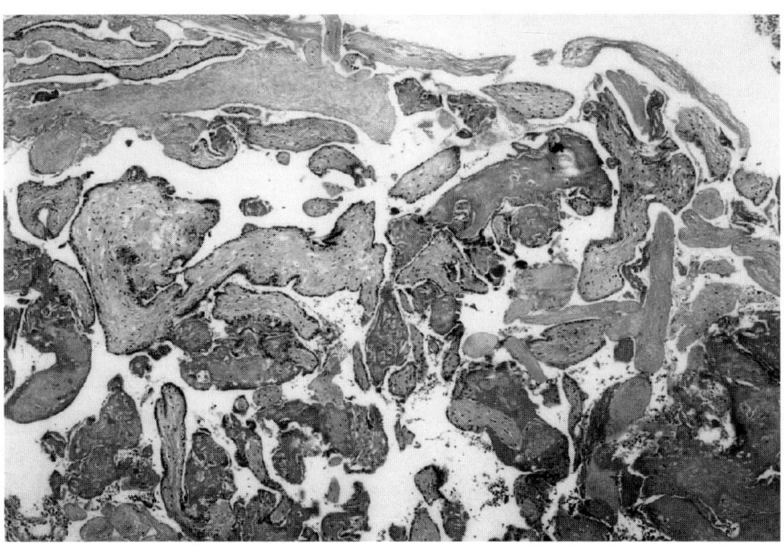

Figure 37–2. Overall smaller chorionic villi with surface irregularity, admixed with normal-sized villi characterize partial hydatidiform mole. Flow cytometry on villous DNA was triploid (40x). (Courtesy of Julianne S. Sandstad, MD.)

Shapiro, 1985; and their colleagues). If, for example, there is a 5 percent cross-reactivity with 40 mIU/mL of LH, the LH can then be expected to contribute as much as 2 mIU/mL to the measurement of hCG. This lack of complete specificity can result in treating patients with cytotoxic chemotherapy longer than necessary. Furthermore, elevations in the zero point of the assay may result in failure to appreciate small residual foci of trophoblastic disease (Borek and co-workers, 1983).

Epidemiology

The incidence of hydatidiform mole in the United States, based on population studies, is about 1/1000 pregnancies. Higher rates are reported, primarily from Asian countries, by hospital-based studies. These data tend to exaggerate the rate because of the smaller number of hospital-based deliveries in these countries. Population-based studies in these countries indicate that the incidence probably approaches the 1/1000 reported in the United States. Based on this rate, 126,000 cases of hydatidiform mole can be expected annually worldwide (WHO, 1983).

The most significant risk factor for developing a molar pregnancy is a prior history of hydatidiform mole (Sand and colleagues, 1984). A maternal age of less than 20 years or greater than 45 years significantly increases the risk. Other factors reported include race, ethnicity, and paternal age greater than 45 years (Miller and associates, 1989).

Signs and Symptoms

Vaginal bleeding is the most common presenting symptom in hydatidiform mole, occurring in over 90 percent of patients. As the uterus enlarges, molar tissue separates from the decidua, disrupting maternal vessels and causing vaginal bleeding. A dark serosanguineous discharge may result from chronic low-grade hemorrhage and necrosis of molar contents. Half of the patients with molar pregnancies have hemoglobin values less than 10 g/dL. This anemia may be dilutional and not secondary to a decrease in the red cell mass. Pritchard (1965) found that most women with hydatidiform mole have blood volume expansions of 25–50 percent above nonpregnant levels. Fifty percent of patients have a uterus larger than expected, and the rest have a uterine size appropriate (25%) or small (25%) for gestational age.

Preeclampsia occurring in the first or early second trimester is seen in approximately one-fourth of patients with hydatidiform mole, although eclampsia is rarely seen (Newman and Eddy, 1989). This correlates with excessive uterine enlargement and markedly elevated hCG levels. Excessive nausea and vomiting also occur in approximately one-fourth of the patients. Ovarian enlargement due to theca lutein cysts is seen in about half of the patients, occurring almost exclusively in patients with markedly elevated hCG levels. Occasionally, these patients may have torsion or cystic rupture. Rarely, patients have trophoblastic pulmonary embolization or signs and symptoms of hyperthyroidism (Lurain, 1987a).

Diagnosis

The definitive diagnosis of hydatidiform mole can be made easily when spontaneous expulsion of typical molar tissue occurs. Ultrasonography allows visualization of the pathognomonic inhomogeneous high- and low-level echoes and sonolucency pattern of molar vesicles, generally not seen until the second trimester (Fig. 37–3) (Santos-Ramos and colleagues, 1980). A concomitant gestational sac or fetus is indicative of a partial hydatidiform mole or the rare dizygotic twins of mole and fetus. Ultrasound has replaced previous diagnostic methods, such as amniography or abdominal x-rays.

Isolated hCG levels alone are insufficient to make the diagnosis of gestational trophoblastic disease. However, any hCG level >1,000,000 mIU/mL at any time in pregnancy or >320,000 mIU/mL after 100 days of amenorrhea is suggestive of hydatidiform mole. Criteria have been proposed for the diagnosis of hydatidiform mole using hCG levels in conjunction with ultrasound. The absence of fetal cardiac activity on ultrasound when the hCG level was above 82,350 mIU/mL correctly diagnosed 89 percent of early moles examined (Romero and co-workers, 1985). Other useful sonographic criteria for excluding a normal intrauterine pregnancy include (1) failure to visualize the sac of a normal intrauterine pregnancy by ultrasound when the hCG level reached 7500 mIU/mL and (2) failure to detect fetal heart motion when the hCG concentration is about 71,000 mIU/mL (Miller and Seifer, 1990).

Patients with partial hydatidiform mole typically have signs and symptoms of a threat-

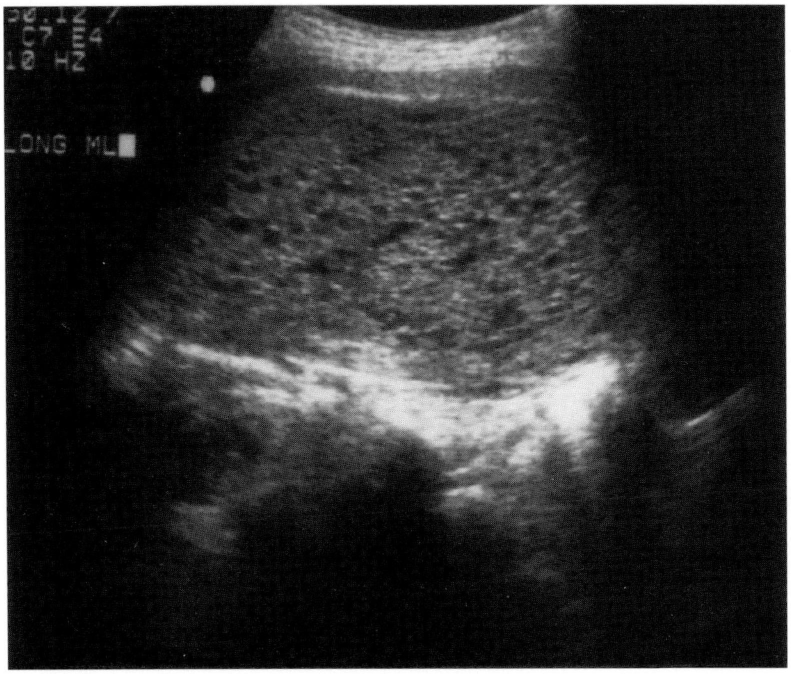

Figure 37–3. Ultrasound of hydatidiform mole. (Courtesy of Diane M. Twickler, MD.)

ened, inevitable, or missed abortion. Uterine size is usually small for gestational age, and the diagnosis is typically made by the pathologist after dilatation and curettage (Watson and associates, 1987).

Evaluation

Pretreatment diagnostic tests should include chest x-ray, liver enzyme studies, and coagulation studies to rule out occult metastatic disease. A baseline β-hCG level should be obtained (Lurain, 1982).

Treatment

The most effective treatment for hydatidiform mole is hysterectomy (Bahar and colleagues, 1989). Hysterectomy reduces the risk of progression to gestational trophoblastic tumor to 3 percent compared to 20 percent with evacuation and curettage (Curry and colleagues, 1975). Hysterectomy is appropriate treatment in patients who desire permanent sterilization. Since most patients with hydatidiform mole desire further fertility, they are best treated by suction evacuation of the uterus, followed by sharp curettage (Tow, 1966; Hankins and colleagues, 1987). Adequate blood and fluid replacement should be available for administration through large-bore intravenous infusions. Since the Rh D antigen has been demonstrated in trophoblast cells from molar pregnancies, it is advisable to administer anti-D immune globulin to Rh-negative patients who are not already sensitized. There is no place in the modern management of hydatidiform mole for hysterotomy (Tow, 1967). Following evacuation of the uterus, the successful outcome of most molar pregnancies is contingent on the careful monitoring of β-hCG levels and the avoidance of pregnancy.

Preoperative Preparation

Prior to operative management of hydatidiform mole, the patient should have a chest x-ray to rule out occult metastasis, which would make the patient more susceptible to developing pulmonary complications from overly aggressive fluid resuscitation. The patient should also be typed and cross-matched for at least two units of packed red blood cells. An hCG level should be drawn in addition to the usual preoperative laboratory studies.

Operative Technique

Hysterectomy. The most effective treatment for hydatidiform mole is hysterectomy; however, most patients are of reproductive age and desire future fertility. Thus, hysterectomy is usually reserved for patients prepared for sterilization. The operative technique is similar to that for nontrophoblastic diseases; however, certain points of technique are critical to minimize the potential for trophoblastic deportation and maximize preparation in case hemorrhagic complications are encountered. An adequate incision should be used, which will allow for exploratory laparotomy with special attention paid to inspection and palpation of the liver and kidneys. Following packing of the intestines, the uterus should be mobilized by bilateral atraumatic clamps placed across the round and ovarian ligaments. The clamps should be without points, with the tips placed in the avascular plain of the broad ligament. Next, the retroperitoneum and ureter should be exposed by a peritoneal incision lateral to the infundibulo-pelvic ligaments prior to or following ligation of the round ligaments. With exposure of the ureter and the hypogastric vessels, immediate measures can be applied should any hemorrhagic sequela develop. In addition, exposure of the ureter will allow its identification as it passes through the parametria since the softening of the cervix may make it more difficult to identify during parametrial dissection. Hysterotomy should be avoided, unless it is required to allow adequate exposure.

Dilatation and Evacuation. The technique for evacuation of hydatidiform moles is similar to that used for therapeutic abortion, but again with some specifics of technique that will allow the surgeon to limit intraoperative complications. General anesthesia is not absolutely required; however, if local sedation is used, it must be sufficient to allow the complete cooperation of the patient without extraneous motions. The patient should have a 14–16-gauge IV catheter placed. Oxytocin in a piggyback bottle should be connected to the main IV line but not started until indicated by the surgeon. The surgeon should have instruments arranged or an assistant available so that the surgeon will never have to take eyes off of the operating field or turn his or her back to the patient. Following gentle but thorough manual pelvic examination, cervical dilation is carried out by leaving the cervical dilator in place and not removing it until the succeeding dilator can be placed immediately into the cervical os. Dilation is carried out to the point that the cervix will easily accommodate a suction catheter whose size roughly equals the number-of-weeks size of the uterus. The last dilator is not removed until the suction catheter is hooked up and ready to commence the evacuation. The uterine contents are evacuated by rotating the suction cannula. Molar contents should be visualized passing through the tubing. The uterine contents in the evacuation bottle should be considered by the anesthesiologist and surgeon as isolated from the circulation and not count it as blood loss (Cotton, 1980; Hankins, 1987; and their associates). Evacuation is continued until no more molar tissue can be seen passing through the tubing and only bubbles are visible. Following suction curettage a gentle sharp curettage with a large curette is carried out, and oxytocin is started. Any further bleeding after this point should be considered as coming from the intravascular compartment and counted as blood loss. If the uterus appears to be completely evacuated, as confirmed by the gentle sharp curettage, then uterine compression and massage should be carried out by grasping the uterus firmly with the abdominal hand. The other hand is placed into the vagina with fingers lateral to the cervix, such that they can compress the uterine arterial blood supply to the cervix. In this way one can completely evaluate the uterus for tone and simultaneously tamponade any further bleeding.

Follow-up

A quantitative hCG level should be obtained every 2 weeks until it is below the limit of detection of the hormone. Levels are then obtained at 1 month, and then every 3 months for 1 year. Pregnancy may be permitted after 1 year of undetectable hCG levels (ACOG, 1993).

Oral Contraceptives

Early reports indicated that patients who received oral contraceptives after evacuation of hydatidiform mole had an increased risk of developing gestational trophoblastic tumors. Only 11 percent of the patients studied received oral contraceptives, however, and the increased risk was not statistically significant. One subsequent study confirmed this finding only in women who received oral contraceptives with greater than 50 μg of estrogen (Miller and Seifer, 1990). These findings were not confirmed in a well-controlled clinical study by Gal and colleagues (1981). In fact, the hCG levels declined to undetectable levels sooner in patients receiving oral contraceptives than in those who did not. At the John I. Brewer Trophoblastic Disease Center of the Northwestern University Cancer Center, patients who used oral contraceptives were less likely to develop gestational trophoblastic tumors than those who did not (Deicas and co-workers, 1991). Thus, the use of oral contraceptives after molar evacuation is an option unless there are other contraindications to their use. There is no substantial evidence that the use of oral contraceptives increases the risk of developing gestational trophoblastic tumors.

Outcome

The natural history of hydatidiform mole is regression after evacuation. From 1962 to 1978, 738 patients with hydatidiform mole were referred to the Brewer Center for follow-up and hCG testing after uterine evacuation. There was spontaneous regression of the disease in 596 (81%) patients and no further treatment was required. Gestational trophoblastic tumors developed in 142 (19%) patients; of these, 125 (17%) had invasive mole and 17 (2%) had choriocarcinoma. All of the 142 patients with gestational trophoblastic tumor subsequently were cured by chemotherapy and/or surgery (Lurain and co-workers, 1983).

Postevacuation Reproductive Endocrinology

Human Chorionic Gonadotropin. After a hydatidiform mole is evacuated, hCG levels fall progressively. Several laboratories have generated regression curves for the disappearance of hCG from the serum. Of the patients whose hCG levels spontaneously regress after uterine evacuation, 65 percent will have undetectable hCG levels by 60 days, and 100 percent by 170 days after evacuation (Lurain and associates, 1983). Serum hCG levels typically return to normal nonpregnant concentrations 10–20 days after term delivery. Since the clearance rate of hCG is constant, with a half-life of 6 days, the time to reach a negative value is determined by the initial level of hCG. This period is shorter in patients with partial hydatidiform mole as they have lower initial levels than do women with complete hydatidiform mole (Miller and Seifer, 1990). The time to undetectable levels is not dependent on the method of evacuation.

Ovulation. The time to the return of normal integrated function by the hypothalamic-pituitary-ovarian axis after molar evacuation also is dependent on the initial level of hCG and upon its normalization. Ovulation can occur in 5 percent of patients when hCG is less than 100 mIU/mL but greater than 20 mIU/mL; usually, ovulation does not occur until hCG levels are less than 20 mIU/mL (approximately 60% of patients). After evacuation, 30 percent of the first menses will be from ovulatory cycles, and the median time to ovulation is 9 weeks (Miller and Seifer, 1990). The quick return of ovulation emphasizes the need for prompt contraception even before the hCG values reach undetectable levels.

Reproductive Outcome. After successful treatment of a molar pregnancy, the incidence of secondary infertility is 2.5 percent. Of conceptions, 67 percent deliver at term, 19 percent spontaneously abort, 8 percent deliver prematurely, 1.3 percent develop gestational trophoblastic disease, of which 68 percent is hydatidiform mole, 1 percent develop ectopic pregnancies, and 0.5 percent have stillbirths (Sand and colleagues, 1984). After two gestational trophoblastic disease (GTD) events, only 44 percent of such patients will ever deliver viable infants and the risk of subsequent GTD is 28 percent (Lurain and associates, 1982d).

GESTATIONAL TROPHOBLASTIC TUMORS

Gestational trophoblastic tumor encompasses clinical evidence of invasive mole, gestational choriocarcinoma, and placental site trophoblastic tumor. The diagnosis often is made on the basis of plateauing or rising hCG levels after evacuation of a hydatidiform mole. Treatment usually is initiated without the benefit or requirement of any further tissue diagnosis (WHO, 1983; Lurain, 1990a).

Pathogenesis—Invasive Mole

Invasive mole, as the name implies, is the invasive phase of hydatidiform mole characterized histologically by the extension of the formed villus, with its hyperplastic and often anaplastic trophoblast, directly into the myometrium or into myometrial venous channels (Fig. 37–4). Metastases may occur to the lung, vagina, cervix, vulva, and broad liga-

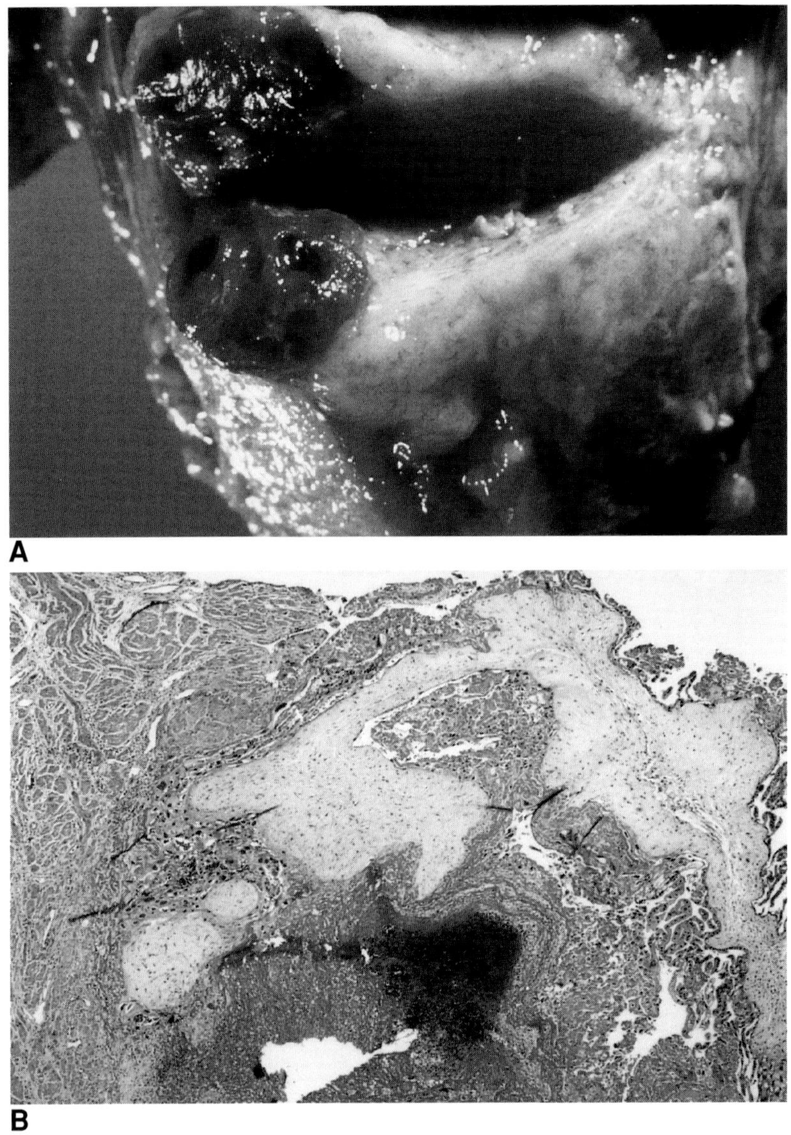

Figure 37–4 **A.** A single nodule (left) of invasive mole is bisected at the uterine fundus to show the depth of corpus penetration. **B.** Chorionic villi are seen (right) penetrating the myometrium (left) in invasive mole. (Courtesy of Julianne S. Sandstad, MD.)

ment. The biologic distinction between hydatidiform mole and invasive mole is not clear-cut. Studies of the natural history of gestational trophoblastic disease based on lung computed tomography (CT) scan, hysterectomy specimens, and prolonged hCG regression curves indicate that about 40 percent of patients with presumed hydatidiform mole have occult invasion or metastases that usually undergo spontaneous regression (Brewer and co-workers, 1978; Lurain, 1987a). The incidence of clinically apparent metastases in diagnosed invasive mole is 15 percent (Lurain and Brewer, 1982). Metastatic invasive mole, as in the uterus, tends to undergo spontaneous regression and rarely causes death. Morbidity and mortality are the result of uterine perforation, hemorrhage, embolic phenomena, and sepsis.

The invasive potential of partial hydatidiform mole remains to be delineated, since most studies of the natural history of hydatidiform mole do not differentiate between partial and complete hydatidiform mole (Watson and colleagues, 1987). Preliminary reports indicate that 3 percent will require further treatment after evacuation (Goto and associates, 1993). These patients probably have invasive moles, since no cases of choriocarcinoma have been reported.

Epidemiology

The incidence of invasive mole is estimated at 1/15,000 pregnancies (Lurain and Brewer,

1982). After treatment of hydatidiform mole, approximately 15 percent of patients will develop invasive mole (Lurain and colleagues, 1983). Several factors have been identified that are associated with a higher risk of persistent trophoblastic disease or gestational trophoblastic tumor. These include preevacuation uterine size larger than expected for gestational age or above the umbilicus, bilateral theca lutein cysts greater than 5 cm, age greater than 40 years, and abnormal postevacuation uterine bleeding (Murad and associates, 1990).

Signs and Symptoms

In virtually all cases, invasive mole follows a hydatidiform mole. Occasionally, patients will develop invasive mole after a purported spontaneous or therapeutic abortion; these gestations were, however, more likely to have been unrecognized hydatidiform moles. The diagnosis of invasive mole usually is made in asymptomatic patients who manifest plateauing or rising hCG levels after hydatidiform mole evacuation. Occasionally, the diagnosis is made when metastases are detected in the course of workup of a presumed hydatidiform mole. Those patients developing symptoms from invasive mole usually note persistent uterine bleeding after evacuation of a hydatidiform mole. Metastatic lesions may present as hemorrhage from vaginal lesions or hemoptysis and pleuritic pain from lung metastases (Lurain and Brewer, 1982).

Pathogenesis—Gestational Choriocarcinoma

These malignancies may arise from any type of gestational event; 50 percent follow hydatidiform mole, 25 percent follow abortions or ectopic pregnancies, and 25 percent follow term gestation. Gestational choriocarcinoma will complicate 1/40,000 pregnancies (Olive, 1984; Lurain, 1986; and their colleagues) and develops in 2 percent of patients with hydatidiform mole (Lurain and co-workers, 1983). To date, no cases have been reported following partial hydatidiform mole. A gestational trophoblastic tumor arising after a term pregnancy is virtually always choriocarcinoma. Gestational choriocarcinoma was once thought to arise from retained or metastatic secundines following gestational events; however, careful studies of placentas from patients developing choriocarcinoma indicate that the tumor arises within the cytotrophoblastic cell layer covering the stromal portion of the chorionic villi of the placenta (Brewer and associates, 1966, 1978, 1981).

Gestational choriocarcinoma is recognized histologically by its lack of villus structures. It is characterized by a core of pleomorphic cytotrophoblastic cells surrounded by a ring of syncytiotrophoblastic cells with extensive hemorrhage and necrosis (Fig. 37–5) (Brewer and Mazur, 1981). There is direct invasion of myometrium and vascular spread to the myometrium and distant sites. Metastases occur early and most commonly to the

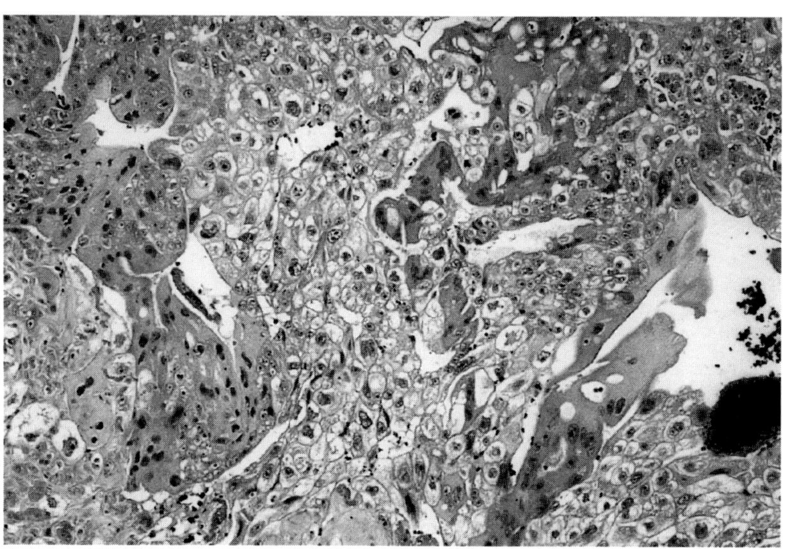

Figure 37–5. Choriocarcinoma is diagnosed when multinucleated syncytotrophoblastic cells cap or cover cytotrophoblasts in a setting of hemorrhage and necrosis (40x). (Courtesy of Julianne S. Sandstad, MD.)

lung, followed by the brain, liver, gastrointestinal tract, and kidney (Veridiano and colleagues, 1980). Death occurs mainly from hemorrhage at metastatic sites, pulmonary insufficiency from tumor infiltration and hemorrhage, and treatment sequelae. Choriocarcinoma accounts for virtually all disease-related deaths from gestational trophoblastic tumors (Brewer, 1971; Mazur, 1982; Lurain, 1982a, 1984, 1987b, 1991; and their colleagues). Transplacental metastasis of gestational choriocarcinoma rarely occurs. Affected infants also present with signs of hemorrhage and of gonadotropin stimulation to include hemoptysis, melena, and anemia. Lung and liver metastasis are common and most of the reported fetal cases have been fatal. Infants of gestational choriocarcinoma patients should have prompt hCG testing (Flam, 1989; Christopherson, 1992; Fraser, 1992; and their co-workers).

Risk Factors

The most significant risk factor for choriocarcinoma is a previous hydatidiform mole. Other risk factors include age greater than 40 years and ABO blood group discrepancies between the mother and her biologic partner (Miller and colleagues, 1989).

Signs and Symptoms

Signs and symptoms of choriocarcinoma most commonly consist of abnormal uterine bleeding after a gestational event or bleeding from metastatic sites, manifested by hemoptysis, melena, hemoperitoneum, or intracerebral hemorrhage. Choriocarcinoma is one of the "great masqueraders" and should always be considered in the differential diagnosis of a reproductive age woman who presents with hemorrhage from any site, particularly if it is catastrophic hemorrhage. Forty-five percent of patients with central nervous system choriocarcinoma die without receiving therapy (Yordan and associates, 1987). Failure to make the antemortem diagnosis of choriocarcinoma has resulted in choriocarcinoma developing in transplant recipients whose organs were procured from these undiagnosed patients (Baquero and colleagues, 1988).

Diagnosis

Based on the natural history of gestational trophoblastic diseases, the following criteria for active therapy of gestational trophoblastic tumors have been established by WHO (1983): (1) high levels of hCG more than 4 weeks after evacuation of a hydatidiform mole (serum level >20,000 mIU/mL; urine level >30,000 IU/L), (2) progressively increasing hCG values at any time after evacuation (minimum of three values in 1 month), (3) histologic evidence of choriocarcinoma at any site, or (4) evidence of central nervous system, renal, hepatic, or gastrointestinal metastases, or pulmonary metastases >2 cm in diameter or more than three in number. In addition to the WHO criteria, most American centers treat patients with plateauing hCG levels (three nondecreasing levels in 1 month) or with any clinically evident metastases (Miller and Lurain, 1988). Using these criteria, 7–20 percent of patients will receive chemotherapy after molar evacuation (Lurain and colleagues, 1983).

Staging

To achieve uniformity in reporting of data and to make the results of treatment more comparable, a clinical staging system for gestational trophoblastic tumors was proposed and tentatively adopted by the FIGO Cancer Committee in 1982 (Miller and Lurain, 1988). This system is based on anatomic criteria and conforms to the staging systems used for all other gynecologic cancers (Table 37–1). This system is limited in that it does not take into consideration the possible influences of antecedent pregnancy, tumor morphology, and prior chemotherapeutic failure. Since identification of patients at high risk of failing chemotherapy is important in determining the appropriate treatment regimen, a prognostic scoring system has been proposed. It is based on the type of and time interval between an antecedent pregnancy and a trophoblastic tumor event, serum hCG value, ABO blood

TABLE 37–1. FIGO TROPHOBLASTIC TUMOR STAGING

Stage	Tumor Status
I	The lesion is confined to the uterus without metastases.
II	The lesion extends outside the uterus but is confined to the genital organs.
III	The lesion has metastasized the lung.
IV	All other metastatic sites.

TABLE 37–2. WHO TROPHOBLASTIC TUMOR SCORING SYSTEM

Prognostic Factor	Score[a]			
	0	*1*	*2*	*4*
Age (yr)	< 39	> 39		
Antecedent pregnancy	HM	Abortion	Term	
Interval (mo)[b]	< 4	4–6	7–12	> 12
hCG (mIU/L)	< 10^3	10^3–10^4	10^4–10^5	> 10^5
ABO groups (female × male)	—	O × A A × O	B AB	—
Largest tumor, including uterine tumor	—	3–5 cm	> 5 cm	
Metastatic sites	—	Spleen, kidney	GI tract liver	Brain
No. metastases identified	—	1–4	4–8	> 8
Prior chemotherapy	—	—	1 drug	≥ 2 drugs

[a]Total patient score is obtained by adding individual scores for each prognostic factor. Total score ≤4 = low risk; 5–7 = middle risk; ≥ 8 = high risk.
[b]Interval between end of antecedent pregnancy and start of chemotherapy.
HM = hydatidiform mole.

type, tumor diameter, site and number of metastases, and previous chemotherapy (Table 37–2) (WHO, 1983).

Most treatment centers in the United States determine therapy and report results of gestational trophoblastic tumors based on the presence of metastases and the risk of failed chemotherapy, using a system proposed in 1965 and later modified (Miller and Lurain, 1988). Patients with gestational trophoblastic tumors are divided into three groups: nonmetastatic, low-risk metastatic, and high-risk metastatic. "High-risk" refers to those patients with metastatic gestational trophoblastic tumors that are not likely to be cured by single-agent methotrexate or actinomycin therapy. This high-risk group is identified by any one of the following: (1) immediate pretreatment hCG level in excess of 100,000 IU/24-hour urine or 40,000 mIU/mL serum (β-subunit assay), (2) greater than 4 months from antecedent pregnancy event or onset of symptoms to treatment, (3) metastases to sites other than the lungs or vagina, (4) antecedent term gestation, or (5) prior unsuccessful chemotherapy (Lurain and associates, 1982b, 1987b). In one study, metastatic gestational trophoblastic tumor following an antecedent term gestation was not found to be an independent risk factor (Olive and colleagues, 1984).

The Brewer Center developed a scoring system that identifies patients at risk for treatment failure. Clinicopathologic diagnosis of choriocarcinoma, metastasis to sites other than lung or vagina, number of metastases, and previous failed chemotherapy were strongly associated with treatment failure (Lurain and Sciarra, 1991).

Staging evaluation of these patients should include a complete history, physical and pelvic examination, complete blood count, platelet count, liver and renal function studies, quantitative serum β-hCG, chest x-ray, and CT of the abdomen and pelvis. CT scans of the lung and brain should be obtained as clinically indicated (Lurain, 1982).

Treatment

Nonmetastatic Gestational Trophoblastic Tumors. Patients with nonmetastatic gestational trophoblastic tumors (GTT) have no clinical evidence of spread beyond the uterus. If they desire sterility, they should be treated with hysterectomy and adjuvant single-agent chemotherapy at the time of operation. Hammond and colleagues (1980) reported that all 17 patients with nonmetastatic GTT treated with primary hysterectomy and chemotherapy were cured, while 13 percent of 122 patients treated with chemotherapy alone failed to achieve remission and required salvage hysterectomy to accomplish cure. Patients treated with primary surgery required an average of 2 cycles of chemotherapy and 33 days to achieve remission, compared to 4 cycles and 51 days for patients treated with chemotherapy alone. Hysterectomy alone cured 40 percent of patients with nonmetastatic choriocarcinoma (Brewer and co-workers, 1963), whereas uterine evacuation or curettage is therapeutic in only 20 percent of these patients (Schlaerth and associates, 1990). Patient desiring to retain fertility can be treated adequately with chemotherapy alone. The standard chemotherapeutic agents include methotrexate, 0.4 mg/kg (25 mg maximum dose) IV or IM every day for 5 days. Actinomycin-D, 10–13 μg/kg IV every day for 5 days is an alternative in patients with hepatic or renal disease that precludes the use of methotrexate. Chemotherapy courses are repeated every 12–14 days providing there is no unacceptable toxicity. Serum β-hCG levels, a complete blood count, and renal and liver function studies are obtained before each course of chemotherapy. If β-hCG levels plateau or rise or if unacceptable toxicity develops despite dosage adjustments, chemotherapy should be switched to the alternate agent. Two to ten percent of patients will have a resistant focus of trophoblastic tumor within the uterus and may then require hysterectomy. Localized uterine resection has been described but its role remains unclear (Wilson, 1965; Kanazawa, 1988; and their colleagues). With proper management, cure should approach 100 percent in these patients. At the Brewer Trophoblastic Disease Center, 323 patients with nonmetastatic gestational trophoblastic tumor were treated between 1962 and 1989 and all patients were cured (Lurain and Sciarra, 1991). Of the 264 patients treated before 1985, 86 percent were cured by their initial chemotherapeutic regime, 11 percent required secondary agents, and 3 percent underwent hysterectomy to achieve remission (Lurain, 1990a).

Low-Risk Metastatic Gestational Trophoblastic Tumor. Patients with low-risk metastatic gestational trophoblastic tumors typically have metastatic disease in the lung or vagina. If the patient is medically stable and desires sterility, she should be treated with hysterectomy and single-agent chemotherapy. Hammond and colleagues (1980) reported that all 15 patients who underwent primary hysterectomy at the start of chemotherapy achieved remission, whereas only 87 percent of 40 patients treated initially with chemotherapy alone achieved remission and the remainder required salvage hysterectomy to be cured. Patients treated with primary surgery required an average of 4 cycles of chemotherapy over 57 days to achieve remission, compared with 6 cycles and 77 days in patients receiving chemotherapy alone. The medical treatment of choice in these patients is single-agent chemotherapy, as outlined for nonmetastatic gestational trophoblastic tumor. These patients, however, are more likely to develop drug resistance (40–50%) and require a change to an alternate agent (Lurain and associates, 1982c). Ten to fifteen percent of these patients subsequently will require triple-agent chemotherapy or surgery to achieve complete remission (Hammond and co-workers, 1980). Almost all patients with low-risk metastatic gestational trophoblastic tumor should be cured. This was again the experience of the Brewer Center, where all 69 patients with low-risk metastatic disease achieved remission (Lurain and Brewer, 1984).

High-Risk Metastatic Gestational Trophoblastic Tumor. In high-risk metastatic gestational trophoblastic tumor, patients are at significant risk of failing single-agent chemotherapy and should be treated with multiagent, combination chemotherapy. Methotrexate, actinomycin, and cyclophosphamide (MAC) was the traditional combination chemotherapeutic regimen recommended, with reported cure rates of 50–80 percent. Of the 73 patients with high-risk metastatic gestational trophoblastic tumor treated with MAC at the Brewer Center from 1968 to 1982, 51 percent achieved remission. Twenty-nine of 46 (63%) receiving MAC as first-line therapy and 8 of 27 (30%) receiving MAC as a secondary treatment after failing initial therapy were cured (Lurain and Brewer, 1985).

Several other multidrug regimens have been proposed; the most useful employs etoposide with methotrexate, actinomycin, cyclophosphamide, and vincristine (EMA-CO) and has induced remission in 83 percent of high-risk patients (Schink and co-workers, 1992). While primary hysterectomy or other operations do not appear to improve outcome in these patients (Hammond and colleagues, 1980), they are likely to develop resistant foci of GTT that will require salvage hysterectomy (Lurain and colleagues, 1982c). Thoracotomy may be therapeutic in patients who have solitary pulmonary lesions, no other metastases, and hCG levels less than 100 mIU/mL (Tomada and colleagues, 1980). Craniotomy may be required to treat intracranial hemorrhage but rarely contributes toward remission (Hammond and colleagues, 1980). If central nervous system metastases are detected, whole brain irradiation with 3000 rad is given concurrently with chemotherapy (Stilp and coworkers, 1972). The outcome for patients with liver metastasis is particularly ominous, since remissions are obtained in only 0–40 percent. There appears to be no advantage to adjuvant radiation therapy for patients with liver metastasis. Still, some patients with resistant disease will have an identifiable focus or foci of choriocarcinoma for which surgical excision will facilitate a cure (Lurain, 1987b).

Follow-up

Treatment is continued with one of the stated regimens until three consecutive negative hCG levels are obtained. hCG level determinations are then repeated at 3-week intervals for 3 months, every month for 3 months, every 2 months for 6 months, and then every 6 months for life (ACOG, 1993). Contraception is required for at least 1 year; oral contraceptives are the method of choice, unless there are contraindications to their use. After 1 year of undetectable hCG levels, pregnancy can be permitted. This allows for the theoretical elimination of germ cells that have been damaged by chemotherapy and enables the clinician to use the β-hCG assay to document cure throughout the year. The risk of recurrent gestational trophoblastic disease after chemotherapy for gestational trophoblastic tumor is 0.67 percent (Sand and associates, 1984).

Prophylaxis Against Gestational Trophoblastic Tumors

A reduction in the rate of development of gestational trophoblastic tumors has been attempted by the administration of prophylactic single-agent chemotherapy at the time of evacuation of hydatidiform mole. Unfortunately, prophylaxis does not prevent gestational trophoblastic tumor development in all patients, and several deaths have resulted from the toxic effects of such treatment. Prophylaxis requires the administration of potentially mutagenic and toxic agents to the majority of patients who would normally never require therapy to prevent tumor progression in only 10 percent of patients. Furthermore, these patients would have been cured using standard treatment protocols without prophylaxis. Other investigators have administered chemotherapy to patients whose β-hCG levels after molar evacuation deviate from normal regression curves. This results in 27 percent of patients being treated, but not all patients achieve remission. The result is again less satisfactory than standard treatment algorithms (Miller and colleagues, 1989).

Reproductive Outcome

Gonadal function after chemotherapy for gestational trophoblastic tumors has not been fully studied. Based on experience acquired from chemotherapy administered for other tumors, gonadal dysfunction as a result of cytotoxic therapy has been reported with alkylating agents (eg, cyclophosphamide, chlorambucil, busulfan, nitrogen mustard), the vinca alkaloids (eg, vinblastine), and mitomycin C. These drugs can cause oocyte depletion and consequent ovarian failure. Similar results have been reported with etoposide. Ovarian failure as evidenced by hypergonadotrophic, hypoestrogenic amenorrhea developed in 32 percent of these patients. Successful pregnancy outcomes after chemotherapy for trophoblastic tumors have been reported. These studies indicate that 73 percent of patients have term deliveries, 2 percent premature deliveries, 16 percent spontaneous abortions, 8 percent therapeutic abortions, and 1 percent hydatidiform mole. Major congenital malformations occurred in 1 percent of cases. A large, long-term, follow-up study showed no unexpected second malignancies following chemotherapy for gestational trophoblastic tumors (Lurain, 1990b).

Pathogenesis—Placental Site Trophoblastic Tumor

Placental site trophoblastic tumor is a very rare neoplasm, with fewer than 50 reported cases (Lathrop and co-workers, 1988). It appears to arise from the placental implantation site after term pregnancy or nonmolar abortions. Histologically, placental site trophoblastic tumor is characterized by pleomorphic, hyperchromatic trophoblastic cells containing prominent nuclei that are predominantly cytotrophoblastic, with only a few multinucleated syncytial cells. This probably accounts for the low serum levels of hCG. Most placental site trophoblastic tumors have an immunohistochemical staining pattern that is positive for many HPL cells and a few hCG or SP_1 cells. The neoplastic cells infiltrate the myometrium, invade vascular spaces, and occasionally metastasize to the liver, lungs, and brain. The aggressiveness of the tumor appears to be correlated with the number of mitotic figures per 10 high-power fields.

Signs and Symptoms

Patients usually have vaginal bleeding after a period of amenorrhea, not necessarily following a recognized pregnancy event. hCG levels range from normal to elevated. Several patients have developed a nephrotic syndrome that may be due to humoral factors released by the tumor.

Treatment

The optimal treatment of placental site trophoblastic tumor is uncertain. Most patients should undergo hysterectomy and HPL and hCG levels should be monitored. Tumors with >5 mitoses per 10 high-power fields may require systemic chemotherapy for a potential cure. Oophorectomy may not contribute to the treatment outcome (Berkowitz and colleagues, 1990). Chemotherapy is indicated if metastases are documented. Unfortunately, placental site trophoblastic tumors are not as responsive to chemotherapy as other gestational trophoblastic tumors, and several deaths have been reported.

SUMMARY

Surgical therapy is a vital modality for the treatment of GTD. Operations are useful to remove known foci of disease, control hemorrhage, relieve obstruction, treat infection, or treat other life-threatening complication so that these patients can survive to be treated and ultimately cured by chemotherapy (Lewis, 1966; Hammond, 1980; Jones, 1988; and associates).

REFERENCES

American College of Obstetricians and Gynecologists. Management of Gestational Trophoblastic Neoplasia. ACOG Technical Bulletin No. 178, Washington, DC: The American College of Obstetricians and Gynecologists, 1993.

Bahar AM, el-Ashnehi MS, Senthilselvan A. Hydatidiform mole in the elderly: hysterectomy or evacuation? Intl J Gynecol Obstet 1989; 29:233.

Baquero A, Bannett A, Werner DJ, Kim P. Misdiagnosis of metastatic cerebral choriocarcinoma in female cadaver donors. Transplantation Proc 1988; 20:776.

Berkowitz BJ, Jones JG, Merkatz IR, Runowicz CD. Ovarian conservation in placental site trophoblastic tumor. Gynecol Oncol 1990; 37:239.

Block, MF, Merrill JA. Hydatidiform mole with coexistent fetus. Obstet Gynecol 1982; 60:129.

Borek E, Sharma OK, Brewer JI. Urinary nucleic acid breakdown products as markers for trophoblastic diseases. Am J Obstet Gynecol 1983; 146:906.

Brewer JI, Gerbie AB. Early development of choriocarcinoma. Am J Obstet Gynecol 1966; 94:692.

Brewer JI, Mazur MT. Gestational choriocarcinoma. Its origin in the placenta during seemingly normal pregnancy. Am J Surg Pathol 1981; 5:267.

Brewer JI, Smith RT, Pratt GB. Choriocarcinoma. Absolute 5-year survival rates of 122 patients treated by hysterectomy. Am J Obstet Gynecol 1963; 85:841.

Brewer JI, Eckman TR, Dolkart RE, et al. Gestational trophoblastic disease. A comparative study of the results of therapy in patients with invasive mole and with choriocarcinoma. Am J Obstet Gynecol 1971; 109:335.

Brewer JI, Torok EE, Kahan BD, et al. Gestational trophoblastic disease: Origin of choriocarcinoma, invasive mole and choriocarcinoma associated with hydatidiform mole, and some immunologic aspects. Adv Cancer Res 1978; 27:89.

Brewer JI, Halpern B, Torok EE. Gestational trophoblastic disease: selected clinical aspects and chorionic gonadotropin test methods. Curr Probl Cancer 1979; 3:1.

Christopherson WA, Kanbour A, Szulman AE. Choriocarcinoma in a term placenta with maternal metastases. Gynecol Oncol 1992; 46:239.

Cotton DB, Bernstein SG, Read JA, et al. Hemodynamic observations in evacuation of molar pregnancy. Am J Obstet Gynecol 1980; 138:6.

Curry SL, Hammond CB, Tyrey L, et al. Hydatidiform mole: diagnosis, management, and long-term follow-up of 347 patients. Obstet Gynecol 1975; 45:1.

Deicas RE, Miller DS, Rademaker AW, Lurain JR. The role of contraception in the development of postmolar gestational trophoblastic tumor. Obstet Gynecol 1991; 78:221.

Flam F, Lundstrom V, Silversward C. Choriocarcinoma in mother and child. Br J Obstet Gynecol 1989; 96:241.

Fraser GC, Blair GK, Hemming A, et al. The treatment of simultaneous choriocarcinoma in mother and baby. J Pediatr Surg 1992; 27:1318.

Gal D, Simpson ER, Porter JC, et al. Failure of contraceptive steroids to modify human chorionic gonadotrophin secretion by hydatidiform mole tissue and choriocarcinoma cells in culture. Steroids 1981; 37:663.

Goto S, Yamada A, Ishizuka T, Tomoda Y. Development of postmolar trophoblastic disease after partial molar pregnancy. Gynecol Oncol 1993; 48:165.

Hammond CB, Weed JC Jr, Currie JL. The role of operation in the current therapy of gestational trophoblastic disease. Am J Obstet Gynecol 1980; 136:844.

Hankins GD, Wendel GD, Snyder RR, Cunningham FG. Trophoblastic embolization during molar evacuation: central hemodynamic observations. Obstet Gynecol 1987; 69:368.

Jones WB, Lewis JL Jr. Integration of surgery and other techniques in the management of trophoblastic malignancy. Obstet Gynecol Clin North Am 1988; 15:565.

Kanazawa K, Sasagawa M, Suzuki T, Takeuchi S. Clinical evaluation of focal excision of myometrial lesion for treatment of invasive hydatidiform mole. Acta Obstet Gynecol Scand 1988; 67:487.

Lathrop JC, Lauchlan S, Nayak R, Ambler M. Clinical characteristics of placental site trophoblastic tumor (PSTT). Gynecol Oncol 1988; 31:32.

Lewis JL Jr, Ketcham AS, Hertz R. Surgical intervention during chemotherapy of gestational trophoblastic neoplasms. Cancer 1966; 19:1517.

Lurain JR. Newer diagnostic approaches to the evaluation of gynecologic malignancies. Obstet Gynecol Surv 1982; 37:437.

Lurain JR. The trophoblast. In: Phillip E, Barnes J, Newton M, eds. Scientific Foundations of Obstetrics and Gynecology. 3rd ed. London: Heinemann, 1986.

Lurain JR. The natural history of gestational trophoblastic diseases. In: Schulman AE, Buchsbaum HJ, eds. Gestational Trophoblastic Disease. New York: Springer-Verlag, 1987a.

Lurain JR. Causes of treatment failure in gestational trophoblastic disease. J Repro Med 1987b; 32:675.

Lurain JR. Chemotherapy of gestational trophoblastic disease. In: Deppe G, ed. Chemotherapy of Gynecologic Cancer. New York: Alan R Liss, 1990a.

Lurain JR. Gestational trophoblastic tumors. Semin Surg Oncol 1990b; 6:347.

Lurain JR, Brewer JI. Invasive mole. Semin Oncol 1982; 9:174.

Lurain JR, Brewer JI. The study and treatment of gestational trophoblastic diseases at the Brewer Trophoblastic Disease Center, 1962–1979. In: Patillo RA, ed. Human Trophoblast Neoplasms. New York: Plenum, 1984.

Lurain JR, Brewer JI. Treatment of high-risk gestational trophoblastic disease with methotrexate, actinomycin and cyclophosphamide chemotherapy. Obstet Gynecol 1985; 65:830.

Lurain JR, Sciarra JJ. Study and treatment of gestational trophoblastic diseases at the John I. Brewer Trophoblastic Disease Center, 1962–1990. Eur J Gynecol Oncol 1991; 12:425.

Lurain JR, Brewer JI, Mazur MT, Halpern B. Fatal gestational choriocarcinoma: clinico-pathologic study of patients treated at a trophoblastic disease center. Cancer 1982a; 50:1833.

Lurain JR, Brewer JI, Torok EE, Halpern B. Gestational trophoblastic disease: effect of duration of disease and hCG titer on response to therapy. J Reprod Med 1982b; 27:401.

Lurain JR, Brewer JI, Torok EE, Halpern B. Gestational trophoblastic disease: treatment results at the Brewer Trophoblastic Disease Center. Obstet Gynecol 1982c; 60:354.

Lurain JR, Sand PK, Carson SA, et al. Pregnancy outcome subsequent to consecutive hydatidiform moles. Am J Obstet Gynecol 1982d; 142:1060.

Lurain JR, Brewer JI, Torok EE, Halpern B. Natural history of hydatidiform mole after primary evacuation. Am J Obstet Gynecol 1983;145:591.

Lurain JR, Sand PK, Brewer JI. Choriocarcinoma associated with ectopic pregnancy. Obstet Gynecol 1986; 68:286.

Lurain JR, Casanova LA, Miller DS, Rademaker AW. Prognostic factors in gestational trophoblastic tumors: a proposed new scoring system based on multivariate analysis. Am J Obstet Gynecol 1991; 164:611.

Mazur MT, Lurain JR, Brewer JI. Fatal gestational choriocarcinoma: clinico-pathologic study of patients treated at a trophoblastic disease center: an analysis of treatment failures. Am J Obstet Gynecol 1982; 144:391.

Miller DS, Lurain JR. Classification and staging of gestational trophoblastic tumors. Obstet Gynecol Clin North Am 1988; 15:477.

Miller DS, Seifer DB. Endocrinologic aspects of gestational trophoblastic diseases. Intl J Fertil 1990; 35:137.

Miller DS, Teng NNH, Ballon SC. Gestational trophoblastic disease. In: Brody SA, Ueland K, eds. Endocrine Disorders in Pregnancy. New York: Appleton-Century-Crofts, 1989.

Mittal KK, Kachru RB, Brewer JI. The HL-A and ABO antigens in trophoblastic disease. Tissue Antigens 1975; 6:57.

Murad TM, Longley JV, Lurain JR, Brewer JI. Hydatidiform mole: clinicopathologic associations with the development of postevacuation trophoblastic disease. Intl J Gynecol Obstet 1990; 32:359.

Newman RB, Eddy GL. Eclampsia as a possible risk factor for persistent trophoblastic disease. Gynecol Oncol 1989; 34:212.

Olive DL, Lurain JR, Brewer J. Choriocarcinoma

associated with term gestation. Am J Obstet Gynecol 1984; 148:711.

Pritchard JA. Blood volume changes in pregnancy and the puerperium. IV: Anemia associated with hydatidiform mole. Am J Obstet Gynecol 1965; 91:621.

Romero R, Horgan JG, Kohorn EI, et al. New criteria for the diagnosis of gestational trophoblastic disease. Obstet Gynecol 1985; 66:553.

Sand PK, Lurain JR, Brewer JI. Repeat gestational trophoblastic disease. Obstet Gynecol 1984; 63:140.

Santos-Ramos R, Forney JP, Schwarz BE. Sonographic findings and clinical correlations in molar pregnancy. Obstet Gynecol 1980; 56:186.

Sarto GE, Stubblefield PA, Lurain JR, Therman E. Mechanisms of growth in hydatidiform moles. Am J Obstet Gynecol 1984; 148:1014.

Schink JC, Singh DK, Rademaker AW, et al. Etoposide, methotrexate, actinomycin D, cyclophosphamide, and vincristine for the treatment of metastatic, high-risk gestational trophoblastic disease. Obstet Gynecol 1992; 80:817.

Schlaerth JB, Morrow CP, Rodriguez M. Diagnostic and therapeutic curettage in gestational trophoblastic disease. Am J Obstet Gynecol 1990; 162:1465.

Shapiro AI, Wu TF, Ballon SC, et al. Use of an immunoradiometric assay and a radioimmunoassay for the detection of free beta human chorionic gonadotropin. Obstet Gynecol 1985; 65:545.

Stilp TJ, Bucy PC, Brewer JI. Cure of metastatic choriocarcinoma of the brain. JAMA 1972; 221:276.

Teng NNH, Ballon SC. Partial hydatidiform mole with diploid karyotype: report of three cases. Am J Obstet Gynecol 1984; 150:961.

Tomoda Y, Aril Y, Kaseki S, et al. Surgical indications for resection in pulmonary metastasis of choriocarcinoma. Cancer 1980; 46:2723.

Tow WSH. The influence of the primary treatment of hydatidiform mole on its subsequent course. J Obstet Gynaecol Br Commonw 1966; 73:544.

Tow WS. The place of hysterotomy in the treatment of hydatidiform mole. Aust NZ J Obstet Gynaecol 1967; 7:97.

Veridiano NP, Gal D, Delke I, et al. Gestational choriocarcinoma of the ovary. Gynecol Oncol 1980; 10:235.

Watson EJ, Hernandez E, Miyazaw K. Partial hydatidiform moles: a review. Obstet Gynecol Surv 1987; 42:540.

Wilson RB, Beecham CT, Symmonds RE. Conservative surgical management of chorioadenoma destruens. Obstet Gynecol 1965; 26:814.

World Health Organization Scientific Group on Gestational Trophoblastic Diseases. Gestational Trophoblastic Disease, Technical Report Series 692. Geneva: World Health Organization, 1983.

Wu TF, Ballon SC, Teng NNH. Monoclonal vs polyclonal antibody radioimmunoassay against β-subunit of human chorionic gonadotropin in patients with gestational trophoblastic neoplasia. Am J Obstet Gynecol 1983; 147:821.

Yordan EL Jr, Schlaerth JB, Gaddis O Jr, Morrow CP. Radiation therapy in the management of gestational choriocarcinoma metastatic to the central nervous stem. Obstet Gynecol 1987; 69:627.

CHAPTER 38

Prophylactic Antibiotics

Infection is the most common complication associated with obstetric surgery. Accordingly, obstetricians have been intensely interested in assessing methods to reduce the likelihood of infection following selected surgical procedures. Most of the effort in clinical research has been devoted to developing and refining protocols for the administration of prophylactic antibiotics.

The first portion of this chapter reviews the pathophysiology of postoperative pelvic infections, criteria for use of prophylactic antibiotics, and mechanism of action and objectives of antibiotic administration. The second portion summarizes the results of clinical trials of antibiotic prophylaxis for cesarean delivery, pregnancy termination, cervical cerclage, and repair of episiotomy disruptions.

PATHOPHYSIOLOGY OF POSTOPERATIVE INFECTIONS

Postoperative infections usually are caused by multiple microorganisms that are part of the normal vaginal flora. The principal aerobic pathogens are group B and group D streptococci and gram negative bacilli such as *E. coli, Klebsiella pneumoniae,* and *Proteus* species. The most common anaerobic organisms are Peptococci and Peptostreptococci species, *Gardnerella vaginalis,* and *Bacteroides* species. Although they are of great importance in the pathogenesis of pelvic inflammatory disease, *Neisseria gonorrhoeae* and *Chlamydia trachomatis* do not typically cause immediate postoperative infections. When postoperative infections are complicated by bacteremia, the most common isolates are group B streptococci, aerobic gram-negative bacilli, and anaerobes (Duff, 1986).

The multiple aerobic and anaerobic organisms of the vagina are very well adapted for causing serious infections when they are inoculated into the upper genital tract coincident with labor, vaginal examination, or surgery. Most of the bacteria have specialized fimbriae, which enable them to adhere tightly to the columnar epithelium of the genital tract. Many of the organisms, such as group B streptococci, *Bacteroides* species, and the aerobic gram-negative bacilli, have capsules or specialized cell walls that impair phagocytosis by host white blood cells. Some bacteria produce a variety of proteolytic enzymes that facilitate infection of host cells. Still others have the capacity to produce beta-lactamase enzymes, which degrade many of the beta-lactam antibiotics used to treat infections.

In women having cesarean delivery, the most important risk factors for postoperative infection are low socioeconomic status, extended duration of labor and ruptured membranes, multiple vaginal examinations, and preexisting lower genital tract infection (Hawrylyshyn and associates, 1981). In women having pregnancy termination, cerclage, or episiotomy repair, the principal risk factors are preexisting lower tract infection and/or gestational age. Each of these risk factors increases the probability that a large number of potentially virulent microorganisms will be inoculated into the upper genital tract during the course of labor and/or surgery (Duff and Park, 1980).

CRITERIA FOR USE OF ANTIBIOTIC PROPHYLAXIS

Prophylactic administration of antibiotics is distinguished from therapeutic administration by both duration of therapy and selection of specific drugs. To be considered prophylaxis, antibiotic use should be confined to the first 24 hours in the perioperative period. In addition, as a general rule, the drugs selected for prophylaxis should have the following characteristics: They should be relatively inexpensive and easy to administer. They should have fairly broad coverage against most, but not necessarily all, of the bacteria likely to be encountered in the operative site. They also should be drugs that are not ordinarily used for treatment of an established infection (Ledger and colleagues, 1975).

Three clinical criteria should be fulfilled to justify the use of prophylactic antibiotics. First, the procedure must be performed through a contaminated operative field. Second, in the absence of prophylaxis, the incidence of postoperative infection should be unacceptably high, usually above 15–20 percent. Third, patients who develop primary infections of the operative site should be at risk for potentially serious complications such as abdominal or pelvic abscess, septic pelvic vein thrombophlebitis, or septic shock (Duff, 1987).

MECHANISM OF ACTION OF PROPHYLACTIC ANTIBIOTICS

Prophylactic antibiotics exert their effect in several ways. By destroying some bacteria and slowing the growth of others, they reduce the size of the bacterial inoculum present at the surgical site. Antibiotics alter the characteristics of the serosanguinous fluid that collects in or near the operative site and make this medium less suitable to support the growth of pathogenic microorganisms. When administered in prophylactic doses, antibiotics also interfere with production of bacterial proteases and impair the attachment of bacteria to the mucosal surfaces of the genital tract. Finally, when absorbed and concentrated within white blood cells, antibiotics enhance the host's endogenous phagocytic capacity (Duff, 1987; Kaiser, 1986).

The landmark studies of Burke (1961, 1973) have demonstrated that the timing of antibiotic delivery to injured tissue is of critical importance in determining the overall effect of prophylaxis. The optimal therapeutic effect occurs when antibiotics are administered to the patient just before, or coincident with, the start of surgery, when maximal bacterial contamination and tissue trauma occur.

OBJECTIVES OF PROPHYLAXIS

The first objective of prophylaxis is to reduce the frequency of infection of the operative site, that is, metritis after cesarean delivery or abortion, chorioamnionitis after cerclage, and deep perineal infection after repair of a disrupted episiotomy. A second objective is to reduce the frequency of abdominal wound infection after procedures such as cesarean delivery. Wound infections are even more likely than endometritis to cause serious morbidity and thereby increase the duration and expense of hospitalization. The third objective of prophylaxis is to reduce the risk of the rare, life-threatening complications of operative site infection (Duff, 1987).

RESULTS OF CLINICAL TRIALS OF PROPHYLAXIS

Cesarean Delivery

To date, more than 25 prospective, randomized, placebo-controlled trials of systemic prophylaxis for cesarean delivery have been published. The results of these investigations have been consistently impressive and may be summarized as follows:

Essentially without exception, all studies have shown that prophylaxis decreases the frequency of metritis in women having unscheduled cesarean after an extended duration of labor and ruptured membranes. In most investigations, the rate of postcesarean metritis has been reduced by 50–60 percent (Duff 1987; Cartwright and colleagues, 1984; Swartz and Grolle, 1981).

The benefit of prophylaxis is less profound in women having scheduled cesarean delivery.

In patient populations where the baseline incidence of infection approaches 10 percent after even low-risk procedures, prophylaxis usually will be cost effective (Duff and co-workers, 1982b). If the baseline risk of infection is less than 5 percent, prophylaxis probably should be withheld, and antibiotic administration should be limited to patients who have evidence of overt infection.

The drugs most frequently used for prophylaxis have been the cephalosporins. Although the newer, extended spectrum cephalosporins have also been used for prophylaxis, there is no convincing evidence that these agents are superior to a first-generation drug such as cefazolin. In fact, the broader spectrum cephalosporins are considerably more expensive, and their injudicious use for prophylaxis may ultimately limit their usefulness as single agents for the treatment of an established infection (Duff, 1987; Carlson and Duff, 1990; Stiver and associates, 1983; Duff and colleagues, 1987).

Most investigators have used three doses of antibiotics for prophylaxis. However, several recent reports have been published demonstrating that a single dose of drug is comparable in efficacy to multidose regimens and offers a distinct cost savings (Gonik, 1985; McGregor, 1986; Padilla, 1983; and their colleagues). Accordingly, multiple doses appear to be warranted only if surgery is unduly prolonged or the patient is at exceptionally high risk of infection (Duff, 1987).

Several investigators have tried to determine if selected patients would benefit from "extended early treatment" rather than simple prophylaxis. Their efforts have been based on the premise that some high-risk patients may be so heavily colonized with bacteria at the time of cesarean that they approach a 100 percent probability of becoming infected despite prophylaxis. Unfortunately, there are no laboratory or clinical criteria that are sufficiently reliable in identifying patients as prophylaxis "successes" vs "failures" (Elliott and associates, 1982; D'Angelo and Sokol, 1980). Accordingly, until a simple test with high sensitivity and predictive value is available, extended prophylactic or early treatment regimens cannot be recommended.

For most operative procedures, antibiotic prophylaxis should be administered immediately prior to surgery. However, in women having cesarean delivery, delay in administration of drug until after the umbilical cord is clamped does not compromise the efficacy of prophylaxis and avoids exposure of the fetus to antibiotics prior to delivery (Duff, 1987; Gordon and associates, 1979).

In the majority of investigations, antibiotic prophylaxis has not significantly reduced the frequency of postoperative wound and urinary tract infections. Investigators who have been able to document beneficial effects have usually been caring for patients with a relatively high baseline frequency of infection (Swartz and Grolle, 1981).

Several investigators have studied the effect of topical antibiotics as prophylaxis against postcesarean infection. In general, topical antibiotics have been administered by irrigating the lower uterine segment, uterine incision, peritoneal cavity, and abdominal wound at appropriate intervals during surgery. Irrigation exerts its primary effect by providing a high concentration of antibiotic directly to the site of injured tissue. Systemic absorption of the antibiotic occurs, however, especially when both intrauterine and intraperitoneal irrigation is performed (Duff and colleagues, 1982a).

Unlike systemic prophylaxis, not all antibiotics have been equally effective when administered by irrigation. Observed differences in treatment effect appear to be due to differences in irrigation technique and pharmacokinetic properties of individual antibiotics. Moreover, although irrigation is effective, it offers no therapeutic or economic advantage over systemic administration of the same antibiotic. In addition, the use of irrigation in conjunction with systemic antibiotics does not enhance the efficacy of prophylaxis. Therefore, combining the two modalities is not justified (Swarz and Grolle, 1981; Elliott and Flaherty, 1986).

No randomized controlled trials of antibiotic prophylaxis in women having cesarean hysterectomy have been published. However, the frequency of pelvic infection after this procedure is similar to that after simple cesarean delivery. Accordingly, antibiotic prophylaxis is indicated when cesarean hysterectomy is performed, particularly on an emergency basis.

To date, serious maternal side effects of antibiotic prophylaxis have been exceedingly uncommon. Alterations in the vaginal flora clearly occur after prophylaxis. In particular, women who develop metritis despite receiving prophylaxis are at increased risk for having enterococcal infections (Carlson and Duff, 1990; Gibbs and colleagues, 1981). In addition, a small number of women who receive prophylaxis have developed antibiotic-associated diarrhea and, in isolated instances, pseudomembranous enterocolitis (Arsura and coworkers, 1985). Fortunately, these complications have not been refractory to conventional therapy. These observations underline the importance of restricting the administration of antibiotics to those patients who clearly benefit from prophylaxis and limiting the number of infusions to a maximum of one to three doses. Table 38–1 summarizes current recommendations for the use of prophylactic antibiotics in women having cesarean delivery.

TABLE 38–1. RECOMMENDATIONS FOR ANTIBIOTIC PROPHYLAXIS IN WOMEN HAVING CESAREAN DELIVERY

- Administer prophylaxis to all women having unscheduled cesarean delivery or cesarean hysterectomy.
- Consider use of prophylaxis for scheduled cesarean delivery in populations where the baseline frequency of postoperative infection is greater than 10%.
- Use a limited spectrum cephalosporin such as cefazolin (1–2 gs) or ampicillin (2 gs) for prophylaxis. Cefazolin provides better coverage against staphylococci and is preferable to ampicillin in patients at high risk of wound infection.
- Avoid use of the extended spectrum cephalosporins and penicillins for prophylaxis.
- As a general rule, limit prophylaxis to one dose, administered immediately after the infant's umbilical cord is clamped. In certain indigent patient populations, and in selected instances where surgery is prolonged, administration of two additional doses of antibiotic, 4–6 and 8–12 hours after the first dose, may enhance the effect of prophylaxis.
- In patients who have an immediate hypersensitivity reaction to beta-lactam antibiotics, two options are possible. The first is to refrain from administering antibiotics unless the patient becomes infected. The second is to administer a drug such as metronidazole (500 mg × one dose) or a combination of clindamycin (900 mg × one dose) and gentamicin (1.5 mg/kg × one dose).
- When prophylactic antibiotics are routinely used on an obstetric service, maintain appropriate surveillance for resistant microorganisms and superinfections.

Pregnancy Termination Procedures

The frequency of endometritis after first-trimester suction curettage is approximately 1 percent. The rate of infection is higher after second-trimester procedures, ranging from 5 to 10 percent in most investigations (Grimes and associates, 1984). Aside from gestational age at the time of surgery, the principal risk factors for postabortal infection are prior history of pelvic inflammatory disease and presence of a sexually transmitted disease such as gonorrhea, chlamydia, or bacterial vaginosis at the time of the surgical procedure (Grimes, 1984; Sonne-Holm, 1981; Darj, 1987; and their colleagues).

The scientific literature concerning antibiotic prophylaxis for abortion is confusing for the following reasons: First, several antibiotics have been used in clinical trials, and they vary somewhat in their pharmacokinetic properties. Second, definitions of postoperative morbidity used by clinical investigators have not been consistent. Third, some authors have failed to control for confounding variables that may have influenced the rate of infection. Fourth, many studies have had relatively small sample sizes and thus have lacked adequate statistical power to identify clinically significant differences in treatment outcome. Fifth, and perhaps most important, not all authors have used antibiotics in a truly prophylactic manner. Some investigators continued antibiotics for 48–96 hours and thus may have provided actual treatment rather than simple prophylaxis.

With these caveats in mind, the outcome of published clinical trials may be summarized as follows. As a general rule, antibiotic prophylaxis is of value in decreasing the frequency of postabortal pelvic infection by approximately 50–70 percent (Grimes and colleagues, 1984). The benefit of prophylaxis has been most convincingly established for women having first-trimester suction curettage and second-trimester intraamnionic instillation procedures (Darj, 1987; Spence, 1982; and their colleagues). Although extensive data are lacking, since second-trimester dilation and evacuation (D&E) procedures are so similar to suction curettage procedures, prophylaxis also should be of value in women choosing this method of abortion. There is insufficient information regarding the value of prophylaxis in women having abortions with RU486 or intravaginal prostaglandins to justify the routine use of antibiotics for these procedures.

The greatest reduction in the risk of infection will usually be in women with a prior history of pelvic inflammatory disease (Grimes and colleagues, 1984). Women who are known to have a sexually transmitted disease at the time of surgery are candidates for full therapeutic courses of antibiotics rather than simple prophylaxis.

Several antibiotics, including tetracycline, doxycycline, metronidazole, tinidazole, cephalothin, and penicillin and its derivatives, have proven to be effective when administered for prophylaxis (Grimes and colleagues, 1984). Of these, tetracycline and doxycycline have been the most extensively tested. Doxycycline has particular utility in this clinical situation because of its relatively low cost, ease of administration, and extended duration of action. It can be given in a single oral dose of 100–200 mg at bedtime on the evening prior to surgery.

If other drugs with shorter durations of action are selected for prophylaxis in first-trimester abortions, a single dose of drug administered just prior to surgery should still be effective for prophylaxis unless the procedure is unduly prolonged. In that case, a second dose of antibiotic should be administered 4–6 hours after the first. For second-trimester instillation procedures, up to three doses of antibiotic may be administered at 4–6 hour intervals during the patient's labor.

CERVICAL CERCLAGE

Firm recommendations regarding use of antibiotics in patients having cervical cerclage are difficult to make for several reasons. There essentially are no prospective, randomized controlled trials of prophylaxis. Many published reports describing use of antibiotics include relatively small numbers of patients and do not consistently distinguish between emergency and scheduled cerclage procedures. Moreover, in virtually every study where antibiotics have been administered, the drugs were given for extended periods of time, usually 5–7 days, rather than prophylactically.

With these caveats in mind, the following two conclusions appear to be warranted. First, in patients having a scheduled cerclage prior to 18 weeks' gestation and before cervical dilation has occurred, the risk of chorioamnionitis as a result of the procedure is very low, 2–5 percent (Harger, 1980; Thomason, 1982; Schwartz, 1984; and their associates). In this situation, prophylactic antibiotics are not justified. However, therapeutic antibiotics are indicated if the patient has a lower genital tract infection due to gonorrhea, chlamydia, group B streptococci, or bacterial vaginosis.

Second, in patients having an emergency cerclage for a partially dilated cervix, especially beyond 18–20 weeks of gestation, the risk of chorioamnionitis subsequent to surgery is much higher. Presumably, infection is primarily due to contact between prolapsed membranes and the multiple pathogens present in the vagina. Charles and Edwards (1981) noted that 10 of 69 patients (14.5%) who had a cerclage between 14 and 18 weeks' gestation developed chorioamnionitis compared to 18 of 46 (39.1%) who had surgery between 19 and 26 weeks ($p < .01$). Similarly, Treadwell and co-workers (1991) observed a significant increase in the risk of postoperative chorioamnionitis in patients having emergent versus elective surgery (12.7% vs 4.7%, $p < .005$) and in patients with cervical dilation >2 cm versus ≤2 cm (5.7% vs 41.7%, $p < .005$).

In an excellent review, Romero and associates (1992) also confirmed the increased prevalence of intraamnionic infection in patients with an incompetent cervix and advanced cervical dilation. They performed amniocentesis in 33 patients between 14 and 24 weeks' gestation who had intact membranes and cervical dilation ≥2 cm. Seventeen patients (51.5%) had positive amnionic fluid cultures. All patients with positive cultures aborted or had rupture of membranes or clinical chorioamnionitis.

The reports discussed above certainly raise the question of whether antibiotic therapy may be of value in patients undergoing emergency cerclage for a partially dilated cervix. Several investigators have employed broad-spectrum antibiotic treatment in conjunction with emergency cerclage and described successful clinical outcomes. Regrettably, the use of antibiotics in these reports, was, in general, not systematically defined.

In nine patients who had cervical dilation of 3–4 cm, Goodlin (1979) performed an amniocentesis to reduce amnionic fluid volume and then instilled 1 g of ampicillin into the amniotic cavity. The patients then had a Wurm procedure. Four of the nine carried their pregnancies to term; the other five aborted within 48 hours of the amniocentesis.

Olatunbosun and Dyck (1981) performed emergency cerclages in 12 women who had cervical effacement of at least 50 percent, dilation of at least 4 cm, and hourglassing membranes. The membranes were reduced by gentle pressure, and both circumferential and vertical sutures were placed to close the cervical os. In addition to tocolytics, patients received ampicillin for 5 days, but the dose and method of administration of the antibiotic were not specified. Ten of the 12 women had liveborn infants that survived. Scheerer and co-workers (1989) operated on four women at 21–23 weeks' gestation who had cervical dilation of 3–5 cm and prolapsed membranes. Patients received antibiotics for 3 days, but, again, the names and doses of the antibiotics were not specified.

Based on the previously cited data regarding the increased prevalence of infection in women undergoing emergency cerclage, the following plan of management appears to be prudent. If a patient has clinical evidence of chorioamnionitis, cerclage is contraindicated and the patient should be delivered. If the patient is asymptomatic but cervical dilation is ≥2 cm, an amniocentesis for Gram stain, culture, and glucose determination can be considered. If the Gram stain is positive or the amnionic fluid glucose concentration is decreased (< 15 mg%), subclinical infection should be suspected, and delivery should be considered. If there is no evidence of subclinical infection, cerclage may be performed. A broad-spectrum antibiotic, active against both aerobes and anaerobes, should be administered for 3–5 days until the patient is clearly stable. In addition, cultures of the lower genital tract also should be performed. If a specific pathogen such as *N. gonorrhoeae* or *C. trachomatis* is identified, antibiotic selection and duration of therapy should be modified to be certain that the lower tract infection is eradicated.

REPAIR OF EPISIOTOMY DEHISCENCE

The traditional approach to repair of an episiotomy dehiscence has been delay in surgical intervention until 2–6 months postpartum. The avowed purpose of this extended delay was to allow all signs of infection to resolve and permit onset of spontaneous healing. Unfortunately, this conservative plan of management often has produced considerable debilitation, frustration, and even anger on the part of the patient. Accordingly, within recent years, several investigators have advocated earlier surgical intervention as a means of reducing the patient's anxiety and morbidity (see Chap. 7).

In all of the recent clinical trials, investigators have administered broad-spectrum antibiotics in conjunction with surgical repair of the episiotomy dehiscence. These drugs have consistently been given for extended periods of time postoperatively rather than simply in the immediate perioperative period. Accordingly, antibiotic administration should more precisely be characterized as therapeutic rather than prophylactic. These studies include relatively small numbers of patients, and, with one exception, they have not included a placebo control group.

The success rate of early closure of episiotomy dehiscence under cover of antibiotics has been quite impressive. For example, Hauth and colleagues (1986) initially described their approach to eight women with fourth degree lacerations that dehisced in the immediate puerperium. All women received a mechanical bowel preparation and a 7-day course of broad-spectrum antibiotics. The exact drug regimens were not specified. Seven of the eight women had successful repairs; the eighth developed a small rectovaginal fistula. These authors subsequently expanded their series to include 31 women with episiotomy dehiscences following a fourth degree laceration (22), third degree laceration (4), or mediolateral incision (5). Twenty-nine women had successful repairs; two formed fistulae (Hankins and co-workers, 1990).

Monberg and Hammen (1987) were the only authors to compare two different methods of dehiscence repair. Their study group included 35 women with infected or "ruptured" episiotomies. Twenty women had early surgical repair and received clindamycin orally for 5 days. In 15 women, the episiotomy wound was cleansed with a topical antiseptic and then allowed to heal spontaneously. Women in the former group had shorter durations of hospitalization, fewer return appointments as an outpatient, and a more rapid return of coital function.

Finally, Ramin and co-workers (1992) reported the results of early surgical repair in

34 patients with dehiscences due to infection of the episiotomy site. All but one patient received intravenous antibiotics in the "perioperative and postoperative periods." The name and dose of the drugs and exact duration of administration were not specified in the report. Thirty-two of the patients (94%) had successful repairs. Two experienced another dehiscence, and their wounds were allowed to heal by secondary intention.

On the basis of these published reports, the following conclusions seem appropriate: Early surgical repair of an episiotomy dehiscence virtually always must be performed through an infected field. In fact, infection of the episiotomy site is the principal cause of the dehiscence. Accordingly, administration of broad-spectrum antibiotics with activity against the polymicrobial pelvic flora is justified. In this clinical setting, the drugs should be administered as therapy for an established infection rather than as prophylaxis. Parenteral antibiotics should be started prior to surgery and continued until the patient is clinically stable. Thereafter, oral antibiotics may be administered until the patient is completely afebrile and the surgical wound is well approximated and free of obvious infection. Table 38–2 lists several parenteral and oral regimens that are suitable for treatment of episiotomy infections.

TABLE 38–2. SELECTED ANTIBIOTICS OF VALUE IN TREATMENT OF EPISIOTOMY-SITE INFECTIONS

Drug	Dose
Parenteral	
Timentin-clavulanic acid	3.1 g Q6h
Ampicillin-sulbactam	3 g Q6h
Cefotaxime	2 g Q8-12h
Cefotetan	2 g Q12h
Cefoxitin	2 g Q6h
Ceftizoxime	2 g Q12h
Imipenem-cilastatin	500 mg Q6h
Clindamycin plus	900 mg Q8h
gentamicin	1.5 mg/kg Q8h
Metronidazole plus	500 mg Q6h
penicillin plus	5 million units Q6h
gentamicin	1.5 mg/kg Q8h
Oral	
Amoxicillin-clavulanic acid	500 mg Q8h

SUMMARY

Prophylactic antibiotics for surgery are indicated when a procedure must be performed through a contaminated operative field and, accordingly, the risk of postoperative infection is unacceptably high. In obstetrics, unscheduled cesarean delivery, suction curettage, and dilation and evacuation are the procedures that most clearly warrant prophylaxis. Drugs selected for prophylaxis should provide reasonable coverage against the broad range of pelvic pathogens, but they should not be first-line agents for treatment of established infections. They should be relatively nontoxic, inexpensive, and easy to administer. Their use should be restricted to one to three doses in the immediate perioperative period. When prophylaxis is used routinely on an obstetric service, surveillance must be maintained to detect the emergence of drug-resistant organisms.

REFERENCES

Arsura EL, Fazio RA, Wickremesinghe PC. Pseudomembranous colitis following prophylactic antibiotic use in primary cesarean section. Am J Obstet Gynecol 1985; 151:87.

Burke JF. The effective period of preventive antibiotic action in experimental incisions and dermal lesions. Surgery 1961; 50:161.

Burke JF. Preventive antibiotic management in surgery. Ann Rev Med 1973; 24:289.

Carlson C, Duff P. Antibiotic prophylaxis for cesarean delivery: Is an extended-spectrum agent necessary? Obstet Gynecol 1990; 76:343.

Cartwright PS, Pittaway DE, Jones HW, Entman SS. The use of prophylactic antibiotics in obstetrics and gynecology. A review. Obstet Gynecol Surv 1984; 39:537.

Charles D, Edwards WR. Infectious complications of cervical cerclage. Am J Obstet Gynecol 1981; 141:1065.

D'Angelo LJ, Sokol RJ. Short- versus long-course prophylactic antibiotic treatment in cesarean section. Obstet Gynecol 1980; 55:583.

Darj E, Stralin EB, Nilsson S. The prophylactic effect of doxycycline on postoperative infection rate after first-trimester abortion. Obstet Gynecol 1987; 70:755.

Duff P. Pathophysiology and management of postcesarean endometritis. Obstet Gynecol 1986; 67:269.

Duff P. Prophylactic antibiotics for cesarean delivery: a simple cost-effective strategy for prevention of postoperative morbidity. Am J Obstet Gynecol 1987; 157:794.

Duff P, Park RC. Antibiotic prophylaxis in vaginal hysterectomy: a review. Obstet Gynecol 1980; 55:193S.

Duff P, Gibbs RS, Jorgensen JH, Alexander G. The pharmacokinetics of prophylactic antibiotics administered by intraoperative irrigation at the time of cesarean section. Obstet Gynecol 1982a; 60:409.

Duff P, Smith PN, Keiser JF. Antibiotic prophylaxis in low-risk cesarean section. J Reprod Med 1982b; 27:133.

Duff P, Robertson AW, Read JA. Single-dose cefazolin versus cefonicid for antibiotic prophylaxis in cesarean delivery. Obstet Gynecol 1987; 70:718.

Elliott JP, Flaherty JF. Comparison of lavage or intravenous antibiotics at cesarean section. Obstet Gynecol 1986; 67:29.

Elliott JP, Freeman RK, Dorchester W. Short versus long course of prophylactic antibiotics in cesarean section. Am J Obstet Gynecol 1982; 143:740.

Gibbs RS, St Clair PJ, Castillo MS, Castaneda YS. Bacteriologic effects of antibiotic prophylaxis in high-risk cesarean section. Obstet Gynecol 1981; 57:277.

Gonik B. Single versus three-dose cefotaxime prophylaxis for cesarean section. Obstet Gynecol 1985; 65:189.

Goodlin RC. Cervical incompetence, hourglass membranes, and amniocentesis. Obstet Gynecol 1979; 54:748.

Gordon HR, Phelps D, Blanchard K. Prophylactic cesarean section antibiotics: maternal and neonatal morbidity before or after cord clamping. Obstet Gynecol 1979; 53:151.

Grimes DA, Schulz KF, Cates W. Prophylactic antibiotics for curettage abortion. Am J Obstet Gynecol 1984; 150:689.

Hankins GDV, Hauth JC, Gilstrap LC, et al. Early repair of episiotomy dehiscence. Obstet Gynecol 1990; 75:48.

Harger JH. Comparison of success and morbidity in cervical cerclage procedures. Obstet Gynecol 1980; 56:543.

Hauth JC, Gilstrap LC, Ward SC, Harkins GDV. Early repair of an external sphincter ani muscle and rectal mucosal dehiscence. Obstet Gynecol 1986; 67:806.

Hawrylyshyn PA, Bernstein P, Papsin FR. Risk factors associated with infection following cesarean section. Am J Obstet Gynecol 1981; 139:294.

Kaiser AB. Antimicrobial prophylaxis in surgery. N Engl J Med 1986; 315:1129.

Ledger WJ, Gee C, Lewis WP. Guidelines for antibiotic prophylaxis in gynecology. Am J Obstet Gynecol 1975; 121:1038.

McGregor JA, French JI, Makowski E. Single-dose cefotetan versus multidose cefoxitin for prophylaxis in cesarean section in high-risk patients. Am J Obstet Gynecol 1986; 154:955.

Monberg J, Hammen S. Ruptured episiotomia resutured primarily. Acta Obstet Gynecol Scand 1987; 66:163.

Olatunbosun OA, Dyck F. Cervical cerclage operation for a dilated cervix. Obstet Gynecol 1981; 57:166.

Padilla SL, Spence MR, Beauchamp PJ. Single-dose ampicillin for cesarean section prophylaxis. Obstet Gynecol 1983; 61:463.

Ramin SM, Ramus RM, Little BB, Gilstrap LC. Early repair of episiotomy dehiscence associated with infection. Am J Obstet Gynecol 1992; 167:1104.

Romero R, Gonzalez R, Sepulveda W, et al. Infection and labor. VIII. Microbial invasion of the amniotic cavity in patients with suspected cervical incompetence: prevalence and clinical significance. Am J Obstet Gynecol 1992; 167:1086.

Scheerer LJ, Lam F, Bartolucci L, Katz M. A new technique for reduction of prolapsed fetal membranes for emergency cervical cerclage. Obstet Gynecol 1989; 74:408.

Schwartz RP, Chatwani A, Sullivan P. Cervical cerclage. A review of 74 cases. J Reprod Med 1984; 29:103.

Sonne-Holm S, Heisterberg L, Hebjorn S, et al. Prophylactic antibiotics in first-trimester abortions: a clinical controlled trial. Am J Obstet 1981; 139:693.

Spence MR, King TM, Burkman RT, Atienza MF. Cephalothin prophylaxis for midtrimester abortion. Obstet Gynecol 1982; 60:502.

Stiver HG, Forward KR, Livingstone RA, et al. Multicenter comparison of cefoxitin versus cefazolin for prevention of infectious morbidity after nonelective cesarean section. Am J Obstet Gynecol 1983; 45:158.

Swartz WH, Grolle K. The use of prophylactic antibiotics in cesarean section. A review of the literature. J Reprod Med 1981; 26:595.

Thomason JL, Sampson MB, Beckmann CR, Spellacy WN. The incompetent cervix. A 1982 update. J Reprod Med 1982; 27:187.

Treadwell MC, Bronsteen RA, Bottoms SF. Prognostic factors and complication rates for cervical cerclage: a review of 482 cases. Am J Obstet Gynecol 1991; 165:555.

CHAPTER 39

The Fetus as a Surgical Patient

The evaluation and treatment of the fetus should, under ideal circumstances have no more limitations than that of the newborn. In reality, however, the fetus is relatively inaccessible. The limitations posed by the intrauterine-intraamniotic location of the fetus are amplified by our relative lack of understanding of the factors responsible for the onset of normal and pathologic labor, and by concern for the intact preservation of the fetal membranes. Because intrusion into this protected environment can result in pregnancy loss, indirect or minimally invasive diagnostic and therapeutic approaches to the fetus have traditionally been preferred.

Despite these limitations, the prenatal diagnosis and surgical treatment of selected fetal anomalies has become a reality as a result of advances in ultrasound technology, reproductive genetics, and basic research using animal models (Harrison, 1982, 1983, 1990; Kleiner, 1987; Clark, 1987; Adzick, 1989; Thorup, 1985; Shalev, 1984; and their associates).

Several considerations are essential prior to contemplation of any form of invasive fetal procedure. First, the potential risks to the mother of any fetal procedure must be of paramount concern. Only those procedures that can be performed with minimal maternal risk warrant consideration. The risks to the fetus depend upon the likelihood that the condition will either disappear, remain stable, or worsen during the course of pregnancy. Given our limited diagnostic capabilities, and our finite knowledge regarding the natural history and prognosis of most pathologic fetal conditions, invasive therapy is generally restricted to fetuses with conditions likely to be fatal in the absence of in utero intervention. Thus, conditions such as mild pleural effusions or unilateral hydronephrosis are generally not treated in-utero, even though such therapy is technically possible.

There are several categories of invasive fetal procedures. Chapter 30 describes cordocentesis for diagnosis and therapy of fetal anemia. In this chapter we focus on ultrasound guided fetal shunt procedures, open fetal surgery and endoscopic approaches to fetal therapy.

FETAL SHUNT PROCEDURES

The use of real-time sonography to guide placement of short plastic catheters into various fetal compartments is the most widespread form of fetal surgery. The goal of these procedures is to establish a shunt from an abnormal fluid-filled fetal compartment such as an obstructed fetal bladder or pulmonary cyst into the amniotic cavity. Such procedures have been used in the prenatal management of select cases of fetal hydrocephalus, hydronephrosis, hydrothorax and cystic adenomatoid malformation of the lung.

Fetal Hydrocephalus

The first procedure for the in-utero treatment of isolated fetal hydrocephalus involved serial needle aspiration of the enlarged lateral ventricles (Birnholtz and Frigaletto, 1981). Thereafter, the placement of valved shunts from lateral ventricle to amniotic cavity was introduced and carried out in several centers (Clewell and co-workers, 1982) (Fig. 39–1). The rationale for such treatment was based upon an extrapolation from newborn data indicating both improved survival and long-term neurologic outcome with aggressive and early neonatal shunting in infants with aquaductal stenosis (Elvidge, 1966; Lorber, 1969; Young and colleagues, 1973). Initial enthusiasm for this procedure waned, however, following the establishment of a National Fetal Surgery Registry and systematic analyses of newborn outcome in fetuses undergoing shunt procedures (Clewell, 1990). Although such shunting may improve overall survival to birth, a number of fetuses have died as a direct result of such surgery (Glick, 1984a; Chervenak, 1984; Clewell 1985a,b; and their associates). Of more concern, however, are data documenting long-term outcome in survivors of ventricular shunting procedures. In a recent analysis of data from the National Registry, 32 fetuses with presumed aquaductal stenosis who were shunted in-utero demonstrated an 87 percent survival rate, compared to 40 percent of 20 untreated fetuses in a separate combined series. However, only 38% of treated fetuses were felt to be neurologically normal at follow-up, compared to 30 percent of un-treated fetuses, a difference which is probably not significant (Manning, 1990).

Most importantly, with improvement in neonatal surgical approaches to ventriculomegaly, that group of infants who survive to birth without in utero treatment and are shunted *following* birth have a 75-80 percent survival rate, with over three-quarters of these children demonstrating no intellectual impairment (Elvidge, 1966; Lorber, 1969; Young and co-workers, 1973). Thus, it is possible that in utero shunting may result in survival of abnormal infants who would otherwise expire prior to birth. Because the outcome of infants treated following birth is generally good, and no criteria exist which would allow selection of those fetuses likely to benefit from in utero shunting, the value of ventriculoamniotic shunting is doubtful. This procedure is not presently being performed in the United States.

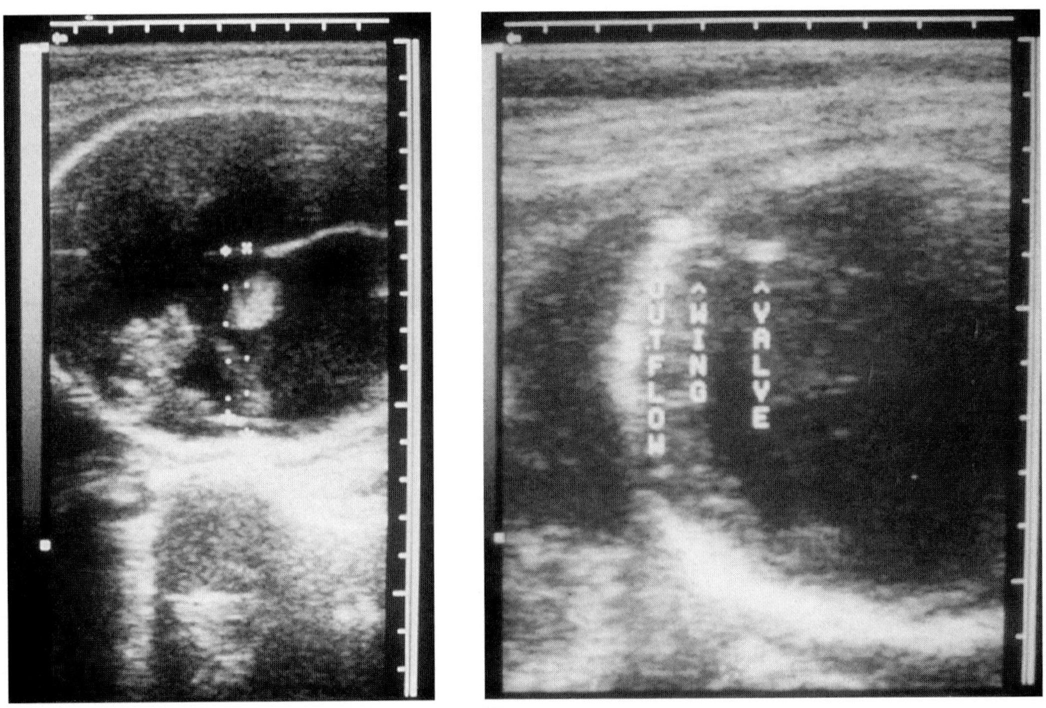

A B

Figure 39–1 A. Enlarged lateral fetal ventricles. **B.** Fetal scan following placement of an early valved shunt. (Courtesy of Lawrence D. Platt, MD)

Obstructive Uropathy

During fetal development, the urinary tract may be obstructed at any level, with varying degrees of resultant, pressure-induced renal injury. Experimental work in fetal sheep has demonstrated that prolonged, severe obstruction leads to hydronephrosis, renal fibrosis and, eventually, cystic dysplasia (Johnson and associates, 1994). In severe cases involving bilateral obstruction of renal outflow, residual renal function at birth may be insufficient to sustain life. Of equal concern is the fact that the fetal kidneys are the source of amniotic fluid beyond the early second trimester. Such fluid is essential to normal pulmonary development. Thus the prolonged oligohydramnios associated with bilateral obstructive uropathy commonly leads to fatal pulmonary hypoplasia, in addition to varying degrees of renal insufficiency (Harrison, 1983; Adzick, 1987; and their co-workers).

Although ureteropelvic junction obstruction is the most common etiology of fetal hydronephrosis, this condition is generally unilateral and thus is uncommonly associated with marked oligohydramnios. On the other hand, untreated posterior urethral valve syndrome, a condition confined almost exclusively to male fetuses, generally results in both permanent renal failure and severe oligohydramnios with secondary pulmonary hypoplasia (Fig. 39–2). Following a classic series of investigations into mechanisms of renal and pulmonary injury in obstructive uropathy and the effects of shunting procedures in the animal model, the concept of vesicoamniotic shunting was introduced in the treatment of human fetuses (Harrison, 1983; Kleiner, 1987; Thorup, 1985; Shalev, 1984; Adzick, 1984, 1987; Glick, 1983; and their colleagues). This technique has now become well-established as potentially beneficial in carefully selected patients with posterior urethral valve syndrome, or rarely, urethral atresia.

Patient Selection

Vesicoamniotic shunting procedures are generally restricted to fetuses with a sonographic diagnosis of urinary outlet obstruction meeting four criteria, (1) bilateral hydronephrosis, (2) megacystitis, (3) oligohydramnios, and (4) no additional anomalies detected by careful sonographic examination. Because oligohy-

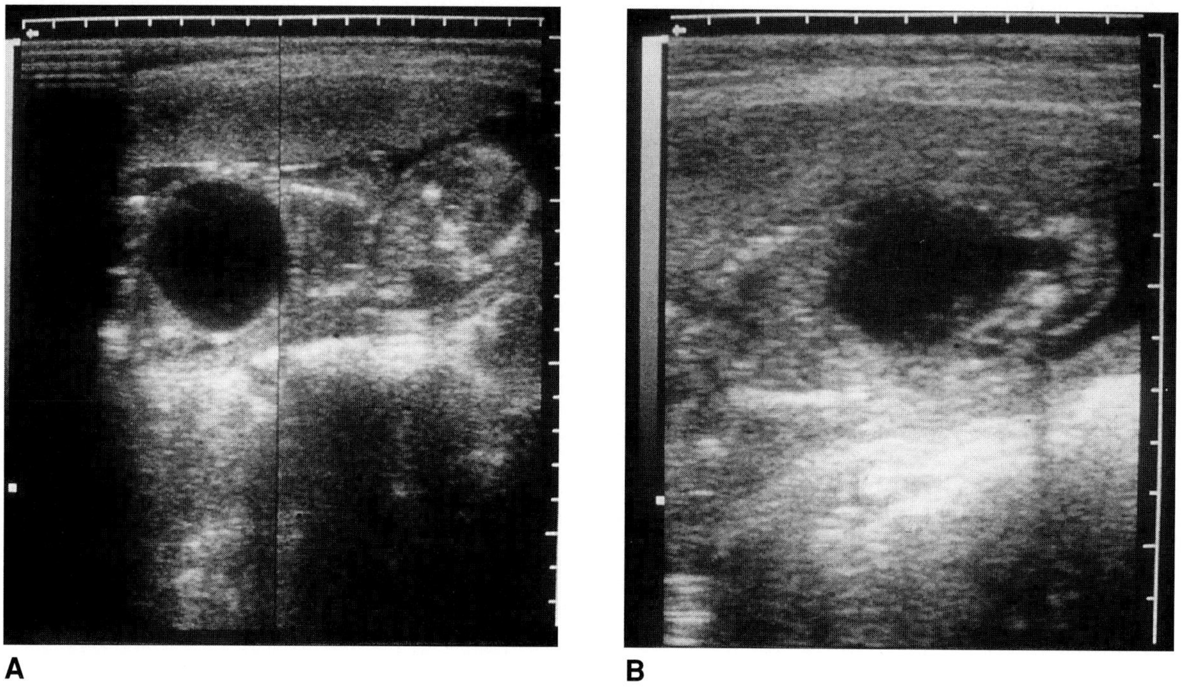

Figure 39–2 A. Fetus with posterior urethral valve syndrome demonstrating megacystitis. Marked bilateral hydronephrosis was also present. **B.** Enlarged image of fetal bladder, demonstrating dilated proximal urethra. (Courtesy of Lawrence D. Platt, MD)

dramnios often hampers precise sonographic fetal assessment, transabdominal saline amnioinfusion may be used to improve the precision of imaging (Haeusler, 1993; Gembruch, 1988; and their associates).

Initial series involving vesicoamniotic shunting of these fetuses yielded mixed results (Wilkins, 1987; Elder, 1990; Drugan, 1989; and their associates). Subsequent studies have focused upon refinement of selection criteria in an effort to identify those fetuses most likely to benefit from such procedures, and exclude those in whom renal failure is so far advanced as to render shunting of no value.

Most such investigations have focused upon analysis of urinary indices of fetal renal function, including sodium, calcium, creatinine, osmolality, total protein, and beta-2 microglobulin. Such analyses are obtained by ultrasound-guided fetal bladder aspiration (Nicolaides, 1992; Lipitz, 1993; Johnson, 1994; and their colleagues). It appears that a single analysis of fetal urine in these fetuses may be misleading; thus, most authorities presently advocate serial bladder aspiration in the preoperative work-up of fetuses with obstructive uropathy (Johnson and co-workers, 1994).

Once a fetus has been identified as meeting the above ultrasound criteria, serial urinalysis is performed. Johnson and associates proposed a series of at least 3 vesicocenteses performed at 48–72 hour intervals (Johnson and associates, 1994). Fetuses exhibiting criteria outlined in Table 39–1 are considered to be good candidates for vesicoamniotic shunting (Johnson and colleagues, 1994). These criteria are based upon the observation that with irreversible renal damage secondary to obstruction, renal tubular function is impaired, resulting in increased loss of sodium, calcium and various proteins into the urine (Nicolaides, 1992; Lipitz, 1993; Johnson, 1994; and their colleagues). Using these criteria, Johnson and co-workers (1994) reported a 100 percent success rate in predicting the absence of significant renal fibrosis or dysplasia. In a similar manner, Lipitz and associates (1993) reported that 100 percent of fetuses in whom elevated urinary levels of sodium and calcium were present showed histologic renal dysplasia on postmortem examination.

TABLE 39–1. FETAL VESICOCENTESIS—GOOD PROGNOSTIC FINDINGS

Urine sodium	< 100 mg/dL
Urine calcium	< 8 mg/dL
Urine osmolality	< 200 mOsm/L
Beta-2 microglobulin	< 4 mg/L
Total protein	< 20 mg/dL
Decreasing values of above indices on serial examination	

Shunting Procedure

The technique of vesicoamniotic shunting is presented as a prototype of current fetal shunting procedures. Minor variations allow this technique to be applied to other indications.

Initially, the patient is brought to the procedure room. Fetal position is confirmed. Because the anterior or anterolateral abdominal wall of the fetus will be entered, a spine-anterior fetal position precludes shunt placement. If the fetus is found to be in a favorable position, the patient is prepped and draped in a sterile manner. Some authorities recommend fetal paralysis using neuromuscular blocking agents (De Crispigny and associates, 1985). However, such paralysis is not always necessary, and the procedure may have to be abandoned if a fetus in an initially favorable presentation changes position before the paralysis takes effect.

In cases of severe oligohydramnios, shunt placement may be facilitated by the instillation of warmed saline within the uterus, thereby creating an artificial fluid pocket between the maternal uterine wall and the fetus.

The apparatus for vesicoamniotic shunting is described in Fig. 39–3. A similar device is available commercially (Rodeck double pigtail shunt, Rocket of London, Watford, UK), although it has not been approved by the FDA and remains investigational. Shunting may be carried out under local or conduction anesthesia depending upon maternal tolerance.

A small incision is made into the maternal anterior abdominal wall and the needle/shunt apparatus is directed under continuous ultrasound guidance through the maternal tissues into the neoamniotic cavity. The needle is then rapidly advanced through the anterior abdominal wall of the fetus into the distended bladder. Using the "pusher" tube apparatus, the distal end of the pigtail shunt is advanced off the end of the needle into the bladder. As the needle is withdrawn, the proximal end of the shunt coils within the amniotic cavity, thus

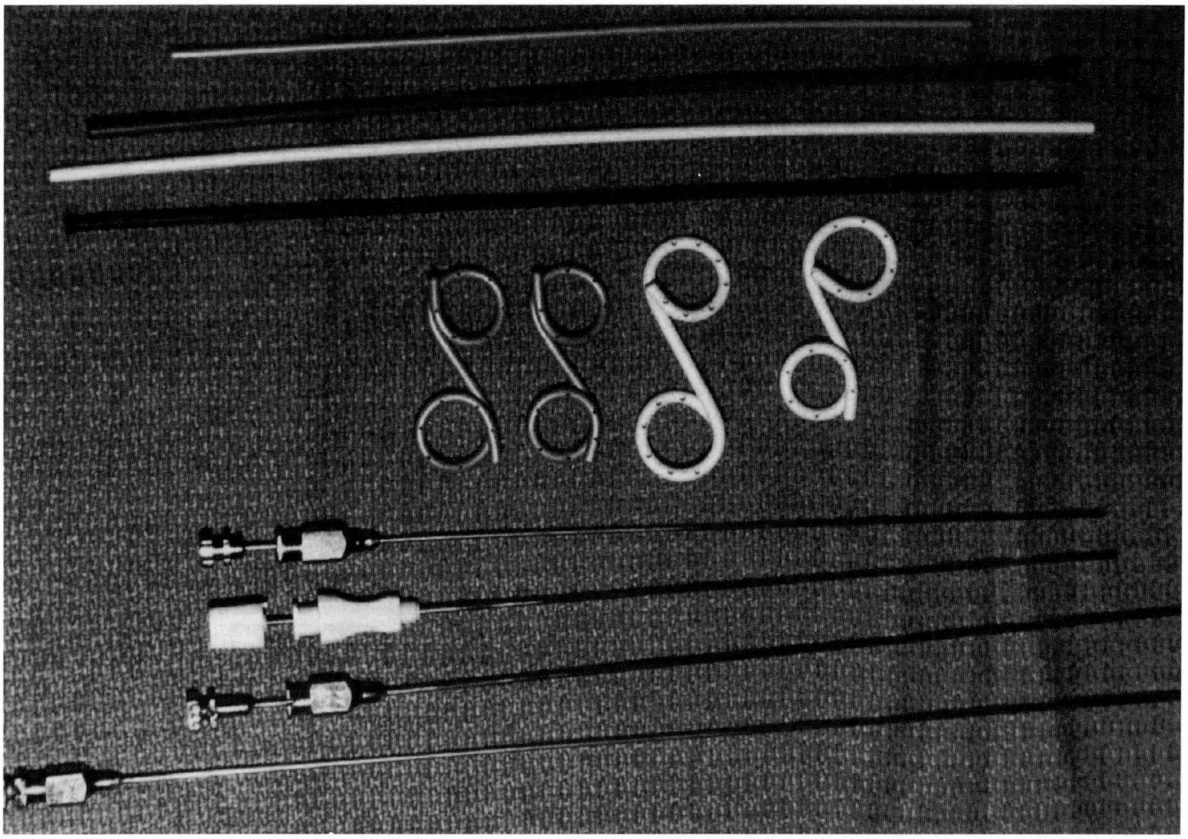

A

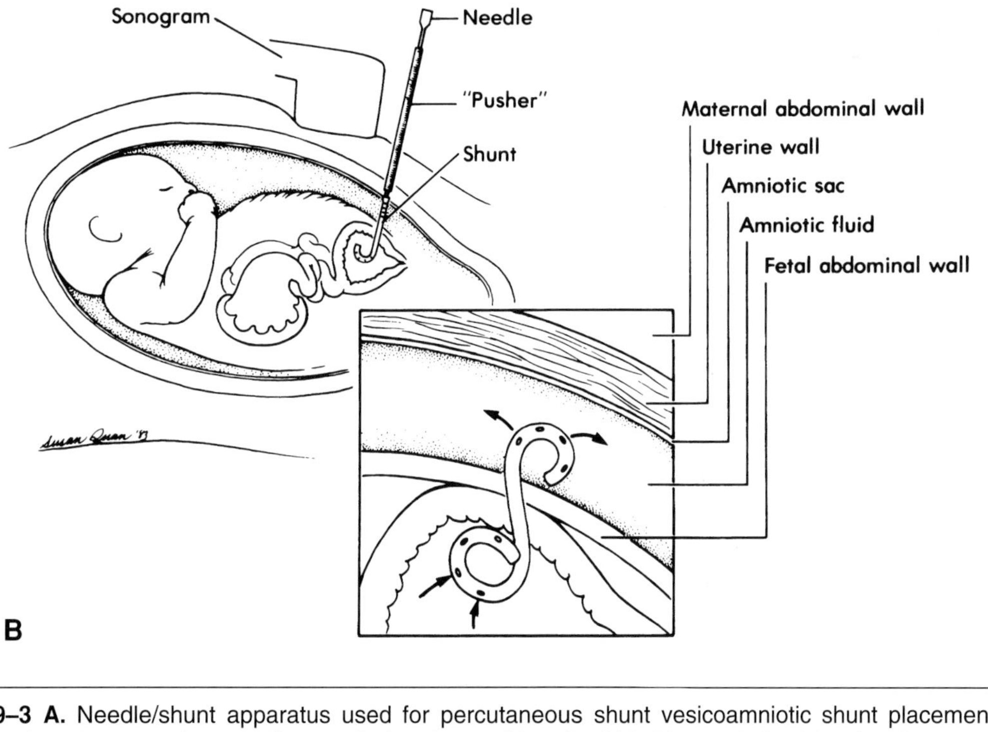

B

Figure 39–3 A. Needle/shunt apparatus used for percutaneous shunt vesicoamniotic shunt placement. Pigtail catheter is placed over trochar needle, needle is advanced into fetal bladder, and distal tip of catheter is then displaced with "pusher" tubing. **B.** Schematic diagram showing details of shunt placement. (Reproduced with permission from Harrison MR, Golbus MS, Filly RA (eds): *The Unborn Patient* 2nd ed., WB Saunders Company, Philadelphia, 1990) establishing a vesicoamniotic pathway for egress of urine (Fig. 39–3). Prophylactic antibiotics may be administered, although no evidence exists to demonstrate their value. Depending upon the gestational age of the fetus, prophylactic administration of tocolytic agents may also be elected. After a period of observation, the patient is discharged to careful follow-up.

Complications

Maternal complications are rare. Amnionitis is occasionally seen and mandates delivery. Preterm contractions are generally responsive to standard tocolytic therapy. Shunt blockage by vernix or other fetal debris is common and may necessitate shunt replacement. The shunt may also become dislodged from the fetal bladder, necessitating replacement. If the distal end of the shunt becomes internalized within the body of the fetus, a vesicoperitoneal passage may be created, giving rise to urinary ascites. This complication may be dealt with by placement of a secondary peritoneal-amniotic shunt.

Following discharge, the fetus is followed carefully for continued shunt function, and the mother is observed for evidence of infection or labor. Delivery is ideally delayed until term. Cesarean section is reserved for standard obstetric indications.

Results

Shunt placement has been performed as early as 14.5 weeks' gestation, with most shunts being performed in the late second trimester (Johnson and co-workers, 1994). Renal function appears to be better in those fetuses shunted prior to 19 weeks, compared to later shunt placement.

Roughly half of fetuses evaluated for possible shunt placement will be candidates for a shunt procedure, in the other half, the identification of more extensive anomalies, or the desire of the mother for pregnancy termination, excluded the fetus from consideration (Johnson and associates, 1994).

In an initial analysis of the Fetal Surgery Registry, shunt placement was successful on the first attempt in only 10 percent of cases, with up to 7 attempts sometimes necessary for adequate placement (Manning, 1990). After successful placement, dislodgement occurs in 25–30 percent of fetuses, necessitating shunt replacement (Johnson and colleagues, 1994). Half of these cases involve fetal intraperitoneal shunt positioning and urinary ascites, treated by placement of a secondary peritoneal-amniotic shunt.

Procedure-related fetal mortality is 7 percent in the Registry data; however, in series from individual institutions with extensive experience in shunt placement mortality is rare (Manning, 1990a; Johnson and associates, 1994). Long-term neonatal survival of treated fetuses is generally reported in the range of 50 percent. Small series of fetuses with favorable preoperative renal function indices (Table 39–1) have demonstrated survival in the range of 70 percent, with mortality generally due to associated undetected anomalies and complications of premature birth. Survivors generally have normal or near normal renal function. Although mortality in poor-prognosis cases is not inevitable, the occasional survivor is very likely to suffer renal failure requiring dialysis or transplant.

A comparison of the results of treated fetuses with those of unmatched historical controls suggests a benefit in appropriately selected fetuses. However, neither randomized prospective trials nor retrospective case-control series are available. Therefore, while in utero shunting of urinary outflow tract obstruction is a well established procedure in maternal–fetal medicine, definitive claims regarding efficacy await the result of properly conducted trials.

Pulmonary Lesions

Congenital adenomatoid malformation (CAM) is a unilateral, hamartomatous lesion which may result in compression of normal lung tissue and pulmonary hypoplasia (Adzick and co-workers, 1985) (Fig. 39–4). In addition, this space occupying lesion may interfere with fetal cardiovascular function, resulting in hydrops and antenatal death. Clark and associates, using a procedure similar to that previously described for bladder outlet obstruction, initially demonstrated successful thoracic placement of a double pigtail shunt in a 22-week fetus with severe hydrops and macrocystic (type I) CAM (Clark and colleagues, 1987) (Fig. 39–4). Following shunt placement, the hydrops resolved and the fetus was born near term with normal long-term outcome. Since this initial description, other investigators have described similar procedures, with mixed outcome (Nico-

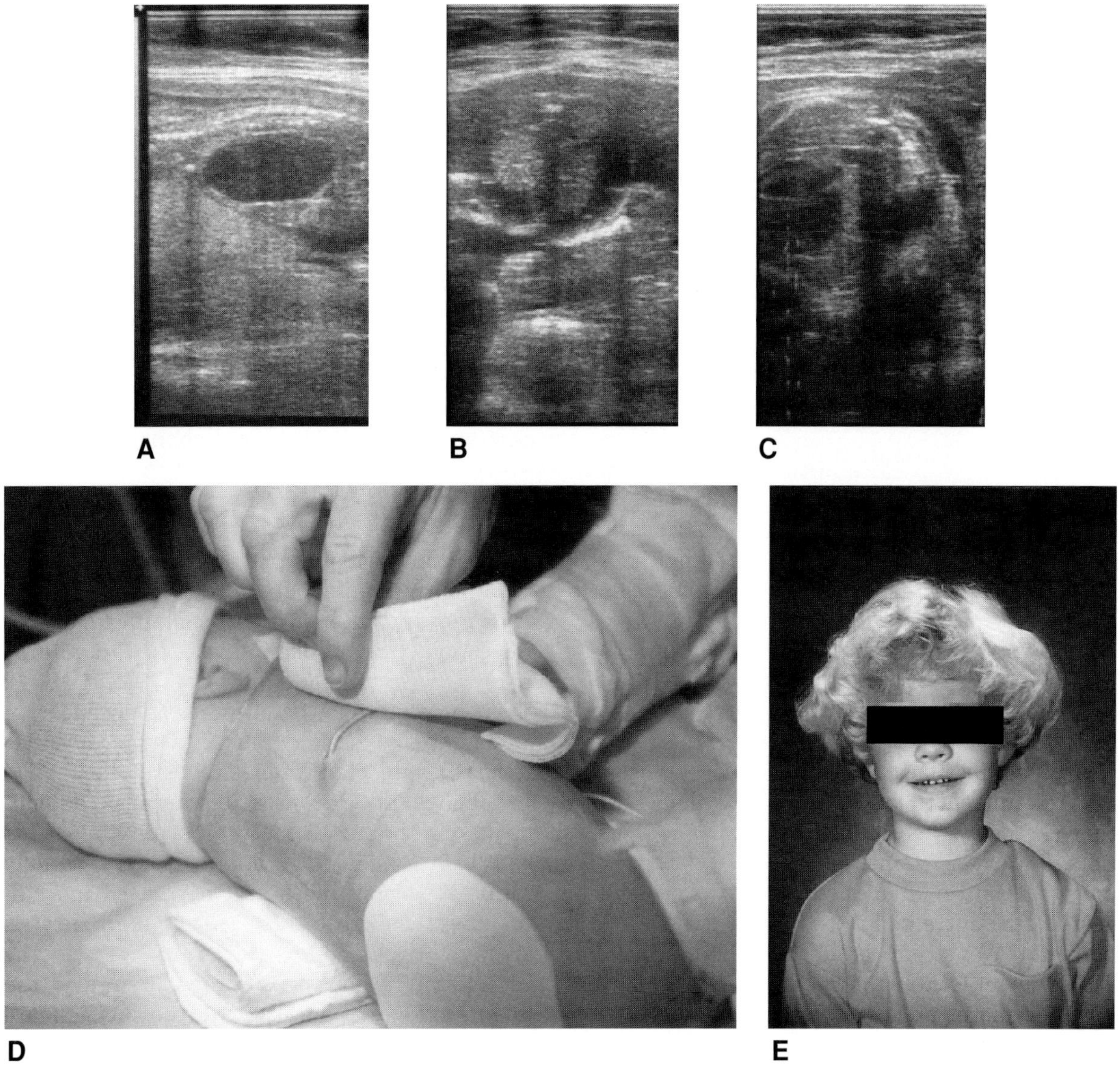

Figure 39–4 **A.** Cystic adenomatoid malformation (CAM) of the lung in a 22-week fetus. **B.** Gross ascites is demonstrated, secondary to vascular compression by the thoracic lesion. **C.** CAM has been decompressed following placement of a thoracoamniotic shunt. Shunt walls are seen. **D.** Infant at birth, demonstrating shunt location. **E.** Normal child, age 6.

laides, 1987; Kuller, 1992; and their associates). Repetitive cyst aspiration has also been described (Kuller, 1992; Nugent, 1989; Obwegeser, 1993; and their colleagues).

Similar procedures have been described for fetuses with pleural effusions (Mandelbrot and associates, 1992; Weber and Philipson, 1992). However, such effusions may be transient, and are often manifestations of more generalized pathologic processes. Thus, while they may be aspirated or permanently drained, indications for these invasive procedures are less well-established than for type I CAM with pulmonary compression or hydrops (Weber and Philipson, 1992).

OPEN FETAL SURGERY

Following extensive investigation in animal models, Harrison, Adzick, and associates introduced the concept of open surgery for human fetal malformations (Adzick, 1989; Harrison, 1990; and their co-workers). Their efforts were initially directed at prenatal management of diaphragmatic hernia, a lesion not amenable to treatment by simple shunt placement. This lesion results from failure of the pleuroperitoneal membrane to fuse by the eighth week of fetal life, thus allowing free communication between thoracic and abdominal cavities (Wenstrom and associates, 1991). Diaphragmatic hernia is not generally fatal during the prenatal period; however, overall neonatal mortality is 50–75 percent, primarily due to severe pulmonary hypoplasia from longstanding lung compression by abdominal organs (Wenstrom, 1991; Sharland, 1992; and their colleagues).

Harrison, Adzick, and co-workers demonstrated that it is possible to open the second-trimester human uterus, partially extract the fetus, replace bowel into the abdomen and close the diaphragmatic defect, while allowing the pregnancy to continue (Harrison and associates, 1990). Although theoretically impressive, clinical results have been disappointing, and long term survivors of this procedure are rare. Although initially justified on the basis of a presumed mortality rate of up to 95 percent in untreated patients, the rationale for this procedure has more recently been questioned after a systematic analysis of diaphragmatic hernia-related neonatal deaths suggested an untreated mortality closer to 50 percent (Wenstrom and co-workers, 1991). Thus, open fetal surgery for diaphragmatic hernia remains an investigational procedure.

Open fetal surgery for treatment of cystic adenomatoid malformation and bladder outlet obstruction has also been described, but in a similar manner remains investigational, with no evidence to suggest actual fetal benefit compared to more conservative approaches. However, in a hydropic fetus with microcystic CAM, such an open approach appears to be the only therapeutic option (Adzick and associates, 1993).

ENDOSCOPIC FETAL SURGERY

Historically, fetal endoscopy preceded the widespread use of ultrasound in fetal medicine. Originally described in 1954 in an isolated case report, the popularity of fetoscopy reached its apex in the late 1970s and early 1980s as a technique to visualize the fetus, and as a diagnostic aid in obtaining tissue samples or fetal blood (Westin, 1954). Despite its initial promise, fetoscopy was performed only in selected centers throughout the world and its limitations were quickly realized. With the development and widespread use of high resolution diagnostic sonography, ultrasound-guided invasive procedures quickly replaced fetoscopy in fetal diagnosis and therapy.

Beginning in 1980, an endoscopic revolution began to take place in medicine as a result of the advances made in fiberoptics and operating instrument technologies. The use of bipolar electrocoagulation, the addition of video imaging, and the development of endoscopic surgical instruments changed virtually every surgical specialty. These advances have been particularly prominent in general surgery, where the successful performance of laparoscopic cholecystectomy demonstrated that even complex operations could be performed endoscopically with significantly less morbidity than with the classic laparotomy approach (Southern Surgeons Club, 1991). Such progress has been more slowly incorporated into gynecologic surgery and continues to be the subject of intense investigation.

The same potential advantages demonstrated with endoscopic surgery in other fields can be extrapolated into fetal surgery, namely minimal invasiveness and decreased morbidity. Because in fetal surgery morbidity is strongly related to the response of the myometrium and membranes to injury, the advantages of a smaller uterine incision are especially important.

Animal Investigation

Potential applications and limitation of endoscopic fetal surgery have been demonstrated in several animal models. De Lia and associates first demonstrated the possibility of photocoagulating the placental surface vessels in a nonhuman primate model using YAG laser (De Lia and associates, 1989). This experience has been extrapolated to justify the use of YAG laser in the management of select pregnancies affected by twin–twin transfusion syndrome (De Lia, 1990; Ville, 1994; Quintero, 1994a; and their associates).

Estes and co-workers have examined the use of endoscopic techniques to repair cleft lip in the fetal lamb (Estes, 1992). Scarring of the lip incision was virtually unnoticeable at birth.

Endoscopic fetal cystotomies and laryngoscopies have also been described following the creation of animal models for posterior urethral valve syndrome and diaphragmatic hernia (Estes, 1992; Luks, 1994b,c; and their coworkers). In addition to the physiologic importance of these experiments, a number of technical concepts were introduced, including the use of balloon trochars, amniotic fluid exchange pumps, and small fetal monitoring devices. These experiments require the use of 5 mm instruments with 7 mm sheaths. The use of 2 mm instruments in a fluid medium has more recently been described by Quintero and colleagues and may facilitate the extrapolation of these animal experiments into clinical investigation (Quintero and associates, 1994b,c).

Technical Considerations

Entry into the amniotic cavity can be performed percutaneously, or through a small laparotomy. The percutaneous approach is less traumatic and can be performed as an outpatient procedure, provided that the size of the instruments is less than 3 mm. The use of a minilaparotomy, while increasing somewhat the maternal morbidity, eliminates the possibility of uncontrolled uterine bleeding or amniotic fluid leakage. In the technique described by De Lia, a 2–3 cm incision is made in the maternal abdomen (De Lia and coworkers, 1990). The trocar (3.5 mm) is introduced through the myometrium, and a purse string is tied around the entry site.

Currently available trocars for adult or pediatric laparoscopy are at least 5 mm in inner diameter (6-7 mm outer diameter). Similarly, most rigid endoscopes are equipped with thick protecting sheaths that keep them from bending. In order to facilitate work in fetuses 2–3 mm trocars have been developed in varying lengths that can be inserted percutaneously through a 1 mm skin incision (Quintero and associates, 1994c). A checkflow valve at the hub prevents amniotic fluid leakage. In addition, a plastic sidearm with a valve allows the infusion of saline or removal of amniotic fluid as desired (Fig. 39–5).

The Working Environment: Fluid or Gas

Laparoscopy uses gas as a distension medium. Fetoscopes that work within a gaseous as opposed to a liquid medium would have several advantages. First, the techniques used in laparo-scopy would be more easily translated into operative fetoscopy. Second, visualization

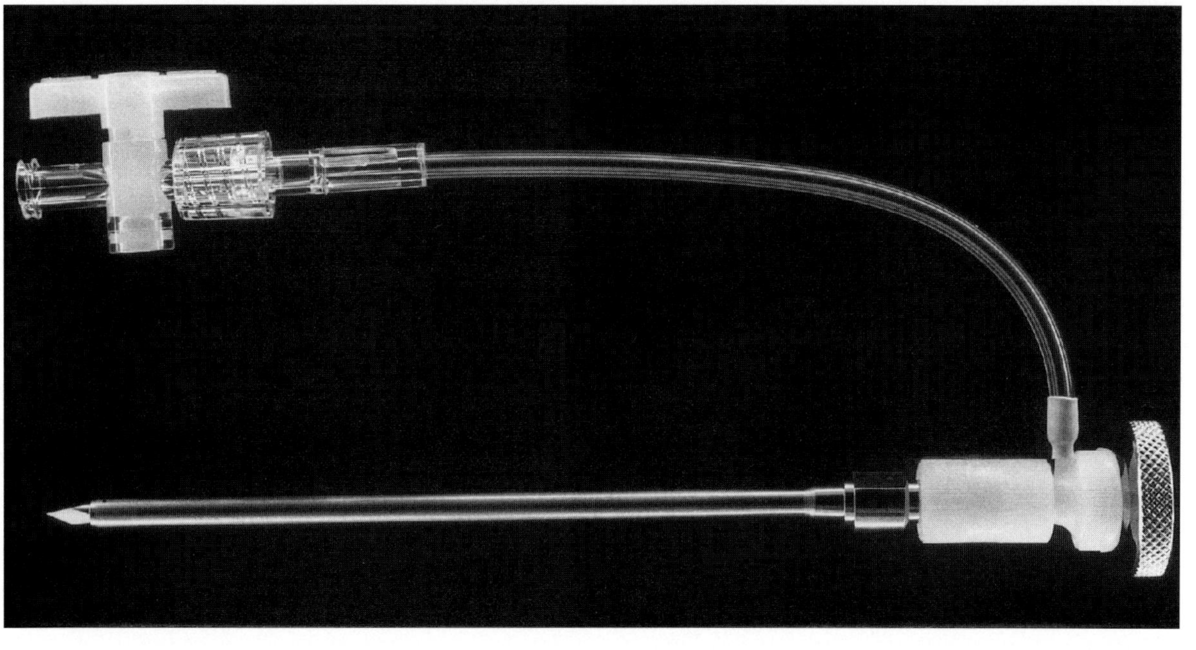

Figure 39–5. Custom-designed 2-mm trochar for use in operative fetoscopy. The checkflow valve prevents amniotic fluid leakage, while retaining the endoscope. The sidearm plastic tubing allows removal of amniotic fluid or instillation of fluid for better visualization.

under gas is superior to that under amniotic fluid, especially in the presence of intraamniotic bleeding. Unfortunately, the development of fetal acidosis using a CO_2/fluid medium in fetal lambs has precluded the use of this technique in humans (Estes, 1992; Luks, 1994a; and their associates). Additionally, the use of gas in the amniotic cavity would preclude the concomitant use of ultrasound. Therefore, a fluid environment ap-pears to be necessary and mandates the use of unique operative techniques.

Visualization

For several reasons, it is necessary to replace amniotic fluid with a crystalloid solution during fetal endoscopy. First, light transmission through human amniotic fluid is significantly less than through air or physiologic solution (Quintero and associates, 1993; Vanderberghe, 1994). The transmission of light decreases further with advancing gestational age. In addition to these baseline limitations, visualization through amniotic fluid may be further limited from blood staining after preoperative cordocentesis, by vernix, or from intraamniotic bleeding during surgery. Initial clinical experience with amnioinfusion was gained as part of protocols designed to decrease the incidence of abnormal fetal heart rate patterns in labor (Miyazaki and Neverez, 1985). The technique currently used in endoscopic fetal surgery involves a suction/irrigation pump with manual pressure calibration, attached to the sideports of the trocars (Fig. 39–6). This system can rapidly clear the amniotic fluid in cases of intraamniotic bleeding, without altering the total amniotic fluid volume. Ideally, different ports are used for irrigation and suction, although the exchange can also be performed in an alternate fashion through a single port.

Image Display

Ultrasound is used to guide the insertion of the instruments into the amniotic cavity, and for orientation during surgery. This is particularly important because the panoramic view

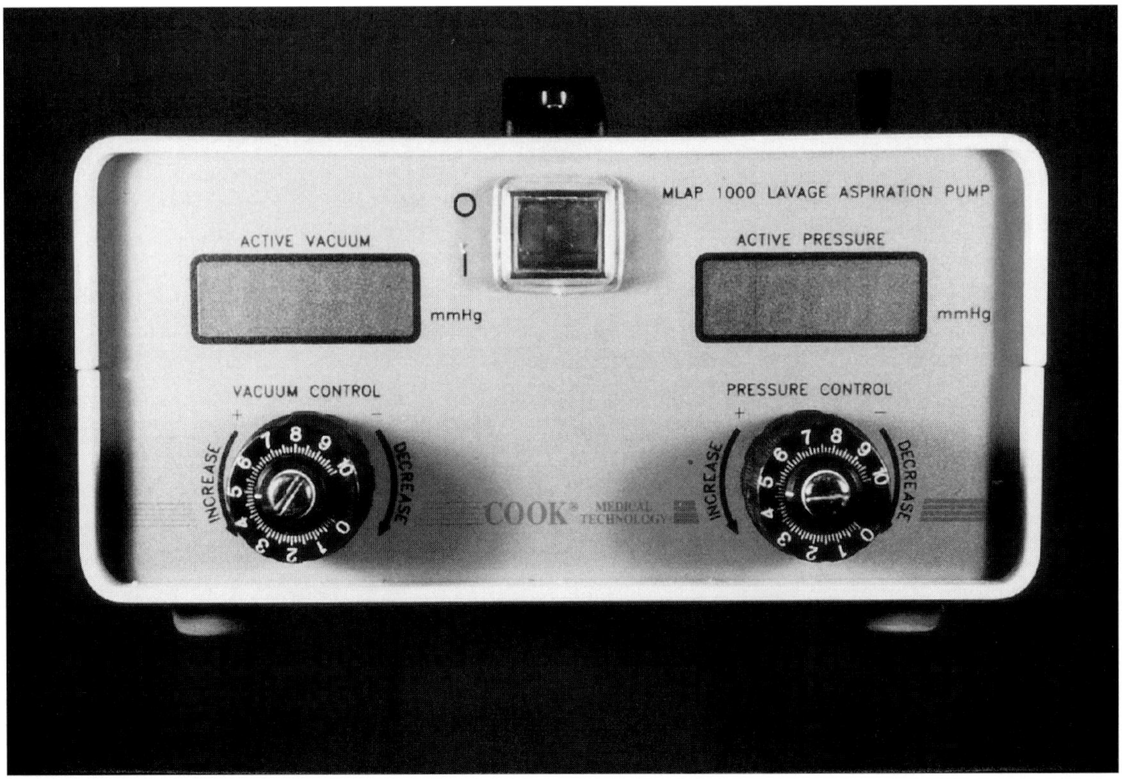

Figure 39–6. Vacuum-pressure pump used for amniotic fluid exchange (Cook, Ob/Gyn, Sydney, Australia). Both pressures can be independently regulated.

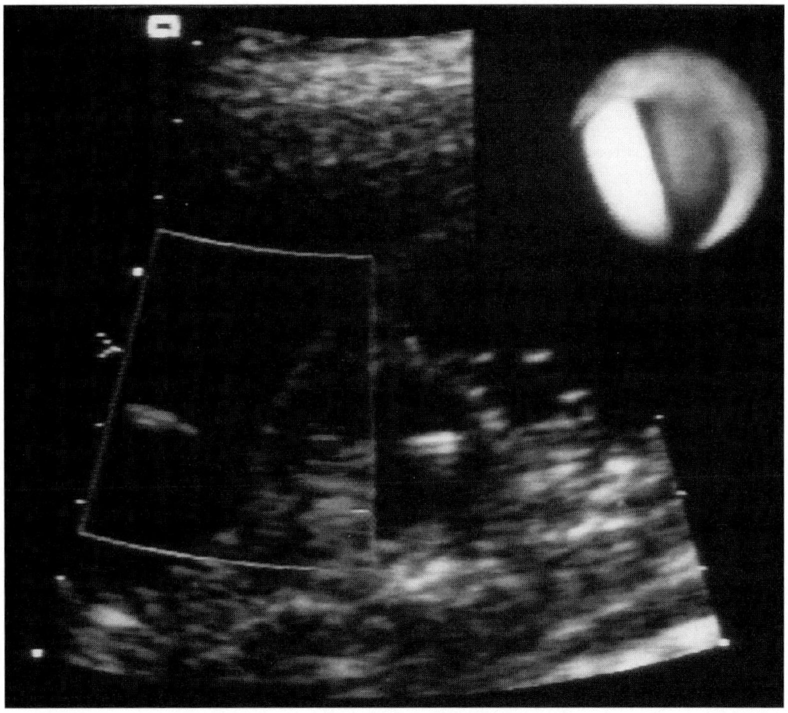

Figure 39–7. Simultaneous display of sonographic and endoscopic image in a single monitor using a videomixer. Coordination of the operating instruments is greatly facilitated.

provided by larger endoscopes (eg, 10 mm) is not available with the smaller devices. To improve the orientation, we use a videomixer, a device that can simultaneously or selectively display the endoscopic and the sonographic image on a single monitor (Fig. 39–7). As with videolaparoscopy, we place a monitor on each side of the patient's bed so that all members of the surgical team can monitor the procedure adequately.

Endoscopes

One of the most important aspects of performing endoscopic fetal surgery is the type of endoscope used. With advances in fiberoptic imaging, a number of endoscopes are currently available; however there is no commercially available endoscope specifically designed for fetoscopic surgery at the present time. Different endoscopes are necessary for different procedures, and the smallest endoscope is generally chosen whenever possible. For diagnostic procedures we prefer to use either a 0.7 mm flexible endoscope (Intramed), or a 1.9 mm rigid scope (Wolf). Wider fiberoptic endoscopes are not necessarily associated with a better image.

The length of the endoscope is also important. It must be longer than the trocars, so that it can reach the amniotic cavity, and preferably be able to span the length of the cavity. This is particularly important if the fetus changes position during the operation. An additional advantage of long fiberoptic endoscopes is that the eyepiece can be placed outside the working field and the operator can concentrate on moving the endoscope without holding the camera. Figure 39–8 demonstrates endoscopic umbilical cord ligation technique, while Figure 39–9 depicts ablation of posterior urethral valves.

Surgical Instruments

As with the endoscopes, there are currently no instruments specifically designed for operative fetoscopy. Therefore, a significant amount of research time has been devoted both to identifying available products that may be adapted to operative fetoscopy, and to designing new instruments (Table 39–2). Currently, there is only a small selection of instruments available less than 3 mm in diameter. Instruments 1 mm or less in diameter can be introduced through the working channel of some endoscopes (operating endoscopes), thus eliminating the need for a second port. Although a wider variety of instruments is available for use through 5 mm ports, the inherent disad-

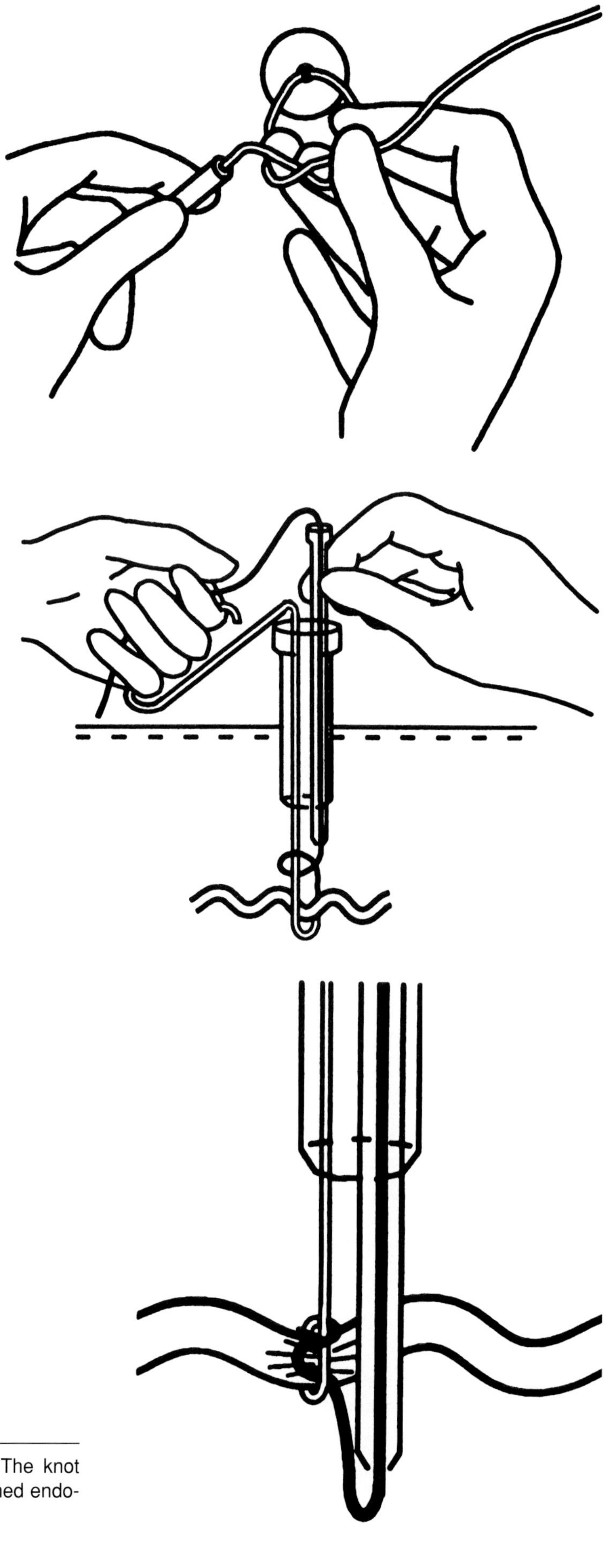

Figure 39–8. Endoscopic knot placement. The knot has been tied extracorporeally, and is tightened endoscopically.

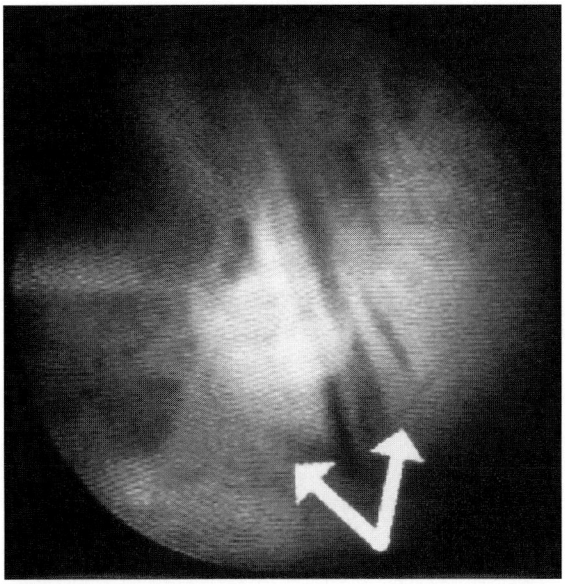

A

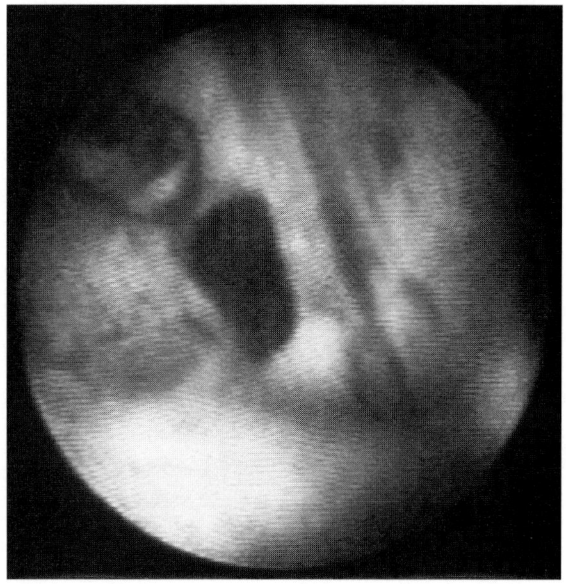

B

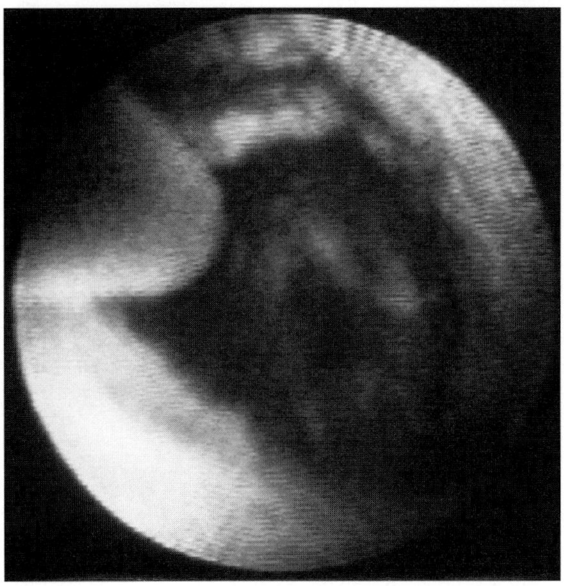

C

Figure 39–9. In utero endoscopic ablation of posterior urethral valves. **A.** The leaflets of the valves are identified (arrows). **B.** The electrode has been fired against the valve, and a small opening has been created. **C.** Completion of the ablation of the valves is accomplished with gentle rotation of the endoscope. Urethral patency has been established.

TABLE 39–2. INSTRUMENTS DESIGNED AND ADAPTED FOR OPERATIVE FETOSCOPY

Designed	Adapted
Trocars	Forceps
Blunt probe	Scissors
Knot pushers	Electrodes
Knot cutters	Wire guides
Bipolar electrocautery scapel	Laser fibers
Bipolar forceps	
Monopolar electrodes	

vantage of these larger endoscopes limits their usefulness in fetal surgery.

Pressure/Volume Regulation

Data from amnioinfusion studies suggests that the intraamniotic pressure may rise significantly with as little as 300 cc of fluid (Fisk and associates, 1991). Thus, we maintain a baseline level of amniotic fluid, unless it is abnormally high or low to begin with. In our initial cases we monitored the intraamniotic pressure several times during the operation. However, because we did not notice variations exceeding 1–2 mm Hg, over time, we have not continued this practice, and currently perform a simple even volume exchange of amniotic fluid for saline.

Safety

The potential for maternal and fetal injury exists, particularly when wide trocars (eg, 3.5 mm) are used. To avoid such complications, some investigators perform minilaparotomy when using these relatively large endoscopes to avoid injuring uterine vessels, and in addition place a purse string stitch around the endoscope to prevent fluid leakage. Data regarding the pregnancy loss rate associated with fetoscopy is limited to the few series performed in ongoing pregnancies. Hobbins and Mahoney reported 2 losses among 65 patients (3 percent) in continuing pregnancies (Hobbins and Mahoney, 1976). These investigators used an endoscope 1.7 mm in diameter inserted transabdominally through a 2.2 × 2.7 mm cannula in patients at risk for hemoglobinopathies and other genetic disorders. Rodeck (1980), using a similar endoscope, had a 3.7 percent pregnancy loss rate among 108 patients who underwent transabdominal fetoscopy for fetal blood sampling, skin biopsy, or evaluation for suspected anomalies. An additional 37 patients underwent pregnancy termination based on the results of the examination. These data suggest a corrected pregnancy loss rate of 3–4 percent associated with transabdominal fetoscopy. An additional 5–7 percent of patients in these series experienced transient amniotic fluid leakage, albeit with successful pregnancy outcome.

Human Applications

In specialized centers, endoscopic techniques have been applied to human fetuses in a few, carefully selected patients with presumed twin–twin transfusion syndrome, acardiac twinning, posterior urethral valve syndrome and chorioangioma (De Lia, 1990; Quintero, 1994d, 1995; Hirata, 1993; Hubinont, 1994; and their associates). Fig. 39–8 demonstrates the technique of in-utero umbilical cord ligation of an acardiac twin. In Fig. 39–9, in utero endoscopic ablation of posterior urethral valves is seen.

The effects of light and heat on the developing fetus during such procedures remain under investigation, and definite clinical benefit has yet to be established.

SUMMARY

Fetal surgery is a rapidly developing discipline now in its infancy. In addition to the approaches described in this chapter, a variety of innovative case reports continue to be published describing novel approaches to conditions previously untreatable prior to birth. While all of these techniques remain investigational, sonographic-guided shunt placement for urinary tract outflow obstruction and select cases of cystic adenomatoid malformation are now well established in specialized centers with expertise in these areas. However, no prospective studies presently exist to document the actual clinical benefit of any of these techniques. It is anticipated that additional research into pathophysiology, surgical technique, and methods of tocolysis will clarify and perhaps broaden the indications for these procedures in the unborn child.

REFERENCES

Adzick NS, Harrison MR, Glick PL, et al. Experimental pulmonary hypoplasia and oligohydramnios: relative contribution of lung fluid and fetal breathing movements. J Pediatr Surg 1984; 19:658.

Adzick NS, Harrison MR, Glick PL, et al. Fetal cystic adenomatoid malformation: prenatal diagnosis and natural history. J Pediatr Surg 1985; 20:483.

Adzick NS, Harrison MR, Hu LM, et al. Pulmonary hypoplasia and renal dysplasia in a fetal urinary tract obstruction model. Surg Forum 1987; 38: 666.

Adzick NS, Vacanti JP, Lillehie CW, et al. Fetal diaphragmatic hernia: ultrasound diagnosis and clinical outcome in 38 cases from a single medical center. J Pediatr Surg 1989; 24:654.

Adzick NS, Harrison MR, Flake AW. Fetal surgery for cystic adenomatoid malformation of the lung. J Pediatr Surg 1993; 28:806.

Birnholz JC, Frigoletto FD. Antenatal treatment of hydrocephalus. N Engl J Med 1981; 303:1021.

Chervenak FA, Duncan C, Mert LR, et al. Outcome of fetal ventriculomegaly. Lancet 1984; 2:179.

Clark SL, Vitale DJ, Minton SD, et al. Successful fetal therapy for cystic adenomatoid malformation associated with second trimester hydrops. Am J Obstet Gynecol 1987; 157:294.

Clewell WH, Johnson ML, Meier PR, et al. A surgical approach to the treatment of fetal hydrocephalus. N Engl J Med 1982; 306:1320.

Clewell WH, Meier PR, Manchester DK, et al. Ventriculomegaly: evaluation and management. Semin Perinatol 1985; 9:98.

Clewell WH. The fetus with ventriculomegaly: selection and treatment. In Harrison MR, Golbus MS, Filly RA (eds): The Unborn Patient, Philadelphia: WB Saunders, 1990; 444.

De Lia JE, Cukierski MA, Lundergan DK, et al. Neodymium: yttrium-aluminum-garnet laser occlusion of rhesus placental vasculature via fetoscopy. Am J Obstet Gynecol 1989; 160:485.

De Lia JE, Cruikshank DP, Keye WR. Fetoscopic neodymium: YAG laser occlusion of placental vessels in severe twin–twin transfusion syndrome. Obstet Gynecol 1990; 75:1046.

De Crispigny LC, Robinson HP, Quinn M, et al. Ultrasound guided fetal blood transfusion for severe rhesus isoimmunization. Obstet Gynecol 1985; 66:529.

Drugan A, Zador IE, Bhatia RK, et al. First trimester diagnosis and early treatment of obstructive uropathy. Acta Obstet Gynecol Scand 1989; 68:645.

Elder JS, O'Grady JP, Ashmead G. Evaluation of fetal renal function: unreliability of fetal urinary electrolytes. J Urol 1990; 144:574.

Elvidge AR. Treatment of obstructive lesion of the aqueduct of Sylvius and fourth ventricle by interventriculostomy. J Neurosurg 1966; 24:11.

Estes JM, Szabo Z, Harrison MR. Techniques for in utero endoscopic surgery. Surg Endoscopy 1992; 6:215.

Fisk NM, Giussani DA, Parkes MJ, et al. Amnioinfusion increases amniotic pressure in pregnant sheep but does not alter fetal acid-base status. Am J Obstet Gynecol 1991; 165:1459.

Gembruch V, Hansmann M. Artificial instillation of amniotic fluid as a new technique for the diagnostic evaluation of cases of oligohydramnios. Prenat Diagn 1988; 8:33.

Glick PL, Harrison MR, Noall RA, et al. Correction of congenital hydronephrosis in utero. III: Early mid-trimester obstruction produces renal dysplasia. J Pediatr Surg 1983; 18:681.

Glick PL, Harrison MR, Nakayama DK, et al. Management of ventriculomegaly in the fetus. J Pediatr 1984a; 105:97.

Glick PL, Harrison MR, Adzick NS, et al. Correction of congenital hydronephrosis in utero IV: In utero decompression prevents renal dysplasia. J Pediatr Surg 1984b; 19:649.

Haeusler MCH, Ryan G, Robson SC, et al. The use of saline solution as a contrast medium in suspected diaphragmatic hernia and renal agenesis. Am J Obstet Gynecol 1993; 168:1486.

Harrison MR, Anderson J, Rosen MA, et al. Fetal surgery in the primate. I. Anesthetic, surgical and tocolytic management to maximize fetal-neonatal survival. J. Pediatr. Surg 1982; 17:115.

Harrison MR, Ross NA, Noall RA, et al. Correction of congenital hydronephrosis in utero. I: The model: fetal urethral obstruction produces hydronephrosis and pulmonary hypoplasia in fetal lambs. J Pediatr Surg 1983; 18:247.

Harrison MR, Langer JC, Adzick NS, et al. Correction of congenital diaphragmatic hernia in utero. V. Initial clinical experience. J Pediatr. Surg 1990; 25:47.

Hirata GI, Masaki DI, O'Toole M, et al. Color flow mapping and doppler velocimetry in the diagnosis and management of a placental chorioangioma associated with nonimmune fetal hydrops. Obstet Gynecol 1993; 81:850.

Hobbins JC, Mahoney MJ. Clinical experience with fetoscopy and fetal blood sampling. In Kaback MM (ed): Intrauterine fetal visualization, a multidisciplinary approach. Amsterdam: Exerpta Medica 1976; 164.

Hubinont C, Bernard P, Khalil N, et al. Fetal liver hemangioma and chorioangioma: two unusual cases of severe fetal anemia detected by ultrasonography and it perinatal management. Ultrasound Obstet Gynecol 1994; 4:330.

Johnson MP, Bukowski TP, Reitleman MD, et al. In utero surgical treatment of fetal obstructive uropathy: a new comprehensive approach to identify appropriate candidates for vesicoamniotic shunt therapy. Am J Obstet Gynecol 1994; 170:1770.

Kleiner B, Callen PW, Filley RA. Sonographic analysis of the fetus with ureteropelvic junction obstruction. AJR 1987; 148:359.

Kuller JA, Yankowitz J, Goldberg JD, et al. Outcome of antenatally diagnosed cystic adenomatoid malformations. Am J Obstet Gynecol 1992; 167:1038.

Lipitz S, Ryan G, Samuell C. Fetal urine analysis for the assessment of renal function in obstructive uropathy. Am J Obstet Gynecol 1993; 168:174.

Lorber J. Ventriculocardiac shunts in the first week of life. Dev Med Child Neurol 1969; 20:13.

Luks FI, Deprest JA, Marcus M, et al. Carbon dioxide pneumoamnios causes acidosis in fetal lambs. Fetal Diagn Ther 1994a; 9:105.

Luks FI, Deprest JA, Vanderberghe K, et al. A model for fetal surgery through intrauterine endoscopy. J Pediatr Surg 1994b; 29:1007.

Luks FI, Deprest JA, Vanderberghe K, et al. Fetoscopy-guided fetal endoscopy in a sheep model. J Am Coll Surg 1994c; 178:609.

Mandelbrot L, Dommergues M, Aubry MC, et al. Reversal of fetal distress by emergency in utero decompression of hydrothorax. Am J Obstet Gynecol 1992; 167:1278.

Manning FA. The fetus with obstructive uropathy: the fetal surgery registry. In Harrison MR, Golbus MS, Filly RA (eds); The Unborn Patient. Philadelphia: WB Saunders, 1990a; 394.

Manning FA. The fetus with ventriculomegaly: the fetal surgery registry. In Harrison MR, Golus MS, Filly RA (eds). The Unborn Patient. Philadelphia: WB Saunders, 1990b: 448.

Miyazaki FS, Neverez F. Saline amnioinfusion for relief of repetitive variable decelerations: a prospective randomized study. Am J Obstet Gynecol 1985; 153:301.

Nicolaides KH, Blott M, Greenough A. Chronic drainage of fetal pulmonary cyst. Lancet 1987; 1:618.

Nicolaides KH, Cheng HH, Snijdes MSc, et al. Fetal urine biochemistry in the assessment of obstructive uropathy. Am J Obstet Gynecol 1992; 166:932.

Nugent CE, Hayashi RH, Rubin J. Prenatal treatment of type I congenital cystic adenomatoid malformation by intrauterine fetal thoracentesis. JCU 1989; 17:675.

Obwegeser R, Deutinger J, Bernaschek G. Fetal pulmonary cyst treated by repeated thoracocentesis. Am J Obstet Gynecol 1993; 169:1622.

Quintero RA, Puder KS, Cotton DB. Embroyoscopy and fetoscopy. Obstet Gynecol Clin North Am 1993; 20:563.

Quintero RA, Goncalves LF, Guevara F, et al. Color-Doppler guided coagulation of abnormal communicating vessels in twin–twin transfusion. Abstract Ultrasound Obstet Gynecol 1994a; 4:93.

Quintero RA, Reich H, Puder KS, et al. Umbilical cord ligation of an acardiac twin by fetoscopy at 19 weeks of gestation. N Engl J Med 1994b; 330:469.

Quintero RA, Reich H, Puder KS, et al. Operative fetoscopy: a new frontier in fetal medicine. Abstract Am J Obstet Gynecol 1994c; 179:297.

Quintero RA, Puder KS, Bardicef M, et al. Hydrolaparoscopy in the rabbit: a fine model for the development of operative fetoscopy. Am J Obstet Gynecol 1994d; 171:1139.

Quintero RA, Hume R, Smith C, et al. Percutaneous fetal cystoscopy and endoscopic fulguration of posterior urethral valves. Am J Obstet Gynecol 1995 (in press).

Rodeck CH. Fetoscopy guided by real-time ultrasound for pure fetal samples, fetal skin samples and examination of the fetus in utero. Br J Obstet Gynecol 1980; 87:449.

Shalev E, Weiner E, Feldman E, et al. External bladder-amniotic fluid shunt for fetal urinary tract obstruction. Obstet Gynecol 1984; 63:315.

Sharland GK, Lockhart SM, Heward AJ, et al. Prognosis in fetal diaphragmatic hernia. Am J Obstet Gynecol 1992; 166:9.

The Southern Surgeons Club. A prospective analysis of 1518 laparoscopic cholecystectomies. N Engl J Med 1991; 324:1073.

Thorup J, Mortensen T, Diemer H, et al. The prognosis of surgically treated congenital hydronephrosis after diagnosis in utero. J Urol 1985; 134:914.

Vanderberghe K. Fetal endoscopic surgery, lessons from animal experiment. Ultrasound Obstet Gynecol 1994; 4:129.

Ville Y, Hyett J, Hecher K, et al. Management of severe twin–twin transfusion: amniodrainage compared to endoscopic surgery. Ultrasound Obstet Gynecol 1994; 4:130.

Weber AM, Philipson EH. Fetal pleural effusion: a review and meta-analysis for prognostic indicators. Obstet Gynecol 1992; 79:281.

Wenstrom K, Weiner CP, Hanson JW. A five year statewide experience with congenital diaphragmatic hernia. Am J Obstet Gynecol 1991; 165:838.

Westin B. Hysteroscopy in early pregnancy. Lancet 1954; 2:872.

Wilkins IA, Chitkara U, Lynch L, et al. The nonpredictive value of fetal urinary electrolytes: preliminary report of outcomes and correlations with pathologic diagnosis. Am J Obstet Gynecol 1987; 157:694.

Young HF, Nulsen FE, Weiss HM, et al. The relationship of intelligence and cerebral matter in treated infantile hydrocephalus. Pediatrics 1973; 52:38.

CHAPTER 40

Circumcision

Newborn circumcision has been performed for centuries and been described in the Book of Genesis (17:10–14, 34:14–16). Few surgical procedures generate as much controversy as the removal of this small free fold of skin. In fact, one could suggest that more has been spent in effort, frustration, and expense in researching and arguing for or against routine neonatal circumcision than the cost of either the benefits or complications of the procedure. For at least half a century the majority of male newborns in America have been circumcised. It is somewhat surprising and disheartening that with this apparent plethora of data the academic community has been inconsistent in its recommendations.

Parents often seek the advice of obstetricians regarding circumcision during the course of their antenatal care. Furthermore, in many clinical settings obstetricians perform newborn circumcision. Although as with most surgical procedures, teachers relay the technique to their students, information in obstetric texts has been scant. In this chapter therefore, we review the anatomy, embryology, and surgical history of newborn circumcision, summarize the data and debate regarding neonatal circumcision, and describe acceptable techniques for performing the procedure.

HISTORY

Circumcision is one of the oldest and most widely performed operations known to man. For Jews and Moslems newborn circumcision remains a religious requirement. Circumcision is accomplished on all male Jews on the eighth day after birth in a ceremony called a *bris*. In orthodox Judaism, an official known as a *mohel* performs the circumcision, while reform Jews allow the procedure to be accomplished by a physician (Allan, 1989). In an excellent review, Grossman and Posner (1981) detail the development of surgical techniques used for circumcision. The Bible describes the use of flint knives as instruments. The codes of Maimonides describes the basic steps of excision of the prepuce, tearing of the mucosa with a thumbnail, and exposure of the glans (Maimonides, 1947). Early surgical improvements involved preventing trauma. Sharp knives negated the need for tearing the skin. In the 1700s a metal plate was used that prevented damage to the glans (Karo, 1960). In the early 1900s a Moslem physician protected the glans by tying two sutures around the stretched prepuce and cutting between the two knots (Bryk, 1934). Topical antibiotics and various surgical clamps led to a reduction in bleeding and infection. Hence, by the 1930s complications of the procedure were minimal.

Urologic research in the 1930s revealed that circumcision prevents cancer of the penis. Wolbarst, in a review of over 1100 cases of penile cancer, found none in men who were circumcised as newborns (Wolbarst, 1932). Schoen analyzed penile cancer and noted that there have been 750–1000 cases annually in the United States, yet only 3 cases of penile cancer have been reported in the last 20 years in men circumcised as newborns (Schoen, 1990). During World War II both US and Canadian studies suggested that circumcision promoted genital hygiene, prevented balanitis, balanoposthitis, phimosis, and paraphimosis, and decreased the incidence of sexually transmitted disease (Wilson, 1947; Gellis, 1978). Thus, in the 1940s physicians prescribed newborn circumcision as a simple, minor procedure that promoted hygiene and prevented genital disease.

The disadvantages of newborn circumcision are rare and short-term and the advantages are long-term. Pediatricians who dealt with the immediate complications, however, began to question the advantages of newborn circumcision. In 1971 and 1975 the Committee on the Fetus and Newborn of the American Academy of Pediatrics (AAP) recommended that routine circumcision of newborn males not be performed (Committee of Fetus and Newborn, 1975). They stated that penile hygiene could and should be taught to parents and penile cancer thereby avoided. Furthermore, the task force concluded that the data suggesting that newborn circumcision had any impact on cancer of the prostate or cervix or on venereal disease was inconclusive. Thus, the 1975 AAP task force concluded that there is "no absolute medical indication for routine newborn circumcision."

In 1988 the AAP task force on circumcision fell just short of a full reversal of their predecessor's opinion (American Academy of Pediatrics, 1989). They stated that newborn circumcision prevents phimosis, paraphimosis, and balanoposthitis. They recognized that circumcision would be necessary in childhood, adolescence, and adulthood in greater than 2–10 percent of males who would otherwise develop phimosis or balanitis. They cited five major series reported since the 1930s that found no cases of penile cancer in men circumcised as newborns and that the lifetime risk of an uncircumcised man in the United States developing penile cancer was 1 in 600 (Kochen and McCurdy, 1980). Additionally, research revealed that human papilloma virus types 16 and 18 may be present in greater than 60 percent of cases of penile carcinoma (McCance and co-workers, 1986), and human papilloma virus on the penis has been linked to sexual and hygienic practice. Thus, poor hygiene, lack of circumcision, and certain sexually transmitted diseases all appeared to correlate with the incidence of penile carcinoma.

Perhaps the major reason for the AAP's shift in opinion related to data on urinary tract infections. Circumcised boys are 10–39 times less likely than noncircumcised boys to have urinary tract infections during infancy (Wiswell, 1990). Wiswell and colleagues (1987) studied over 400,000 infants and found a predominance of urinary tract infections in uncircumcised males. It has been estimated that over 20,000 additional cases of pyelonephritis would result if newborn circumcision were not performed in the United States (Wiswell, 1990). Furthermore, 36 percent of male infants with a urinary tract infection had concomitant bacteremia with the same organism, 3 percent had meningitis, greater than 2 percent had renal failure, and more than 2 percent died (Wiswell and Geschke, 1989). The studies on urinary tract disease, although significant, were retrospective. Thus in 1988, the AAP credited newborn circumcision with prevention of phimosis, paraphimosis, balanoposthitis, and reduction in penile cancer (American Academy of Pediatrics, 1989). The AAP stated circumcision may reduce urinary tract infections and recognized a possible association of penile and cervical cancer in uncircumcised men and their partners infected with human papilloma virus. Recently proponents of newborn circumcision cited studies from Africa and North America that suggested a link between noncircumcision and the human immunodeficiency virus (Simonsen and colleagues, 1988; Cameron and associates, 1989). Thus, newborn circumcision has potential medical benefits and advantages as well as risks. As with any surgical procedure, circumcision should only be performed after first obtaining informed consent from the parents.

ANATOMY AND EMBRYOLOGY

In order to master any surgical technique, the operator should understand the pertinent anatomy and embryology. Circumcision is no exception to this dictum. The epithelium of the spongy urethra, except the glandular portion, emanates from cells of the urogenital sinus (Fig. 40–1A). The epithelium of the na-

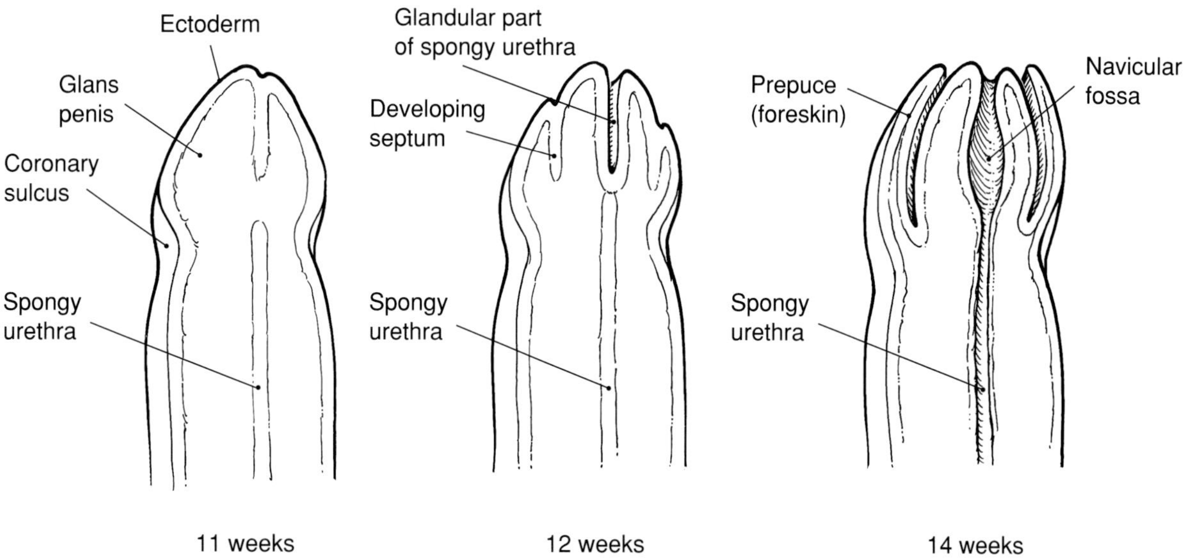

Figure 40–1. Development of the penis with prepuce and glandular portion of spongy urethra. (Adapted from Moore, 1982, with permission).

vicular fossa (Fig. 40–1B, C) develops by canalization of ectodermal cells known as the glandular plate, which extends from the tip of the penis. Splanchnic mesenchyme is the source of the connective tissue and smooth muscle of the penis. The prepuce develops as a circular ingrowth of ectoderm at the periphery of the glans penis during the twelfth week of development (Fig. 40–1) (Moore, 1982). This in-growth forms a septum, which then breaks down except for the area vertical to the glans that forms the frenulum. Subsequently, a double layer or free fold of skin exists as the prepuce.

The normal anatomy of the foreskin or prepuce is shown in Figure 40–2. The prepuce, also known as the foreskin, is the freefold of skin that covers the glans penis. The preputial space denotes the area between the glans penis and the prepuce. The preputial ring consists of the opening of the preputial space to outside the prepuce. The corona refers to the base of the glans penis, and the coronal sulcus lies between the glans and the penile shaft. In newborn males, the foreskin fully retracts in 4 percent, the glans recedes to see the urethral meatus in 54 percent, and the tip of the glans cannot be seen in 42 percent (Anderson, 1989). If retractability has not occurred naturally after 3 years of age, steps should be taken to render the prepuce of all boys retractable and capable of being cleaned. By puberty, daily hygiene includes cleansing of the preputial space.

Circumcision is defined as the surgical excision of the foreskin to the level of the coronal sulcus. Circumcision may be done in the newborn period or later in life as treatment for several conditions. Phimosis is a stenosis

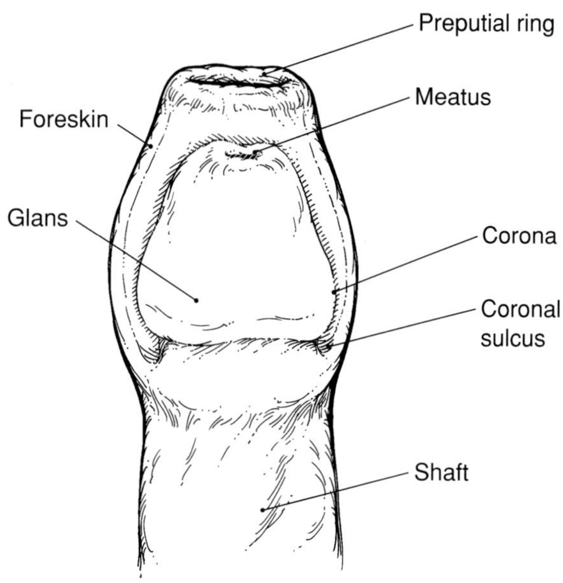

Figure 40–2. The normal anatomy of the penis and foreskin.

of the preputial ring, which prevents retraction of the foreskin. Paraphimosis consists of a partial stenosis with retraction usually blocked at the level of the corona. Balanitis and posthitis signify inflammation or infection of the glans and prepuce, respectively. Phimosis, paraphimosis, and recurrent balanoposthitis are indications for circumcision. Five to 10 percent of uncircumcised males require circumcision for these conditions (McKim, 1947; Warner and Streskin, 1981).

SURGICAL TECHNIQUE

Circumcision is a safe surgical procedure if performed by a trained operator using sterile technique. Newborn circumcision should be performed only on a healthy, stable infant. Contraindications to circumcision are listed in Table 40–1. We do not recommend circumcision on infants weighing less than 2500 g. It should also not be done on infants with evidence of a coagulopathy or penile anomalies. Furthermore, if a family history of a coagulopathy exists, it should be ruled out in the infant prior to the procedure. The most commonly used instruments include the Gomco and Mogen clamps, and the Plastibell device (Fig. 40–3). In a review of nearly six thousand patients (Gee and Ansell, 1976), complications with the Gomco clamp and Plastibell were rare and minor (Table 40–2). The AAP estimated the postoperative complication rate to be 0.2–0.6 percent (American Academy of Pediatrics, 1989). The most common complications are bleeding and local infection.

TABLE 40–1. CONTRAINDICATIONS AND RELATIVE CONTRAINDICATIONS TO ROUTINE NEWBORN CIRCUMCISION

Low birthweight (< 2500 g)
Bleeding abnormality
Family history of bleeding disorder not ruled out in infant
Infection
Unstable infant
Hypospadias and outer genitourinary anomalies
Abnormal body temperature
Abnormal feeding

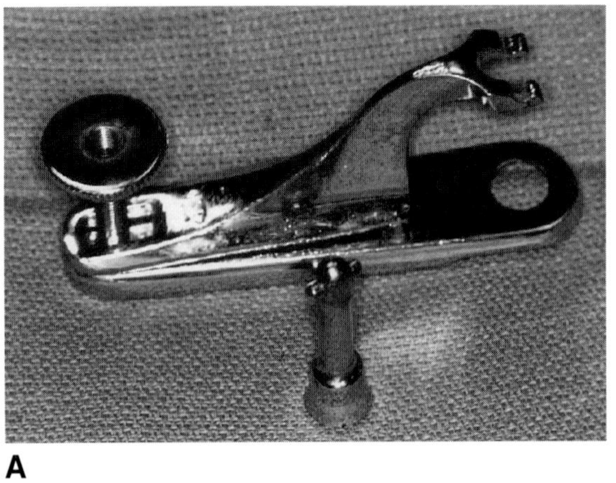

A

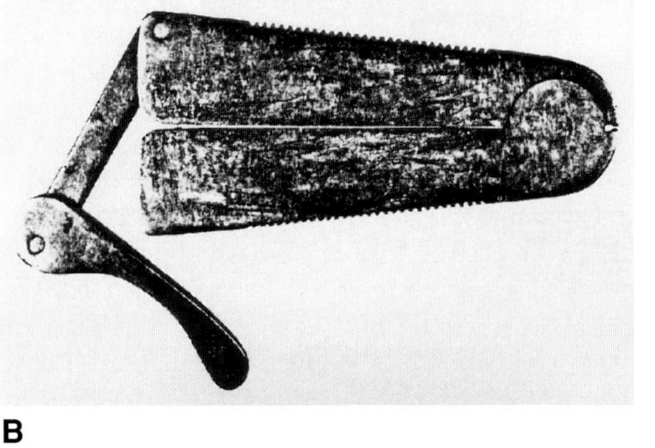

B

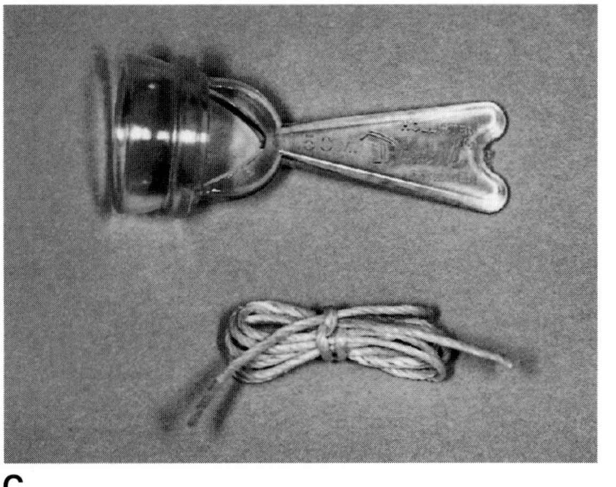

C

Figure 40–3. The Gomco **(A)** and Mogen **(B)** clamps and the Plastibell device **(C)** are the most common instruments used to perform newborn circumcision in the United States.

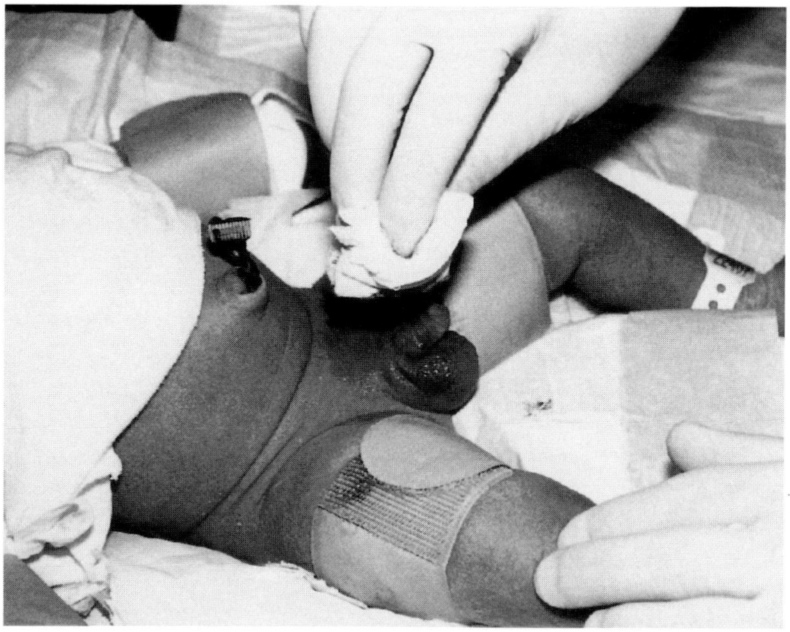

Figure 40–4. After the infant is identified and restrained, the penis and surrounding area are cleaned with betadine.

Regardless of surgical instruments employed for circumcision, some principles are uniform and include identification of the infant, aseptic technique, adequate but not excessive excision of the prepuce to the level of the coronal sulcus, hemostasis, and cosmetics. Upon obtaining informed consent from the parents, the infant should be identified and adequately restrained. The operator uses an iodine based or other antiseptic solution to prepare the surgical field (Fig. 40–4) and employs strict aseptic technique (Fig. 40–5). If an anesthetic block is used, it is administered at this time. Some surgeons may choose to mark the location of the coronal sulcus on the skin shaft with a surgical marking pen. The preputial ring is dilated with a hemostat and the urethral meatus is identified, thus ruling out hypospadias. The foreskin is grasped at 10 and 2 o'clock positions (Fig. 40–6). A hemostat or probe is used to separate the foreskin off the surface of the glans (Fig. 40–7). The hemostat is then clamped in the midline, one third the distance down the dorsal foreskin (Fig. 40–8). After 10 seconds the hemostat is removed (Fig. 40–9) and a straight blunt-tipped scissors cuts the crushed foreskin (Fig. 40–10). The foreskin is then bluntly freed off

TABLE 40–2. COMPLICATIONS OF NEWBORN CIRCUMCISION

	Number of Newborns (%)		
Complications	*Gomco*	*Plastibell*	*Total*
Hemorrhage	29 (1.00)	30 (1.14)	59 (1.07)
Infection	4 (0.14)	19 (0.72)	23 (0.42)
Dehiscence	8 (0.28)	1 (0.04)	9 (0.16)
Injury to glans	0 (0.00)	1 (0.04)	1 (0.02)
Excess skin removed	3 (0.10)	0 (0.00)	3 (0.05)
Plastibell ring too tight	—	7 (0.27)	7 (0.13)
Urinary retention	1 (0.04)	0 (0.00)	1 (0.02)

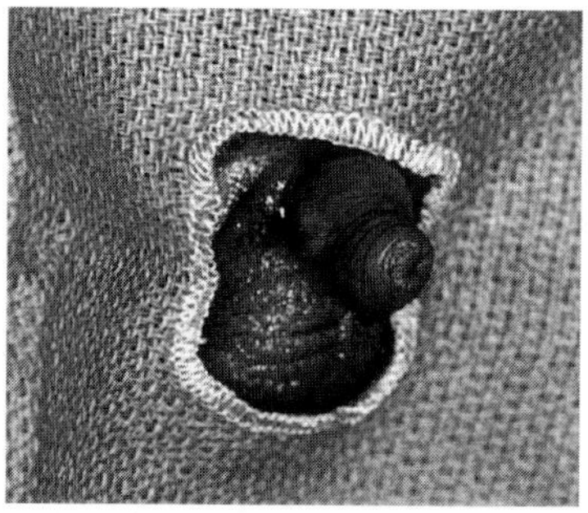

Figure 40–5. As with other surgical procedures, a sterile field is created with surgical towels.

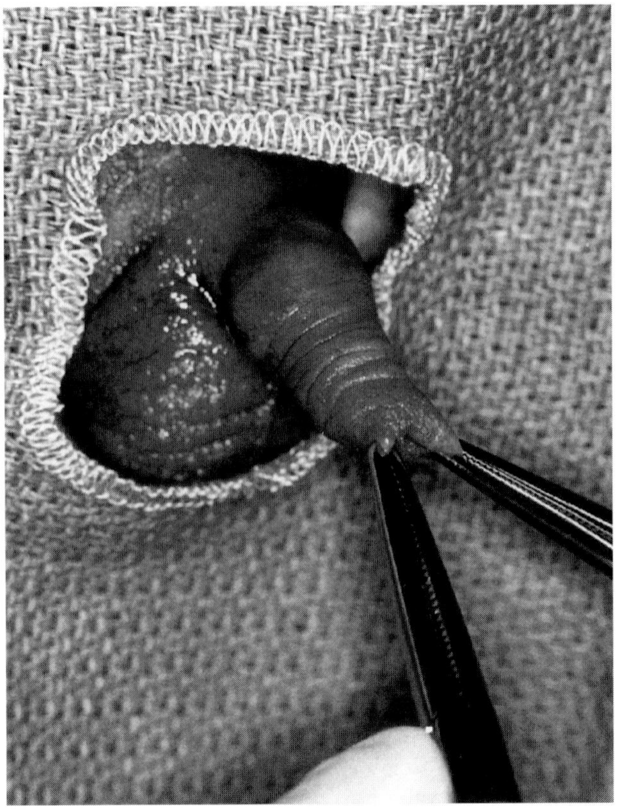

Figure 40–6. After identifying the urethral meatus, the foreskin is grasped with hemostats at 10 o'clock and 2 o'clock.

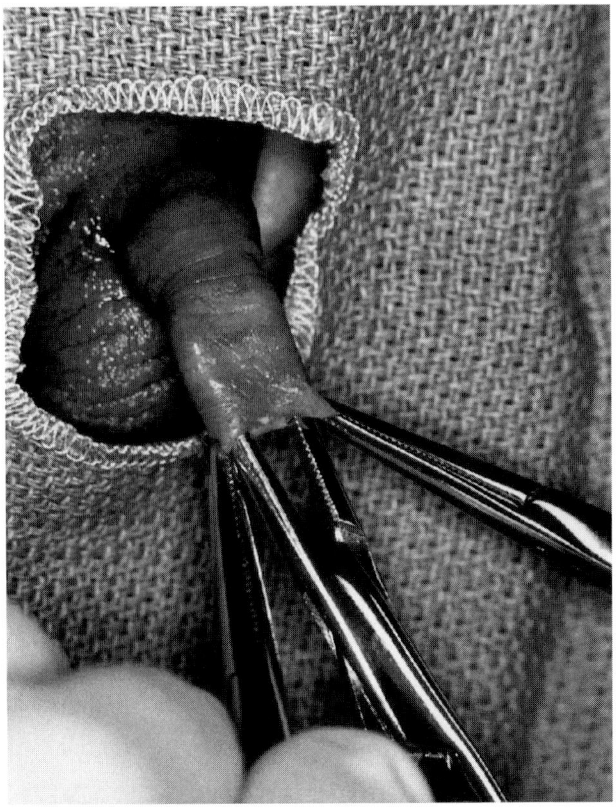

Figure 40–7. A hemostat is spread bluntly, separating the foreskin and glans penis.

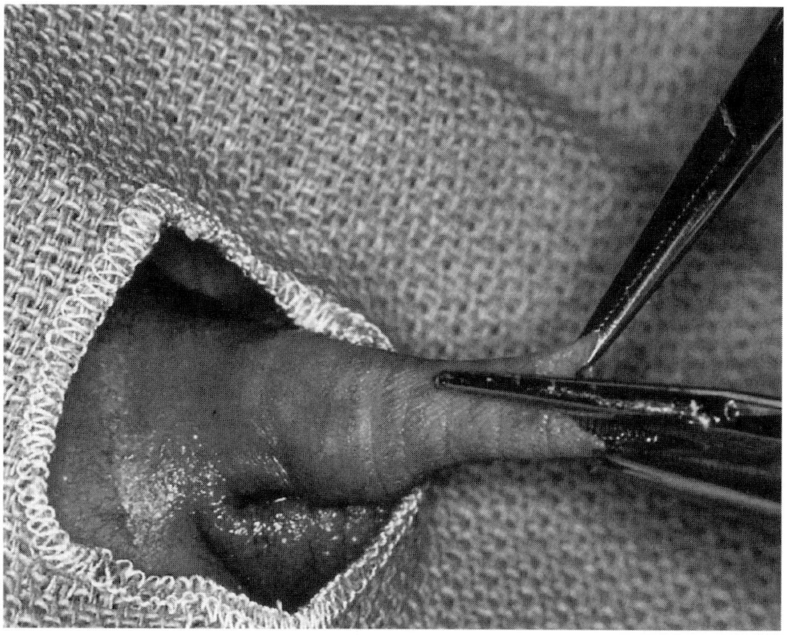

Figure 40–8. Once the foreskin is separated from the glans, a straight hemostat is clamped down the midline approximately one third the distance down the dorsal foreskin.

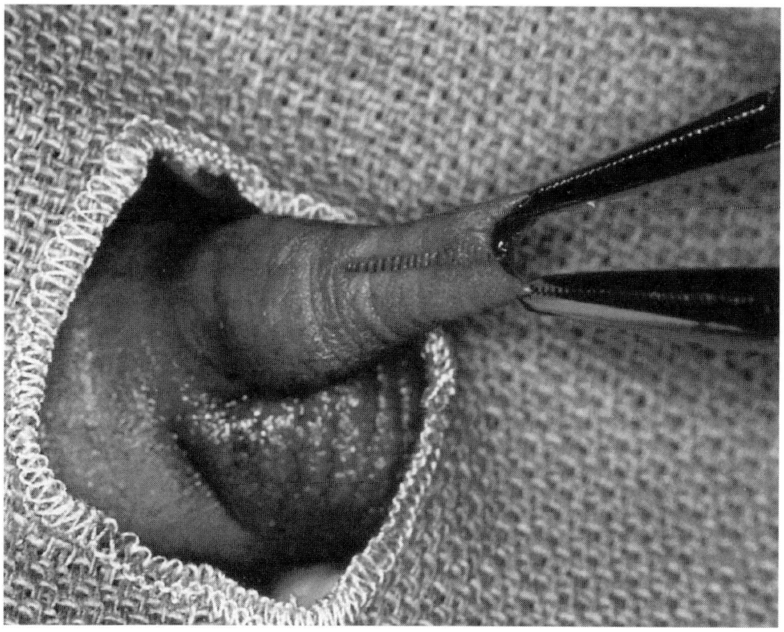

Figure 40–9. The hemostat should be left in place 5–10 seconds and will leave a crushed area when removed.

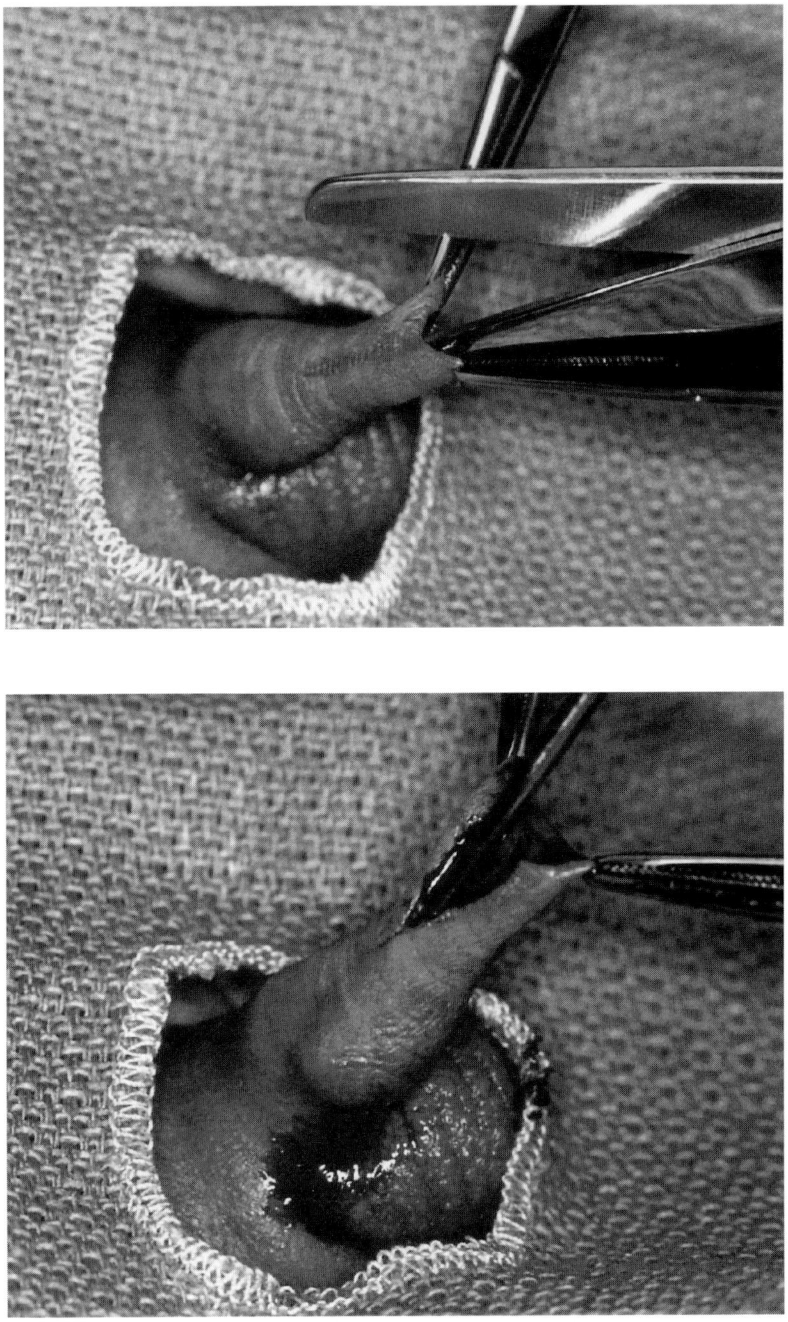

Figure 40–10. The surgeon cuts through the crushed area with a blunt-tipped scissors.

the glans with a hemostat or probe and retracted off the glans (Fig. 40–11). When using a Gomco device, a Gomco bell is chosen that fits over the entire corona. The bell distends the foreskin (Fig. 40–12) and the foreskin is regrasped with a hemostat over the bell of the Gomco (Fig. 40–13). The Gomco bell and overlying foreskin are now pulled through the Gomco plate (Fig. 40–14). The foreskin should be pulled through so that the level of the coronal sulcus is even with the top of the clamp. The bell is seated in the yolk, which is seated in the plate (Fig. 40–15). The clamp is screwed down on the bell as tight as possible.

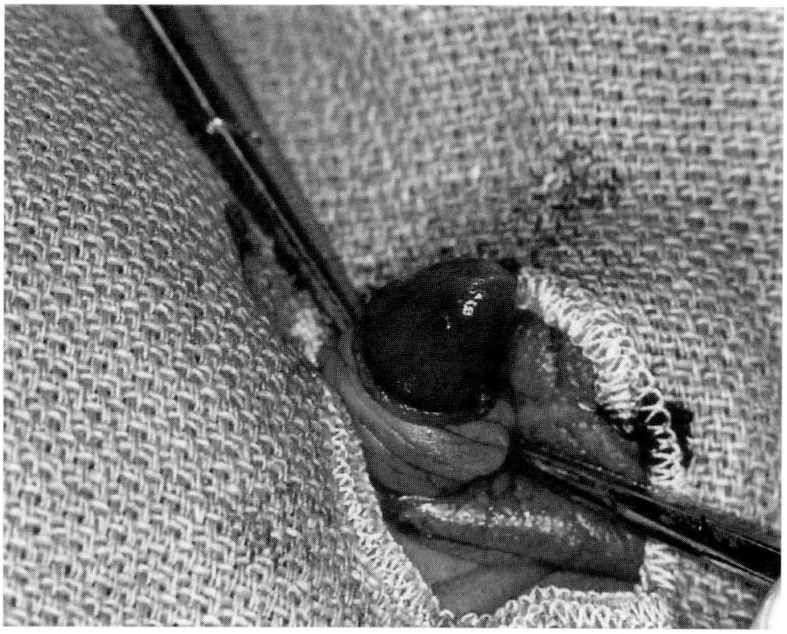

Figure 40–11. The foreskin is retracted off the glans penis.

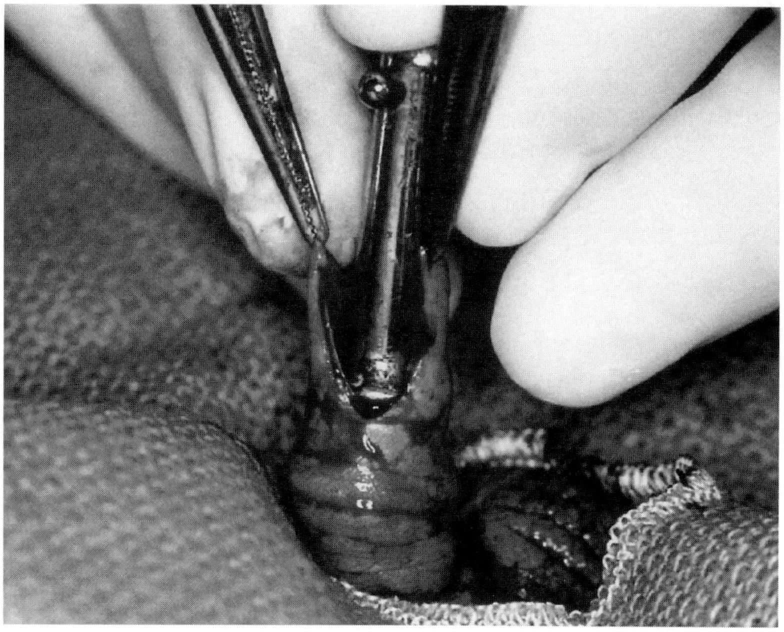

Figure 40–12. A Gomco bell large enough to extend over the corona and distend the foreskin is placed.

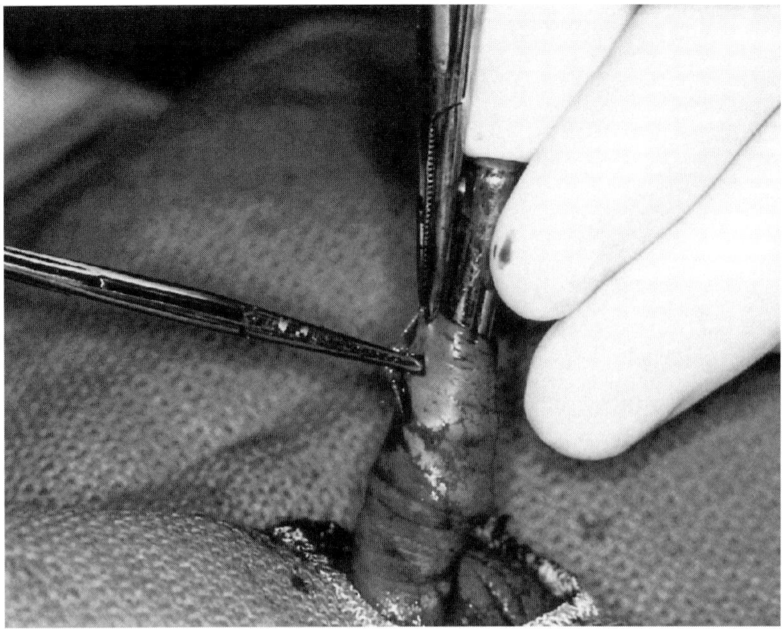

Figure 40–13. The surgeon re-grasps the cut edges of the foreskin, securing them over the neck of the Gomco bell.

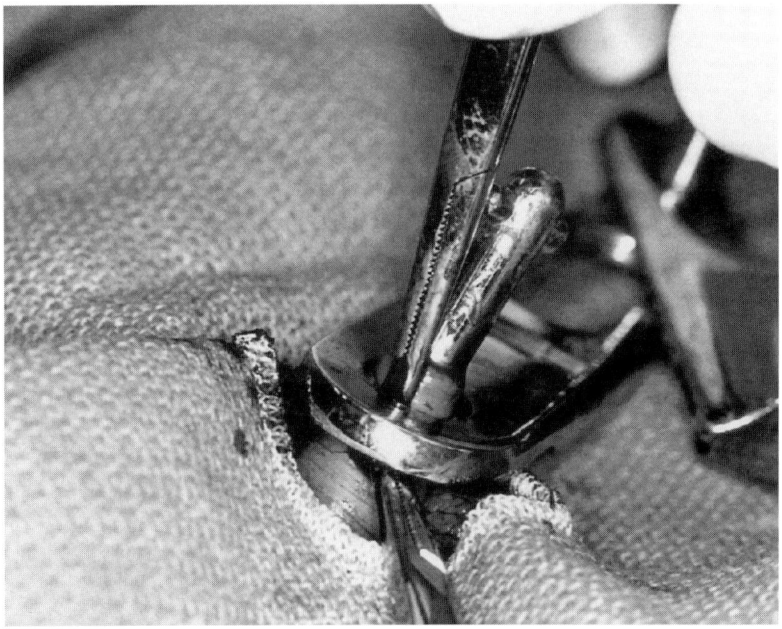

Figure 40–14. Sometimes a second hemostat is helpful in pulling the bell and surrounding foreskin through the Gomco plate.

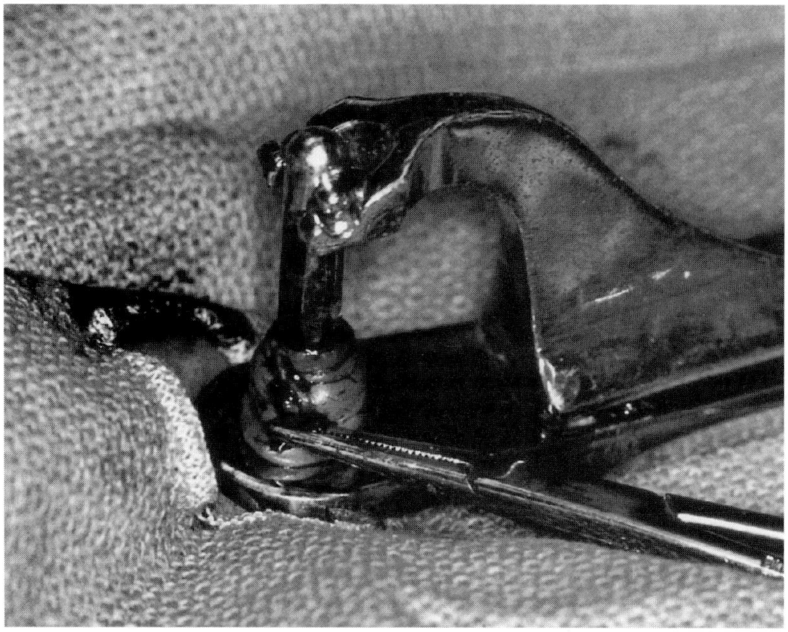

Figure 40–15. The bell is seated in the yolk and the yolk seated in the groove on the Gomco plate. Care must be taken to ensure that the foreskin is pulled all the way through and the coronal sulcus is even with the top of the clamp.

The clamp, bell, and excised foreskin are removed (Fig. 40–16) and the glans is dressed with petroleum gel or antiseptic ointment and a clean dressing (Fig. 40–17A and B).

If the Plastibell device (Fig. 40–3C) is used, the initial steps are similar to those with the Gomco clamp. Once the foreskin is bluntly freed off the glans and retracted (Fig. 40–11), a Plastibell is chosen that completely covers the corona and distends the foreskin similarly as the Gomco bell. The foreskin is drawn over the Plastibell until the coronal sulcus lies over the groove in the Plastibell. The surgeon secures an absorbable suture as tight as possible in the groove in the Plastibell. The distal end of the foreskin past the outermost groove is excised and the neck of the Plastibell is detached. The plastic rim usually drops off 5–8 days after circumcision. No special dressing is required. It is important to inform the parents that a dark brown or black ring may encircle the plastic rim and this will disappear when the rim falls off.

The initial steps for newborn circumcision are similar when the Mogen clamp (Fig. 40–3B) is used as well. The foreskin must be bluntly freed off the glans penis and be able to be retracted (Fig. 40–7). The foreskin is then pulled through the narrow slit in the clamp. The extremely small slit allows the foreskin to pass through while the glans retracts beneath the clamp. The clamp is then closed, crushing the foreskin, and after a brief waiting period a scalpel is used to excise the foreskin above the clamp.

Postoperative bleeding is rare, and usually may be controlled with pressure. However, sometimes in order to achieve hemostasis, ligation of a vessel or the application of silver nitrate, thrombin, or gelfoam may be necessary. Importantly, electrocautery should never be used when a metal clamp is on the surgical field. Rare cases of penile necrosis necessitating sex reassignment have been reported (Du Toit and Villet, 1979).

Anesthesia

It is generally agreed that infants undergoing circumcision feel pain, as documented by physiologic changes involving increases in heart rate, blood pressure, and oxygen saturation (Poland, 1990). These responses are short term with no evidence of long-term sequelae. Several methods of anesthesia have been suggested to render the procedure painless. Kirya and Werthmann introduced the technique of dorsal penile block (Kirya and Werthman, 1978). The dorsal penile nerves are paired and

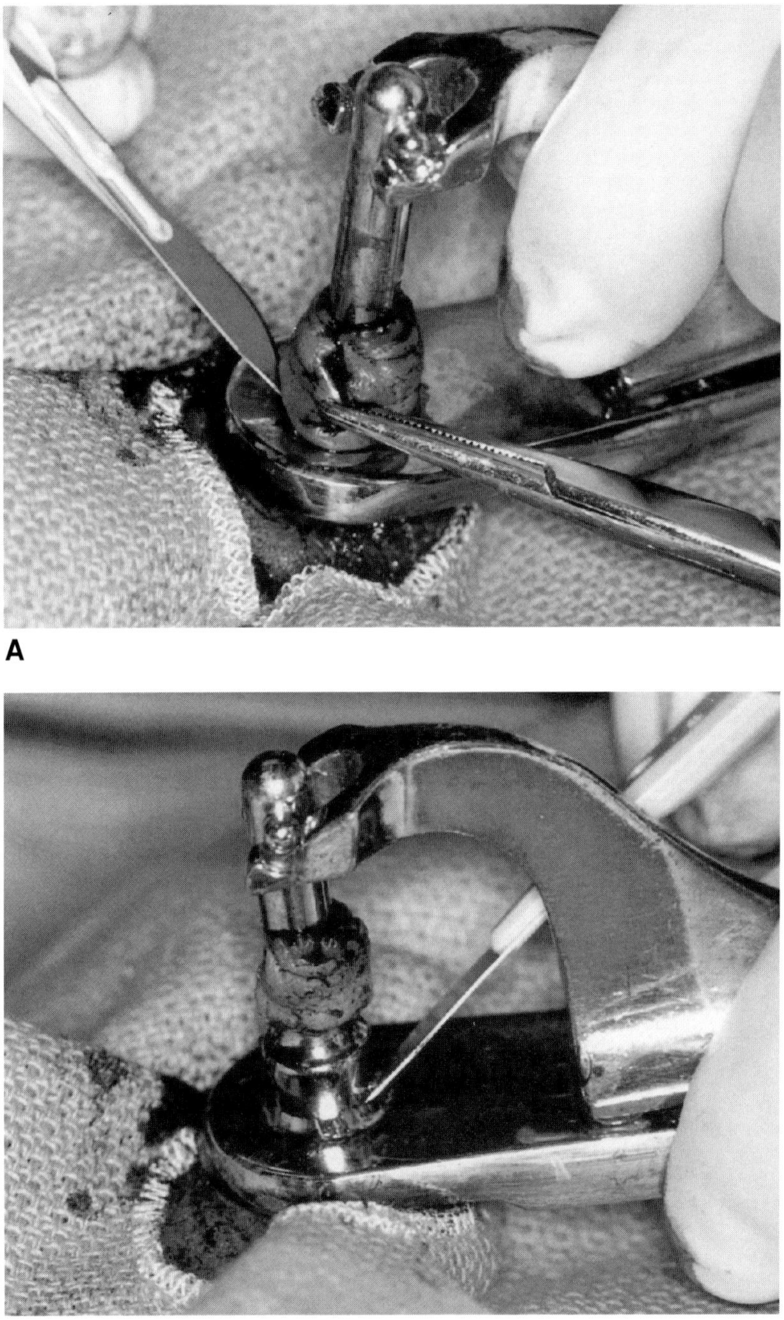

A

B

Figure 40–16. A. The foreskin is removed with a scalpel circumferentially. **B.** Prior to disassembling the Gomco clamp, the scalpel is used to remove the remaining tissue and ensure a clean excision line.

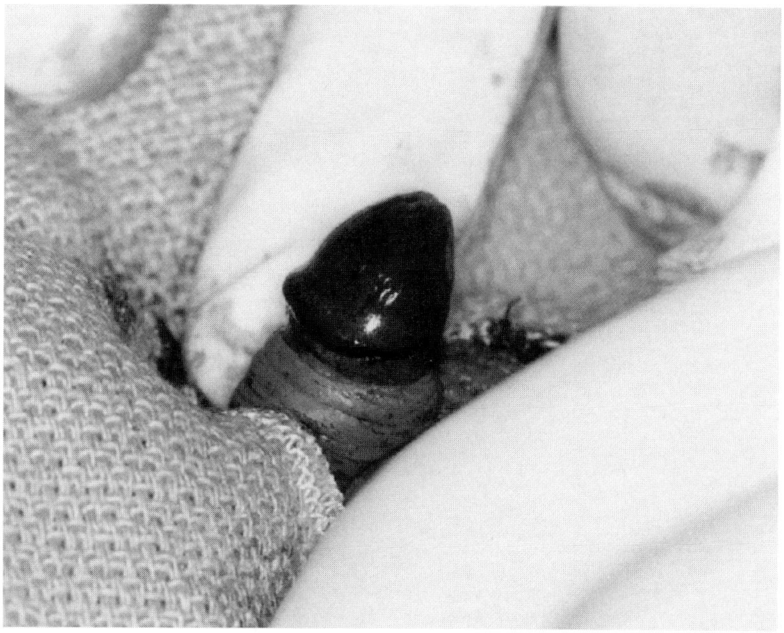

A

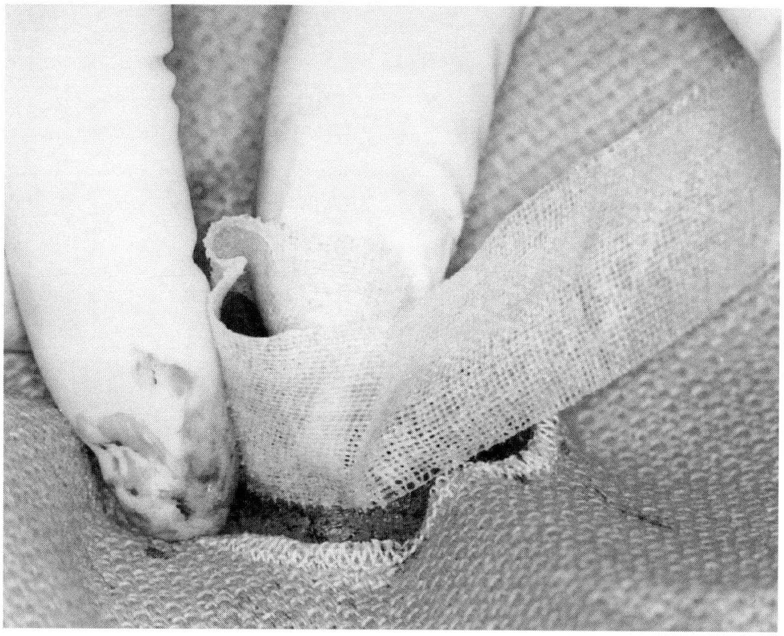

B

Figure 40–17. **(A)** The exposed glans post procedure is **(B)** dressed with petroleum jelly and clean gauze and the infant returned to the mother for feeding.

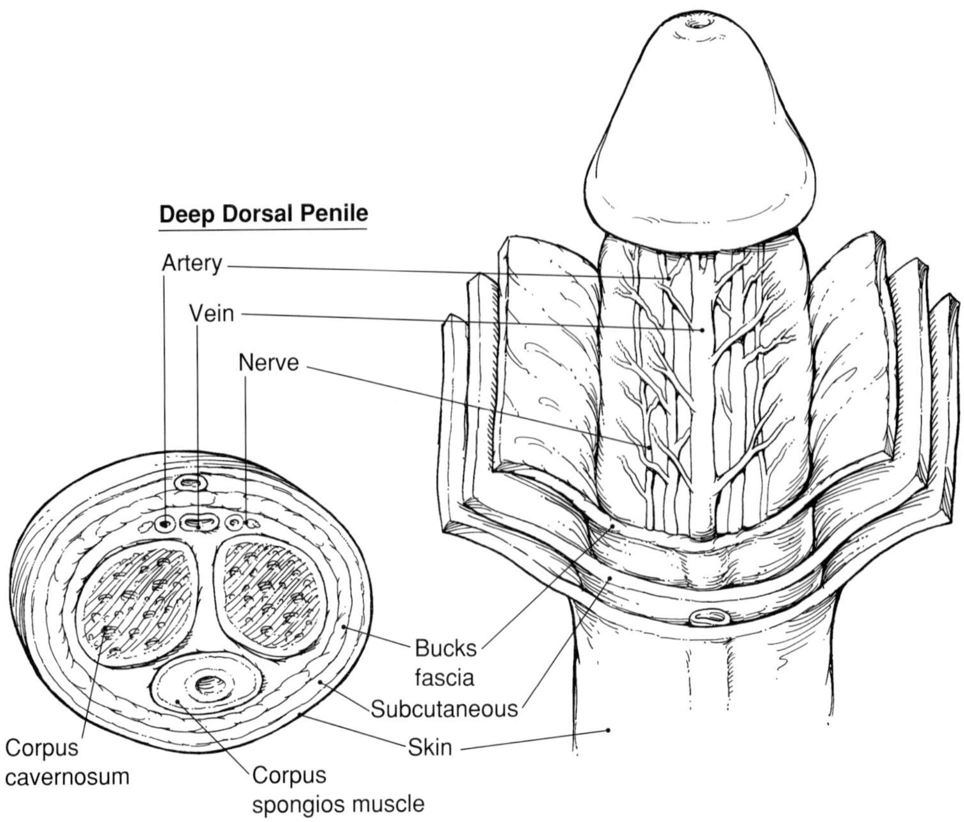

Figure 40–18. The blood and nerve supply of the penis in cross and longitudinal section.

run in the Buck fascia at the 10 and 2 o'clock positions (Fig. 40–18). The operator identifies the penile root and inserts a 26-gauge needle 0.5 cm distal to the root at the 10 and 2 o'clock positions (Fig. 40–19). The needle is inserted posteromedially no deeper than 0.5 cm, and assuming there is no blood return on aspiration, 0.2–0.4 mL of 1% lidocaine without epinephrine is injected bilaterally into the subcutaneous tissue. Masciello described a technique in which local anesthesia is administered by injecting 0.4 mL of 1% lidocaine without epinephrine subcutaneously into the foreskin at both 10 and 2 o'clock positions (Fig. 40–19) (Masciello, 1990). Benini and colleagues (1993) reported success with a topical anesthetic. They administered a eutectic mixture (1:1 oil/water emulsion) of lidocaine and prilocaine hydrochloride bases. The cream was applied on the outside of the prepuce and wrapped with gauze for approximately an hour. The topical agent appeared to reduce the pain response in

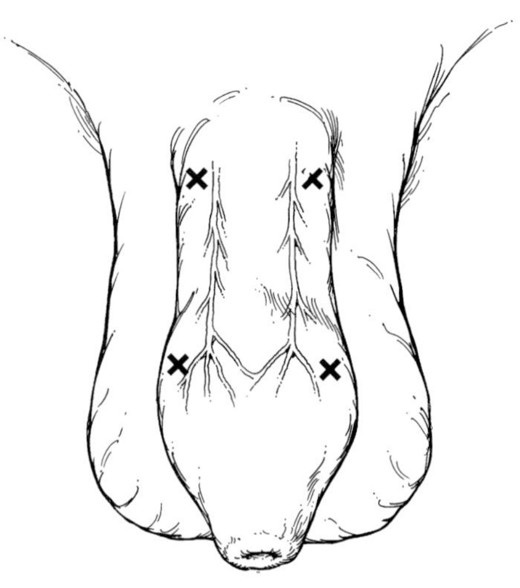

Figure 40–19. Injection sites for dorsal nerve block and local anesthesia for newborn circumcision.

this small cohort. Blass and Hoffmeyer maintain that even a sucrose-flavored pacifier proves adequate anesthesia for newborn circumcision (Blass and Hoffmeyer, 1991). Indeed for centuries *mohels* performing circumcision have allowed the infant to suck on a pacifier dipped with wine. The AAP task force on circumcision concluded that complications due to local anesthesia are rare and consist mainly of hematomas and local skin necrosis (American Academy of Pediatrics, 1989). They concluded that local anesthesia adds an element of risk and that it would be prudent to obtain more data before advocating local anesthesia for newborn circumcision.

SUMMARY

Circumcision is performed on a majority of newborn males in the United States. Although complications are rare, they may be significant. The obstetrician must make sense of the emotional rhetoric on both sides of the circumcision debate and inform parents of potential advantages and disadvantages. Obstetricians are often called on to perform newborn circumcision, and the procedure should not be taken lightly. We have described acceptable techniques for performing newborn circumcision in this text in the hope it will serve as a reference for those performing and learning to perform circumcision.

REFERENCES

Allan N. A Polish Rabbi's Circumcision Manual—Illustrations from the Wellcome Institute Library. Medical History 1989; 33:247.

American Academy of Pediatrics Task Force on Circumcision. Report of the Task Force on Circumcision. Pediatrics 1989; 84:388.

Anderson GF: Circumcision. Pediatr Ann 1989; 18:205.

Blass EM, Hoffmeyer LB. Sucrose as an analgesic for newborn infants. Pediatrics 1991; 87:215.

Benini F, Johnston C, Faucher D, Aranda JV. Topical anesthesia during circumcision in newborn infants. JAMA 1993; 270:850.

Bryk F. Circumcision in man and woman. New York: American Ethnological Press, 1934.

Cameron DW, Simonsen JN, D'Costa LJ, et al. Female to male transmission of human immunodeficiency virus type 1: risk factors for seroconversion in men. Lancet 1989; 2:403.

Committee on Fetus and Newborn. Report of the Ad Hoc Task Force on Circumcision. Pediatrics 1975; 56:610.

Du Toit DF, Villet WT. Gangrene of the penis after circumcision. S Afr Med J 1979; 55:521.

Gee WF, Ansell JS. Neonatal circumcision: a ten-year overview: with comparison of the Gomco clamp and the Plastibell device. Pediatrics 1976; 58:824.

Gellis SS. Circumcision. Am J Dis Child 1978; 132:1168.

Grossman E, Posner NA. Surgical circumcision of neonates: a history of its development. Obstet Gynecol 1981; 58:241.

Karo J. Shulchan Oruch, Code of Jewish Law, Yoreh Deah 264:13. Reprinted by Ozar Halacha Publishing, New York, 1960.

Kirya C, Werthmann MW Jr. Neonatal circumcision and penile dorsal nerve block—a painless procedure. Pediatrics 1978; 92:998.

Kochen M, McCurdy S. Circumcision and the risk of cancer of the penis. Am J Dis Child 1980; 134:484.

Maimonides M. Laws of circumcision 2:2, Mishne Torah. Reprinted by Binah Publishing, New York, 1947.

Masciello AL. Anesthesia for neonatal circumcision: local anesthesia is better than dorsal penile nerve block. Obstet Gynecol 1990; 75:834.

McCance DJ, Kalache A, Ashdown K, et al. Human papillomavirus types 16 and 18 in carcinomas of the penis from Brazil. Int J Cancer 1986; 37:55.

McKim JS. Neonatal circumcision. Can Med Assoc J 1947; 56:54.

Moore KL. The Developing Human—Clinically Oriented Embryology. 3rd ed. Philadelphia: Saunders, 1982.

Poland RL. The question of routine neonatal circumcision. N Engl J Med 1990; 322:1312.

Schoen EJ. The status of newborn circumcisions. N Engl J Med 1990; 322:1308.

Simonsen JN, Cameron W, Gakinya MN, et al. Human immunodeficiency virus infection among men with sexually transmitted diseases: experience from a center in Africa. N Engl J Med 1988; 319:274.

Warner E, Streskin E. Benefits and risks of circumcision. Med Assoc J 1981; 125:967.

Wilson RA. Circumcision and venereal disease. Can Med Assoc J 1947; 56:54.

Wiswell TE. Routine neonatal circumcision: a reappraisal. Am Fam Physician 1990; 41:859.

Wiswell TE, Geschke DW. Risks from circumcision during the first month of life compared with those for uncircumcised boys. Pediatrics 1989; 83:1011.

Wiswell TE, Enzenauer RW, Cornish JD, Hankins CT. Declining frequency of circumcision: Implications for changes in the absolute incidence and male to female sex ratio of urinary tract infections in early infancy. Pediatrics 1987; 79:338.

Wolbarst AL. Circumcision and penile cancer. Lancet 1932; 1:150.

INDEX